HARRISON'S Endocrinology

Derived from Harrison's Principles of Internal Medicine, 16th Edition

Editors

DENNIS L. KASPER, MD
William Ellery Channing Professor of Medicine, Professor of Microbiology and Molecular Genetics, Harvard Medical School; Director, Channing Laboratory, Department of Medicine, Brigham and Women's Hospital, Boston

ANTHONY S. FAUCI, MD
Chief, Laboratory of Immunoregulation; Director, National Institute of Allergy and Infectious Diseases, National Institutes of Health, Bethesda

DAN L. LONGO, MD
Scientific Director, National Institute on Aging, National Institutes of Health, Bethesda and Baltimore

EUGENE BRAUNWALD, MD
Distinguished Hersey Professor of Medicine, Harvard Medical School; Chairman, TIMI Study Group, Brigham and Women's Hospital, Boston

STEPHEN L. HAUSER, MD
Robert A. Fishman Distinguished Professor and Chairman, Department of Neurology, University of California San Francisco, San Francisco

J. LARRY JAMESON, MD, PhD
Irving S. Cutter Professor and Chairman, Department of Medicine, Northwestern University Feinberg School of Medicine; Physician-in-Chief, Northwestern Memorial Hospital, Chicago

HARRISON'S Endocrinology

EDITOR

J. Larry Jameson, MD, PhD
Irving S. Cutter Professor and Chairman
Department of Medicine
Northwestern University Feinberg School of Medicine
Physician-in-Chief, Northwestern Memorial Hospital, Chicago

McGraw-Hill
Medical Publishing Division

New York Chicago San Francisco Lisbon London Madrid
Mexico City Milan New Delhi Seoul Singapore Sydney Toronto

The McGraw-Hill Companies

Dr. Fauci's and Dr. Longo's works were performed outside the scope of their employment as U.S. government employees. These works represent their personal and professional views and not necessarily those of the U.S. government.

Harrison's Endocrinology

1234567890 DOWDOW 09876

ISBN 0-07-145744-5

This book was set in Bembo by Progressive Information Technologies. The editors were James Shanahan and Mariapaz Ramos Englis. The production supervisor was Catherine Saggese. The Index was prepared by Barbara Littlewood. Illustration manager was Charissa Baker; cover design was by Janice Bielawa; additional text design was by Alan Barnett.

Medical Illustrator: Dragonfly Media Group, Pennsylvania.
Illustration for Section and chapter openers was done by Emantras, Inc.

RR Donnelley was printer and binder.

Library of Congress Cataloging-in-Publication Data

Harrison's endocrinology / editors, J. Larry Jameson ... [et al.].
p. ; cm.
Expansion of the endocrinology section of Harrison's principles of internal medicine.
Includes bibliographical references and index.
ISBN 0-07-145744-5 (softcover : alk. paper)
1. Endocrinology. 2. Endocrine glands—Diseases. 3. Metabolism—Disorders.
[DNLM: 1. Endocrine System Diseases. 2. Metabolic Diseases. WK 140 H323 2006]
I. Title: Edocrinology. II. Jameson, J. Larry. III. Harrison's principles of internal medicine.
RC648.H27 2006
616.4—dc22

2005058005

CONTENTS

CONTRIBUTORS

Numbers in brackets refer to the Sectional chapters written or co-written by the contributor.

JOHN C. ACHERMANN, MRCP, MRCPCH, MD
Wellcome Trust Clinician Scientist, Department of Medicine and Institute of Child Health, University College London, London, UK [7]

SHARI S. BASSUK, ScD
Epidemiologist, Division of Preventive Medicine, Brigham and Women's Hospital Boston [11]

SHALENDAR BHASIN, MD
Professor of Medicine, University of California-Los Angeles School of Medicine; Chief, Division of Endocrinology, Charles R. Drow University, Los Angeles [8]

GEORGE J. BOSL, MD
Chairman, Department of Medicine, Memorial Sloan-Kettering Cancer Center; Professor of Medicine, Weill Medical College of Cornell University, New York [9]

KAREN D. BRADSHAW, MD
Professor of Obstetrics/Gynecology and Surgery, Helen J. and Robert S. Strauss and Diana K. and Richard C. Strauss Distinguished Professor in Women's Health, The University of Texas Southwestern Medical Center, Dallas [10]

F. RICHARD BRINGHURST, MD
Associate Professor of Medicine, Harvard Medical School, Boston [23]

CYNTHIA D. BROWN, MD
Department of Internal Medicine
The Johns Hopkins University School of Medicine
Baltimore (Review and Self-Assessment)

BRUCE R. CARR, MD
Professor and Director, Division of Reproductive Endocrinology and Infertility; Holder, Paul C. MacDonald Distinguished Chair in Obstetrics and Gynecology, The University of Texas Southwestern Medical Center, Dallas [10]

PHILIP E. CRYER, MD
Irene E. and Michael M. Karl Professor of Endocrinology and Metabolism in Medicine, Washington University School of Medicine, St. Louis [19]

MARIE B. DEMAY, MD
Associate Professor of Medicine, Harvard Medical School, Boston [23]

ROBERT G. DLUHY, MD
Professor of Medicine, Harvard Medical School, Brigham and Women's Hospital, Boston [5]

DAVID A. EHRMANN, MD
Associate Professor, Section of Endocrinology, Department of Medicine, University of Chicago Pritzker School of Medicine, Chicago [12]

MURRAY J. FAVUS, MD
Professor of Medicine, University of Chicago Pritzker School of Medicine, Division of Biological Sciences, Chicago [26]

JEFFREY S. FLIER, MD
Chief Academic Officer, Beth Israel Deaconess Medical Center; George C. Reisman Professor of Medicine, Harvard Medical School, Boston [16]

JANET E. HALL, MD
Associate Professor of Medicine, Harvard Medical School; Assistant Physician, Massachusetts General Hospital, Boston [15]

ANNA R. HEMNES, MD
Department of Internal Medicine
The Johns Hopkins University School of Medicine
Baltimore (Review and Self-Assessment)

HELEN HASKELL HOBBS, MD
Investigator, Howard Hughes Medical Institute; Professor of Internal Medicine and Molecular Genetics, University of Texas Southwestern Medical Center, Dallas [18]

J. LARRY JAMESON, MD, PhD
Irving S. Cutter Professor and Chair, Department of Medicine, Northwestern University Feinberg School of Medicine; Physician-in-Chief, Northwestern Memorial Hospital, Chicago [1, 2, 4, 7, 8, 22]

JAMES L. JANUZZI, JR., MD
Assistant Professor of Medicine, Harvard Medical School; Assistant Physician, Division of Cardiology and Department of Medicine, Massachusetts General Hospital, Boston [Appendix]

ROBERT T. JENSEN, MD
Chief, Digestive Diseases Branch, National Institute of Diabetes and Digestive and Kidney Diseases, National Institutes of Health, Bethesda [20]

STEPHEN M. KRANE, MD
Persis, Cyrus, and Marlow B. Harrison Professor of Medicine, Harvard Medical School; Physician and Chief, Arthritis Unit, Massachusetts General Hospital, Boston [23]

ALEXANDER KRATZ, MD, PhD, MPH
Assistant Professor of Pathology, Harvard Medical School; Director, Clinical Hematology Laboratory, Massachusetts General Hospital [Appendix]

HENRY M. KRONENBERG, MD
Professor of Medicine, Harvard Medical School; Chief, Endocrine Unit, Massachusetts General Hospital, Boston [23]

LEWIS LANDSBERG, MD
Professor of Medicine, Dean and Vice President for Medical Affairs, Northwestern University Feinberg School of Medicine, Chicago [6]

KENT B. LEWANDROWSKI, MD
Associate Chief of Pathology, Director, Core Laboratory, Massachusetts General Hospital; Associate Professor, Harvard Medical School, Boston [Appendix]

ROBERT LINDSAY, MD, PhD
Professor of Clinical Medicine, Columbia University College of Physicians and Surgeons; Chief, Internal Medicine, Helen Hayes Hospital, West Haverstraw, New York [25]

JOANN E. MANSON, MD, DRPH
Professor of Medicine and the Elizabeth F. Brigham Professor of Women's Health, Harvard Medical School; Chief, Division of Preventive Medicine, Brigham and Women's Hospital, Boston [11]

ELEFTHERIA MARATOS-FLIER, MD
Associate Professor of Medicine, Harvard Medical School; Chief, Obesity Section, Joslin Diabetes Center, Boston [16]

KEVIN T. McVARY, MD
Associate Professor of Urology, Northwestern University Feinberg School of Medicine, Chicago [14]

SHLOMO MELMED, MD
Professor and Associate Dean, David Geffen School of Medicine at University of California-Los Angeles; Senior Vice President and Chief Academic Officer at Cedars-Sinai Medical Center, Los Angeles [2]

ROBERT J, MOTZER, MD
Attending Physician, Memorial Sloan-Kettering Cancer Center; Professor of Medicine, Weill Medical College of Cornell University, New York [9]

PHILIP J. NIVATPUMIN, MD
Department of Internal Medicine
The Johns Hopkins University School of Medicine
Baltimore (Review and Self-Assessment)

JOHN T. POTTS, Jr., MD
Jackson Distinguished Professor of Clinical Medicine, Harvard Medical School, Boston [24]

ALVIN C. POWERS, MD
Ruth K. Scoville Professor of Medicine, Division of Diabetes, Endocrinology, and Metabolism, Vanderbilt University Medical Center; Chief, Diabetes and Endocrinology Section, VA Tennessee Valley Healthcare System, Nashville [17]

DANIEL J. RADER, MD
Associate Professor, Department of Medicine, University of Pennsylvania School of Medicine, Philadelphia [18]

GARY L. ROBERTSON, MD
Professor of Medicine and Neurology, Northwestern University Feinberg School of Medicine, Chicago [3]

STEVEN I. SHERMAN, MD
Associate Professor, University of Texas M.D. Anderson Cancer Center; Adjunct Associate Professor, Baylor College of Medicine, Houston [21]

PATRICK M. SLUSS, PhD
Director, Immunodiagnostics Laboratory, Department of Pathology, Massachusetts General Hospital; Assistant Professor, Harvard Medical School, Boston [Appendix]

EVERETT E. VOKES, MD
Director, Section of Hematology/Oncology; John E. Ultmann Professor of Medicine and Radiation Oncology, University of Chicago, Chicago [26]

ANTHONY P. WEETMAN, MD, DSc
Professor of Medicine and Dean, University of Sheffield Medical School; Consultant Physician, Northern General Hospital, Sheffield, UK [4]

CHARLES WIENER, MD
Vice-Chair, Department of Medicine
The Johns Hopkins University School of Medicine
Baltimore (Review and Self-Assessment)

GORDON H. WILLIAMS, MD
Professor of Medicine, Harvard Medical School; Chief, Cardiovascular Endocrinology Section, Brigham and Women's Hospital, Boston [5]

JAMES B. YOUNG, MD
Professor of Medicine, Executive Associate Dean for Faculty Affairs, Northwestern University Feinberg School of Medicine, Chicago [6]

ROBERT C. YOUNG, MD
President, Fox Chase Cancer Center, Philadelphia [13]

PREFACE

The Editor's of *Harrison's Principles of Internal Medicine* refer to it as the "Mother Book," a description that confers respect but also acknowledges its size and its ancestral status among the growing list of Harrison's products, which now include *Harrison's Manual of Medicine, Harrison's Online*, and *Harrison's On Hand* PDA. This book, *Harrison's Endocrinology and Metabolism*, is the latest progeny of the Mother Book, and consists of a compilation of chapters related to the specialty of endocrinology.

Our readers consistently note the sophistication of the material in the specialty sections of *Harrison's*. Our goal was to bring this information to readers in a more compact and usable form. Because the topic is more focused, it was possible to increase the presentation of the material by enlarging the text and the tables. The figures have undergone major revisions. In addition to being updated, they have been redrawn using state-of-the-art graphics. We have also added Questions & Answers at the end of the book to provoke reflection on the topic and to provide additional teaching points.

The clinical manifestations of endocrine disorders can usually be explained by considering the physiologic role of hormones, which are either deficient or excessive. Thus, a thorough understanding of hormone action, and principles of feedback control, arms the clinician with a logical diagnostic approach and a conceptual framework for treatment approaches. The first chapter of the book, Principles of Endocrinology, provides this type of "systems" overview. Using numerous examples of translational research, this introduction links genetics, cell biology, and physiology with pathophysiology and treatment. The integration of pathophysiology with clinical management is a hallmark of *Harrison's* and can be found throughout each of the subsequent disease-oriented chapters. The book is divided into five main sections that reflect the physiologic roots of endocrinology: (I) Pituitary, Thyroid, and Adrenal Disorders; (II) Reproductive Endocrinology; (III) Diabetes Mellitus, Obesity, and Lipoprotein Metabolism; (IV) Disorders Affecting Multiple Endocrine Systems; (V) Disorders of Bone and Calcium Metabolism.

While *Harrison's Endocrinology and Metabolism* is classic in its organization, readers will sense the impact of our current scientific renaissance as they explore the individual chapters in each section. In addition to the dramatic advances emanating from genetics and molecular biology, the introduction of an unprecedented number of new drugs, particularly for the management of diabetes and osteoporosis, is transforming the field of endocrinology. Numerous recent clinical studies involving common diseases like diabetes, obesity, hypothyroidism, osteoporosis, and polycystic ovarian syndrome provide powerful evidence for medical decision-making and treatment. These rapid changes in endocrinology are exciting for new students of medicine and underscore the need for practicing physicians to continuously update their knowledge base and clinical skills.

Our access to information through web-based journals and data bases is remarkably efficient. While these sources of information are invaluable, the daunting body of data creates an even greater need for synthesis and for highlighting important facts. Thus, the preparation of these chapters is a special craft that requires the ability to distill core information from the ever-expanding knowledge base. The Editors are therefore indebted to our authors, a group of internationally recognized authorities who are masters at providing a comprehensive overview while being able to distill a topic into a concise and interesting chapter. We are also grateful to our assistants, Karl Cremieux, Sue Anne Tae, and Amy Camponeschi, who patiently kept this project on schedule. Our colleagues at McGraw-Hill continue to innovate in health care publishing. This new product was championed by Jim Shanahan and Marty Wonsiewicz and impeccably managed in production by Mariapaz Ramos Englis, Catherine Saggese, and Charissa Baker.

We hope you find this book useful in your effort to achieve continuous learning on behalf of your patients.

NOTICE

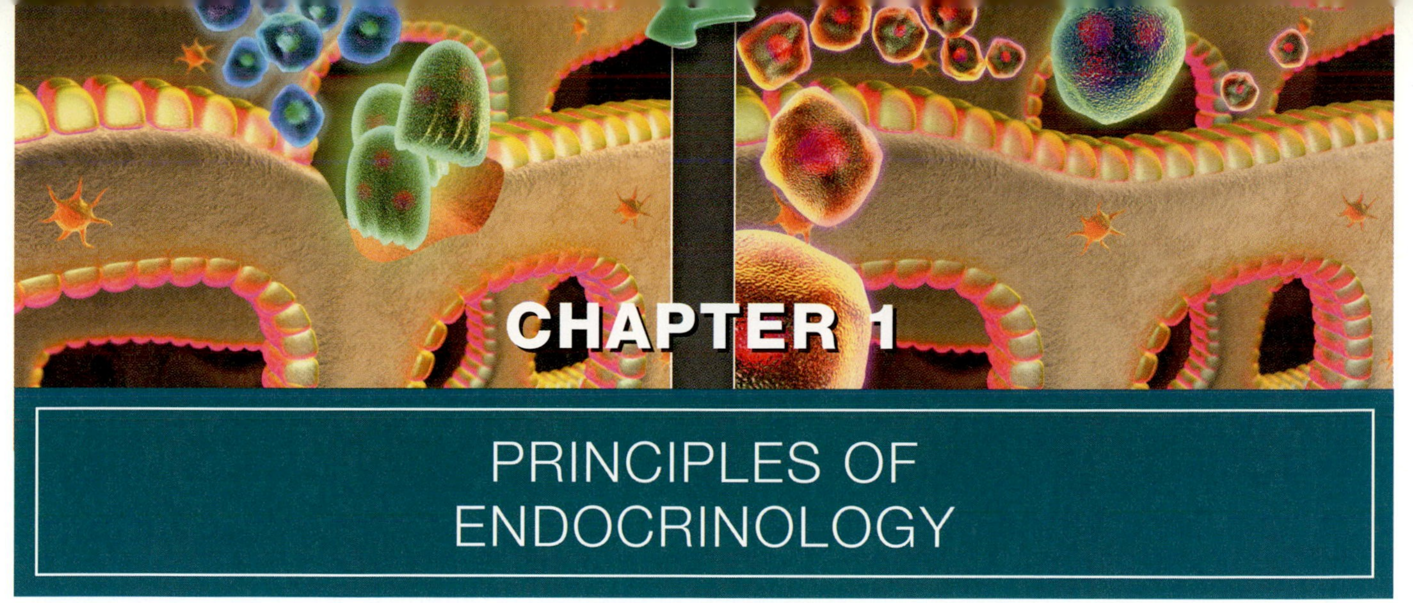

PRINCIPLES OF ENDOCRINOLOGY

J. Larry Jameson

The management of endocrine disorders requires an understanding of such disparate areas as intermediary metabolism, reproductive physiology, bone metabolism, and growth. Accordingly, the practice of endocrinology is intimately linked to a conceptual framework for understanding hormone secretion, hormone action, and principles of feedback control systems. The endocrine system is evaluated primarily by measuring hormone concentrations, thereby arming the clinician with valuable diagnostic information. Most disorders of the endocrine system are amenable to effective treatment, once the correct diagnosis is determined. Endocrine deficiency disorders are treated with physiologic hormone replacement; hormone excess conditions, usually due to benign glandular adenomas, are managed by removing tumors surgically or by reducing hormone levels medically.

SCOPE OF ENDOCRINOLOGY

The specialty of endocrinology encompasses the study of glands and the hormones they produce. The term *endocrine* was coined by Starling to contrast the actions of hormones secreted internally (endocrine) with those secreted externally (*exocrine*) or into a lumen, such as the gastrointestinal tract. The term *hormone,* derived from a Greek phrase meaning "to set in motion," aptly describes the dynamic actions of hormones as they elicit cellular responses and regulate physiologic processes through feedback mechanisms.

Unlike many other specialties in medicine, it is not possible to define endocrinology strictly along anatomical lines. The classic endocrine glands—pituitary, thyroid, parathyroid, pancreatic islets, adrenal, and gonads—communicate broadly with other organs through the nervous system, hormones, cytokines, and growth factors. In addition to its traditional synaptic functions, the brain produces a vast array of peptide hormones, spawning the discipline of neuroendocrinology. Through the production of hypothalamic releasing factors, the central nervous system (CNS) exerts a major regulatory influence over pituitary hormone secretion (Chap. 2). The peripheral nervous system modulates adrenal medulla and pancreatic islet hormone production. The immune and endocrine systems are also intimately intertwined. The adrenal glucocorticoid, cortisol, is a powerful immunosuppressant. Cytokines and interleukins (ILs) have profound effects on the functions of the pituitary, adrenal, thyroid, and gonads. Common endocrine diseases, such as autoimmune thyroid disease and type 1 diabetes mellitus, are caused by dysregulation of immune surveillance and tolerance. Less common diseases such as polyglandular failure, Addison's disease, and lymphocytic hypophysitis also have an immunologic basis.

The interdigitation of endocrinology with physiologic processes in other specialties sometimes blurs the role of hormones. For example, hormones play an important role in maintenance of blood pressure, intravascular volume, and peripheral resistance in the cardiovascular system. Vasoactive substances such as catecholamines, angiotensin II, endothelin, and nitric oxide are involved in dynamic changes of vascular tone, in addition to their multiple roles in other tissues. The heart is the principal source of atrial natriuretic peptide, which acts in classic endocrine fashion to induce natriuresis at a distant target organ (the kidney). Erythropoietin, a traditional circulating hormone, is made in the kidney and stimulates erythropoiesis in the bone marrow. The kidney is also integrally involved in the renin-angiotensin axis (Chap. 5) and is a primary target of several hormones including parathyroid hormone (PTH), mineralocorticoids, and vasopressin. The gastrointestinal tract produces a surprising number of peptide hormones such as cholecystokinin, ghrelin, gastrin, secretin, and vasoactive intestinal peptide, among many others. Carcinoid and islet tumors can secrete excessive amounts of these hormones, leading to specific clinical syndromes (Chap. 20). Many of these gastrointestinal hormones are also produced in the CNS, where their functions remain poorly understood. As new hormones such as inhibin, ghrelin, and leptin are discovered, they become integrated into the science and practice of medicine on the basis of their functional roles rather than their tissues of origin or their structures or mechanisms of action.

Characterization of hormone receptors frequently reveals unexpected relationships to factors in nonendocrine disciplines. The growth hormone (GH) receptor, for example, is a member of the cytokine receptor family. The G protein–coupled receptors (GPCRs), which mediate the actions of many peptide hormones, are used in numerous physiologic processes including vision, smell, and neurotransmission.

It is apparent that hormones and growth factors play an important functional role in all organ systems. Though endocrinologists are not usually involved in the administration of the hormones or growth factors used to treat diseases in other specialties (e.g., cardiology, hematology), the principles of endocrinology can be applied in these cases, thus emphasizing the impact of endocrinology across multiple disciplines.

NATURE OF HORMONES

Hormones can be divided into five major classes: (1) *amino acid derivatives* such as dopamine, catecholamines, and thyroid hormone; (2) *small neuropeptides* such as gonadotropin-releasing hormone (GnRH), thyrotropin-releasing hormone (TRH), somatostatin, and vasopressin; (3) *large proteins* such as insulin, luteinizing hormone (LH), and PTH produced by classic endocrine glands; (4) *steroid hormones* such as cortisol and estrogen that are synthesized from cholesterol-based precursors; and (5) *vitamin derivatives* such as retinoids (vitamin A) and vitamin D. A variety of *peptide growth factors,* most of which act locally, share actions with hormones. As a rule, amino acid derivatives and peptide hormones interact with cell-surface membrane receptors. Steroids, thyroid hormones, vitamin D, and retinoids are lipid-soluble and interact with intracellular nuclear receptors.

HORMONE AND RECEPTOR FAMILIES

Many hormones and receptors can be grouped into families, reflecting their structural similarities (**Table 1-1**). The evolution of these families generates diverse but highly selective pathways of hormone action. Recognizing these relationships allows extrapolation of information gleaned from one hormone or receptor to other family members.

The glycoprotein hormone family, consisting of thyroid-stimulating hormone (TSH), follicle-stimulating hormone (FSH), LH, and human chorionic gonadotropin (hCG), illustrates many features of related hormones. The glycoprotein hormones are heterodimers that share the α subunit in common; the β subunits are distinct and confer specific biologic actions. The overall three-dimensional architecture of the β subunits is similar, reflecting the locations of conserved disulfide bonds that restrain protein conformation. The cloning of the β-subunit genes from multiple species suggests that this family arose from a common ancestral gene, probably by gene duplication and subsequent divergence to evolve new biologic functions.

As the hormone families enlarge and diverge, their receptors must co-evolve, if new biologic functions are to be derived. Related GPCRs, for example, have evolved for each of the glycoprotein hormones. These receptors are structurally similar, and each is coupled to the $G_s\alpha$ signaling pathway. However, there is minimal overlap of hormone binding. For example, TSH binds with high specificity to the TSH receptor but interacts minimally with the LH or the FSH receptor. Nonetheless, there can be subtle physiologic consequences of hormone cross-reactivity with other receptors. Very high levels of hCG during pregnancy stimulate the TSH receptor and increase thyroid hormone levels.

Insulin, insulin-like growth factor (IGF) I, and IGF-II share structural similarities that are most apparent when precursor forms of the proteins are compared. In contrast to the high degree of specificity seen with the glycoprotein hormones, there is moderate cross-talk among the members of the insulin/IGF family. High concentrations of an IGF-II precursor produced by certain tumors (e.g., sarcomas) can cause hypoglycemia, partly because of binding to insulin and IGF-I receptors (Chap. 22). High concentrations of insulin also bind to the IGF-I

TABLE 1-1

MEMBRANE RECEPTOR FAMILIES AND SIGNALING PATHWAYS

RECEPTORS	EFFECTORS	SIGNALING PATHWAYS
G protein-coupled seven-transmembrane (GPCR)		
β-Adrenergic LH, FSH, TSH Glucagon PTH, PTHrP ACTH, MSH GHRH, CRH	$G_s\alpha$, adenylate cyclase Ca^{2+} channels	Stimulation of cyclic AMP production, protein kinase A Calmodulin, Ca^{2+}-dependent kinases
α-Adrenergic	$G_i\alpha$	Inhibition of cyclic AMP production
Somatostatin		Activation of K^+, Ca^{2-} channels
TRH, GnRH	G_q, G_{11}	Phospholipase C, diacylglycerol-IP_3, protein kinase C, voltage-dependent Ca^{2+} channels
Receptor tyrosine kinase		
Insulin, JGF-1	Tyrosine kinases, IRS-1 to IRS-4	MAP kinases, PI 3-kinase, RSK
EGF, NGF	Tyrosine kinases, ras	Raf, MAP kinases, RSK
Cytokine receptor–linked kinase		
GH, PRL	JAK, tyrosine kinases	STAT, MAP kinase, PI 3-kinase, IRS-1, IRS-2
Serine kinase		
Activin, TGF-β, MIS	Serine kinase	Smads

Note: IP_3, inositol triphosphate; IRS, insulin receptor substrates; MAP, mitogen-activated protein; MSH, melanocyte-stimulating hormone; NGF, nerve growth factor; PI, phosphatidylinositol; RSK, ribosomal S6 kinase; TGF-β, transforming growth factor β. For all other abbreviations, see text.

receptor, perhaps accounting for some of the clinical manifestations seen in severe insulin resistance.

Another important example of receptor cross-talk is seen with PTH and parathyroid hormone–related peptide (PTHrP) (Chap. 24). PTH is produced by the parathyroid glands, whereas PTHrP is expressed at high levels during development and by a variety of tumors (Chap. 22). These hormones share amino acid sequence similarity, particularly in their amino-terminal regions. Both hormones bind to a single PTH receptor that is expressed in bone and kidney. Hypercalcemia and hypophosphatemia may therefore result from excessive production of either hormone, making it difficult to distinguish hyperparathyroidism from hypercalcemia of malignancy solely on the basis of serum chemistries. However, sensitive and specific assays for PTH and PTHrP now allow these disorders to be separated more readily.

Based on their specificities for DNA-binding sites, the nuclear receptor family can be subdivided into type 1 receptors (GR, MR, AR, ER, PR) that bind steroids and type 2 receptors (TR, VDR, RAR, PPAR) that bind thyroid hormone, vitamin D, retinoic acid, or lipid derivatives. Certain functional domains in nuclear receptors, such as the zinc finger DNA-binding domains, are highly conserved. However, selective amino acid differences within this domain confer DNA sequence specificity. The hormone-binding domains are more variable, providing great diversity in the array of small molecules that can bind to different nuclear receptors. With few exceptions, hormone binding is highly specific for a single type of nuclear receptor. One exception involves the highly related glucocorticoid and mineralocorticoid receptors. Because the mineralocorticoid receptor also binds glucocorticoids with high affinity, an enzyme (11β-hydroxysteroid dehydrogenase) located in renal tubular cells inactivates glucocorticoids, allowing selective responses to mineralocorticoids such as aldosterone. However, when very high glucocorticoid concentrations occur, as in Cushing's syndrome, the glucocorticoid degradation pathway becomes saturated, allowing excessive cortisol levels to exert mineralocorticoid effects (sodium retention, potassium wasting). This phenomenon is particularly pronounced in ectopic adrenocorticotropic hormone (ACTH) syndromes (Chap. 5). Another example of relaxed nuclear receptor specificity involves the estrogen receptor, which can bind an array of compounds, some of which share little structural similarity to the high-affinity ligand estradiol. This feature of the estrogen receptor makes it susceptible to activation by "environmental estrogens" such as resveratrol, octylphenol, and many other aromatic hydrocarbons. On the other hand, this lack of specificity provides an opportunity to synthesize a remarkable series of clinically useful antagonists (e.g., tamoxifen) and selective estrogen response modulators (SERMs), such as raloxifene. These compounds generate distinct conformations that alter receptor interactions with components of the transcription machinery (see below), thereby conferring their unique actions.

HORMONE SYNTHESIS AND PROCESSING

The synthesis of peptide hormones and their receptors occurs through a classic pathway of gene expression: transcription → mRNA → protein → posttranslational protein processing → intracellular sorting, membrane integration, or secretion. Though endocrine genes contain regulatory DNA elements similar to those found in many other genes, their exquisite control by other hormones also necessitates the presence of specific hormone response elements. For example, the TSH genes are repressed directly by thyroid hormones acting through the thyroid hormone receptor, a member of the nuclear receptor family. Steroidogenic enzyme gene expression requires specific transcription factors such as steroidogenic factor-1 (SF-1), acting in conjunction with signals transmitted by trophic hormones (e.g., ACTH or LH). For some hormones, substantial regulation occurs at the level of translational efficiency. Insulin biosynthesis, while requiring ongoing gene transcription, is regulated primarily at the translational level in response to elevated levels of glucose or amino acids.

Many hormones are embedded within larger precursor polypeptides that are proteolytically processed to yield the biologically active hormone. Examples include: proopiomelanocortin (POMC) → ACTH; proglucagon → glucagon; proinsulin → insulin; pro-PTH → PTH, among others. In many cases, such as POMC and proglucagon, these precursors generate multiple biologically active peptides. It is provocative that hormone precursors are typically inactive, presumably adding an additional level of regulatory control. This is true not only for peptide hormones but also for certain steroids (testosterone → dihydrotestosterone) and thyroid hormone ($T_4 \rightarrow T_3$).

Hormone precursor processing is intimately linked to intracellular sorting pathways that transport proteins to appropriate vesicles and enzymes, resulting in specific cleavage steps, followed by protein folding and translocation to secretory vesicles. Hormones destined for secretion are translocated across the endoplasmic reticulum under the guidance of an amino-terminal signal sequence that is subsequently cleaved. Cell-surface receptors are inserted into the membrane via short segments of hydrophobic amino acids that remain embedded within the lipid bilayer. During translocation through the Golgi and endoplasmic reticulum, hormones and receptors are also subject to a variety of posttranslational modifications, such as glycosylation and phosphorylation, which can alter protein conformation, modify circulating half-life, and alter biologic activity.

Synthesis of most steroid hormones is based on modifications of the precursor, cholesterol. Multiple regulated enzymatic steps are required for the synthesis of testosterone (Chap. 8), estradiol (Chap. 10), cortisol (Chap. 5), and vitamin D (Chap. 23). This large number of synthetic steps predisposes to multiple genetic and acquired disorders of steroidogenesis.

HORMONE SECRETION, TRANSPORT, AND DEGRADATION

The circulating level of a hormone is determined by its rate of secretion and its circulating half-life. After protein processing, peptide hormones (GnRH, insulin, GH) are stored in secretory granules. As these granules mature, they are poised beneath the plasma membrane for imminent release into the circulation. In most instances, the stimulus for hormone secretion is a releasing factor or neural signal that induces rapid changes in intracellular calcium concentrations, leading to secretory granule fusion with the plasma membrane and release of its contents into the extracellular environment and bloodstream. Steroid hormones, in contrast, diffuse into the circulation as they are synthesized. Thus, their secretory rates are closely aligned with rates of synthesis. For example, ACTH and LH induce steroidogenesis by stimulating the activity of *st*eroidogenic *a*cute *r*egulatory (StAR) protein (transports cholesterol into the mitochondrion) along with other rate-limiting steps (e.g., cholesterol side-chain cleavage enzyme, CYP11A1) in the steroidogenic pathway.

Hormone transport and degradation dictate the rapidity with which a hormonal signal decays. Some hormonal signals are evanescent (e.g., somatostatin), whereas others are longer lived (e.g., TSH). Because somatostatin exerts effects in virtually every tissue, a short half-life allows its concentrations and actions to be controlled locally. Structural modifications that impair somatostatin degradation have been useful for generating long-acting therapeutic analogues, such as octreotide (Chap. 2). On the other hand, the actions of TSH are highly specific for the thyroid gland. Its prolonged half-life accounts for relatively constant serum levels, even though TSH is secreted in discrete pulses.

An understanding of circulating hormone half-life is important for achieving physiologic hormone replacement, as the frequency of dosing and the time required to reach steady state are intimately linked to rates of hormone decay. T_4, for example, has a circulating half-life of 7 days. Consequently, >1 month is required to reach a new steady state, but single daily doses are sufficient to achieve constant hormone levels. T_3, in contrast, has a half-life of 1 day. Its administration is associated with more dynamic serum levels and it must be administered two to three times per day. Similarly, synthetic glucocorticoids vary widely in their half-lives; those with longer half-lives (e.g., dexamethasone) are associated with greater suppression of the hypothalamic-pituitary-adrenal (HPA) axis. Most protein hormones [e.g., ACTH, GH, prolactin (PRL); PTH, LH] have relatively short half-lives (<20 min), leading to sharp peaks of secretion and decay. The only accurate way to profile the pulse frequency and amplitude of these hormones is to measure levels in frequently sampled blood (every 10 min) over long durations (8 to 24 h). Because this is not practical in a clinical setting, an alternative strategy is to pool three to four samples drawn at about 30-min intervals, recognizing that pulsatile secretion makes it difficult to establish a narrow normal range. Rapid hormone decay is useful in certain clinical settings. For example, the short half-life of PTH allows the use of intraoperative PTH determinations to confirm successful removal of an adenoma. This is particularly valuable diagnostically when there is a possibility of multicentric disease or parathyroid hyperplasia, as occurs with multiple endocrine neoplasia (MEN) or renal insufficiency.

Many hormones circulate in association with serum-binding proteins. Examples include: (1) T_4 and T_3 binding to thyroxine-binding globulin (TBG), albumin, and thyroxine-binding prealbumin (TBPA); (2) cortisol binding to cortisol-binding globulin (CBG); (3) androgen and estrogen binding to sex hormone–binding globulin (SHBG) (also called testosterone-binding globulin, TeBG); (4) IGF-I and -II binding to multiple IGF-binding proteins (IGF-BPs); (5) GH interactions with GH-binding protein (GHBP), a circulating fragment of the GH receptor extracellular domain; and (6) activin binding to follistatin. These interactions provide a hormonal reservoir, prevent otherwise rapid degradation of unbound hormones, restrict hormone access to certain sites (e.g., IGFBPs), and modulate the unbound, or "free," hormone concentrations. Although a variety of binding protein abnormalities have been identified, most have little clinical consequence, aside from creating diagnostic problems. For example, TBG deficiency can greatly reduce total thyroid hormone levels, but the free concentrations of T_4 and T_3 remain normal. Liver disease and certain medications can also influence binding protein levels (e.g., estrogen increases TBG) or cause displacement of hormones from binding proteins (e.g., salsalate displaces T_4 from TBG). Only unbound hormone is available to interact with receptors and thereby elicit a biologic response. Short-term perturbations in binding proteins change the free hormone concentration, which in turn induces compensatory adaptations through feedback loops. SHBG changes in women are an exception to this self-correcting mechanism. When SHBG decreases because of insulin resistance or androgen excess, the unbound testosterone concentration is increased, potentially leading to hirsutism (Chap. 12). The increased unbound testosterone level does not result in an adequate compensatory feedback correction because estrogen, and not testosterone, is the primary regulator of the reproductive axis.

HORMONE ACTION THROUGH RECEPTORS

Receptors for hormones are divided into two major classes—membrane and nuclear. *Membrane receptors* primarily bind peptide hormones and catecholamines. *Nuclear receptors* bind small molecules that can diffuse across the cell membrane, such as thyroid hormone, steroids, and vitamin D. Certain general principles apply to hormone-receptor interactions, regardless of the class of receptor. Hormones bind to receptors with specificity and a high affinity that generally coincides with the dynamic range of circulating hormone concentrations. Low concentrations of free hormone (usually 10^{-12} to 10^{-9} *M*) rapidly associate and dissociate from receptors in a bimolecular reaction, such that the occupancy of the receptor at any given moment is a function of hormone concentration and the receptor's affinity for the hormone. Receptor numbers vary greatly in different target tissues, providing one of the major determinants of specific cellular responses to circulating hormones. For example, ACTH receptors are located almost exclusively in the adrenal cortex, and FSH receptors are found only in the gonads. In contrast, insulin and thyroid hormone receptors are widely distributed, reflecting the need for metabolic responses in all tissues.

MEMBRANE RECEPTORS

Membrane receptors for hormones can be divided into several major groups: (1) seven transmembrane GPCRs, (2) tyrosine kinase receptors, (3) cytokine receptors, and (4) serine kinase receptors (**Fig. 1-1**). The *seven transmembrane GPCR family* binds a remarkable array of hormones including large proteins (e.g., LH, PTH), small peptides (e.g., TRH, somatostatin), catecholamines (epinephrine, dopamine), and even minerals (e.g., calcium).

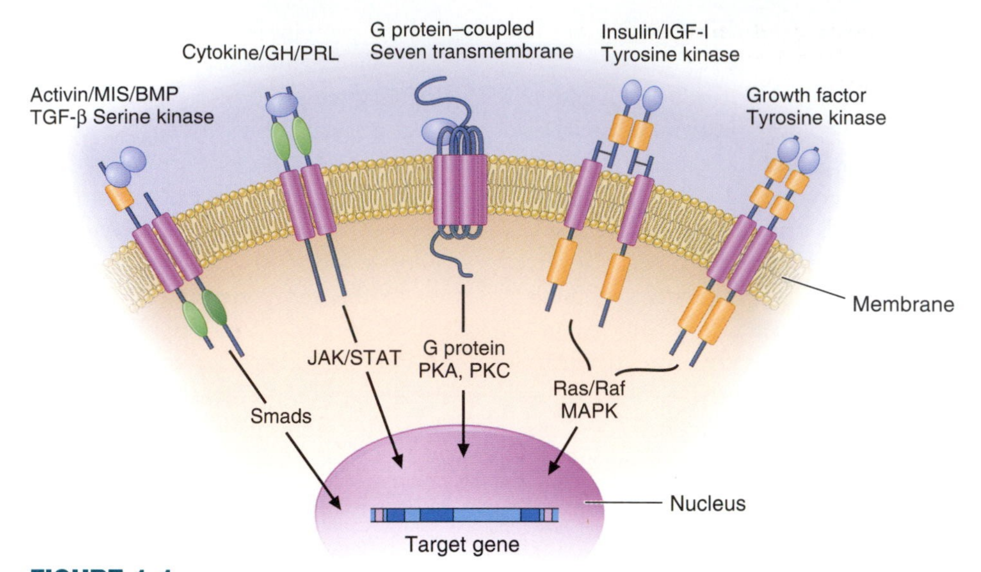

FIGURE 1-1

Membrane receptor signaling. MAPK, mitogen-activated protein kinase; PKA, -C, protein kinase A, C; TGF, transforming growth factor. For other abbreviations, see text.

The extracellular domains of GPCRs vary widely in size and are the major binding site for large hormones. The transmembrane-spanning regions are composed of hydrophobic α-helical domains that traverse the lipid bilayer. Like some channels, these domains are thought to circularize and form a hydrophobic pocket into which certain small ligands fit. Hormone binding induces conformational changes in these domains, transducing structural changes to the intracellular domain, which is a docking site for G proteins.

The large family of G *proteins*, so named because they bind guanine nucleotides (GTP, GDP), provides great diversity for coupling signaling pathways to different receptors. G proteins form a heterotrimeric complex that is composed of various α and $\beta\gamma$ subunits. The α subunit contains the guanine nucleotide–binding site and hydrolyzes GTP $\rightarrow$ GDP. The $\beta\gamma$ subunits are tightly associated and modulate the activity of the α subunit, as well as mediating their own effector signaling pathways. G protein activity is regulated by a cycle that involves GTP hydrolysis and dynamic interactions between the α and $\beta\gamma$ subunits. Hormone binding to the receptor induces GDP dissociation, allowing Gα to bind GTP and dissociate from the $\beta\gamma$ complex. Under these conditions, the Gα subunit is activated and mediates signal transduction through various enzymes such as adenylate cyclase or phospholipase C. GTP hydrolysis to GDP allows reassociation with the $\beta\gamma$ subunits and restores the inactive state. As described below, a variety of endocrinopathies result from G protein mutations or from mutations in receptors that modify their interactions with G proteins.

There are more than a dozen isoforms of the Gα subunit. $G_s\alpha$ stimulates, whereas $G_i\alpha$ inhibits adenylate cyclase, an enzyme that generates the second messenger, cyclic AMP, leading to activation of protein kinase A (Table 1-1). G_q subunits couple to phospholipase C, generating diacylglycerol and inositol triphosphate, leading to activation of protein kinase C and the release of intracellular calcium.

The *tyrosine kinase receptors* transduce signals for insulin and a variety of growth factors, such as IGF-I, epidermal growth factor (EGF), nerve growth factor, platelet-derived growth factor, and fibroblast growth factor. The cysteine-rich extracellular ligand-binding domains contain growth factor–binding sites. After ligand binding, this class of receptors undergoes autophosphorylation, inducing interactions with intracellular adaptor proteins such as Shc and insulin receptor substrates 1 to 4. In the case of the insulin receptor, multiple kinases are activated including the Raf-Ras-MAPK and the Akt/protein kinase B pathways. The tyrosine kinase receptors play a prominent role in cell growth and differentiation as well as in intermediary metabolism.

The GH and PRL receptors belong to the *cytokine receptor* family. Analogous to the tyrosine kinase receptors, ligand binding induces receptor interaction with intracellular kinases—the Janus kinases (JAKs), which phosphorylate members of the signal transduction and activators of transcription (STAT) family—as well as other signaling pathways (Ras, PI3-K, MAPK). The activated STAT proteins translocate to the nucleus and stimulate expression of target genes (Chap. 2).

The *serine kinase receptors* mediate the actions of activins, transforming growth factor β, müllerian-inhibiting sub-

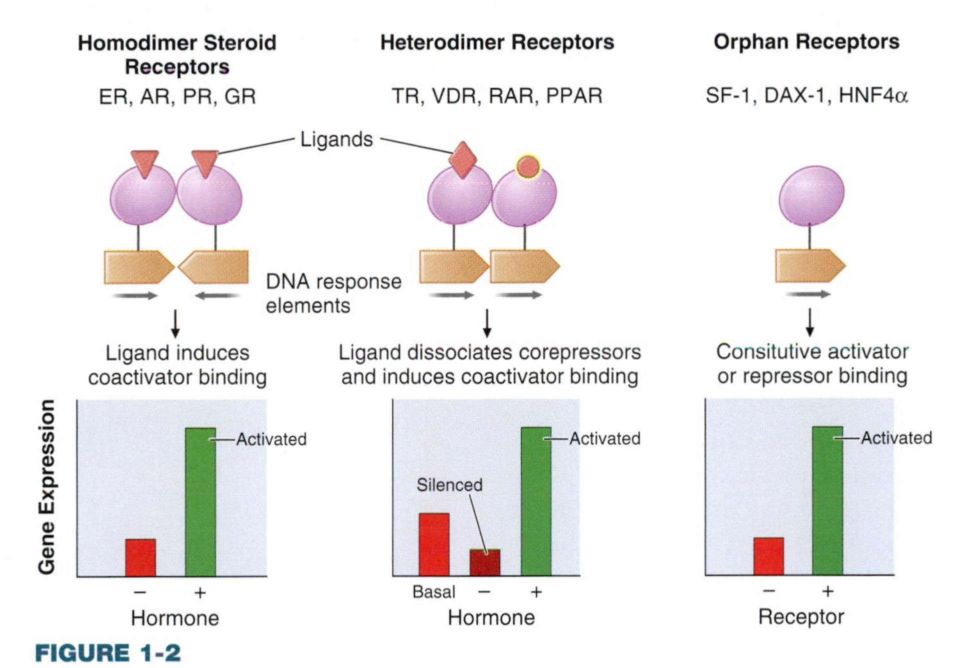

FIGURE 1-2

Nuclear receptor signaling. ER, estrogen receptor; AR, androgen receptor; PR, progesterone receptor; GR, glucocorticoid receptor; TR, thyroid hormone receptor; VDR, vitamin D receptor; RAR, retinoic acid receptor; PPAR, peroxisome proliferator activated receptor; SF-1, steroidogenic factor-1; DAX, *d*osage sensitive sex-reversal, *a*drenal hypoplasia congenita, *X*-chromosome; HNF4α, hepatic nuclear factor 4α.

stance (MIS, also known as anti-müllerian hormone, AMH), and bone morphogenic proteins (BMPs). This family of receptors (consisting of type I and II subunits) signal through proteins termed *smads* (fusion of terms for *Caenorhabditis elegans* sma + mammalian mad). Like the STAT proteins, the smads serve a dual role of transducing the receptor signal and acting as transcription factors. The pleomorphic actions of these growth factors dictate that they act primarily in a local (paracrine or autocrine) manner. Binding proteins, such as follistatin (which binds activin and other members of this family), function to inactivate the growth factors and restrict their distribution.

NUCLEAR RECEPTORS

The family of nuclear receptors has grown to nearly 100 members, many of which are still classified as orphan receptors because their ligands, if they exist, remain to be identified (**Fig. 1-2**). Otherwise, most nuclear receptors are classified based on the nature of their ligands. Though all nuclear receptors ultimately act to increase or decrease gene transcription, some (e.g., glucocorticoid receptor) reside primarily in the cytoplasm, whereas others (e.g., thyroid hormone receptor) are always located in the nucleus. After ligand binding, the cytoplasmically localized receptors translocate to the nucleus. There is growing evidence that certain nuclear receptors (e.g., glucocorticoid, estrogen) can also activate or repress signal transduction pathways, providing a mechanism for cross-talk between membrane and nuclear receptors.

The structures of nuclear receptors have been extensively studied, including by x-ray crystallography. The DNA binding domain, consisting of two zinc fingers, contacts specific DNA recognition sequences in target genes. Most nuclear receptors bind to DNA as dimers. Consequently, each monomer recognizes an individual DNA motif, referred to as a "half-site." The steroid receptors, including the glucocorticoid, estrogen, progesterone, and androgen receptors, bind to DNA as homodimers. Consistent with this twofold symmetry, their DNA recognition half-sites are palindromic. The thyroid, retinoid, peroxisome proliferator-activated, and vitamin D receptors bind to DNA preferentially as heterodimers in combination with retinoid X receptors (RXRs). Their DNA half-sites are arranged as direct repeats. Receptor specificity for DNA sequences is determined by (1) the sequence of the half-site, (2) the orientation of the half-sites (palindromic, direct repeat), and (3) the spacing between the half-sites. For example, vitamin D, thyroid, and retinoid receptors recognize similar tandemly repeated half-sites (TAAGTCA), but these DNA repeats are spaced by three, four, and five nucleotides, respectively.

The carboxy-terminal hormone-binding domain mediates transcriptional control. For type II receptors, such as thyroid hormone receptor (TR) and retinoic acid receptor (RAR), co-repressor proteins bind to the receptor in the absence of ligand and silence gene transcription. Hormone binding induces conformational changes, triggering the release of co-repressors and inducing the recruitment of coactivators that stimulate transcription. Thus, these receptors are capable of mediating dramatic changes in the level of gene activity. Certain disease states are associated with defective regulation of these events. For example, mutations in the TR prevent co-repressor dissociation, resulting in a dominant form of hormone resistance (Chap. 4). In promyelocytic leukemia, fusion of RAR to other nuclear proteins causes aberrant gene silencing and prevents normal cellular differentiation. Treatment with retinoic acid reverses this repression and allows cellular differentiation and apoptosis to occur. Most type 1 steroid receptors do not interact with co-repressors, but ligand binding still mediates interactions with an array of coactivators. X-ray crystallography shows that various SERMs induce distinct receptor conformations. The tissue-specific responses caused by these agents in breast, bone, and uterus appear to reflect distinct interactions with coactivators. The receptor-coactivator complex stimulates gene transcription by several pathways including (1) recruitment of enzymes (histone acetyl transferases) that modify chromatin structure, (2) interactions with additional transcription factors on the target gene, and (3) direct interactions with components of the general transcription apparatus to enhance the rate of RNA polymerase II–mediated transcription.

FUNCTIONS OF HORMONES

The functions of individual hormones are described in detail in subsequent chapters. Nevertheless, it is useful to illustrate how most biologic responses require integration of several different hormonal pathways. The physiologic functions of hormones can be divided into three general areas: (1) growth and differentiation, (2) maintenance of homeostasis, and (3) reproduction.

GROWTH

Multiple hormones and nutritional factors mediate the complex phenomenon of growth (Chap. 2). Short stature may be caused by GH deficiency, hypothyroidism, Cushing's syndrome, precocious puberty, malnutrition or chronic illness, or genetic abnormalities that affect the epiphyseal growth plates (e.g., *FGFR3* or *SHOX* mutations). Many factors (GH, IGF-I, thyroid hormone) stimulate growth, whereas others (sex steroids) lead to epiphyseal closure. Understanding these hormonal interactions is important in the diagnosis and management of growth disorders. For example, delaying exposure to high levels of sex steroids may enhance the efficacy of GH treatment.

MAINTENANCE OF HOMEOSTASIS

Though virtually all hormones affect homeostasis, the most important among these are the following:

1. Thyroid hormone—controls about 25% of basal metabolism in most tissues
2. Cortisol—exerts a permissive action for many hormones in addition to its own direct effects
3. PTH—regulates calcium and phosphorus levels
4. Vasopressin—regulates serum osmolality by controlling renal free water clearance
5. Mineralocorticoids—control vascular volume and serum electrolyte (Na^+, K^+) concentrations
6. Insulin—maintains euglycemia in the fed and fasted states

The defense against hypoglycemia is an impressive example of integrated hormone action (Chap. 19). In response to the fasted state and falling blood glucose, insulin secretion is suppressed, resulting in decreased glucose uptake and enhanced glycogenolysis, lipolysis, proteolysis, and gluconeogenesis to mobilize fuel sources. If hypoglycemia develops (usually from insulin administration or sulfonylureas), an orchestrated counterregulatory response occurs—glucagon and epinephrine rapidly stimulate glycogenolysis and gluconeogenesis, whereas GH and cortisol act over several hours to raise glucose levels and antagonize insulin action.

Although free water clearance is primarily controlled by vasopressin, cortisol and thyroid hormone are also important for facilitating renal tubular responses to vasopressin (Chap. 3). PTH and vitamin D function in an interdependent manner to control calcium metabolism (Chap. 23). PTH stimulates renal synthesis of 1,25 dihydroxyvitamin D, which increases calcium absorption in the gastrointestinal tract and enhances PTH action in bone. Increased calcium, along with vitamin D, feeds back to suppress PTH, thereby maintaining calcium balance.

Depending on the severity of a given stress and whether it is acute or chronic, multiple endocrine and cytokine pathways are activated to mount an appropriate physiologic response. In severe acute stress such as trauma or shock, the sympathetic nervous system is activated and catecholamines are released, leading to increased cardiac output and a primed musculoskeletal system. Catecholamines also increase mean blood pressure and stimulate glucose production. Multiple stress-induced pathways converge on the hypothalamus, stimulating several hormones including vasopressin and corticotropin-releasing hormone (CRH). These hormones, in addition to cytokines (tumor necrosis factor α, IL-2, IL-6), increase

ACTH and GH production. ACTH stimulates the adrenal gland, increasing cortisol, which in turn helps to sustain blood pressure and dampen the inflammatory response. Increased vasopressin acts to conserve free water.

REPRODUCTION

The stages of reproduction include: (1) sex determination during fetal development (Chap. 7); (2) sexual maturation during puberty (Chaps. 8 and 10); (3) conception, pregnancy, lactation, and child-rearing (Chap. 10); and (4) cessation of reproductive capability at menopause (Chap. 11). Each of these stages involves an orchestrated interplay of multiple hormones, a phenomenon well illustrated by the dynamic hormonal changes that occur during each 28-day menstrual cycle. In the early follicular phase, pulsatile secretion of LH and FSH stimulates the progressive maturation of the ovarian follicle. This results in gradually increasing estrogen and progesterone levels, leading to enhanced pituitary sensitivity to GnRH, which, when combined with accelerated GnRH secretion, triggers the LH surge and rupture of the mature follicle. Inhibin, a protein produced by the granulosa cells, enhances follicular growth and feeds back to the pituitary to selectively suppress FSH, without affecting LH. Growth factors such as EGF and IGF-I modulate follicular responsiveness to gonadotropins. Vascular endothelial growth factor and prostaglandins play a role in follicle vascularization and rupture.

During pregnancy, the increased production of prolactin, in combination with placentally derived steroids (e.g., estrogen and progesterone), prepares the breast for lactation. Estrogens induce the production of progesterone receptors, allowing for increased responsiveness to progesterone. In addition to these and other hormones involved in lactation, the nervous system and oxytocin mediate the suckling response and milk release.

HORMONAL FEEDBACK REGULATORY SYSTEMS

Feedback control, both negative and positive, is a fundamental feature of endocrine systems. Each of the major hypothalamic-pituitary-hormone axes is governed by negative feedback, a process that maintains hormone levels within a relatively narrow range. Examples of hypothalamic-pituitary negative feedback include (1) thyroid hormones on the TRH-TSH axis, (2) cortisol on the CRH-ACTH axis, (3) gonadal steroids on the GnRH-LH/FSH axis, and (4) IGF-I on the growth hormone–releasing hormone (GHRH)-GH axis (**Fig. 1-3**). These regulatory loops include both positive (e.g., TRH, TSH) and negative components (e.g., T_4, T_3), allowing for exquisite control of hormone levels. As an example, a small reduction of thyroid hormone triggers a rapid increase of TRH and TSH

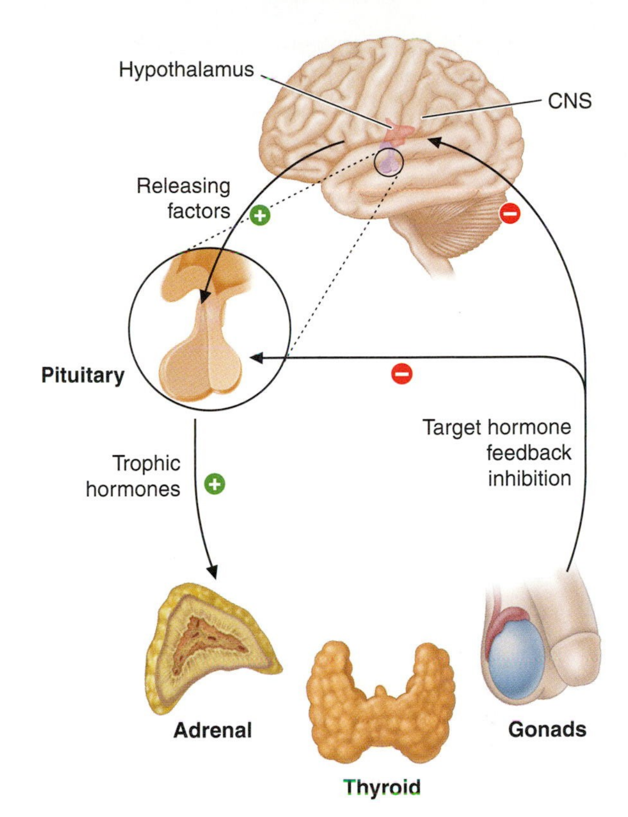

FIGURE 1-3
Feedback regulation of endocrine axes. CNS, central nervous system.

secretion, resulting in thyroid gland stimulation and increased thyroid hormone production. When the thyroid hormone reaches a normal level, it feeds back to suppress TRH and TSH, and a new steady state is attained. Feedback regulation also occurs for endocrine systems that do not involve the pituitary gland, such as calcium feedback on PTH, glucose inhibition of insulin secretion, and leptin feedback on the hypothalamus. An understanding of feedback regulation provides important insights into endocrine testing paradigms (see below).

Positive feedback control also occurs but is not well understood. The primary example is estrogen-mediated stimulation of the midcycle LH surge. Though chronic low levels of estrogen are inhibitory, gradually rising estrogen levels stimulate LH secretion. This effect, which is illustrative of an endocrine rhythm (see below), involves activation of the hypothalamic GnRH pulse generator. In addition, estrogen-primed gonadotropes are extraordinarily sensitive to GnRH, leading to a 10- to 20-fold amplification of LH release.

PARACRINE AND AUTOCRINE CONTROL

The aforementioned examples of feedback control involve classic endocrine pathways in which hormones are released by one gland and act on a distant target gland.

However, local regulatory systems, often involving growth factors, are increasingly recognized. *Paracrine regulation* refers to factors released by one cell that act on an adjacent cell in the same tissue. For example, somatostatin secretion by pancreatic islet δ cells inhibits insulin secretion from nearby β cells. *Autocrine regulation* describes the action of a factor on the same cell from which it is produced. IGF-I acts on many cells that produce it, including chondrocytes, breast epithelium, and gonadal cells. Unlike endocrine actions, paracrine and autocrine control are difficult to document because local growth factor concentrations cannot be readily measured.

Anatomical relationships of glandular systems also greatly influence hormonal exposure—the physical organization of islet cells enhances their intercellular communication; the portal vasculature of the hypothalamic-pituitary system exposes the pituitary to high concentrations of hypothalamic releasing factors; testicular seminiferous tubules gain exposure to high testosterone levels produced by the interdigitated Leydig cells; the pancreas receives nutrient information from the gastrointestinal tract; and the liver is the proximal target of insulin action because of portal drainage from the pancreas.

HORMONAL RHYTHMS

The feedback regulatory systems described above are superimposed on hormonal rhythms that are used for adaptation to the environment. Seasonal changes, the daily occurrence of the light-dark cycle, sleep, meals, and stress are examples of the many environmental events that affect hormonal rhythms. The *menstrual cycle* is repeated on average every 28 days, reflecting the time required to follicular maturation and ovulation (Chap. 10). Essentially all pituitary hormone rhythms are entrained to sleep and the *circadian cycle*, generating reproducible patterns that are repeated approximately every 24 h. The HPA axis, for example, exhibits characteristic peaks of ACTH and cortisol production in the early morning, with a nadir during the night. Recognition of these rhythms is important for endocrine testing and treatment. Patients with Cushing's syndrome characteristically exhibit increased midnight cortisol levels when compared to normal individuals (Chap. 5). In contrast, morning cortisol levels are similar in these groups, as cortisol is normally high at this time of day in normal individuals. The HPA axis is more susceptible to suppression by glucocorticoids administered at night as they blunt the early-morning rise of ACTH. Understanding these rhythms allows glucocorticoid replacement that mimics diurnal production by administering larger doses in the morning than in the afternoon (Chap. 5). Disrupted sleep rhythms can alter hormonal regulation. For example, sleep deprivation causes mild insulin resistance and hypertension, which are reversible at least in the short term.

Other endocrine rhythms occur on a more rapid time scale. Many peptide hormones are secreted in discrete bursts every few hours. LH and FSH secretion are exquisitely sensitive to GnRH pulse frequency. Intermittent pulses of GnRH are required to maintain pituitary sensitivity, whereas continuous exposure to GnRH causes pituitary gonadotrope desensitization. This feature of the hypothalamic-pituitary-gonadotrope (HPG) axis forms the basis for using long-acting GnRH agonists to treat central precocious puberty or to decrease testosterone levels in the management of prostate cancer.

It is important to be aware of the pulsatile nature of hormone secretion and the rhythmic patterns of hormone production when relating serum hormone measurements to normal values. For some hormones, integrated markers have been developed to circumvent hormonal fluctuations. Examples include 24-h urine collections for cortisol, IGF-I as a biologic marker of GH action, and HbA1c as an index of long-term (weeks to months) blood glucose control.

Often, one must interpret endocrine data only in the context of other hormonal results. For example, PTH levels are typically assessed in combination with serum calcium concentrations. A high serum calcium level in association with elevated PTH is suggestive of hyperparathyroidism, whereas a suppressed PTH in this situation is more likely to be caused by hypercalcemia of malignancy or other causes of hypercalcemia. Similarly, TSH should be elevated when T_4 and T_3 concentrations are low, reflecting reduced feedback inhibition. When this is not the case, it is important to consider other abnormalities in the hormonal axis, such as secondary hypothyroidism, which is caused by a defect at the level of the pituitary.

PATHOLOGIC MECHANISMS OF ENDOCRINE DISEASE

Endocrine diseases can be divided into three major types of conditions: (1) hormone excess, (2) hormone deficiency, and (3) hormone resistance (**Table 1-2**).

CAUSES OF HORMONE EXCESS

Syndromes of hormone excess can be caused by neoplastic growth of endocrine cells, autoimmune disorders, and excess hormone administration. Benign endocrine tumors, including parathyroid, pituitary, and adrenal adenomas, often retain the capacity to produce hormones, perhaps reflecting the fact that they are relatively well differentiated. Many endocrine tumors exhibit subtle defects in their "set

TABLE 1-2

CAUSES OF ENDOCRINE DYSFUNCTION

TYPE OF ENDOCRINE DISORDER	EXAMPLES
Hyperfunction	
Neoplastic	
Benign	Pituitary adenomas, hyperparathyroidism, autonomous thyroid or adrenal nodules, pheochromocytoma
Malignant	Adrenal cancer, medullary thyroid cancer, carcinoid
Ectopic	Ectopic ACTH, SIADH secretion
Multiple endocrine neoplasia	MEN 1, MEN 2
Autoimmune	Graves' disease
Iatrogenic	Cushing's syndrome, hypoglycemia
Infectious/inflammatory	Subacute thyroiditis
Activating receptor mutations	LH, TSH, Ca^{2+} and PTH receptors, $G_s\alpha$
Hypofunction	
Autoimmune	Hashimoto's thyroiditis, type 1 diabetes mellitus, Addison's disease, polyglandular failure
Iatrogenic	Radiation-induced hypopituitarism, hypothyroidism, surgical
Infectious/inflammatory	Adrenal insufficiency, hypothalamic sarcoidosis
Hormone mutations	GH, LHβ, FSHβ, vasopressin
Enzyme defects	21-Hydroxylase deficiency
Developmental defects	Kallmann syndrome, Turner syndrome, transcription factors
Nutritional/vitamin deficiency	Vitamin D deficiency, iodine deficiency
Hemorrhage/infarction	Sheehan's syndrome, adrenal insufficiency
Hormone resistance	
Receptor mutations	
Membrane	GH, vasopressin, LH, FSH, ACTH, GnRH, GHRH, PTH, leptin, Ca^{2+}
Nuclear	AR, TR, VDR, ER, GR, $PPAR_\gamma$
Signaling pathway mutations	Albright's hereditary osteodystrophy
Postreceptor	Type 2 diabetes mellitus, leptin resistance

Note: AR, androgen receptor; ER, estrogen receptor; GR, glucocorticoid receptor; PPAR, peroxisome proliferator activated receptor; SIADH, syndrome of inappropriate antidiuretic hormone; TR, thyroid hormone receptor; VDR, vitamin D receptor. For all other abbreviations, see text.

points" for feedback regulation. For example, in Cushing's disease, impaired feedback inhibition of ACTH secretion is associated with autonomous function. However, the tumor cells are not completely resistant to feedback, as evidenced by ACTH suppression by higher doses of dexamethasone (e.g., high-dose dexamethasone test) (Chap. 5). Similar set point defects are also typical of parathyroid adenomas and autonomously functioning thyroid nodules.

The molecular basis of some endocrine tumors, such as the MEN syndromes (MEN 1, 2A, 2B), have provided important insights into tumorigenesis (Chap. 21). MEN 1 is characterized primarily by the triad of parathyroid, pancreatic islet, and pituitary tumors. MEN 2 predisposes to medullary thyroid carcinoma, pheochromocytoma, and hyperparathyroidism. The *MEN1* gene, located on chromosome 11q13, encodes a putative tumor-suppressor gene, menin. Analogous to the paradigm first described for retinoblastoma, the affected individual inherits a mutant copy of the *MEN1* gene, and tumorigenesis ensues after a somatic "second hit" leads to loss of function of the normal *MEN1* gene (through deletion or point mutations).

In contrast to inactivation of a tumor-suppressor gene, as occurs in MEN 1 and most other inherited cancer syndromes, MEN 2 is caused by activating mutations in a single allele. In this case, activating mutations of the *RET* proto-oncogene, which encodes a receptor tyrosine kinase, leads to thyroid C-cell hyperplasia in childhood before the development of medullary thyroid carcinoma. Elucidation of the pathogenic mechanism has allowed early genetic screening for *RET* mutations in individuals at risk for MEN 2, permitting identification of those who may benefit from prophylactic thyroidectomy and biochemical screening for pheochromocytoma and hyperparathyroidism.

Mutations that activate hormone receptor signaling have been identified in several GPCRs. For example, activating mutations of the LH receptor cause a dominantly transmitted form of male-limited precocious puberty, reflecting premature stimulation of testosterone synthesis in Leydig cells (Chap. 8). Activating mutations in these GPCRs are predominantly located in the transmembrane domains and induce receptor coupling to $G_s\alpha$, even in the absence of hormone. Consequently, adenylate cyclase is activated and cyclic AMP levels increase in a manner that mimics hormone action. A similar phenomenon results from activating mutations in $G_s\alpha$. When these occur early in development, they cause McCune-Albright syndrome. When they occur only in somatotropes, the activating $G_s\alpha$ mutations cause GH-secreting tumors and acromegaly (Chap. 2).

In autoimmune Graves' disease, antibody interactions with the TSH receptor mimic TSH action, leading to hormone overproduction (Chap. 4). Analogous to the effects of activating mutations of the TSH receptor, these stimulating autoantibodies induce conformational changes that release the receptor from a constrained state, thereby triggering receptor coupling to G proteins.

CAUSES OF HORMONE DEFICIENCY

Most examples of hormone deficiency states can be attributed to glandular destruction caused by autoimmunity, surgery, infection, inflammation, infarction, hemorrhage, or tumor infiltration (Table 1-2). Autoimmune damage to the thyroid gland (Hashimoto's thyroiditis) and pancreatic islet β cells (type 1 diabetes mellitus) is a prevalent cause of endocrine disease. Mutations in a number of hormones, hormone receptors, transcription factors, enzymes, and channels can also lead to hormone deficiencies.

HORMONE RESISTANCE

Most severe hormone resistance syndromes are due to inherited defects in membrane receptors, nuclear receptors, or in the pathways that transduce receptor signals. These disorders are characterized by defective hormone action, despite the presence of increased hormone levels. In complete androgen resistance, for example, mutations in the androgen receptor cause genetic (XY) males to have a female phenotypic appearance, even though LH and testosterone levels are increased (Chap. 7). In addition to these relatively rare genetic disorders, more common acquired forms of functional hormone resistance include insulin resistance in type 2 diabetes mellitus, leptin resistance in obesity, and GH resistance in catabolic states. The pathogenesis of functional resistance involves receptor downregulation and postreceptor desensitization of signaling pathways; functional forms of resistance are generally reversible.

APPROACH TO THE PATIENT WITH ENDOCRINE DISORDERS

Because endocrinology interfaces with numerous physiologic systems, there is no standard endocrine history and examination. Moreover, because most glands are relatively inaccessible, the examination usually focuses on the manifestations of hormone excess or deficiency, as well as direct examination of palpable glands, such as the thyroid and gonads. For these reasons, it is important to evaluate patients in the context of their presenting symptoms, review of systems, family and social history, and exposure to medications that may affect the endocrine system. Astute clinical skills are required to detect subtle symptoms and signs suggestive of underlying endocrine disease. For example, a patient with Cushing's syndrome may manifest specific findings, such as central fat redistribution, striae, and proximal muscle weakness, in addition to features seen commonly in the general population, such as obesity, plethora, hypertension, and glucose intolerance. Similarly, the insidious onset of hypothyroidism—with mental slowing, fatigue, dry skin, and other features—can be difficult to distinguish from similar, nonspecific findings in the general population. Clinical judgment, based on knowledge of disease prevalence and pathophysiology, is required to decide when to embark on more extensive evaluation of these disorders. Laboratory testing plays an essential role in endocrinology by allowing quantitative assessment of hormone levels and dynamics. Radiologic imaging tests, such as computed tomography (CT) scan, magnetic resonance imaging (MRI), thyroid scan, and ultrasound, are also used for the diagnosis of endocrine disorders. However, these tests are generally employed only after a hormonal abnormality has been established by biochemical testing.

Hormone Measurements and Endocrine Testing

Radioimmunoassays are the most important diagnostic tool in endocrinology, as they allow sensitive, specific, and quantitative determination of steady-state and dynamic changes in hormone concentrations. Radioimmunoassays use antibodies to detect specific hormones. For many peptide hormones, these measurements are now configured as immunoradiometric assays (IRMAs), which use two different antibodies to increase binding affinity and specificity. There are many variations of these assays—a common format involves using one antibody to capture the antigen (hormone) onto an immobilized surface and a second antibody, labeled with a fluorescent or radioactive tag, to detect the antigen. These assays are sensitive enough to detect plasma hormone concentrations in the picomolar to nanomolar range, and they can readily distinguish structurally related proteins, such as PTH from PTHrP. A variety of other techniques are used to measure specific hormones, including mass spectroscopy, various forms of chromatography, and enzymatic methods; bioassays are now rarely used.

Most hormone measurements are based on plasma or serum samples. However, urinary hormone determinations remain useful for the evaluation of some conditions. Urinary collections over 24 h provide an integrated assessment of the production of a hormone or metabolite, many of which vary during the day. It is important to assure complete collections of 24-h urine samples; simultaneous measurement of creatinine provides an internal control for the adequacy of collection and can be used to normalize some hormone measurements. A 24-h urine free cortisol measurement largely reflects the amount of unbound cortisol, thus providing a reasonable index of biologically available hormone. Other commonly used urine determinations include: 17-hydroxycorticosteroids, 17-ketosteroids, vanillylmandelic acid (VMA), metanephrine, catecholamines, 5-hydroxyindoleacetic acid (5-HIAA), and calcium.

The value of quantitative hormone measurements lies in their correct interpretation in a clinical context. The normal range for most hormones is relatively broad, often varying by a factor of two- to tenfold. The normal ranges for many hormones are gender- and age-specific. Thus, using the correct normative database is an essential part of interpreting hormone tests. The pulsatile nature of hormones, and factors that can affect their secretion such as sleep, meals, and medications, must also be considered. Cortisol values increase fivefold between midnight and dawn; reproductive hormone levels vary dramatically during the female menstrual cycle.

For many endocrine systems, much information can be gained from basal hormone testing, particularly when different components of an endocrine axis are assessed simultaneously. For example, low testosterone and elevated LH levels suggest a primary gonadal problem, whereas a hypothalamic-pituitary disorder is likely if both LH and testosterone are low. Because TSH is a sensitive indicator of thyroid function, it is generally recommended as a first-line test for thyroid disorders. An elevated TSH level is almost always the result of primary hypothyroidism, whereas a low TSH is most often caused by thyrotoxicosis. These predictions can be confirmed by determining the free thyroxine level. Elevated calcium and PTH levels suggest hyperparathyroidism, whereas PTH is suppressed in hypercalcemia caused by malignancy or granulomatous diseases. A suppressed ACTH in the setting of hypercortisolemia, or increased urine free cortisol, is seen with hyperfunctioning adrenal adenomas.

It is not uncommon, however, for baseline hormone levels associated with pathologic endocrine conditions to overlap with the normal range. In this circumstance, dynamic testing is useful to further separate the two groups. There are a multitude of dynamic endocrine tests, but all are based on principles of feedback regulation, and most responses can be remembered based on the pathways that govern endocrine axes. *Suppression tests* are used in the setting of suspected endocrine hyperfunction. An example is the dexamethasone suppression test used to evaluate Cushing's syndrome (Chaps. 2 and 5). *Stimulation tests* are generally used to assess endocrine hypofunction. The ACTH stimulation test, for example, is used to assess the adrenal gland response in patients with suspected adrenal insufficiency. Other stimulation tests use hypothalamic-releasing factors such as TRH, GnRH, CRH, and GHRH to evaluate pituitary hormone reserve (Chap. 2). Insulin-induced hypoglycemia evokes pituitary ACTH and GH responses. Stimulation tests based on reduction or inhibition of endogenous hormones are now used infrequently. Examples include metyrapone inhibition of cortisol synthesis and clomiphene inhibition of estrogen feedback.

Screening and Assessment of Common Endocrine Disorders

Because many endocrine disorders are prevalent in the adult population (**Table 1-3**), most are diagnosed and managed by general internists, family practitioners, or other primary health care providers. The high prevalence and clinical impact of certain endocrine diseases justifies vigilance for features of these disorders during routine physical examinations; laboratory screening is indicated in selected high-risk populations.

TABLE 1-3

EXAMPLES OF PREVALENT ENDOCRINE AND METABOLIC DISORDERS IN THE ADULT

DISORDER	APPROX. PREVALENCE IN ADULTS[a]	SCREENING/TESTING RECOMMENDATIONS[b]	SPECIFIC GUIDELINES
Obesity	23% BMI > 30 50% BMI > 25	Calculate BMI Measure waist circumference Exclude secondary causes Consider comorbid complications	NHLBI Clinical Guidelines on the Identification, Evaluation, and Treatment of Overweight and Obesity
Type 2 diabetes mellitus	>6%	Test every 3 years or more often in high-risk groups: Fasting plasma glucose (FPG) > 126 mg/dL Random plasma glucose > 200 mg/dL An elevated HbA1c Consider comorbid complications	Expert Committee on the Diagnosis and Classification of Diabetes Mellitus
Hyperlipidemia	15–20%	Cholesterol screening at least every 5 years; more often in high-risk groups Lipoprotein analysis (LDL, HDL) for increased cholesterol, CAD, diabetes Consider secondary causes	Expert Panel of the National Cholesterol Education Program (NCEP)
Hypothyroidism	5–10%, women 0.5–2%, men	TSH; confirm with free T_4 Screen women after age 35 and every 5 years thereafter	American Thyroid Association
Graves' disease	1–3%, women 0.1%, men	TSH, free T_4	
Thyroid nodules and neoplasia	5%	Physical examination of thyroid Fine-needle aspiration biopsy	American Thyroid Association
Osteoporosis	5%, women 1%, men	Bone mineral density measurements in women >65 years or in postmenopausal women or men at risk Exclude secondary causes	World Health Organization National Osteoporosis Foundation
Hyperparathyroidism	0.1–0.5%, women > men	Serum calcium PTH, if calcium is elevated Assess comorbid conditions	NIH Consensus Conference on Diagnosis and Management of Asymptomatic Primary Hyperparathyroidism
Infertility	10%, couples	Investigate both members of couple Semen analysis in male Assess ovulatory cycles in female Specific tests as indicated	
Polycystic ovarian syndrome	4–7% women	Free testosterone, DHEAS Consider comorbid conditions	
Hirsutism	Variable	Free testosterone, DHEAS Exclude secondary causes Additional tests as indicated	
Menopause	Median age, 51	FSH	
Hyperprolactinemia	Common in women with amenorrhea or galactorrhea	PRL level MRI, if not medication-related	
Erectile dysfunction	10–15%	PRL, testosterone Consider secondary causes (e.g., diabetes)	
Gynecomastia	Common in older men	Often, no tests are indicated Consider Klinefelter syndrome Consider medications, hypogonadism, liver disease	
Klinefelter syndrome	0.2%, men	Karyotype Testosterone	
Turner syndrome	0.03%, women	Karyotype Consider comorbid conditions	

[a]The prevalence of most disorders varies among ethnic groups and with aging.

[b]See individual chapters for additional information on evaluation and treatment. Early testing is indicated in patients with signs and symptoms of disease or in those at increased risk.

Note: BMI, body mass index; CAD, coronary artery disease; DHEAS, dehydroepiandrosterone; HDL, high-density lipoprotein; LDL, low-density lipoprotein. For other abbreviations, see text.

FURTHER READINGS

DeGroot LJ, Jameson JL (eds): *Endocrinology*, 5th ed. Philadelphia, Elsevier, 2006

A comprehensive textbook of endocrinology that contains both basic science and clinical chapters.

Kopchick JJ: History and future of growth hormone research. Horm Res 60:103, 2003

A review of the growth hormone field, including the development of GH receptor antagonists, and animal models that reveal mechanisms of GH action.

Larsen PR et al (eds): *Textbook of Endocrinology*, 10th ed. Philadelphia, Saunders, 2002

This text contains in-depth discussions of endocrine topics.

Leo CP et al: Hormonal genomics. Endocr Rev 23:369, 2002

An overview of how bioinformatics is used to better understand genetic regulatory networks and endocrine signaling.

McKenna NJ, O'Malley BW: Combinatorial control of gene expression by nuclear receptors and coregulators. Cell 108:465, 2002

A summary of the importance of transcriptional coregulators as mediators of biologic responses.

Nakae J et al: Distinct and overlapping functions of insulin and IGF-I receptors. Endocr Rev 22:818, 2001

Comprehensive summary of the relative roles of insulin, IGF-I, IGF-II, and their receptors, with particular focus on new insights derived using murine knockout models.

Riggs BL et al: Selective estrogen-receptor modulators—mechanisms of action and application to clinical practice. N Engl J Med 348:618, 2003

The development of selective estrogen receptor modulators (SERMs) represents a major conceptual and therapeutic advance. This article summarizes how SERMs exert mixed agonist and antagonist actions and defines their current and future use in clinical practice.

Smith CL et al: Coregulator function: A key to understanding tissue specificity of selective receptor modulators. Endocr Rev 25:45, 2004

Transcriptional coregulators include coactivators and corepressors that interact with other components of the active transcription complex. This extensive review classifies these factors and explains their mechanisms of action, particularly with respect to nuclear receptors.

Weinstein LS et al: Minireview: GNAS: Normal and abnormal functions. Endocrinology 145:5459, 2004

An excellent review that summarizes the complex genetic imprinting of the GNAS gene in the context of disease states like Albright hereditary osteodystrophy.

SECTION I

PITUITARY, THYROID, AND ADRENAL DISORDERS

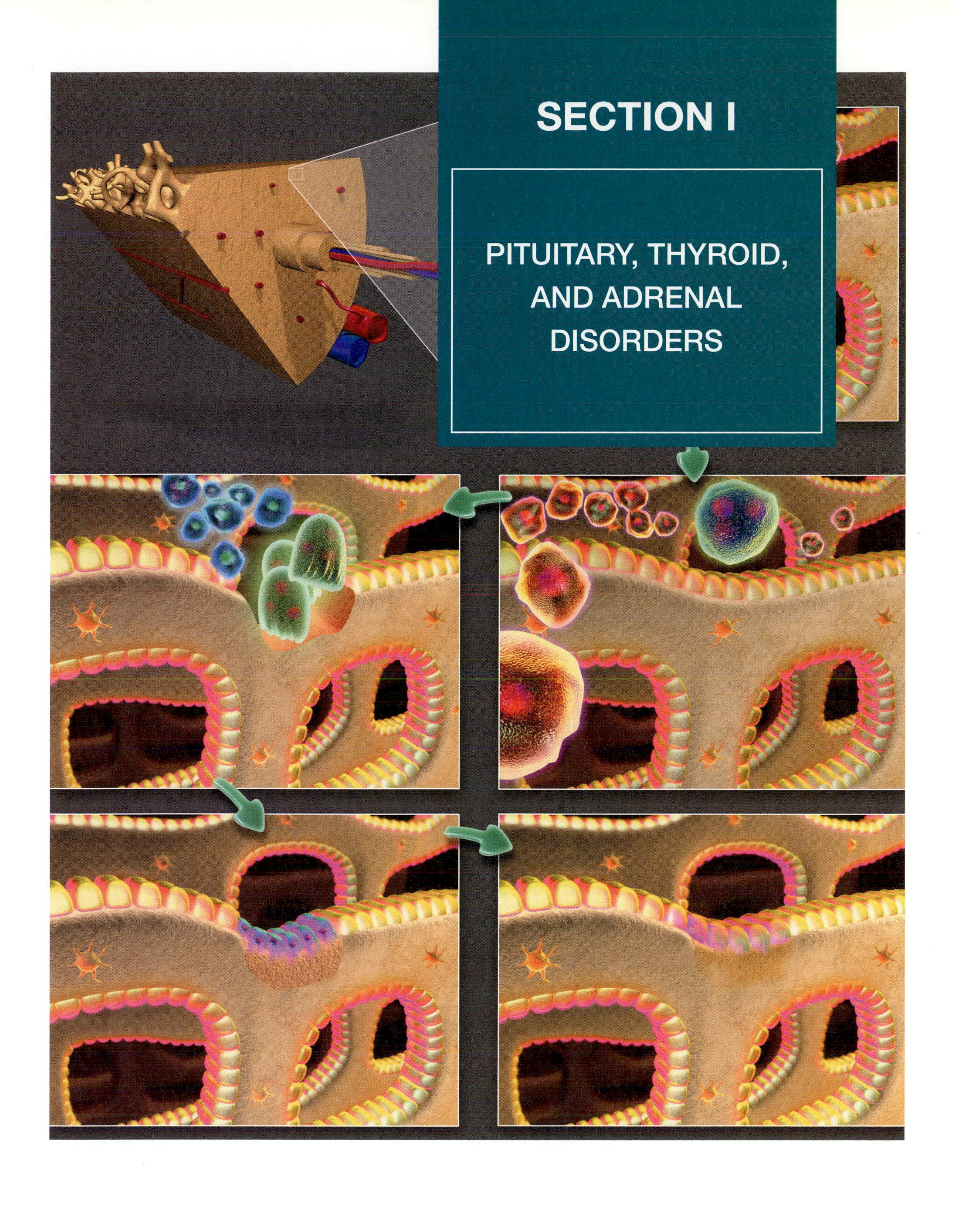

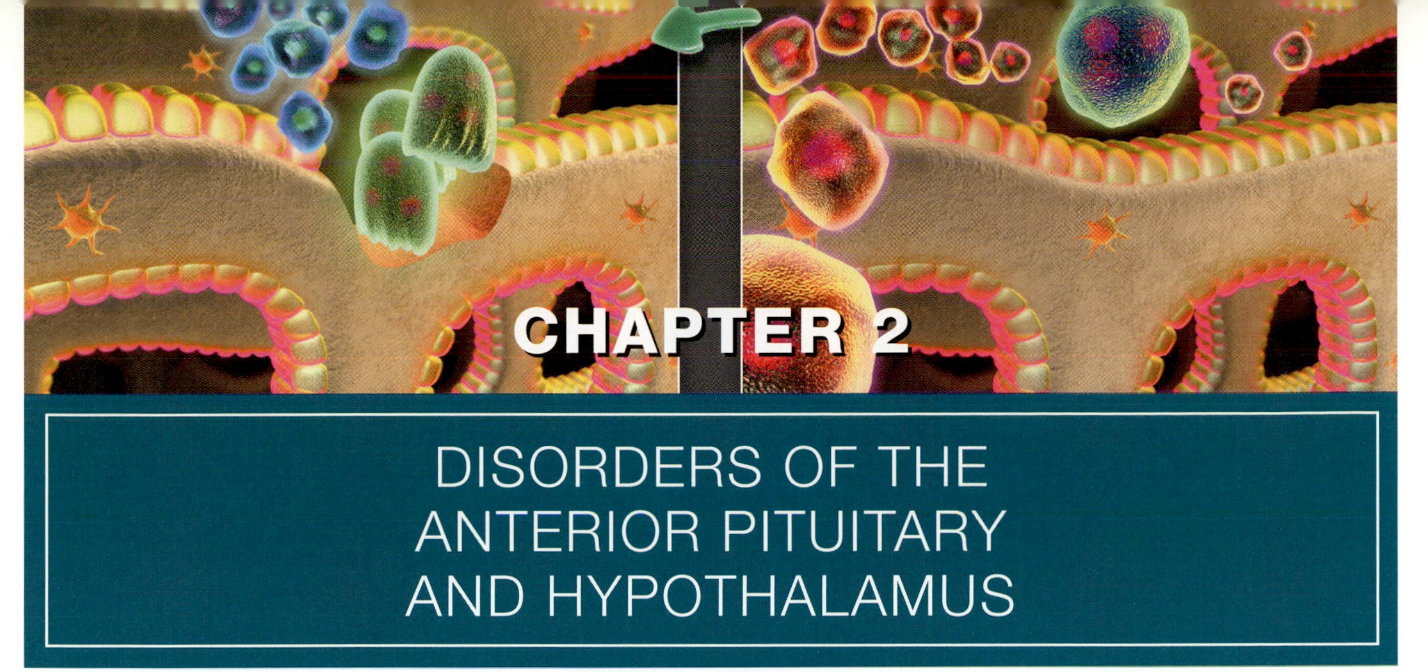

DISORDERS OF THE ANTERIOR PITUITARY AND HYPOTHALAMUS

Shlomo Melmed
J. Larry Jameson

The anterior pituitary is often referred to as the "master gland" because, together with the hypothalamus, it orchestrates the complex regulatory functions of multiple other endocrine glands. The anterior pituitary gland produces six major hormones: (1) prolactin (PRL), (2) growth hormone (GH), (3) adrenocorticotropin hormone (ACTH), (4) luteinizing hormone (LH), (5) follicle-stimulating hormone (FSH), and (6) thyroid-stimulating hormone (TSH) (**Table 2-1**). Pituitary hormones are secreted in a pulsatile manner, reflecting stimulation by an array of specific hypothalamic releasing factors. Each of these pituitary hormones elicits specific responses in peripheral target tissues. The hormonal products of these peripheral glands, in turn, exert feedback control at the level of the hypothalamus and pituitary to modulate pituitary function (**Fig. 2-1**). Pituitary tumors cause characteristic hormone excess syndromes. Hormone deficiency may be inherited or acquired. Fortunately, efficacious treatments exist for the various pituitary hormone excess and deficiency syndromes. Nonetheless, these diagnoses are often elusive, emphasizing the importance of recognizing subtle clinical manifestations and performing the correct laboratory

TABLE 2-1

ANTERIOR PITUITARY HORMONE EXPRESSION AND REGULATION

CELL	CORTICOTROPE	SOMATOTROPE	LACTOTROPE	THYROTROPE	GONADOTROPE
Tissue-specific transcription factor	PTX-1, CUTE	Prop-1, Pit-1	Prop-1, Pit-1	Prop-1, Pit-1, TEF	SF-1, DAX-1
Fetal appearance	6 weeks	8 weeks	12 weeks	12 weeks	12 weeks
Hormone	POMC	GH	PRL	TSH	FSH LH
Chromosomal locus	2p	17q	6	α −6q, β-1p	β-11p; β-19q
Protein	Polypeptide	Polypeptide	Polypeptide	Glycoprotein α, β subunits	Glycoprotein α, β subunits
Amino acids	266 (ACTH 1–39)	191	199	211	210 204
Stimulators	CRH, AVP, gp-130 cytokines	GHRH, GHRP	Estrogen, TRH, VIP	TRH	GnRH, activins, estrogen
Inhibitors	Glucocorticoids	Somatostatin, IGF-I	Dopamine	T_3, T_4, dopamine somatostatin, glucocorticoids	Sex steroids, inhibin
Target gland	Adrenal	Liver, other tissues	Breast, other tissues	Thyroid	Ovary, testis
Trophic effect	Steroid production	IGF-I production, growth induction, insulin antagonism	Milk production	T_4 synthesis and secretion	Sex steroid production, follicle growth, germ cell maturation
Normal range	ACTH, 4–22 pg/L	<0.5 μg/L[a]	M $<$ 15; F $<$ 20 μg/L	0.1–5, mU/L	M, 5–20 IU/L, F (basal) 5–20 IU/L

[a] Hormone secretion integrated over 24 h.

Note: M, male; F, female. For other abbreviations, see text.

Source: Adapted from I Shimon, S Melmed, in P Conn, S Melmed (eds): *Endocrinology: Basic and Clinical Principles*. Totowa, NJ, Humana, 1996.

diagnostic tests. For discussion of disorders of the posterior pituitary, or neurohypophysis, see Chap. 3.

ANATOMY AND DEVELOPMENT

ANATOMY

The pituitary gland weighs ~600 mg and is located within the sella turcica ventral to the diaphragma sella; it comprises anatomically and functionally distinct anterior and posterior lobes. The sella is contiguous to vascular and neurologic structures, including the cavernous sinuses, cranial nerves, and optic chiasm. Thus, expanding intrasellar pathologic processes may have significant central mass effects in addition to their endocrinologic impact.

Hypothalamic neural cells synthesize specific releasing and inhibiting hormones that are secreted directly into the portal vessels of the pituitary stalk. Blood supply of the pituitary gland is derived from the superior and inferior hypophyseal arteries (**Fig. 2-2**). The hypothalamic-pituitary portal plexus provides the major blood source for the anterior pituitary, allowing reliable transmission of hypothalamic peptide pulses without significant systemic dilution; consequently, pituitary cells are exposed to sharp spikes of releasing factors and in turn release their hormones as discrete pulses (**Fig. 2-3**).

The posterior pituitary is supplied by the inferior hypophyseal arteries. In contrast to the anterior pituitary, the posterior lobe is directly innervated by hypothalamic neurons (supraopticohypophyseal and tuberohypophyseal nerve tracts) via the pituitary stalk (Chap. 3). Thus, posterior pituitary production of vasopressin (antidiuretic hormone; ADH) and oxytocin is particularly sensitive to neuronal damage by lesions that affect the pituitary stalk or hypothalamus.

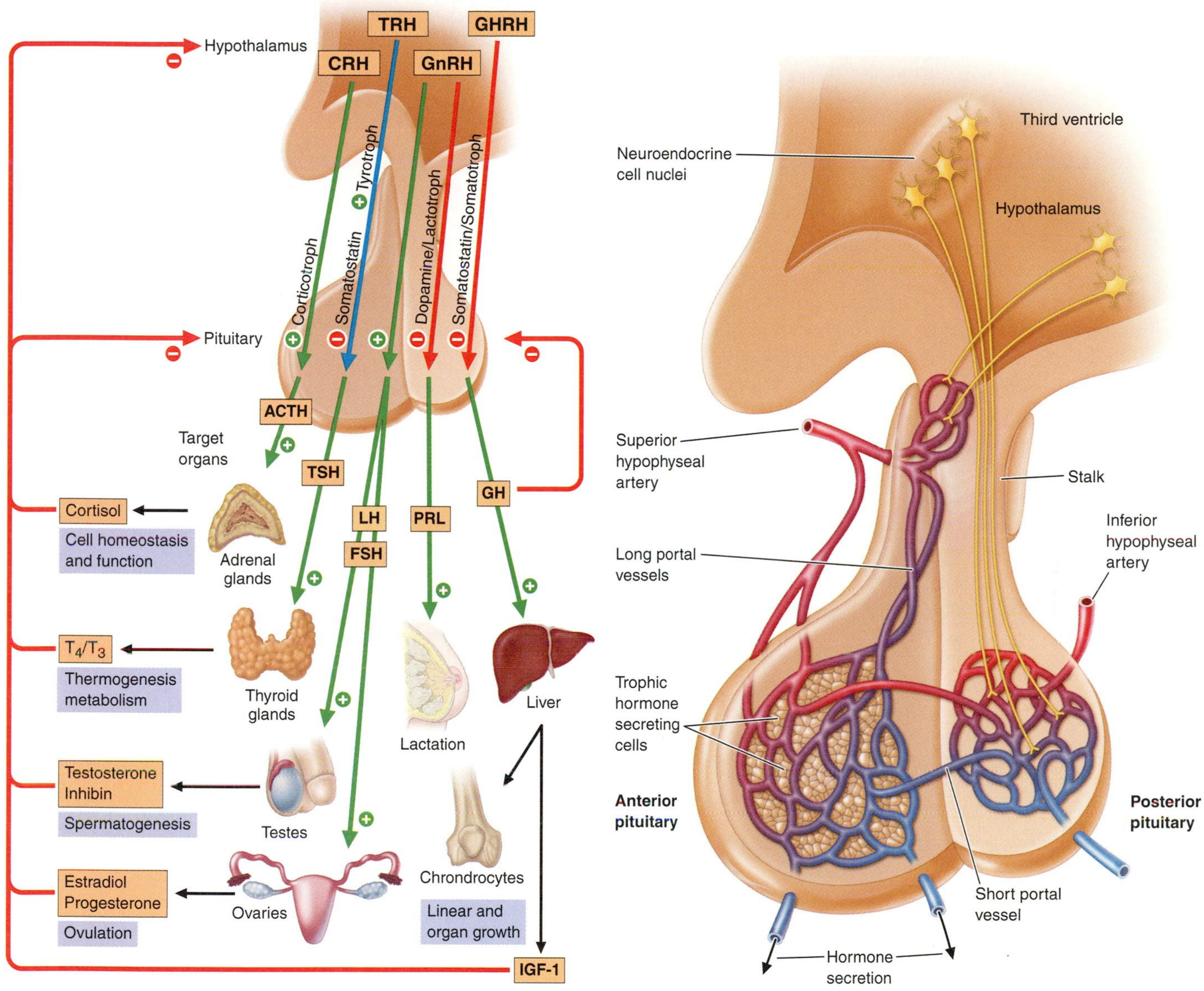

FIGURE 2-1

Diagram of pituitary axes. Hypothalamic hormones regulate anterior pituitary trophic hormones that, in turn, determine target gland secretion. Peripheral hormones feed back to regulate hypothalamic and pituitary hormones. For abbreviations, see text.

FIGURE 2-2

Diagram of hypothalamic-pituitary vasculature: The hypothalamic nuclei produce hormones that traverse the portal system and impinge on anterior pituitary cells to regulate pituitary hormone secretion. Posterior pituitary hormones are derived from direct neural extensions.

PITUITARY DEVELOPMENT

The embryonic differentiation and maturation of anterior pituitary cells have been elucidated in considerable detail. Pituitary development from Rathke's pouch involves a complex interplay of lineage-specific transcription factors expressed in pluripotential stem cells and gradients of locally produced growth factors (Table 2-1). The transcription factor Pit-1 determines cell-specific expression of GH, PRL, and TSH in somatotropes, lac-

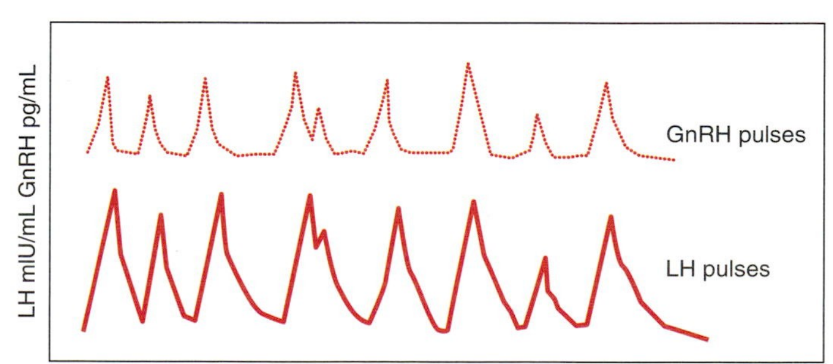

FIGURE 2-3

Hypothalamic gonadotropin-releasing hormone (GnRH) pulses induce secretory pulses of luteinizing hormone (LH).

totropes, and thyrotropes. Expression of high levels of estrogen receptors in cells that contain Pit-1 favors PRL expression, whereas thyrotrope embryonic factor (TEF) induces TSH expression. Pit-1 binds to GH, PRL, and TSH gene regulatory elements, as well as to recognition sites on its own promoter, providing a mechanism for perpetuating selective pituitary phenotypic stability. The transcription factor Prop-1 induces the pituitary development of Pit-1-specific lineages, as well as gonadotropes. Gonadotrope cell development is further defined by the cell-specific expression of the nuclear receptors, steroidogenic factor (SF-1) and DAX-1. Development of corticotrope cells, which express the proopiomelanocortin (POMC) gene, requires corticotropin upstream transcription element (CUTE) and the PTX-1 transcription factor. Abnormalities of pituitary development caused by mutations of Pit-1, Prop-1, SF-1, and DAX-1 result in a series of rare, selective or combined, pituitary hormone deficits.

HYPOTHALAMIC AND ANTERIOR PITUITARY INSUFFICIENCY

Hypopituitarism results from impaired production of one or more of the anterior pituitary trophic hormones. Reduced pituitary function can result from inherited disorders; more commonly, it is acquired and reflects the mass effects of tumors or the consequences of inflammation or vascular damage. These processes may also impair synthesis or secretion of hypothalamic hormones, with resultant pituitary failure (**Table 2-2**).

TABLE 2-2

ETIOLOGY OF HYPOPITUITARISM[a]
Development/structural
Transcription factor defect
Pituitary dysplasia/aplasia
Congenital CNS mass, encephalocele
Primary empty sella
Congenital hypothalamic disorders (septo-optic dysplasia, Prader-Willi syndrome, Laurence-Moon-Biedl-syndrome, Kallmann syndrome)
Traumatic
Surgical resection
Radiation damage
Head injuries
Neoplastic
Pituitary adenoma
Parasellar mass (meningioma, germinoma, ependymoma, glioma)
Rathke's cyst
Craniopharyngioma
Hypothalamic hamartoma, gangliocytoma
Pituitary metastases (breast, lung, colon carcinoma)
Lymphoma and leukemia
Meningioma
Infiltrative/inflammatory
Hemochromatosis
Lymphocytic hypophysitis
Sarcoidosis
Histiocytosis X
Granulomatous hypophysitis
Vascular
Pituitary apoplexy
Pregnancy-related (infarction with diabetes; postpartum necrosis)
Sickle cell disease
Arteritis
Infections
Fungal (histoplasmosis)
Parasitic (toxoplasmosis)
Tuberculosis
Pneumocystis carinii

[a] Trophic hormone failure associated with pituitary compression or destruction usually occurs sequentially GH > FSH > LH > TSH > ACTH. During childhood, growth retardation is often the presenting feature, and in adults hypogonadism is the earliest symptom.

DEVELOPMENTAL AND GENETIC CAUSES OF HYPOPITUITARISM

Pituitary Dysplasia

Pituitary dysplasia may result in aplastic, hypoplastic, or ectopic pituitary gland development. Because pituitary development requires midline cell migration from the nasopharyngeal Rathke's pouch, midline craniofacial disorders may be associated with pituitary dysplasia. Acquired pituitary failure in the newborn can also be caused by birth trauma, including cranial hemorrhage, asphyxia, and breech delivery.

Septo-Optic Dysplasia

Hypothalamic dysfunction and hypopituitarism may result from dysgenesis of the septum pellucidum or corpus callosum. Affected children have mutations in the *HESX1* gene, which is involved in early development of the ventral prosencephalon. These children exhibit variable combinations of cleft palate, syndactyly, ear deformities, hypertelorism, optic atrophy, micropenis, and anosmia. Pituitary dysfunction leads to diabetes insipidus, GH deficiency and short stature, and, occasionally, TSH deficiency.

Tissue-Specific Factor Mutations

Several pituitary cell–specific transcription factors, such as Pit-1 and Prop-1, are critical for determining the development and function of specific anterior pituitary cell lineages. Autosomal dominant or recessive Pit-1 mutations cause combined GH, PRL, and TSH deficiencies. These patients present with growth failure and varying degrees of hypothyroidism. The pituitary may appear hypoplastic on magnetic resonance imaging (MRI).

Prop-1 is expressed early in pituitary development and appears to be required for Pit-1 function. Familial and sporadic *PROP1* mutations result in combined GH, PRL, TSH, and gonadotropin deficiency, with preservation of ACTH. Over 80% of these patients have growth retardation and, by adulthood, all are deficient in TSH and gonadotropins. Because of gonadotropin deficiency, they do not enter puberty spontaneously. In some cases, the pituitary gland is enlarged.

Developmental Hypothalamic Dysfunction

Kallmann Syndrome This syndrome results from defective hypothalamic gonadotropin-releasing hormone (GnRH) synthesis and is associated with anosmia or hyposmia due to olfactory bulb agenesis or hypoplasia (Chap. 8). The syndrome may also be associated with color blindness, optic atrophy, nerve deafness, cleft palate, renal abnormalities, cryptorchidism, and neurologic abnormalities such as mirror movements. Defects in the *KAL* gene, which maps to chromosome Xp22.3, prevent embryonic migration of GnRH neurons from the hypothalamic olfactory placode to the hypothalamus. Genetic abnormalities, in addition to *KAL* mutations, can also cause isolated GnRH deficiency, as autosomal recessive and dominant modes of transmission have been described. GnRH deficiency prevents progression through puberty. Males present with delayed puberty and pronounced hypogonadal features, including micropenis, probably the result of low testosterone levels during infancy. Female patients present with primary amenorrhea and failure of secondary sexual development.

Kallmann syndrome and other causes of congenital GnRH deficiency are characterized by low LH and FSH levels and low concentrations of sex steroids (testosterone or estradiol). In sporadic cases of isolated gonadotropin deficiency, the diagnosis is often one of exclusion after eliminating other causes of hypothalamic-pituitary dysfunction. Repetitive GnRH administration restores normal pituitary gonadotropin responses, pointing to a hypothalamic defect.

Long-term treatment of males with human chorionic gonadotropin (hCG) or testosterone restores pubertal development and secondary sex characteristics; females can be treated with cyclic estrogen and progestin. Fertility may also be restored by the administration of gonadotropins or by using a portable infusion pump to deliver subcutaneous, pulsatile GnRH.

Laurence-Moon-Bardet-Biedl Syndrome This rare autosomal recessive disorder is characterized by mental retardation; obesity; and hexadactyly, brachydactyly, or syndactyly. Central diabetes insipidus may or may not be associated. GnRH deficiency occurs in 75% of males and half of affected females. Retinal degeneration begins in early childhood, and most patients are blind by age 30.

Fröhlich Syndrome (Adipose Genital Dystrophy) A broad spectrum of hypothalamic lesions may be associated with hyperphagia, obesity, and central hypogonadism. Decreased GnRH production in these patients results in attenuated pituitary FSH and LH synthesis and release. Deficiencies of leptin, or its receptor, cause these clinical features (Chap. 16).

Prader-Willi Syndrome Chromosome 15q deletions are associated with hypogonadotropic hypogonadism, hyperphagia-obesity, chronic muscle hypotonia, mental retardation, and adult-onset diabetes mellitus. Multiple somatic defects also involve the skull, eyes, ears, hands, and feet. Diminished hypothalamic oxytocin- and vasopressin-producing nuclei have been reported. Deficient GnRH synthesis is suggested by the observation that chronic GnRH treatment restores pituitary LH and FSH release.

ACQUIRED HYPOPITUITARISM

Hypopituitarism may be caused by accidental or neurosurgical trauma; vascular events such as apoplexy; pituitary or hypothalamic neoplasms such as pituitary adenomas, craniopharyngiomas, or metastatic tumors; inflammatory disease such as lymphocytic hypophysitis; infiltrative disorders such as sarcoidosis, hemochromatosis and tuberculosis; or irradiation.

Hypothalamic Infiltration Disorders

These disorders—including sarcoidosis, histiocytosis X, amyloidosis, and hemochromatosis—frequently involve both hypothalamic and pituitary neuronal and neurochemical tracts. Consequently, diabetes insipidus occurs in half of patients with these disorders. Growth retardation is seen if attenuated GH secretion occurs before pubertal epiphyseal closure. Hypogonadotropic hypogonadism and hyperprolactinemia are also common.

Inflammatory Lesions

Pituitary damage and subsequent dysfunction can be seen with chronic infections such as tuberculosis, opportunistic fungal infections associated with AIDS, and in tertiary syphilis. Other inflammatory processes, such as granulomas or sarcoidosis, may mimic a pituitary adenoma. These lesions may cause extensive hypothalamic and pituitary damage, leading to trophic hormone deficiencies.

Cranial Irradiation

Cranial irradiation may result in long-term hypothalamic and pituitary dysfunction, especially in children and adolescents, as they are more susceptible to damage following whole-brain or head and neck therapeutic irradiation. The development of hormonal abnormalities correlates strongly with irradiation dosage and the time interval after completion of radiotherapy. Up to two-thirds of patients ultimately develop hormone insufficiency afer a median dose of 50 Gy (5000 rad) directed at the skull base. The development of hypopituitarism occurs over 5 to 15 years and usually reflects hypothalamic damage rather than absolute destruction of pituitary cells. Though the pattern of hormone loss is variable, GH deficiency is most common, followed by gonadotropin and ACTH deficiency. When deficiency of one or more hormones is documented, the possibility of diminished reserve of other hormones is likely. Accordingly, anterior pituitary function should be evaluated over the long term in previously irradiated patients, and replacement therapy instituted when appropriate (see below).

Lymphocytic Hypophysitis

This occurs mainly in pregnant or post-partum women; it usually presents with hyperprolactinemia and MRI evidence of a prominent pituitary mass resembling an adenoma, with mildly elevated PRL levels. Pituitary failure caused by diffuse lymphocytic infiltration may be transient or permanent but requires immediate evaluation and treatment. Rarely, isolated pituitary hormone deficiencies have been described, suggesting a selective autoimmune process targeted to specific cell types. Most patients manifest symptoms of progressive mass effects with headache and visual disturbance. The erythrocyte sedimentation rate is often elevated. As the MRI image may be indistinguishable from that of a pituitary adenoma, hypophysitis should be considered in a postpartum woman with a newly diagnosed pituitary mass before embarking on unnecessary surgical intervention. The inflammatory process often resolves after several months of glucocorticoid treatment, and pituitary function may be restored, depending on the extent of damage.

Pituitary Apoplexy

Acute intrapituitary hemorrhagic vascular events can cause substantial damage to the pituitary and surrounding sellar structures. Pituitary apoplexy may occur spontaneously in a preexisting adenoma (usually nonfunctioning); postpartum (Sheehan's syndrome); or in association with diabetes, hypertension, sickle cell anemia, or acute shock. The hyperplastic enlargement of the pituitary during pregnancy increases the risk for hemorrhage and infarction. Apoplexy is an endocrine emergency that may result in severe hypoglycemia, hypotension, central nervous system (CNS) hemorrhage, and death. Acute symptoms may include severe headache with signs of meningeal irritation, bilateral visual changes, ophthalmoplegia, and, in severe cases, cardiovascular collapse and loss of consciousness. Pituitary computed tomography (CT) or MRI may reveal signs of intratumoral or sellar hemorrhage, with deviation of the pituitary stalk and compression of pituitary tissue.

Patients with no evident visual loss or impaired consciousness can be observed and managed conservatively with high-dose glucocorticoids. Those with significant or progressive visual loss or loss of consciousness require urgent surgical decompression. Visual recovery after surgery is inversely correlated with the length of time after the acute event. Therefore, severe ophthalmoplegia or visual deficits are indications for early surgery. Hypopituitarism is very common after apoplexy.

Empty Sella

A partial or apparently totally empty sella is often an incidental MRI finding. These patients usually have normal pituitary function, implying that the surrounding rim of pituitary tissue is fully functional. Hypopituitarism, however, may develop insidiously. Pituitary masses may undergo clinically silent infarction with development of a partial or totally empty sella by cerebrospinal fluid (CSF) filling the dural herniation. Rarely, functional pituitary adenomas may arise within the rim of pituitary tissue, and these are not always visible on MRI.

PRESENTATION AND DIAGNOSIS

The clinical manifestations of hypopituitarism depend on which hormones are lost and the extent of the hormone deficiency. GH deficiency causes growth disorders in children and leads to abnormal body composition in adults (see below). Gonadotropin deficiency causes menstrual disorders and infertility in women and decreased sexual function, infertility, and loss of secondary sexual characteristics in men. TSH and ACTH deficiency usually develop later in the course of pituitary failure. TSH deficiency causes growth retardation in children and features of hypothyroidism in children and in adults. The secondary form of adrenal insufficiency caused by ACTH deficiency leads to hypocortisolism with relative preservation of mineralocorticoid production. PRL deficiency causes failure of lactation. When lesions involve the posterior pituitary, polyuria and polydipsia reflect loss of vasopressin secretion. Epidemiologic studies have documented an increased mortality rate in patients with longstanding pituitary damage, primarily from increased cardiovascular and cerebrovascular disease.

LABORATORY INVESTIGATION

Biochemical diagnosis of pituitary insufficiency is made by demonstrating low levels of trophic hormones in the setting of low target hormone levels. For example, low free thyroxine in the setting of a low or inappropriately normal TSH level suggests secondary hypothyroidism. Similarly, a low testosterone level without elevation of gonadotropins suggests hypogonadotropic hypogonadism. Provocative tests may be required to assess pituitary reserve (**Table 2-3**). GH responses to insulin-induced hypoglycemia, arginine, L-dopa, growth hormone–releasing hormone (GHRH), or growth hormone–releasing peptides (GHRPs) can be used to assess GH reserve. PRL and TSH responses to thyrotropin-releasing hormone (TRH) reflect lactotrope and thyrotrope function. Corticotropin-releasing hormone (CRH) administration induces ACTH release, and administration of synthetic ACTH (cortrosyn) evokes adrenal cortisol release as an indirect indicator of pituitary ACTH reserve (Chap. 5). ACTH reserve is most reliably assessed during insulin-induced hypoglycemia. However, this test should be performed cautiously in patients with suspected adrenal insufficiency because of increased risk of hypoglycemia and hypotension. Insulin-induced hypoglycemia is contraindicated in patients with coronary heart disease or seizure disorders.

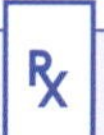

TREATMENT FOR HYPOPITUITARISM

Hormone replacement therapy, including glucocorticoids, thyroid hormone, sex steroids, growth hormone, and vasopressin, is usually free of complications. Treatment regimens that mimic physiologic hormone production allow for maintenance of satisfactory clinical homeostasis. Effective dosage schedules are outlined in **Table 2-4**. Patients in need of glucocorticoid replacement require careful dose adjustments during stressful events such as acute illness, dental procedures, trauma, and acute hospitalization (Chap. 5).

HYPOTHALAMIC, PITUITARY, AND OTHER SELLAR MASSES

PITUITARY TUMORS

Pituitary adenomas are the most common cause of pituitary hormone hypersecretion and hyposecretion syndromes in adults. They account for ~10% of all intracranial neoplasms. At autopsy, up to a quarter of all pituitary glands harbor an unsuspected microadenoma (<10 mm diameter). Similarly, pituitary imaging detects small pituitary lesions in at least 10% of normal individuals.

Pathogenesis

Pituitary adenomas are benign neoplasms that arise from one of the five anterior pituitary cell types. The clinical and biochemical phenotype of pituitary adenomas depend on the cell type from which they are derived. Thus, tumors arising from lactotrope (PRL), somatotrope (GH), corticotrope (ACTH), thyrotrope (TSH), or gonadotrope (LH, FSH) cells hypersecrete their respective hormones (**Table 2-5**). Plurihormonal tumors that

TABLE 2-3

TESTS OF PITUITARY INSUFFICIENCY

HORMONE	TEST	BLOOD SAMPLES	INTERPRETATION
Growth hormone	Insulin tolerance test: Regular insulin (0.05–0.15 U/kg IV)	−30, 0, 30, 60, 120 min for glucose and GH	Glucose <2.2 mmol/L (<40 mg/dL); GH should be >3 μg/L
	GHRH test: 1μ/kg IV	0, 15, 30, 45, 60, 120 min for GH	Normal response is GH >3 μg/L
	L-Arginine test: 30 g IV over 30 min	0, 30, 60, 120 min for GH	Normal response is GH >3 μg/L
	L-dopa test: 500 mg PO	0, 30, 60, 120 min for GH	Normal response is >3 μg/L
Prolactin	TRH test: 200–500 μg IV	0, 20, and 60 min for TSH and PRL	Normal prolactin is >2 μg/L and increase >200% of baseline
ACTH	Insulin tolerance test: Regular insulin (0.05–0.15 U/kg IV)	−30, 0, 30, 60, 90 min for glucose and cortisol	Glucose <2.2 mmol/L (<40 mg/dL) Cortisol should increase by >7 μg/dL or to >20 μg/dL
	CRH test: 1 μg/kg ovine CRH IV at 0800 h	0, 15, 30, 60, 90, 120 min for ACTH and cortisol	Basal ACTH increases 2- to 4-fold and peaks at 20–100 pg/mL Cortisol levels >20–25 μg/dL
	Metyrapone test: Metyrapone (30 mg/kg) at midnight	Plasma 11-deoxycortisol and cortisol at 8 A.M.; ACTH can also be measured	Plasma cortisol should be <4 μg/dL to assure an adequate response Normal response is 11-deoxycortisol >7.5 μg/dL or ACTH >75 pg/mL
	Standard ACTH stimulation test: ACTH 1-24 (Cosyntropin), 0.25 mg IM or IV	0, 30, 60 min for cortisol and aldosterone	Normal response is cortisol >21 μg/dL and aldosterone response of >4 ng/dL above baseline
	Low-dose ACTH test: ACTH 1-24 (Cosyntropin), 1 μg IV	0, 30, 60 min for cortisol	Cortisol should be >21 μg/dL
	3-day ACTH stimulation test consists of 0.25 mg ACTH 1-24 given IV over 8 h each day		Cortisol >21 μg/dL
TSH	Basal thyroid function tests: T_4, T_3, TSH	Basal tests	Low free thyroid hormone levels in the setting of TSH levels that are not appropriately increased
	TRH test: 200–500 μg IV	0, 20, 60 min for TSH and PRL	TSH should increase by >5 mU/L unless thyroid hormone levels are increased
LH, FSH	LH, FSH, testosterone, estrogen	Basal tests	Basal LH and FSH should be increased in postmenopausal women Low testosterone levels in the setting of low LH and FSH
	GnRH test: GnRH (100 μg) IV	0, 30, 60 min for LH and FSH	In most adults, LH should increase by 10 IU/L and FSH by 2 IU/L Normal responses are variable
Multiple hormones	Combined anterior pituitary test:GHRH (1 μg/kg), CRH (1 μg/kg), GnRH (100 μg), TRH (200 μg) are given IV	−30, 0, 15, 30, 60, 90, 120 min for GH, ACTH, cortisol, LH, FSH, and TSH	Combined or individual releasing hormone responses must be elevated in the context of basal target gland hormone values and may not be diagnostic (see text)

Note: For abbreviations, see text.

TABLE 2-4

HORMONE REPLACEMENT THERAPY FOR ADULT HYPOPITUITARISM[a]

TROPHIC HORMONE DEFICIT	HORMONE REPLACEMENT
ACTH	Hydrocortisone (10–20 mg A.M.; 10 mg P.M.) Cortisone acetate (25 mg A.M.; 12.5 mg P.M.) Prednisone (5 mg A.M.; 2.5 mg P.M.)
TSH	L-Thyroxine (0.075–0.15 mg daily)
FSH/LH	Males Testosterone enanthate (200 mg IM every 2 weeks) Testosterone skin patch (5 mg/d) Testosterone gel (5–10 g/d) Females Conjugated estrogen (0.65–1.25 mg qd for 25 days) Progesterone (5–10 mg qd) on days 16–25 Estradiol skin patch (0.5 mg, every other day) For fertility: Menopausal gonadotropins, human chorionic gonadotropins
GH	Adults: Somatotropin (0.3–1.0 mg SC qd) Children: Somatotropin [0.02–0.05 (mg/kg per day)]
Vasopressin	Intranasal desmopressin (5–20 μg twice daily) Oral 300–600 μg qd

[a] All doses shown should be individualized for specific patients and should be reassessed during stress, surgery, or pregnancy. Male and female fertility requirements should be managed as discussed in Chaps. 8 and 10.

Note: For abbreviations, see text.

express combinations of GH, PRL, TSH, ACTH, and the glycoprotein hormone α subunit may be diagnosed by careful immunocytochemistry or may manifest as clinical syndromes that combine features of these hormonal hypersecretory syndromes. Morphologically, these tumors may arise from a single polysecreting cell type or consist of cells with mixed function within the same tumor.

Hormonally active tumors are characterized by autonomous hormone secretion with diminished responsiveness to the normal physiologic pathways of in-

TABLE 2-5

CLASSIFICATION OF PITUITARY ADENOMAS[a]

ADENOMA CELL ORIGIN	HORMONE PRODUCT	CLINICAL SYNDROME
Lactotrope	PRL	Hypogonadism, galactorrhea
Gonadotrope	FSH, LH, subunits	Silent or hypogonadism
Somatotrope	GH	Acromegaly/gigantism
Corticotrope	ACTH	Cushing's disease
Mixed growth hormone and prolactin cell	GH, PRL	Acromegaly, hypogonadism, galactorrhea
Other plurihormonal cell	Any	Mixed
Acidophil stem cell	PRL, GH	Hypogonadism, galactorrhea, acromegaly
Mammosomatotrope	PRL, GH	Hypogonadism, galactorrhea, acromegaly
Thyrotrope	TSH	Thyrotoxicosis
Null cell	None	Pituitary failure
Oncocytoma	None	Pituitary failure

[a] Hormone-secreting tumors are listed in decreasing order of frequency. All tumors may cause local pressure effects, including visual disturbances, cranial nerve palsy, and headache.

Note: For abbreviations, see text.

Source: Adapted from S Melmed, in JL Jameson (ed.). *Principles of Molecular Medicine*, Totowa, Humana Press, 1998.

hibition. Hormone production does not always correlate with tumor size. Small hormone-secreting adenomas may cause significant clinical perturbations, whereas larger adenomas that produce less hormone may be clinically silent and remain undiagnosed (if no central compressive effects occur). About one-third of all adenomas are clinically nonfunctioning and produce no distinct clinical hypersecretory syndrome. Most of these arise from gonadotrope cells and may secrete small amounts of α- and β-glycoprotein hormone subunits or, very rarely, intact circulating gonadotropins. True pituitary carcinomas with documented extracranial metastases are exceedingly rare.

Almost all pituitary adenomas are monoclonal in origin, implying the acquisition of one or more somatic mutations that confer a selective growth advantage. In addition to direct studies of oncogene mutations, this idea is supported by X-chromosomal inactivation analyses of tumors in female patients heterozygous for X-linked genes. Consistent with their clonal origin, complete surgical resection of small pituitary adenomas usually cures hormone hypersecretion. Nevertheless, hypothalamic hormones, such as GHRH or CRH, also enhance the mitotic activity of their respective pituitary target cells, in addition to their role in pituitary hormone regulation. Thus, patients harboring rare abdominal or chest tumors elaborating ectopic GHRH or CRH may present with somatotrope or corticotrope hyperplasia.

Several etiologic genetic events have been implicated in the development of pituitary tumors. The pathogenesis of sporadic forms of acromegaly has been particularly informative as a model of tumorigenesis. GHRH, after binding to its G protein–coupled somatotrope receptor, utilizes cyclic AMP as a second messenger to stimulate GH secretion and somatotrope proliferation. A subset (~35%) of GH-secreting pituitary tumors contain sporadic mutations in Gsα (Arg 201 → Cys or His; Gln 227 → Arg). These mutations inhibit intrinsic GTPase activity, resulting in constitutive elevation of cyclic AMP, Pit-1 induction, and activation of cyclic AMP response element binding protein (CREB), thereby promoting somatotrope cell proliferation.

Characteristic loss of heterozygosity (LOH) in various chromosomes has been documented in large or invasive macroadenomas, suggesting the presence of putative tumor-suppressor genes at these loci. LOH of chromosome region on 11q13, 13, and 9 is present in up to 20% of sporadic pituitary tumors including GH-, PRL-, and ACTH-producing adenomas and in some nonfunctioning tumors.

Compelling evidence also favors growth factor promotion of pituitary tumor proliferation. Basic fibroblast growth factor (bFGF) is abundant in the pituitary and has been shown to stimulate pituitary cell mitogenesis. Other factors involved in initiation and promotion of pituitary tumors include loss of negative-feedback inhibition (as seen with primary hypothyroidism or hypogonadism) and estrogen-mediated or paracrine angiogenesis. Growth characteristics and neoplastic behavior may also be influenced by several activated oncogenes, including *RAS* and pituitary tumor transforming gene (*PTTG*).

Genetic Syndromes Associated with Pituitary Tumors

Several familial syndromes are associated with pituitary tumors, and the genetic mechanisms for some of these have been unraveled.

Multiple endocrine neoplasia (MEN) 1 is an autosomal dominant syndrome characterized primarily by a genetic predisposition to parathyroid, pancreatic islet, and pituitary adenomas (Chap. 21). MEN 1 is caused by inactivating germline mutations in *MENIN*, a constitutively expressed tumor-suppressor gene located on chromosome 11q13. Loss of heterozygosity, or a somatic mutation of the remaining normal *MENIN* allele, leads to tumorigenesis. About half of affected patients develop prolactinomas; acromegaly and Cushing's syndrome are less commonly encountered.

Carney syndrome is characterized by spotty skin pigmentation, myxomas, and endocrine tumors including testicular, adrenal, and pituitary adenomas. Acromegaly occurs in about 20% of patients. A subset of patients have mutations in the R1α regulatory subunit of protein kinase A (*PRKAR1A*).

McCune-Albright syndrome consists of polyostotic fibrous dysplasia, pigmented skin patches, and a variety of endocrine disorders, including GH-secreting pituitary tumors, adrenal adenomas, and autonomous ovarian function (Chap. 10). Hormonal hypersecretion is due to constitutive cyclic AMP production caused by inactivation of the GTPase activity of $G_s\alpha$. The $G_s\alpha$ mutations occur postzygotically, leading to a mosaic pattern of mutant expression.

Familial acromegaly is a rare disorder in which family members may manifest either acromegaly or gigantism. The disorder is associated with LOH at a chromosome 11q13 locus distinct from that of *MENIN*.

OTHER SELLAR MASSES

Craniopharyngiomas are derived from Rathke's pouch. They arise near the pituitary stalk and commonly extend into the suprasellar cistern. These tumors are often large, cystic, and locally invasive. Many are partially calcified, providing a characteristic appearance on skull x-ray and CT images. More than half of all patients present before age 20, usually with signs of increased intracranial pressure, including headache, vomiting, papilledema, and hydrocephalus. Associated symptoms include visual field abnormalities, personality changes and cognitive deterioration, cranial nerve damage, sleep difficulties, and weight gain. Anterior pituitary dysfunction and diabetes insipidus are common. About half of affected children present with growth retardation.

Treatment usually involves transcranial or transsphenoidal surgical resection followed by postoperative radiation of residual tumor. This approach can result in long-term survival and ultimate cure, but most patients require lifelong pituitary hormone replacement. If the pituitary stalk is uninvolved and can be preserved at the time of surgery, the incidence of subsequent anterior pituitary dysfunction is significantly diminished.

Developmental failure of Rathke's pouch obliteration may lead to *Rathke's cysts*, which are small (<5 mm) cysts entrapped by squamous epithelium; these cysts are found in about 20% of individuals at autopsy. Although Rathke's cleft cysts do not usually grow and are often diagnosed incidentally, about a third present in adulthood with compressive symptoms, diabetes insipidus, and hyperprolactinemia due to stalk compression. Rarely, internal hydrocephalus develops. The diagnosis is suggested preoperatively by visualizing the cyst wall on MRI, which distinguishes these lesions from craniopharyngiomas. Cyst contents range from CSF-like fluid to mucoid material. *Arachnoid cysts* are rare and generate an MRI image isointense with cerebrospinal fluid.

Sella chordomas usually present with bony clival erosion, local invasiveness, and, on occasion, calcification. Normal pituitary tissue may be visible on MRI, distinguishing chordomas from aggressive pituitary adenomas. Mucinous material may be obtained by fine-needle aspiration.

Meningiomas arising in the sellar region may be difficult to distinguish from nonfunctioning pituitary adenomas. Meningiomas typically enhance on MRI and may show evidence of calcification or bony erosion. Meningiomas may cause compressive symptoms.

Histiocytosis X comprises a variety of syndromes associated with foci of eosinophilic granulomas. Diabetes insipidus, exophthalmos, and punched-out lytic bone lesions (*Hand-Schüller-Christian disease*) are associated with granulomatous lesions visible on MRI, as well as a characteristic axillary skin rash. Rarely, the pituitary stalk may be involved.

Pituitary metastases occur in ~3% of cancer patients. Blood-borne metastatic deposits are found almost exclusively in the posterior pituitary. Accordingly, diabetes insipidus can be a presenting feature of lung, gastrointestinal, breast, and other pituitary metastases. About half of pituitary metastases originate from breast cancer; about 25% of patients with breast cancer have such deposits. Rarely, pituitary stalk involvement results in anterior pituitary insufficiency. The MRI diagnosis of a metastatic lesion may be difficult to distinguish from an aggressive pituitary adenoma; the diagnosis may require histologic examination of excised tumor tissue. Primary or metastatic lymphoma, leukemias, and plasmacytomas also occur within the sella.

Hypothalamic hamartomas and ***gangliocytomas*** may arise from astrocytes, oligodendrocytes, and neurons with varying degrees of differentiation. These tumors may overexpress hypothalamic neuropeptides including GnRH, GHRH, or CRH. In GnRH-producing tumors, children present with precocious puberty, psychomotor delay, and laughing-associated seizures. Medical treatment of GnRH-producing hamartomas with long-acting GnRH analogues effectively suppresses gonadotropin secretion and controls premature pubertal development. Rarely, hamartomas are also associated with craniofacial abnormalities; imperforate anus; cardiac, renal, and lung disorders; and pituitary failure (*Pallister-Hall syndrome*). Hypothalamic hamartomas are often contiguous with the pituitary, and preoperative MRI diagnosis may not be possible. Histologic evidence of hypothalamic neurons in tissue resected at transsphenoidal surgery may be the first indication of a primary hypothalamic lesion.

Hypothalamic gliomas and ***optic gliomas*** occur mainly in childhood and usually present with visual loss. Adults have more aggressive tumors; about a third are associated with neurofibromatosis.

Brain germ cell tumors may arise within the sellar region. These include *dysgerminomas*, which are frequently associated with diabetes insipidus and visual loss. They rarely metastasize. *Germinomas, embryonal carcinomas, teratomas*, and *choriocarcinomas* may arise in the parasellar region and produce hCG. These germ cell tumors present with precocious puberty, diabetes insipidus, visual field defects, and thirst disorders. Many patients are GH-deficient with short stature.

METABOLIC EFFECTS OF HYPOTHALAMIC LESIONS

Lesions involving the anterior and preoptic hypothalamic regions cause paradoxical vasoconstriction, tachycardia, and hyperthermia. Acute hyperthermia is usually due to a hemorrhagic insult, but poikilothermia may also occur. Central disorders of thermoregulation result from posterior hypothalamic damage. The *periodic hypothermia syndrome* comprises episodic attacks of rectal temperatures <30°C, sweating, vasodilation, vomiting, and bradycardia. Damage to the ventromedial nuclei by craniopharyngiomas, hypothalamic trauma, or inflammatory disorders may be associated with *hyperphagia* and *obesity*. This region appears to contain an energy-satiety center where melanocortin receptors are influenced by leptin, insulin, POMC products, and gastrointestinal peptides (Chap. 16). Hypothalamic gliomas in early childhood may be associated with a diencephalic syndrome characterized by progressive severe emaciation and growth failure. Polydipsia and hypodipsia are associated with damage to central osmo-receptors located in preoptic nuclei (Chap. 3). Slow-growing hypothalamic lesions can cause increased somnolence and disturbed sleep cycles as well as obesity, hypothermia, and emotional outbursts. Lesions of the central hypothalamus may stimulate sympathetic neurons, leading to elevated serum catecholamine and cortisol levels. These patients are predisposed to cardiac arrhythmias, hypertension, and gastric erosions.

EVALUATION

Local Mass Effects

Clinical manifestations of sellar lesions vary, depending on the anatomical location of the mass and direction of its extension (**Table 2-6**). The dorsal roof of the sella presents the least resistance to soft tissue expansion from within the confines of the sella; consequently, pituitary adenomas frequently extend in a suprasellar direction. Bony invasion may ultimately occur as well.

Headaches are common features of small intrasellar tumors, even with no demonstrable suprasellar extension. Because of the confined nature of the pituitary, small changes in intrasellar pressure stretch the dural plate; however, the severity of the headache correlates poorly with adenoma size or extension.

Suprasellar extension can lead to visual loss by several mechanisms, the most common being compression of the optic chiasm, but direct invasion of the optic nerves or obstruction of CSF flow leading to secondary visual disturbances also occurs. Pituitary stalk compression by a hormonally active or inactive intrasellar mass may compress the portal vessels, disrupting pituitary access to the hypothalamic hormones and dopamine; this results in hyperprolactinemia and concurrent loss of other pituitary hormones. This "stalk section" phenomenon may also be caused by trauma, whiplash injury with posterior clinoid stalk compression, or skull base fractures. Lateral mass invasion may impinge on the cavernous sinus and compress its neural contents, leading to cranial nerve III, IV, and VI palsies as well as effects on the ophthalmic and maxillary branches of the fifth cranial nerve. Patients may present with diplopia, ptosis, ophthalmoplegia, and decreased facial sensation, depending on the extent of neural damage. Extension into the sphenoid sinus indicates that the pituitary mass has eroded through the sellar floor. Aggressive tumors rarely invade the palate roof and cause nasopharyngeal obstruction, infection, and CSF leakage. Both temporal and frontal lobes may be invaded, leading to uncinate seizures, personality disorders, and anosmia. Direct hypothalamic encroachment by an invasive pituitary mass may cause important metabolic sequelae, precocious puberty or hypogonadism, diabetes insipidus, sleep disturbances, dysthermia, and appetite disorders.

TABLE 2-6

FEATURES OF SELLAR MASS LESIONS[a]

IMPACTED STRUCTURE	CLINICAL IMPACT
Pituitary	Hypogonadism Hypothyroidism Growth failure and adult hyposomatotropism Hypoadrenalism
Optic chiasm	Loss of red perception Bitemporal hemianopia Superior or bitemporal field defect Scotoma Blindness
Hypothalamus	Temparature dysregulation Appetite and thirst disorders Obesity Diabetes insipidus Sleep disorders Behavioral dysfunction Autonomic dysfunction
Cavernous sinus	Opthalmoplegia ± ptosis or diplopia Facial numbness
Frontal lobe	Personality disorder Anosmia
Brain	Headache Hydrocephalus Psychosis Dementia Laughing seizures

[a] As the intrasellar mass expands, it first compresses intrasellar pituitary tissue, then usually invades dorsally through the dura to lift the optic chiasm or laterally to the cavernous sinuses. Bony erosion is rare, as is direct brain compression. Microadenomas may present with headache.

MRI

Sagittal and coronal T1-weighted spin-echo MRI imaging, before and after administration of gadolinium, allow precise visualization of the pituitary gland with clear delineation of the hypothalamus, pituitary stalk, pituitary tissue and surrounding suprasellar cisterns, cavernous sinuses, sphenoid sinus, and optic chiasm. Pituitary gland height ranges from 6 mm in children to 8 mm in adults; during pregnancy and puberty, the height may reach 10 to 12 mm. The upper aspect of the adult pituitary is flat or slightly concave, but in adolescent and pregnant individuals, this surface may be convex, reflecting physiologic pituitary enlargement. The stalk should be vertical. CT scan is indicated to define the extent of bony erosion or the presence of calcification.

The soft tissue consistency of the pituitary gland is slightly heterogeneous on MRI. Anterior pituitary signal intensity resembles that of brain matter on T1-imaging (**Fig. 2-4**). Adenoma density is usually lower than that of surrounding normal tissue on T1-weighted imaging, and the signal intensity increases with T2-weighted images. The high phospholipid content of the posterior pituitary results in a "pituitary bright spot."

Sellar masses are commonly encountered as incidental findings on MRI, and most of these are pituitary adenomas (incidentalomas). In the absence of hormone hypersecretion, these small lesions can be safely monitored by MRI, which is performed annually and then less often if there is no evidence of growth. Resection should be considered for incidentally discovered macroadenomas, as about one-third become invasive or cause local pressure effects. If hormone hypersecretion is evident, specific therapies are indicated. When larger masses (>1 cm) are encountered, they should also be distinguished from nonadenomatous lesions. Meningiomas are often associated with bony hyperostosis; craniopharyngiomas may be calcified and are usually hypodense, whereas gliomas are hyperdense on T2-weighted images.

Ophthalmologic Evaluation

Because optic tracts may be contiguous to an expanding pituitary mass, reproducible visual field assessment that uses perimetry techniques should be performed on all patients with sellar mass lesions that abut the optic chiasm. Bitemporal hemianopia or superior bitemporal defects are classically observed, reflecting the location of these tracts within the inferior and posterior part of the chiasm. Homonymous cuts are postchiasmal and monocular field cuts are prechiasmal. Loss of red perception is an early sign of optic tract pressure. Early diagnosis reduces the risk of blindness, scotomas, or other visual disturbances.

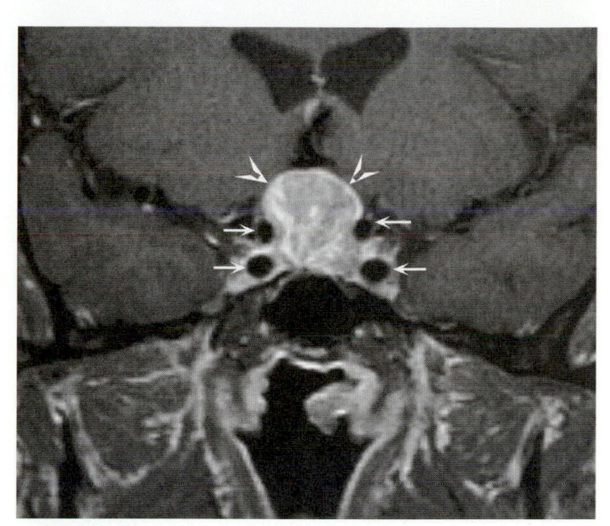

FIGURE 2-4

Pituitary adenoma. Coronal T1-weighted postcontrast MR image shows a homogeneously enhancing mass (*arrowheads*) in the sella turcica and suprasellar region compatible with a pituitary adenoma; the small arrows outline the carotid arteries.

Laboratory Investigation

The presenting clinical features of functional pituitary adenomas (e.g., acromegaly, prolactinomas, or Cushing's disease) should guide the laboratory studies (**Table 2-7**). However, for a sellar mass with no obvious clinical features of hormone excess, laboratory studies are geared towards determining the nature of the tumor and assessing the possible presence of hypopituitarism. When a pituitary adenoma is suspected based on MRI, initial hormonal evaluation usually includes: (1) basal PRL; (2) insulin-like growth factor (IGF) I; (3) 24-h urinary free cortisol (UFC) and/or overnight oral dexamethasone (1 mg) suppression test; (4) α-subunit, FSH, and LH levels; and (5) thyroid function tests. Additional hormonal evaluation may be indicated based on the results of these tests. Pending more detailed assessment of hypopituitarism, a menstrual history, testosterone level, 8 A.M. cortisol, and thyroid function tests usually identify patients with pituitary hormone deficiencies that require hormone replacement before further testing or surgery.

Histologic Evaluation

Immunohistochemical staining of pituitary tumor specimens obtained at transsphenoidal surgery confirms clinical and laboratory studies and provides a histologic diagnosis when hormone studies are equivocal and in cases of clinically nonfunctioning tumors. Occasionally, ultrastructural assessment by electron microscopy is required for diagnosis.

TABLE 2-7

SCREENING TESTS FOR FUNCTIONAL PITUITARY ADENOMAS

	TEST	COMMENTS
Acromegaly	Serum IGF-I	Interpret IGF-I relative to age- and gender-matched controls
	Oral glucose tolerance test with GH obtained at 0, 30, and 60 min	Normal subjects should suppress growth hormone to <1 μg/L
Prolactinoma	Exclude medications	MRI of the sella should be ordered if prolactin is elevated
Cushing's disease	24-h urinary free cortisol	Ensure urine collection is total and accurate
	Dexamethasone (1 mg) at 11 P.M. and fasting plasma cortisol measured at 8 A.M.	Normal subjects suppress to <5 μg/dL
	ACTH assay	Distinguishes adrenal adenoma (ACTH suppressed) from ectopic ACTH or Cushing's disease (ACTH normal or elevated)

Note: For abbreviations, see text.

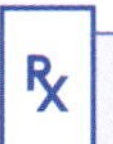

TREATMENT FOR SELLAR MASSES

Overview

Successful management of sellar masses requires accurate diagnosis as well as selection of optimal therapeutic modalities. Most pituitary tumors are benign and slow-growing. Clinical features result from local mass effects and hormonal hypo- or hypersecretion syndromes caused directly by the adenoma or as a consequence of treatment. Thus, lifelong management and follow-up are necessary for these patients.

MRI technology with gadolinium enhancement for pituitary visualization, new advances in transsphenoidal surgery and in stereotactic radiotherapy (including gamma-knife radiotherapy), and novel therapeutic agents have improved pituitary tumor management. The goals of pituitary tumor treatment include normalization of excess pituitary secretion, amelioration of symptoms and signs of hormonal hypersecretion syndromes, and shrinkage or ablation of large tumor masses with relief of adjacent structure compression. Residual anterior pituitary function should be preserved and can sometimes be restored by removing tumor mass. Ideally, adenoma recurrence should be prevented.

Transsphenoidal Surgery

Transsphenoidal rather than transfrontal resection is the desired surgical approach for pituitary tumors, except for the rare invasive suprasellar mass surrounding the frontal or middle fossa, the optic nerves, or invading posteriorly behind the clivus. Intraoperative microscopy facilitates visual distinction between adenomatous and normal pituitary tissue, as well as microdissection of small tumors that may not be visible by MRI (**Fig. 2-5**). Transsphenoidal surgery also avoids the cranial invasion and manipulation of brain tissue required by subfrontal surgical approaches. Endoscopic techniques with three-dimensional intraoperative localization have improved visualization and access to tumor tissue. The endoscopic approach is also less traumatic, as the technique is endonasal and does not require a transsphenoidal retractor.

In addition to correction of hormonal hypersecretion, pituitary surgery is indicated for mass lesions that impinge on surrounding structures. Surgical decompression and resection are required for an expanding pituitary mass accompanied by persistent headache, progressive visual field defects, cranial nerve palsies, internal hydrocephalus, and, occasionally, intrapituitary hemorrhage and apoplexy.

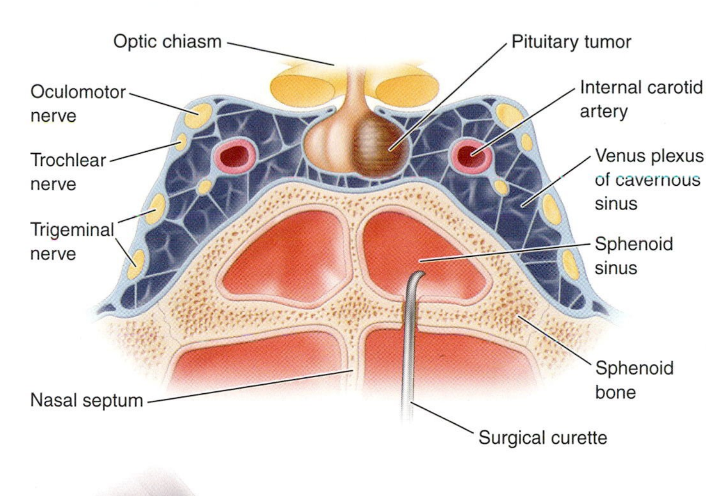

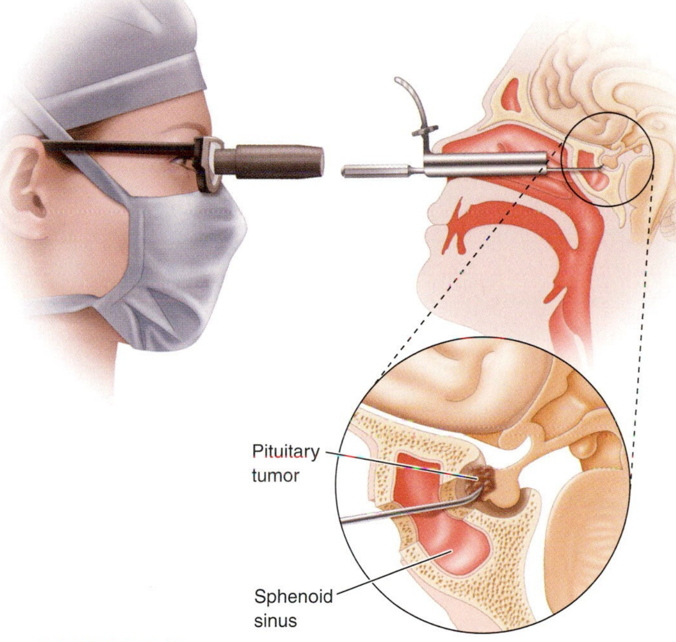

FIGURE 2-5

Transsphenoidal resection of pituitary mass via the endonasal approach. (*Adapted from Fahlbusch R: Endocrinol Metab Clin North Am 21:669, 1992.*)

Transsphenoidal surgery is sometimes used for pituitary tissue biopsy and histologic diagnosis.

Whenever possible, the pituitary mass lesion should be selectively excised; normal tissue should be manipulated or resected only when critical for effective dissection. Nonselective hemihypophysectomy or total hypophysectomy may be indicated if no mass lesion is clearly discernible, multifocal lesions are present, or the remaining nontumorous pituitary tissue is obviously necrotic. This strategy increases the likelihood of hypopituitarism and the need for lifelong hormonal replacement.

Preoperative local compression signs, including visual field defects or compromised pituitary function, may be reversed by surgery, particularly when these deficits are not long-standing. For large and invasive tumors, it is necessary to determine the optimal balance between maximal tumor resection and preservation of anterior pituitary function, especially for preserving growth and reproductive function in younger patients. Similarly, tumor invasion outside of the sella is rarely amenable to surgical cure; the surgeon must judge the risk:benefit ratio of extensive tumor resection.

SIDE EFFECTS

Tumor size and the degree of invasiveness largely determine the incidence of surgical complications. Operative mortality is about 1%. Transient diabetes insipidus and hypopituitarism occur in up to 20% of patients. Permanent diabetes insipidus, cranial nerve damage, nasal septal perforation, or visual disturbances may be encountered in up to 10% of patients. CSF leaks occur in 4% of patients. Less common complications include carotid artery injury, loss of vision, hypothalamic damage, and meningitis. Permanent side effects are rarely encountered after surgery for microadenomas.

Radiation

Radiation is used either as a primary therapy for pituitary or parasellar masses or, more commonly, as an adjunct to surgery or medical therapy. Focused megavoltage irradiation is achieved by precise MRI localization, using a high-voltage linear accelerator and accurate isocentric rotational arcing. A major determinant of accurate irradiation is to reproduce the patient's head position during multiple visits and to maintain absolute head immobility. A total of <50 Gy (5000 rad) is given as 180-cGy (180 rad) fractions split over about 6 weeks. Stereotactic radiosurgery delivers a large single high-energy dose from a cobalt 60 source (gamma knife), linear accelerator, or cyclotron. Long-term effects of gamma-knife surgery are as yet unknown.

The role of radiation therapy in pituitary tumor management depends on multiple factors including the nature of the tumor, age of the patient, and the availability of surgical and radiation expertise.

Because of its relatively slow onset of action, radiation therapy is usually reserved for postsurgical management. As an adjuvant to surgery, radiation is used to treat residual tumor and in an attempt to prevent regrowth. Irradiation offers the only effective means for ablating significant residual tumor tissue derived from nonfunctioning tumors. PRL-, GH-, and ACTH-secreting tumor tissues are also amenable to medical therapy.

SIDE EFFECTS

In the short term, radiation may cause transient nausea and weakness. Alopecia and loss of taste and smell may be more long-lasting. Failure of pituitary hormone synthesis is common in patients who have undergone head and neck or pituitary-directed irradiation. More than 50% of patients develop failure of GH, ACTH, TSH, and/or gonadotropin secretion within 10 years, usually due to hypothalamic damage. Lifelong follow-up with testing of anterior pituitary hormone reserve is therefore necessary after radiation treatment. Optic nerve damage with impaired vision due to optic neuritis is reported in about 2% of patients who undergo pituitary irradiation. Cranial nerve damage is uncommon now that radiation doses are ≤2 Gy (200 rad) at any one treatment session and the maximum dose is <50 Gy (5000 rad). The advent of stereotactic radiotherapy may reduce damage to adjacent structures. The cumulative risk of developing a secondary tumor after conventional radiation is 1.3% after 10 years and 1.9% after 20 years.

Medical

Medical therapy for pituitary tumors is highly specific and depends on tumor type. For prolactinomas, dopamine agonists are the treatment of choice. For acromegaly and TSH-secreting tumors, somatostatin analogues and, occasionally, dopamine agonists are indicated. ACTH-secreting tumors and nonfunctioning tumors are generally not responsive to medication and require surgery and/or irradiation.

PROLACTIN

SYNTHESIS

PRL consists of 198 amino acids and has a molecular mass of 21,500 kDa; it is weakly homologous to GH and human placental lactogen (hPL), reflecting the duplication and divergence of a common GH-PRL-hPL precursor gene on chromosome 6. PRL is synthesized in lactotropes, which comprise about 20% of anterior pituitary cells. Lactotropes and somatotropes are derived from a common precursor cell that may give rise to a tumor secreting both PRL and GH. Marked lactotrope cell hyperplasia develops during the last two trimesters of pregnancy and the first few months of lactation. These transient adaptive changes in the lactotrope population are induced by estrogen.

SECRETION

Normal adult serum PRL levels are about 10 to 25 μg/L in women and 10 to 20 μg/L in men. PRL secretion is pulsatile, with the highest secretory peaks occurring during rapid eye movement sleep. Peak serum PRL levels (up to 30 μg/L) occur between 4:00 and 6:00 A.M. The circulating half-life of PRL is about 50 min.

PRL is unique among the pituitary hormones in that the predominant central control mechanism is inhibitory, reflecting dopamine-mediated suppression of PRL release. This regulatory pathway accounts for the spontaneous PRL hypersecretion that occurs after pituitary stalk section, often a consequence of mass lesions at the skull base. Pituitary, dopamine type 2 (D_2) receptors mediate PRL inhibition. Targeted disruption (gene knockout) of the murine D_2 receptor results in hyperprolactinemia and lactotrope proliferation. As discussed below, dopamine agonists play a central role in the management of hyperprolactinemic disorders.

TRH (pyro Glu-His-Pro-NH2) is a hypothalamic tripeptide that releases prolactin within 15 to 30 min after intravenous injection. The physiologic relevance of TRH for PRL regulation is unclear, as it appears primarily to regulate TSH (Chap. 4). *Vasoactive intestinal peptide* (VIP) also induces PRL release, whereas glucocorticoids and thyroid hormone weakly suppress PRL secretion.

Serum PRL levels rise after exercise, meals, sexual intercourse, minor surgical procedures, general anesthesia, acute myocardial infarction, and other forms of acute stress. PRL levels also increase significantly (approximately tenfold) during pregnancy and decline rapidly within 2 weeks of parturition. If breastfeeding is initiated, basal PRL levels remain elevated; suckling stimulates reflex increases in PRL levels that last for about 30 to 45 min. Breast suckling activates neural afferent pathways in the hypothalamus that induce PRL release. With time, the suckling-induced responses diminish and interfeeding PRL levels return to normal.

ACTION

The PRL receptor is a member of the type I cytokine receptor family that also includes GH and interleukin (IL) 6 receptors. Ligand binding leads to receptor dimerization followed by intracellular signaling mediated by Janus kinase (JAK) and components of the signal transduction and activators of transcription (STAT) family that translocate to the nucleus, where they act as transcription factors on target genes. In the breast, the lobuloalveolar epithelium proliferates in response to PRL, placental lactogens, estrogen, progesterone, and local paracrine growth factors.

PRL acts to induce and maintain lactation, decrease reproductive function, and suppress sexual drive. These functions are geared towards ensuring that maternal lactation is sustained and not interrupted by pregnancy. PRL inhibits reproductive function by suppressing hypothalamic GnRH and pituitary gonadotropin secretion and by impairing gonadal steroidogenesis in both female and male subjects. In the ovary, PRL blocks folliculogenesis and inhibits granulosa cell aromatase activity, leading to hypoestrogenism and anovulation. PRL also has a luteolytic effect, generating a shortened, or inadequate, luteal phase of the menstrual cycle. In males, attenuated LH secretion leads to low testosterone levels and decreased spermatogenesis. These hormonal changes decrease libido and reduce fertility in patients with hyperprolactinemia.

HYPERPROLACTINEMIA

Etiology

Hyperprolactinemia is the most common pituitary hormone hypersecretion syndrome in both males and females. PRL-secreting pituitary adenomas (prolactinomas) are the most common cause of PRL levels >100 μg/L (see below). Less pronounced PRL elevation can also be seen with microprolactinomas but is more commonly caused by drugs, pituitary stalk compression, hypothyroidism, or renal failure (**Table 2-8**).

Pregnancy and lactation are the important physiologic causes of hyperprolactinemia. Sleep-associated hyperprolactinemia reverts to normal within an hour of

TABLE 2-8

ETIOLOGY OF HYPERPROLACTINEMIA[a]

I. Physiologic hypersecretion
- A. Pregnancy
- B. Lactation
- C. Chest wall stimulation
- D. Sleep
- E. Stress

II. Hypothalamic–pituitary stalk damage
- A. Tumors
  1. Craniopharyngioma
  2. Suprasellar pituitary mass extension
  3. Meningioma
  4. Dysgerminoma
  5. Metastases
- B. Empty sella
- C. Lymphocytic hypophysitis
- D. Adenoma with stalk compression
- E. Granulomas
- F. Rathke's cyst
- G. Irradiation
- H. Trauma
  1. Pituitary stalk section
  2. Suprasellar surgery

III. Pituitary hypersecretion
- A. Prolactinoma
- B. Acromegaly

IV. Systemic disorders
- A. Chronic renal failure
- B. Hypothyroidism
- C. Cirrhosis
- D. Pseudocyesis
- E. Epileptic seizures

V. Drug-induced hypersecretion
- A. Dopamine receptor blockers
  1. Phenothiazines: chlorpromazine, perphenazine
  2. Butyrophenones: haloperidol
  3. Thioxanthenes
  4. Metoclopramide
- B. Dopamine synthesis inhibitors
  1. α-Methyldopa
- C. Catecholamine depletors
  1. Reserpine
- D. Opiates
- E. H_2 antagonists
  1. Cimetidine, ranitidine
- F. Imipramines
  1. Amitriptyline, amoxapine
- G. Serotonin-reuptake inhibitors
  1. Fluoxetine
- H. Calcium channel blockers
  1. Verapamil
- I. Hormones
  1. Estrogens
  2. Antiandrogens

[a] Hyperprolactinemia >100 μg/L almost invariably is indicative of a prolactin-secreting pituitary adenoma. Physiologic causes, hypothyroidism, and drug-induced hyperprolactinemia should be excluded before extensive evaluation.

awakening. Nipple stimulation and sexual orgasm may also cause acute PRL increases. Chest wall stimulation or trauma (including chest surgery and herpes zoster) invoke the reflex suckling arc with resultant hyperprolactinemia. Chronic renal failure elevates PRL by decreasing peripheral PRL clearance. Primary hypothyroidism is associated with mild hyperprolactinemia, probably because of enhanced TRH secretion.

Lesions of the hypothalamic-pituitary region that disrupt hypothalamic dopamine synthesis, portal vessel delivery, or lactotrope responses are associated with hyperprolactinemia. Thus, hypothalamic tumors, cysts, infiltrative disorders, and radiation-induced damage cause elevated PRL levels, usually in the range of 30 to 100 μg/L. Plurihormonal adenomas (including GH and ACTH tumors) may directly hypersecrete PRL. Clinically nonfunctioning pituitary tumors commonly compress the pituitary stalk to cause hyperprolactinemia.

Drug-induced inhibition or disruption of dopaminergic receptor function is a common cause of hyperprolactinemia (Table 2-8). Thus, many antipsychotics and antidepressants cause hyperprolactinemia. Methyldopa inhibits dopamine synthesis and verapamil blocks dopamine release, also leading to hyperprolactinemia. Hormonal agents that induce PRL include estrogens, antiandrogens, and TRH.

Presentation and Diagnosis

Amenorrhea, galactorrhea, and infertility are the hallmarks of hyperprolactinemia in women. If hyperprolactinemia develops prior to the menarche, primary amenorrhea results. More commonly, hyperprolactinemia develops later in life and leads to oligomenorrhea and, ultimately, to amenorrhea. If hyperprolactinemia is sustained, vertebral bone mineral density can be reduced compared to age-matched controls, particularly when associated with pronounced hypoestrogenemia. Galactorrhea is present in up to 80% of hyperprolactinemic women. Though usually bilateral and spontaneous, it may be unilateral or only expressed manually. Patients may also complain of decreased libido, weight gain, and mild hirsutism.

In men with hyperprolactinemia, diminished libido or visual loss (from optic nerve compression) are the usual presenting symptoms. Gonadotropin suppression leads to reduced testosterone, impotence, and oligospermia. True galactorrhea is uncommon in men with hyperprolactinemia. If the disorder is long-standing, secondary effects of hypogonadism are evident, including osteopenia, reduced muscle mass, and decreased beard growth.

The diagnosis of idiopathic hyperprolactinemia is made by exclusion of known causes of hyperprolactinemia in the setting of a normal pituitary MRI. Some of these patients may have small microadenomas below MRI sensitivity (~2 mm).

Laboratory Investigation

Basal, fasting morning PRL levels (normally <20 μg/L) should be measured to assess hypersecretion. Because hormone secretion is pulsatile and levels vary widely in some individuals with hyperprolactinemia, it may be necessary to measure levels on several different occasions when clinical suspicion is high. Both false-positive and false-negative results may be encountered. In patients with markedly elevated PRL levels (>1000 μg/L), results may be falsely lowered because of assay artifacts; sample dilution is required to measure these high values accurately. Falsely elevated values may be caused by aggregated forms of circulating PRL, which are biologically inactive (macroprolactinemia). Hypothyroidism should be excluded by measuring TSH and T_4 levels.

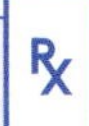

TREATMENT FOR HYPERPROLACTINEMIA

Treatment of hyperprolactinemia depends on the cause of elevated PRL levels. Regardless of the etiology, however, treatment should be aimed at normalizing PRL levels to alleviate suppressive effects on gonadal function, halt galactorrhea, and preserve bone mineral density. Dopamine agonists are effective for many different causes of hyperprolactinemia (see "Treatment" for "Prolactinoma," below).

If the patient is taking a medication known to cause hyperprolactinemia, the drug should be withdrawn, if possible. For psychiatric patients who require neuroleptic agents, dose titration or the addition of a dopamine agonist can help restore normoprolactinemia and alleviate reproductive symptoms. However, dopamine agonists sometimes worsen the underlying psychiatric condition, especially at high doses. Hyperprolactinemia usually resolves after adequate thyroid hormone replacement in hypothyroid patients or after renal transplantation in patients receiving dialysis. Resection of hypothalamic or sellar mass lesions can reverse hyperprolactinemia caused by reduced dopamine tone. Granulomatous infiltrates occasionally respond to glucocorticoid administration. In patients with irreversible hypothalamic damage, no treatment may be warranted. In up to 30% of patients with hyperprolactinemia—with or without a visible pituitary microadenoma—the condition resolves spontaneously.

GALACTORRHEA

Galactorrhea, the inappropriate discharge of milk-containing fluid from the breast, is considered abnormal if it persists for longer than 6 months after childbirth or discontinuation of breastfeeding. Post-partum galactorrhea associated with amenorrhea is a self-limiting disorder usually associated with moderately elevated PRL levels. Galactorrhea may occur spontaneously, or be elicited by nipple pressure. In both males and females, galactorrhea may vary in color and consistency (transparent, milky, or bloody) and arise either unilaterally or bilaterally. Mammography or ultrasound is indicated for bloody discharges (particularly from a single duct), which may be caused by breast cancer. Galactorrhea is commonly associated with hyperprolactinemia caused by any of the conditions listed in Table 2-8. Acromegaly is associated with galactorrhea in about one-third of patients. Treatment of galactorrhea usually involves managing the underlying disorder (e.g., replacing T_4 for hypothyroidism; discontinuing a medication; treating prolactinoma).

PROLACTINOMA

Etiology and Prevalence

Tumors arising from lactotrope cells account for about half of all functioning pituitary tumors, with an annual incidence of ~3/100,000 population. Mixed tumors secreting combinations of GH and PRL, ACTH and PRL, and rarely TSH and PRL, are also seen. These plurihormonal tumors are usually recognized by immunohistochemistry, without apparent clinical manifestations from the production of additional hormones. Microadenomas are classified as <1 cm in diameter and do not usually invade the parasellar region. Macroadenomas are >1 cm in diameter and may be locally invasive and impinge on adjacent structures. The female:male ratio for microprolactinomas is 20:1, whereas the gender ratio is near 1:1 for macroadenomas. Tumor size generally correlates directly with PRL concentrations; values >100 μg/L are usually associated with macroadenomas. Males tend to present with larger tumors than females, possibly because the features of hypogonadism are less readily evident. PRL levels remain stable in most patients, reflecting the slow growth of these tumors. About 5% of microadenomas progress in the long term to macroadenomas. Hyperprolactinemia resolves spontaneously in about 30% of microadenomas.

Presentation and Diagnosis

Women usually present with amenorrhea, infertility, and galactorrhea. If the tumor extends outside of the sella, visual field defects or other mass effects may be seen. Men often present with impotence, loss of libido, infertility, or signs of central CNS compression including headaches and visual defects. Assuming that known physiologic and medication-induced causes of hyperprolactinemia are excluded (Table 2-8), the diagnosis of prolactinoma is likely with a PRL level >100 μg/L. PRL levels <100 μg/L may be caused by microadenomas, other sellar lesions that decrease dopamine inhibition, or nonneoplastic causes of hyperprolactinemia. For this reason, an MRI should be performed in all patients with hyperprolactinemia. It is important to remember that hyperprolactinemia caused by the mass effects of nonlactotrope lesions is also corrected by treatment with dopamine agonists. Consequently, PRL suppression by dopamine agonists does not necessarily indicate that the lesion is a prolactinoma.

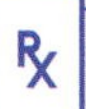

TREATMENT FOR GALACTORRHEA

As microadenomas rarely progress to become macroadenomas, no treatment may be needed if fertility is not desired. Estrogen replacement is indicated to prevent bone loss and other consequences of hypoestrogenemia and does not appear to increase the risk of tumor enlargement. These patients should be monitored by regular serial PRL and MRI measurements.

For symptomatic microadenomas, therapeutic goals include control of hyperprolactinemia, reduction of tumor size, restoration of menses and fertility, and improvement of galactorrhea. Dopamine agonists should be titrated to achieve maximal PRL suppression and restoration of reproductive function (**Fig. 2-6**). A normalized PRL level does not assure reduced tumor size. However, tumor shrinkage is not usually seen in those who do not respond with lowered PRL levels. For macroadenomas, formal visual field testing should be performed before initiating dopamine agonists. MRI and visual fields should be assessed at 6- to 12-month intervals until the mass shrinks and annually thereafter until maximum size reduction has occurred.

Medical

Oral dopamine agonists (cabergoline or bromocriptine) are the mainstay of therapy for patients with micro- or macroprolactinomas. Dopamine agonists suppress PRL secretion and synthesis as well as lactotrope cell proliferation. About 20% of patients are resistant to dopaminergic treatment; they may have decreased D_2 dopamine receptor numbers or a postreceptor defect. D_2 receptor gene mutations in the pituitary have not been reported.

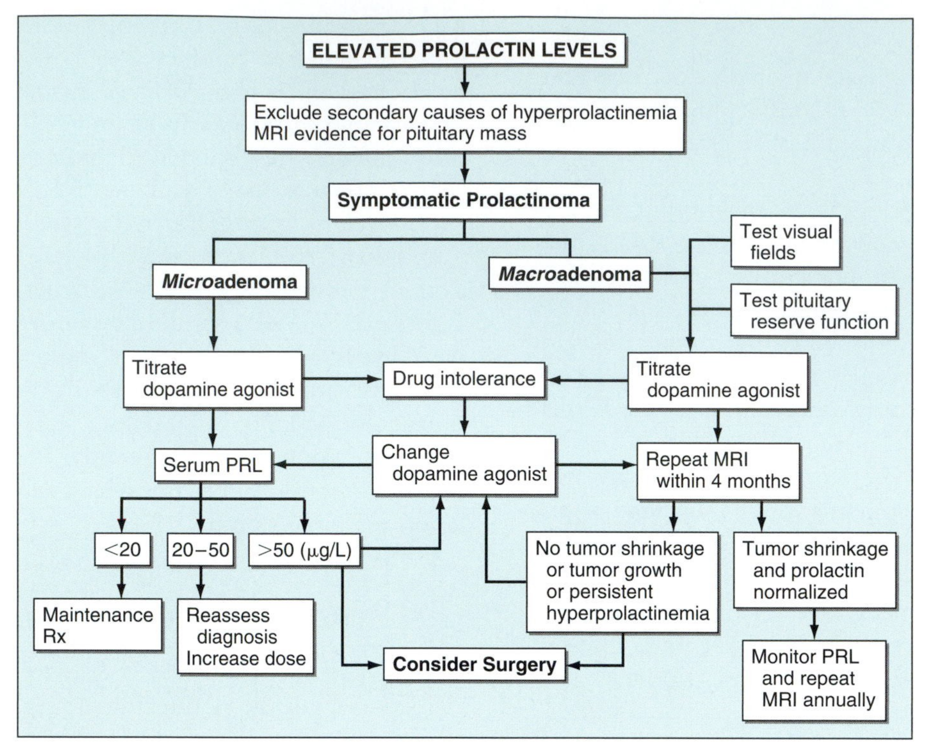

FIGURE 2-6

Management of prolactinoma. MRI, magnetic resonance imaging; PRL, prolactin.

CABERGOLINE

An ergoline derivative, cabergoline is a long-acting dopamine agonist with high D_2 receptor affinity. The drug effectively suppresses PRL for >14 days after a single oral dose and induces prolactinoma shrinkage in most patients. Cabergoline (0.5 to 1.0 mg twice weekly) achieves normoprolactinemia and resumption of normal gonadal function in (~80% of patients with microadenomas; galactorrhea improves or resolves in 90% of patients. Cabergoline normalizes PRL and shrinks ~70% of macroprolactinomas. Mass effect symptoms, including headaches and visual disorders, usually improve dramatically within days after cabergoline initiation; improvement of sexual function requires several weeks of treatment but may occur before complete normalization of prolactin levels. Drug withdrawal usually results in recurrent hyperprolactinemia and tumor reexpansion, with the risk of visual compromise. After initial control of PRL levels has been achieved, cabergoline should be reduced to the lowest effective maintenance dose. In ~5% of treated patients, hyperprolactinemia may resolve and not recur when dopamine agonists are discontinued after long-term treatment. Cabergoline may also be effective in patients resistant to bromocriptine. Adverse effects and drug intolerance are encountered less commonly than with bromocriptine.

BROMOCRIPTINE

The ergot alkaloid bromocriptine mesylate is a dopamine receptor agonist that suppresses prolactin secretion. Because it is short-acting, the drug is preferred when pregnancy is desired. In microadenomas the drug rapidly lowers serum prolactin levels to normal in up to 70% of patients, decreases tumor size, and restores gonadal function. In patients with macroadenomas, prolactin levels are also normalized in 70% of patients and tumor mass shrinkage (≥50%) is achieved in up to 40% of patients.

Therapy is initiated by administering a low bromocriptine dose (0.625 to 1.25 mg) at bedtime with a snack, followed by gradually increasing the dose. Most patients are successfully controlled with a daily dose of ≤7.5 mg (2.5 mg tid).

Nausea, vomiting, and postural hypotension with faintness may occur in ~25% of patients after the initial dose. These symptoms may persist in some patients.

OTHER DOPAMINE AGONISTS

These include *pergolide mesylate*, an ergot derivative with dopaminergic properties; *lisuride*, an ergot derivative; and *quinagolide* (CV 205-502, Norprolac), a nonergot oral dopamine agonist with specific D_2 receptor activity.

SIDE EFFECTS

Side effects of dopamine agonists include constipation, nasal stuffiness, dry mouth, nightmares, insomnia, and vertigo; decreasing the dose usually alleviates these problems. For the approximately 15% of patients who are intolerant of oral bromocriptine, dostinex may be better tolerated. Intravaginal administration of bromocriptine is often efficacious. Auditory hallucinations, delusions, and mood swings have been reported in up to 5% of patients and may be due to the dopamine agonist properties or to the lysergic acid derivative of the compounds. Rare reports of leukopenia, thrombocytopenia, pleural fibrosis, cardiac arrhythmias, and hepatitis have been described with bromocriptine.

Surgery

Indications for surgical debulking include dopamine resistance or intolerance or the presence of an invasive macroadenoma with compromised vision that fails to improve rapidly after drug treatment. Initial PRL normalization is achieved in about 70% of microprolactinomas after surgical resection, but only 30% of macroadenomas can be successfully resected. Follow-up studies have shown that recurrence of hyperprolactinemia occurs in up to 20% of patients within the first year after surgery; long-term recurrence rates exceed 50% for macroadenomas. Radiotherapy for prolactinomas is reserved for patients with aggressive tumors that do not respond to maximally tolerated dopamine agonists and/or surgery.

Pregnancy

The pituitary increases in size during pregnancy, reflecting the stimulatory effects of estrogen and perhaps other growth factors. About 5% of microadenomas significantly increase in size, but 15 to 30% of macroadenomas grow during pregnancy. Bromocriptine has been used for over 25 years to restore fertility in women with hyperprolactinemia, without evidence of untoward teratogenic effects. Nonetheless, most authorities recommend strategies to minimize fetal exposure to the drug. For women taking bromocriptine who desire pregnancy, mechanical contraception should be used through three regular menstrual cycles to allow for conception timing. When pregnancy is confirmed, bromocriptine should be discontinued and PRL levels followed serially, especially if headaches or visual symptoms occur. For women harboring macroadenomas, regular visual field testing is recommended, and the drug should be reinstituted if tumor growth is apparent. Although pituitary MRI may be safe during pregnancy, this procedure should be reserved for symptomatic patients with severe headache and/or visual field defects. Alternatively, surgical decompression may be indicated if vision is threatened. Though comprehensive data support the efficacy and relative safety of bromocriptine-facilitated fertility, patients should be advised of potential unknown deleterious effects and the risk of tumor growth during pregnancy. As cabergoline is long-acting with a high D_2-receptor affinity, it is not approved for routine use when fertility is desired.

GROWTH HORMONE

SYNTHESIS

GH is the most abundant anterior pituitary hormone, and GH-secreting somatotrope cells constitute up to 50% of the total anterior pituitary cell population. Mammosomatotrope cells, which coexpress PRL with GH, can be identified using double immunostaining techniques. Somatotrope development and GH transcription are determined by expression of the cell-specific Pit-1 nuclear transcription factor. Five distinct genes on chromosome 17q22 encode GH and related proteins. The pituitary GH gene (*hGH-N*) produces two alternatively spliced products that give rise to 22-kDa GH (191 amino acids) and a less abundant, 20-kDa GH molecule, with similar biologic activity. Placental syncytiotrophoblast cells express a GH variant (*hGH-V*) gene; the related hormone human chorionic somatotropin (HCS) is expressed by distinct members of the gene cluster.

SECRETION

GH secretion is controlled by complex hypothalamic and peripheral factors. *GHRH* is a 44-amino-acid hypothalamic peptide that stimulates GH synthesis and release. Ghrelin, or octonoylated gastric-derived peptide, as well as synthetic agonists of the *GHRP* receptor stimulate

GHRH and also directly stimulate GH release. *Somatostatin* [somatotropin-release inhibiting factor (SRIF)] is synthesized in the medial preoptic area of the hypothalamus and inhibits GH secretion. GHRH is secreted as discrete spikes that elicit GH pulses, whereas SRIF sets basal GH tone. SRIF is also expressed in many extrahypothalamic tissues, including the CNS, gastrointestinal tract, and pancreas, where it also acts to inhibit islet hormone secretion. *IGF-I,* the peripheral target hormone for GH, feeds back to inhibit GH; estrogen induces GH, whereas glucocorticoid excess suppresses GH release.

Surface receptors on the somatotrope regulate GH synthesis and secretion. The GHRH receptor is a G protein–coupled receptor (GPCR) that signals through the intracellular cyclic AMP pathway. Activation of this receptor stimulates somatotrope cell proliferation as well as hormone production. Inactivating mutations of the GHRH receptor cause profound dwarfism (see below). A distinct surface receptor for ghrelin, a gastric-derived GH secretagogue, is expressed in the hypothalamus and pituitary. Somatostatin binds to five distinct receptor subtypes (SSTR1 to SSTR5); SSTR2 and SSTR5 subtypes preferentially suppress GH (and TSH) secretion.

GH secretion is pulsatile, with greatest levels at night, generally correlating with the onset of sleep. GH secretory rates decline markedly with age so that hormone production in middle age is about 15% of production during puberty. These changes are paralleled by an age-related decline in lean muscle mass. GH secretion is also reduced in obese individuals, though IGF-I levels are usually preserved, suggesting a change in the setpoint for feedback control. Elevated GH levels occur within an hour of deep sleep onset as well as after exercise, physical stress, trauma, and during sepsis. Integrated 24-h GH secretion is higher in women and is also enhanced by estrogen replacement. Using standard assays, random GH measurements are undetectable in ~50% of daytime samples obtained from healthy subjects and are undetectable in most obese and elderly subjects. Thus, single random GH measurements do not distinguish patients with adult GH deficiency from normal persons.

GH secretion is profoundly influenced by nutritional factors. Using newer ultrasensitive chemiluminescence-based GH assays with a sensitivity of 0.002 μg/L, a glucose load can be shown to suppress GH to <0.7 μg/L in female and to <0.07 μg/L in male subjects. Increased GH pulse frequency and peak amplitudes occur with chronic malnutrition or prolonged fasting. GH is stimulated by high-protein meals and by L-arginine. GH secretion is induced by dopamine and apomorphine (a dopamine receptor agonist), as well as by α-adrenergic pathways. β-Adrenergic blockage induces basal GH and enhances GHRH- and insulin-evoked GH release.

ACTION

The pattern of GH secretion may affect tissue responses. The higher GH pulsatility observed in males, as compared to the relatively continuous GH secretion in females, may be an important biologic determinant of linear growth patterns and liver enzyme induction.

The 70-kDa peripheral GH receptor protein shares structural homology with the cytokine/hematopoietic superfamily. A fragment of the receptor extracellular domain generates a soluble GH-binding protein (GHBP) that interacts with GH in the circulation. The liver contains the greatest number of GH receptors. GH binding induces receptor dimerization, followed by signaling through the JAK/STAT pathway. The activated STAT proteins translocate to the nucleus, where they modulate expression of GH-regulated target genes. GH analogues that bind to the receptor, but are incapable of mediating receptor dimerization, are potent antagonists of GH action and are being investigated for potential use in the treatment of acromegaly and diabetic microangiopathy.

GH induces protein synthesis and nitrogen retention and impairs glucose tolerance by antagonizing insulin action. GH also stimulates lipolysis, leading to increased circulating fatty acid levels, reduced omental fat mass, and enhanced lean body mass. GH promotes sodium, potassium, and water retention and elevates serum levels of inorganic phosphate. Linear bone growth occurs as a result of complex hormonal and growth factor actions, including those of IGF-I. GH stimulates epiphyseal prechondrocyte differentiation. These precursor cells produce IGF-I locally and are also responsive to the growth factor.

INSULIN-LIKE GROWTH FACTORS

Though GH exerts direct effects in target tissues, many of its physiologic effects are mediated indirectly through IGF-I, a potent growth and differentiation factor. The major source of circulating IGF-I is hepatic in origin. Peripheral tissue IGF-I exerts local paracrine actions that appear to be both dependent and independent of GH. Thus, GH administration induces circulating IGF-I as well as stimulating IGF-I expression in multiple tissues.

Both IGF-I and -II are bound to high-affinity circulating IGF-binding proteins (IGFBPs) that regulate IGF bioactivity. Levels of IGFBP3 are GH-dependent, and it serves as the major carrier protein for circulating IGF-I. GH deficiency and malnutrition are associated with low IGFBP3 levels. IGFBP1 and −2 regulate local tissue IGF action but do not bind appreciable amounts of circulating IGF-I.

Serum IGF-I concentrations are profoundly affected by various physiologic factors. Levels increase during puberty, peak at 16 years, and subsequently decline by

>80% during the aging process. IGF-I concentrations are higher in females than in males. Because GH is the major determinant of hepatic IGF-I synthesis, abnormalities of GH synthesis or action (e.g., pituitary failure, GHRH receptor defect, or GH receptor defect) reduce IGF-I levels. Hypocaloric states are associated with GH resistance; IGF-I levels are therefore low with cachexia, malnutrition, and sepsis. In acromegaly, IGF-I levels are invariably high and reflect a log-linear relationship with GH concentrations.

IGF-I Physiology

Though IGF-I is not an approved drug, investigational studies provide insight into its physiologic effects. Injected IGF-I (100 μg/kg) induces hypoglycemia, and lower doses improve insulin sensitivity in patients with severe insulin resistance and diabetes. In cachectic subjects, IGF-I infusion (12 μg/kg per hour) enhances nitrogen retention and lowers cholesterol levels. Longer-term subcutaneous IGF-I injections exert a marked anabolic effect with enhanced protein synthesis. Although bone formation markers are induced, bone turnover may also be stimulated by IGF-I.

IGF-I side effects are dose-dependent, and overdose may result in hypoglycemia, hypotension, fluid retention, temporomandibular jaw pain, and increased intracranial pressure, all of which are reversible. Avascular femoral head necrosis has been reported. Chronic excess IGF-I would presumably result in features of acromegaly.

DISORDERS OF GROWTH AND DEVELOPMENT

Skeletal Maturation and Somatic Growth

The growth plate is dependent on a variety of hormonal stimuli including GH, IGF-I, sex steroids, thyroid hormones, paracrine growth factors, and cytokines. The growth-promoting process also requires caloric energy, amino acids, vitamins, and trace metals and consumes about 10% of normal energy production. Malnutrition impairs chondrocyte activity and reduces circulating IGF-I and IGFBP3 levels.

Bone age is delayed in patients with all forms of true GH deficiency or GH receptor defects that result in attenuated GH action. Rarely, GH excess accelerates growth, particularly in the setting of delayed bone age from concomitant hypogonadism. Bone age is delayed by thyroid hormone deficiency. Consequently, congenital or acquired hypothyroidism is associated with stunted growth, which is partially reversed by thyroid hormone replacement (Chap. 4). Elevated pubertal sex steroid levels (especially estrogen) induce the GHRH-GH-IGF-I axis and also directly stimulate epiphyseal growth. High doses of estrogen lead to epiphyseal closure. A mutation of the estrogen receptor α prevented epiphyseal closure, confirming the important role of this pathway in bone maturation. Several pathologic conditions accompanied by increased levels of sex steroids, including precocious puberty, androgen exposure (exogenous or endogenous), congenital adrenal hyperplasia, and obesity, are associated with accelerated bone maturation. Thus, children with these conditions have accelerated early growth, but end up with reduced final height. In contrast to sex steroids, glucocorticoid excess inhibits linear growth.

Linear bone growth rates are very high in infancy and are pituitary-dependent. Mean growth velocity is ~6 cm/year in later childhood and is usually maintained within a given range on a standardized percentile chart. Peak growth rates occur during midpuberty when bone age is 12 (girls) or 13 (boys). Secondary sexual development is associated with elevated sex steroids that cause progressive epiphyseal growth plate closure.

Short stature may occur as a result of constitutive intrinsic growth defects or because of acquired extrinsic factors that impair growth. In general, delayed bone age in a child with short stature is suggestive of a hormonal or systemic disorder, whereas normal bone age in a short child is more likely to be caused by a genetic cartilage dysplasia or growth plate disorder.

GH Deficiency in Children

GH Deficiency Isolated GH deficiency is characterized by short stature, micropenis, increased fat, high-pitched voice, and a propensity to hypoglycemia. Familial modes of inheritance are seen in one-third of these individuals and may be autosomal dominant, recessive, or X-linked. About 10% of children with GH deficiency have mutations in the *GH-N* gene, including gene deletions and a wide range of point mutations. Mutations in transcription factors Pit-1 and Prop-1, which control somatotrope development, cause GH deficiency in combination with other pituitary hormone deficiencies, which may only become manifest in adulthood. The diagnosis of *idiopathic GH deficiency* (IGHD) should be made only after known molecular defects have been excluded.

GHRH Receptor Mutations Recessive mutations of the GHRH receptor gene in subjects with severe proportionate dwarfism are associated with low basal GH levels that cannot be stimulated by exogenous GHRH, GHRP, or insulin-induced hypoglycemia. The syndrome exemplifies the importance of the GHRH receptor for somatotrope cell proliferation and hormonal responsiveness.

Growth Hormone Insensitivity This is caused by defects of GH receptor structure or signaling. Homozygous or heterozygous mutations of the GH receptor are associated with partial or complete GH insensitivity and growth failure (*Laron syndrome*). The diagnosis is based on normal or high GH levels, with decreased circulating GHBP, and low IGF-I levels. Very rarely, defective IGF-I, IGF-I receptor, or IGF-I signaling defects are also encountered.

Nutritional Short Stature Caloric deprivation and malnutrition, uncontrolled diabetes, and chronic renal failure represent secondary causes of abrogated GH receptor function. These conditions also stimulate production of proinflammatory cytokines, which can block GH-mediated signal transduction. Children with these conditions typically exhibit features of acquired short stature with elevated GH and low IGF-I levels. Circulating GH receptor antibodies may rarely cause peripheral GH insensitivity.

Psychosocial Short Stature Emotional and social deprivation lead to growth retardation accompanied by delayed speech, discordant hyperphagia, and attenuated response to administered GH. A nurturing environment restores growth rates.

Presentation and Diagnosis Short stature is commonly encountered in clinical practice, and the decision to evaluate these children requires clinical judgment in association with auxologic data and family history. Short stature should be comprehensively evaluated if a patient's height is >3 SD below the mean for age or if the growth rate has decelerated. Skeletal maturation is best evaluated by measuring a radiologic bone age, which is based mainly on the degree of growth plate fusion. Final height can be predicted using standardized scales (Bayley-Pinneau or Tanner-Whitehouse) or estimated by adding 6.5 cm (boys) or subtracting 6.5 cm (girls) from the midparental height.

Laboratory Investigation Because GH secretion is pulsatile, GH deficiency is best assessed by examining the response to provocative stimuli including exercise, insulin-induced hypoglycemia, and other pharmacologic tests which normally increase GH to >7 μg/L in children. Random GH measurements do not distinguish normal children from those with true GH deficiency. Adequate adrenal and thyroid hormone replacement should be assured before testing. Age- and gender-matched IGF-I levels are not sufficiently sensitive or specific to make the diagnosis but can be useful to confirm GH deficiency. Pituitary MRI may reveal pituitary mass lesions or structural defects.

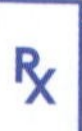

TREATMENT FOR GH DISORDERS

Replacement therapy with recombinant GH (0.02 to 0.05 mg/kg per day subcutaneously) restores growth velocity in GH-deficient children to ~10 cm/year. If pituitary insufficiency is documented, other associated hormone deficits should be corrected—especially adrenal steroids. GH treatment is also moderately effective for accelerating growth rates in children with Turner syndrome and chronic renal failure.

In patients with GH insensitivity and growth retardation due to mutations of the GH receptor, treatment with IGF-I bypasses the dysfunctional GH receptor. Growth rates have been maintained for several years, and this therapy now portends improved final adult stature in this group of patients.

ADULT GH DEFICIENCY (AGHD)

This disorder is usually caused by hypothalamic or pituitary somatotrope damage. Acquired pituitary hormone deficiency follows a typical sequential pattern whereby loss of adequate GH reserve foreshadows subsequent hormone deficits. The sequential order of hormone loss is usually GH → FSH/LH → TSH → ACTH.

Presentation and Diagnosis

The clinical features of AGHD include changes in body composition, lipid metabolism, and quality of life and cardiovascular dysfunction (**Table 2-9**). Body composition changes are common and include reduced lean body mass, increased fat mass with selective deposition of intraabdominal visceral fat, and increased waist-to-hip ratio. Hyperlipidemia, left ventricular dysfunction, hypertension, and increased plasma fibrinogen levels may also be present. Bone mineral content is reduced, with resultant increased fracture rates. Patients may experience social isolation, depression, and difficulty in maintaining gainful employment. Adult hypopituitarism is associated with a threefold increased cardiovascular mortality rate in comparison to age- and sex-matched controls, and this may be due to GH deficiency.

Laboratory Investigation

AGHD is rare, and in light of the nonspecific nature of associated clinical symptoms, patients appropriate for testing should be carefully selected on the basis of well-defined criteria. With few exceptions, testing should be restricted to patients with the following predisposing

TABLE 2-9

FEATURES OF ADULT GROWTH HORMONE DEFICIENCY

Clinical

- Impaired quality of life
  - Decreased energy and drive
  - Poor concentration
  - Low self-esteem
  - Social isolation
- Body composition changes
  - Increased body fat mass
  - Central fat deposition
  - Increased waist-hip ratio
  - Decreased lean body mass
- Reduced exercise capacity
  - Reduced maximum O_2 uptake
  - Impaired cardiac function
  - Reduced muscle mass
- Cardiovascular risk factors
  - Impaired cardiac structure and function
  - Abnormal lipid profile
  - Decreased fibrinolytic activity
  - Atherosclerosis
  - Omental obesity

Imaging

- Pituitary: Mass or structural damage
  - Bone: Reduced bone mineral density
  - Abdomen: Excess omental adiposity

Laboratory

- Evoked GH <3 ng/mL
- IGF-I and IGFBP3 low or normal
- Increased LDL-cholesterol
- Concomitant gonadotropin, TSH, and/or ACTH reserve deficits may be present

Note: LDL, low-density lipoprotein; for other abbreviations, see text.

factors: (1) pituitary surgery, (2) pituitary or hypothalamic tumor or granulomas, (3) cranial irradiation, (4) radiologic evidence of a pituitary lesion, (5) childhood requirement for GH replacement therapy, or, rarely, (6) unexplained low age- and sex-matched IGF-I level. The transition of the GH-deficient adolescent to adulthood requires retesting to document adult GH deficiency. Up to 20% of patients treated for childhood-onset GH deficiency are found to be GH-sufficient on repeat testing as adults.

A significant proportion (~25%) of truly GH-deficient adults have low-normal IGF-I levels. Thus, as in the evaluation of GH deficiency in children, valid age- and gender-matched IGF-I measurements provide a useful index of therapeutic responses but are not sufficiently sensitive for diagnostic purposes. The most validated test to distinguish pituitary-sufficient patients from those with AGHD is insulin-induced (0.05 to 0.1 U/kg) hypoglycemia. After glucose reduction to ~40 mg/dL (2.2 mmol/L), most individuals experience neuroglycopenic symptoms (Chap. 19), and peak GH release occurs at 60 min and remains elevated for up to 2 h. About 90% of healthy adults exhibit GH responses >5 μg/L; AGHD is defined by a peak GH response to hypoglycemia of <3 μg/L. Although insulin-induced hypoglycemia is safe when performed under appropriate supervision, it is contraindicated in patients with diabetes, ischemic heart disease, cerebrovascular disease, or epilepsy, and in elderly patients. Alternative stimulatory tests include intravenous arginine (30 g), GHRH (1 μg/kg), and GHRP-6 (90 μg). Combinations of these tests may evoke GH secretion in subjects not responsive to a single test.

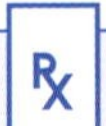

TREATMENT FOR AGHD

Once the diagnosis of AGHD is unequivocally established, replacement of GH may be indicated. Contraindications to therapy include the presence of an active neoplasm, intracranial hypertension, or uncontrolled diabetes and retinopathy. The starting dose of 0.15 to 0.3 mg/d should be titrated (up to a maximum of 1.25 mg/d) to maintain IGF-I levels in the mid-normal range for age- and gender-matched controls (**Fig. 2-7**). Women require higher doses than men, and elderly patients require less GH. Long-term GH maintenance sustains normal IGF-I levels and is associated with persistent body composition changes (e.g., enhanced lean body mass and lower body fat). High-density lipoprotein cholesterol increases, but total cholesterol and insulin levels do not change significantly. Lumbar spine bone mineral density increases, but this response is gradual (>1 year). Many patients

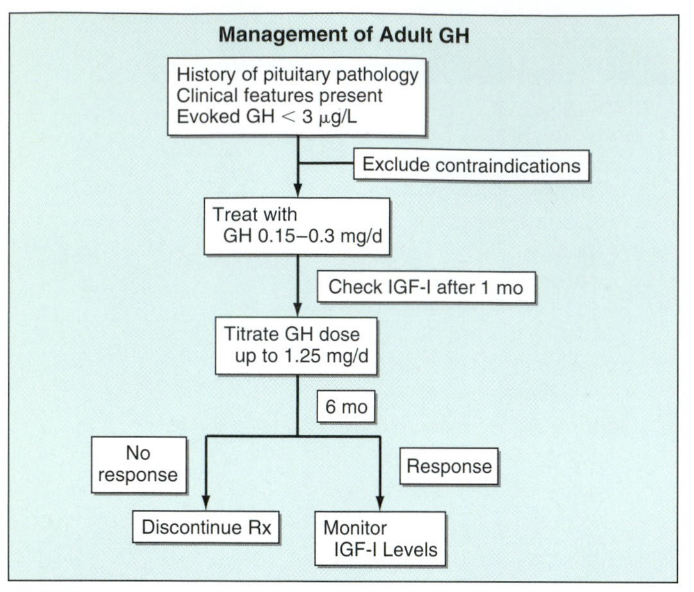

FIGURE 2-7
Management of adult growth hormone (GH) deficiency. IGF, insulin-like growth factor.

note significant improvement in quality of life when evaluated by standardized questionnaires. The effect of GH replacement on mortality rates in GH-deficient patients is currently the subject of long-term prospective investigation.

About 30% of patients exhibit reversible dose-related fluid retention, joint pain, and carpal tunnel syndrome, and up to 40% exhibit myalgias and paresthesia. Patients receiving insulin require careful monitoring for dosing adjustments, as GH is a potent counterregulatory hormone for insulin action. Patients with type 2 diabetes mellitus initially develop further insulin resistance. However, glycemic control improves with the sustained loss of abdominal fat associated with long-term GH replacement. Headache, increased intracranial pressure, hypertension, atrial fibrillation, and tinnitus occur rarely. Prevalence of pituitary tumor regrowth and potential progression of skin lesions are currently being assessed in long-term surveillance programs. To date, development of these potential side effects does not appear significant.

ACROMEGALY

Etiology

GH hypersecretion is usually the result of somatotrope adenomas but is also rarely caused by extrapituitary lesions (**Table 2-10**). In addition to typical GH-secreting somatotrope adenomas, mixed mammosomatotrope tumors and acidophilic stem cell adenomas can secrete

TABLE 2-10

CAUSES OF ACROMEGALY

	PREVALENCE, %
Excess growth hormone secretion	
Pituitary	98
Densely or sparsely granulated GH cell adenoma	60
Mixed GH cell and PRL cell adenoma	25
Mammosomatrope cell adenoma	10
Plurihormonal adenoma	
GH cell carcinoma or metastases	
Multiple endocrine neoplasia-1 (GH cell adenoma)	
McCune-Albright syndrome	
Ectopic sphenoid or parapharyngeal sinus pituitary adenoma	
Extrapituitary tumor	
Pancreatic islet cell tumor	<1
Excess growth hormone–releasing hormone secretion	
Central	<1
Hypothalamic hamartoma, choristoma, ganglioneuroma	<1
Peripheral	<1
Bronchial carcinoid, pancreatic islet cell tumor, small cell lung cancer, adrenal adenoma, medullary thyroid carcinoma, pheochromocytoma	

Source: Adapted from S Melmed: N Engl J Med 322:966, 1990.

both GH and PRL. In patients with acidophilic stem cell adenomas, features of hyperprolactinemia (hypogonadism and galactorrhea) predominate over the less clinically evident signs of acromegaly. Occasionally, mixed plurihormonal tumors are encountered that secrete ACTH, the glycoprotein hormone α subunit, or TSH, in addition to GH. Patients with partially empty sella may present with GH hypersecretion due to a small GH-secreting adenoma within the compressed rim of pituitary tissue; some of these may reflect the spontaneous necrosis of tumors that were previously larger. GH-secreting tumors rarely arise from ectopic pituitary tissue remnants in the nasopharynx or midline sinuses.

There are case reports of ectopic GH secretion by tumors of pancreatic, ovarian, or lung origin. Excess GHRH production may cause acromegaly because of chronic stimulation of somatotropes. These patients present with classic features of acromegaly, elevated GH levels, pituitary enlargement on MRI, and pathologic characteristics of pituitary hyperplasia. The most common cause of GHRH-mediated acromegaly is a chest or abdominal carcinoid tumor. Although these tumors usually express positive GHRH immunoreactivity, clinical features of acromegaly are evident in only a minority of patients with carcinoid disease. Excessive GHRH may also be elaborated by hypothalamic tumors, usually choristomas or neuromas.

Presentation and Diagnosis

Protean manifestations of GH and IGF-I hypersecretion are indolent and often are not clinically diagnosed for 10 years or more. Acral bony overgrowth results in frontal bossing, increased hand and foot size, mandibular enlargement with prognathism, and widened space between the lower incisor teeth. In children and adolescents, initiation of GH hypersecretion prior to epiphyseal long bone closure is associated with the development of pituitary gigantism (**Fig. 2-8**). Soft tissue swelling results in increased heel pad thickness, increased shoe or glove size, ring tightening, characteristic coarse facial features, and a large fleshy nose. Other commonly encountered clinical features include hyperhidrosis, deep and hollow-sounding voice, oily skin, arthropathy, kyphosis, carpal tunnel syndrome, proximal muscle weakness and fatigue, acanthosis nigricans, and skin tags. Generalized visceromegaly occurs, including cardiomegaly, macroglossia, and thyroid gland enlargement.

The most significant clinical impact of GH excess occurs with respect to the cardiovascular system. Coronary

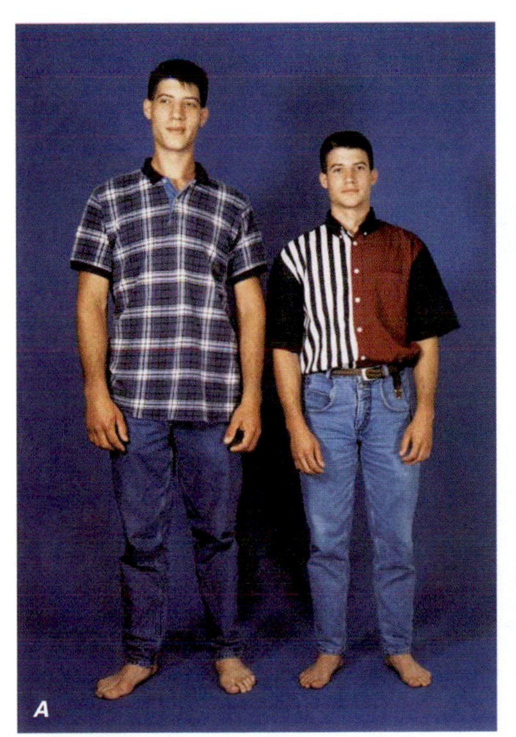

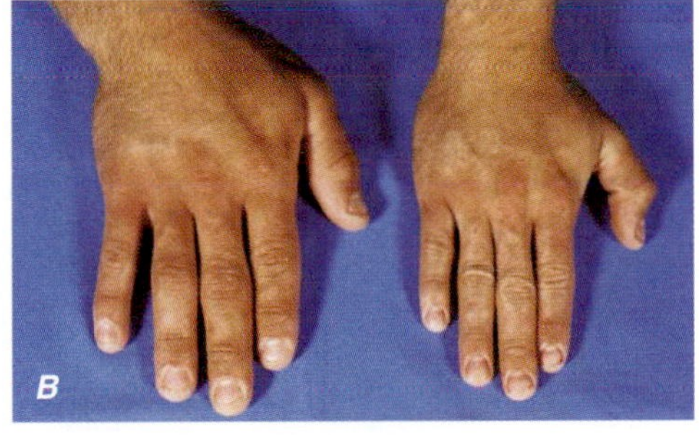

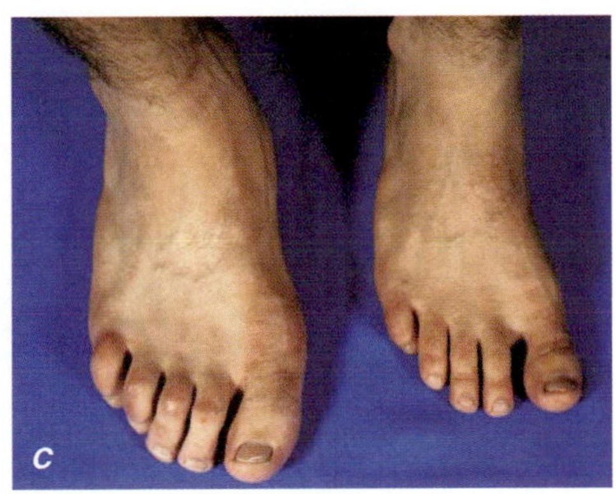

FIGURE 2-8

Features of acromegaly/gigantism. A 22-year-old man with gigantism due to excess growth hormone is shown to the left of his identical twin. The increased height and prognathism (*A*) and enlarged hand (*B*) and foot (*C*) of the affected twin are apparent. Their clinical features began to diverge at the age of approximately 13 years. (*Reproduced from R Gagel, IE McCutcheon: N Engl J Med 340:524, 1999, with permission. Copyright © Massachusetts Medical Society. All rights reserved.*)

heart disease, cardiomyopathy with arrhythmias, left ventricular hypertrophy, decreased diastolic function, and hypertension occur in about 30% of patients. Upper airway obstruction with sleep apnea occurs in about 60% of patients and is associated with both soft tissue laryngeal airway obstruction and central sleep dysfunction. Diabetes mellitus develops in 25% of patients with acromegaly, and most patients are intolerant of a glucose load (as GH counteracts the action of insulin). Acromegaly is associated with an increased risk of colon polyps and colonic malignancy; polyps are diagnosed in up to one-third of acromegalic patients. Overall mortality is increased about threefold and is due primarily to cardiovascular and cerebrovascular disorders, malignancy, and respiratory disease. Unless GH levels are controlled, survival is reduced by an average of 10 years compared with an age-matched control population.

Laboratory Investigation

Age- and gender-matched serum IGF-I levels are elevated in acromegaly. Consequently, an IGF-I level provides a useful laboratory screening measure when clinical features raise the possibility of acromegaly. Due to the pulsatility of GH secretion, measurement of a single random GH level is not useful for the diagnosis or exclusion of acromegaly and does not correlate with disease severity. The diagnosis of acromegaly is confirmed by demonstrating the failure of GH suppression to <1 μg/L within 1 to 2 h of an oral glucose load (75 g). About 20% of patients exhibit a paradoxical GH rise after glucose. About 60% of patients with GH-secreting tumors may exhibit paradoxical GH responses to TRH administration. PRL should be measured as it is elevated in ~25% of patients with acromegaly. Thyroid function, gonadotropins, and sex steroids may be attenuated because of tumor mass effects. Because most patients will undergo surgery with glucocorticoid coverage, tests of ACTH reserve in asymptomatic patients are more efficiently deferred until after surgery.

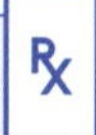

TREATMENT FOR ACROMEGALY

Surgical resection of GH-secreting adenomas is the initial treatment for most patients (**Fig. 2-9**). Somatostatin analogues are used as adjuvant treatment for preoperative shrinkage of large invasive macroadenomas, immediate relief of debilitating symptoms, and reduction of GH hypersecretion, in elderly patients experiencing morbidity, in patients who decline surgery, or, when surgery fails, to

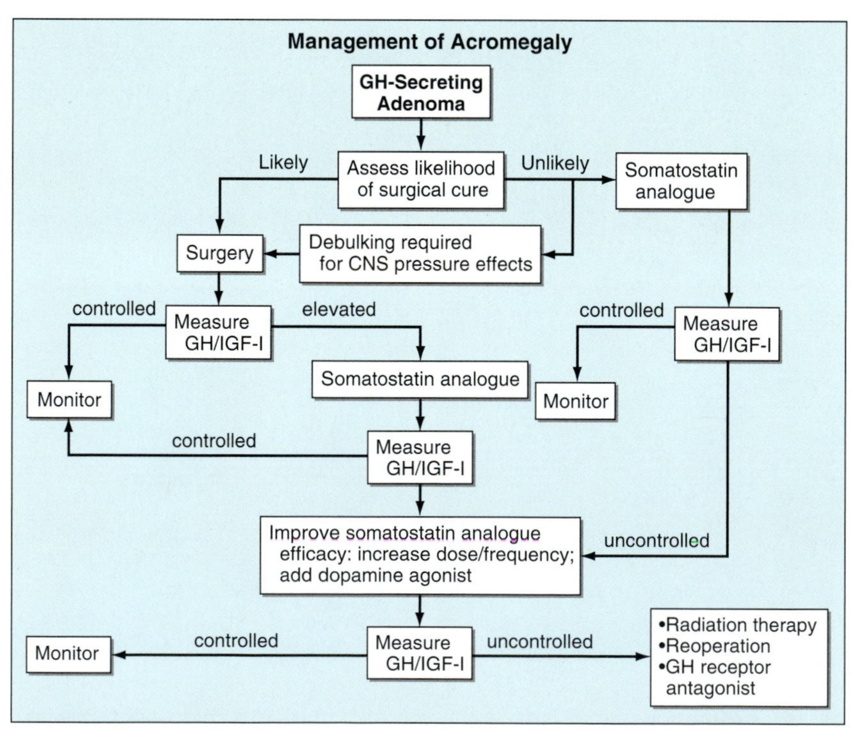

FIGURE 2-9

Management of acromegaly. GH, growth hormone; CNS, central nervous system; IGF, insulin-like growth factor. (*Adapted from S. Melmed et al: J Clin Endocrinol Metab 83:2646, 1998; © The Endocrine Society.*)

achieve biochemical control. Irradiation or repeat surgery may be required for patients who cannot tolerate or do not respond to adjunctive medical therapy. The high rate of late hypopituitarism and the slow rate (5 to 15 years) of biochemical response are the main disadvantages of radiotherapy. Irradiation is relatively ineffective in normalizing IGF-I levels. Stereotactic ablation of GH-secreting adenomas by gamma-knife radiotherapy is promising, but long-term results are not available and the side effects have not been clearly delineated. Somatostatin analogues may be given while awaiting the full effect of radiotherapy. Systemic sequelae of acromegaly, including cardiovascular disease, diabetes, and arthritis, should also be managed aggressively. Maxillofacial surgery for mandibular repair may also be indicated.

Surgery

Transsphenoidal surgical resection by an experienced surgeon is the preferred primary treatment for both microadenomas (cure rate ~70%) and macroadenomas (<50% cured). Soft tissue swelling improves immediately after tumor resection. GH levels return to normal within an hour, and IGF-I levels are normalized within 3 to 4 days. In ~10% of patients, acromegaly may recur several years after apparently successful surgery; hypopituitarism develops in up to 15% of patients.

Somatostatin Analogues

Somatostatin analogues exert their therapeutic effects through SSTR2 and -5 receptors, both of which are expressed by GH-secreting tumors. Octreotide acetate is an 8-amino-acid synthetic somatostatin analogue. In contrast to native somatostatin, the analogue is relatively resistant to plasma degradation. It has a 2-h serum half-life and possesses 40-fold greater potency than native somatostatin to suppress GH. Octreotide is administered by subcutaneous injection, beginning with 50 μg tid; the dose can be gradually increased up to 1500 μg/d. Fewer than 10% of patients do not respond to the analogue. Octreotide suppresses integrated GH levels to <5 μg/L in ~70% of patients and to <2 μg/L in up to 60% of patients. It normalizes IGF-I levels in ~75% of treated patients. Prolonged use of the analogue is not associated with desensitization, even after ≥10 years of treatment. Rapid relief of headache and soft tissue swelling occurs in ~75% of patients within days to weeks of treatment initiation. Subjective clinical benefits of octreotide therapy occur more frequently than biochemical remission, and most patients report symptomatic improvement, including amelioration of headache, perspiration, obstructive apnea, and cardiac failure. Modest pituitary tumor size reduction occurs in about 40% of patients, but this effect is reversed when treatment is stopped.

Two long-acting somatostatin depot formulations, octreotide and lanreotide, are becoming the preferred medical treatment for acromegalic patients. *Sandostatin-LAR* is a sustained-release, long-acting formulation of octreotide incorporated into microspheres that sustain drug level s for several weeks after intramuscular injection. GH suppression occurs for as long as 6 weeks after a 30-mg injection; long-term monthly treatment sustains GH and IGF-I suppression and reduction of pituitary tumor size. *Lanreotide*, a slow-release depot somatostatin preparation, is a cyclic somatostatin octapeptide analogue that suppresses GH and IGF-I hypersecretion for 10 to 14 days after a 30-mg intramuscular injection. Long-term administration controls GH hypersecretion in two-thirds of treated patients and improves patient compliance because of the long interval required between drug injections.

SIDE EFFECTS

Somatostatin analogues are well tolerated in most patients. Adverse effects are short-lived and mostly relate to drug-induced suppression of gastrointestinal motility and secretion. Nausea, abdominal discomfort, fat malabsorption, diarrhea, and flatulence occur in one-third of patients, though these symptoms usually remit within 2 weeks. Octreotide suppresses postprandial gallbladder contractility and delays gallbladder emptying; up to 30% of patients treated long-term develop echogenic sludge or asymptomatic cholesterol gallstones. Other side effects include mild glucose intolerance due to transient insulin suppression, asymptomatic bradycardia, hypothyroxinemia, and local pain at the injection site.

Dopamine Agonists

Bromocriptine may suppress GH secretion in some acromegalic patients, particularly those with cosecretion of PRL. High doses (≥20 mg/d), administered as three to four daily doses, are usually required to lower GH, and therapeutic efficacy is modest. GH levels are suppressed to <5 μg/L in ~20% of patients, and IGF-I levels are normalized in only 10% of patients. Cabergoline also suppresses GH and decreases adenoma size when given at a relatively high dose of 0.5 mg/d. Combined treatment with octreotide and bromocriptine induces additive biochemical control compared to either drug alone.

GH Antagonists

GH analogues (e.g., pegvisomant) antagonize endogenous GH action by blocking peripheral GH binding to its receptor. Consequently, serum IGF-I levels are suppressed, potentially reducing the deleterious effects of excess endogenous GH.

Radiation

External radiation therapy or high-energy stereotactic techniques are used as adjuvant therapy for acromegaly. An advantage of radiation is that patient compliance with long-term treatment is not required. Tumor mass is reduced, and GH levels are attenuated over time. However, 50% of patients require at least 8 years for GH levels to be suppressed to <5 μg/L; this level of GH reduction is achieved in about 90% of patients after 18 years but represents suboptimal GH suppression. Patients may require interim medical therapy for several years prior to attaining maximal radiation benefits. Most patients also experience hypothalamic-pituitary damage, leading to gonadotropin, ACTH, and/or TSH deficiency within 10 years of therapy.

In summary, surgery is the preferred primary treatment for GH-secreting microadenomas (Fig. 2-9). The high frequency of GH hypersecretion after macroadenoma resection usually necessitates adjuvant or primary medical therapy for these larger tumors. Patients unable to receive or respond to medical treatment can be offered radiation.

ADRENOCORTICOTROPIN HORMONE

(See also Chap. 5)

SYNTHESIS

ACTH-secreting corticotrope cells constitute about 20% of the pituitary cell population. ACTH (39 amino acids) is derived from the POMC precursor protein (266 amino acids) that also generates several other peptides, including β-lipotropin, β-endorphin, met-enkephalin, α melanocyte-stimulating hormone (MSH), and corticotropin-like intermediate lobe protein (CLIP). The POMC gene is powerfully suppressed by glucocorticoids and induced by CRH, arginine vasopressin (AVP), and proinflammatory cytokines, including IL-6, and leukemia inhibitory factor.

CRH, a 41-amino-acid hypothalamic peptide synthesized in the paraventricular nucleus as well as in higher brain centers, is the predominant stimulator of ACTH synthesis and release. The CRH receptor is a GPCR that is expressed on the corticotrope and induces POMC transcription.

SECRETION

ACTH secretion is pulsatile and exhibits a characteristic circadian rhythm, peaking at 6 A.M. and reaching a nadir about midnight. Adrenal glucocorticoid secretion, which is driven by ACTH, follows a parallel diurnal pattern. ACTH circadian rhythmicity is determined by variations in secretory pulse amplitude rather than changes in pulse frequency. Superimposed on this endogenous rhythm, ACTH levels are increased by AVP, physical stress, exercise, acute illness, and insulin-induced hypoglycemia.

Loss of cortisol feedback inhibition, as occurs in primary adrenal failure, results in extremely high ACTH levels. Glucocorticoid-mediated negative regulation of the hypothalamo-pituitary-adrenal (HPA) axis occurs as a consequence of both hypothalamic CRH suppression and direct attenuation of pituitary POMC gene expression and ACTH release.

Acute inflammatory or septic insults activate the HPA axis through the integrated actions of proinflammatory cytokines, bacterial toxins, and neural signals. The overlapping cascade of ACTH-inducing cytokines [tumor necrosis factor (TNF); IL-1, -2, and -6; and leukemia inhibitory factor] activates hypothalamic CRH and AVP secretion, pituitary POMC gene expression, and local paracrine pituitary cytokine networks. The resulting cortisol elevation restrains the inflammatory response and provides host protection. Concomitantly, cytokine-mediated central glucocorticoid receptor resistance impairs glucocorticoid suppression of the HPA. Thus, the neuroendocrine stress response reflects the net result of highly integrated hypothalamic, intrapituitary, and peripheral hormone and cytokine signals.

ACTION

The major function of the HPA axis is to maintain metabolic homeostasis and to mediate the neuroendocrine stress response. ACTH induces cortical steroidogenesis by maintaining adrenal cell proliferation and function. The receptor for ACTH, designated *melanocortin-2 receptor,* is a GPCR that induces steroidogenesis by stimulating a cascade of steroidogenic enzymes (Chap. 5).

ACTH DEFICIENCY

Presentation and Diagnosis

Secondary adrenal insufficiency occurs as a result of pituitary ACTH deficiency. It is characterized by fatigue, weakness, anorexia, nausea, vomiting, and, occasionally, hypoglycemia (due to diminished insulin counterregulation). In contrast to primary adrenal failure, hypocortisolism associated with pituitary failure is not usually accompanied by pigmentation changes or mineralocorticoid deficiency. ACTH deficiency is commonly due to glucocorticoid withdrawal following treatment-associated suppression of the HPA axis. Isolated ACTH deficiency may occur after surgical resection of an ACTH-secreting pituitary adenoma that has suppressed the HPA axis; this phenomenon is suggestive of a surgical cure. The mass effects of other pituitary adenomas or sellar lesions may lead to ACTH deficiency, but usually in combination with other pituitary hormone deficiencies. Partial ACTH deficiency may be unmasked in the presence of an acute medical or surgical illness, when clinically significant hypocortisolism reflects diminished ACTH reserve.

Laboratory Diagnosis

Inappropriately low ACTH levels in the setting of low cortisol levels are characteristic of diminished ACTH reserve. Low basal serum cortisol levels are associated with blunted cortisol responses to ACTH stimulation and impaired cortisol response to insulin-induced hypoglycemia, or testing with metyrapone or CRH. For description of provocative ACTH tests, see "Tests of Pituitary-Adrenal Responsiveness" in Chap. 5.

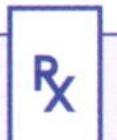

TREATMENT FOR ACTH DEFICIENCY

Glucocorticoid replacement therapy improves most features of ACTH deficiency. The total daily dose of hydrocortisone replacement should not exceed 30 mg daily, divided into two or three doses. Prednisone (5 mg each morning; 2.5 mg each evening) is longer acting and has fewer mineralocorticoid effects than hydrocortisone. Some authorities advocate lower maintenance doses in an effort to avoid cushingoid side effects. Doses should be increased several-fold during periods of acute illness or stress.

CUSHING'S DISEASE (ACTH-PRODUCING ADENOMA) (See also Chap. 5)

Etiology and Prevalence

Pituitary corticotrope adenomas account for 70% of patients with endogenous causes of Cushing's syndrome. However, it should be recalled that iatrogenic hypercortisolism is the most common cause of cushingoid features. Ectopic tumor ACTH production, cortisol-producing adrenal adenomas, carcinoma, and hyperplasia account for the other causes; rarely, ectopic tumor CRH production is encountered.

ACTH-producing adenomas account for about 10 to 15% of all pituitary tumors. Because the clinical features of Cushing's syndrome often lead to early diagnosis, most ACTH-producing pituitary tumors are relatively small microadenomas. However, macroadenomas are also seen, and some ACTH-secreting adenomas are clinically silent. Cushing's disease is 5 to 10 times more common in women than in men. These pituitary adenomas exhibit unrestrained ACTH secretion, with resultant hypercortisolemia. However, they retain partial suppressibility in the presence of high doses of administered glucocorticoids, providing the basis for dynamic testing to distinguish pituitary and nonpituitary causes of Cushing's syndrome.

Presentation and Diagnosis

The diagnosis of Cushing's syndrome presents two great challenges: (1) to distinguish patients with pathologic cortisol excess from those with physiologic or other disturbances of cortisol production; and (2) to determine the etiology of cortisol excess.

Typical features of chronic cortisol excess include thin, brittle skin, central obesity, hypertension, plethoric moon facies, purple striae and easy bruisability, glucose intolerance or diabetes mellitus, gonadal dysfunction, osteoporosis, proximal muscle weakness, signs of hyperandrogenism (acne, hirsutism), and psychological disturbances (depression, mania, and psychoses) (**Table 2-11**). Hematopoietic features of hypercortisolism include leukocytosis, lymphopenia, and eosinopenia. Immune suppression includes delayed hypersensitivity. The protean manifestations of hypercortisolism make it challenging to decide which patients mandate formal laboratory evaluation. Certain features make pathologic causes of hypercortisolism more likely—these include characteristic central redistribution of fat, thin skin with striae and bruising, and proximal muscle weakness. In children and in young females, early osteoporosis may be particularly prominent. The primary cause of death is cardiovascular disease, but infections and risk of suicide are also increased.

Rapid development of features of hypercortisolism associated with skin hyperpigmentation and severe myopathy suggests the possibility of ectopic sources of ACTH. Hypertension, hypokalemic alkalosis, glucose intolerance, and edema are also more pronounced in these patients. Serum potassium levels <3.3 mmol/L are evident in ~70% of patients with ectopic ACTH secretion but are seen in $<10\%$ of patients with pituitary-dependent Cushing's disease.

TABLE 2-11

CLINICAL FEATURES OF CUSHING'S SYNDROME (ALL AGES)

SYMPTOMS/SIGNS	FREQUENCY, %
Obesity or weight gain (>115% ideal body weight)	80
Thin skin	80
Moon facies	75
Hypertension	75
Purple skin striae	65
Hirsutism	65
Abnormal glucose tolerance	55
Impotence	55
Menstrual disorders (usually amenorrhea)	60
Plethora	60
Proximal muscle weakness	50
Truncal obesity	50
Acne	45
Bruising	45
Mental changes	45
Osteoporosis	40
Edema of lower extremities	30
Hyperpigmentation	20
Hypokalemic alkalosis	15
Diabetes mellitus	15

Source: Adapted from MA Magiokou et al, in ME Wierman (ed), *Diseases of the Pituitary.* Totowa, NJ, Humana, 1997.

Laboratory Investigation

The diagnosis of Cushing's syndrome is based on laboratory documentation of endogenous hypercortisolism. Measurements of 24-h urine free cortisol (UFC) is a precise and cost-effective screening test. Alternatively, the failure to suppress plasma cortisol after an overnight 1-mg dexamethasone suppression test can be used to identify patients with hypercortisolism. As nadir levels of cortisol occur at night, elevated midnight samples of cortisol are suggestive of Cushing's syndrome. Basal plasma ACTH levels often distinguish patients with ACTH-independent (adrenal or exogenous glucocorticoid) from those with ACTH-dependent (pituitary, ectopic ACTH) Cushing's disease. Mean basal ACTH levels are about eightfold higher in patients with ectopic ACTH secretion compared to those with pituitary ACTH-secreting adenomas. However, extensive overlap of ACTH levels in these two disorders precludes using ACTH to make the distinction. Instead, dynamic testing, based on differential sensitivity to glucocorticoid feedback, or ACTH stimulation in response to CRH or cortisol reduction is used to discriminate ectopic versus pituitary sources of excess ACTH (**Table 2-12**). Very rarely, circulating CRH levels are elevated, reflecting ectopic tumor-derived secretion of CRH and often ACTH. For discussion of dynamic testing for Cushing's syndrome, see Chap. 5.

Most ACTH-secreting pituitary tumors are <5 mm in diameter, and about half are undetectable by sensitive MRI. The high prevalence of incidental pituitary microadenomas diminishes the ability to distinguish ACTH-secreting pituitary tumors accurately by MRI.

Inferior Petrosal Venous Sampling

Because pituitary MRI with gadolinium enhancement is insufficiently sensitive to detect small (<2 mm) pituitary ACTH-secreting adenomas, bilateral inferior petrosal sinus ACTH sampling before and after CRH administration may be required to distinguish these lesions from ectopic ACTH-secreting tumors that may have similar clinical and biochemical characteristics. Simultaneous assessment of ACTH concentrations in each inferior petrosal vein and in the peripheral circulation provides a strategy for confirming and localizing pituitary ACTH production. Sampling is performed at baseline and 2, 5, and 10 min after intravenous ovine CRH (1 μg/kg) injection. An increased ratio (>2) of inferior petrosal:peripheral vein ACTH confirms pituitary Cushing's disease. After CRH injection, peak petrosal:peripheral ACTH ratios of ≥3 confirm the presence of a pituitary ACTH-secreting tumor. The sensitivity of this test is >95%, with very rare false-positive results. False-negative results may be encountered in patients with aberrant venous anatomical drainage. Petrosal sinus catheterizations are technically difficult, and about 0.05% of patients develop neurovascular complications. The procedure should not be performed in patients with hypertension or in the presence of a well-visualized pituitary adenoma on MRI.

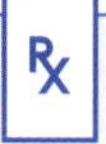

TREATMENT FOR CUSHING'S DISEASE

Selective transsphenoidal resection is the treatment of choice for Cushing's disease (**Fig. 2-10**). The remission rate for this procedure is ~80% for microadenomas but <50% for macroadenomas. After successful tumor resection, most patients experience a postoperative period of adrenal insufficiency that lasts for up to 12 months. This usually requires low-dose cortisol replacement, as patients experience steroid withdrawal symptoms as well as having a suppressed HPA axis. Biochemical recurrence occurs in approximately 5% of patients in whom surgery was initially successful.

When initial surgery is unsuccessful, repeat surgery is sometimes indicated, particularly when a pituitary source for ACTH is well documented. In

TABLE 2-12

DIFFERENTIAL DIAGNOSIS OF ACTH-DEPENDENT CUSHING'S SYNDROME[a]

	ACTH-SECRETING PITUITARY TUMOR	ECTOPIC ACTH SECRETION
Etiology	Pituitary corticotrope adenoma Plurihormonal adenoma	Bronchial, abdominal carcinoid Small cell lung cancer Thymoma
Gender	F > M	M > F
Clinical features	Slow onset	Rapid onset Pigmentation Severe myopathy
Serum potassium <3.3 μ/gL	<10%	75%
24-h urinary free cortisol (UFC)	High	High
Basal ACTH level	Inappropriately high	Very high
Dexamethasone suppression		
1 mg overnight		
Low dose (0.5 mg q6h)	Cortisol >5 μg/dL	Cortisol >5 μ/dL
High dose (2 mg q6h)	Cortisol >5 μg/dL	Cortisol >5 μ/dL
UFC > 80% suppressed	Microadenomas: 90% Macroadenomas: 50%	10%
Inferior petrosal sinus sampling (IPSS)		
Basal		
IPSS: peripheral	>2	<2
CRH-induced		
IPSS: peripheral	>3	<3

[a] ACTH-independent causes of Cushing's syndrome are diagnosed by suppressed ACTH levels and an adrenal mass in the setting of hypercortisolism. Iatrogenic Cushing's syndrome is excluded by history.
Note: ACTH, adrenocorticotropin hormone; F, female; M, male; CRH corticotropin-releasing hormone.

older patients when growth and fertility are no longer important, hemi- or total hypophysectomy may be necessary if an adenoma is not recognized. Pituitary irradiation may be used after unsuccessful surgery, but it cures only about 15% of patients. Because radiation is slow and only partially effective in adults, steroidogenic inhibitors are used in combination with pituitary irradiation to block the adrenal effects of persistently high ACTH levels.

Ketoconazole, an imidazole derivative antimycotic agent, inhibits several P450 enzymes and effectively lowers cortisol in most patients with Cushing's disease when administered twice daily (600 to 1200 mg/d). Elevated hepatic transaminases, gynecomastia, impotence, gastrointestinal upset, and edema are common side effects. *Metyrapone* (2 to 4 g/d) inhibits 11β-hydroxylase activity and normalizes plasma cortisol in up to 75% of patients. Side effects include nausea and vomiting, rash, and exacerbation of acne or hirsutism. *Mitotane* (*o,p'*-DDD; 3 to 6 g/d orally in four divided doses) suppresses cortisol hypersecretion by inhibiting 11β-hydroxylase and cholesterol side-chain cleavage enzymes and by destroying adrenocortical cells. Side effects of mitotane include gastrointestinal symptoms, dizziness, gynecomastia, hyperlipidemia, skin rash, and hepatic enzyme elevation. It may also lead to hypoaldosteronism. Other agents include *aminoglutethimide* (250 mg tid), *trilostane* (200 to 1000 mg/d), *cyproheptadine* (24 mg/d), and IV *etomidate* (0.3 mg/kg per hour). Glucocorticoid insufficiency is a potential side effect of agents used to block steroidogenesis.

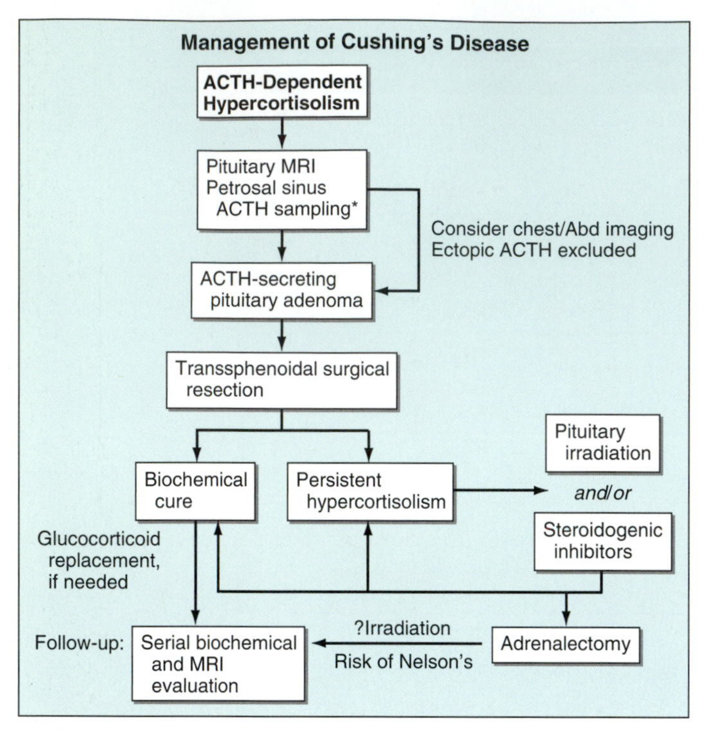

FIGURE 2-10

Management of Cushing's disease. ACTH, adrenocorticotropin hormone; MRI, magnetic resonance imaging. *, Not usually required.

The use of steroidogenic inhibitors has decreased the need for bilateral adrenalectomy. Removal of both adrenal glands corrects hypercortisolism but may be associated with significant morbidity and necessitates permanent glucocorticoid and mineralocorticoid replacement. Adrenalectomy in the setting of residual corticotrope adenoma tissue predisposes to the development of *Nelson's syndrome*, a disorder characterized by rapid pituitary tumor enlargement and increased pigmentation secondary to high ACTH levels. Radiation therapy may be indicated to prevent the development of Nelson's syndrome after adrenalectomy.

GONADOTROPINS: FSH AND LH

SYNTHESIS AND SECRETION

Gonadotrope cells comprise about 10% of anterior pituitary cells and produce two gonadotropins—LH and FSH. Like TSH and hCG, LH and FSH are glycoprotein hormones consisting of α and β subunits. The α subunit is common to these glycoprotein hormones; specificity is conferred by the β subunits, which are expressed by separate genes.

Gonadotropin synthesis and release are dynamically regulated. This is particularly true in females, in whom the rapidly fluctuating gonadal steroid levels vary throughout the menstrual cycle. Hypothalamic GnRH, a 10-amino-acid peptide, regulates the synthesis and secretion of both LH and FSH. GnRH is secreted in discrete pulses every 60 to 120 min, which in turn elicit LH and FSH pulses (Fig. 2-3). The pulsatile mode of GnRH input is essential to its action; pulses prime gonadotrope responsiveness, whereas continuous GnRH exposure induces desensitization. Based on this phenomenon, long-acting GnRH agonists are used to suppress gonadotropin levels in children with precocious puberty and in men with prostate cancer and are used in some ovulation-induction protocols to reduce endogenous gonadotropins (Chap. 15). Estrogens act at the hypothalamic and pituitary levels to control gonadotropin secretion. Chronic estrogen exposure is inhibitory, whereas rising estrogen levels, as occurs during the preovulatory surge, exert positive feedback to increase gonadotropin pulse frequency and amplitude. Progesterone slows GnRH pulse frequency but enhances gonadotropin responses to GnRH. Testosterone feedback in males also occurs at the hypothalamic and pituitary levels and partially reflects its conversion to estrogens.

Though GnRH is the main regulator of LH and FSH secretion, FSH synthesis is also under separate control by the gonadal peptides inhibin and activin, which are members of the transforming growth factor β (TGF-β) family. Inhibin selectively suppresses FSH, whereas activin stimulates FSH synthesis (Chap. 10).

ACTION

The gonadotropin hormones interact with their respective GPCRs expressed in the ovary and testis, evoking germ cell development and maturation and steroid hormone biosynthesis. In women, FSH regulates ovarian follicle development and stimulates ovarian estrogen production. LH mediates ovulation and maintenance of the corpus luteum. In men, LH induces Leydig cell testosterone synthesis and secretion and FSH stimulates seminiferous tubule development and regulates spermatogenesis.

GONADOTROPIN DEFICIENCY

Hypogonadism is the most common presenting feature of adult hypopituitarism, even when other pituitary hormones are also deficient. It is often a harbinger of hypothalamic or pituitary diseases that impair GnRH production or delivery through the pituitary stalk. As noted above, hypogonadotropic hypogonadism is a common presenting feature of hyperprolactinemia.

A variety of inherited and acquired disorders are associated with *isolated hypogonadotropic hypogonadism* (IHH) (Chap. 8). Hypothalamic defects associated with GnRH deficiency include two X-linked disorders, Kallmann syndrome (see above) and mutations in the *DAX1* gene. GnRH receptor mutations and inactivating mutations of the LH β and FSH β subunit genes are rare causes of selective gonadotropin deficiency. Acquired forms of GnRH deficiency leading to hypogonadotropism are seen in association with anorexia nervosa, stress, starvation, and extreme exercise, but may also be idiopathic. Hypogonadotropic hypogonadism in these disorders is reversed by removal of the stressful stimulus.

Presentation and Diagnosis

In premenopausal women, hypogonadotropic hypogonadism presents as diminished ovarian function leading to oligomenorrhea or amenorrhea, infertility, decreased vaginal secretions, decreased libido, and breast atrophy. In hypogonadal adult males, secondary testicular failure is associated with decreased libido and potency, infertility, decreased muscle mass with weakness, reduced beard and body hair growth, soft testes, and characteristic fine facial wrinkles. Osteoporosis occurs in both untreated hypogonadal females and males.

Laboratory Investigation

Central hypogonadism is associated with low or inappropriately normal serum gonadotropin levels in the setting of low sex hormone concentrations (testosterone in males, estradiol in females). Three pooled serum samples drawn 20 min apart are used for accurate measurement of serum LH and FSH levels, thus allowing for the effects of hormone secretory pulses. Male patients have abnormal semen analysis.

Intravenous GnRH (100 μg) stimulates gonadotropes to secrete LH (which peaks within 30 min) and FSH (which plateaus during the ensuing 60 min). Normal responses vary according to menstrual cycle stage, age, and sex of the patient. Generally, LH levels increase about threefold, whereas FSH responses are less pronounced. In the setting of gonadotropin deficiency, a normal gonadotropin response to GnRH indicates intact gonadotrope function and suggests a hypothalamic abnormality. An absent response, however, cannot reliably distinguish pituitary from hypothalamic causes of hypogonadism. For this reason, GnRH testing usually adds little to the information gained from baseline evaluation of the hypothalamic-pituitary-gonadotrope axis, except in cases of isolated GnRH deficiency (e.g., Kallmann syndrome).

MRI examination of the sellar region and assessment of other pituitary functions are usually indicated in patients with documented central hypogonadism.

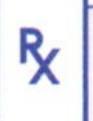

TREATMENT FOR GONADOTROPIN DEFICIENCY

In males, testosterone replacement is necessary to achieve and maintain normal growth and development of the external genitalia, secondary sex characteristics, male sexual behavior, and androgenic anabolic effects including maintenance of muscle function and bone mass. Testosterone may be administered by intramuscular injections every 1 to 4 weeks or using patches that are replaced daily (Chap. 8). Testosterone creams are also available. Gonadotropin injections [hCG or human menopausal gonadotropin (hMG)] over 12 to 18 months are used to restore fertility. Pulsatile GnRH therapy (25 to 150 ng/kg every 2 h), administered by a subcutaneous infusion pump, is also effective for treatment of hypothalamic hypogonadism when fertility is desired.

In premenopausal women, cyclical replacement of estrogen and progesterone maintains secondary sexual characteristics and genitourinary tract integrity and prevents premature osteoporosis (Chap. 10). Gonadotropin therapy is used for ovulation induction. Follicular growth and maturation are initiated using hMG or recombinant FSH; hCG is subsequently injected to induce ovulation. As in men, pulsatile GnRH therapy can be used to treat hypothalamic causes of gonadotropin deficiency.

NONFUNCTIONING AND GONADOTROPIN-PRODUCING PITUITARY ADENOMAS

Etiology and Prevalence

Nonfunctioning pituitary adenomas include those that secrete little or no pituitary hormones, as well as tumors that produce too little hormone to result in recognizable clinical features. They are the most common type of pituitary adenoma and are usually macroadenomas at the time of diagnosis because clinical features are inapparent until tumor mass effects occur. Based on immunohistochemistry, most clinically nonfunctioning adenomas can be shown to originate from gonadotrope cells. These tumors typically produce small amounts of intact gonadotropins (usually FSH) as well as uncombined α and LH β and FSH β subunits. Tumor secretion may lead to elevated α and FSH β subunits and, rarely, to increased LH β subunit levels. Some adenomas express α subunits without FSH or LH. TRH administration often induces an atypical increase of tumor-derived gonadotropins or subunits.

Presentation and Diagnosis

Clinically nonfunctioning tumors may present with optic chiasm pressure and other symptoms of local expansion or be incidentally discovered on an MRI performed for another indication. Menstrual disturbances or ovarian hyperstimulation rarely occur in women with large tumors that produce FSH and LH. More commonly, adenoma compression of the pituitary stalk or surrounding pituitary tissue leads to attenuated LH and features of hypogonadism. PRL levels are usually slightly increased, also because of stalk compression. It is important to distinguish this circumstance from true prolactinomas, as most nonfunctioning tumors respond poorly to treatment with dopamine agonists.

Laboratory Investigation

The goal of laboratory testing in clinically nonfunctioning tumors is to classify the type of the tumor, to identify hormonal markers of tumor activity, and to detect possible hypopituitarism. Free α subunit levels may be elevated in 10 to 15% of patients with nonfunctioning tumors. In female patients, peri- or postmenopausal basal FSH concentrations are difficult to distinguish from tumor-derived FSH elevation. Premenopausal women have cycling FSH levels, also preventing clear-cut diagnostic distinction from tumor-derived FSH. In men, gonadotropin-secreting tumors may be diagnosed because of slightly increased gonadotropins (FSH > LH) in the setting of a pituitary mass. Testosterone levels are usually low, despite the normal or increased LH level, perhaps reflecting reduced LH bioactivity or the loss of normal LH pulsatility. Because this pattern of hormone tests is also seen in primary gonadal failure and, to some extent, with aging (Chap. 8), the increased gonadotropins alone are insufficient for the diagnosis of a gonadotropin-secreting tumor. In the majority of patients with gonadotrope adenomas, TRH administration stimulates LH β subunit secretion; this response is not seen in normal individuals. GnRH testing is not helpful for making the diagnosis. For nonfunctioning and gonadotropin-secreting tumors, the diagnosis usually rests on immunohistochemical analyses of resected tumor tissue, as the mass effects of these tumors usually necessitate resection.

Although acromegaly or Cushing's syndrome usually presents with unique clinical features, clinically inapparent somatotrope or corticotrope adenomas can be excluded by a normal IGF-I value and normal 24-h urinary free cortisol levels. If PRL levels are <100 μg/L in a patient harboring a pituitary mass, a nonfunctioning adenoma causing pituitary stalk compression should be considered.

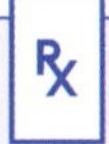

TREATMENT FOR MACROADENOMAS

Asymptomatic small nonfunctioning adenomas with no threat to vision may be followed with regular MRI and visual field testing without immediate intervention. However, for larger macroadenomas, transsphenoidal surgery is the only effective way to reduce tumor size and relieve mass effects (**Fig. 2-11**). Although it is not usually possi-

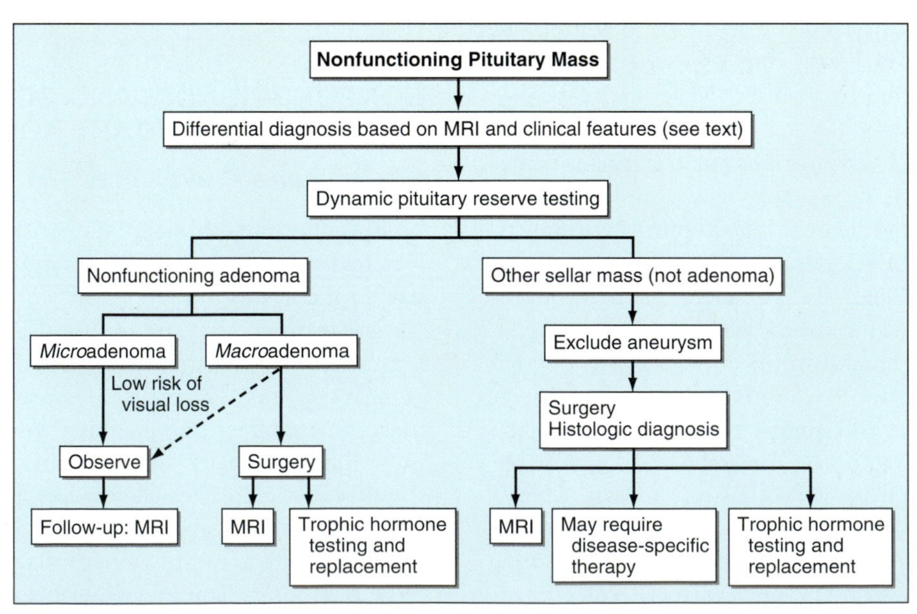

FIGURE 2-11
Management of a nonfunctioning pituitary mass.

ble to remove all adenoma tissue surgically, vision improves in 70% of patients with preoperative visual field defects. Preexisting hypopituitarism that results from tumor mass effects commonly improves or may resolve completely. Beginning about 6 months postoperatively, MRI scans should be performed yearly to detect tumor regrowth. Within 5 to 6 years following successful surgical resection, ~15% of nonfunctioning tumors recur. When substantial tumor remains after transsphenoidal surgery, adjuvant radiotherapy may be indicated to prevent tumor growth. Radiotherapy may be deferred if no postoperative residual mass is evident.

Nonfunctioning pituitary tumors respond poorly to dopamine agonist treatment, with modest tumor shrinkage occurring in <10% of patients. Although SSTR subtypes 2 and 5 have been identified on nonfunctioning pituitary adenomas, octreotide does not shrink these tumors and only modestly suppresses gonadotropin and α subunit levels. Visual improvement sometimes occurs without evident reduction of tumor size by MRI, presumably reflecting relief of pressure on the optic tracts. The selective GnRH antagonist, Nal-Glu GnRH, suppresses FSH hypersecretion but has no effect on adenoma size.

THYROID-STIMULATING HORMONE

SYNTHESIS AND SECRETION

TSH-secreting thyrotrope cells comprise 5% of the anterior pituitary cell population. TSH is structurally related to LH and FSH. It shares a common α subunit with these hormones but contains a specific TSH β subunit. TRH is a hypothalamic tripeptide (pyroglutamyl histidylprolinamide) that acts through a GPCR to stimulate TSH synthesis and secretion; it also stimulates the lactotrope cell to secrete PRL. TSH secretion is stimulated by TRH, whereas thyroid hormones, dopamine, SRIF, and glucocorticoids suppress TSH by overriding TRH induction.

The thyrotrope is stimulated by a release from the negative feedback inhibition by thyroid hormones. Thus, thyroid damage (including surgical thyroidectomy), radiation-induced hypothyroidism, chronic thyroiditis, or prolonged goitrogen exposure are associated with increased TSH. Long-standing untreated hypothyroidism can lead to thyrotrope hyperplasia and pituitary enlargement, which may be evident on MRI.

ACTION

TSH is secreted in pulses, though the excursions are modest in comparison to other pituitary hormones because of the relatively low amplitude of the pulses and the relatively long half-life of TSH. Consequently, single determinations of TSH suffice to assess its circulating levels. TSH binds to a GPCR on thyroid follicular cells to stimulate thyroid hormone synthesis and release (Chap. 4).

TSH DEFICIENCY

Features of central hypothyroidism caused by TSH deficiency mimic those seen with primary hypothyroidism but are generally less severe. Pituitary hypothyroidism is characterized by low basal TSH levels in the setting of low free thyroid hormone. In contrast, patients with hypothyroidism of hypothalamic origin (presumably due to a lack of endogenous TRH) may exhibit normal or even slightly elevated TSH levels. There is evidence that the TSH produced in this circumstance has reduced biologic activity because of altered glycosylation.

TRH (200 μg) injected intravenously causes a two- to threefold increase in TSH (and PRL) levels within 30 min. Although TRH testing can be used to assess TSH reserve, abnormalities of the thyroid axis can usually be detected based on basal free T_4 and TSH levels, without the need for TRH testing.

Thyroid-replacement therapy should be initiated after establishing adequate adrenal function. Dose adjustment is based on thyroid hormone levels and clinical parameters rather than the TSH level.

TSH-SECRETING ADENOMAS

TSH-producing macroadenomas are rare but are often large and locally invasive when they occur. Patients usually present with thyroid goiter and hyperthyroidism, reflecting overproduction of TSH. Diagnosis is based on demonstrating elevated serum free T_4 levels, inappropriately normal or high TSH secretion, and MRI evidence of a pituitary adenoma.

It is important to exclude other causes of inappropriate TSH secretion, such as resistance to thyroid hormone, an autosomal dominant disorder caused by mutations in the thyroid hormone β receptor (Chap. 4). The presence of a pituitary mass and elevated α subunit levels are suggestive of a TSH-secreting tumor. Dysalbuminemic hyperthyroxinemia syndromes, caused by various mutations in serum thyroid hormone–binding proteins, are also characterized by elevated thyroid hormone levels, but with normal rather than suppressed TSH levels. Moreover, free thyroid hormone levels are normal in these disorders, most of which are familial.

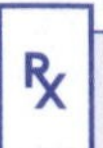

TREATMENT FOR TSH-SECRETING ADENOMAS

The initial therapeutic approach is to remove or debulk the tumor mass surgically, using either a transsphenoidal or subfrontal approach. Total resection is not often achieved as most of these adenomas are large and locally invasive. Normal circulating thyroid hormone levels are achieved in about two-thirds of patients after surgery. Thyroid ablation or antithyroid drugs (methimazole or propylthiouracil) can be used to reduce thyroid hormone levels. Dopamine agonists are rarely effective for suppressing TSH secretion from these tumors. However, somatostatin analogue treatment effectively normalizes TSH and α subunit hypersecretion, shrinks the tumor mass in 50% of patients, and improves visual fields in 75% of patients; euthyroidism is restored in most patients. In some patients, octreotide markedly suppresses TSH, causing biochemical hypothyroidism that requires concomitant thyroid hormone replacement. Lanreotide (30 mg intramuscularly), a long-acting somatostatin analogue (see above), effectively suppresses TSH and thyroid hormone in patients treated every 14 days.

DIABETES INSIPIDUS

See Chap. 3 for diagnosis and treatment of diabetes insipidus.

FURTHER READINGS

Arnaldi G et al: Diagnosis and complications of Cushing's syndrome: A consensus statement. J Clin Endocrinol Metab 88:5593, 2003

Attanusio AF et al: Human growth hormone replacement in adult hypopituitary patients. J Clin Endocrinol Metab 87:1600, 2002

Broglio F et al: Ghrelin, a natural GH secretagogue produced by the stomach, induces hyperglycemia and reduces insulin secretion in humans. J Clin Endocrinol Metab 86:5083, 2001

Ghrelin is one of several recently discovered hormones. Though initially identified as a growth hormone secretagogue, ghrelin exerts multiple biologic effects, and provides a physiologic link between the stomach, the hypothalamus, and various metabolic pathways.

Clemmons DR et al: Optimizing control of acromegaly: Integrating a growth hormone receptor antagonist into the treatment algorithm. J Clin Endocrinol Metab 88:4759, 2003

Colao A: Long-term effects of depot long-acting somatostatin analog octreotide on hormone levels and tumor mass in acromegaly. J Clin Endocrinol Metab 86:2779, 2001

Because the half-lives of somatostatin and its analogues are relatively short, there has been interest in developing depot formulations for convenience and better suppression of growth hormone secretion. This study demonstrates efficacy of a depot formulation of Octreotide-LAR.

Colao A et al: Systemic complications of acromegaly: epidemiology, pathogenesis, and management. Endocr Rev 25:102, 2004

With the advent of new medical therapies, such as somatostatin analogues and growth hormone receptor antagonists, the indications and strategies for managing acromegaly are evolving. This review objectively evaluates the long-term complications associated with growth hormone excess.

Cummings DE et al: Plasma ghrelin levels after diet-induced weight loss or gastric bypass surgery. N Engl J Med 346:1623, 2002

This study documents that ghrelin levels are higher in diet-induced weight loss than after gastric bypass surgery, supporting the hypothesis that the relative efficacy of gastric bypass may involve loss of compensatory production of gut factors, such as ghrelin, that stimulate appetite.

Dattani MT: Novel insights into the aetiology and pathogenesis of hypopituitarism. Horm Res 62 (Suppl 3)1, 2004

Findling JW et al: Screening and diagnosis of Cushing's syndrome. Endocrinol Metab Clin North Am 34:385, 2005

Melmed S et al: Consensus. Guidelines for acromegaly management. J Clin Endocrinol Metab 87:4054, 2002

Millar RP et al: Gonadotropin-releasing hormone receptors. Endocr Rev 25:235, 2004

Mullis PE: Genetic control of growth. Eur J Endocrinol 152:11, 2005

Olson LE, Rosenfeld MG: Perspective: Genetic and genomic approaches in elucidating mechanisms of pituitary development. Endocrinology 143:2007, 2002

Prezant TP, Melmed S: Molecular pathogenesis of pituitary disorders. Curr Opinion Endocrinol Diabetes 9:61, 2002

Genetic causes of pituitary tumors, whether inherited or acquired, are summarized in this review.

Valdes-Socin H et al: Hypogonadism in a patient with a mutation in the luteinizing hormone β-subunit gene. N Engl J Med 351:2619, 2004

Vella A, Young WF: Pituitary apoplexy. Endocrinologist 11:282, 2001

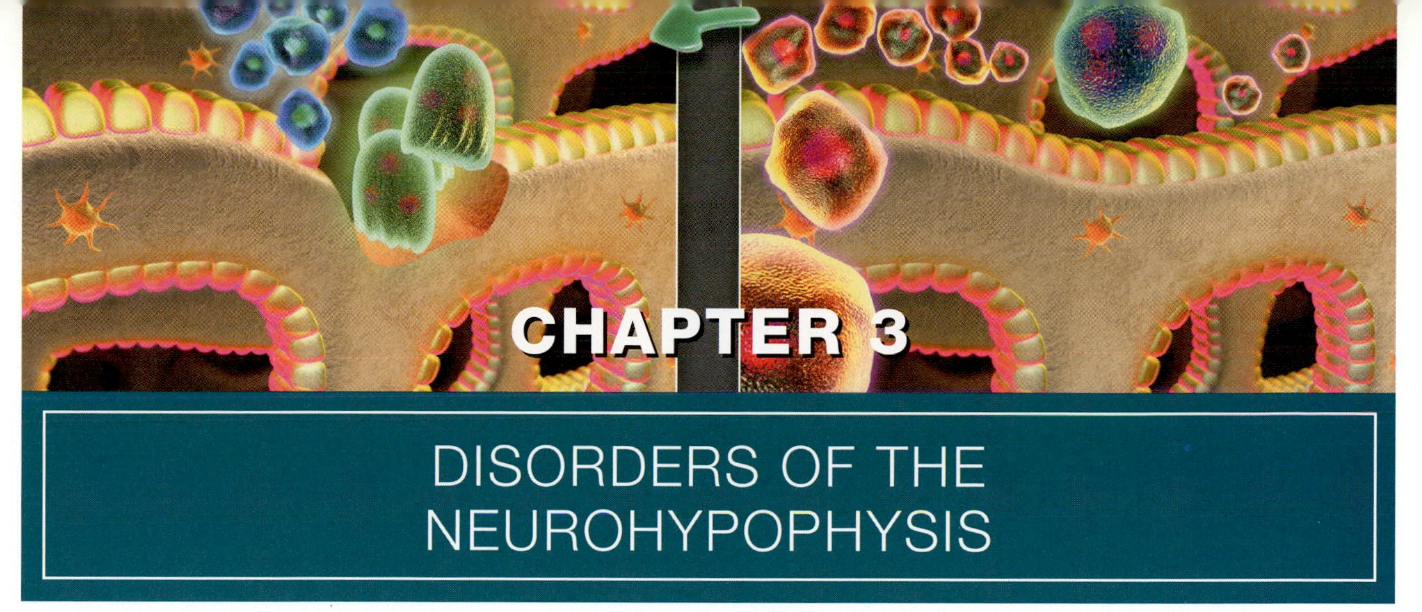

CHAPTER 3

DISORDERS OF THE NEUROHYPOPHYSIS

Gary L. Robertson

The neurohypophysis, or posterior pituitary gland, is formed by axons that originate in large cell bodies in the supraoptic and paraventricular nuclei of the hypothalamus. It produces two hormones: (1) arginine vasopressin (AVP), also known as antidiuretic hormone; and (2) oxytocin. AVP acts on the renal tubules to reduce water loss by concentrating the urine. Oxytocin stimulates postpartum milk letdown in response to suckling. AVP deficiency causes diabetes insipidus (DI), characterized by the production of large amounts of dilute urine. Excessive or inappropriate AVP production predisposes to hyponatremia if water intake is not reduced in parallel with urine output.

VASOPRESSIN

ACTION

AVP is a nonapeptide composed of a six-membered disulfide ring and a tripeptide tail (**Fig. 3-1**). The most important, if not the only, physiologic action of AVP is to reduce water excretion by promoting concentration of urine. This antidiuretic effect is achieved by increasing the hydroosmotic permeability of cells that line the distal tubule and medullary collecting ducts of the kidney (**Fig. 3-2**). In the absence of AVP, these cells are impermeable to water and reabsorb little, if any, of the relatively large volume of dilute filtrate that enters from the proximal nephron. This results in the excretion of very large volumes (as much as 0.2 mL/kg per min) of maximally dilute urine (specific gravity and osmolarity ~1.000 and 50 mosmol/L, respectively), a condition known as a *water diuresis.* In the presence of AVP, these cells become selectively permeable to water, allowing it to diffuse back down the osmotic gradient created by the hypertonic renal medulla. As a result, the dilute fluid passing through the tubules is concentrated and the rate of urine flow decreases. The magnitude of this effect varies in direct proportion to the plasma AVP concentration and, at maximum levels, approximates a urine flow rate as low as 0.35 mL/min and a urine osmolarity as high as 1200 mosmol/L. AVP action is mediated via binding to G protein–coupled V_2 receptors on the serosal surface of the cell, activation of adenyl cyclase, and insertion into the luminal surface of water channels composed of a protein known as *aquaporin 2.*

At high concentrations, AVP also causes contraction of smooth muscle in blood vessels and in the gastrointestinal tract, induces glycogenolysis in the liver, and potentiates adrenocorticotropic hormone (ACTH) release by corticotropin-releasing factor. These effects are mediated by V_{1a} or V_{1b} receptors that are coupled to phospholipase C. Their role, if any, in human physiology/pathophysiology is still uncertain.

SYNTHESIS AND SECRETION

AVP secretion is synthesized via a polypeptide precursor that includes AVP, neurophysin, and copeptin. After preliminary processing and folding, the precursor is packaged in neurosecretory vesicles where it is transported down the axon, further processed to AVP, and stored until the hormone and other components are released by exocytosis into peripheral blood.

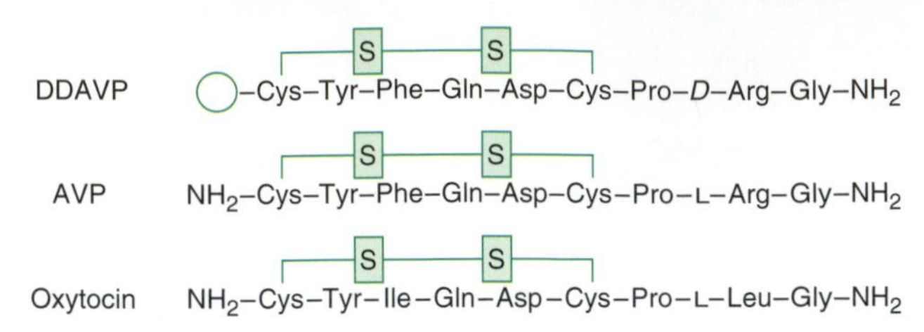

FIGURE 3-1
Primary structures of arginine vasopressin (AVP), oxytocin, and DDAVP.

AVP secretion is regulated primarily by the "effective" osmotic pressure of body fluids. This control is mediated by specialized hypothalamic cells, known as *osmoreceptors,* which are extremely sensitive to small changes in the plasma concentration of sodium and certain other solutes but are insensitive to other solutes such as urea or glucose. The osmoreceptors appear to include inhibitory as well as stimulatory components that function in concert to form a threshold, or set point, control system for AVP release. Below this threshold, plasma AVP is suppressed to levels that permit the development of a maximum water diuresis. Above it, plasma AVP rises steeply in direct proportion to plasma osmolarity, quickly reaching levels sufficient to effect a maximum antidiuresis. The absolute levels of plasma osmolarity/sodium at which minimally and maximally effective levels of plasma AVP occur vary appreciably from person to person, owing apparently to genetic influences on the set and sensitivity of the system. However, the average threshold, or set point, for AVP release corresponds to a plasma osmolarity or sodium of about 280 mosmol/L or 135 meq/L, respectively; levels only 2 to 4% higher nor-

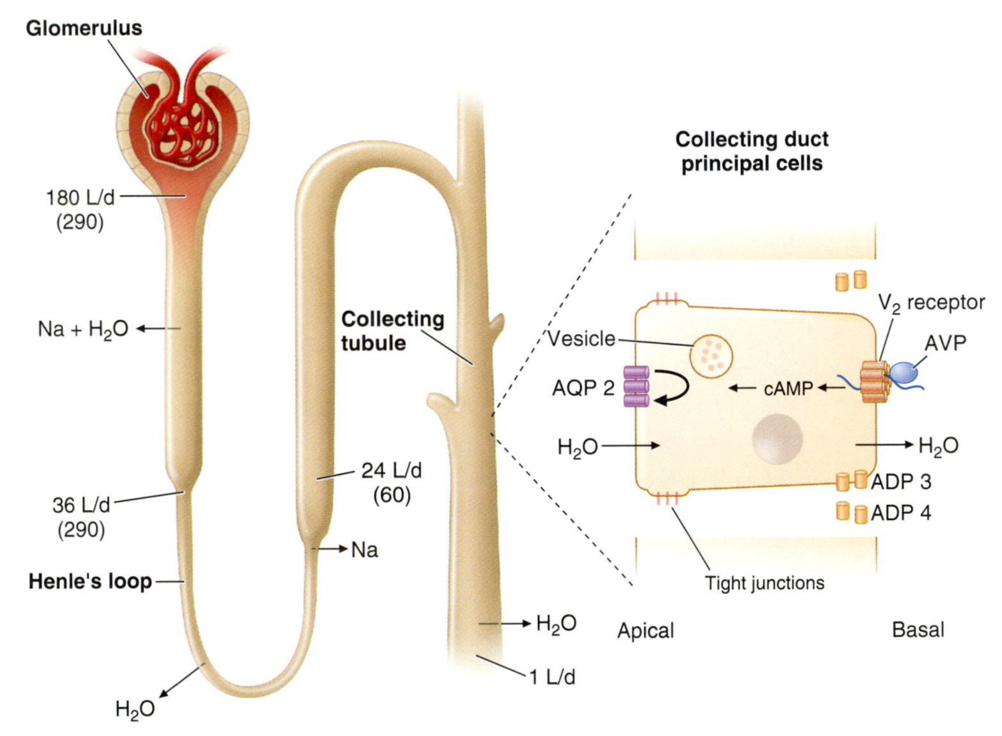

FIGURE 3-2
Antidiuretic effect of arginine vasopressin (AVP) in the regulation of urine volume. In a typical 70-kg adult, the kidney filters about 180 L/d of plasma. Of this, ~144 L (80%) is reabsorbed isosmotically in the proximal tubule and another 8 L (4 to 5%) is reabsorbed without solute in the descending limb of Henle's loop. The remainder is diluted to an osmolarity of about 60 mmol/kg by selective reabsorption of sodium and chloride in the ascending limb. In the absence of AVP, the urine issuing from the loop passes largely unmodified through the distal tubules and collecting ducts, resulting in a maximum water diuresis. In the presence of AVP, solute-free water is reabsorbed osmotically through the principal cells of the collecting ducts, resulting in the excretion of a much smaller volume of concentrated urine. This antidiuretic effect is mediated via a G protein–coupled V_2 receptor that increases intracellular cyclic AMP, thereby inducing translocation of aquaporin 2 (AQP 2) water channels into the apical membrane. The resultant increase in permeability permits an influx of water that diffuses out of the cell through AQP 3 and AQP 4 water channels on the basal-lateral surface. The net rate of flux across the cell is determined by the number of AQP 2 water channels in the apical membrane and the strength of the osmotic gradient between tubular fluid and the renal medulla. Tight junctions on the lateral surface of the cells serve to prevent unregulated water flow.

mally result in maximum antidiuresis. Though relatively stable in a healthy adult, the set of the osmoregulatory system can also be lowered by pregnancy, the menstrual cycle, and relatively large, acute reductions in blood pressure or volume.

The effects of acute changes in blood volume or pressure are mediated largely by neuronal afferents that originate in transmural pressure receptors of the heart and large arteries and project via the vagus and glossopharyngeal nerves to the brainstem, from whence postsynaptic projections ascend to the hypothalmus. These pathways maintain a tonic inhibitory tone that decreases when blood volume or pressure falls by >10 to 20%. This baroregulatory system is probably of minor importance in the physiology of AVP secretion because the hemodynamic changes required to affect it do not usually occur during normal activities. However, the baroregulatory system undoubtedly plays an important role in AVP secretion in patients with large, acute disturbances of hemodynamic function.

AVP secretion can also be stimulated by nausea, acute hypoglycemia, glucocorticoid deficiency, smoking, and, possibly, hyperangiotensinemia. The emetic stimuli are extremely potent since they typically elicit immediate, 50- to 100-fold increases in plasma AVP, even when the nausea is transient and unassociated with vomiting or other symptoms. They appear to act via the emetic center in the medulla and can be completely blocked by treatment with antiemetics such as fluphenazine. There is no evidence that pain or other noxious stresses have any affect on AVP unless they elicit a vasovagal reaction with its associated nausea and hypotension.

METABOLISM

AVP distributes rapidly into a space roughly equal to the extracellular fluid volume. It is cleared irreversibly with a $t_{1/2}$ of 10 to 30 min. Most AVP clearance is due to degradation in the liver and kidneys. During pregnancy, the metabolic clearance of AVP is increased three- to fourfold due to placental production of an N-terminal peptidase.

THIRST

Because AVP cannot reduce water loss below a certain minimum level obligated by urinary solute load and evaporation from skin and lungs, a mechanism for ensuring adequate intake is essential for preventing dehydration. This vital function is performed by the thirst mechanism. Like AVP, thirst is regulated primarily by an osmostat that is located in the anteromedial hypothalamus and is able to detect very small changes in the plasma concentration of sodium and certain other effective solutes. The thirst osmostat appears to be "set" about 5% higher than the AVP osmostat. This arrangement ensures that thirst, polydipsia, and dilution of body fluids do not occur until plasma osmolarity/sodium start to exceed the defensive capacity of the antidiuretic mechanism.

OXYTOCIN

Oxytocin is also a nonapeptide and differs from AVP only at positions 3 and 8 (Fig. 3-1). However, it has relatively little antidiuretic effect and seems to act mainly on mammary ducts to facilitate milk letdown during nursing. It may also help to initiate or facilitate labor by stimulating contraction of uterine smooth muscle, but it is not yet clear if this action is physiologic or necessary for normal delivery.

DEFICIENCIES OF VASOPRESSIN SECRETION AND ACTION

DIABETES INSIPIDUS

Clinical Characteristics

Decreased secretion or action of AVP usually manifests as DI, a syndrome characterized by the production of abnormally large volumes of dilute urine. The 24-h urine volume is >50 mL/kg body weight and the osmolarity is <300 mosmol/L. The polyuria produces symptoms of urinary frequency, enuresis, and/or nocturia, which may disturb sleep and cause mild daytime fatigue or somnolence. It is also associated with thirst and a commensurate increase in fluid intake (polydipsia). Clinical signs of dehydration are uncommon unless fluid intake is impaired.

Etiology

Deficient secretion of AVP can be primary or secondary. The primary form usually results from agenesis or irreversible destruction of the neurohypophysis and is variously referred to as *neurohypophyseal DI, pituitary DI,* or *central DI.* It can be caused by a variety of congenital, acquired, or genetic disorders but almost half the time it is idiopathic (**Table 3-1**). The genetic form of neurohypophyseal DI is usually transmitted in an autosomal dominant mode and is caused by diverse mutations in the coding region of the AVP–neurophysin II (or AVP-NPII) gene. In this type, the AVP deficiency and DI begin several months to several years after birth and appear to be a result of selective degeneration of AVP-producing magnocellular neurons. An autosomal recessive form, due to inactivating mutations in the AVP gene, and an X-linked recessive form, due to an unidentified gene on Xq28, have also been described. A primary deficiency of plasma AVP can also result from increased metabolism by an N-terminal aminopeptidase produced by the placenta. It is referred to as *gestational DI* since the signs and symptoms manifest during pregnancy and usually remit several weeks after delivery. However, a subclinical deficiency in AVP secretion can often be demonstrated in the nonpregnant state, indicating that damage to the neurohypophysis may also contribute to the AVP deficiency. Finally, a primary deficiency of AVP can also result from malformation or destruction of the neurohypophysis by a variety of diseases or toxins (Table 3-1).

TABLE 3-1

CAUSES OF DIABETES INSIPIDUS

PITUITARY DIABETES INSIPIDUS

- **Acquired**
  - Head trauma (closed and penetrating)
  - Neoplasms
    - Primary
      - Craniopharyngioma
      - Pituitary adenoma (suprasellar)
      - Dysgerminoma
      - Meningioma
    - Metastatic (lung, breast)
    - Hematologic (lymphoma, leukemia)
  - Granulomas
    - Neurosarcoid
    - Histiocytosis
    - Xanthoma disseminatum
  - Infectious
    - Chronic meningitis
    - Viral encephalitis
    - Toxoplasmosis
  - Inflammatory
    - Lymphocytic infundibuloneurohypophysitis
    - Wegener's granulomatosis
    - Lupus erythematosus
    - Scleroderma
  - Chemical toxins
    - Tetrodotoxin
    - Snake venom
  - Vascular
    - Sheehan's syndrome
    - Aneurysm (internal carotid)
    - Aortocoronary bypass
    - Hypoxic encephalopathy
  - Pregnancy (vasopressinase)
  - Idiopathic
- **Congenital malformations**
  - Septooptic dysplasia
  - Midline craniofacial defects
  - Holoprosencephaly
  - Hypogenesis, ectopia of pituitary
- **Genetic**
  - Autosomal dominant (AVP-neurophysin gene)
  - Autosomal recessive (AVP-neurophysin gene)
  - Autosomal recessive-Wolfram-(4p–WFS 1 gene)
  - X-linked recessive (Xq28)
  - Deletion chromosome 7q

NEPHROGENIC DIABETES INSIPIDUS

- **Acquired**
  - Drugs
    - Lithium
    - Demeclocycline
    - Methoxyflurane
    - Amphotericin B
    - Aminoglycosides
    - Cisplatin
    - Rifampin
    - Foscarnet
  - Metabolic
    - Hypercalcemia, hypercalciuria
    - Hypokalemia
  - Obstruction (ureter or urethra)
  - Vascular
    - Sickle cell disease and trait
    - Ischemia (acute tubular necrosis)
  - Granulomas
    - Neurosarcoid
  - Neoplasms
    - Sarcoma
  - Infiltration
    - Amyloidosis
  - Pregnancy
  - Idiopathic
- **Genetic**
  - X-linked recessive (AVP receptor-2 gene)
  - Autosomal recessive (aquaporin-2 gene)
  - Autosomal dominant (aquaporin-2 gene)

PRIMARY POLYDIPSIA

- **Acquired**
  - Psychogenic
    - Schizophrenia
    - Obsessive-compulsive disorder
  - Dipsogenic (abnormal thirst)
    - Granulomas
      - Neurosarcoid
    - Infectious
      - Tuberculous meningitis
    - Head trauma (closed and penetrating)
    - Demyelination
      - Multiple sclerosis
    - Drugs
      - Lithium
      - Carbamazepine
    - Idiopathic
  - Iatrogenic

Secondary deficiencies of AVP result from inhibition of secretion by excessive intake of fluids. They are referred to as *primary polydipsia* and can be divided into three subcategories. One of them, called *dipsogenic DI,* is characterized by an inappropriate increase in thirst caused by a reduction in the "set" of the osmoregulatory mechanism. It sometimes occurs in association with multifocal diseases of the brain such as neurosarcoid, tuberculous meningitis, or multiple sclerosis but is often idiopathic. The second subtype, called *psychogenic polydipsia,* is not associated with thirst, and the polydipsia seems to be a feature of psychosis. The third subtype, which may be referred to as *iatrogenic polydipsia,* results from recommendations of health professionals or the popular media to increase fluid intake for its presumed preventive or therapeutic benefits for other disorders.

Primary deficiencies in the antidiuretic action of AVP result in *nephrogenic DI* (Table 3-1). It can be genetic, acquired, or caused by exposure to various drugs. The genetic form is usually transmitted in an X-linked mode and is caused by mutations in the coding region of the V_2 receptor gene. Autosomal recessive or dominant forms result from mutations in the gene encoding the aquaporin protein that forms the water channels in the distal nephron.

Secondary deficiencies in the antidiuretic response to AVP result from polyuria per se. They are caused by washout of the medullary concentration gradient and/or suppression of aquaporin function. They usually resolve 24 to 48 h after the polyuria is corrected but often complicate interpretation of tests commonly used for differential diagnosis.

Pathophysiology

When the secretion or action of AVP is reduced to <80 to 85% of normal, urine concentration ceases and the rate of output increases to symptomatic levels. If the defect is primary (e.g., the patient has pituitary, gestational, or nephrogenic DI), the polyuria results in a small (1 to 2%) decrease in body water and a commensurate increase in plasma osmolarity and sodium concentration that stimulate thirst and a compensatory increase in water intake. As a result, *overt physical or laboratory signs of dehydration do not develop unless the patient also has a defect in thirst* (see below) *or fails to drink for some other reason.*

The severity of the antidiuretic defect varies markedly among patients with pituitary, gestational, or nephrogenic DI. In some, the deficiencies in AVP secretion or action are so severe that basal urine output approximates the maximum (10 to 15 mL/min); even an intense stimulus such as nausea or severe dehydration does not raise plasma AVP enough to concentrate the urine. In others, however, the deficiency in AVP secretion or action is incomplete, and a modest stimulus such as a few hours of fluid deprivation, smoking, or a vasovagal reaction increases plasma AVP sufficiently to produce a profound antidiuresis. The maximum urine osmolarity achieved in these patients is usually less than normal, largely because their maximal concentrating capacity is temporarily impaired by chronic polyuria. However, in a few patients with partial pituitary or nephrogenic DI, it can reach levels as high as 800 mosmol/L.

In primary polydipsia, the pathogenesis of the polydipsia and polyuria is the reverse of that in pituitary, nephrogenic, and gestational DI. Thus, the excessive intake of fluids slightly increases body water, thereby reducing plasma osmolarity, AVP secretion, and urinary concentration. The latter results in a compensatory increase in urinary free-water excretion that varies in direct proportion to intake. Therefore, clinically appreciable overhydration is uncommon unless the compensatory water diuresis is impaired by a drug or disease that stimulates or mimics endogenous AVP.

In the dipsogenic form of primary polydipsia, fluid intake is excessive because the osmotic threshold for thirst appears to be reset to the left, often well below that for AVP release. When deprived of fluids or subjected to some other acute osmotic or nonosmotic stimulus, these individuals invariably increase plasma AVP normally, but the resultant increase in urine concentration is usually subnormal because their renal capacity to concentrate the urine is also blunted by chronic polyuria. Thus, their antidiuretic response to these stimuli may be indistinguishable from that in patients with partial pituitary, partial gestational, or partial nephrogenic DI. Patients with psychogenic or iatrogenic polydipsia respond similarly to fluid restriction but do not complain of thirst and usually offer other explanations for their high fluid intake.

Differential Diagnosis

When symptoms of urinary frequency, enuresis, nocturia, and/or persistent thirst are present, the presence of polyuria should be verified by documenting a 24-h urine output >50 mL/kg per day (>3500 mL in a 70-kg man). If the osmolarity of the 24-h urine is >300 mosmol/L, the polyuria is due to a solute diuresis and the patient should be evaluated for uncontrolled diabetes mellitus or other less common causes of excessive solute excretion. However, if the 24-h urine osmolarity is <300 mosmol/L, the patient has a water diuresis and should be evaluated further to determine which type of DI is present.

In differentiating between the various types of DI,

the history, physical examination, and routine laboratory tests may be helpful but are rarely sufficient because few, if any, of the findings are pathognomonic. Except in the rare patient who is clearly dehydrated under basal conditions of *ad libitum* fluid intake, this evaluation should begin with a *fluid deprivation test*. To minimize patient discomfort, avoid excessive dehydration, and maximize the information obtained, the test should be started in the morning and water balance should be monitored closely with hourly measurements of body weight, plasma osmolarity and/or sodium concentration, and urine volume and osmolarity.

If fluid deprivation does not result in urine concentration (osmolarity > 300 mosmol/L, specific gravity > 1.010) before body weight decreases by 5% or plasma osmolarity/sodium exceed the upper limit of normal, primary polydipsia or a partial defect in AVP secretion or action are largely excluded. In these patients, severe pituitary or nephrogenic DI are the only remaining possibilities, and they can usually be distinguished by administering desmopressin (DDAVP, 0.03 μg/kg subcutaneously or intravenously) and repeating the measurement of urine osmolarity 1 to 2 h later. An increase of >50% indicates severe pituitary DI, whereas a smaller or absent response is strongly suggestive of nephrogenic DI.

However, in patients who concentrate their urine during fluid deprivation, the change in urine osmolarity after administration of desmopressin is not useful for differential diagnosis because the values vary widely and over the same range in primary polydipsia, partial pituitary DI, and partial nephrogenic DI. The best way to differentiate these three conditions is to measure plasma or urine AVP before and during the fluid deprivation test and analyze the result in relation to the concurrent plasma or urine osmolarity (**Fig. 3-3**). This approach invariably differentiates partial nephrogenic DI from partial pituitary DI and primary polydipsia. It also differentiates pituitary DI from primary polydipsia if the hormone is measured when plasma osmolarity or sodium is clearly above the normal range. However, the requisite level of hypertonic dehydration is difficult to produce by fluid deprivation alone when urine concentration occurs. Therefore, it is usually necessary to add an infusion of hypertonic (3%) saline and repeat the AVP measurements when plasma osmolarity rises to >300 mosmol/L (Na^+ > 145 mmol/L). This endpoint is usually reached within 30 to 120 min if the hypertonic saline is infused at a rate of 0.1 mL/kg per min and the fluid deprivation is maintained.

The differential diagnosis of DI may also be facilitated by magnetic resonance imaging (MRI) of the pituitary and hypothalamus. In most healthy adults and children, the posterior pituitary emits a hyperintense signal in T1-weighted mid-saggital images. This "bright spot" is almost invariably absent or abnormally small in patients with pituitary DI but is present in 80 to 90% of patients with primary polydipsia. Thus, the presence of a normal bright spot virtually excludes pituitary DI, whereas its absence supports but does not prove this diagnosis. Therefore, the MRI findings must be interpreted with caution and only in conjunction with other diagnostic studies based on assays of AVP or the differential responses to treatment.

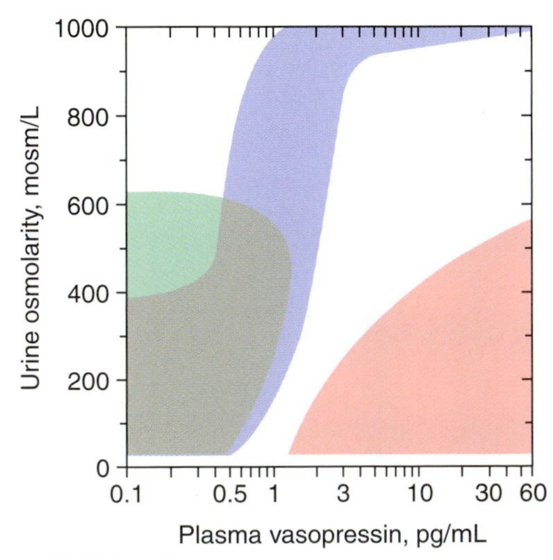

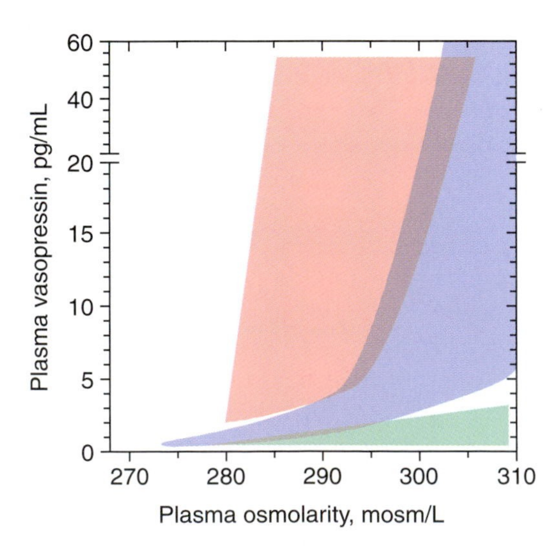

FIGURE 3-3
Relationship of plasma AVP to urine osmolarity (*left*) and plasma osmolarity (*right*) before and during fluid deprivation–hypertonic saline infusion test in patients who are normal or have primary polydipsia (■), pituitary diabetes insipidus (■), or nephrogenic diabetes insipidus (■).

Rx TREATMENT FOR PITUITARY DI

The signs and symptoms of uncomplicated pituitary DI can be eliminated completely by treatment with desmopressin (**Fig. 3-4**). It is a synthetic analogue of AVP (Fig. 3-1) that acts selectively at V_2 receptors to increase urine concentration and decrease urine flow in a dose-dependent manner. It is also more resistant to degradation than AVP and has a three- to fourfold longer duration of action. Desmopressin can be given by intravenous or subcutaneous injection, nasal inhalation, or oral tablet. The doses required to completely control pituitary DI vary widely, depending on the patient and the route of administration. However, they usually range from 1 to 2 μg qd or bid by injection, 10 to 20 μg bid or tid by nasal spray, or 100 to 400 μg bid or tid orally. The onset of action is rapid, ranging from as little as 15 min after injection to 60 min after oral administration. When given in doses sufficient to completely normalize urinary osmolarity and flow, desmopressin produces a slight (1 to 3%) increase in total-body water and a commensurate decrease in plasma osmolarity and sodium concentration that rapidly eliminate thirst and polydipsia. Consequently, water balance is maintained and hyponatremia does not develop unless the patient has an associated abnormality in the osmoregulation of thirst or ingests/receives excessive amounts of fluid for some other reason. Fortunately, abnormal thirst occurs in <10% of patients with pituitary DI, and the other causes of excessive intake can usually be eliminated by educating the patient about the risks of drinking for reasons other than thirst. Therefore, most patients with pituitary DI can take desmopressin in doses sufficient to maintain a normal urine output continuously and do not need to endure the inconvenience and discomfort of allowing intermittent escape to prevent water intoxication.

Pituitary DI can also be treated with chlorpropamide (Diabinese). The mechanism of its antidiuretic action is uncertain but may involve potentiation of the effect of small amounts of AVP or direct activation of the V_2 receptor. In patients with severe or partial pituitary DI, doses of chlorpropamide similar to those used in the treatment of diabetes mellitus (125 to 500 mg once daily) increase urine concentration and decrease urine flow, thirst, and polydipsia in a manner similar to desmopressin. The antidiuresis is almost always sufficient to reduce urine output by 30 to 70%. Moreover, its antidiuretic effect can be enhanced appreciably by cotreatment with a thiazide diuretic. Side effects of chlorpropamide include hypoglycemia, which can be precipitated by severe reductions in caloric intake or heavy exercise, and it may cause a disulfiram (Antabuse)-like reaction to ethanol. Chlorpropamide is contraindicated in the treatment of gestational DI because its teratogenicity is unknown.

Primary polydipsia cannot be treated with desmopressin because a sustained inhibition of the compensatory water diuresis almost invariably results in the development of water intoxication within 24 to 48 h. Iatrogenic polydipsia can often be corrected by patient counseling; however, there is no effective treatment for either psychogenic or dipsogenic DI. In the latter, nocturia or nocturnal enuresis can often be controlled safely by administering a single small dose of desmopressin at bedtime. If the dose is adjusted carefully to provide no

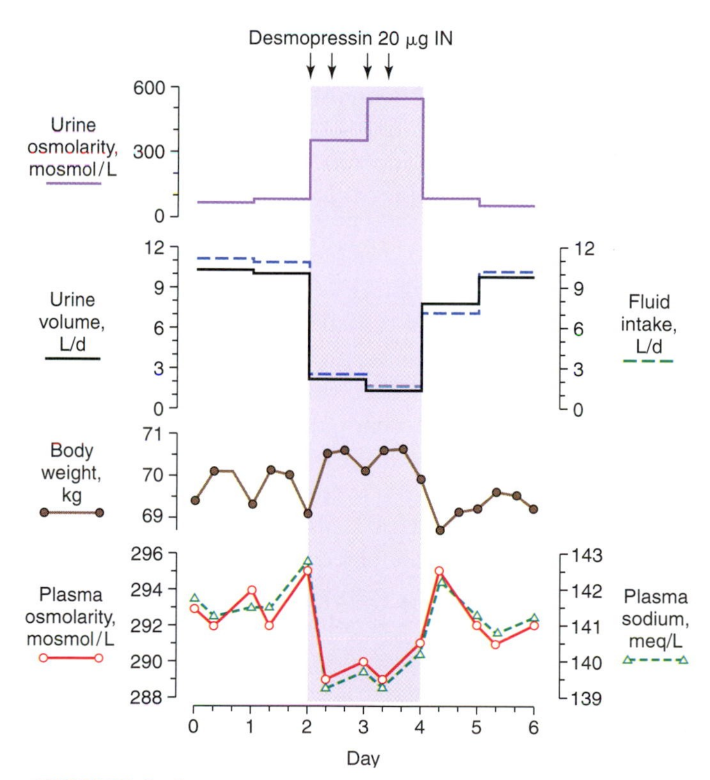

FIGURE 3-4

Effect of desmopressin therapy on water balance in patient with uncomplicated pituitary diabetes insipidus. Note that treatment rapidly reduces thirst and fluid intake as well as urine output to normal, with only a slight increase in body water (weight) and decrease in plasma osmolarity/sodium. [*From Endocrinology and Metabolism, 4th ed, P Felig, L Frohman (eds). New York, McGraw-Hill, 2001, with permission.*]

more than 8 to 10 h of antidiuresis, it will not result in water intoxication, because patients with dipsogenic, as well as other forms of DI, tend to drink less fluid at night than during the day.

The symptoms and signs of nephrogenic DI are not affected by treatment with desmopressin or chlorpropamide but may be reduced by treatment with a thiazide diuretic and/or amiloride in conjunction with a low-sodium diet. Inhibitors of prostaglandin synthesis (e.g., indomethacin) are also effective in some patients.

ADIPSIC HYPERNATREMIA

Clinical Characteristics

Adipsic hypernatremia is characterized by chronic or recurrent hypertonic dehydration and a deficient AVP response to osmotic stimulation. Despite hypertonic dehydration, these patients have little or no thirst and may even resist efforts to increase their oral intake of fluids. The hypernatremia varies in severity and usually is associated with commensurate signs of hypovolemia such as tachycardia, postural hypotension, azotemia, hyperuricemia, and hypokalemia. Muscle weakness, pain, rhabdomyolysis, hyperglycemia, hyperlipidemia, and acute renal failure may also occur.

Pathophysiology

Adipsic hypernatremia is caused by agenesis or destruction of the hypothalamic osmoreceptors that normally regulate thirst and AVP secretion (**Fig. 3-5**). Lack of thirst and failure to drink enough water to replenish renal and extrarenal losses decrease total-body water and increase plasma osmolarity/sodium. Plasma renin activity and aldosterone secretion also increase, and plasma potassium falls due to increased urinary excretion. The osmoreceptor deficiency can usually be traced to an identifiable congenital or acquired disease in the hypothalamus but is sometimes idiopathic (**Table 3-2**). An MRI typically shows a normal posterior pituitary bright spot, and the AVP response to nonosmotic stimuli is also normal. Occasionally, the neurohypophysis is also affected, resulting in a combined defect in water balance that is particularly severe and difficult to manage.

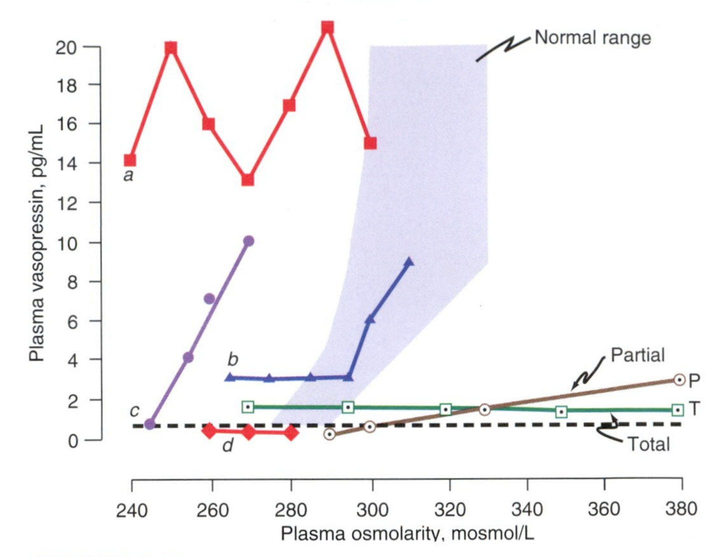

FIGURE 3-5

Heterogeneity of osmoregulatory dysfunction in adipsic hypernatremia (AH) and the syndrome of inappropriate antidiuretic hormone (SIADH). Each line depicts schematically the relationship of plasma arginine vasopressin (AVP) to plasma osmolarity during water loading and/or infusion of 3% saline in a patient with either AH (open symbols) or SIADH (closed symbols). The shaded area indicates the normal range of the relationship. The horizontal broken line indicates the plasma AVP level below which the hormone is undetectable and urinary concentration usually does not occur. Lines P and T represent patients with a selective deficiency in the osmoregulation of thirst and AVP that is either partial (○) or total (□). In the latter, plasma AVP does not change in response to increases or decreases in plasma osmolarity but remains within a range sufficient to concentrate the urine even if overhydration produces hypotonic hyponatremia. In contrast, if the osmoregulatory deficiency is partial (○), rehydration of the patient suppresses plasma AVP to levels that result in urinary dilution and polyuria before plasma osmolarity and sodium are reduced to normal. Lines *a–d* represent different defects in the osmoregulation of plasma AVP observed in patients with SIADH. In *a* (■), plasma AVP is markedly elevated and fluctuates widely without relation to changes in plasma osmolarity, indicating complete loss of osmoregulation. In *b* (▲), plasma AVP remains fixed at a slightly elevated level until plasma osmolarity reaches the normal range at which point it begins to rise appropriately, indicating a selective defect in the inhibitory component of the osmoregulatory mechanism. In *c* (●), plasma AVP rises in close correlation with plasma osmolarity before the latter reaches the normal range, indicating downward resetting of the osmostat. In *d* (◆), plasma AVP appears to be osmoregulated normally, suggesting that the inappropriate antidiuresis is caused by some other abnormality.

Differential Diagnosis

Adipsic hypernatremia should be distinguished from the hypernatremia that results from various other causes. These distinctions can usually be made from the history, physical examination, and routine laboratory tests. If a conscious patient denies thirst and/or does not drink vigorously in the presence of significant hypernatremia,

TABLE 3-2

CAUSES OF ADIPSIC HYPERNATREMIA

CAUSES OF ADIPSIC HYPERNATREMIA
Acquired
Vascular: Occlusion anterior communicating artery
Tumors
Primary
Craniopharyngioma
Pinealoma, germinoma
Meningioma
Glioma
Metastatic: (lung, breast)
Granulomas: Neurosarcoid
Histiocytosis
Trauma: Closed
Penetrating (pituitary-hypothalamic surgery)
Psychogenic: Psychotic depression
Other: Hydrocephalus
Neurodegenerative
AIDS, cytomegalovirus encephalitis
Idiopathic
Congenital
Midline malformation (septum and corpus callosum)
Microcephaly
Genetic: Autosomal recessive (Schinzel-Giedion syndrome)

the diagnosis of hypodipsia or adipsia can be made with confidence. This diagnosis is supported by physical laboratory evidence of hypovolemia (postural hypotension, azotemia, hypokalemia, hyperuricemia, hyperreninemia) and a relative deficiency of plasma AVP. During rehydration, patients may develop either DI or the syndrome of inappropriate antidiuretic hormone (SIADH) depending on whether they have partial or total deficiency of the osmoregulation of AVP (Fig. 3-5). If the patient is obtunded or otherwise unable to answer questions or drink at the time of presentation, the possibility of adipsic hypernatremia can be evaluated after rehydration by assessing the thirst and plasma AVP response to a controlled fluid deprivation–hypertonic saline infusion test similar to that described for evaluation of DI.

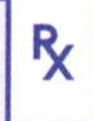

TREATMENT FOR ADIPSIC HYPERNATREMIA

Adipsic hypernatremia should be treated by administering water by mouth, if the patient is alert, or 0.45% saline intravenously, if the patient is obtunded or uncooperative. The number of liters of free water that will be required to correct the deficit (ΔFW) can be estimated from body weight in kg (BW) and the serum sodium concentration in mmol/L (S_{Na}) by the formula $\Delta FW = 0.5BW \times [(S_{Na} - 140)/140]$. If serum glucose ($S_{Glu}$) is elevated, the measured S_{Na} should be corrected (S_{Na}^*) by the formula $S_{Na}^* = S_{Na} + [(S_{Glu} - 90)/36]$. This amount plus an allowance for continuing insensible and urinary losses should be given over a 24- to 48-h period. If DI is present or develops before rehydration is complete, desmopressin should also be given in standard doses to minimize urinary losses. If hyperglycemia and/or hypokalemia are present, insulin and/or potassium supplements should be given with the expectation that both can be discontinued after rehydration is complete. These variables plus urine output and plasma urea/creatinine should be monitored closely during treatment for signs of emerging DI, SIADH, or acute renal failure.

Once the acute fluid and electrolyte imbalances are corrected, an MRI of the brain and tests of anterior pituitary function should be performed. A long-term management plan to prevent or minimize recurrence of the fluid and electrolyte imbalance should also be developed. This should include a practical method that the patient can use to regulate fluid intake in accordance with day-to-day variations in water balance. The most effective way to accomplish these objectives is to prescribe desmopressin or chlorpropamide to completely control DI, if it is present, and teach the patient how to use day-to-day changes in body weight as a guide for adjusting fluid intake. Prescribing a constant fluid intake is less satisfactory because it does not take into account the large, uncontrolled variations in insensible loss that inevitably occur.

EXCESS VASOPRESSIN SECRETION AND ACTION

HYPONATREMIA

Clinical Characteristics

Excessive secretion or action of AVP results in the production of decreased volumes of more highly concentrated urine. If not accompanied by a commensurate reduction in fluid intake, the reduced suppressibility of AVP results in water retention and a decrease in plasma osmolarity/sodium. If the hyponatremia develops gradually or has been present for more than a few days, it may be asymptomatic. However, if it develops acutely, it is almost always accompanied by symptoms and signs of water intoxication that may include mild headache, confusion, anorexia, nausea, vomiting, coma, and convulsions. Severe hyponatremia may be lethal. Depending on the cause of the antidiuresis, osmotically inappropriate thirst and/or fluid intake and other disturbances of fluid and electrolyte balance may also be present.

Etiology

Osmotically inappropriate antidiuresis can be caused by a primary defect in AVP secretion or action or can be secondary to a recognized nonosmotic stimulus such as hypovolemia, hypotension, or glucocorticoid deficiency. The primary forms are generally referred to as SIADH or euvolemic (type III) hyponatremia. They have many different causes, including ectopic production of AVP by lung cancer or other neoplasms, eutopic release by various diseases or drugs, and exogenous administration of AVP, desmopressin, or large doses of oxytocin (**Table 3-3**). The ectopic forms result from abnormal expression of the AVP-NPII gene by primary or metastatic malignancies. They do not usually remit unless the ectopic source is eliminated. The eutopic forms manifest most often in patients with acute infections or strokes, but the mechanisms by which these diseases disrupt osmoregulation are not known. A form of acute or chronic euvolemic hyponatremia very similar to SIADH can also result from stimulation of AVP secretion by protracted nausea or isolated glucocorticoid deficiency. In these patients the excess AVP secretion can be corrected quickly and completely by specific treatments (antiemetics or glucocorticoids) that are not useful in other forms of SIADH.

The secondary forms of osmotically inappropriate antidiuresis are usually divided into two groups: type I (hypervolemic) and type II (hypovolemic) hyponatremia. Type I occurs in sodium-retaining, edema-forming states such as congestive heart failure, cirrhosis, or nephrosis and is thought to be due to a reduction in "effective" blood volume. Type II occurs in sodium-depleted states

TABLE 3-3

CAUSES OF SYNDROME OF INAPPROPRIATE ANTIDIURETIC HORMONE (SIADH)

- **Neoplasms**
  - Carcinomas
    - Lung
    - Duodenum
    - Pancreas
    - Ovary
    - Bladder, ureter
  - Other neoplasms
    - Thymoma
    - Mesothelioma
    - Bronchial adenoma
    - Carcinoid
    - Gangliocytoma
    - Ewing's sarcoma
- **Head trauma** (closed and penetrating)
- **Infections**
  - Pneumonia, bacterial or viral
  - Abscess, lung or brain
  - Cavitation (aspergillosis)
  - Tuberculosis, lung or brain
  - Meningitis, bacterial or viral
  - Encephalitis
  - AIDS
- **Vascular**
  - Cerebrovascular occlusions, hemorrhage
  - Cavernous sinus thrombosis
- **Neurologic**
  - Guillain-Barré syndrome
  - Multiple sclerosis
  - Delirium tremens
  - Amyotrophic lateral sclerosis
  - Hydrocephalus
  - Psychosis
  - Peripheral neuropathy
- **Congenital malformations**
  - Agenesis corpus callosum
  - Cleft lip/palate
  - Other midline defects
- **Metabolic**
  - Acute intermittent porphyria
  - Pulmonary
  - Asthma
  - Pneumothorax
  - Positive-pressure respiration
- **Drugs**
  - Vasopressin or desmopressin
  - Chlorpropamide
  - Oxytocin, high dose
  - Vincristine
  - Carbamazepine
  - Nicotine
  - Phenothiazines
  - Cyclophosphamide
  - Tricyclic antidepressants
  - Monoamine oxidase inhibitors
  - Serotonin reuptake inhibitors

such as severe gastroenteritis, diuretic abuse, or mineralocorticoid deficiency and is probably a result of reduction in extracellular volume as well as blood volume and/or pressure.

Pathophysiology

In SIADH, interference with the osmotic suppression of AVP release results in significant expansion and dilution of body fluids only if water intake exceeds the rate of insensible and urinary output. The excess water intake often results from an associated defect in the osmoregulation of thirst but can also be due to psychogenic or iatrogenic factors, including the administration of intravenous fluids.

In SIADH, the abnormal osmoregulation of antidiuretic function can take any of four distinct forms (Fig. 3-5). For example, AVP secretion remains fully responsive to changes in plasma osmolarity/sodium, but the threshold, or set point, of the osmoregulatory system is abnormally low. Patients with this type of downward resetting of the osmostat differ from those with the other types of osmoregulatory defect in that they are able to maximally suppress plasma AVP and dilute their urine if their fluid intake is high enough to reduce their plasma osmolarity/sodium to the new set point. Another, smaller subgroup (about 10% of the total) does not have a demonstrable defect in the osmoregulation of AVP (Fig. 3-5). Thus, their inappropriate antidiuresis may be due to other abnormalities such as enhanced renal sensitivity to the antidiuretic effect of normally low levels of AVP or activation of aquaporin 2 water channels by a mechanism that is independent of AVP and V_2 receptors.

The extracellular volume expansion that results from excessive retention of water in SIADH also produces an increase in atrial natriuretic hormone, suppression of plasma renin activity, and a compensatory increase in urinary sodium excretion that serves to reduce the hypervolemia but aggravates the hyponatremia. Thus, hyponatremia is due to a decrease in total-body sodium as well as an increase in total-body water. The acute retention of water and fall in plasma sodium also increase intracellular volume. The resultant brain swelling increases intracranial pressure and probably causes the acute symptoms of water intoxication. After several days, this intracellular volume expansion may be reduced by inactivation or elimination of intracellular solutes, resulting in the remission of symptoms that often occur with hyponatremia of longer duration.

In type I (edematous) or type II (hypovolemic) hyponatremia, the osmotic inhibition of AVP and urine concentration is counteracted by a hemodynamic stimulus that results from a substantial reduction in effective or absolute blood volume. In both cases, the reduced suppression of AVP appears to be due to downward resetting of the osmostat. The resultant antidiuresis is usually enhanced by decreased distal delivery of filtrate that results from increased reabsorption of sodium in proximal nephrons secondary to the hypovolemia. If it is not associated with a commensurate reduction in water intake, the marked reduction in urine output that ensues also leads to expansion and dilution of body fluids with symptoms of hyponatremia. This attenuates, but does not completely eliminate, the antidiuresis because the amount of water retained is usually insufficient to fully correct the effective or absolute hypovolemia. Unlike in SIADH, therefore, plasma renin activity is elevated, causing secondary hyperaldosteronism and hypokalemia. The disturbance in salt and water balance that underlies the hyponatremia also differs from SIADH in that total-body sodium and water are increased in type I but decreased in type II.

Differential Diagnosis

SIADH is a diagnosis of exclusion that can usually be accomplished with routine historic, physical, and laboratory information. In a patient with hyponatremia, the possibility of simple dilution caused by an osmotically driven shift of water from the intracellular to the extracellular space should be excluded by measuring plasma glucose and/or plasma osmolarity. If the glucose is not elevated enough to account for the hyponatremia [serum sodium decreases ~1 meq/L for each 2.0 mmol/L (36 mg/dL) rise in glucose] and/or plasma osmolarity is reduced in proportion to sodium (each decrease in serum sodium of 1 meq/L should reduce plasma osmolarity by about 2 mosmol/L), the hyponatremia is "true" and can be typed or classified by standard clinical indicators of the extracellular fluid volume (**Table 3-4**). If these findings are ambiguous or contradictory, measuring the rate of urinary sodium excretion or plasma renin activity may be helpful. These measurements can be misleading, however, if SIADH is stable or resolving or if the patient has type II hyponatremia due to a primary defect in renal conservation of sodium, surreptitious diuretic abuse, or hyporeninemic hypoaldosteronism. The latter may be suspected if serum potassium is elevated instead of low as is usually seen in types I and II hyponatremia. Measurements of plasma AVP are currently of no diagnostic value since they exhibit the same wide variation in abnormalities in all three types of hyponatremia. In patients who fulfill the clinical criteria for type III (euvolemic) hyponatremia, plasma cortisol should also be measured to rule out unsuspected secondary adrenal insufficiency. If this is normal and there is no other obvious cause for SIADH, a careful search for occult lung cancer should also be undertaken.

TABLE 3-4

DIFFERENTIAL DIAGNOSIS OF HYPONATREMIA BASED ON CLINICAL ASSESSMENT OF EXTRACELLULAR FLUID VOLUME (ECFV)

CLINICAL FINDINGS	TYPE I, HYPERVOLEMIC	TYPE II, HYPOVOLEMIC	TYPE IIIA, EUVOLEMIC	TYPE IIIB, EUVOLEMIC (SIADH)
History				
CHF, cirrhosis, or nephrosis	Yes	No	No	No
Salt and water loss	No	Yes	No	No
ACTH-cortisol deficiency and/or nausea and vomiting	No	No	Yes	No
Physical Examination				
Generalized edema, ascites	Yes	No	No	No
Postural hypotension	Maybe	Maybe	Maybe[a]	No
Laboratory				
BUN, creatinine	High-normal	High-normal	Low-normal	Low-normal
Uric acid	High-normal	High-normal	Low-normal	Low-normal
Serum potassium	Low-normal	Low-normal[b]	Normal[c]	Normal
Serum albumin	Low-normal	High-normal	Normal	Normal
Serum cortisol	Normal-high	Normal-high[d]	Low[e]	Normal
Plasma renin activity	High	High	Low[f]	Low
Urinary sodium (meq unit of time)[g]	Low	Low[h]	High[i]	High[i]

[a]Postural hypotension may occur in secondary (ACTH-dependent) adrenal insufficiency even though ECFV and aldosterone are usually normal.
[b]Serum potassium may be high if hypovolemia is due to aldosterone deficiency.
[c]Serum potassium may be low if vomiting causes alkalosis.
[d]Serum cortisol is low if hypovolemia is due to primary adrenal insufficiency (Addison's disease).
[e]Serum cortisol will be normal or high if the cause is nausea and vomiting rather than secondary (ACTH-dependent) adrenal insufficiency.
[f]Plasma renin activity may be high if the cause is secondary (ACTH) adrenal insufficiency.
[g]Urinary sodium should be expressed as the *rate of excretion* rather than the concentration. In a hyponatremic adult, an excretion rate $>$25 meq/day (or 25 μeq/mg of creatinine) could be considered high.
[h]The rate of urinary sodium excretion may be high if the hypovolemia is due to diuretic abuse, primary adrenal insufficiency, or other causes of renal sodium wasting.
[i]The rate of urinary sodium excretion may be low if intake is curtailed by symptoms or treatment.
Note: SIADH, syndrome of inappropriate antidiuretic hormone; CHF, congestive heart failure; ACTH, adrenocorticotropic hormone; BUN, blood urea nitrogen

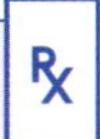

TREATMENT FOR HYPONATREMIA

In acute SIADH, the keystone to treatment of hyponatremia is to restrict total fluid intake to less than the sum of insensible losses and urinary output. Total intake should include the water derived from food (300 to 500 mL/d). Because insensible losses in adults usually approximate 500 mL/d, total discretionary intake (all water in liquid form) should be at least 500 mL less than urinary output. If achieved, this deficit usually reduces body water and increases serum sodium by about 1 to 2% per day. If more rapid correction of the hyponatremia is desired to eliminate severe symptoms or signs, the fluid restriction can be supplemented by intravenous infusion of hypertonic (3%) saline. This treatment has the advantage of correcting the sodium deficiency that is partly responsible for the hyponatremia as well as producing a solute diuresis that serves to remove some of the excess water. However, if the hyponatremia has been present for more than 24 to 48 h, correction that is too rapid has the potential to produce central pontine myelinolysis, an acute, potentially fatal neurologic syndrome characterized by quadriparesis, ataxia, and abnormal extraocular movements. The following guidelines appear to minimize, if not eliminate, the risk of this complication: the 3% saline should be infused at a rate $\leq$0.05 mL/kg body weight per min; the effect should be monitored continuously by STAT measurements of serum sodium at least once every 2 h; and the infusion should be stopped as soon as serum sodium increases by 12 mmol/L or to 130 mmol/L, whichever comes first. Urinary output should also be monitored continuously since spontaneous remission of the SIADH can occur at any time and can result in an acute water diuresis that greatly accelerates the rate of rise in serum sodium produced by fluid restriction and 3% saline infusion.

In chronic SIADH, the hyponatremia can be corrected by treatment with demeclocycline, 150 to 300 mg orally three or four times a day, or fludrocortisone, 0.05 to 0.2 mg orally twice a day. The effect of the demeclocycline manifests in 7 to 14 days and is due to production of a reversible form of nephrogenic DI. Potential side effects include phototoxicity and azotemia. The effect of fludrocortisone also requires 1 to 2 weeks and is partly due to increased retention of sodium and possibly inhibition of thirst. It also increases urinary potassium excretion, which may require replacement through dietary adjustments or supplements. Fludrocortisone may induce hypertension, occasionally necessitating discontinuation of the treatment.

One or more nonpeptide AVP antagonists that block the antidiuretic effect of AVP may soon be approved for use in the United States. Preliminary studies with these antagonists in acute or chronic SIADH indicate that they produce a dose-dependent increase in urinary free-water excretion, which, if combined with a modest restriction of fluid intake, gradually reduces body water and corrects the hyponatremia without any recognized adverse effect. Thus, they may become the treatment of choice for those forms of SIADH in which there is inappropriate secretion of AVP that cannot be corrected by other, more specific therapy such as antiemetics or glucocorticoids.

When an SIADH-like syndrome is due to protracted nausea and vomiting or isolated glucocorticoid deficiency, all abnormalities can be corrected quickly and completely by giving an antiemetic or hydrocortisone. As with other treatments, care must be taken to ensure that serum sodium does not rise too quickly or too far.

In type I hyponatremia, the only treatment currently available is severe fluid restriction, administration of urea or mannitol to produce a solute diuresis, and/or administration of cardiotonics or serum albumin to correct the effective hypovolemia. None of these treatments is particularly effective, and some (e.g., administration of mannitol or albumin) carry significant risks. Infusion of hypertonic saline is contraindicated because it worsens the sodium retention and edema and may precipitate cardiovascular decompensation. However, preliminary studies indicate that the AVP antagonists may be almost as effective and safe in type I hyponatremia as they are in SIADH. Thus, they may become the treatment of choice for this form of hyponatremia also.

In type II hyponatremia, the defect in AVP secretion and water balance can usually be corrected easily and quickly by stopping the loss of sodium and water and/or replacing the deficits by mouth or intravenous infusion of normal or hypertonic saline. As with the treatment of other forms of hyponatremia, care must be taken to ensure that plasma sodium does not increase too rapidly. Fluid restriction or administration of AVP antagonists is contraindicated as they would only aggravate the underlying volume depletion and could result in cardiovascular decompensation.

FURTHER READINGS

Adrogue HJ: Hypernatremia. N Engl J Med 342:1493, 2000

———, Madias NE: Hyponatremia. N Engl J Med 342:1581, 2000

Ball SG et al: Tests of posterior pituitary function. J Endocrinol Invest 26:15, 2003

King LS et al: From structure to disease: The evolving tale of aquaporin biology. Nat Rev Mol Cell Biol 5:687, 2004

Aquaporins, the channels that regulate water permeability across membranes, play a critical role in physiology, including renal responses to vasopressin. This review, written by the Nobel prize–winning scientist, provides a broad perspective of the roles of aquaporins physiology and disease.

Nguyen MK et al: Molecular pathogenesis of nephrogenic diabetes insipidus. Clin Exp Nephrol 7:9, 2003

This review focuses on genetic causes of nephrogenic DI and uses this new understanding to elucidate the normal physiology of vasopressin-induced water reabsorption.

Russell TA et al: A murine model of autosomal dominant neurohypophyseal diabetes insipidus reveals progressive loss of vasopressin-producing neurons. J Clin Invest 112:1697, 2003

This study documents that vasopressin gene mutations cause neurohypophyseal DI by inducing neuronal cell death.

Verbalis JG: Vasopressin V_2 receptor antagonists. J Mol Endocrinol 29:1, 2002

The high prevalence of hyponatremia in hospitalized patients has led to a search for vasopressin receptor antagonists. This paper reviews early clinical trials.

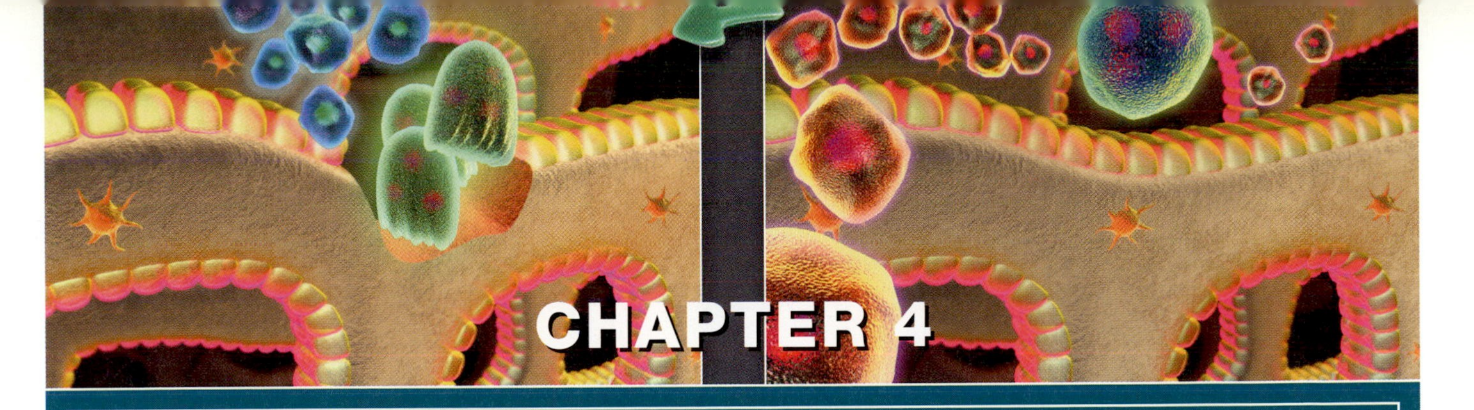

DISORDERS OF THE THYROID GLAND

J. Larry Jameson
Anthony P. Weetman

The thyroid gland produces two related hormones, thyroxine (T_4) and triiodothyronine (T_3) (**Fig. 4-1**). Acting through nuclear receptors, these hormones play a critical role in cell differentiation during development and help maintain thermogenic and metabolic homeostasis in the adult. Disorders of the thyroid gland result primarily from autoimmune processes that either stimulate the overproduction of thyroid hormones (*thyrotoxicosis*) or cause glandular destruction and hormone deficiency (*hypothyroidism*). In addition, benign nodules and various forms of thyroid cancer are relatively common and amenable to detection by physical examination.

ANATOMY AND DEVELOPMENT

The thyroid gland is located in the neck, anterior to the trachea, between the cricoid cartilage and the suprasternal notch. The thyroid (Greek *thyreos,* shield, plus *eidos,* form) consists of two lobes that are connected by an isthmus. It is normally 12 to 20 g in size, highly vascular, and soft in consistency. Four parathyroid glands, which produce parathyroid hormone (Chap. 24), are located in the posterior region of each pole of the thyroid. The recurrent laryngeal nerves traverse the lateral borders of the thyroid gland and must be identified during thyroid surgery to avoid vocal cord paralysis.

The thyroid gland develops from the floor of the primitive pharynx during the third week of gestation. The gland migrates from the foramen cecum, at the base of the tongue, along the thyroglossal duct to reach its final location in the neck. This feature accounts for the rare ectopic location of thyroid tissue at the base of the tongue (lingual thyroid), as well as for the presence of thyroglossal duct cysts along this developmental tract. Thyroid hormone synthesis normally begins at about 11 weeks' gestation.

The parathyroid glands migrate from the third (inferior glands) and fourth (superior glands) pharyngeal pouches and become embedded in the thyroid gland. Neural crest derivatives from the ultimobranchial body

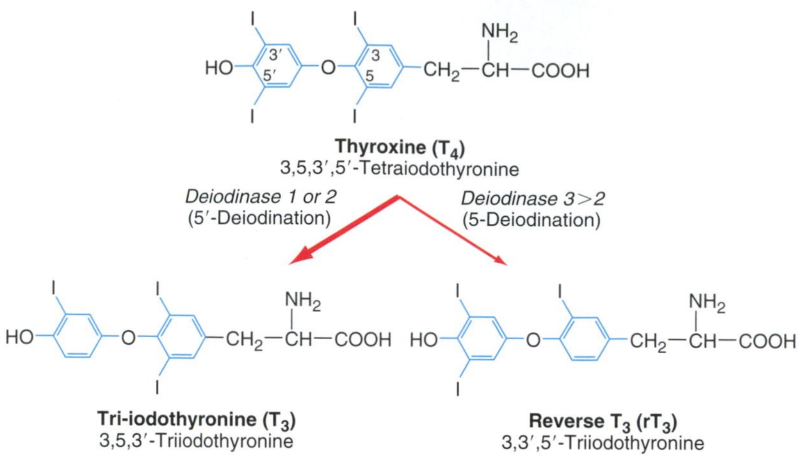

Thyroxine (T_4)
3,5,3′,5′-Tetraiodothyronine

Deiodinase 1 or 2
(5′-Deiodination)

Deiodinase 3>2
(5-Deiodination)

Tri-iodothyronine (T_3)
3,5,3′-Triiodothyronine

Reverse T_3 (rT_3)
3,3′,5′-Triiodothyronine

FIGURE 4-1

Structures of thyroid hormones. Thyroxine (T_4) contains four iodine atoms. Deiodination leads to production of the potent hormone, triiodothyronine (T_3), or the inactive hormone, reverse T_3.

give rise to thyroid medullary C cells that produce calcitonin, a calcium-lowering hormone. The C cells are interspersed throughout the thyroid gland, although their density is greatest in the juncture of the upper one-third and lower two-thirds of the gland.

Thyroid gland development is controlled by a series of developmental transcription factors. Thyroid transcription factor (TTF) 1 (also known as NKX2A), TTF-2 (also known as FKHL15), and paired homeobox-8 (PAX-8) are expressed selectively, but not exclusively, in the thyroid gland. In combination, they orchestrate thyroid cell development and the induction of thyroid-specific genes such as thyroglobulin (Tg), thyroid peroxidase (TPO), the sodium iodide symporter (NIS), and the thyroid-stimulating hormone receptor (TSH-R). Mutations in these developmental transcription factors or their downstream target genes are rare causes of thyroid agenesis or dyshormonogenesis and can cause congenital hypothyroidism (**Table 4-1**). Congenital hypothyroidism is common enough (approximately 1 in 4000 newborns) that neonatal screening is performed in most industrialized countries (see below). Though the underlying causes of most cases of congenital hypothyroidism are unknown, early treatment with thyroid hormone replacement precludes potentially severe developmental abnormalities.

The mature thyroid gland contains numerous spherical follicles composed of thyroid follicular cells that surround secreted colloid, a proteinaceous fluid that

TABLE 4-1

GENETIC CAUSES OF CONGENITAL HYPOTHYROIDISM

DEFECTIVE GENE PROTEIN	INHERITANCE	CONSEQUENCES
PROP-1	Autosomal recessive	Combined pituitary hormone deficiencies with preservation of adrenocorticotropic hormone
PIT-1	Autosomal recessive Autosomal dominant	Combined deficiencies of growth hormone, prolactin, thyroid-stimulating hormone (TSH)
TSHβ	Autosomal recessive	TSH deficiency
TTF-1	Autosomal dominant	Variable thyroid hypoplasia, choreoathetosis, pulmonary problems
TTF-2	Autosomal recessive	Thyroid agenesis, choanal atresia, spiky hair
PAX-8	Autosomal dominant	Thyroid dysgenesis
TSH-receptor	Autosomal recessive	Resistance to TSH
$G_{s\alpha}$ (Albright hereditary osteodystrophy)	Autosomal dominant	Resistance to TSH
Na^+/I^- symporter	Autosomal recessive	Inability to transport iodide
THOX2	Autosomal dominant	Organification defect
Thyroid peroxidase	Autosomal recessive	Defective organification of iodide
Thyroglobulin	Autosomal recessive	Defective synthesis of thyroid hormone
Pendrin	Autosomal recessive	Pendred's syndrome: sensorineural deafness and partial organification defect in thyroid
Dehalogenase	Autosomal recessive	Loss of iodide reutilization

contains large amounts of thyroglobulin, the protein precursor of thyroid hormones (**Fig. 4-2**). The thyroid follicular cells are polarized—the basolateral surface is apposed to the bloodstream and an apical surface faces the follicular lumen. Increased demand for thyroid hormone, usually signaled by thyroid-stimulating hormone (TSH) binding to its receptor on the basolateral surface of the follicular cells, leads to Tg reabsorption from the follicular lumen and proteolysis within the cell to yield thyroid hormones for secretion into the bloodstream.

REGULATION OF THE THYROID AXIS

TSH, secreted by the thyrotrope cells of the anterior pituitary, plays a pivotal role in control of the thyroid axis and serves as the most useful physiologic marker of thyroid hormone action. TSH is a 31-kDa hormone composed of α and β subunits; the α subunit is common to the other glycoprotein hormones [luteinizing hormone, follicle-stimulating hormone, human chorionic gonadotropin (hCG)], whereas the TSH β subunit is unique to TSH. The extent and nature of carbohydrate modification are modulated by thyrotropin-releasing hormone (TRH) stimulation and influence the biologic activity of the hormone.

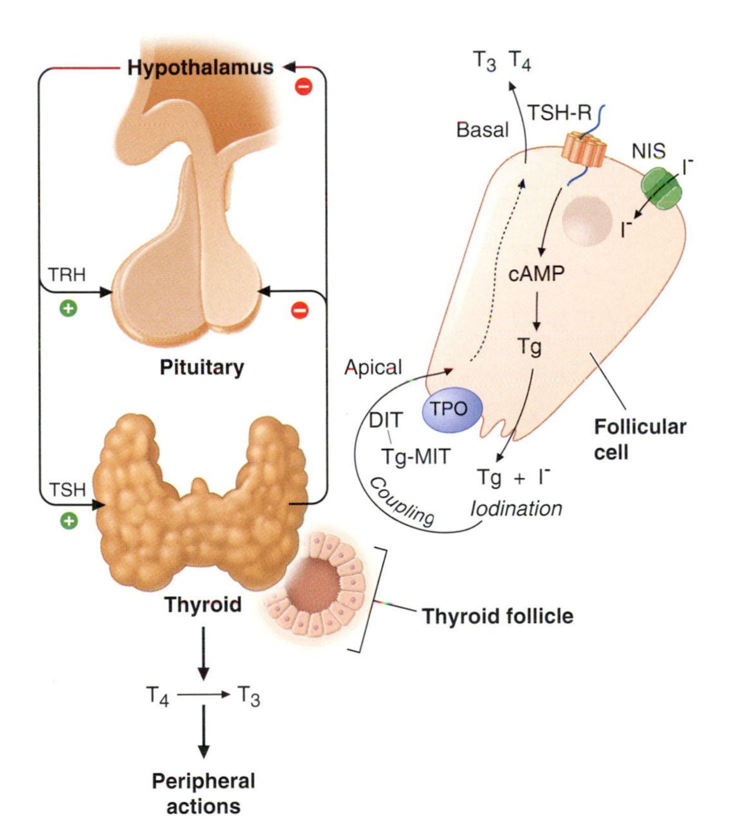

FIGURE 4-2

Regulation of thyroid hormone synthesis. ***Left.*** Thyroid hormones T_4 and T_3 feed back to inhibit hypothalamic production of thyrotropin-releasing hormone (TRH) and pituitary production of thyroid-stimulating hormone (TSH). TSH stimulates thyroid gland production of T_4 and T_3. ***Right.*** Thyroid follicles are formed by thyroid epithelial cells surrounding proteinaceous colloid, which contains thyroglobulin. Follicular cells, which are polarized, synthesize thyroglobulin and carry out thyroid hormone biosynthesis (see text for details). TSH-R, thyroid-stimulating hormone receptor; Tg, thyroglobulin; NIS, sodium-iodide symporter; TPO, thyroid peroxidase; DIT, diiodotyrosine; MIT, monoiodotyrosine

The thyroid axis is a classic example of an endocrine feedback loop. Hypothalamic TRH stimulates pituitary production of TSH, which, in turn, stimulates thyroid hormone synthesis and secretion. Thyroid hormones feed back negatively to inhibit TRH and TSH production (Fig. 4-2). The "set-point" in this axis is established by TSH. TRH is the major positive regulator of TSH synthesis and secretion. Peak TSH secretion occurs ~15 min after administration of exogenous TRH. Dopamine, glucocorticoids, and somatostatin suppress TSH but are not of major physiologic importance except when these agents are administered in pharmacologic doses. Reduced levels of thyroid hormone increase basal TSH production and enhance TRH-mediated stimulation of TSH. High thyroid hormone levels rapidly and directly suppress TSH and inhibit TRH-mediated stimulation of TSH, indicating that thyroid hormones are the dominant regulator of TSH production. Like other pituitary hormones, TSH is released in a pulsatile manner and exhibits a diurnal rhythm; its highest levels occur at night. However, these TSH excursions are modest in comparison to those of other pituitary hormones, in part because TSH has a relatively long plasma half-life (50 min). Consequently, single measurements of TSH are adequate for assessing its circulating level. TSH is measured using immunoradiometric assays that are highly sensitive and specific. These assays readily distinguish between normal and suppressed TSH values; thus, TSH can be used for the diagnosis of hyperthyroidism (low TSH) as well as hypothyroidism (high TSH).

THYROID HORMONE SYNTHESIS, METABOLISM, AND ACTION

THYROID HORMONE SYNTHESIS

Thyroid hormones are derived from Tg, a large iodinated glycoprotein. After secretion into the thyroid follicle, Tg is iodinated on selected tyrosine residues that are subsequently coupled via an ether linkage. Reuptake of Tg into the thyroid follicular cell initiates proteolysis and the release of newly synthesized T_4 and T_3.

Iodine Metabolism and Transport

Iodide uptake is a critical first step in thyroid hormone synthesis. Ingested iodine is bound to serum proteins, particularly albumin. Unbound iodine is excreted in the urine. The thyroid gland extracts iodine from the circulation in a highly efficient manner. For example, 10 to 25% of radioactive tracer (e.g., ^{123}I) is taken up by the normal thyroid gland over 24 h; this value can rise to 70 to 90% in Graves' disease. Iodide uptake is mediated by the Na^+/I^- symporter (NIS), which is expressed at the basolateral membrane of thyroid follicular cells. NIS is most highly expressed in the thyroid gland but low levels are present in the salivary glands, lactating breast, and placenta. The iodide transport mechanism is highly regulated, allowing adaptation to variations in dietary supply. Low iodine levels increase the amount of NIS and stimulate uptake, whereas high iodine levels suppress NIS expression and uptake. The selective expression of the NIS in the thyroid allows isotopic scanning, treatment of hyperthyroidism, and ablation of thyroid cancer with radioisotopes of iodine, without significant effects on other organs. Mutation of the *NIS* gene is a rare cause of congenital hypothyroidism, underscoring its importance in thyroid hormone synthesis. Another iodine transporter, pendrin, is located on the apical surface of thyroid cells and mediates iodine efflux into the lumen. Mutation of the *PENDRIN* gene causes *Pendred syndrome,* a disorder characterized by defective organification of iodine, goiter, and sensorineural deafness.

Iodine deficiency is prevalent in many mountainous regions and in central Africa, central South America, and northern Asia. In areas of relative iodine deficiency, there is an increased prevalence of goiter and, when deficiency is severe, hypothyroidism and cretinism. *Cretinism* is characterized by mental and growth retardation and occurs when children who live in iodine-deficient regions are not treated with iodine or thyroid hormone to restore normal thyroid hormone levels during early childhood. These children are often born to mothers with iodine deficiency, and it is likely that maternal thyroid hormone deficiency worsens the condition. Concomitant selenium deficiency may also contribute to the neurologic manifestations of cretinism. Iodine supplementation of salt, bread, and other food substances has markedly reduced the prevalence of cretinism. Unfortunately, however, iodine deficiency remains the most common cause of preventable mental deficiency, often because of resistance to the use of food additives or the cost of supplementation. In addition to overt cretinism, mild iodine deficiency can lead to subtle reduction of IQ. Oversupply of iodine, through supplements or foods enriched in iodine (e.g., shellfish, kelp), is associated with an increased incidence of autoimmune thyroid disease. The recommended average daily intake of iodine is 150 μg/d for adults, 90 to 120 μg/d for children, and 200 μg/d for pregnant women. Urinary iodine is >10 μg/dL in iodine-sufficient populations.

Organification, Coupling, Storage, Release

After iodide enters the thyroid, it is trapped and transported to the apical membrane of thyroid follicular cells where it is oxidized in an organification reaction that involves TPO and hydrogen peroxide. The reactive iodine atom is added to selected tyrosyl residues within Tg, a large (660 kDa) dimeric protein that consists of 2769 amino acids. The iodotyrosines in Tg are then coupled via an ether linkage in a reaction that is also catalyzed by TPO. Either T_4 or T_3 can be produced by this reaction, depending on the number of iodine atoms present in the iodotyrosines. After coupling, Tg is taken back into the thyroid cell where it is processed in lysosomes to release T_4 and T_3. Uncoupled mono- and diiodotyrosines (MIT, DIT) are deiodinated by the enzyme dehalogenase, thereby recycling any iodide that is not converted into thyroid hormones.

Disorders of thyroid hormone synthesis are rare causes of congenital hypothyroidism. The vast majority of these disorders are due to recessive mutations in TPO or Tg, but defects have also been identified in the TSH-R, NIS, pendrin, hydrogen peroxide generation, and in dehalogenase. Because of the biosynthetic defect, the gland is incapable of synthesizing adequate amounts of hormone, leading to increased TSH and a large goiter.

TSH Action

TSH regulates thyroid gland function through the TSH-R, a seven-transmembrane G protein–coupled receptor (GPCR). The TSH-R is coupled to the α subunit of stimulatory G protein ($G_s\alpha$), which activates adenylyl cyclase, leading to increased production of cyclic AMP. TSH also stimulates phosphatidylinositol turnover by activating phospholipase C. The functional roles of the TSH-R are exemplified by the consequences of naturally occurring mutations. Recessive loss-of-function mutations are a rare cause of thyroid hypoplasia and congenital hypothyroidism. Dominant gain-of-function mutations cause sporadic or familial nonautoimmune hyperthyroidism that is characterized by goiter, thyroid cell hyperplasia, and autonomous function. Most of these activating mutations occur in the transmembrane domain of the receptor. They are thought to mimic conformational changes similar to those induced by TSH binding or the interactions of thyroid-stimulating immunoglobulins (TSI) in Graves' disease. Activating TSH-R mutations also occur as somatic events and lead to clonal selection and expansion of the affected thyroid follicular cell (see below).

Other Factors that Influence Hormone Synthesis and Release

Although TSH is the dominant hormonal regulator of thyroid gland growth and function, a variety of growth factors, most produced locally in the thyroid gland, also influence thyroid hormone synthesis. These include insulin-like growth factor I (IGF-I), epidermal growth factor, transforming growth factor β (TGF-β), endothelins, and various cytokines. The quantitative roles of these factors are not well understood, but they are important in selected disease states. In acromegaly, for example, increased levels of growth hormone and IGF-I are associated with goiter and predisposition to multinodular goiter. Certain cytokines and interleukins (ILs) produced in association with autoimmune thyroid disease induce thyroid growth, whereas others lead to apoptosis. Iodine deficiency increases thyroid blood flow and upregulates the NIS, stimulating more efficient uptake. Excess iodide transiently inhibits thyroid iodide organification, a phenomenon known as the *Wolff-Chaikoff effect*. In individuals with a normal thyroid, the gland escapes from this inhibitory effect and iodide organification resumes; the suppressive action of high iodide may persist, however, in patients with underlying autoimmune thyroid disease.

THYROID HORMONE TRANSPORT AND METABOLISM

Serum Binding Proteins

T_4 is secreted from the thyroid gland in at least 20-fold excess over T_3 (**Table 4-2**). Both hormones are bound to plasma proteins, including thyroxine-binding globulin (TBG), transthyretin (TTR), formerly known as thyroxine-binding prealbumin, or TBPA), and albumin. The plasma-binding proteins increase the pool of circulating hormone, delay hormone clearance, and may modulate hormone delivery to selected tissue sites. The concentration of TBG is relatively low (1 to 2 mg/dL), but because of its high affinity for thyroid hormones ($T_4 > T_3$), it carries about 80% of the bound hormones. Albumin has relatively low affinity for thyroid hormones but has a high plasma concentration (~3.5 g/dL), and it binds up to 10% of T_4 and 30% of T_3. TTR carries about 10% of T_4 but little T_3.

When the effects of the various binding proteins are combined, ~99.98% of T_4 and 99.7% of T_3 are protein-bound. Because T_3 is less tightly bound than T_4, the amount of unbound T_3 is greater than unbound T_4, even though there is less total T_3 in the circulation. The unbound, or free, concentrations of the hormones are $\sim 2 \times 10^{-11}$ *M* for T_4 and $\sim 6 \times 10^{-12}$ *M* for T_3, which roughly correspond to the thyroid hormone receptor binding constants for these hormones (see below). Only the unbound hormone is biologically available to tissues. Therefore, homeostatic mechanisms that regulate the thyroid axis are directed towards maintenance of normal concentrations of unbound hormones.

Dysalbuminemic Hyperthyroxinemia

A number of inherited and acquired abnormalities affect thyroid hormone binding proteins. X-linked TBG deficiency is associated with very low levels of total T_4 and T_3. However, because unbound hormone levels are normal, patients are euthyroid and TSH levels are normal. The importance of recognizing this disorder is to avoid efforts to normalize total T_4 levels, as this leads to thyrotoxicosis and is futile because of rapid hormone clearance in the absence of TBG. TBG levels are elevated by estrogen, which increases sialylation and delays TBG clearance. Consequently, in women who are pregnant or taking estrogen-containing contraceptives, elevated TBG increases total T_4 and T_3 levels; however, unbound T_4 and T_3 levels are normal. Mutations in TBG, TTR, and albumin that increase binding affinity for T_4 and/or T_3 cause disorders known as *euthyroid hyperthyroxinemia* or *familial dysalbuminemic hyperthyroxinemia* (FDH) (**Table 4-3**). These disorders result in increased total T_4 and/or T_3, but unbound hormone levels are normal. The

TABLE 4-2

CHARACTERISTICS OF CIRCULATING T_4 AND T_3

HORMONE PROPERTY	T_4	T_3
Serum concentrations		
Total hormone	8 μg/dL	0.14 μg/dL
Fraction of total hormone in the free form	0.02 %	0.3 %
Free (unbound) hormone	21×10^{-12} *M*	6×10^{-12} *M*
Serum half-life	7 d	0.75 d
Fraction directly from the thyroid	100%	20%
Production rate, including peripheral conversion	90 μg/d	32 μg/d
Intracellular hormone fraction	~20 %	~70 %
Relative metabolic potency	0.3	1
Receptor binding	10^{-10} *M*	10^{-11} *M*

TABLE 4-3

CONDITIONS ASSOCIATED WITH EUTHYROID HYPERTHYROXINEMIA

DISORDER	CAUSE	TRANSMISSION	CHARACTERISTICS
Familial dysalbuminemic hyperthyroxinemia (FDH)	Albumin mutations, usually R218 H	AD	Increased T_4 Normal unbound T_4 Rarely increased T_3
TBG			
Familial excess	Increased TBG production	XL	Increased total T_4, T_3 Normal unbound T_4, T_3
Acquired excess	Medications (estrogen), pregnancy, cirrhosis, hepatitis	Acquired	Increased total T_4, T_3 Normal unbound T_4, T_3
Transthyretin[a]			
Excess	Islet tumors	Acquired	Usually normal T_4, T_3
Mutations	Increased affinity for T_4 or T_3	AD	Increased total T_4, T_3 Normal unbound T_4, T_3
Medications: propranolol, ipodate, iopanoic acid, amiodarone	Decreased $T_4 \rightarrow T_3$ conversion	Acquired	Increased T_4 Decreased T_3 Normal or increased TSH
Sick-euthyroid syndrome	Acute illness, especially psychiatric disorders	Acquired	Transiently increased unbound T_4 Decreased TSH T_4 and T_3 may also be decreased (see text)
Resistance to thyroid hormone (RTH)	Thyroid hormone receptor β mutations	AD	Increased unbound T_4, T_3 Normal or increased TSH Some patients clinically thyrotoxic

[a]Also known as thyroxine-binding prealbumin, TBPA.

Note: AD, autosomal dominant; TBG, thyroxine-binding globulin; TSH, thyroid-stimulating hormone; XL, X-linked.

familial nature of the disorders, and the fact that TSH levels are normal rather than suppressed, suggest this diagnosis. Unbound hormone levels (ideally measured by dialysis) are normal in FDH. The diagnosis can be confirmed by using tests that measure the affinities of radiolabeled hormone binding to specific transport proteins or by performing DNA sequence analyses of the abnormal transport protein genes.

Certain medications, such as salicylates and salsalate, can displace thyroid hormones from circulating binding proteins. Although these drugs transiently perturb the thyroid axis by increasing free thyroid hormone levels, TSH is suppressed until a new steady state is reached, thereby restoring euthyroidism. Circulating factors associated with acute illness may also displace thyroid hormone from binding proteins (see "Sick Euthyroid Syndrome," below).

Deiodinases

T_4 may be thought of as a precursor for the more potent T_3. T_4 is converted to T_3 by the deiodinase enzymes (Fig. 4-1). Type I deiodinase, which is located primarily in thyroid, liver, and kidney, has a relatively low affinity for T_4. Type II deiodinase has a higher affinity for T_4 and is found primarily in the pituitary gland, brain, brown fat, and thyroid gland. The presence of type II deiodinase allows it to regulate T_3 concentrations locally, a property that may be important in the context of levothyroxine (T_4) replacement. Type II deiodinase is also regulated by thyroid hormone—hypothyroidism induces the enzyme, resulting in enhanced $T_4 \rightarrow T_3$ conversion in tissues such as brain and pituitary. $T_4 \rightarrow T_3$ conversion is impaired by fasting, systemic illness or acute trauma, oral contrast agents, and a variety of medications (e.g., propylthiouracil, propranolol, amiodarone, glucocorticoids). Type III deiodinase inactivates T_4 and T_3 and is the most important source of reverse T_3 (rT_3). Massive hemangiomas that express type III deiodinase are a rare cause of hypothyroidism in infants.

THYROID HORMONE ACTION

Nuclear Thyroid Hormone Receptors

Thyroid hormones act by binding to nuclear *thyroid hormone receptors* (TRs) α and β. Both TRα and TRβ are expressed in most tissues, but their relative levels of expression vary among organs; TRα is particularly abundant in brain, kidney, gonads, muscle, and heart, whereas TRβ expression is relatively high in the pituitary and liver. Both receptors are variably spliced to form unique isoforms. The TRβ2 isoform, which has a unique amino terminus, is selectively expressed in the hypothalamus and pituitary, where it plays a role in feedback control of the thyroid axis. The TRα2 isoform contains a unique carboxy terminus that prevents thyroid hormone binding; it may function to block the action of other TR isoforms.

The TRs contain a central DNA-binding domain and a C-terminal ligand-binding domain. They bind to specific DNA sequences, termed *thyroid response elements* (TREs), in the promoter regions of target genes (**Fig. 4-3**). The receptors bind as homodimers or as heterodimers with retinoic acid X receptors (RXRs) (Chap. 1). The activated receptor can either stimulate gene transcription (e.g., myosin heavy chain α) or inhibit transcription (e.g., TSH β-subunit gene), depending on the nature of the regulatory elements in the target gene.

Thyroid hormones bind with similar affinities to TRα and TRβ. However, T_3 is bound with 10 to 15 times greater affinity than T_4, which explains its increased hormonal potency. Though T_4 is produced in excess of T_3, receptors are occupied mainly by T_3, reflecting $T_4 \rightarrow T_3$ conversion by peripheral tissues, greater T_3 bioavailability in the plasma, and receptors' greater affinity for T_3. After binding to TRs, thyroid hormone induces conformational changes in the receptors that modify its interactions with accessory transcription factors. In the absence of thyroid hormone binding, the aporeceptors bind to co-repressor proteins that inhibit gene transcription. Hormone binding dissociates the co-repressors and allows the recruitment of coactivators that enhance transcription. The discovery of TR interactions with co-repressors explains the fact that TR silences gene expression in the absence of hormone binding. Consequently, hormone deficiency has a profound effect on gene expression because it causes gene repression as well as loss of hormone-induced stimulation. This concept has been corroborated by the finding that targeted deletion of the TR genes in mice has a less pronounced phenotypic effect than hormone deficiency.

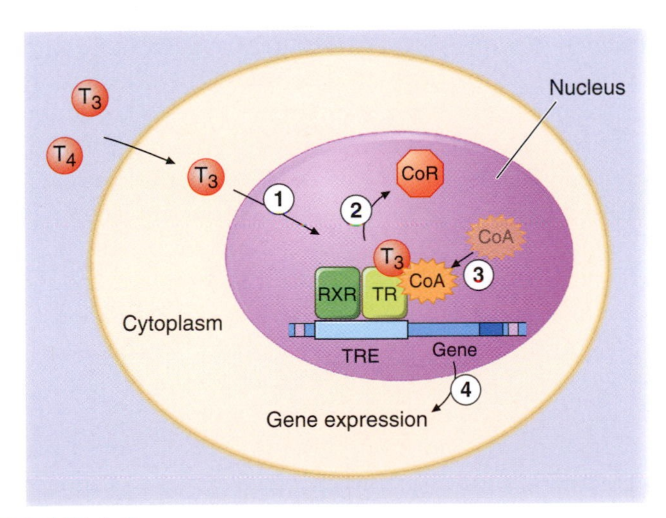

FIGURE 4-3

Mechanism of thyroid hormone receptor action. The thyroid hormone receptor (TR) and retinoid X receptor (RXR) form heterodimers that bind specifically to thyroid hormone response elements (TRE) in the promoter regions of target genes. In the absence of hormone, TR binds co-repressor (CoR) proteins that silence gene expression. The numbers refer to a series of ordered reactions that occur in response to thyroid hormone: **(1)** T_4 or T_3 enters the nucleus; **(2)** T_3 binding dissociates CoR from TR; **(3)** coactivators (CoA) are recruited to the T_3-bound receptor; **(4)** gene expression is altered.

Thyroid Hormone Resistance

Resistance to thyroid hormone (RTH) is an autosomal dominant disorder characterized by elevated thyroid hormone levels and inappropriately normal or elevated TSH. Individuals with RTH do not, in general, exhibit signs and symptoms that are typical of hypothyroidism because hormone resistance is partial and is compensated by increased levels of thyroid hormone. The clinical features of RTH can include goiter, attention deficit disorder, mild reduction in IQ, delayed skeletal maturation, tachycardia, and impaired metabolic responses to thyroid hormone.

The disorder is caused by mutations in the TRβ receptor gene. These mutations, located in restricted regions of the ligand-binding domain, cause loss of receptor function. However, because the mutant receptors retain the capacity to dimerize with RXRs, bind to DNA, and recruit co-repressor proteins, they function as antagonists of the remaining, normal TRβ and TRα receptors. This property, referred to as "dominant negative" activity, explains the autosomal dominant mode of transmission. The diagnosis is suspected when unbound thyroid hormone levels are increased without suppression of TSH. Similar hormonal abnormalities are found in other affected family members, although the TRβ mutation arises de novo in about 20% of patients. DNA sequence analysis of the TRβ gene provides a definitive diagnosis. RTH must be distinguished from other causes of euthyroid hyperthyroxinemia (e.g., FDH) and inappropriate secretion of TSH by TSH-secreting pituitary adenomas (Chap. 2). In most patients, no treatment is indicated; the importance of making the diagnosis is to avoid inappropriate treatment of mistaken hyperthyroidism and to provide genetic counseling.

PHYSICAL EXAMINATION

In addition to the examination of the thyroid itself, the physical examination should include a search for signs of abnormal thyroid function and the extrathyroidal features of ophthalmopathy and dermopathy (see below). Examination of the neck begins by inspecting the seated patient from the front and side, and noting any surgical scars, obvious masses, or distended veins. The thyroid can be palpated with both hands from behind or while facing the patient, using the thumbs to palpate each lobe. It is best to use a combination of these methods, especially when the nodules are small. The patient's neck should be slightly flexed to relax the neck muscles. After locating the cricoid cartilage, the isthmus can be identified and followed laterally to locate either lobe (normally the right lobe is slightly larger than the left). By asking the patient to swallow sips of water, thyroid consistency can be better appreciated as the gland moves beneath the examiner's fingers.

Features to be noted include thyroid size, consistency, nodularity, and any tenderness or fixation. An estimate of thyroid size (normally 12 to 20 g) should be made, and a drawing is often the best way to record findings. However, ultrasound is the method of choice when it is important to determine thyroid size accurately. The size, location, and consistency of any nodules should also be defined. A bruit over the gland indicates increased vascularity, as occurs in hyperthyroidism. If the lower borders of the thyroid lobes are not clearly felt, a goiter may be retrosternal. Large retrosternal goiters can cause venous distention over the neck and difficulty breathing, especially when the arms are raised (Pemberton's sign). With any central mass above the thyroid, the tongue should be extended, as thyroglossal cysts then move upward. The thyroid examination is not complete without assessment for lymphadenopathy in the supraclavicular and cervical regions of the neck.

LABORATORY EVALUATION

Measurement of Thyroid Hormones

The enhanced sensitivity and specificity of *TSH assays* have greatly improved laboratory assessment of thyroid function. Because TSH levels change dynamically in response to alterations of T_4 and T_3, a logical approach to thyroid testing is to first determine whether TSH is suppressed, normal, or elevated. With rare exceptions (see below), a normal TSH level excludes a primary abnormality of thyroid function. This strategy depends on the use of immunoradiometric assays (IRMAs) for TSH that are sensitive enough to discriminate between the lower limit of the reference range and the suppressed values that occur with thyrotoxicosis. Extremely sensitive (fourth generation) assays can detect TSH levels ≤ 0.004 mU/L, but for practical purposes assays sensitive to ≤ 0.1 mU/L are sufficient. The widespread availability of the TSH IRMA has rendered the TRH stimulation test obsolete, as the failure of TSH to rise after an intravenous bolus of 200 to 400 μg TRH has the same implications as a suppressed basal TSH measured by IRMA.

The finding of an abnormal TSH level must be followed by measurements of circulating thyroid hormone levels to confirm the diagnosis of hyperthyroidism (suppressed TSH) or hypothyroidism (elevated TSH). Radioimmunoassays are widely available for serum *total* T_4 and *total* T_3. T_4 and T_3 are highly protein-bound, and numerous factors (illness, medications, genetic factors) can influence protein binding. It is useful, therefore, to measure the free, or unbound, hormone levels, which correspond to the biologically available hormone pool. Two direct methods are used to measure *unbound thyroid hormones*: (1) unbound thyroid hormone competition with radiolabeled T_4 (or an analogue) for binding to a solid-phase antibody, and (2) physical separation of the unbound hormone fraction by ultracentrifugation or equilibrium dialysis. Though early unbound hormone immunoassays suffered from artifacts, newer assays correlate well with the results of the more technically demanding and expensive physical separation methods. An indirect method to estimate unbound thyroid hormone levels is to calculate the free T_3 or free T_4 index from the total T_4 or T_3 concentration and the *thyroid hormone binding ratio* (THBR). The latter is derived from the *T_3-resin uptake test,* which determines the distribution of radiolabeled T_3 between an absorbent resin and the unoccupied thyroid hormone binding proteins in the sample. The binding of the labeled T_3 to the resin is increased when there is reduced unoccupied protein binding sites (e.g., TBG deficiency) or increased total thyroid hormone in the sample; it is decreased under the opposite circumstances. The product of THBR and total T_3 or T_4 provides the *free T_3 or T_4 index*. In effect, the index corrects for anomalous total hormone values caused by abnormalities in hormone-protein binding.

Total thyroid hormone levels are *elevated* when TBG is increased due to estrogens (pregnancy, oral contraceptives, hormone replacement therapy, tamoxifen), and *decreased* when TBG binding is reduced (androgens, the nephrotic syndrome). Genetic disorders and acute illness can also cause abnormalities in thyroid hormone binding proteins, and various drugs (phenytoin, carbamazepine, salicylates, and nonsteroidal anti-inflammatory drugs) can interfere with thyroid hormone binding. Because unbound thyroid hormone levels are normal and the patient is euthyroid in all of these circumstances, assays that measure unbound hormone are preferable to those for total thyroid hormones.

For most purposes, the unbound T_4 level is sufficient to confirm thyrotoxicosis, but 2 to 5% of patients have only an elevated T_3 level (T_3 toxicosis). Thus, unbound T_3 levels should be measured in patients with a suppressed TSH but normal unbound T_4 levels.

There are several clinical conditions in which the use of TSH as a screening test may be misleading, particularly without simultaneous unbound T_4 determinations. Any severe nonthyroidal illness can cause abnormal TSH levels (see below). Although hypothyroidism is the most common cause of an elevated TSH level, rare causes include a TSH-secreting pituitary tumor (Chap. 2), thyroid hormone resistance, and assay artifact. Conversely, a suppressed TSH level, particularly <0.1 mU/L, usually indicates thyrotoxicosis but may also be seen during the first trimester of pregnancy (due to hCG secretion), after treatment of hyperthyroidism (because TSH remains suppressed for several weeks), and in response to certain medications (e.g., high doses of glucocorticoids or dopamine). Importantly, secondary hypothyroidism, caused by hypothalamic-pituitary disease, is associated with a variable (low to high-normal) TSH level, which is inappropriate for the low T_4 level. Thus, *TSH should not be used to assess thyroid function in patients with suspected or known pituitary disease.*

Tests for the end-organ effects of thyroid hormone excess or depletion, such as estimation of basal metabolic rate, tendon reflex relaxation rates, or serum cholesterol, are not useful as clinical determinants of thyroid function.

Tests to Determine the Etiology of Thyroid Dysfunction

Autoimmune thyroid disease is detected most easily by measuring circulating antibodies against TPO and Tg. As antibodies to Tg alone are uncommon, it is reasonable to measure only TPO antibodies. About 5 to 15% of euthyroid women and up to 2% of euthyroid men have thyroid antibodies; such individuals are at increased risk of developing thyroid dysfunction. Almost all patients with autoimmune hypothyroidism, and up to 80% of those with Graves' disease, have TPO antibodies, usually at high levels.

TSI are antibodies that stimulate the TSH-R in Graves' disease. They can be measured in bioassays or indirectly in assays that detect antibody binding to the receptor. The main use of these assays is to predict neonatal thyrotoxicosis caused by high maternal levels of TSI in the last trimester of pregnancy.

Serum Tg levels are increased in all types of thyrotoxicosis except *thyrotoxicosis factitia* caused by self-administration of thyroid hormone. The main role for Tg measurement, however, is in the follow-up of thyroid cancer patients. After total thyroidectomy and radioablation, Tg levels should be undetectable; measurable levels (>1 to 2 ng/mL) suggest incomplete ablation or recurrent cancer.

Radioiodine Uptake and Thyroid Scanning

The thyroid gland selectively transports radioisotopes of iodine (^{123}I, ^{125}I, ^{131}I) and ^{99m}Tc pertechnetate, allowing thyroid imaging and quantitation of radioactive tracer fractional uptake.

Nuclear imaging of Graves' disease is characterized by an enlarged gland and increased tracer uptake that is distributed homogeneously. Toxic adenomas appear as focal areas of increased uptake, with suppressed tracer uptake in the remainder of the gland. In toxic multinodular goiter, the gland is enlarged—often with distorted architecture—and there are multiple areas of relatively increased or decreased tracer uptake. Subacute thyroiditis is associated with very low uptake because of follicular cell damage and TSH suppression. Thyrotoxicosis factitia is also associated with low uptake.

Although the use of fine-needle aspiration (FNA) biopsy has diminished the use of thyroid scans in the evaluation of solitary thyroid nodules, the functional features of thyroid nodules have some prognostic significance. So-called cold nodules, which have diminished tracer uptake, are usually benign. However, these nodules are more likely to be malignant (~5 to 10%) than so-called hot nodules, which are almost never malignant.

Thyroid scanning is also used in the follow-up of thyroid cancer. After thyroidectomy and ablation using ^{131}I, there is diminished radioiodine uptake in the thyroid bed, allowing the detection of metastatic thyroid cancer deposits that retain the ability to transport iodine. Whole-body scans using 111 to 185 MBq (3 to 5 mCi) ^{131}I are typically performed after thyroid hormone withdrawal to raise the TSH level or after the administration of recombinant human TSH.

Thyroid Ultrasound

Ultrasonography is used increasingly to assist in the diagnosis of nodular thyroid disease, a reflection of the limitations of the physical examination and improvements in ultrasound technology. Using 10-MHz instruments, spatial resolution and image quality are excellent, allowing the detection of nodules and cysts >3 mm. In addition to detecting thyroid nodules, ultrasound is useful for monitoring nodule size, for guiding FNA biopsies, and for the aspiration of cystic lesions. Ultrasound is also used in the evaluation of recurrent thyroid cancer, including possible spread to cervical lymph nodes.

HYPOTHYROIDISM

Iodine deficiency remains the most common cause of hypothyroidism worldwide. In areas of iodine sufficiency, autoimmune disease (Hashimoto's thyroiditis) and iatrogenic causes (treatment of hyperthyroidism) are most common (**Table 4-4**).

CONGENITAL HYPOTHYROIDISM

Prevalence

Hypothyroidism occurs in about 1 in 4000 newborns. It may be transient, especially if the mother has TSH-R blocking antibodies or has received antithyroid drugs, but permanent hypothyroidism occurs in the majority. Neonatal hypothyroidism is due to thyroid gland dysgenesis in 80 to 85%, inborn errors of thyroid hormone synthesis in 10 to 15%, and is TSH-R antibody-mediated in 5% of affected newborns. The developmental abnormalities are twice as common in girls. Mutations that cause congenital hypothyroidism are being increasingly recognized, but the vast majority remain idiopathic (Table 4-1).

Clinical Manifestations

The majority of infants appear normal at birth, and <10% are diagnosed based on clinical features, which include prolonged jaundice, feeding problems, hypotonia, enlarged tongue, delayed bone maturation, and umbilical hernia. Importantly, permanent neurologic damage results if treatment is delayed. Typical features of adult hypothyroidism may also be present (**Table 4-5**). Other congenital malformations, especially cardiac, are four times more common in congenital hypothyroidism.

Diagnosis and Treatment

Because of the severe neurologic consequences of untreated congenital hypothyroidism, neonatal screening programs have been established in developed countries. These are generally based on measurement of TSH or T_4 levels in heel-prick blood specimens. When the diagnosis is confirmed, T_4 is instituted at a dose of 10 to 15 μg/kg per day and the dosage is adjusted by close monitoring of TSH levels. T_4 requirements are relatively great during the first year of life, and a high circulating T_4 level is usually needed to normalize TSH. Early treatment with T_4 results in normal IQ levels, but subtle neurodevelopmental abnormalities may occur in those with the most severe hypothyroidism at diagnosis or when treatment is suboptimal.

AUTOIMMUNE HYPOTHYROIDISM

Classification

Autoimmune hypothyroidism may be associated with a goiter (Hashimoto's, or *goitrous thyroiditis*) or, at the later stages of the disease, minimal residual thyroid tissue (*atrophic thyroiditis*). Because the autoimmune process

TABLE 4-4

CAUSES OF HYPOTHYROIDISM
Primary
Autoimmune hypothyroidism: Hashimoto's thyroiditis, atrophic thyroiditis
Iatrogenic: ^{131}I treatment, subtotal or total thyroidectomy, external irradiation of neck for lymphoma or cancer
Drugs: iodine excess (including iodine-containing contrast media and amiodarone), lithium, antithyroid drugs, *p*-aminosalicyclic acid, interferon-α and other cytokines, aminoglutethimide
Congenital hypothyroidism: absent or ectopic thyroid gland, dyshormonogenesis, TSH-R mutation
Iodine deficiency
Infiltrative disorders: amyloidosis, sarcoidosis, hemochromatosis, scleroderma, cystinosis, Riedel's thyroiditis
Overexpression of type 3 deoiodinase in infantile hemangioma
Transient
Silent thyroiditis, including postpartum thyroiditis
Subacute thyroiditis
Withdrawal of thyroxine treatment in individuals with an intact thyroid
After ^{131}I treatment or subtotal thyroidectomy for Graves' disease
Secondary
Hypopituitarism: tumors, pituitary surgery or irradiation, infiltrative disorders, Sheehan's syndrome, trauma, genetic forms of combined pituitary hormone deficiencies
Isolated TSH deficiency or inactivity
Bexarotene treatment
Hypothalamic disease: tumors, trauma, infiltrative disorders, idiopathic

Note: TSH, thyroid-stimulating hormone; TSH-R, TSH receptor.

TABLE 4-5

SIGNS AND SYMPTOMS OF HYPOTHYROIDISM (DESCENDING ORDER OF FREQUENCY)

Symptoms	Signs
Tiredness, weakness	Dry coarse skin; cool peripheral extremities
Dry skin	Puffy face, hands, and feet (myxedema)
Feeling cold	Diffuse alopecia
Hair loss	Bradycardia
Difficulty concentrating and poor memory	Peripheral edema
Constipation	Delayed tendon reflex relaxation
Weight gain with poor appetite	Carpal tunnel syndrome
Dyspnea	Serous cavity effusions
Hoarse voice	
Menorrhagia (later oligomenorrhea or amenorrhea)	
Paresthesia	
Impaired hearing	

gradually reduces thyroid function, there is a phase of compensation when normal thyroid hormone levels are maintained by a rise in TSH. Though some patients may have minor symptoms, this state is called *subclinical hypothyroidism* or *mild hypothyroidism*. Later, free T_4 levels fall and TSH levels rise further; symptoms become more readily apparent at this stage (usually TSH > 10 mU/L), which is referred to as *clinical hypothyroidism* or *overt hypothyroidism*.

Prevalence

The mean annual incidence rate of autoimmune hypothyroidism is up to 4 per 1000 women and 1 per 1000 men. It is more common in certain populations, such as the Japanese, probably because of genetic factors and chronic exposure to a high-iodine diet. The mean age at diagnosis is 60 years, and the prevalence of overt hypothyroidism increases with age. Subclinical hypothyroidism is found in 6 to 8% of women (10% over the age of 60) and 3% of men. The annual risk of developing clinical hypothyroidism is about 4% when subclinical hypothyroidism is associated with positive TPO antibodies.

Pathogenesis

In Hashimoto's thyroiditis, there is a marked lymphocytic infiltration of the thyroid with germinal center formation, atrophy of the thyroid follicles accompanied by oxyphil metaplasia, absence of colloid, and mild to moderate fibrosis. In atrophic thyroiditis, the fibrosis is much more extensive, lymphocyte infiltration is less pronounced, and thyroid follicles are almost completely absent. Atrophic thyroiditis likely represents the end stage of Hashimoto's thyroiditis rather than a distinct disorder.

As with most autoimmune disorders, susceptibility to autoimmune hypothyroidism is determined by a combination of genetic and environmental factors, and the risk of either autoimmune hypothyroidism or Graves' disease is increased among siblings. HLA-DR polymorphisms are the best documented genetic risk factors for autoimmune hypothyroidism, especially HLA-DR3, -DR4, and -DR5 in Caucasians. A weak association also exists between polymorphisms in *CTLA-4,* a T cell–regulating gene, and autoimmune hypothyroidism. Both of these genetic associations are shared by other autoimmune diseases, which may explain the relationship between autoimmune hypothyroidism and other autoimmune diseases, especially type 1 diabetes mellitus, Addison disease, pernicious anemia, and vitiligo (Chap. 21). HLA-DR and *CTLA*-4 polymorphisms account for approximately half of the genetic susceptibility to autoimmune hypothyroidism. The other contributory loci remain to be identified. A gene on chromosome 21 may be responsible for the association between autoimmune hypothyroidism and Down syndrome. The female preponderance of thyroid autoimmunity is most likely due to the effects of sex steroids on the immune response, but an X chromosome—related genetic factor is also possible, which may account for the high frequency of autoimmune hypothyroidism in Turner syndrome. Environmental susceptibility factors are also poorly defined at present. A high iodine intake may increase the risk of autoimmune hypothyroidism by immunologic effects or direct thyroid toxicity. There is no convincing evidence for a role of infection, except for the congenital rubella syndrome, in which there is a high frequency of autoimmune hypothyroidism. Viral thyroiditis does not induce subsequent autoimmune thyroid disease.

The thyroid lymphocytic infiltrate in autoimmune hypothyroidism is composed of activated CD4+ and CD8+ T cells, as well as B cells. Thyroid cell destruction is believed to be primarily mediated by the CD8+ cytotoxic T cells, which destroy their targets by either perforin-induced cell necrosis or granzyme B–induced apoptosis. In addition, local T cell production of cytokines, such as tumor necrosis factor (TNF), IL-1, and interferon (IFN) γ, may render thyroid cells more susceptible to apoptosis mediated by death receptors, such as Fas, which are activated by their respective ligands on T cells. These cytokines also impair thyroid cell function directly, and induce the expression of other proinflammatory molecules by the thyroid cells themselves, such as cytokines, HLA class I and class II molecules, adhesion molecules, CD40, and nitric oxide. Administration of high concentrations of cytokines for therapeutic purposes (especially IFN-α) is associated with increased autoimmune thyroid disease, possibly through mechanisms similar to those in sporadic disease.

Antibodies to Tg and TPO are clinically useful markers of thyroid autoimmunity, but any pathogenic effect is restricted to a secondary role in amplifying an ongoing autoimmune response. TPO antibodies fix complement, and complement membrane attack complexes are present in the thyroid in autoimmune hypothyroidism. However, transplacental passage of Tg or TPO antibodies has no effect on the fetal thyroid, which suggests that T cell–mediated injury is required to initiate autoimmune damage to the thyroid. Up to 20% of patients with autoimmune hypothyroidism have antibodies against the TSH-R, which, in contrast to TSI, do not stimulate the receptor but prevent the binding of TSH. These TSH-R-blocking antibodies therefore cause hypothyroidism and, especially in Asian patients, thyroid atrophy. Their transplacental passage may induce transient neonatal hypothyroidism. Rarely, patients have a mixture of TSI- and TSH-R-blocking antibodies, and thyroid function can oscillate between hyperthyroidism and hypothyroidism as one or the other antibody becomes dominant. Predicting the course of disease in such individuals is difficult, and they require close monitoring of thyroid function. Bioassays can be used to document that TSH-R-blocking antibodies reduce the cyclic AMP–inducing effect of TSH on cultured TSH-R-expressing cells, but these assays are difficult to perform. Assays that measure the binding of antibodies to the receptor by competition with radiolabeled TSH [TSH-binding inhibiting immunoglobulins (TBII)] do not distinguish between TSI- and TSH-R-blocking antibodies, but a positive result in a patient with spontaneous hypothyroidism is strong evidence for the presence of blocking antibodies. The use of these assays does not generally alter clinical management, although they may be useful to confirm the cause of transient neonatal hypothyroidism.

Clinical Manifestations

The main clinical features of hypothyroidism are summarized in Table 4-5. The onset is usually insidious, and the patient may become aware of symptoms only when euthyroidism is restored. Patients with Hashimoto's thyroiditis may present because of goiter rather than symptoms of hypothyroidism. The goiter may not be large but is usually irregular and firm in consistency. It is often possible to palpate a pyramidal lobe, normally a vestigial remnant of the thyroglossal duct. Rarely, uncomplicated Hashimoto's thyroiditis is associated with pain.

Patients with atrophic thyroiditis, or the late stage of Hashimoto's thyroiditis, present with symptoms and signs of hypothyroidism. The skin is dry, and there is decreased sweating, thinning of the epidermis, and hyperkeratosis of the stratum corneum. Increased dermal glycosaminoglycan content traps water, giving rise to skin thickening without pitting (*myxedema*). Typical features include a puffy face with edematous eyelids and nonpitting pretibial edema (**Fig. 4-4**). There is pallor, often with a yellow tinge to the skin due to carotene accumulation. Nail growth is retarded, and hair is dry, brittle, difficult to manage, and falls out easily. In addition to diffuse alopecia, there is thinning of the outer third of the eyebrows, although this is not a specific sign of hypothyroidism.

Other common features include constipation and weight gain (despite a poor appetite). In contrast to popular perception, the weight gain is usually modest and due

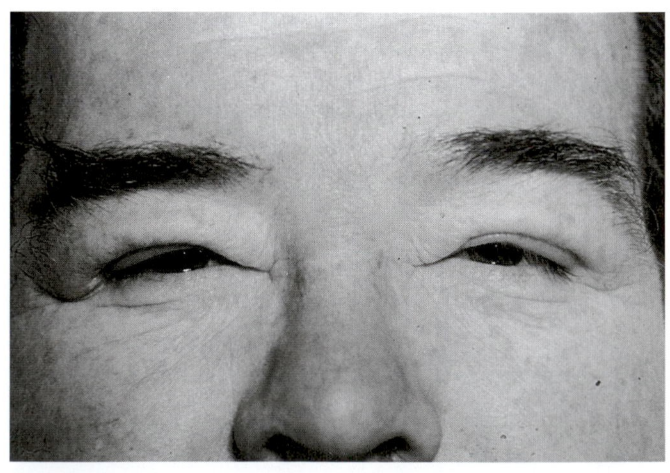

FIGURE 4-4

Facial appearance in hypothyroidism. Note puffy eyes and thickened, pale skin.

mainly to fluid retention in the myxedematous tissues. Libido is decreased in both sexes, and there may be oligomenorrhea or amenorrhea in long-standing disease, but menorrhagia is also common. Fertility is reduced and the incidence of miscarriage is increased. Prolactin levels are often modestly increased (Chap. 2) and may contribute to alterations in libido and fertility and cause galactorrhea.

Myocardial contractility and pulse rate are reduced, leading to a reduced stroke volume and bradycardia. Increased peripheral resistance may be accompanied by hypertension, particularly diastolic. Blood flow is diverted from the skin, producing the cool extremities. Pericardial effusions occur in up to 30% of patients but rarely compromise cardiac function. Though alterations in myosin heavy chain isoform expression have been documented, cardiomyopathy is unusual. Fluid may also accumulate in other serous cavities and in the middle ear, giving rise to conductive deafness. Pulmonary function is generally normal, but dyspnea may be caused by pleural effusion, impaired respiratory muscle function, diminished ventilatory drive, or sleep apnea.

Carpal tunnel and other entrapment syndromes are common, as is impairment of muscle function with stiffness, cramps, and pain. On examination, there may be slow relaxation of tendon reflexes and pseudomyotonia. Memory and concentration are impaired. Rare neurologic problems include reversible cerebellar ataxia, dementia, psychosis, and myxedema coma. *Hashimoto's encephalopathy* is a rare and distinctive syndrome associated with myoclonus and slow-wave activity on electroencephalography, which can progress to confusion, coma, and death. It is steroid-responsive and may occur in the presence of autoimmune thyroiditis, without hypothyroidism. The hoarse voice and occasionally clumsy speech of hypothyroidism reflect fluid accumulation in the vocal cords and tongue.

The features described above are the consequence of thyroid hormone deficiency. However, autoimmune hypothyroidism may be associated with signs or symptoms of other autoimmune diseases, particularly vitiligo, pernicious anemia, Addison disease, alopecia areata, and type 1 diabetes mellitus. Less common associations include celiac disease, dermatitis herpetiformis, chronic active hepatitis, rheumatoid arthritis, systemic lupus erythematosus (SLE), and Sjögren's syndrome. Thyroid-associated ophthalmopathy, which usually occurs in Graves' disease (see below), occurs in about 5% of patients with autoimmune hypothyroidism.

Autoimmune hypothyroidism is uncommon in children and usually presents with slow growth and delayed facial maturation. The appearance of permanent teeth is also delayed. Myopathy, with muscle swelling, is more common in children than in adults. In most cases, puberty is delayed, but precocious puberty sometimes occurs. There may be intellectual impairment if the onset is before 3 years and the hormone deficiency is severe.

Laboratory Evaluation

A summary of the investigations used to determine the existence and cause of hypothyroidism is provided in **Fig. 4-5**. A normal TSH level excludes primary (but not

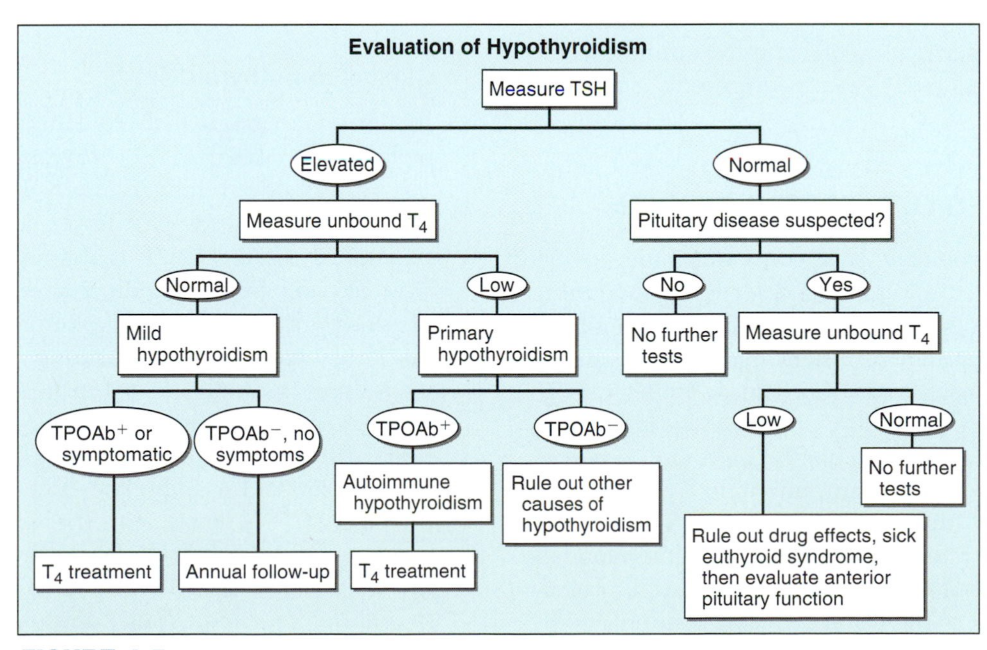

FIGURE 4-5

Evaluation of hypothyroidism. $TPOAb^+$, thyroid peroxidase antibodies present; $TPOAb^-$, thyroid peroxidase antibodies not present. TSH, thyroid-stimulating hormone.

secondary) hypothyroidism. If the TSH is elevated, an unbound T_4 level is needed to confirm the presence of clinical hypothyroidism, but T_4 is inferior to TSH when used as a screening test, as it will not detect subclinical or mild hypothyroidism. Circulating unbound T_3 levels are normal in about 25% of patients, reflecting adaptive responses to hypothyroidism. T_3 measurements are therefore not indicated.

Once clinical or subclinical hypothyroidism is confirmed, the etiology is usually easily established by demonstrating the presence of TPO antibodies, which are present in 90 to 95% of patients with autoimmune hypothyroidism. TBII can be found in 10 to 20% of patients, but these determinations are not needed routinely. If there is any doubt about the cause of a goiter associated with hypothyroidism, FNA biopsy can be used to confirm the presence of autoimmune thyroiditis. Other abnormal laboratory findings in hypothyroidism may include increased creatine phosphokinase, elevated cholesterol and triglycerides, and anemia (usually normocytic or macrocytic). Except when accompanied by iron deficiency, the anemia and other abnormalities gradually resolve with thyroxine replacement.

Differential Diagnosis

An asymmetric goiter in Hashimoto's thyroiditis may be confused with a multinodular goiter or thyroid carcinoma, in which thyroid antibodies may also be present. Ultrasound can be used to show the presence of a solitary lesion or a multinodular goiter, rather than the heterogeneous thyroid enlargement typical of Hashimoto's thyroiditis. FNA biopsy is useful in the investigation of focal nodules. Other causes of hypothyroidism are discussed below but rarely cause diagnostic confusion (Table 4-4).

OTHER CAUSES OF HYPOTHYROIDISM

Iatrogenic hypothyroidism is a common cause of hypothyroidism and can often be detected by screening before symptoms develop. In the first 3 to 4 months after radioiodine treatment, transient hypothyroidism may occur due to reversible radiation damage rather than to cellular destruction. Low-dose thyroxine treatment can be withdrawn if recovery occurs. Because TSH levels are suppressed by hyperthyroidism, unbound T_4 levels are a better measure of thyroid function than TSH in the months following radioiodine treatment. Mild hypothyroidism after subtotal thyroidectomy may also resolve after several months, as the gland remnant is stimulated by increased TSH levels.

Iodine deficiency is responsible for endemic goiter and cretinism but is an uncommon cause of adult hypothyroidism unless the iodine intake is very low or there are complicating factors, such as the consumption of thiocyanates in cassava or selenium deficiency. Though hypothyroidism due to iodine deficiency can be treated with thyroxine, public health measures to improve iodine intake should be advocated to eliminate this problem. Iodized salt or bread or a single bolus of oral or intramuscular iodized oil have all been used successfully.

Paradoxically, chronic iodine excess can also induce goiter and hypothyroidism. The intracellular events that account for this effect are unclear, but individuals with autoimmune thyroiditis are especially susceptible. Iodine excess is responsible for the hypothyroidism that occurs in up to 13% of patients treated with amiodarone (see below). Other drugs, particularly lithium, may also cause hypothyroidism. Transient hypothyroidism caused by thyroiditis is discussed below.

Secondary hypothyroidism is usually diagnosed in the context of other anterior pituitary hormone deficiencies; isolated TSH deficiency is very rare (Chap. 2). TSH levels may be low, normal, or even slightly increased in secondary hypothyroidism; the latter is due to secretion of immunoactive but bioinactive forms of TSH. The diagnosis is confirmed by detecting a low unbound T_4 level. The goal of treatment is to maintain unbound T_4 levels in the upper half of the reference range, as TSH levels cannot be used to monitor therapy.

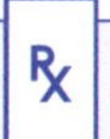

TREATMENT FOR HYPOTHYROIDISM

Clinical Hypothyroidism

If there is no residual thyroid function, the daily replacement dose of levothyroxine is usually 1.6 μg/kg body weight (typically 100 to 150 μg). In many patients, however, lower doses suffice until residual thyroid tissue is destroyed. In patients who develop hypothyroidism after the treatment of Graves' disease, there is often underlying autonomous function, necessitating lower replacement doses (typically 75 to 125 μg/d).

Adult patients under 60 without evidence of heart disease may be started on 50 to 100 μg levothyroxine (T_4) daily. The dose is adjusted on the basis of TSH levels, with the goal of treatment being a normal TSH, ideally in the lower half of the reference range. TSH responses are gradual and should be measured about 2 months after instituting treatment or after any subsequent change in levothyroxine dosage. The clinical effects of levothyroxine replacement are often slow to appear. Patients may not experience full relief from symptoms until 3 to 6 months after normal TSH levels are restored. Adjustment of levothyroxine dosage is made in 12.5- or 25-μg increments if the TSH is high; decrements of the same magnitude should be made if the TSH is suppressed. Patients with a suppressed TSH of any cause, including T_4 overtreatment, have an increased risk of atrial fibrillation and reduced bone density.

Although dessicated animal thyroid preparations (thyroid extract USP) are available, they are not recommended as potency and composition vary between batches. Interest in using levothyroxine combined with liothyronine (triiodothyronine, T_3) has been revived, based on studies suggesting that patients feel better when taking the T_4/T_3 combination compared to T_4 alone. However, a long-term benefit from this combination is not established. There is no place for liothyronine alone as long-term replacement, because the short half-life necessitates three or four daily doses and is associated with fluctuating T_3 levels.

Once full replacement is achieved and TSH levels are stable, follow-up measurement of TSH is recommended at annual intervals and may be extended to every 2 to 3 years, if a normal TSH is maintained over several years. It is important to ensure ongoing compliance, however, as patients do not feel any difference after missing a few doses of levothyroxine, and this sometimes leads to self-discontinuation.

In patients of normal body weight who are taking $\geq$200 μg of levothyroxine per day, an elevated TSH level is often a sign of poor compliance. This is also the likely explanation for fluctuating TSH levels, despite a constant levothyroxine dosage. Such patients often have normal or high unbound T_4 levels, despite an elevated TSH, because they remember to take medication for a few days before testing; this is sufficient to normalize T_4, but not TSH, levels. It is important to consider variable compliance, as this pattern of thyroid function tests is otherwise suggestive of disorders associated with inappropriate TSH secretion (Table 4-3). Because T_4 has a long half-life (7 days), patients who miss doses can be advised to take up to three doses of the skipped tablets at once. Other causes of increased levothyroxine requirements must be excluded, particularly malabsorption (e.g., celiac disease, small-bowel surgery), estrogen therapy, and drugs that interfere with T_4 absorption or clearance such as cholestyramine, ferrous sulfate, calcium supplements, lovastatin, aluminum hydroxide, rifampicin, amiodarone, carbamazepine, and phenytoin.

Mild Hypothyroidism

By definition, subclinical or mild hypothyroidism refers to biochemical evidence of thyroid hormone deficiency in patients who have few or no apparent clinical features of hypothyroidism. There are no universally accepted guidelines for the treatment of mild hypothyroidism. As long as excessive treatment is avoided, there is little risk in correcting a slightly increased TSH, and some patients likely derive modest clinical benefit from treatment. Moreover, there is some risk that patients will progress to overt hypothyroidism, particularly when the TSH level is >6 mU/L and TPO antibodies are present. Treatment is administered by starting with a low dose of levothyroxine (25 to 50 μg/d) with the goal of normalizing TSH. If thyroxine is not given, thyroid function should be evaluated annually.

Special Treatment Considerations

Rarely, levothyroxine replacement is associated with pseudotumor cerebri in *children*. Presentation appears to be idiosyncratic and occurs months after treatment has begun. Women with a history or high risk of hypothyroidism should ensure that they are euthyroid prior to conception and during early pregnancy as maternal hypothyroidism may adversely affect fetal neural development. Thyroid function should be evaluated once pregnancy is confirmed and at the beginning of the second and third trimesters. The dose of levothyroxine may need to be increased by $\geq$50% during pregnancy and returned to previous levels after delivery. *Elderly* patients may require up to 20% less thyroxine than younger patients. In the elderly, especially patients with known coronary artery disease, the starting dose of levothyroxine is 12.5 to 25 μg/d with similar increments every 2 to 3 months until TSH is normalized. In some patients it may be impossible to achieve full replacement, despite optimal antianginal treatment. *Emergency surgery* is generally safe in patients with untreated hypothyroidism, although routine surgery in a hypothyroid patient should be deferred until euthyroidism is achieved.

Myxedema coma still has a high mortality rate, despite intensive treatment. Clinical manifestations include reduced level of consciousness, sometimes associated with seizures, as well as the other features of hypothyroidism (Table 4-5). Hypothermia can reach 23°C (74°F). There may be a history of treated hypothyroidism with poor compliance, or the patient may be previously undiagnosed. Myxedema coma almost always occurs in the elderly and is usually precipitated by factors that impair respiration, such as drugs (especially sedatives, anesthetics, antidepressants), pneumonia, congestive heart failure, myocardial infarction, gastrointestinal bleeding, or cerebrovascular accidents. Sepsis should also be suspected. Exposure to cold may also be a risk factor. Hypoventilation, leading to hypoxia and hypercapnia, plays a major role in pathogenesis; hypoglycemia and dilutional hyponatremia also contribute to the development of myxedema coma.

Levothyroxine can initially be administered as a single intravenous bolus of 500 μg, which serves as a loading dose. Although further levothyroxine is not strictly necessary for several days, it is usually continued at a dose of 50 to 100 μg/d. If suitable intravenous preparation is not available, the same initial dose of levothyroxine can be given by nasogastric tube (though absorption may be impaired in myxedema). An alternative is to give liothyronine (T_3) intravenously or via nasogastric tube, in doses ranging from 10 to 25 μg every 8 to 12 h. This treatment has been advocated because $T_4 \rightarrow T_3$ conversion is impaired in myxedema coma. However, excess liothyroxine has the potential to provoke arrhythmias. Another option is to combine levothyroxine (200 μg) and liothyronine (25 μg) as a single, initial intravenous bolus followed by daily treatment with levothyroxine (50 to 100 μg/d) and liothyronine (10 μg every 8 h).

Supportive therapy should be provided to correct any associated metabolic disturbances. External warming is indicated only if the temperature is <30°C, as it can result in cardiovascular collapse. Space blankets should be used to prevent further heat loss. Parenteral hydrocortisone (50 mg every 6 h) should be administered, as there is impaired adrenal reserve in profound hypothyroidism. Any precipitating factors should be treated, including the early use of broad-spectrum antibiotics, pending the exclusion of infection. Ventilatory support with regular blood gas analysis is usually needed during the first 48 h. Hypertonic saline or intravenous glucose may be needed if there is hyponatremia or hypoglycemia; hypotonic intravenous fluids should be avoided because they may exacerbate water retention secondary to reduced renal perfusion and inappropriate vasopressin secretion. The metabolism of most medications is impaired, and sedatives should be avoided if possible or used in reduced doses. Medication blood levels should be monitored, when available, to guide dosage.

THYROTOXICOSIS

Thyrotoxicosis is defined as the state of thyroid hormone excess and is not synonymous with *hyperthyroidism,* which is the result of excessive thyroid function. However, the major etiologies of thyrotoxicosis are hyperthyroidism caused by Graves' disease, toxic multinodular goiter, and toxic adenomas. Other causes are listed in **Table 4-6**.

GRAVES' DISEASE

Epidemiology

Graves' disease accounts for 60 to 80% of thyrotoxicosis, but the prevalence varies among populations, depending mainly on iodine intake (high iodine intake is associated with an increased prevalence of Graves' disease). Graves' disease occurs in up to 2% of women but is one-tenth as frequent in men. The disorder rarely begins before adolescence and typically occurs between 20 and 50 years of age, but it also occurs in the elderly.

Pathogenesis

As in autoimmune hypothyroidism, a combination of genetic factors, including HLA-DR and *CTLA-4* polymorphisms, and environmental factors contribute to Graves' disease susceptibility. The concordance for Graves' disease in monozygotic twins is 20 to 30%, compared to <5% in dizygotic twins. Indirect evidence suggests that stress is an important environmental factor, presumably operating through neuroendocrine effects on the immune system. Smoking is a minor risk factor for Graves' disease and a major risk factor for the development of ophthalmopathy. Sudden increases in iodine intake may precipitate Graves' disease, and there is a threefold increase in the occurrence of Graves' disease in the postpartum period.

The hyperthyroidism of Graves' disease is caused by TSI that are synthesized in the thyroid gland as well as in bone marrow and lymph nodes. Such antibodies can be detected by bioassays or using the more widely available

TABLE 4-6

CAUSES OF THYROTOXICOSIS
Primary hyperthyroidism
Graves' disease
Toxic multinodular goiter
Toxic adenoma
Functioning thyroid carcinoma metastases
Activating mutation of the TSH receptor
Activating mutation of $G_{s\alpha}$ (McCune-Albright syndrome)
Struma ovarii
Drugs: iodine excess (Jod-Basedow phenomenon)
Thyrotoxicosis without hyperthyroidism
Subacute thyroiditis
Silent thyroiditis
Other causes of thyroid destruction: amiodarone, radiation, infarction of adenoma
Ingestion of excess thyroid hormone (thyrotoxicosis factitia) or thyroid tissue
Secondary hyperthyroidism
TSH-secreting pituitary adenoma
Thyroid hormone resistance syndrome: occasional patients may have features of thyrotoxicosis
Chorionic gonadotropin-secreting tumors[a]
Gestational thyrotoxicosis[a]

[a]Circulating TSH levels are low in these forms of secondary hyperthyroidism.
Note: TSH, thyroid-stimulating hormone.

TBII assays. The presence of TBII in a patient with thyrotoxicosis is strong indirect evidence for the existence of TSI, and these assays are useful in monitoring pregnant Graves' patients in whom high levels of TSI can cross the placenta and cause neonatal thyrotoxicosis. Other thyroid autoimmune responses, similar to those in autoimmune hypothyroidism (see above), occur concurrently in patients with Graves' disease. In particular, TPO antibodies occur in up to 80% of cases and serve as a readily measurable marker of autoimmunity. Because T cell–mediated cytotoxicity can also affect thyroid function, there is no direct correlation between the level of TSI and thyroid hormone levels. In the long term, spontaneous autoimmune hypothyroidism may develop in up to 15% of Graves' patients.

Cytokines appear to play a major role in thyroid-associated ophthalmopathy. There is infiltration of the extraocular muscles by activated T cells; the release of cytokines such as IFN-γ, TNF, and IL-1 results in fibroblast activation and increased synthesis of glycosaminoglycans that trap water, thereby leading to characteristic muscle swelling. Late in the disease, there is fibrosis and only then do the muscle cells show evidence of injury. Orbital fibroblasts may be uniquely sensitive to cytokines, perhaps explaining the anatomical localization of the immune response. Though the pathogenesis of thyroid-associated ophthalmopathy remains unclear, there is mounting evidence that expression of the TSH-R may provide an important orbital autoantigen. In support of this idea, injection of TSH-R into certain strains of mice induces autoimmune hyperthyroidism, as well as features of ophthalmopathy. A variety of autoantibodies against orbital muscle and fibroblast antigens have been detected in patients with ophthalmopathy, but these antibodies most likely arise as a secondary phenomenon, dependent on T cell–mediated autoimmune responses. Similar mechanisms are involved in dermopathy.

Clinical Manifestations

Signs and symptoms include features that are common to any cause of thyrotoxicosis (**Table 4-7**) as well as those specific for Graves' disease. The clinical presentation depends on the severity of thyrotoxicosis, the duration of disease, individual susceptibility to excess thyroid hormone, and the patient's age. In the elderly, features of thyrotoxicosis may be subtle or masked, and patients may present mainly with fatigue and weight loss, leading to *apathetic hyperthyroidism*.

Thyrotoxicosis may cause unexplained weight loss, despite an enhanced appetite, due to the increased metabolic rate. Weight gain occurs in 5% of patients, however, because of increased food intake. Other prominent features include hyperactivity, nervousness, and irritability, ultimately leading to a sense of easy fatiguability in some patients. Insomnia and impaired concentration are common; apathetic thyrotoxicosis may be mistaken for depression in the elderly. Fine tremor is a frequent

TABLE 4-7

SIGNS AND SYMPTOMS OF THYROTOXICOSIS (DESCENDING ORDER OF FREQUENCY)

Symptoms	Signs[a]
Hyperactivity, irritability, dysphoria	Tachycardia; atrial fibrillation in the elderly
Heat intolerance and sweating	Tremor
Palpitations	Goiter
Fatigue and weakness	Warm, moist skin
Weight loss with increased appetite	Muscle weakness, proximal myopathy
Diarrhea	Lid retraction or lag
Polyuria	Gynecomastia
Oligomenorrhea, loss of libido	

[a]Excludes the signs of ophthalmopathy and dermopathy specific for Graves' disease.

finding, best elicited by having patients stretch out their fingers and feeling the fingertips with the palm. Common neurologic manifestations include hyperreflexia, muscle wasting, and proximal myopathy without fasciculation. Chorea is a rare feature. Thyrotoxicosis is sometimes associated with a form of hypokalemic periodic paralysis; this disorder is particularly common in Asian males with thyrotoxicosis.

The most common cardiovascular manifestation is sinus tachycardia, often associated with palpitations, occasionally caused by supraventricular tachycardia. The high cardiac output produces a bounding pulse, widened pulse pressure, and an aortic systolic murmur and can lead to worsening of angina or heart failure in the elderly or those with preexisting heart disease. Atrial fibrillation is more common in patients >50 years. Treatment of the thyrotoxic state alone reverts atrial fibrillation to normal sinus rhythm in fewer than half of patients, suggesting the existence of an underlying cardiac problem in the remainder.

The skin is usually warm and moist, and the patient may complain of sweating and heat intolerance, particularly during warm weather. Palmar erythema; onycholysis; and, less commonly, pruritus, urticaria, and diffuse hyperpigmentation may be evident. Hair texture may become fine, and a diffuse alopecia occurs in up to 40% of patients, persisting for months after restoration of euthyroidism. Gastrointestinal transit time is decreased, leading to increased stool frequency, often with diarrhea and occasionally mild steatorrhea. Women frequently experience oligomenorrhea or amenorrhea; in men there may be impaired sexual function and, rarely, gynecomastia. The direct effect of thyroid hormones on bone resorption leads to osteopenia in long-standing thyrotoxicosis; mild hypercalcemia occurs in up to 20% of patients, but hypercalciuria is more common. There is a small increase in fracture rate in patients with a previous history of thyrotoxicosis.

In Graves' disease the thyroid is usually diffusely enlarged to two to three times its normal size. The consistency is firm, but less so than in multinodular goiter. There may be a thrill or bruit due to the increased vascularity of the gland and the hyperdynamic circulation.

Lid retraction, causing a staring appearance, can occur in any form of thyrotoxicosis and is the result of sympathetic overactivity. However, Graves' disease is associated with specific eye signs that comprise *Graves' ophthalmopathy* (**Fig. 4-6***A*). This condition is also called *thyroid-associated ophthalmopathy,* as it occurs in the absence of Graves' disease in 10% of patients. Most of these individuals have autoimmune hypothyroidism or thyroid antibodies. The onset of Graves' ophthalmopathy occurs within the year before or after the diagnosis of thyrotoxicosis in 75% of patients but can sometimes precede or follow thyrotoxicosis by several years, accounting for some cases of euthyroid ophthalmopathy.

Many patients with Graves' disease have little clinical evidence of ophthalmopathy. However, the enlarged extraocular muscles typical of the disease, and other subtle features, can be detected in almost all patients when investigated by ultrasound or computed tomography (CT) imaging of the orbits. Unilateral signs are found in up to 10% of patients. The earliest manifestations of ophthalmopathy are usually a sensation of grittiness, eye discomfort, and excess tearing. About a third of patients have proptosis, best detected by visualization of the sclera between the lower border of the iris and the lower eyelid, with the eyes in the primary position. Proptosis can be measured using an exophthalmometer. In severe cases, proptosis may cause corneal exposure and damage, especially if the lids fail to close during sleep. Periorbital edema, scleral injection, and chemosis are also frequent. In 5 to 10% of patients, the muscle swelling is so severe that diplopia results, typically but not exclusively when the patient looks up and laterally. The most serious manifestation is compression of the

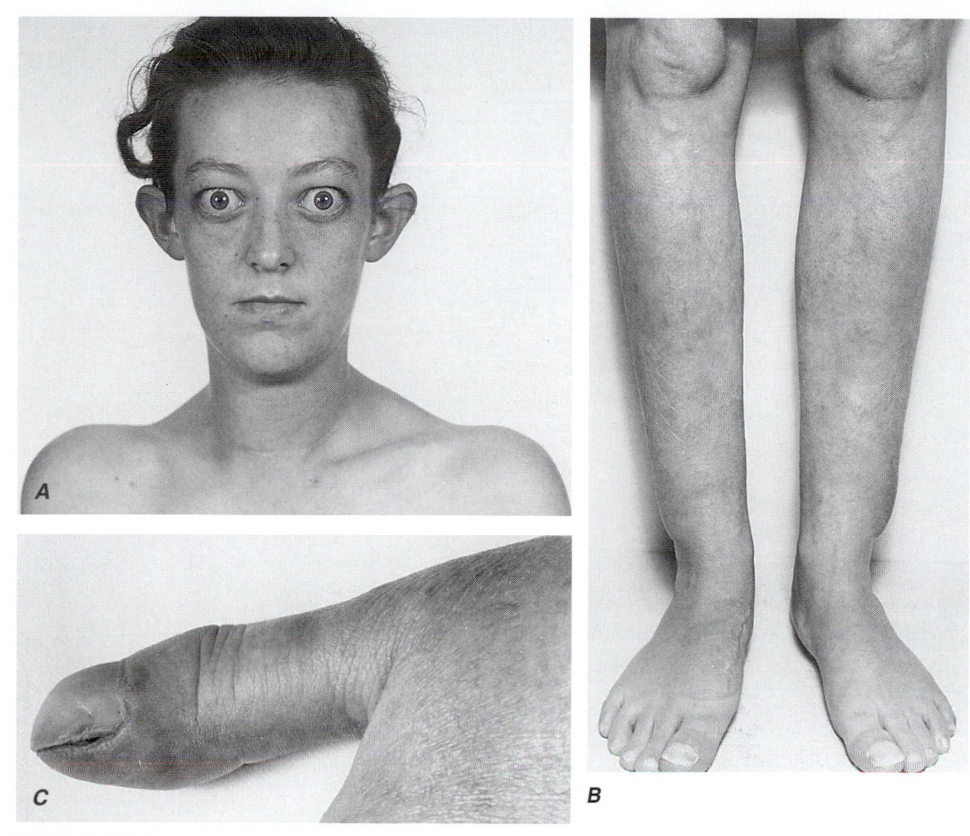

FIGURE 4-6

Features of Graves' disease. ***A***. Facial appearance in Graves' disease; lid retraction, periorbital edema, and proptosis are marked. ***B***. Thyroid dermopathy over the lateral aspects of the shins. ***C***. Thyroid acropachy.

optic nerve at the apex of the orbit, leading to papilledema, peripheral field defects, and, if left untreated, permanent loss of vision.

Many scoring systems have been used to gauge the extent and activity of the orbital changes in Graves' disease. The "NO SPECS" scheme is an acronym derived from the following classes of eye change:

0 = **N**o signs or symptoms
1 = **O**nly signs (lid retraction or lag), no symptoms
2 = **S**oft tissue involvement (periorbital edema)
3 = **P**roptosis (>22 mm)
4 = **E**xtraocular muscle involvement (diplopia)
5 = **C**orneal involvement
6 = **S**ight loss

Although useful as a mnemonic, the NO SPECS scheme is inadequate to describe the eye disease fully, and patients do not necessarily progress from one class to another. When Graves' eye disease is active and severe, referral to an ophthalmologist is indicated and objective measurements are needed, such as lid fissure width; corneal staining with fluorescein; and evaluation of extraocular muscle function (e.g., Hess chart), intraocular pressure and visual fields, acuity, and color vision.

Thyroid dermopathy occurs in <5% of patients with Graves' disease (Fig. 4-6*B*), almost always in the presence of moderate or severe ophthalmopathy. Although most frequent over the anterior and lateral aspects of the lower leg (hence the term *pretibial myxedema*), skin changes can occur at other sites, particularly after trauma. The typical lesion is a noninflamed, indurated plaque with a deep pink or purple color and an "orange-skin" appearance. Nodular involvement can occur, and the condition can rarely extend over the whole lower leg and foot, mimicking elephantiasis. *Thyroid acropachy* refers to a form of clubbing found in <1% of patients with Graves' disease (Fig. 4-6*C*). It is so strongly associated with thyroid dermopathy that an alternative cause of clubbing should be sought in a Graves' patient without coincident skin and orbital involvement.

Laboratory Evaluation

Investigations used to determine the existence and cause of thyrotoxicosis are summarized in **Fig. 4-7**. In Graves' disease, the TSH level is suppressed and total and unbound thyroid hormone levels are increased. In 2 to 5%

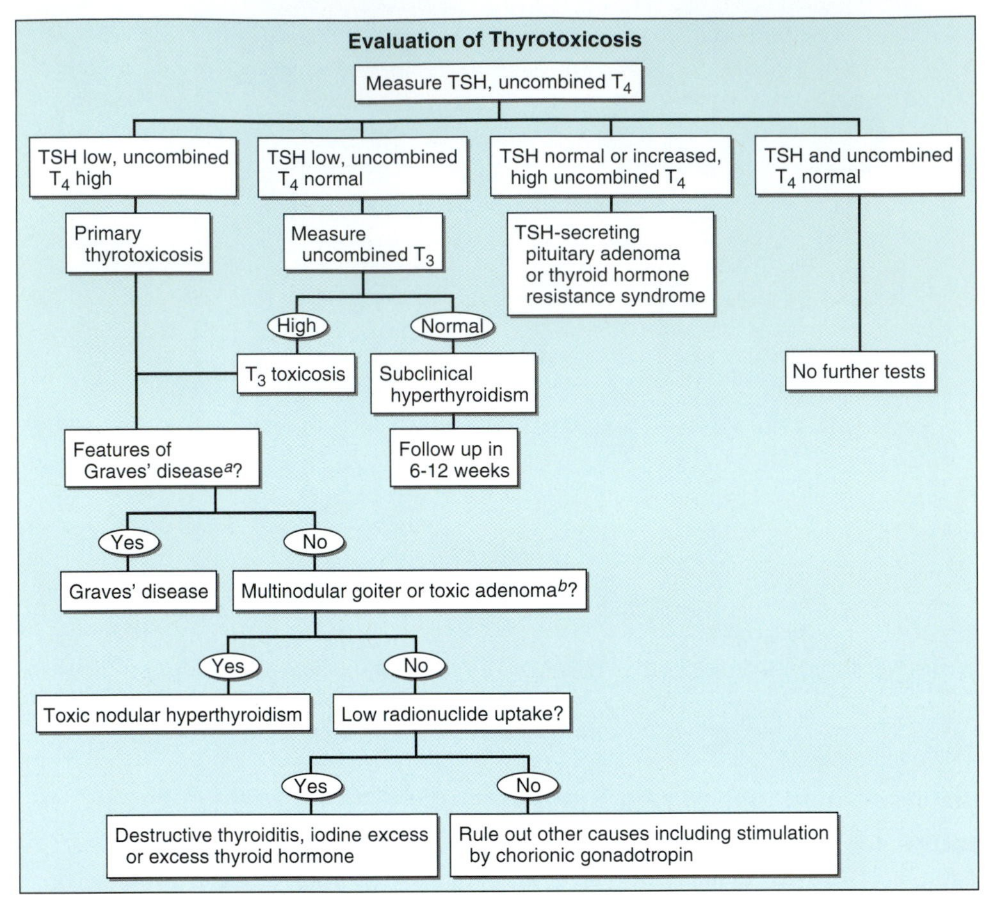

FIGURE 4-7

Evaluation of thyrotoxicosis. [a]Diffuse goiter, positive TPO antibodies, ophthalmopathy, dermopathy; [b]can be confirmed by radionuclide scan. TSH, thyroid-stimulating hormone.

of patients (and more in areas of borderline iodine intake), only T_3 is increased (T_3 toxicosis). The converse state of T_4 toxicosis, with elevated total and unbound T_4 and normal T_3 levels, is occasionally seen when hyperthyroidism is induced by excess iodine, providing surplus substrate for thyroid hormone synthesis. Measurement of TPO antibodies is useful in differential diagnosis. Measurement of TBII or TSI will confirm the diagnosis but is not needed routinely. Associated abnormalities that may cause diagnostic confusion in thyrotoxicosis include elevation of bilirubin, liver enzymes, and ferritin. Microcytic anemia and thrombocytopenia may occur.

Differential Diagnosis

Diagnosis of Graves' disease is straightforward in a patient with biochemically confirmed thyrotoxicosis, diffuse goiter on palpation, ophthalmopathy, positive TPO antibodies, and often a personal or family history of autoimmune disorders. For patients with thyrotoxicosis who lack these features, the most reliable diagnostic method is a radionuclide (^{99m}Tc, ^{123}I, or ^{131}I) scan of the thyroid, which will distinguish the diffuse, high uptake of Graves' disease from nodular thyroid disease, destructive thyroiditis, ectopic thyroid tissue, and factitious thyrotoxicosis. In secondary hyperthyroidism due to a TSH-secreting pituitary tumor, there is also a diffuse goiter. The presence of a nonsuppressed TSH level and the finding of a pituitary tumor on CT or magnetic resonance imaging (MRI) scan readily identify such patients.

Clinical features of thyrotoxicosis can mimic certain aspects of other disorders including panic attacks, mania, pheochromocytoma, and the weight loss associated with malignancy. The diagnosis of thyrotoxicosis can be easily excluded if the TSH and T_3 levels are normal. A normal TSH also excludes Graves' disease as a cause of diffuse goiter.

Clinical Course

Clinical features generally worsen without treatment; mortality was 10 to 30% before the introduction of satisfactory therapy. Some patients with mild Graves' disease experience spontaneous relapses and remissions. Rarely, there may be fluctuation between hypo- and hyperthyroidism due to changes in the functional activity of

TSH-R antibodies. About 15% of patients who enter remission after treatment with antithyroid drugs develop hypothyroidism 10 to 15 years later as a result of the destructive autoimmune process. The clinical course of ophthalmopathy does not follow that of the thyroid disease. Ophthalmopathy typically worsens over the initial 3 to 6 months, followed by a plateau phase over the next 12 to 18 months, with spontaneous improvement, particularly in the soft tissue changes. However, the course is more fulminant in up to 5% of patients, requiring intervention in the acute phase if there is optic nerve compression or corneal ulceration. Diplopia may appear late in the disease due to fibrosis of the extraocular muscles. Some studies suggest that radioiodine treatment for hyperthyroidism worsens the eye disease in a small proportion of patients (especially smokers). Antithyroid drugs or surgery have no adverse effects on the clinical course of ophthalmopathy. Thyroid dermopathy, when it occurs, usually appears 1 to 2 years after the development of Graves' hyperthyroidism; it may improve spontaneously.

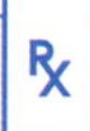

TREATMENT FOR HYPERTHYROIDISM

The *hyperthyroidism* of Graves' disease is treated by reducing thyroid hormone synthesis, using antithyroid drugs, or by reducing the amount of thyroid tissue with radioiodine (^{131}I) treatment or by subtotal thyroidectomy. Antithyroid drugs are the predominant therapy in many centers in Europe and Japan, whereas radioiodine is more often the first line of treatment in North America. These differences reflect the fact that no single approach is optimal and that patients may require multiple treatments to achieve remission.

The main *antithyroid drugs* are the thionamides, such as propylthiouracil, carbimazole, and the active metabolite of the latter, methimazole. All inhibit the function of TPO, reducing oxidation and organification of iodide. These drugs also reduce thyroid antibody levels by mechanisms that remain unclear, and they appear to enhance rates of remission. Propylthiouracil inhibits deiodination of $T_4 \rightarrow T_3$. However, this effect is of minor benefit, except in the most severe thyrotoxicosis, and is offset by the much shorter half-life of this drug (90 min) compared to methimazole (6 h).

There are many variations of antithyroid drug regimens. The initial dose of carbimazole or methimazole is usually 10 to 20 mg every 8 or 12 h, but once-daily dosing is possible after euthyroidism is restored. Propylthiouracil is given at a dose of 100 to 200 mg every 6 to 8 h, and divided doses are usually given throughout the course. Lower doses of each drug may suffice in areas of low iodine intake. The starting dose of antithyroid drugs can be gradually reduced (titration regimen) as thyrotoxicosis improves. Alternatively, high doses may be given combined with levothyroxine supplementation (block-replace regimen) to avoid drug-induced hypothyroidism. Initial reports suggesting superior remission rates with the block-replace regimen have not been reproduced in several other trials. The titration regimen is often preferred to minimize the dose of antithyroid drug and provide an index of treatment response.

Thyroid function tests and clinical manifestations are reviewed 3 to 4 weeks after starting treatment, and the dose is titrated based on unbound T_4 levels. Most patients do not achieve euthyroidism until 6 to 8 weeks after treatment is initiated. TSH levels often remain suppressed for several months and therefore do not provide a sensitive index of treatment response. The usual daily maintenance doses of antithyroid drugs in the titration regimen are 2.5 to 10 mg of carbimazole or methimazole and 50 to 100 mg of propylthiouracil. In the block-replace regimen, the initial dose of antithyroid drug is held constant and the dose of levothyroxine is adjusted to maintain normal unbound T_4 levels. When TSH suppression is alleviated, TSH levels can also be used to monitor therapy.

Maximum remission rates (up to 30 to 50% in some populations) are achieved by 18 to 24 months. For unclear reasons, remission rates appear to vary in different geographic regions. Patients with severe hyperthyroidism and large goiters are most likely to relapse when treatment stops, but outcome is difficult to predict. All patients should be followed closely for relapse during the first year after treatment and at least annually thereafter.

The common side effects of antithyroid drugs are rash, urticaria, fever, and arthralgia (1 to 5% of patients). These may resolve spontaneously or after substituting an alternative antithyroid drug. Rare but major side effects include hepatitis, an SLE-like syndrome, and, most importantly, agranulocytosis (<1%). It is essential that antithyroid drugs are stopped and not restarted if a patient develops major side effects. Written instructions should be provided regarding the symptoms of possible agranulocytosis (e.g., sore throat, fever, mouth ulcers) and the need to stop treatment pending a complete blood count to confirm that agranulocytosis is not present. It is not useful to monitor blood counts prospectively, as the onset of agranulocytosis is idiosyncratic and abrupt.

Propranolol (20 to 40 mg every 6 h) or longer-acting beta blockers, such as atenolol, may be helpful to control adrenergic symptoms, especially in the early stages before antithyroid drugs take effect. The need for anticoagulation with warfarin should be considered in all patients with atrial fibrillation. If digoxin is used, increased doses are often needed in the thyrotoxic state.

Radioiodine causes progressive destruction of thyroid cells and can be used as initial treatment or for relapses after a trial of antithyroid drugs. There is a small risk of thyrotoxic crisis (see below) after radioiodine, which can be minimized by pretreatment with antithyroid drugs for at least a month before treatment. Antecedent treatment with antithyroid drugs should be considered for all elderly patients or for those with cardiac problems, to deplete thyroid hormone stores before administration of radioiodine. Antithyroid drugs must be stopped at least 3 days before radioiodine administration to achieve optimum iodine uptake.

Efforts to calculate an optimal dose of radioiodine that achieves euthyroidism, without a high incidence of relapse or progression to hypothyroidism, have not been successful. Some patients inevitably relapse after a single dose because the biologic effects of radiation vary between individuals, and hypothyroidism cannot be uniformly avoided even using accurate dosimetry. A practical strategy is to give a fixed dose based on clinical features, such as the severity of thyrotoxicosis, the size of the goiter (increases the dose needed), and the level of radioiodine uptake (decreases the dose needed). ^{131}I dosage generally ranges between 185 MBq (5 mCi) to 555 MBq (15 mCi). Incomplete treatment or early relapse is more common in males and in patients <40 years of age. Many authorities favor an approach aimed at thyroid ablation (as opposed to euthyroidism), given that levothyroxine replacement is straightforward and most patients ultimately progress to hypothyroidism over 5 to 10 years, frequently with some delay in the diagnosis of hypothyroidism.

Certain radiation safety precautions are necessary in the first few days after radioiodine treatment, but the exact guidelines vary depending on local protocols. In general, patients need to avoid close, prolonged contact with children and pregnant women for several days because of possible transmission of residual isotope and excessive exposure to radiation emanating from the gland. Rarely there may be mild pain due to radiation thyroiditis 1 to 2 weeks after treatment. Hyperthyroidism can persist for 2 to 3 months before radioiodine takes full effect. For this reason, β-adrenergic blockers or antithyroid drugs can be used to control symptoms during this interval. Persistent hyperthyroidism can be treated with a second dose of radioiodine, usually 6 months after the first dose. The risk of hypothyroidism after radioiodine depends on the dosage but is at least 10 to 20% in the first year and 5% per year thereafter. Patients should be informed of this possibility before treatment and require close follow-up during the first year and annual thyroid function testing.

Pregnancy and breast feeding are absolute contraindications to radioiodine treatment, but patients can conceive safely 6 months after treatment. The presence of severe ophthalmopathy requires caution, and some authorities advocate the use of prednisone, 40 mg/d, at the time of radioiodine treatment, tapered over 2 to 3 months to prevent exacerbation of ophthalmopathy. The overall risk of cancer after radioiodine treatment in adults is not increased, but many physicians avoid radioiodine in children and adolescents because of the theoretical risks of malignancy.

Subtotal thyroidectomy is an option for patients who relapse after antithyroid drugs and prefer this treatment to radioiodine. Some experts recommend surgery in young individuals, particularly when the goiter is very large. Careful control of thyrotoxicosis with antithyroid drugs, followed by potassium iodide (3 drops SSKI orally tid), is needed prior to surgery to avoid thyrotoxic crisis and to reduce the vascularity of the gland. The major complications of surgery—i.e., bleeding, laryngeal edema, hypoparathyroidism, and damage to the recurrent laryngeal nerves—are unusual when the procedure is performed by highly experienced surgeons. Recurrence rates in the best series are <2%, but the rate of hypothyroidism is only slightly less than that following radioiodine treatment.

The titration regimen of antithyroid drugs should be used to manage Graves' disease in *pregnancy,* as blocking doses of these drugs produce fetal hypothyroidism. Propylthiouracil is usually used because of relatively low transplacental transfer and its ability to block $T_4 \rightarrow T_3$ conversion. Also, carbimazole and methimazole have been associated with rare cases of fetal *aplasia cutis* and other defects, such as choanal atresia. The lowest effective dose of propylthiouracil should be given, and it is often possible to stop treatment in the last trimester since TSH-R antibodies tend to decline in pregnancy. Nonetheless, the transplacental transfer of these antibodies rarely causes *fetal thyrotoxicosis* or *neonatal thyrotoxicosis.* Poor intrauterine growth, a fetal heart rate of >160 beats/min, and high levels of maternal TSH-R antibodies in the last trimester may herald this complication. Antithyroid drugs given to the mother can be used to treat the fetus and may be needed for 1 to 3 months after delivery, until the maternal antibodies disappear from the baby's circulation. The postpartum period is a time of major risk for relapse of Graves' disease. Breast feeding is safe with low doses of antithyroid drugs. Graves' disease in *children* is best managed with antithyroid drugs, often given as a prolonged course of the titration regimen. Surgery may be indicated for severe disease. Radioiodine can also be used in children, although most experts defer this treatment until adolescence or later.

Thyrotoxic crisis, or ***thyroid storm,*** is rare and presents as a life-threatening exacerbation of hyperthyroidism, accompanied by fever, delirium, seizures, coma, vomiting, diarrhea, and jaundice. The mortality rate due to cardiac failure, arrhythmia, or hyperthermia is as high as 30%, even with treatment. Thyrotoxic crisis is usually precipitated by acute illness (e.g., stroke, infection, trauma, diabetic ketoacidosis), surgery (especially on the thyroid), or radioiodine treatment of a patient with partially treated or untreated hyperthyroidism. Management requires intensive monitoring and supportive care, identification and treatment of the precipitating cause, and measures that reduce thyroid hormone synthesis. Large doses of propylthiouracil (600-mg loading dose and 200 to 300 mg every 6 h) should be given orally or by nasogastric tube or per rectum; the drug's inhibitory action on $T_4 \rightarrow T_3$ conversion makes it the antithyroid drug of choice. One hour after the first dose of propylthiouracil, stable iodide is given to block thyroid hormone synthesis via the Wolff-Chaikoff effect (the delay allows the antithyroid drug to prevent the excess iodine from being incorporated into new hormone). A saturated solution of potassium iodide (5 drops SSKI every 6 h), or ipodate or iopanoic acid (0.5 mg every 12 h), may be given orally. (Sodium iodide, 0.25 g intravenously every 6 h is an alternative but is not generally available.) Propranolol should also be given to reduce tachycardia and other adrenergic manifestations (40 to 60 mg orally every 4 h; or 2 mg intravenously every 4 h). Although other β-adrenergic blockers can be used, high doses of propranolol decrease $T_4 \rightarrow T_3$ conversion, and the doses can be easily adjusted. Caution is needed to avoid acute negative inotropic effects, but controlling the heart rate is important, as some patients develop a form of high-output heart failure. Additional therapeutic measures include glucocorticoids (e.g., dexamethasone, 2 mg every 6 h), antibiotics if infection is present, cooling, oxygen, and intravenous fluids.

Ophthalmopathy requires no active treatment when it is mild or moderate, as there is usually spontaneous improvement. General measures include meticulous control of thyroid hormone levels, advice about cessation of smoking, and an explanation of the natural history of ophthalmopathy. Discomfort can be relieved with artificial tears (e.g., 1% methylcellulose) and the use of dark glasses with side frames. Periorbital edema may respond to a more upright sleeping position or a diuretic. Corneal exposure during sleep can be avoided by taping the eyelids shut. Minor degrees of diplopia improve with prisms fitted to spectacles. Severe ophthalmopathy, with optic nerve involvement or chemosis resulting in corneal damage, is an emergency requiring joint management with an ophthalmologist. Short-term benefit can be gained in about two-thirds of patients by the use of high-dose glucocorticoids (e.g., prednisone, 40 to 80 mg daily), sometimes combined with cyclosporine. Glucocorticoid doses are tapered by 5 mg every 1 to 2 weeks, but the taper often results in reemergence of congestive symptoms. Pulse therapy with intravenous methylprednisolone (1 g of methylprednisolone in 250 mL of saline infused over 2 h daily for 1 week) followed by an oral regimen is also used. Once the eye disease has stabilized, surgery may be indicated for relief of diplopia and correction of the appearance of the eyes. Orbital decompression can be achieved by removing bone from any wall of the orbit, thereby allowing displacement of fat and swollen extraocular muscles. The transantral route is used most often, as it requires no external incision. Proptosis recedes an average of 5 mm, but there may be residual or even worsened diplopia. Alternatively, retrobulbar tissue can be decompressed without the removal of bony tissue. External beam radiotherapy of the orbits has been used for many years, especially for ophthalmopathy of recent onset, but the objective evidence that this therapy is beneficial remains equivocal.

Thyroid dermopathy does not usually require treatment but can cause cosmetic problems or interfere with the fit of shoes. Surgical removal is not indicated. If necessary, treatment consists of topical, high-potency glucocorticoid ointment under an occlusive dressing. Octreotide may be beneficial.

OTHER CAUSES OF THYROTOXICOSIS

Destructive thyroiditis (subacute or silent thyroiditis) typically presents with a short thyrotoxic phase due to the release of preformed thyroid hormones and catabolism of Tg (see "Subacute Thyroiditis," below). True hyperthyroidism is absent, as demonstrated by a low radionuclide uptake. Circulating Tg and IL-6 levels are usually increased. Other causes of thyrotoxicosis with low or absent thyroid radionuclide uptake include *thyrotoxicosis factitia*; iodine excess and, rarely, ectopic thyroid tissue, particularly teratomas of the ovary (*struma ovarii*); and functional metastatic follicular carcinoma. Whole-body radionuclide studies can demonstrate ectopic thyroid tissue, and thyrotoxicosis factitia can be distinguished from destructive thyroiditis by the clinical features and low levels of Tg. Amiodarone treatment is associated with thyrotoxicosis in up to 10% of patients, particularly in areas of low iodine intake.

TSH-secreting pituitary adenoma is a rare cause of thyrotoxicosis. It can be identified by the presence of an inappropriately normal or increased TSH level in a patient with hyperthyroidism, diffuse goiter, and elevated T_4 and T_3 levels (Chap. 2). Elevated levels of the α subunit of TSH, released by the TSH-secreting adenoma, support this diagnosis, which can be confirmed by demonstrating the pituitary tumor on CT or MRI scan. A combination of transsphenoidal surgery, sella irradiation, and octreotide may be required to normalize TSH, as many of these tumors are large and locally invasive at the time of diagnosis. Radioiodine or antithyroid drugs can be used to control thyrotoxicosis.

Thyrotoxicosis caused by *toxic multinodular goiter* and *hyperfunctioning solitary nodules* is discussed below.

THYROIDITIS

A clinically useful classification of thyroiditis is based on the onset and duration of disease (**Table 4-8**).

ACUTE THYROIDITIS

Acute thyroiditis is rare and due to suppurative infection of the thyroid. In children and young adults, the most common cause is the presence of a piriform sinus, a remnant of the fourth branchial pouch that connects the oropharynx with the thyroid. Such sinuses are predominantly left sided. A long-standing goiter and degeneration in a thyroid malignancy are risk factors in the elderly. The patient presents with thyroid pain, often referred to the throat or ears, and a small, tender goiter that may be asymmetric. Fever, dysphagia, and erythema over the thyroid are common, as are systemic symptoms of a febrile illness and lymphadenopathy.

The differential diagnosis of *thyroid pain* includes subacute or, rarely, chronic thyroiditis, hemorrhage into a cyst, malignancy including lymphoma, and, rarely, amio-

TABLE 4-8

CAUSES OF THYROIDITIS
Acute
Bacterial infection: especially *Staphylcoccus*, *Streptococcus*, and *Enterobacter*
Fungal infection: *Aspergillus*, *Candida*, *Coccidioides*, *Histoplasma*, and *Pneumocystis*
Radiation thyroiditis after ^{131}I treatment
Amiodarone (may also be subacute or chronic)
Subacute
Viral (or granulomatous) thyroiditis
Silent thyroiditis (including postpartum thyroiditis)
Mycobacterial infection
Chronic
Autoimmunity: focal thyroiditis, Hashimoto's thyroiditis, atrophic thyroiditis
Riedel's thyroiditis
Parasitic thyroiditis: echinococcosis, strongyloidiasis, cysticercosis
Traumatic: after palpation

darone-induced thyroiditis or amyloidosis. However, the abrupt presentation and clinical features of acute thyroiditis rarely cause confusion. The erythrocyte sedimentation rate (ESR) and white cell count are usually increased, but thyroid function is normal. FNA biopsy shows infiltration by polymorphonuclear leukocytes; culture of the sample can identify the organism. Caution is needed in immunocompromised patients as fungal, mycobacterial, or *Pneumocystis* thyroiditis can occur in this setting. Antibiotic treatment is guided initially by Gram stain and subsequently by cultures of the FNA biopsy. Surgery may be needed to drain an abscess, which can be localized by CT scan or ultrasound. Tracheal obstruction, septicemia, retropharyngeal abscess, mediastinitis, and jugular venous thrombosis may complicate acute thyroiditis but are uncommon with prompt use of antibiotics.

SUBACUTE THYROIDITIS

This is also termed *de Quervain's thyroiditis, granulomatous thyroiditis,* or *viral thyroiditis.* Many viruses have been implicated, including mumps, coxsackie, influenza, adenoviruses, and echoviruses, but attempts to identify the virus in an individual patient are often unsuccessful and do not influence management. The diagnosis of subacute thyroiditis is often overlooked because the symptoms can mimic pharyngitis. The peak incidence occurs at 30 to 50 years, and women are affected three times more frequently than men.

Pathophysiology

The thyroid shows a characteristic patchy inflammatory infiltrate with disruption of the thyroid follicles and multinucleated giant cells within some follicles. The follicular changes progress to granulomas accompanied by fibrosis. Finally, the thyroid returns to normal, usually several months after onset. During the initial phase of follicular destruction, there is release of Tg and thyroid hormones, leading to increased circulating T_4 and T_3 and suppression of TSH (**Fig. 4-8**). During this destructive phase, radioactive iodine uptake is low or undetectable. After several weeks, the thyroid is depleted of stored thyroid hormone and a phase of hypothyroidism typically occurs, with low unbound T_4 (and sometimes T_3) and moderately increased TSH levels. Radioactive iodine uptake returns to normal or is even increased as a result of the rise in TSH. Finally, thyroid hormone and TSH levels return to normal as the disease subsides.

Clinical Manifestations

The patient usually presents with a painful and enlarged thyroid, sometimes accompanied by fever. There may be

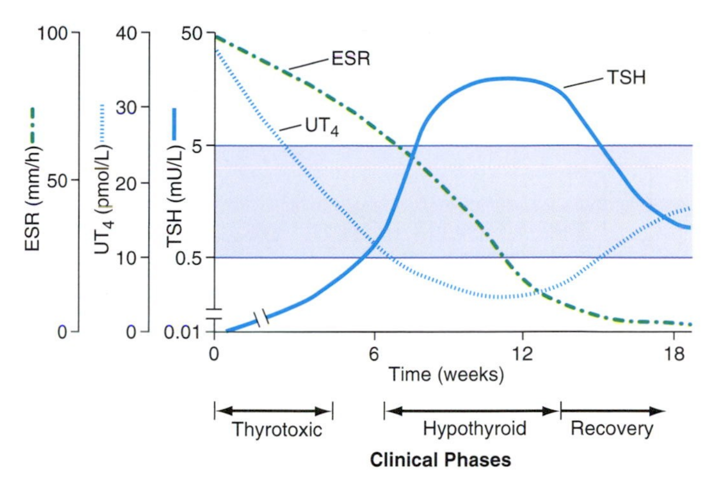

FIGURE 4-8

Clinical course of subacute thyroiditis. The release of thyroid hormones is initially associated with a thyrotoxic phase and suppressed thyroid-stimulating hormone (TSH). A hypothyroid phase then ensues, with low T_4 and TSH levels that are initially low but gradually increase. During the recovery phase, increased TSH levels combined with resolution of thyroid follicular injury leads to normalization of thyroid function, often several months after the beginning of the illness. ESR, erythrocyte sedimentation rate; UT_4, unbound T_4.

features of thyrotoxicosis or hypothyroidism, depending on the phase of the illness. Malaise and symptoms of an upper respiratory tract infection may precede the thyroid-related features by several weeks. In other patients, the onset is acute, severe, and without obvious antecedent. The patient typically complains of a sore throat, and examination reveals a small goiter that is exquisitely tender. Pain is often referred to the jaw or ear. Complete resolution is the usual outcome, but permanent hypothyroidism can occur, particularly in those with coincidental thyroid autoimmunity. A prolonged course over many months, with one or more relapses, occurs in a small percentage of patients.

Laboratory Evaluation

As depicted in Fig. 4-8, thyroid function tests characteristically evolve through three distinct phases over about 6 months: (1) thyrotoxic phase, (2) hypothyroid phase, and (3) recovery phase. In the thyrotoxic phase, T_4 and T_3 levels are increased, reflecting their discharge from the damaged thyroid cells, and TSH is suppressed. The T_4/T_3 ratio is greater than in Graves' disease or thyroid autonomy, in which T_3 is often disproportionately increased. The diagnosis is confirmed by a high ESR and low radioiodine uptake. Serum IL-6 levels increase during the thyrotoxic phase. The white blood cell count may be increased, and thyroid antibodies are negative. If the diagnosis is in doubt, FNA biopsy may be useful, particularly to distinguish unilateral involvement from bleeding into a cyst or neoplasm.

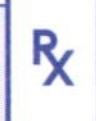

TREATMENT FOR SUBACUTE THYROIDITIS

Relatively large doses of aspirin (e.g., 600 mg every 4 to 6 h) or nonsteroidal anti-inflammatory drugs are sufficient to control symptoms in most cases. If this treatment is inadequate, or if the patient has marked local or systemic symptoms, glucocorticoids should be given. The usual starting dose is 40 to 60 mg prednisone, depending on severity. The dose is gradually tapered over 6 to 8 weeks, in response to improvement in symptoms and the ESR. If a relapse occurs during glucocorticoid withdrawal, treatment should be started again and withdrawn more gradually. In these patients, it is useful to wait until the radioactive iodine uptake normalizes before stopping treatment. Thyroid function should be monitored every 2 to 4 weeks using TSH and unbound T_4 levels. Symptoms of thyrotoxicosis improve spontaneously but may be ameliorated by β-adrenergic blockers; antithyroid drugs play no role in treatment of the thyrotoxic phase. Levothyroxine replacement may be needed if the hypothyroid phase is prolonged, but doses should be low enough (50 to 100 μg daily) to allow TSH-mediated recovery.

SILENT THYROIDITIS

Painless thyroiditis, or *"silent" thyroiditis,* occurs in patients with underlying autoimmune thyroid disease. It has a clinical course similar to that of subacute thyroiditis, except that there is little or no thyroid tenderness. The condition occurs in up to 5% of women 3 to 6 months after pregnancy and is then termed *postpartum thyroiditis.* Typically, patients have a brief phase of thyrotoxicosis, lasting 2 to 4 weeks, followed by hypothyroidism for 4 to 12 weeks, and then resolution; often, however, only one phase is apparent. The condition is associated with the presence of TPO antibodies antepartum, and is three times more common in women with type 1 diabetes mellitus. As in subacute thyroiditis, the radioactive iodine uptake is initially suppressed. In addition to the painless goiter, silent thyroiditis can be distinguished from subacute thyroiditis by the normal ESR and the presence of TPO antibodies. Glucocorticoid treatment is not indicated for silent thyroiditis. Severe thyrotoxic symptoms can be managed with a brief course of propranolol, 20 to 40 mg three or four times daily. Thyroxine replacement may be needed for the hypothyroid phase but should be withdrawn after 6 to 9 months, as recovery is the rule. Annual follow-up thereafter is recommended, as a proportion of these individuals develop permanent hypothyroidism.

DRUG-INDUCED THYROIDITIS

Patients receiving IFN-α, IL-2, or amiodarone may develop painless thyroiditis. IFN-α, which is used to treat chronic hepatitis B or C, causes thyroid dysfunction in up to 5% of treated patients. It has been associated with painless thyroiditis, hypothyroidism, and Graves' disease. IL-2, which has been used to treat various malignancies, has also been associated with thyroiditis and hypothyroidism, though fewer patients have been studied. For discussion of amiodarone, see "Amiodarone Effects on Thyroid Function," below.

CHRONIC THYROIDITIS

Focal thyroiditis is present in 20 to 40% of euthyroid autopsy cases and is associated with serologic evidence of autoimmunity, particularly the presence of TPO antibodies. These antibodies are 4 to 10 times more common in otherwise healthy women than men. The most common clinically apparent cause of chronic thyroiditis is *Hashimoto's thyroiditis,* an autoimmune disorder that often presents as a firm or hard goiter of variable size (see above). *Riedel's thyroiditis* is a rare disorder that typically occurs in middle-aged women. It presents with an insidious, painless goiter with local symptoms due to compression of the esophagus, trachea, neck veins, or recurrent laryngeal nerves. Dense fibrosis disrupts normal gland architecture and can extend outside the thyroid capsule. Despite these extensive histologic changes, thyroid dysfunction is uncommon. The goiter is hard, nontender, often asymmetric and fixed, leading to suspicion of a malignancy. Diagnosis requires open biopsy as FNA biopsy is usually inadequate. Treatment is directed to surgical relief of compressive symptoms. Tamoxifen may also be beneficial. There is an association between Riedel's thyroiditis and idiopathic fibrosis at other sites (retroperitoneum, mediastinum, biliary tree, lung, and orbit).

SICK EUTHYROID SYNDROME

Any acute, severe illness can cause abnormalities of circulating TSH or thyroid hormone levels in the absence of underlying thyroid disease, making these measurements potentially misleading. The major cause of these hormonal changes is the release of cytokines. Unless a thyroid disorder is strongly suspected, the routine testing of thyroid function should be avoided in acutely ill patients.

The most common hormone pattern in sick euthyroid syndrome (SES) is a decrease in total and unbound T_3 levels (low T_3 syndrome) with normal levels of T_4 and TSH. The magnitude of the fall in T_3 correlates with the severity of the illness. T_4 conversion to T_3 via peripheral deiodination is impaired, leading to increased reverse T_3 (rT_3). Despite this effect, decreased clearance rather than increased production is the major basis for increased rT_3. Also, T_4 is alternately metabolized to the hormonally inactive T_3 sulfate. It is generally assumed that this low T_3 state is adaptive, as it can be induced in normal individuals by fasting. Teleologically, the fall in T_3 may limit catabolism in starved or ill patients.

Very sick patients may exhibit a dramatic fall in total T_4 and T_3 levels (low T_4 syndrome). This state has a poor prognosis. A key factor in the fall in T_4 levels is altered binding to TBG. T_4 assays usually demonstrate a normal unbound T_4 level in such patients, depending on the assay method used. Fluctuation in TSH levels also creates challenges in the interpretation of thyroid function in sick patients. TSH levels may range from <0.1 to >20 mU/L; these alterations reverse after recovery, confirming the absence of underlying thyroid disease. A rise in cortisol or administration of glucocorticoids may provide a partial explanation for decreased TSH levels. However, the exact mechanisms underlying the subnormal TSH seen in 10% of sick patients and the increased TSH seen in 5% remain unclear.

Any severe illness can induce changes in thyroid hormone levels, but certain disorders exhibit a distinctive pattern of abnormalities. Acute liver disease is associated with an initial rise in total (but not unbound) T_3 and T_4 levels, due to TBG release; these levels become subnormal with progression to liver failure. A transient increase in total and unbound T_4 levels, usually with a normal T_3 level, is seen in 5 to 30% of acutely ill psychiatric patients. TSH values may be transiently low, normal, or high in these patients. In the early stage of HIV infection, T_3 and T_4 levels rise, even if there is weight loss. T_3 levels fall with progression to AIDS, but TSH usually remains normal. Renal disease is often accompanied by low T_3 concentrations, but with normal rather than increased rT_3 levels, due to an unknown factor that increases uptake of rT_3 into the liver.

The diagnosis of SES is challenging. Historic information may be limited, and patients often have multiple metabolic derangements. Useful features to consider include previous history of thyroid disease and thyroid function tests, evaluation of the severity and time course of the patient's acute illness, documentation of medications that may affect thyroid function or thyroid hormone levels, and measurements of rT_3 together with unbound thyroid hormones and TSH. The diagnosis of SES is frequently presumptive, given the clinical context and pattern of laboratory values; only resolution of the test results with clinical recovery can clearly establish this disorder. Treatment of SES with thyroid hormone (T_4 and/or T_3) is controversial, but most authorities recommend monitoring the patient's thyroid function tests during recovery, without administering thyroid hormone, unless there is historic or clinical evidence suggestive of hypothyroidism. Sufficiently large randomized controlled trials using thyroid hormone are unlikely to resolve this therapeutic controversy in the near future, because clinical presentations and outcomes are highly variable.

AMIODARONE EFFECTS ON THYROID FUNCTION

Amiodarone is a commonly used type III antiarrhythmic agent. It is structurally related to thyroid hormone and contains 39% iodine by weight. Thus, typical doses of amiodarone (200 mg/d) are associated with very high iodine intake, leading to >40-fold increases in plasma and urinary iodine levels. Moreover, because amiodarone is stored in adipose tissue, high iodine levels persist for >6 months after discontinuation of the drug. Amiodarone inhibits deiodinase activity, and its metabolites function as weak antagonists of thyroid hormone action. Amiodarone has the following effects on thyroid function: (1) acute, transient suppression of thyroid function; (2) hypothyroidism in patients susceptible to the inhibitory effects of a high iodine load; and (3) thyrotoxicosis that may be caused by at least three mechanisms—a Jod-Basedow effect from the iodine load in the setting of multinodular goiter, a thyroiditis-like condition, and possibly induction of autoimmune Graves' disease.

The initiation of amiodarone treatment is associated with a transient decrease of T_4 levels, reflecting the inhibitory effect of iodine on T_4 release. Soon thereafter, most individuals escape from iodide-dependent suppression of the thyroid (Wolff-Chaikoff effect), and the inhibitory effects on deiodinase activity and thyroid hormone receptor action become predominant. These events lead to the following pattern of thyroid function tests: increased T_4, decreased T_3, increased rT_3, and a transient increase of TSH (up to 20 mU/L). TSH levels normalize or are slightly suppressed by 1 to 3 months.

The incidence of hypothyroidism from amiodarone varies geographically, apparently correlating with iodine intake. Hypothyroidism occurs in up to 13% of amiodarone-treated patients in iodine-replete countries, such as the United States, but is less common (<6% incidence) in areas of lower iodine intake, such as Italy or Spain. The pathogenesis appears to involve an inability of the thyroid to escape from the high iodine load. Consequently, amiodarone-associated hypothyroidism is more common in women and individuals with positive TPO antibodies. It is usually unnecessary to discontinue amiodarone for this side effect, as levothyroxine can be used to normalize thyroid function. TSH levels should be monitored, because T_4 levels are often increased for the reasons described above.

The management of amiodarone-induced thyrotoxicosis (AIT) is complicated by the fact that there are several causes of thyrotoxicosis and because the increased thyroid hormone levels exacerbate underlying arrhythmias and coronary artery disease. Amiodarone treatment causes thyrotoxicosis in 10% of patients living in areas of low iodine intake and in 2% of patients in regions of high iodine intake. There are two major forms of AIT, although some patients have features of both. Type 1 AIT is associated with an underlying thyroid abnormality (preclinical Graves' disease or nodular goiter). Thyroid hormone synthesis becomes excessive as a result of increased iodine exposure (Jod-Basedow phenomenon). Type 2 AIT occurs in individuals with no intrinsic thyroid abnormalities and is the result of drug-induced lysosomal activation leading to destructive thyroiditis with histiocyte accumulation in the thyroid. Mild forms of type 2 AIT can resolve spontaneously or can occasionally lead to hypothyroidism. Color-flow doppler thyroid scanning shows increased vascularity in type 1 AIT but decreased vascularity in type 2 AIT. Thyroid scans are difficult to interpret in this setting, because the high endogenous iodine levels diminish tracer uptake. However, the presence of normal or increased uptake favors type 1 AIT.

In AIT the drug should be stopped, if possible, although this is often impractical because of the underlying cardiac disorder. Discontinuation of amiodarone will not have an acute effect because of its storage and prolonged half-life. High doses of antithyroid drugs can be used in type 1 AIT but are often ineffective. In type 2 AIT, oral contrast agents, such as sodium ipodate (500 mg/d) or sodium tyropanoate (500 mg, 1 to 2 doses/d), rapidly reduce T_4 and T_3 levels, decrease $T_4 \rightarrow T_3$ conversion, and may block tissue uptake of thyroid hormones. Potassium perchlorate, 200 mg every 6 h, has been used to reduce thyroidal iodide content. Perchlorate treatment has been associated with agranulocytosis, though the risk appears relatively low with short-term use. Glucocorticoids, administered as for subacute thyroiditis, are of variable benefit in type 2 AIT. Lithium blocks thyroid hormone release and can provide modest benefit. Near-total thyroidectomy rapidly decreases thyroid hormone levels and may be the most effective long-term solution, if the patient can undergo the procedure safely.

THYROID FUNCTION IN PREGNANCY

Four factors alter thyroid function in pregnancy: (1) the transient increase in hCG during the first trimester, which stimulates the TSH-R; (2) the estrogen-induced rise in TBG during the first trimester, which is sustained during pregnancy; (3) alterations in the immune system, leading to the onset, exacerbation, or amelioration of an underlying autoimmune thyroid disease (see above); and (4) increased urinary iodide excretion, which can cause impaired thyroid hormone production in areas of marginal iodine sufficiency. Women with a precarious iodine intake (<50 μg/d) are most at risk of developing a goiter during pregnancy, and iodine supplementation should be considered to prevent maternal and fetal hypothyroidism and the development of neonatal goiter.

The rise in circulating hCG levels during the first trimester is accompanied by a reciprocal fall in TSH that persists into the middle of pregnancy. This appears to reflect weak binding of hCG, which is present at very high levels, to the TSH-R. Rare individuals have been described with variant TSH-R sequences that enhance hCG binding and TSH-R activation. hCG-induced changes in thyroid function can result in transient gestational hyperthyroidism and/or *hyperemesis gravidarum,* a condition characterized by severe nausea and vomiting and risk of volume depletion. Antithyroid drugs are rarely needed, and parenteral fluid replacement usually suffices until the condition resolves.

Maternal hypothyroidism occurs in 2 to 3% of women of child-bearing age and is associated with increased risk of developmental delay in the offspring. Thyroid hormone requirements are increased by 25 to 50 μg/d during pregnancy.

GOITER AND NODULAR THYROID DISEASE

Goiter refers to an enlarged thyroid gland. Biosynthetic defects, iodine deficiency, autoimmune disease, and nodular diseases can each lead to goiter, though by different mechanisms. Biosynthetic defects and iodine deficiency are associated with reduced efficiency of thyroid hormone synthesis, leading to increased TSH, which stimulates thyroid growth as a compensatory mechanism to overcome the block in hormone synthesis. Graves' disease and Hashimoto's thyroiditis are also associated with goiter. In Graves' disease, the goiter results mainly from the TSH-R-mediated effects of TSI. The goitrous form of Hashimoto's thyroiditis occurs because of acquired defects in hormone synthesis, leading to elevated levels of TSH and its consequent growth effects. Lymphocytic infiltration and immune system–induced growth factors also contribute to thyroid enlargement in Hashimoto's thyroiditis. Nodular disease is characterized by the disordered growth of thyroid cells, often combined with the gradual development of fibrosis. Because the management of goiter depends on the etiology, the detection of thyroid enlargement on physical examination should prompt further evaluation to identify its cause.

Nodular thyroid disease is common, occurring in about 3 to 7% of adults when assessed by physical examination. Using more sensitive techniques, such as ultrasound, it is present in >25% of adults. Thyroid nodules may be solitary or multiple, and they may be functional or nonfunctional.

DIFFUSE NONTOXIC (SIMPLE) GOITER

Etiology and Pathogenesis

When diffuse enlargement of the thyroid occurs in the absence of nodules and hyperthyroidism, it is referred to as a *diffuse nontoxic goiter.* This is sometimes called *simple goiter,* because of the absence of nodules, or *colloid goiter,* because of the presence of uniform follicles that are filled with colloid. Worldwide, diffuse goiter is most commonly caused by iodine deficiency and is termed *endemic goiter* when it affects >5% of the population. In nonendemic regions, *sporadic goiter* occurs, and the cause is usually unknown. Thyroid enlargement in teenagers is sometimes referred to as *juvenile goiter.* In general, goiter is more common in women than men, probably because of the greater prevalence of underlying autoimmune disease and the increased iodine demands associated with pregnancy.

In *iodine-deficient areas,* thyroid enlargement reflects a compensatory effort to trap iodide and produce sufficient hormone under conditions in which hormone synthesis is relatively inefficient. Somewhat surprisingly, TSH levels are usually normal or only slightly increased, suggesting increased sensitivity to TSH or activation of other pathways that lead to thyroid growth. Iodide appears to have direct actions on thyroid vasculature and may indirectly affect growth through vasoactive substances such as endothelins and nitric oxide. Endemic goiter is also caused by exposure to environmental *goitrogens* such as cassava root, which contains a thiocyanate, vegetables of the Cruciferae family (e.g., brussels sprouts, cabbage, and cauliflower), and milk from regions where goitrogens are present in grass. Though relatively rare, inherited defects in thyroid hormone synthesis lead to a diffuse nontoxic goiter. Abnormalities at each step in hormone synthesis, including iodide transport (NIS), Tg synthesis, organification and coupling (TPO), and the regeneration of iodide (dehalogenase), have been described.

Clinical Manifestations and Diagnosis

If thyroid function is preserved, most goiters are asymptomatic. Spontaneous hemorrhage into a cyst or nodule may cause the sudden onset of localized pain and swelling. Examination of a diffuse goiter reveals a symmetrically enlarged, nontender, generally soft gland without palpable nodules. Goiter is defined, somewhat arbitrarily, as a lateral lobe with a volume greater than the thumb of the individual being examined. If the thyroid is markedly enlarged, it can cause tracheal or esophageal compression. These features are unusual, however, in the absence of nodular disease and fibrosis. *Substernal goiter* may obstruct the thoracic inlet. *Pemberton's sign* refers to symptoms of faintness with evidence of facial congestion and external jugular venous obstruction when the arms are raised above the head, a maneuver that draws the thyroid into the thoracic inlet. Respiratory flow measurements and CT or MRI should be used to evaluate substernal goiter in patients with obstructive signs or symptoms.

Thyroid function tests should be performed in all patients with goiter to exclude thyrotoxicosis or hypothyroidism. It is not unusual, particularly in iodine deficiency, to find a low total T_4, with normal T_3 and TSH, reflecting enhanced $T_4 \rightarrow T_3$ conversion. A low TSH, particularly in older patients, suggests the possibility of thyroid autonomy or undiagnosed Graves' disease, causing subclinical thyrotoxicosis. TPO antibodies may be useful to identify patients at increased risk of autoimmune thyroid disease. Low urinary iodine levels (<10 μg/dL) support a diagnosis of iodine deficiency. Thyroid scanning is not generally necessary but will reveal increased uptake in iodine deficiency and most cases of dyshormonogenesis. Ultrasound is not generally indicated in the evaluation of diffuse goiter, unless a nodule is palpable on physical examination.

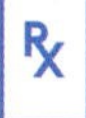

TREATMENT FOR NONDULAR THYROID DISEASE

Iodine or thyroid hormone replacement induces variable regression of goiter in iodine deficiency, depending on how long it has been present and the degree of fibrosis that has developed. Because of the possibility of underlying thyroid autonomy, caution should be exercised when instituting suppressive thyroxine therapy in other causes of diffuse nontoxic goiter, particularly if the baseline TSH is in the low-normal range. In younger patients, the dose of levothyroxine can be started at 100 μg/d and adjusted to suppress the TSH into the low-normal but detectable range. Treatment of elderly patients should be initiated at 50 μg/d. The efficacy of suppressive treatment is greater in younger patients and for those with soft goiters. Significant regression is usually seen within 3 to 6 months of treatment; after this time it is unlikely to occur. In older patients, and in those with some degree of nodular disease or fibrosis, fewer than one-third demonstrate significant shrinkage of the goiter. Surgery is rarely indicated for diffuse goiter. Exceptions include documented evidence of tracheal compression or obstruction of the thoracic inlet, which are more likely to be associated with substernal multinodular goiters (see below). Subtotal or near-total thyroidectomy for these or cosmetic reasons should be performed by an experienced surgeon to minimize complication rates, which occur in up to 10% of cases. Surgery should be followed by mild suppressive treatment with levothyroxine to prevent regrowth of the goiter. Radioiodine reduces goiter size by about 50% in the majority of patients. It is rarely associated with transient acute swelling of the thyroid, which is usually inconsequential unless there is severe tracheal narrowing. If not treated with levothyroxine, patients should be followed after radioiodine treatment for the possible development of hypothyroidism.

NONTOXIC MULTINODULAR GOITER

Etiology and Pathogenesis

Depending on the population studied, multinodular goiter (MNG) occurs in up to 12% of adults. MNG is more common in women than men and increases in prevalence with age. It is more common in iodine-deficient regions but also occurs in regions of iodine sufficiency, reflecting multiple genetic, autoimmune, and environmental influences on the pathogenesis.

There is typically wide variation in nodule size. Histology reveals a spectrum of morphologies ranging from hypercellular regions to cystic areas filled with colloid. Fibrosis is often extensive, and areas of hemorrhage or lymphocytic infiltration may be seen. Using molecular techniques, most nodules within a MNG are polyclonal in origin, suggesting a hyperplastic response to locally produced growth factors and cytokines. TSH, which is usually not elevated, may play a permissive or contributory role. Monoclonal lesions also occur within a MNG, reflecting mutations in genes that confer a selective growth advantage to the progenitor cell.

Clinical Manifestations

Most patients with nontoxic MNG are asymptomic and, by definition, euthyroid. MNG typically develops over many years and is detected on routine physical examination or when an individual notices an enlargement in the neck. If the goiter is large enough, it can ultimately lead to compressive symptoms including difficulty swallowing, respiratory distress (tracheal compression), or plethora (venous congestion), but these symptoms are uncommon. Symptomatic MNGs are usually extraordinarily large and/or develop fibrotic areas that cause compression. Sudden pain in a MNG is usually caused by hemorrhage into a nodule but should raise the possibility of invasive malignancy. Hoarseness, reflecting laryngeal nerve involvement, also suggests malignancy.

Diagnosis

On examination, thyroid architecture is distorted and multiple nodules of varying size can be appreciated. Because many nodules are deeply embedded in thyroid tissue or reside in posterior or substernal locations, it is not possible to palpate all nodules. A TSH level should be measured to exclude subclinical hyper- or hypothyroidism, but thyroid function is usually normal. Tracheal deviation is common, but compression must usually exceed 70% of the tracheal diameter before there is significant airway compromise. Pulmonary function testing can be used to assess the functional effects of compression and to detect tracheomalacia, which characteristically causes inspiratory stridor. CT or MRI can be used to evaluate the anatomy of the goiter and the extent of substernal extension, which is often much greater than is apparent on physical examination. A barium swallow may reveal the extent of esophageal compression. MNG does not appear to predispose to thyroid carcinoma or to more aggressive carcinoma. For this reason, and because it is not possible to biopsy all nodular lesions, thyroid biopsies should be performed only if malignancy is suspected because of a dominant or enlarging nodule.

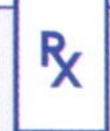

TREATMENT FOR MULTINODULAR GOITER

Most nontoxic MNGs can be managed conservatively. T_4 suppression is rarely effective for reducing goiter size and introduces the risk of thyrotoxicosis, particularly if there is underlying autonomy or if it develops during treatment. If levothyroxine is used, it should be started at low doses (50 μg) and advanced gradually while monitoring the TSH level to avoid excessive suppression. Contrast agents and other iodine-containing substances should be avoided because of the risk of inducing the *Jod-Basedow effect,* characterized by enhanced thyroid hormone production by autonomous nodules. Radioiodine is being used with increasing frequency because it often decreases goiter size and may selectively ablate regions of autonomy. Dosage of ^{131}I depends on the size of the goiter and radioiodine uptake but is usually about 3.7 MBq (0.1 mCi) per gram of tissue, corrected for uptake [typical dose, 370 to 1070 Mbq (10 to 29 mCi)]. Repeat treatment may be needed. It is possible to achieve a 40 to 50% reduction in goiter size in most patients. Earlier concerns about radiation-induced thyroid swelling and tracheal compression have diminished as recent studies have shown this complication to be rare. When acute compression occurs, glucocorticoid treatment or surgery may be needed. Radiation-induced hypothyroidism is less common than after treatment for Graves' disease. However, post-treatment autoimmune thyrotoxicosis may occur in up to 5% of patients treated for nontoxic MNG. Surgery remains highly effective but is not without risk, particularly in older patients with underlying cardiopulmonary disease.

TOXIC MULTINODULAR GOITER

The pathogenesis of toxic MNG appears to be similar to that of nontoxic MNG; the major difference is the presence of functional autonomy in toxic MNG. The molecular basis for autonomy in toxic MNG remains unknown. As in nontoxic goiters, many nodules are polyclonal, while others are monoclonal and vary in their clonal origins. Genetic abnormalities known to confer functional autonomy, such as activating TSH-R or $G_{s\alpha}$ mutations (see below), are not usually found in the autonomous regions of toxic MNG goiter.

In addition to features of goiter, the clinical presentation of toxic MNG includes subclinical hyperthyroidism or mild thyrotoxicosis. The patient is usually elderly and may present with atrial fibrillation or palpitations, tachycardia, nervousness, tremor, or weight loss. Recent exposure to iodine, from contrast dyes or other sources, may precipitate or exacerbate thyrotoxicosis. The TSH level is low. The T_4 level may be normal or minimally increased; T_3 is often elevated to a greater degree than T_4. Thyroid scan shows heterogeneous uptake with multiple regions of increased and decreased uptake; 24-h uptake of radioiodine may not be increased.

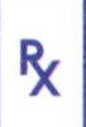

TREATMENT FOR TOXIC MNG

The management of toxic MNG is challenging. Antithyroid drugs, often in combination with beta blockers, can normalize thyroid function and address clinical features of thyrotoxicosis. This treatment, however, often stimulates the growth of the goiter, and, unlike in Graves' disease, spontaneous remission does not occur. Radioiodine can be used to treat areas of autonomy, as well as to decrease the mass of the goiter. Usually, however, some degree of autonomy remains, presumably because multiple autonomous regions emerge as soon as others are treated. Nonetheless, a trial of radioiodine should be considered before subjecting patients, many of whom are elderly, to surgery. Surgery provides definitive treatment of underlying thyrotoxicosis as well as goiter. Patients should be rendered euthyroid using antithyroid drugs before operation.

HYPERFUNCTIONING SOLITARY NODULE

A solitary, autonomously functioning thyroid nodule is referred to as *toxic adenoma*. The pathogenesis of this disorder has been unraveled by demonstrating the functional effects of mutations that stimulate the TSH-R signaling pathway. Most patients with solitary hyperfunctioning nodules have acquired somatic, activating mutations in the TSH-R (**Fig. 4-9**). These mutations, located primarily in the receptor transmembrane domain, induce constitutive receptor coupling to $G_{s\alpha}$, increasing cyclic AMP levels and leading to enhanced thyroid follicular cell proliferation and function. Less commonly, somatic mutations are identified in $G_{s\alpha}$. These mutations, which are similar to those seen in McCune-Albright syndrome (Chap. 10) or in a subset of somatotrope adenomas (Chap. 2), impair GTP hydrolysis, also causing constitutive activation of the cyclic AMP signaling pathway. In most series, activating mutations in either the TSH-R or the $G_{s\alpha}$ subunit genes are identified in >90% of patients with solitary hyperfunctioning nodules.

Thyrotoxicosis is usually mild. The disorder is suggested by the presence of the thyroid nodule, which is generally large enough to be palpable, and by the absence

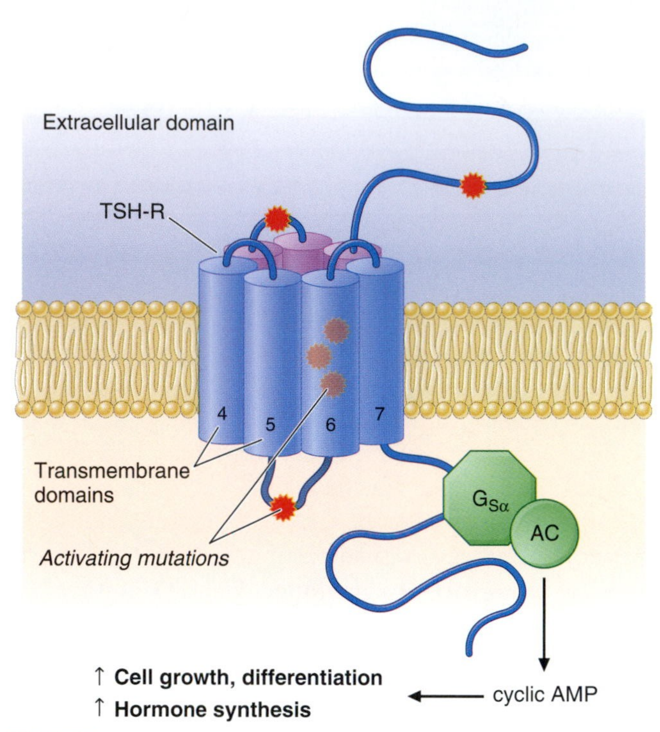

FIGURE 4-9

Activating mutations of the TSH-R. Mutations (*) that activate the thyroid-stimulating hormone receptor (TSH-R) reside mainly in transmembrane 5 and intracellular loop 3, though mutations have occurred in a variety of different locations. The effect of these mutations is to induce conformational changes that mimic TSH binding, thereby leading to coupling to stimulatory G protein ($G_{s\alpha}$) and activation of adenylate cyclase (AC), an enzyme that generates cyclic AMP.

of clinical features suggestive of Graves' disease or other causes of thyrotoxicosis. A thyroid scan provides a definitive diagnostic test, demonstrating focal uptake in the hyperfunctioning nodule and diminished uptake in the remainder of the gland, as activity of the normal thyroid is suppressed.

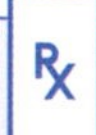

TREATMENT FOR THYROTOXICOSIS

Radioiodine ablation is usually the treatment of choice. Because normal thyroid function is suppressed, ^{131}I is concentrated in the hyperfunctioning nodule with minimal uptake and damage to normal thyroid tissue. Relatively large radioiodine doses [e.g., 370 to 1110 MBq (10 to 29.9 mCi) ^{131}I] have been shown to correct thyrotoxicosis in about 75% of patients within 3 months. Hypothyroidism occurs in <10% of patients over the next 5 years. Surgical resection is also effective and is usually limited to enucleation of the adenoma or lobectomy, thereby preserving thyroid function and minimizing risk of hypoparathyroidism or damage to the recurrent laryngeal nerves. Medical therapy using antithyroid drugs and beta blockers can normalize thyroid function but is not an optimal long-term treatment. Ethanol injection under ultrasound guidance has been used successfully in some centers to ablate hyperfunctioning nodules. Repeated injections (often more than 5 sessions) are required to reduce nodule size. Normal thyroid function can be achieved in most patients using this technique.

BENIGN NEOPLASMS

The various types of benign thyroid nodules are listed in **Table 4-9**. These lesions are common (5 to 10% adults), particularly when assessed by sensitive techniques such as ultrasound. The risk of malignancy is very low for *macrofollicular adenomas* and *normofollicular adenomas. Microfollicular, trabecular,* and *Hürthle cell variants* raise greater concern, and the histology is more difficult to interpret. About one-third of palpable nodules are *thyroid cysts.* These may be recognized by their ultrasound appearance or based on aspiration of large amounts of pink or straw-colored fluid (colloid). Many are mixed cystic/solid lesions, in which case it is desirable to aspirate cellular components under ultrasound or harvest cells after cytospin of cyst fluid. Cysts frequently recur, even after repeated aspiration, and may require surgical excision if they are large or if the cytology is suspicious. Sclerosis has been used with variable success but is often painful and may be complicated by infiltration of the sclerosing agent.

The treatment approach for benign nodules is similar to that for MNG. TSH suppression with levothyroxine decreases the size of about 30% of nodules and may prevent further growth. The TSH level should be suppressed into the low-normal range, assuming there are no contraindications; alternatively, nodule size can be monitored without suppression. If a nodule has not decreased in size after 6 to 12 months of suppressive therapy, treatment should be discontinued as little benefit is likely to accrue from long-term treatment.

THYROID CANCER

Thyroid carcinoma is the most common malignancy of the endocrine system. Malignant tumors derived from the follicular epithelium are classified according to histologic features. Differentiated tumors, such as

TABLE 4-9

CLASSIFICATION OF THYROID NEOPLASMS

BENIGN	
Follicular epithelial cell adenomas	
Macrofollicular (colloid)	
Normofollicular (simple)	
Microfollicular (fetal)	
Trabecular (embryonal)	
Hürthle cell variant (oncocytic)	
MALIGNANT	**APPROXIMATE PREVALENCE, %**
Follicular epithelial cell	
Well-differentiated carcinomas	
Papillary carcinomas	80–90
Pure papillary	
Follicular variant	
Diffuse sclerosing variant	
Tall cell, columnar cell variants	
Follicular carcinomas	5–10
Minimally invasive	
Widely invasive	
Hürthle cell carcinoma (oncocytic)	
Insular carcinoma	
Undifferentiated (anaplastic) carcinomas	
C cell (calcitonin-producing)	
Medullary thyroid cancer	10
Sporadic	
Familial	
MEN 2	
Other malignancies	
Lymphomas	1–2
Sarcomas	
Metastases	
Others	

Note: MEN, multiple endocrine neoplasia.

papillary thyroid cancer (PTC) or follicular thyroid cancer (FTC), are often curable, and the prognosis is good for patients identified with early-stage disease. In contrast, anaplastic thyroid cancer (ATC) is aggressive, responds poorly to treatment, and is associated with a bleak prognosis.

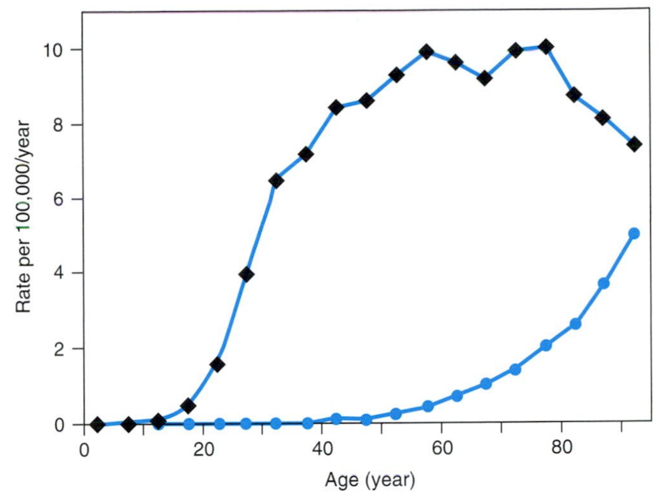

FIGURE 4-10

Age-associated incidence (◆) and mortality (–●–) rates for invasive thyroid cancer. *[Adapted from LAG Ries et al (eds): SEER Cancer Statistics Review, 1973–1996, Bethesda, National Cancer Institute, 1999.]*

The incidence of thyroid cancer (~9/100,000 per year) increases with age, plateauing after about age 50 (**Fig. 4-10**). Age is also an important prognostic factor—thyroid cancer at a young age (<20) or in older persons (>65) is associated with a worse prognosis. Thyroid cancer is twice as common in women as men, but male sex is associated with a worse prognosis. Additional important risk factors include a history of childhood head or neck irradiation, large nodule size (≥4 cm), evidence for local tumor fixation or invasion into lymph nodes, and the presence of metastases (**Table 4-10**).

Several unique features of thyroid cancer facilitate its management: (1) thyroid nodules are readily palpable, allowing early detection and biopsy by FNA; (2) iodine radioisotopes can be used to diagnose (^{123}I) and treat (^{131}I) differentiated thyroid cancer, reflecting the unique uptake of this anion by the thyroid gland; and (3) serum markers allow the detection of residual or recurrent disease, including the use of Tg levels for PTC and FTC and calcitonin for medullary thyroid cancer (MTC).

TABLE 4-10

RISK FACTORS FOR THYROID CARCINOMA IN PATIENTS WITH THYROID NODULE

History of head and neck irradiation	Family history of thyroid cancer or MEN 2
Age <20 or >70 years	Vocal cord paralysis, hoarse voice
Increased nodule size (>4 cm)	Nodule fixed to adjacent structures
New or enlarging neck mass	Suspected lymph node involvement
Male gender	Iodine deficiency (follicular cancer)

Note: MEN, multiple endocrine neoplasia.

TABLE 4-11

AMERICAN JOINT COMMITTEE ON CANCER STAGING SYSTEM FOR THYROID CANCERS USING THE TNM CLASSIFICATION[a]

Papillary or follicular thyroid cancers		
	<45 years	>45 years
Stage I	Any T, any N, M0	T1, N0, M0
Stage II	Any T, any N, M1	T2 or T3, N0, M0
Stage III	—	T4, N0, M0 Any T, N1, M0
Stage IV	—	Any T, any N, M1
Anaplastic thyroid cancer		
Stage IV	All cases are stage IV	
Medullary thyroid cancer		
Stage I	T1, N0, M0	
Stage II	T2–T4, N0, M0	
Stage III	Any T, N1, M0	
Stage IV	Any T, any N, M1	

[a]Criteria include: T, the size and extent of the primary tumor (T1≤ 1 cm; 1 cm <T2 ≤ 4 cm; T3 > 4 cm; T4 direct invasion through the thyroid capsule); N, the absence (N0) or presence (N1) of regional node involvement; M, the absence (M0) or presence (M1) of metastases.

CLASSIFICATION

Thyroid neoplasms can arise in each of the cell types that populate the gland, including thyroid follicular cells, calcitonin-producing C cells, lymphocytes, and stromal and vascular elements, as well as metastases from other sites (Table 4-9). The American Joint Committee on Cancer (AJCC) has designated a staging system using the TNM classification (**Table 4-11**). Several other classification and staging systems are also widely used, some of which place greater emphasis on histologic features or risk factors such as age or gender.

PATHOGENESIS AND GENETIC BASIS

Radiation

Early studies of the pathogenesis of thyroid cancer focused on the role of external radiation, which predisposes to chromosomal breaks, presumably leading to genetic rearrangements and loss of tumor-suppressor genes. External radiation of the mediastinum, face, head, and neck region was administered in the past to treat an array of conditions including acne and enlargement of the thymus, tonsils, and adenoids. Radiation exposure increases the risk of benign and malignant thyroid nodules, is associated with multicentric cancers, and shifts the incidence of thyroid cancer to an earlier age group. Radiation from nuclear fallout also increases the risk of thyroid cancer. Children seem more predisposed to the effects of radiation than adults. Of note, radiation derived from ^{131}I therapy appears to contribute little, if any, increased risk of thyroid cancer.

TSH and Growth Factors

Thyroid growth is regulated primarily by TSH but also by a variety of growth factors and cytokines. Many differentiated thyroid cancers express TSH receptors and, therefore, remain responsive to TSH. This observation provides the rationale for T_4 suppression of TSH in patients with thyroid cancer. Residual expression of TSH receptors also allows TSH-stimulated uptake of ^{131}I therapy (see below).

Oncogenes and Tumor-Suppressor Genes

Thyroid cancers are monoclonal in origin, consistent with the idea that they originate as a consequence of mutations that confer a growth advantage to a single cell. In addition to increased rates of proliferation, some thyroid cancers exhibit impaired apoptosis and features that enhance invasion, angiogenesis, and metastasis. By analogy with the model of multistep carcinogenesis proposed for colon cancer. Thyroid neoplasms have been analyzed for a variety of genetic alterations, but without clear evidence of an ordered acquisition of somatic mutations as they progress from the benign to the malignant state. On the other hand, certain mutations are relatively specific for thyroid neoplasia, some of which correlate with histologic classification (**Table 4-12**). For example, activating mutations of the TSH-R and the $G_{s\alpha}$ subunit are associated with autonomously functioning nodules. Though these mutations induce thyroid cell growth, this type of nodule is almost always benign. A variety of rearrangements involving the *RET* gene on chromosome 10 bring this receptor tyrosine kinase under the control

TABLE 4-12

GENETIC ALTERATIONS IN THYROID NEOPLASIA

GENE/PROTEIN	TYPE OF GENE	CHROMOSOMAL LOCATION	GENETIC ABNORMALITY	TUMOR
TSH receptor	GPCR receptor	14q31	Point mutations	Toxic adenoma, differentiated carcinomas
$G_{s\alpha}$	G protein	20q13.2	Point mutations	Toxic adenoma, differentiated carcinomas
RET/PTC	Receptor tyrosine kinase	10q11.2	Rearrangements PTC1: (inv(10)q11.2q21) PTC2: (t(10;17)(q11.2;q23)) PTC3: ELE1/TK	PTC
RET	Receptor tyrosine kinase	10q11.2	Point mutations	MEN 2, medullary thyroid cancer
TRK	Receptor tyrosine kinase	1q23-24	Rearrangements	Multinodular goiter, papillary thyroid cancer
RAS	Signal transducing p21	Hras 11p15.5 Kras 12p12.1; Nras 1p13.2	Point mutations	Differentiated thyroid carcinoma, adenomas
p53	Tumor suppressor, cell cycle control, apoptosis	17p13	Point mutations Deletion, insertion	Anaplastic cancer
APC	Tumor suppressor, adenomatous polyposis coli gene	5q21-q22	Point mutations	Anaplastic cancer, also associated with familial polyposis coli
p16 (MTS1, CDKN2A)	Tumor suppressor, cell cycle control	9p21	Deletions	Differentiated carcinomas
p21/WAF	Tumor suppressor, cell cycle control	6p21.2	Overexpression	Anaplastic cancer
MET	Receptor tyrosine kinase	7q31	Overexpression	Follicular thyroid cancer
c-MYC	Receptor tyrosine kinase	8q24.12–13	Overexpression	Differentiated carcinoma
PTEN	Phosphatase	10q23	Point mutations	PTC in Cowden's syndrome (multiple hamartomas, breast tumors, gastrointestinal polyps, thyroid tumors)
Loss of heterozygosity (LOH)	?Tumor suppressors	3p; 11q13 Other loci	Deletions	Differentiated thyroid carcinomas, anaplastic cancer
PAX8-PPARγ1	Transcription factor Nuclear receptor fusion	t(2;3)(q13;p25)	Translocation	Follicular adenoma or carcinoma

Note: TSH, thyroid-stimulating hormone; $G_{s\alpha}$, G-protein stimulating α-subunit; RET, rearranged during transfection proto-oncogene; PTC, papillary thyroid cancer; TRK, tyrosine kinase receptor; RAS, rat sarcoma proto-oncogene; p53, p53 tumor suppressor gene; MET, met proto-oncogene (hepatocyte growth factor receptor); c-MYC, cellular homologue of myelocytomatosis virus proto-oncogene; PTEN, phosphatase and tensin homologue; APC, adenomatous polyposis coli; MTS, multiple tumor suppressor; CDKN2A, cyclin-dependent kinase inhibitor 2A; P21, p21 tumor suppressor; WAF, wild-type p53 activated fragment; GPCR, G protein–coupled receptor; ELE1/TK, ret-activating gene ele1/tyrosine kinase; MEN 2, multiple endocrine neoplasia-2; PAX8, Paired domain transcription factor; PPARγ1, peroxisome-proliferator activated receptor γ1.

Source: Adapted with permission from P Kopp, JL Jameson, in JL Jameson (ed): *Principles of Molecular Medicine*. Totowa, NJ, Humana Press, 1998.

of other promoters, leading to receptor overexpression. *RET* rearrangements occur in 20 to 40% of PTCs in different series and were observed with increased frequency in tumors developing after the Chernobyl radiation disaster. Rearrangements in PTC have also been observed for another tyrosine kinase gene, *TRK1,* which is located on chromosome 1. To date, the identification of PTC with *RET* or *TRK1* rearrangements has not proven useful for predicting prognosis or treatment responses. Another rearrangement, linking the thyroid developmental transcription factor PAX8 to the nuclear receptor PPARγ, has been identified in a significance fraction of follicular adenomas and FTCs. *RAS* mutations are found in about 20 to 30% of thyroid neoplasms, including adenomas as well as PTC and FTC, suggesting that these mutations do not strongly affect tumor phenotype. Loss of heterozygosity, consistent with deletions of tumor-suppressor genes, is particularly common in FTC, often involving chromosomes 3p or 11q. Mutations of the tumor suppressor, p53, play an important role in the development of ATC. Because p53 plays a role in cell cycle surveillance, DNA repair, and apoptosis, its loss may contribute to the rapid acquisition of genetic instability as well as poor treatment responses. The role of other tumor-suppressor genes in thyroid cancer is under investigation (Table 4-12).

MTC, when associated with multiple endocrine neoplasia (MEN) type 2, harbors an inherited mutation of the *RET* gene. Unlike the rearrangements of *RET* seen in PTC, the mutations in MEN2 are point mutations that induce constitutive activity of the tyrosine kinase (Chap. 21). MTC is preceded by hyperplasia of the C cells, raising the likelihood that as-yet-unidentified "second hits" lead to cellular transformation. A subset of sporadic MTC contain somatic mutations that activate *RET.*

WELL-DIFFERENTIATED THYROID CANCER

Papillary

PTC is the most common type of thyroid cancer, accounting for 70 to 90% of well-differentiated thyroid malignancies. Microscopic PTC is present in up to 25% of thyroid glands at autopsy, but most of these lesions are very small (several millimeters) and are not clinically significant. Characteristic cytologic features of PTC help make the diagnosis by FNA or after surgical resection; these include psammoma bodies, cleaved nuclei with an "orphan-Annie" appearance caused by large nucleoli, and the formation of papillary structures.

PTC tends to be multifocal and to invade locally within the thyroid gland as well as through the thyroid capsule and into adjacent structures in the neck. It has a propensity to spread via the lymphatic system but can metastasize hematogenously as well, particularly to bone and lung. Because of the relatively slow growth of the tumor, a significant burden of pulmonary metastases may accumulate, sometimes with remarkably few symptoms. The prognostic implication of lymph node spread is debated. Lymph node involvement by thyroid cancer can be remarkably well tolerated but probably increases the risk of recurrence and mortality, particularly in older patients. The staging of PTC by the TNM system is outlined in Table 4-11. Most papillary cancers are identified in the early stages (>80% stages I or II) and have an excellent prognosis, with survival curves similar to expected survival (**Fig. 4-11***A*). Mortality is markedly increased in stage IV disease (distant metastases), but this group comprises only about 1% of patients. The treatment of PTC is described below.

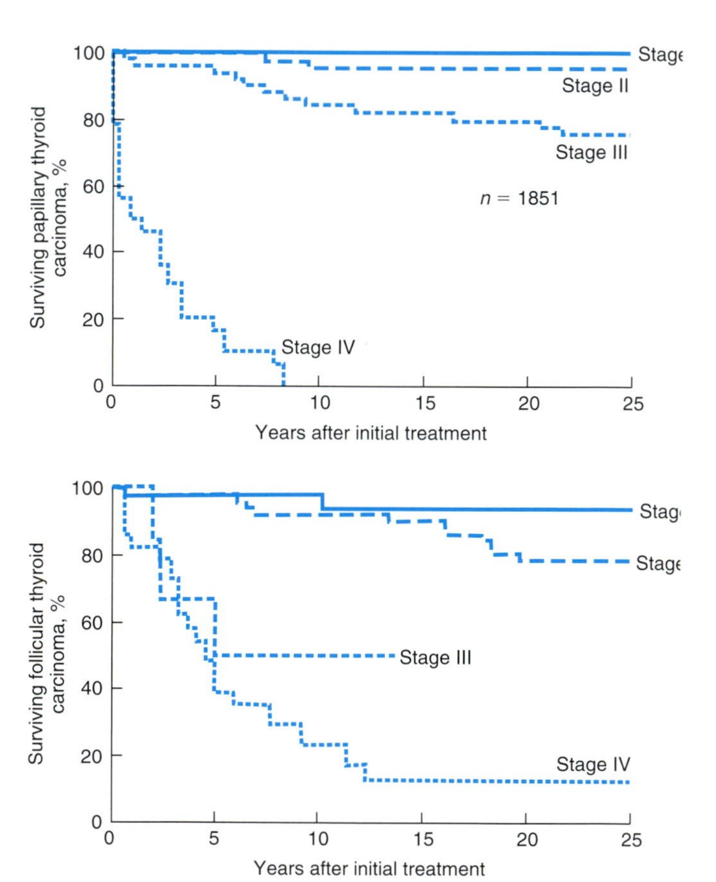

FIGURE 4-11

Survival rates in patients with differentiated thyroid cancer. ***A.*** Papillary cancer, cohort of 1851 patients. I, 1107 (60%), II, 408 (22%), III, 312 (17%), IV, 24 (1%); *n* = 1185. ***B.*** Follicular cancer, cohort of 153 patients. I, 42 (27%), II, 82 (54%), III, 6 (4%); IV, 23 (15%); *n* = 153. *[Adapted from PR Larsen et al: William's Textbook of Endocrinology, 9th ed, JD Wilson et al (eds). Philadelphia, Saunders, 1998, pp 389-575; with permission.]*

Follicular

The incidence of FTC varies widely in different parts of the world; it is more common in iodine-deficient regions. FTC is difficult to diagnose by FNA because the distinction between benign and malignant follicular neoplasms rests largely on evidence of invasion into vessels, nerves, or adjacent structures. FTC tends to spread by hematogenous routes leading to bone, lung, and central nervous system metastases. Mortality rates associated with FTC are less favorable than for PTC, in part because a larger proportion of patients present with stage IV disease (Fig. 4-11*B*). Poor prognostic features include distant metastases, age >50 years, primary tumor size >4 cm, Hürthle cell histology, and the presence of marked vascular invasion.

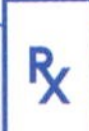

TREATMENT FOR THYROID CANCER

Surgery

All well-differentiated thyroid cancers should be surgically excised. In addition to removing the primary lesion, surgery allows accurate histologic diagnosis and staging, and multicentric disease is commonly found in the contralateral thyroid lobe. Lymph node spread can also be assessed at the time of surgery, and involved nodes can be removed. Recommendations about the extent of surgery vary for stage I disease, as survival rates are similar for lobectomy and near-total thyroidectomy. Lobectomy is associated with a lower incidence of hypoparathyroidism and injury to the recurrent laryngeal nerves. However, it is not possible to monitor Tg levels or to perform whole-body ^{131}I scans in the presence of the residual lobe. Moreover, if final staging or subsequent follow-up indicates the need for radioiodine scanning or treatment, repeat surgery is necessary to remove the remaining thyroid tissue. Therefore, near-total thyroidectomy is preferable in almost all patients; complication rates are acceptably low if the surgeon is highly experienced in the procedure. This approach, in combination with postsurgical radioablation of the remnant thyroid tissue, facilitates the use of radioiodine scanning and Tg determinations to assess disease recurrence.

TSH Suppression Therapy

As most tumors are still TSH-responsive, levothyroxine suppression of TSH is a mainstay of thyroid cancer treatment. Though TSH suppression clearly provides therapeutic benefit, there are no prospective studies that identify the optimal level of TSH suppression. A reasonable goal is to suppress TSH as much as possible without subjecting the patient to unnecessary side effects from excess thyroid hormone, such as atrial fibrillation, osteopenia, anxiety, and other manifestations of thyrotoxicosis. For patients at low risk of recurrence, TSH should be suppressed into the low but detectable range (0.1 to 0.5 IU/L). For patients at high risk of recurrence, or with known metastatic disease, complete TSH suppression is indicated, if there are no strong contraindications to mild thyrotoxicosis. In this instance, unbound T_4 must also be monitored to avoid excessive treatment.

Radioiodine Treatment

Well-differentiated thyroid cancer still incorporates radioiodine, though less efficiently than normal thyroid follicular cells. Radioiodine uptake is determined primarily by expression of the NIS and is stimulated by TSH, requiring expression of the TSH-R. The retention time for radioactivity is influenced by the extent to which the tumor retains differentiated functions such as iodide trapping and organification. After near-total thyroidectomy, substantial thyroid tissue remains, particularly in the thyroid bed and surrounding the parathyroid glands. Consequently, ^{131}I ablation is necessary to eliminate remaining normal thyroid tissue and to treat residual tumor cells.

Indications

The use of therapeutic doses of radioiodine remains an area of controversy in thyroid cancer management. Postoperative thyroid ablation and radiodine treatment of known residual PTC or FTC reduce recurrence rates. For tumors that take up iodine, ^{131}I treatment can reduce or eliminate residual disease with relatively little associated toxicity. However, it is not clear that prophylactic radioiodine treatment reduces mortality for patients at relatively low risk. Most patients with stage 1 PTC with primary tumors <1.5 cm in size can be managed safely with thyroxine suppression, without radiation treatment, as the risk of recurrence and mortality is very low. For patients with larger papillary tumors, spread to the adjacent lymph nodes, FTC, or evidence of metastases, thyroid ablation and radioiodine treatment are generally indicated.

^{131}I THYROID ABLATION AND TREATMENT

As noted above, the decision to use ^{131}I for thyroid ablation should be coordinated with the surgical approach, as radioablation is much more effective when there is minimal remaining normal thyroid tissue. A typical strategy is to treat the patient for several weeks postoperatively with liothyronine (25 μg bid or tid), followed by thyroid hormone withdrawal. Ideally, the TSH level should increase to >50 IU/L over 3 to 4 weeks. The level to which TSH rises is dictated largely by the amount of normal thyroid tissue remaining postoperatively. A scanning dose of ^{131}I [usually 148 to 185 MBq (4 to 5 mCi)] will reveal the amount of residual tissue and provides guidance about the dose needed to accomplish ablation. A maximum outpatient ^{131}I dose is 1110 MBq (29.9 mCi) in the United States, though ablation is often more complete using greater doses [1850 to 2775 MBq (50 to 75 mCi)]. In patients with known residual cancer, the larger doses ensure thyroid ablation and may destroy remaining tumor cells. A whole-body scan following the high-dose radioiodine treatment is useful to identify possible metastatic disease.

FOLLOW-UP WHOLE-BODY THYROID SCANNING AND THYROGLOBULIN DETERMINATIONS

An initial whole-body scan should be performed about 6 months after surgery and thyroid ablation. The strategy for follow-up management of thyroid cancer has been altered by the availability of recombinant human TSH (rhTSH) to stimulate ^{131}I uptake and by the improved sensitivity of Tg assays to detect residual or recurrent disease. A scheme for using either rhTSH or thyroid hormone withdrawal for thyroid scanning is summarized in **Fig. 4-12**. After thyroid ablation, rhTSH can be used to stimulate ^{131}I uptake without subjecting patients to thyroid hormone withdrawal and its associated symptoms of hypothyroidism and the risk of prolonged TSH-stimulated tumor growth. This approach is recommended for patients predicted to be at low risk of disease recurrence, since rhTSH is not currently approved for use in conjunction with therapeutic doses of ^{131}I. Alternatively, in patients who are likely to require ^{131}I treatment, the traditional approach of thyroid hormone withdrawal can be used to increase TSH. This involves switching patients from levothyroxine (T_4) to the more rapidly cleared hormone, liothyronine (T_3), thereby allowing TSH to increase more quickly. If residual disease is detected on the initial whole-body scan [148 to 185 MBq (4 to 5 mCi)], a larger treatment dose, usually between 2775 and 5550 MBq (75 and 150 mCi), can be administered depending on the degree of residual uptake and assessment of cancer risk. Because TSH stimulates Tg

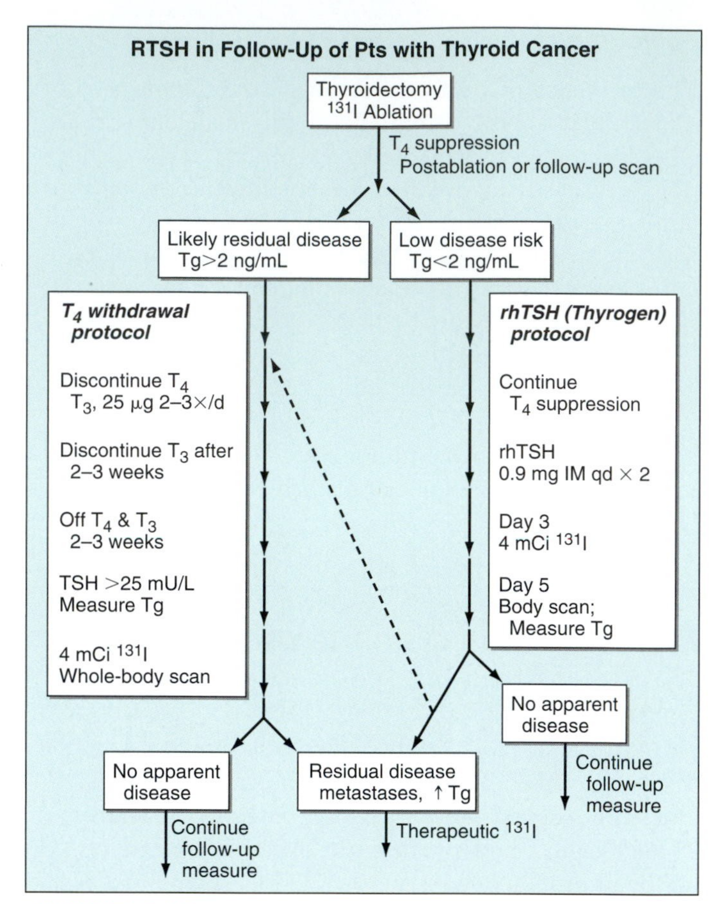

FIGURE 4-12

Use of recombinant thyroid-stimulating hormone (TSH) in the follow-up of patients with thyroid cancer. Tg, thyroglobulin; rhTSH, recombinant human TSH.

levels, Tg measurements should be obtained after administration of rhTSH or when TSH levels have risen after thyroid hormone withdrawal. Investigational protocols are measuring Tg levels after rhTSH stimulation but without radioiodine scanning. If the initial whole-body scan is negative and Tg levels are low, a repeat scan should be performed 1 year later. If still negative, the patient can be managed with suppressive therapy and measurements of Tg every 6 to 12 months. If a second follow-up scan is negative, no further scanning may be necessary if the patient is at low risk and there is no clinical or laboratory evidence of recurrence. Many authorities advocate radioiodine treatment for scan-negative, Tg-positive (Tg >5 to 10 ng/mL) patients, as many derive therapeutic benefit from a large dose of ^{131}I.

In addition to radioiodine, external beam radiotherapy is also used to treat specific metastatic lesions, particularly when they cause bone pain or threaten neurologic injury (e.g., vertebral metastases).

ANAPLASTIC AND OTHER FORMS OF THYROID CANCER

Anaplastic Thyroid Cancer

As noted above, ATC is a poorly differentiated and aggressive cancer. The prognosis is poor, and most patients die within 6 months of diagnosis. Because of the undifferentiated state of these tumors, the uptake of radioiodine is usually negligible, but it can be used therapeutically if there is residual uptake. Chemotherapy has been attempted with multiple agents, including anthracyclines and paclitaxel, but is usually ineffective. External radiation therapy can be attempted and continued if tumors are responsive.

Thyroid Lymphoma

Lymphoma in the thyroid gland often arises in the background of Hashimoto's thyroiditis. A rapidly expanding thyroid mass suggests the possibility of this diagnosis. Diffuse large cell lymphoma is the most common type in the thyroid. Biopsies reveal sheets of lymphoid cells that can be difficult to distinguish from small cell lung cancer or ATC. These tumors are often highly sensitive to external radiation. Surgical resection should be avoided as initial therapy because it may spread disease that is otherwise localized to the thyroid. If staging indicates disease outside of the thyroid, treatment should follow guidelines used for other forms of lymphoma.

MEDULLARY THYROID CARCINOMA

MTC can be sporadic or familial and accounts for about 5 to 10% of thyroid cancers. There are three familial forms of MTC: MEN 2A, MEN 2B, and familial MTC without other features of MEN (Chap. 21). In general, MTC is more aggressive in MEN 2B than in MEN 2A, and familial MTC is more aggressive than sporadic MTC. Elevated serum calcitonin provides a marker of residual or recurrent disease. It is reasonable to test all patients with MTC for *RET* mutations, as genetic counseling and testing of family members can be offered to those individuals who test positive for mutations.

The management of MTC is primarily surgical. Unlike tumors derived from thyroid follicular cells, these tumors do not take up radioiodine. External radiation treatment and chemotherapy may provide palliation in patients with advanced disease (Chap. 21).

APPROACH TO THE PATIENT WITH THYROID CANCER

Patient with a Thyroid Nodule

Palpable thyroid nodules are found in about 5% of adults, but the prevalence varies considerably worldwide. Given this high prevalence rate, it is common for the practitioner to identify thyroid nodules. The main goal of this evaluation is to

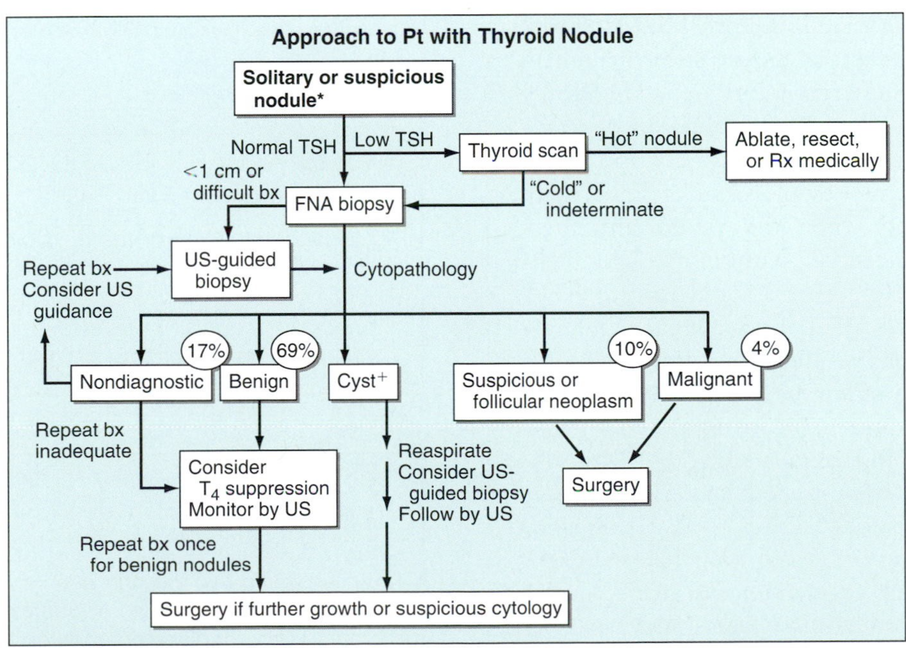

FIGURE 4-13

Approach to the patient with a thyroid nodule. *There are many exceptions to the suggested options. See text and references for details. †About one-third of nodules are cystic or mixed solid-cystic. US, ultrasound; TSH, thyroid-stimulating hormone; FNA, fine-needle aspiration.

identify, in a cost-effective manner, the small subgroup of individuals with malignant lesions.

As described above, nodules are more common in iodine-deficient areas, in women, and with aging. Most palpable nodules are >1 cm in diameter, but the ability to feel a nodule is influenced by its location within the gland (superficial versus deeply embedded), the anatomy of the patient's neck, and the experience of the examiner. More sensitive methods of detection, such as thyroid ultrasound and pathologic studies, reveal thyroid nodules in >20% of glands. These findings have led to much debate about how to detect nodules and which nodules to investigate further. Most authorities still rely on physical examination to detect thyroid nodules, reserving ultrasound for monitoring nodule size or as an aid in thyroid biopsy.

It is important to distinguish whether a patient presents with a solitary thyroid nodule or a prominent nodule in the context of a MNG, as the incidence of malignancy is greater in solitary nodules. An approach to the evaluation of a solitary nodule is outlined in **Fig. 4-13**. Most patients with thyroid nodules have normal thyroid function tests. Nonetheless, thyroid function should be assessed by measuring a TSH level, which may be suppressed by one or more autonomously functioning nodules. If the TSH is suppressed, a radionuclide scan is indicated to determine if the identified nodule is "hot," as lesions with increased uptake are almost never malignant and FNA is unnecessary. Otherwise, FNA biopsy should be the first step in the evaluation of a thyroid nodule. FNA has good sensitivity and specificity when performed by physicians familiar with the procedure and when the results are interpreted by experienced cytopathologists. The technique is particularly accurate for detecting PTC. The distinction of benign and malignant follicular lesions is often not possible using cytology alone.

In several large studies, FNA biopsies yielded the following findings: 70% benign, 10% malignant or suspicious for malignancy, and 20% nondiagnostic or yielding insufficient material for diagnosis. Characteristic features of malignancy mandate surgery. A diagnosis of follicular neoplasm also warrants surgery, as benign and malignant lesions cannot be distinguished based on cytopathology or frozen section. The management of patients with benign lesions is more variable. Many authorities advocate TSH suppression, whereas others monitor nodule size without suppression. With either approach, thyroid nodule size should be monitored, either by palpation or ultrasound. Repeat FNA is indicated if a nodule enlarges, and a second biopsy should be performed within 2 to 5 years to confirm the benign status of the nodule.

Nondiagnostic biopsies occur for many reasons, including a fibrotic reaction with relatively few cells available for aspiration, a cystic lesion in which cellular components reside along the cyst margin, or a nodule that may be too small for accurate aspiration. For these reasons, ultrasound-guided FNA is useful when the FNA is repeated. Ultrasound is also increasingly used for initial biopsies in an effort to enhance nodule localization and the accuracy of sampling.

The evaluation of a thyroid nodule is stressful for most patients. They are concerned about the possibility of thyroid cancer, whether verbalized or not. It is constructive, therefore, to review the diagnostic approach and to reassure patients when malignancy is not found. When a suspicious lesion or thyroid cancer is identified, an explanation of the generally favorable prognosis and available treatment options should be provided.

FURTHER READINGS

Abraham P et al: Antithyroid drug regimen for treating Graves' hyperthyroidism. Cochrane Database Syst Rev:CD003420, 2004

Bianco AC et al: Biochemistry, cellular and molecular biology, and physiological roles of the iodothyronine selenodeiodinases. Endocr Rev 23:38, 2002

Our understanding of the physiologic role of the iodothyronine deiodinases has increased rapidly since the cloning of their cDNAs and the development of murine knockout models. This review summarizes the complex function and biology of this family of enzymes.

Braga M et al: Efficacy of ultrasound-guided fine-needle aspiration biopsy in the diagnosis of complex thyroid nodules. J Clin Endocrinol Metab 86:4089, 2001

An evaluation of the fine needle aspiration in 113 patients with cystic thyroid nodules, demonstrating efficacy in 94% of biopsied nodules.

Cooper DS: Antithyroid drugs. N Engl J Med 352:905, 2005

de Vijlder JJ: Primary congenital hypothyroidism: Defects in iodine pathways. Eur J Endocrinol 149:247, 2003

◪ FAGIN JA: How thyroid tumors start and why it matters: kinase mutants as targets for solid cancer pharmacotherapy. J Endocrinol 183:249, 2004

A review of recent breakthroughs in the pathogenesis of thyroid cancer with a focus on potential new approaches for medical therapy.

◪ GHARIB H et al: Subclinical thyroid dysfunction: A joint statement on management from the American Association of Clinical Endocrinologists, the American Thyroid Association, and the Endocrine Society. J Clin Endocrinol Metab 90:581, 2005

The diagnosis and management of subclinical thyroid dysfunction has been highly controversial. This joint statement represents expert opinion from major U.S. endocrine societies.

GRUTERS A et al: Molecular genetic defects in congenital hypothyroidism. Eur J Endocrinol 151 Suppl 3:U39, 2004

LIN SH: Thyrotoxic periodic paralysis. Mayo Clin Proc 80:99, 2005

◪ MAZZAFERRI EL et al: A consensus report of the role of serum thyroglobulin as a monitoring method for low-risk patients with papillary thyroid carcinoma. J Clin Endocrinol Metab 88:1433, 2003

Based on a comprehensive review of numerous studies, the consensus group recommends a Tg cutoff of 2 microgram/liter (either after thyroid hormone withdrawal or 72 h after rhTSH) in the follow-up management of low-risk patients with differentiated thyroid cancer.

◪ PRABHAKAR BS et al: Current perspective on the pathogenesis of Graves' disease and ophthalmopathy. Endocr Rev 24:802, 2003

An extensive review of immunologic pathways that cause Graves' hyperthyroidism and ophthalmopathy. The article focuses on new insights derived from cloning the TSH receptor.

ROBERTS CG et al: Hypothyroidism. Lancet 363:793, 2004

◪ SMALLRIDGE RC, LADENSON PW: Hypothyroidism in pregnancy: Consequences to neonatal health. J Clin Endocrinol Metab 86:2349, 2001

This review updates concepts of thyroid hormone transfer across the placenta and the consequences of maternal hypothyroidism on the developing fetus.

◪ WHITLEY RJ et al: Thyroglobulin: A specific serum marker for the management of thyroid carcinoma. Clin Lab Med 24:29, 2004

Serum thyroglobulin is an important marker for recurrence of differentiated thyroid cancer. This article summarizes the limitations of this assay, including the formation of autoantibodies.

◪ ZIMMERMANN MB: Assessing iodine status and monitoring progress of iodized salt programs. J Nutr 134:1673, 2004

Iodine deficiency remains a significant global health problem. This review discusses clinical endpoints that should be evaluated to assess the efficacy of iodine supplementation programs.

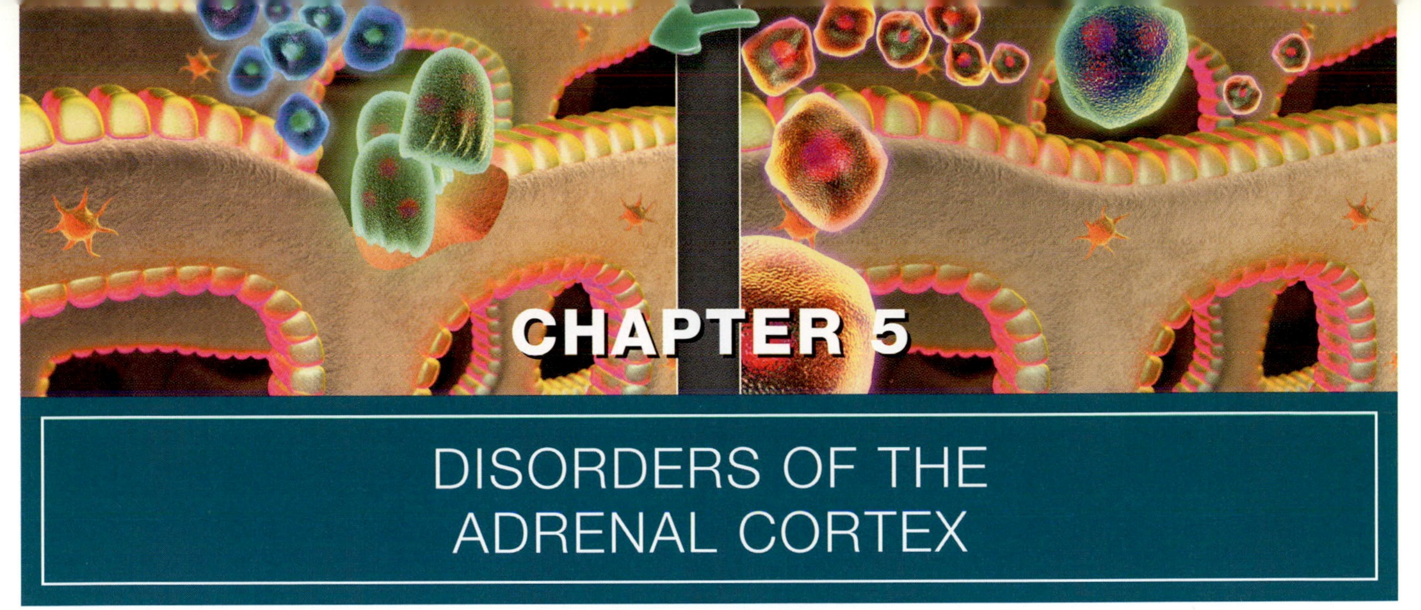

DISORDERS OF THE ADRENAL CORTEX

Gordon H. Williams
Robert G. Dluhy

BIOCHEMISTRY AND PHYSIOLOGY

The adrenal cortex produces three major classes of steroids: (1) glucocorticoids, (2) mineralocorticoids, and (3) adrenal androgens. Consequently, normal adrenal function is important for modulating intermediary metabolism and immune responses through glucocorticoids; blood pressure, vascular volume, and electrolytes through mineralocorticoids; and secondary sexual characteristics (in females) through androgens. The adrenal axis plays an important role in the stress response by rapidly increasing cortisol levels. Adrenal disorders include hyperfunction (Cushing's syndrome) and hypofunction (adrenal insufficiency), as well as a variety of genetic abnormalities of steroidogenesis.

STEROID NOMENCLATURE

The basic structure of steroids is built on a five-ring nucleus (**Fig. 5-1**). The carbon atoms are numbered in a sequence beginning with ring A. Adrenal steroids contain either 19 or 21 carbon atoms. The C_{19} steroids have methyl groups at C-18 and C-19. C_{19} steroids with a ketone group at C-17 are termed *17-ketosteroids*; C_{19} steroids have predominantly androgenic activity. The C_{21} steroids have a 2-carbon side chain (C-20 and C-21) attached at position 17 and methyl groups at C-18 and C-19; C_{21} steroids with a hydroxyl group at position 17 are termed *17-hydroxycorticosteroids*. The C_{21} steroids have either glucocorticoid or mineralocorticoid properties.

BIOSYNTHESIS OF ADRENAL STEROIDS

Cholesterol, derived from the diet and from endogenous synthesis, is the substrate for steroidogenesis. Uptake of cholesterol by the adrenal cortex is mediated by the low-density lipoprotein (LDL) receptor. With long-term stimulation of the adrenal cortex by adrenocorticotropic hormone (ACTH), the number of LDL receptors increases. The three major adrenal biosynthetic pathways lead to the production of glucocorticoids (cortisol),

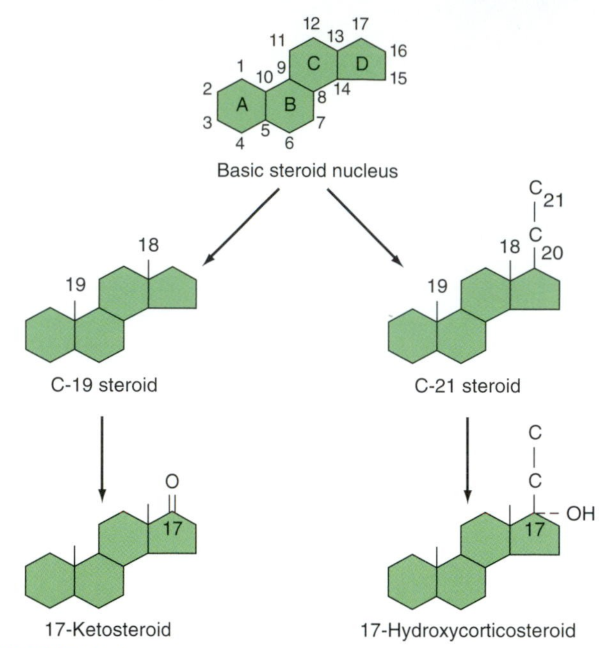

FIGURE 5-1
Basic steroid structure and nomenclature.

mineralocorticoids (aldosterone), and adrenal androgens (dehydroepiandrosterone). Separate zones of the adrenal cortex synthesize specific hormones (**Fig. 5-2**). This zonation is accompanied by the selective expression of the genes encoding the enzymes unique to the formation of each type of steroid: aldosterone synthase is normally expressed only in the outer (glomerulosa) cell layer, whereas 21- and 17-hydroxylase are expressed in the (inner) fasiculata-reticularis cell layers, which are the sites of cortisol and androgen biosynthesis, respectively.

STEROID TRANSPORT

Cortisol circulates in the plasma as free cortisol, protein-bound cortisol, and cortisol metabolites. *Free cortisol* is a physiologically active hormone that is not protein-bound and therefore can act directly on tissue sites. Normally, <5% of circulating cortisol is free. Only the unbound cortisol and its metabolites are filterable at the glomerulus. Increased quantities of free steroid are excreted in the urine in states characterized by hypersecretion of cortisol, because the unbound fraction of plasma cortisol rises. Plasma has two cortisol-binding systems. One is a high-affinity, low-capacity α_2-globulin termed *transcortin* or *cortisol-binding globulin* (CBG), and the other is a low-affinity, high-capacity protein, *albumin*. Cortisol binding to CBG is reduced in areas of inflammation, thus increasing the local concentration of free cortisol. When the concentration of cortisol is >700 nmol/L (25 μg/dL), part of the excess binds to albumin, and a greater proportion than usual circulates unbound. CBG is increased in high-estrogen states (e.g., pregnancy, oral contraceptive administration). The rise in CBG is accompanied by a parallel rise in *protein-bound cortisol,* with the result that the total plasma cortisol concentration is elevated. However, the free cortisol level probably remains normal, and manifestations of glucocorticoid excess are absent. Most synthetic glucocorticoid analogues bind less efficiently to CBG (~70% binding). This may explain the propensity of some synthetic analogues to produce cushingoid effects at low doses. *Cortisol metabolites* are biologically inactive and bind only weakly to circulating plasma proteins.

Aldosterone is bound to proteins to a smaller extent than cortisol, and an ultrafiltrate of plasma contains as much as 50% of circulating aldosterone.

STEROID METABOLISM AND EXCRETION

Glucocorticoids

The daily secretion of cortisol ranges between 40 and 80 μmol (15 and 30 mg; 8–10 mg/m^2), with a pronounced circadian cycle. The plasma concentration of cortisol is determined by the rate of secretion, the rate of inactivation, and the rate of excretion of free cortisol. The liver is the major organ responsible for steroid inactivation. A major enzyme regulating cortisol metabolism is 11β-hydroxysteroid dehydrogenase (11β-HSD). There are two isoforms: 11β-HSD I is primarily expressed in the liver and acts as a reductase, converting the inactive cortisone to the active glucocorticoid, cortisol; the 11β-HSD II isoform is expressed in a number of tissues and converts cortisol to the inactive metabolite, cortisone. Mutations in the *11BHSD1* gene are associated with rapid cortisol turnover, leading to activation of the hypothalamic-pituitary-adrenal (HPA) axis and excessive adrenal androgen production in women. In animal models, excess omental expression of 11β-HSD I increases local glucocorticoid production and is associated with central obesity and insulin resistance. The oxidative reaction of 11β-HSD I is increased in hyperthyroidism. Mutations in the *11BHSD2* gene cause the syndrome of *apparent mineralocorticoid excess,* reflecting insufficient inactivation of cortisol in the kidney, allowing inappropriate cortisol activation of the mineralocorticoid receptor (see below).

Mineralocorticoids

In individuals with normal salt intake, the average daily secretion of aldosterone ranges between 0.1 and 0.7 μmol (50 and 250 μg). During a single passage through the liver, >75% of circulating aldosterone is normally inactivated by conjugation with glucuronic acid. However, under certain conditions, such as congestive failure, this rate of inactivation is reduced.

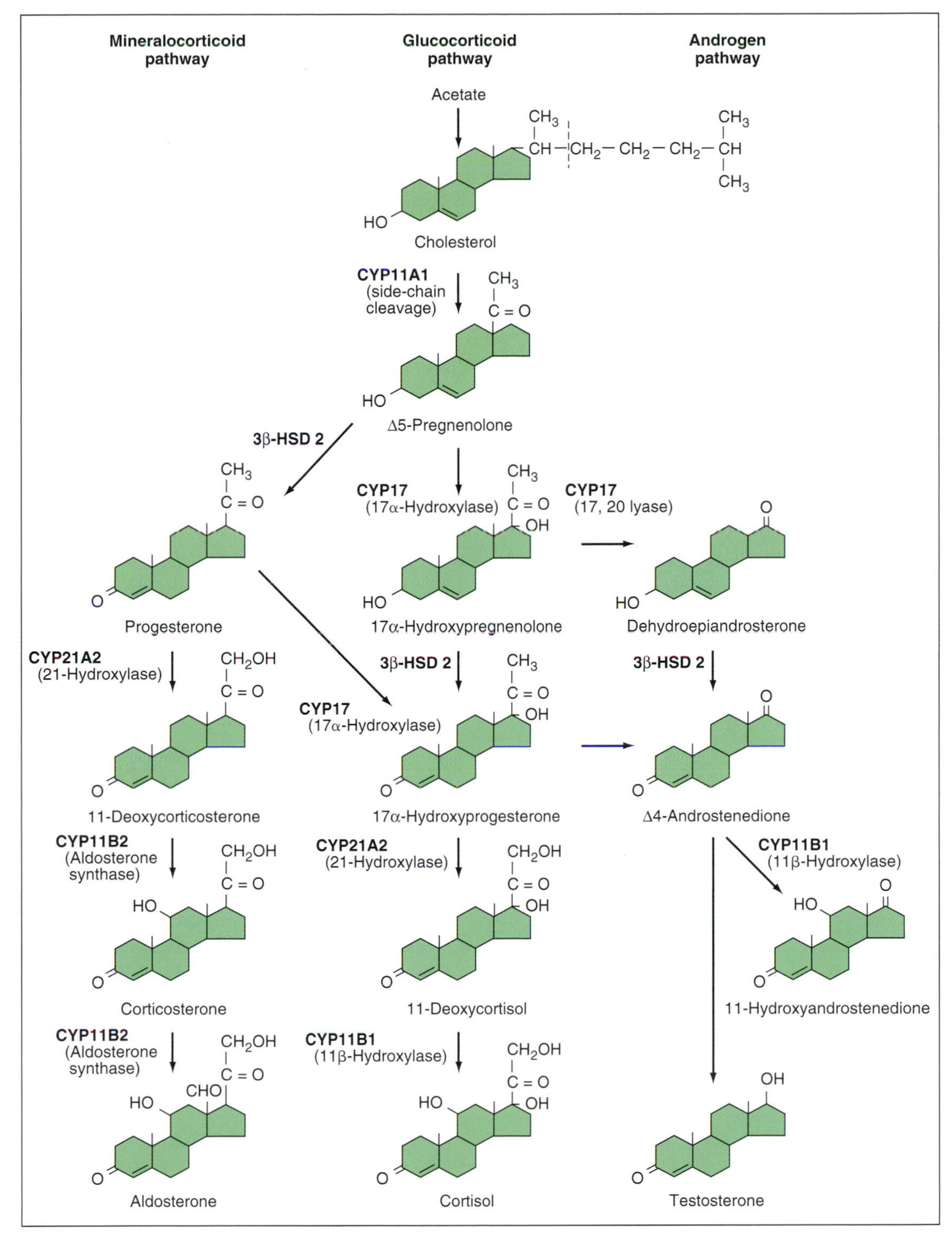

FIGURE 5-2
Biosynthetic pathways for adrenal steroid production; major pathways to mineralocorticoids, glucocorticoids, and androgens. 3β-HSD, 3β-hydroxysteroid dehydrogenase.

Adrenal Androgens

The major androgen secreted by the adrenal is dehydroepiandrosterone (DHEA) and its sulfuric acid ester (DHEAS). Approximately 15 to 30 mg of these compounds is secreted daily. Smaller amounts of androstenedione, 11β-hydroxyandrostenedione, and testosterone are secreted. DHEA is the major precursor of the urinary 17-ketosteroids. Two-thirds of the urine 17-ketosteroids in the male are derived from adrenal metabolites, and the remaining one-third comes from testicular androgens. In the female, almost all urine 17-ketosteroids are derived from the adrenal.

Steroids diffuse passively through the cell membrane and bind to intracellular receptors (Chap. 1). Glucocorticoids and mineralocorticoids bind with nearly equal affinity to the mineralocorticoid receptor (MR). However, only glucocorticoids bind to the glucocorticoid receptor (GR). After the steroid binds to the receptor, the steroid-receptor complex is transported to the nucleus, where it binds to specific sites on steroid-regulated genes, altering levels of transcription. Some actions of glucocorticoids (e.g., anti-inflammatory effects) are mediated by GR-mediated inhibition of other transcription factors, such as activating protein-1 (AP-1) or nuclear factor kappa B (NFκB), which normally stimulate the activity of various cytokine genes. Because cortisol binds to the MR with the same affinity as aldosterone, mineralocorticoid specificity is achieved by local metabolism of cortisol to the inactive compound cortisone by 11β-HSD II. The glucocorticoid effects of other steroids, such as high-dose progesterone, correlate with their relative binding affinities for the GR. Inherited defects in the GR cause glucocorticoid resistance states. Individuals with GR defects have high levels of cortisol but do not have manifestations of hypercortisolism.

ACTH PHYSIOLOGY

ACTH and a number of other peptides (lipotropins, endorphins, and melanocyte-stimulating hormones) are processed from a larger precursor molecule of 31,000 mol wt—proopiomelanocortin (POMC) (Chap. 2). POMC is made in a variety of tissues, including brain, anterior and posterior pituitary, and lymphocytes. The constellation of POMC-derived peptides secreted depends on the tissue. ACTH, a 39-amino-acid peptide, is synthesized and stored in basophilic cells of the anterior pituitary. The *N*-terminal 18-amino-acid fragment of ACTH has full biologic potency, and shorter *N*-terminal fragments have partial biologic activity. Release of ACTH and related peptides from the anterior pituitary gland is stimulated by corticotropin-releasing hormone (CRH), a 41-amino-acid peptide produced in the median eminence of the hypothalamus (**Fig. 5-3**). Urocortin, a neuropeptide related to CRH, mimics many of the central effects of CRH (e.g., appetite suppression, anxiety), but its role in ACTH regulation is unclear. Some related peptides such as β-lipotropin (β-LPT) are released in equimolar concentrations with ACTH, suggesting that they are cleaved enzymatically from the parent POMC before or during the secretory process. However, β-endorphin levels may or may not correlate with circulating levels of ACTH, depending on the nature of the stimulus.

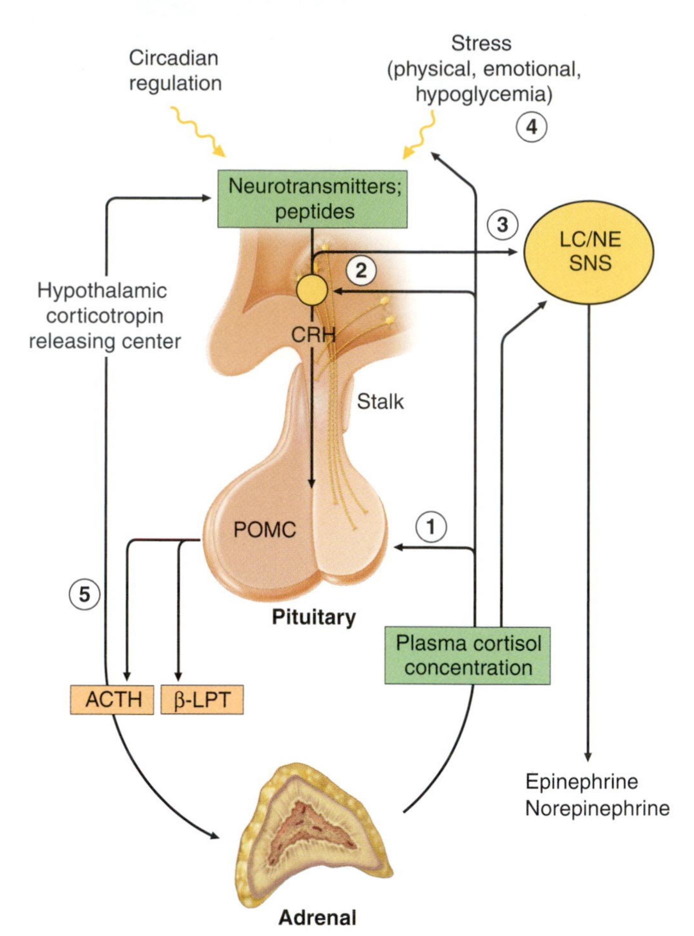

FIGURE 5-3
The hypothalamic-pituitary-adrenal axis. The main sites for feedback control by plasma cortisol are the pituitary gland (**1**) and the hypothalamic corticotropin-releasing center (**2**). Feedback control by plasma cortisol also occurs at the locus coeruleus/sympathetic system (**3**) and may involve higher nerve centers (**4**) as well. There may also be a short feedback loop involving inhibition of corticotropin-releasing hormone (CRH) by adrenocorticotropic hormone (ACTH) (**5**). Hypothalamic neurotransmitters influence CRH release; serotoninergic and cholinergic systems stimulate the secretion of CRH and ACTH; α-adrenergic agonists and γ-aminobutyric acid (GABA) probably inhibit CRH release. The opioid peptides β-endorphin and enkephalin inhibit, and vasopressin and angiotensin II augment, the secretion of CRH and ACTH. β-LPT, β-lipotropin; POMC, proopiomelanocortin; LC, locus coeruleus; NE, norepinephrine; SNS, sympathetic nervous system.

The major factors controlling ACTH release include CRH, the free cortisol concentration in plasma, stress, and the sleep-wake cycle (Fig. 5-3). Plasma ACTH varies during the day as a result of its pulsatile secretion, and follows a circadian pattern with a peak just prior to waking and a nadir before sleeping. If a new sleep-wake cycle is adopted, the pattern changes over several days to conform to it. ACTH and cortisol levels also increase in response to eating. Stress (e.g., pyrogens, surgery, hypoglycemia, exercise, and severe emotional trauma) causes the release of CRH and arginine vasopressin (AVP) and activation of the sympathetic nervous system. These changes in turn enhance ACTH release, acting individually or in concert. For example, AVP release acts synergistically with CRH to amplify ACTH secretion; CRH also stimulates the locus coeruleus/sympathetic system. Stress-related secretion of ACTH abolishes the circadian periodicity of ACTH levels but is, in turn, suppressed by prior high-dose glucocorticoid administration. The normal pulsatile, circadian pattern of ACTH release is regulated by CRH; this mechanism is the so-called open feedback loop. CRH secretion, in turn, is influenced by hypothalamic neurotransmitters including the serotoninergic and cholinergic pathways. The immune system also influences the HPA axis (**Fig. 5-4**). For example, inflammatory cytokines [tumor necrosis factor (TNF) α, interleukin (IL) 1α, IL-1β, and IL-6] produced by monocytes increase ACTH release by stimulating secretion of CRH and/or AVP. Finally, ACTH release is regulated by the level of free cortisol in plasma. Cortisol decreases the responsiveness of pituitary corticotropic cells to CRH; the response of the POMC mRNA to CRH is also inhibited by glucocorticoids. In addition, glucocorticoids inhibit the locus coeruleus/sympathetic system and CRH release. The latter servomechanism establishes the primacy of cortisol in the control of ACTH secretion. The suppression of ACTH secretion that results in adrenal atrophy following *prolonged* glucocorticoid therapy is caused primarily by suppression of hypothalamic CRH release, as exogenous CRH administration in this circumstance produces a rise in plasma ACTH. Cortisol also exerts feedback effects on higher brain centers (hippocampus, reticular system, and septum) and perhaps on the adrenal cortex (Fig. 5-4).

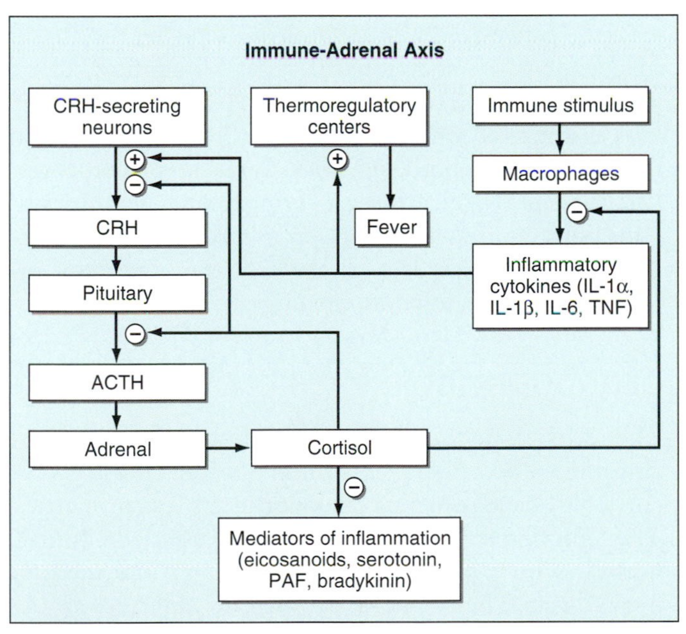

FIGURE 5-4

The immune-adrenal axis. Cortisol has anti-inflammatory properties that include effects on the microvasculature, cellular actions, and the suppression of inflammatory cytokines (the so-called immune-adrenal axis). A stress such as sepsis increases adrenal secretion, and cortisol in turn suppresses the immune response via this system. −, suppression; +, stimulation; CRH, corticotropin-releasing hormone; ACTH, adrenocorticotropic hormone; IL, interleukin; TNF, tumor necrosis factor; PAF, platelet activating factor.

The biologic half-life of ACTH in the circulation is <10 min. The action of ACTH also is rapid; within minutes of its release, the concentration of steroids in the adrenal venous blood increases. ACTH stimulates steroidogenesis via activation of adenyl cyclase. Adenosine-3′,5′-monophosphate (cyclic AMP), in turn, stimulates the synthesis of protein kinase enzymes, thereby resulting in the phosphorylation of proteins that activate steroid biosynthesis.

RENIN-ANGIOTENSIN PHYSIOLOGY

Renin is a proteolytic enzyme that is produced and stored in the granules of the juxtaglomerular cells surrounding the afferent arterioles of glomeruli in the kidney. Renin acts on the basic substrate angiotensinogen (a circulating α_2-globulin made in the liver) to form the decapeptide angiotensin I (**Fig. 5-5**). Angiotensin I is then enzymatically transformed by angiotensin-converting enzyme (ACE), which is present in many tissues (particularly the pulmonary vascular endothelium), to the octapeptide angiotensin II by the removal of the two C-terminal amino acids. Angiotensin II is a potent pressor agent and exerts its action by a direct effect on arteriolar smooth muscle. In addition, angiotensin II stimulates production of aldosterone by the zona glomerulosa of the adrenal cortex; the heptapeptide angiotensin III also may stimulate aldosterone production. The two major classes of angiotensin receptors are termed *AT1* and *AT2*; AT1 may exist as two subtypes-α and β. Most of the effects of angiotensins II and III are mediated by the AT1 receptor. Angiotensinases rapidly destroy angiotensin II (half-life, ~1 min), while the half-life of renin is more prolonged (10 to 20 min). In addition to circulating renin-angiotensin, many tissues have a local renin-angiotensin system and the ability to produce angiotensin II. These tissues include the uterus, placenta, vascular tissue, heart, brain, and, particularly, the adrenal cortex and kidney. Although the role of locally generated angiotensin II is not established, it may modulate the growth and function of the adrenal cortex and vascular smooth muscle.

The amount of renin released reflects the combined effects of four interdependent factors. The *juxtaglomerular*

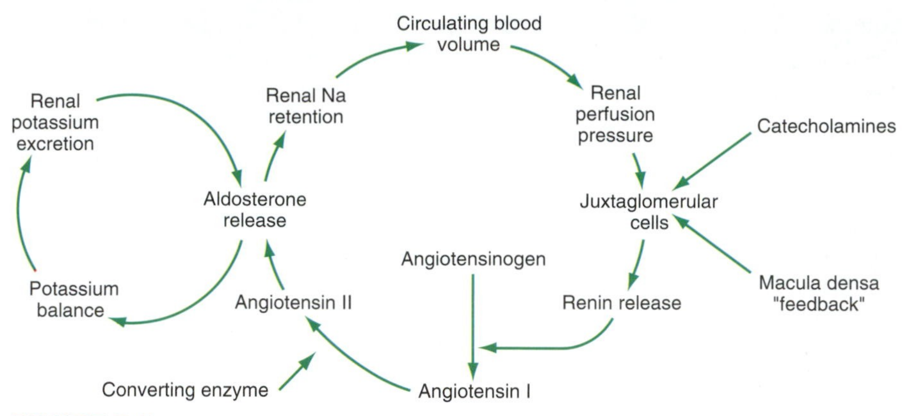

FIGURE 5-5

The interrelationship of the volume and potassium feedback loops on aldosterone secretion. Integration of signals from each loop determines the level of aldosterone secretion.

cells, which are specialized myoepithelial cells that cuff the afferent arterioles, act as miniature pressure transducers, sensing renal perfusion pressure and corresponding changes in afferent arteriolar perfusion pressures. For example, a reduction in circulating blood volume leads to a corresponding reduction in renal perfusion pressure and afferent arteriolar pressure (Fig. 5-5). This change is perceived by the juxtaglomerular cells as a decreased stretch exerted on the afferent arteriolar walls, and the juxtaglomerular cells release more renin into the renal circulation. This results in the formation of angiotensin I, which is converted in the kidney and peripherally to angiotensin II by ACE. Angiotensin II influences sodium homeostasis via two major mechanisms: it changes renal blood flow so as to maintain a constant glomerular filtration rate, thereby changing the filtration fraction of sodium, and it stimulates the adrenal cortex to release aldosterone. Increasing plasma levels of aldosterone enhance renal sodium retention and thus result in expansion of the extracellular fluid volume, which, in turn, dampens the stimulus for renin release. In this context, the renin-angiotensin-aldosterone system regulates volume by modifying renal hemodynamics and tubular sodium transport.

A second control mechanism for renin release is centered in the *macula densa cells,* a group of distal convoluted tubular epithelial cells directly opposed to the juxtaglomerular cells. They may function as chemoreceptors, monitoring the sodium (or chloride) load presented to the distal tubule. Under conditions of increased delivery of filtered sodium to the macula densa, a signal is conveyed to decrease juxtaglomerular cell release of renin, thereby modulating the glomerular filtration rate and the filtered load of sodium.

The *sympathetic nervous system* regulates the release of renin in response to assumption of the upright posture. The mechanism is either a direct effect on the juxtaglomerular cell to increase adenyl cyclase activity or an indirect effect on either the juxtaglomerular or the macula densa cells via vasoconstriction of the afferent arteriole.

Finally, circulating factors influence renin release. Increased dietary intake of potassium decreases renin release, whereas decreased potassium intake increases it. The significance of these effects is unclear. *Angiotensin II* exerts negative feedback control on renin release that is independent of alterations in renal blood flow, blood pressure, or aldosterone secretion. *Atrial natriuretic peptides* also inhibit renin release. Thus, the control of renin release involves both *intrarenal* (pressor receptor and macula densa) and *extrarenal* (sympathetic nervous system, potassium, angiotensin, etc.) mechanisms. Steady-state renin levels reflect all these factors, with the intrarenal mechanism predominating.

GLUCOCORTICOID PHYSIOLOGY

The division of adrenal steroids into glucocorticoids and mineralocorticoids is arbitrary in that most glucocorticoids have some mineralocorticoid-like properties. The descriptive term *glucocorticoid* is used for adrenal steroids whose predominant action is on intermediary metabolism. Their overall actions are directed at enhancing the production of the high-energy fuel, glucose, and reducing all other metabolic activity not directly involved in that process. Sustained activation, however, results in a pathophysiologic state, e.g., Cushing's syndrome. The principal glucocorticoid is cortisol (hydrocortisone). The effect of glucocorticoids on intermediary metabolism is mediated by the GR. Physiologic effects of glucocorticoids include the regulation of protein, carbohydrate, lipid, and nucleic acid metabolism. Glucocorticoids raise the blood glucose level by antagonizing the secretion and actions of insulin, thereby inhibiting peripheral glucose uptake, which promotes hepatic glucose synthesis (gluconeogenesis) and hepatic glycogen content. The actions on protein metabolism are mainly catabolic, resulting in an increase in protein breakdown and nitrogen excretion. In large part, these actions reflect a mobilization of glycogenic amino acid precursors from peripheral supporting structures, such as bone, skin, muscle, and connective tissue, due to protein breakdown and inhibition of protein synthesis and amino acid uptake. Hyperaminoacidemia also facilitates gluconeogenesis by stimulating glucagon secretion. Glucocorticoids act directly on the liver to stimulate the synthesis of certain enzymes, such as tyrosine aminotransferase and tryptophan pyrrolase. Glucocorticoids regulate fatty acid mobilization by enhancing the activation of cellular lipase by lipid-mobilizing hormones (e.g., catecholamines and pituitary peptides).

The actions of cortisol on protein and adipose tissue vary in different parts of the body. For example, pharmacologic doses of cortisol can deplete the protein matrix of the vertebral column (trabecular bone), whereas long bones (which are primarily compact bone) are affected only minimally; similarly, peripheral adipose tissue mass decreases, whereas abdominal and interscapular fat expand.

Glucocorticoids have anti-inflammatory properties, which are probably related to effects on the microvasculature and to suppression of inflammatory cytokines. In this sense, glucocorticoids modulate the immune response via the so-called immune-adrenal axis (Fig. 5-4). This "loop" is one mechanism by which a stress, such as sepsis, increases adrenal hormone secretion, and the elevated cortisol level in turn suppresses the immune response. For example, cortisol maintains vascular responsiveness to circulating vasoconstrictors and opposes the increase in capillary permeability during acute inflammation. Glucocorticoids cause a leukocytosis that reflects release from the bone marrow of mature cells as well as inhibition of their egress through the capillary wall. Glucocorticoids produce a depletion of circulating eosinophils and lymphoid tissue, specifically T cells, by causing a redistribution from the circulation into other compartments. Thus, cortisol impairs cell-mediated immunity. Glucocorticoids also inhibit the production and action of the mediators of inflammation, such as the lymphokines and prostaglandins. Glucocorticoids inhibit the production and action of interferon by T lymphocytes and the production of IL-1 and IL-6 by macrophages. The antipyretic action of glucocorticoids may be explained by an effect on IL-1, which appears to be an endogenous pyrogen (Chap. 16 in HPIM, 16e). Glucocorticoids also inhibit the production of T cell growth factor (IL-2) by T lymphocytes. Glucocorticoids reverse macrophage activation and antagonize the action of migration-inhibiting factor (MIF), leading to reduced adherence of macrophages to vascular endothelium. Glucocorticoids reduce prostaglandin and leukotriene production by inhibiting the activity of phospholipase A_2, thus blocking release of arachidonic acid from phospholipids. Finally, glucocorticoids inhibit the production and inflammatory effects of bradykinin, platelet-activating factor, and serotonin. It is probably only at pharmacologic dosages that antibody production is reduced and lysosomal membranes are stabilized, the latter effect suppressing the release of acid hydrolases.

Cortisol levels respond within minutes to stress, whether physical (trauma, surgery, exercise), psychological (anxiety, depression), or physiologic (hypoglycemia, fever). The reasons why elevated glucocorticoid levels protect the organism under stress are not understood, but in conditions of glucocorticoid deficiency, such stresses may cause hypotension, shock, and death. Consequently, in individuals with adrenal insufficiency, glucocorticoid administration should be increased during stress.

Cortisol has major effects on body water. It helps regulate the extracellular fluid volume by retarding the migration of water into cells and by promoting renal water excretion, the latter effect mediated by suppression of vasopressin secretion, by an increase in the rate of glomerular filtration, and by a direct action on the renal tubule. The consequence is to prevent water intoxication by increasing solute-free water clearance. Glucocorticoids also have weak mineralocorticoid-like properties, and high doses promote renal tubular sodium reabsorption and increased urine potassium excretion. Glucocorticoids can also influence behavior; emotional disorders may occur with either an excess or a deficit of cortisol. Finally, cortisol suppresses the secretion of pituitary POMC and its derivative peptides (ACTH, β-endorphin, and β-LPT) and the secretion of hypothalamic CRH and vasopressin.

MINERALOCORTICOID PHYSIOLOGY

Mineralocorticoids modify function in two classes of cells—epithelial and nonepithelial.

Effects on Epithelia

Classically, mineralocorticoids are considered major regulators of extracellular fluid volume and are the major determinants of potassium metabolism. These effects are mediated by the binding of aldosterone to the MR in epithelial cells, primarily the principal cells in the renal cortical collecting duct. Because of its electrochemical gradient, sodium passively enters these cells from the urine via epithelial sodium channels located on the luminal membrane and is actively extruded from the cell via the Na/K-activated ATPase ("sodium pump") located on the basolateral membrane. The sodium pump also provides the driving force of potassium loss into the urine through potassium-selective luminal channels, again assisted by the electrochemical gradient for potassium in these cells. Aldosterone stimulates all three of these processes by increasing gene expression directly (for the sodium pump and the potassium channels) or via a complex process (for epithelial sodium channels) to increase both the number and activity of the sodium channels. Water passively follows the transported sodium, thus expanding intra- and extravascular volume.

Because the concentration of hydrogen ion is greater in the lumen than in the cell, hydrogen ion is also actively secreted. Mineralocorticoids also act on the epithelium of the salivary ducts, sweat glands, and gastrointestinal tract to cause reabsorption of sodium in exchange for potassium.

When normal individuals are given aldosterone, an initial period of sodium retention is followed by natriuresis, and sodium balance is reestablished after 3 to 5 days. As a result, edema does not develop. This process is referred to as the *escape phenomenon,* signifying an "escape" by the renal tubules from the sodium-retaining action of aldosterone. While renal hemodynamic factors may play a role in the escape, the level of atrial natriuretic peptide also increases. However, it is important to realize that there is no escape from the potassium-losing effects of mineralocorticoids.

Effect on Nonepithelial Cells

The MR has been identified in a number of nonepithelial cells, e.g., neurons in the brain, myocytes, endothelial cells, and vascular smooth-muscle cells. In these cells, the actions of aldosterone differ from those in epithelial cells in several ways:

1. They do not modify sodium-potassium homeostasis.
2. The groups of regulated genes differ, although only a few are known–for example, in nonepithelial cells, aldosterone modifies the expression of several collagen genes and/or genes controlling tissue growth factors, e.g., transforming growth factor (TGF) β and plasminogen activator inhibitor type 1 (PAI-1).
3. In some of these tissues (e.g., myocardium and brain), the MR is not protected by the 11β-HSD II enzyme. Thus, cortisol rather than aldosterone may be activating the MR. In other tissues (e.g., the vasculature), 11β-HSD II is expressed in a manner similar to that of the kidney. Therefore, aldosterone is activating the MR.
4. Some effects on nonepithelial cells may occur via nongenomic mechanisms. These actions are too rapid—occurring within 1 to 2 min and peaking within 5 to 10 min—to be considered genomic, suggesting that they are secondary to activation of a cell-surface receptor. However, no cell-surface MR has been identified, raising the possibility that the same MR is mediating both genomic and nongenomic effects. Rapid, nongenomic effects have also been described for other steroids including estradiol, progesterone, thyroxine, and vitamin D.
5. Some of these tissues—the myocardium and vasculature—may also produce aldosterone, although this theory is controversial.

Regulation of Aldosterone Secretion

Three primary mechanisms control adrenal aldosterone secretion: the renin-angiotensin system, potassium, and ACTH (**Table 5-1**). Whether these are also the primary regulatory mechanisms modifying nonadrenal production is uncertain. The renin-angiotensin system controls extracellular fluid volume via regulation of aldosterone secretion (Fig. 5-5). In effect, the renin-angiotensin system maintains the circulating blood volume constant by causing aldosterone-induced sodium retention during volume deficiency and by decreasing aldosterone-dependent sodium retention when volume is ample. There is an increasing body of evidence indicating that some tissues, in addition to the kidney, produce angiotensin II and may participate in the regulation of aldosterone secretion from either the adrenal or extraadrenal sources. Intriguingly, the adrenal itself is capable of synthesizing angiotensin II. What role(s) the extrarenal production of angiotensin II plays in normal physiology is still largely unknown. However, the tissue renin-angiotensin system is activated in utero in response to growth and development and/or later in life in response to injury.

Potassium ion directly stimulates aldosterone secretion, independent of the circulating renin-angiotensin system, which it suppresses (Fig. 5-5). In addition to a direct effect, potassium also modifies aldosterone secretion indirectly by activating the local renin-angiotensin system in the zona glomerulosa. This effect can be blocked by the administration of ACE inhibitors that reduce the local production of angiotensin II and thereby reduce the acute aldosterone response to potassium. An increase in serum potassium of as little as 0.1 mmol/L increases plasma aldosterone

TABLE 5-1

FACTORS REGULATING ALDOSTERONE BIOSYNTHESIS

FACTOR	EFFECT
Renin-angiotensin system	Stimulation
Sodium ion	Inhibition (?physiologic)
Potassium ion	Stimulation
Neurotransmitters	
Dopamine	Inhibition
Serotonin	Stimulation
Pituitary hormones	
ACTH	Stimulation
Non-ACTH pituitary hormones (e.g., growth hormone)	Permissive (for optimal response to sodium restriction)
β-Endorphin	Stimulation
γ-Melanocyte-stimulating hormone	Permissive
Atrial natriuretic peptide	Inhibition
Ouabain-like factors	Inhibition
Endothelin	Stimulation

Note: ACTH, adrenocorticotropic hormone.

levels under certain circumstances. Oral potassium loading therefore increases aldosterone secretion, plasma levels, and excretion.

Physiologic amounts of ACTH stimulate aldosterone secretion acutely, but this action is not sustained unless ACTH is administered in a pulsatile fashion. Most studies relegate ACTH to a minor role in the control of aldosterone. For example, subjects receiving high-dose glucocorticoid therapy, and with presumed complete suppression of ACTH, have normal aldosterone secretion in response to sodium restriction.

Prior dietary intake of both potassium and sodium can alter the magnitude of the aldosterone response to acute stimulation. This effect results from a change in the expression and activity of aldosterone synthase. Increasing potassium intake or decreasing sodium intake sensitizes the response of the glomerulosa cells to acute stimulation by ACTH, angiotensin II, and/or potassium.

Neurotransmitters (dopamine and serotonin) and some peptides, such as atrial natriuretic peptide, γ-melanocyte-stimulating hormone (γ-MSH), and β-endorphin, also participate in the regulation of aldosterone secretion (Table 5-1). Thus, the control of aldosterone secretion involves both stimulatory and inhibitory factors.

ANDROGEN PHYSIOLOGY

Androgens regulate male secondary sexual characteristics and can cause virilizing symptoms in women (Chap. 12). Adrenal androgens have a minimal effect in males, whose sexual characteristics are predominately determined by gonadal steroids (testosterone). In females, however, several androgen-like effects, e.g., sexual hair, are largely mediated by adrenal androgens. The principal adrenal androgens are DHEA, androstenedione, and 11-hydroxyandrostenedione. DHEA and androstenedione are weak androgens and exert their effects via conversion to the potent androgen testosterone in extraglandular tissues. DHEA also has poorly understood effects on the immune and cardiovascular systems. Adrenal androgen formation is regulated by ACTH, not by gonadotropins. Adrenal androgens are suppressed by exogenous glucocorticoid administration.

LABORATORY EVALUATION OF ADRENOCORTICAL FUNCTION

A basic assumption is that measurements of the plasma or urinary level of a given steroid reflect the rate of adrenal *secretion* of that steroid. However, urine *excretion* values may not truly reflect the secretion rate because of improper collection or altered metabolism. Plasma levels reflect the level of secretion only at the time of measurement. The plasma level (*PL*) depends on two factors: the secretion rate (*SR*) of the hormone and the rate at which it is metabolized, i.e., its metabolic clearance rate (*MCR*). These three factors can be related as follows:

$$PL = SR/MCR \text{ or } SR = MCR \times PL$$

BLOOD LEVELS

Peptides

The plasma levels of ACTH and angiotensin II can be measured by immunoassay techniques. Basal ACTH secretion shows a circadian rhythm, with lower levels in the early evening than in the morning. However, ACTH is secreted in a pulsatile manner, leading to rapid fluctuations superimposed on this circadian rhythm. Angiotensin II levels also vary diurnally and are influenced by dietary sodium and potassium intakes and posture. Both upright posture and sodium restriction elevate angiotensin II levels.

Most clinical determinations of the renin-angiotensin system, however, involve measurements of peripheral *plasma renin activity* (PRA) in which the renin activity is gauged by the generation of angiotensin I during a standardized incubation period. This method depends on the presence of sufficient angiotensinogen in the plasma as substrate. The generated angiotensin I is measured by radioimmunoassay. The PRA depends on the dietary sodium intake and on whether the patient is ambulatory. In normal humans, the PRA shows a diurnal rhythm characterized by peak values in the morning and a nadir in the afternoon. An alternative approach is to measure plasma active renin, which is easier and not dependent on endogenous substrate concentration. PRA and active renin correlate very well on low-sodium diets but less well on high-sodium diets.

Steroids

Cortisol and aldosterone are both secreted episodically, and levels vary during the day, with peak values in the morning and low levels in the evening. In addition, the plasma level of aldosterone, but not of cortisol, is increased by dietary potassium loading, by sodium restriction, or by assumption of the upright posture. Measurement of the sulfate conjugate of DHEA may be a useful index of adrenal androgen secretion, as little DHEA sulfate is formed in the gonads and because the half-life of DHEA sulfate is 7 to 9 h. However, DHEA sulfate levels reflect both DHEA production and sulfatase activity.

URINE LEVELS

For the assessment of glucocorticoid secretion, the urine 17-hydroxycorticosteroid assay has been replaced by measurement of urinary free cortisol. Elevated levels of urinary free cortisol correlate with states of hypercortisolism, reflecting changes in the levels of unbound, physiologically active circulating cortisol. Normally, the rate of excretion is higher in the daytime (7 A.M. to 7 P.M.) than at night (7 P.M. to 7 A.M.).

Urinary 17-ketosteroids originate in either the adrenal gland or the gonad. In normal women, 90% of urinary 17-ketosteroids is derived from the adrenal, and in men 60 to 70% is of adrenal origin. Urine 17-ketosteroid values are highest in young adults and decline with age.

A carefully timed urine collection is a prerequisite for all excretory determinations. Urinary creatinine should be measured simultaneously to determine the accuracy and adequacy of the collection procedure.

STIMULATION TESTS

Stimulation tests are useful in the diagnosis of hormone deficiency states.

Tests of Glucocorticoid Reserve

Within minutes after administration of ACTH, cortisol levels increase. This responsiveness can be used as an index of the functional reserve of the adrenal gland for production of cortisol. Under maximal ACTH stimulation, cortisol secretion increases tenfold, to 800 μmol/d (300 mg/d), but maximal stimulation can be achieved only with prolonged ACTH infusions.

A screening test (the so-called rapid ACTH stimulation test) involves the administration of 25 units (0.25 mg) of cosyntropin intravenously or intramuscularly and measurement of plasma cortisol levels before administration and 30 and 60 min after administration; the test can be performed at any time of the day. The most clear-cut criterion for a normal response is a stimulated cortisol level of >500 nmol/L (>18 μg/dL), and the minimal stimulated normal increment of cortisol is >200 nmol/L (>7 μg/dL) above baseline. Severely ill patients with elevated basal cortisol levels may show no further increases following acute ACTH administration.

Tests of Mineralocorticoid Reserve and Stimulation of the Renin-Angiotensin System

Stimulation tests use protocols designed to create a programmed volume depletion, such as sodium restriction, diuretic administration, or upright posture. A simple, potent test consists of severe sodium restriction and upright posture. After 3 to 5 days of a 10-mmol/d sodium intake, rates of aldosterone secretion or excretion should increase two- to threefold over the control values. Supine morning plasma aldosterone levels are usually increased three- to sixfold, and they increase a further two- to fourfold in response to 2 to 3 h of upright posture.

When the dietary sodium intake is normal, stimulation testing requires the administration of a potent diuretic, such as 40 to 80 mg furosemide, followed by 2 to 3 h of upright posture. The normal response is a two- to fourfold rise in plasma aldosterone levels.

SUPPRESSION TESTS

Suppression tests to document hypersecretion of adrenal hormones involve measurement of the target hormone response after standardized suppression of its tropic hormone.

Tests of Pituitary-Adrenal Suppressibility

The ACTH release mechanism is sensitive to the circulating glucocorticoid level. When blood levels of glucocorticoid are increased in normal individuals, less ACTH is released from the anterior pituitary and less steroid is produced by the adrenal gland. The integrity of this feedback mechanism can be tested clinically by giving a glucocorticoid and judging the suppression of ACTH secretion by analysis of urine steroid levels and/or plasma cortisol and ACTH levels. A potent glucocorticoid such as dexamethasone is used, so that the agent can be given in an amount small enough not to contribute significantly to the pool of steroids to be analyzed.

The best *screening* procedure is the overnight dexamethasone suppression test. This involves the measurement of plasma cortisol levels at 8 A.M. following the oral administration of 1 mg dexamethasone the previous midnight. The 8 A.M. value for plasma cortisol in normal individuals should be <140 nmol/L (5 μg/dL).

The definitive test of adrenal suppressibility involves administering 0.5 mg dexamethasone every 6 h for 2 successive days while collecting urine over a 24-h period for determination of creatinine and free cortisol and/or measuring plasma cortisol levels. In a patient with a normal hypothalamic-pituitary ACTH release mechanism, a fall in the urine free cortisol to <80 nmol/d (30 μg/d) or of plasma cortisol to <140 nmol/L (5 μg/dL) is seen on the second day of administration.

A normal response to either suppression test implies that the glucocorticoid regulation of ACTH and its control of the adrenal glands is physiologically normal. However, an isolated abnormal result, particularly to the overnight suppression test, does not in itself demonstrate pituitary and/or adrenal disease.

Tests of Mineralocorticoid Suppressibility

These tests rely on an expansion of extracellular fluid volume, which should decrease circulating plasma renin activity and decrease the secretion and/or excretion of aldosterone. Various tests differ in the rate at which extracellular fluid volume is expanded. One convenient suppression test involves the intravenous infusion of 500 mL/h of normal saline solution for 4 h, which normally suppresses plasma aldosterone levels to <220 pmol/L (<8 ng/dL) from a sodium-restricted diet or to <140 pmol/L (<5 ng/dL) from a normal sodium intake. Alternatively, a high-sodium diet can be administered for 3 days with 0.2 mg fludrocortisone twice daily. Aldosterone excretion is measured on the third day and should be <28 nmol/d (10 μg/d). These tests should not be performed in potassium-depleted individuals since they carry a risk of precipitating hypokalemia.

TESTS OF PITUITARY-ADRENAL RESPONSIVENESS

Stimuli such as insulin-induced hypoglycemia, AVP, and pyrogens induce the release of ACTH from the pituitary by an action on higher neural centers or on the pituitary itself. Insulin-induced hypoglycemia is particularly useful, because it stimulates the release of both growth hormone and ACTH. In this test, regular insulin (0.05 to 0.1 U/kg body weight) is given intravenously as a bolus to reduce the fasting glucose level to at least 50% below basal. The normal cortisol response is a rise to >500 nmol/L (18 μg/dL). Glucose levels must be monitored during insulin-induced hypoglycemia, and it should be terminated by feeding or intravenous glucose if subjects develop symptoms of hypoglycemia. This test is contraindicated in individuals with coronary artery disease or a seizure disorder.

Metyrapone inhibits 11β-hydroxylase in the adrenal. As a result, the conversion of 11-deoxycortisol (compound S) to cortisol is impaired, causing 11-deoxycortisol to accumulate in the blood and the blood level of cortisol to decrease (Fig. 5-2). The hypothalamic-pituitary axis responds to the declining cortisol blood levels by releasing more ACTH. Note that assessment of the response depends on both an intact hypothalamic-pituitary axis and an intact adrenal gland.

Although modifications of the original metyrapone test have been described, a commonly used protocol involves administering 750 mg of the drug by mouth every 4 h over a 24-h period and comparing the control and postmetyrapone plasma levels of 11-deoxycortisol, cortisol, and ACTH. In normal individuals, plasma 11-deoxycortisol levels should exceed 210 nmol/L (7 μg/dL) and ACTH levels should exceed 17 pmol/L (75 pg/mL) following metyrapone administration. The metyrapone test does not accurately reflect ACTH reserve if subjects are ingesting exogenous glucocorticoids or drugs that accelerate the metabolism of metyrapone (e.g., phenytoin).

A direct and selective test of the pituitary corticotrophs can be achieved with CRH. The bolus injection of ovine

CRH (corticorelin ovine triflutate; 1 μg/kg body weight) stimulates secretion of ACTH and β-LPT in normal human subjects within 15 to 60 min. In normal individuals, the mean increment in ACTH is 9 pmol/L (40 pg/mL). However, the magnitude of the ACTH response is less than that produced by insulin-induced hypoglycemia, implying that additional factors (such as vasopressin) augment stress-induced increases in ACTH secretion.

The rapid ACTH test can often distinguish between primary and secondary adrenal insufficiency, because aldosterone secretion is preserved in secondary adrenal failure by the renin-angiotensin system and potassium. Cosyntropin (25 U) is given intravenously or intramuscularly, and plasma cortisol and aldosterone levels are measured before and at 30 and 60 min after administration. The cortisol response is abnormal in both groups, but patients with secondary insufficiency show an increase in aldosterone levels of at least 140 pmol/L (5 ng/dL). No aldosterone response is seen in patients in whom the adrenal cortex is destroyed. Alternatively, ACTH at a physiologic dose (1 μg), the so-called low-dose ACTH test, may be used to detect secondary adrenal insufficiency. An abnormal response is similar to that in the rapid ACTH test. However, levels need to be measured at 30 min, and the ACTH needs to be directly injected intravenously because it can be absorbed by plastic tubing. Because the use of a bolus of exogenous ACTH does not invariably exclude a diagnosis of secondary adrenocortical insufficiency, direct tests of pituitary ACTH reserve (metyrapone test, insulin-induced hypoglycemia) may be required in the appropriate clinical setting.

HYPERFUNCTION OF THE ADRENAL CORTEX

Excess cortisol is associated with Cushing's syndrome; excess aldosterone causes aldosteronism; and excess adrenal androgens cause adrenal virilism. These syndromes do not always occur in the "pure" form but may have overlapping features.

CUSHING'S SYNDROME

Etiology

Cushing described a syndrome characterized by truncal obesity, hypertension, fatigability and weakness, amenorrhea, hirsutism, purplish abdominal striae, edema, glucosuria, osteoporosis, and a basophilic tumor of the pituitary. As awareness of this syndrome has increased, the diagnosis of Cushing's syndrome has been broadened into the classification shown in **Table 5-2**. Regardless of etiology, all cases of endogenous Cushing's syndrome are due to increased production of cortisol by the adrenal. In most cases the cause is *bilateral adrenal hyperplasia* due to hypersecretion of pituitary ACTH or ectopic production of ACTH by a nonpituitary source. The incidence of pituitary-dependent adrenal hyperplasia is three times greater in women than in men, and the most frequent

TABLE 5-2

CAUSES OF CUSHING'S SYNDROME
Adrenal hyperplasia
Secondary to pituitary ACTH overproduction
Pituitary-hypothalamic dysfunction
Pituitary ACTH-producing micro- or macroadenomas
Secondary to ACTH or CRH-producing nonendocrine tumors (bronchogenic carcinoma, carcinoid of the thymus, pancreatic carcinoma, bronchial adenoma)
Adrenal macronodular hyperplasia (including ectopic expression of GIP receptors in the adrenal cortex)
Adrenal micronodular dysplasia
Sporadic
Familial (Carney's syndrome)
Adrenal neoplasia
Adenoma
Carcinoma
Exogenous, iatrogenic causes
Prolonged use of glucocorticoids
Prolonged use of ACTH

Note: ACTH, adrenocorticotropic hormone; CRH, corticotropin-releasing hormone; GIP, gastric inhibitory peptide.

age of onset is the third or fourth decade. Most evidence indicates that the primary defect is the de novo development of a pituitary adenoma, as tumors are found in >90% of patients with pituitary-dependent adrenal hyperplasia. Alternatively, the defect may occasionally reside in the hypothalamus or in higher neural centers, leading to release of CRH inappropriate to the level of circulating cortisol. This primary defect leads to hyperstimulation of the pituitary, resulting in hyperplasia or tumor formation. In surgical series, most individuals with hypersecretion of pituitary ACTH are found to have a microadenoma (<10 mm in diameter; 50% are ≤5 mm in diameter), but a pituitary macroadenoma (>10 mm) or diffuse hyperplasia of the corticotrope cells may be found. Traditionally, only an individual who has an ACTH-producing pituitary tumor is defined as having *Cushing's disease,* whereas Cushing's syndrome refers to all causes of excess cortisol: exogenous ACTH tumor, adrenal tumor, pituitary ACTH-secreting tumor, or excessive glucocorticoid treatment.

The *ectopic ACTH syndrome* is caused by nonpituitary tumors that secrete either ACTH and/or CRH and cause bilateral adrenal hyperplasia (Chap. 86 in HPIM, 16e). The ectopic production of CRH results in clinical, biochemical, and radiologic features indistinguishable from those caused by hypersecretion of pituitary ACTH. The typical signs and symptoms of Cushing's syndrome may be absent or minimal with ectopic ACTH production, and hypokalemic alkalosis is a prominent manifestation. Most of these cases are associated with the primitive small cell (oat cell) type of bronchogenic carcinoma or with carcinoid tumors of the thymus, pancreas, or ovary; medullary carcinoma of the thyroid; or bronchial adenomas. The onset of Cushing's syndrome may be sudden, particularly in patients with carcinoma of the lung, and this feature accounts in part for the failure of these patients to exhibit the classic manifestations. On the other hand, patients with carcinoid tumors or pheochromocytomas have longer clinical courses and usually exhibit the typical cushingoid features. The ectopic secretion of ACTH is also accompanied by the accumulation of ACTH fragments in plasma and by elevated plasma levels of ACTH precursor molecules. Because such tumors may produce large amounts of ACTH, baseline steroid values are usually very high and increased skin pigmentation may be present.

Approximately 20 to 25% of patients with Cushing's syndrome have an adrenal neoplasm. These tumors are usually unilateral, and about half are malignant. Occasionally, patients have biochemical features both of pituitary ACTH excess and of an adrenal adenoma. These individuals may have *nodular hyperplasia* of both adrenal glands, often the result of prolonged ACTH stimulation in the absence of a pituitary adenoma. Two additional entities cause nodular hyperplasia: a familial disorder in children or young adults (so-called pigmented micronodular dysplasia; see below) and an abnormal cortisol response to gastric inhibitory polypeptide or luteinizing hormone, secondary to ectopic expression of receptors for these hormones in the adrenal cortex.

The most common cause of Cushing's syndrome is *iatrogenic* administration of steroids for a variety of reasons. Although the clinical features bear some resemblance to those seen with adrenal tumors, these patients are usually distinguishable on the basis of history and laboratory studies.

Clinical Signs, Symptoms, and Laboratory Findings

Many of the signs and symptoms of Cushing's syndrome follow logically from the known action of glucocorticoids (**Table 5-3**). Catabolic responses in peripheral supportive tissue causes muscle weakness and fatigability, osteoporosis, broad violaceous cutaneous striae, and easy bruisability. The latter signs are secondary to weakening and rupture of collagen fibers in the dermis. Osteoporosis may cause collapse of vertebral bodies and pathologic fractures of other bones. Decreased bone mineralization is particularly pronounced in children. Increased hepatic gluconeogenesis and insulin resistance can cause impaired glucose tolerance. Overt diabetes mellitus occurs in <20% of patients, who probably are individuals with a predisposition to this disorder. Hypercortisolism promotes the deposition of adipose tissue in characteristic sites, notably the upper face (producing the typical "moon"

TABLE 5-3

FREQUENCY OF SIGNS AND SYMPTOMS IN CUSHING'S SYNDROME

SIGN OR SYMPTOM	PERCENT OF PATIENTS
Typical habitus (centripetal obesity)[a]	97
Increased body weight	94
Fatigability and weakness	87
Hypertension (blood pressure > 150/90)	82
Hirsutism[a]	80
Amenorrhea[a]	77
Broad violaceous cutaneous striae[a]	67
Personality changes	66
Ecchymoses[a]	65
Proximal myopathy[a]	62
Edema	62
Polyuria, polydipsia	23
Hypertrophy of clitoris	19

[a]Features more specific for Cushing's syndrome.

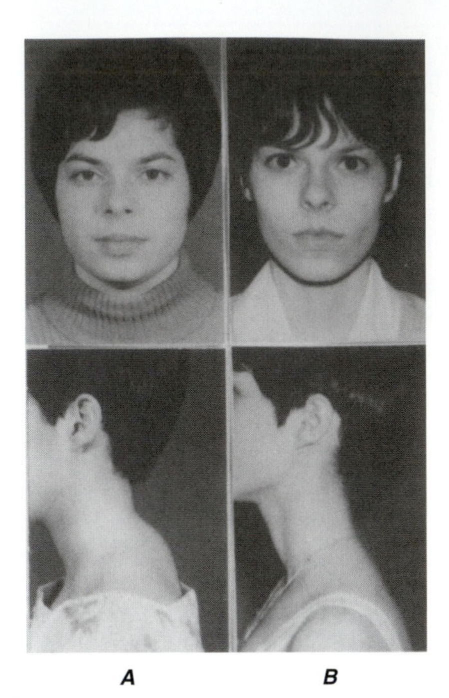

FIGURE 5-6

A woman with Cushing's syndrome due to a right adrenal cortical adenoma. *A*. One month prior to surgery, age 20. ***B***. One year after surgery, age 21.

facies), the interscapular area (producing the "buffalo hump"), supraclavicular fat pads, and the mesenteric bed (producing "truncal" obesity) (**Fig. 5-6**). Rarely, episternal fatty tumors and mediastinal widening secondary to fat accumulation occur. The reason for this peculiar distribution of adipose tissue is not known, but it is associated with insulin resistance and/or elevated insulin levels. The face appears plethoric, even in the absence of any increase in red blood cell concentration. Hypertension is common, and emotional changes may be profound, ranging from irritability and emotional lability to severe depression, confusion, or even frank psychosis. In women, increased levels of adrenal androgens can cause acne, hirsutism, and oligomenorrhea or amenorrhea. Some signs and symptoms in patients with hypercortisolism—i.e., obesity, hypertension, osteoporosis, and diabetes—are nonspecific and therefore are less helpful in diagnosing the condition. On the other hand, easy bruising, typical striae, myopathy, and virilizing signs (although less frequent) are, if present, more suggestive of Cushing's syndrome (Table 5-3).

Except in iatrogenic Cushing's syndrome, plasma and urine cortisol levels are elevated. Occasionally, hypokalemia, hypochloremia, and metabolic alkalosis are present, particularly with ectopic production of ACTH.

Diagnosis

The diagnosis of Cushing's syndrome depends on the demonstration of increased cortisol production and failure to suppress cortisol secretion normally when dexamethasone is administered (Chap. 2). Once the diagnosis is established, further testing is designed to determine the etiology (**Fig. 5-7** and **Table 5-4**).

For initial screening, the overnight dexamethasone suppression test is recommended (see above). In difficult cases (e.g., in obese or depressed patients), measurement

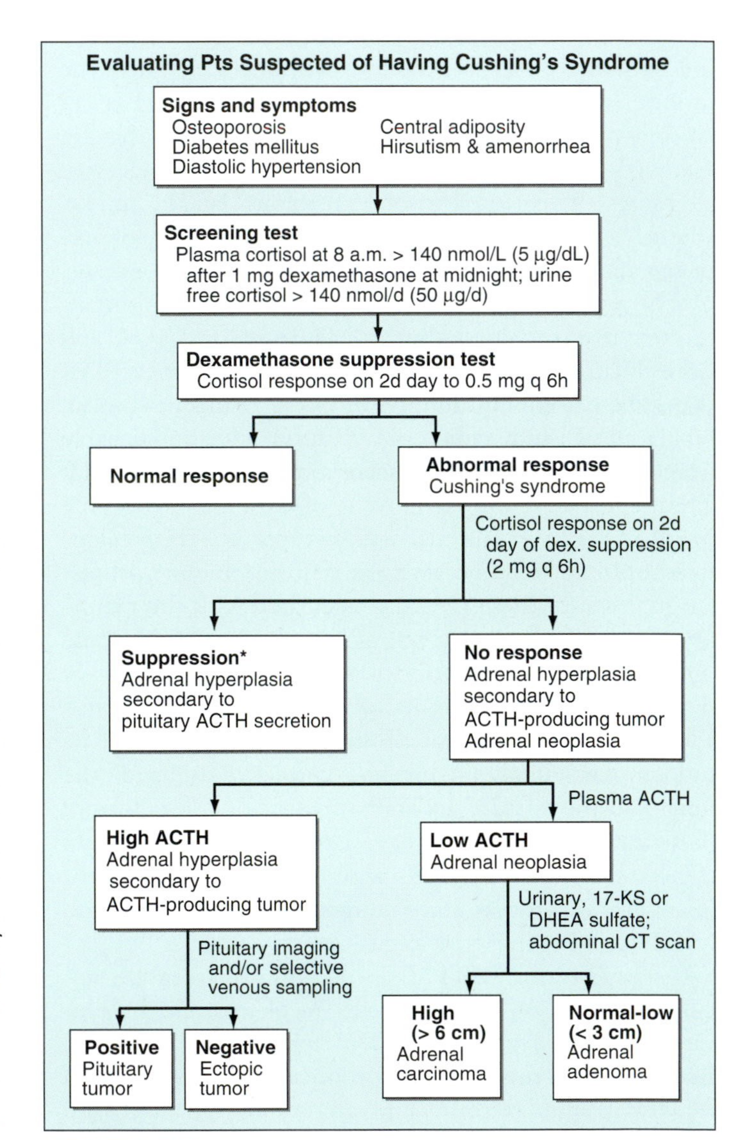

FIGURE 5-7

Diagnostic flowchart for evaluating patients suspected of having Cushing's syndrome. *This group probably includes some patients with pituitary-hypothalamic dysfunction and some with pituitary microadenomas. In some instances, a microadenoma may be visualized by pituitary magnetic resonance scanning. 17-KS, 17-ketosteroids; DHEA, dehydroepiandrosterone; ACTH, adrenocorticotropic hormone; CT, computed tomography.

TABLE 5-4

DIAGNOSTIC TESTS TO DETERMINE THE TYPE OF CUSHING'S SYNDROME

TEST	PITUITARY MACRO-ADENOMA	PITUITARY MICRO-ADENOMA	ECTOPIC ACTH OR CRH PRODUCTION	ADRENAL TUMOR
Plasma ACTH level	↑ to ↑↑	N to ↑	↑ to ↑↑↑	↓
Percent who respond to high-dose dexamethasone	<10	95	<10	<10
Percent who respond to CRH	>90	>90	<10	<10

Note: ACTH, adrenocorticotropic hormone; CRH, corticotropin-releasing hormone; N, normal; ↑, elevated; ↓, decreased. See text for definition of a response.

of a 24-h urine free cortisol also can be used as a screening test. A level >140 nmol/d (50 μg/d) is suggestive of Cushing's syndrome. The definitive diagnosis is then established by failure of urinary cortisol to fall to <25 nmol/d (10 μg/d) or of plasma cortisol to fall to <140 nmol/L (5 μg/dL) after a standard low-dose dexamethasone suppression test (0.5 mg every 6 h for 48 h). Owing to circadian variability, plasma cortisol and, to a certain extent, ACTH determinations are not meaningful when performed in isolation, but the absence of the normal fall of plasma cortisol at midnight is consistent with Cushing's syndrome because there is loss of the diurnal cortisol rhythm.

The task of determining the etiology of Cushing's syndrome is complicated by the fact that all the available tests lack specificity and by the fact that the tumors producing this syndrome are prone to spontaneous and often dramatic changes in hormone secretion (periodic hormonogenesis). No test has a specificity >95%, and it may be necessary to use a combination of tests to arrive at the correct diagnosis.

Plasma ACTH levels can be useful in distinguishing the various causes of Cushing's syndrome, particularly in separating ACTH-dependent from ACTH-independent causes. In general, measurement of plasma ACTH is useful in the diagnosis of ACTH-independent etiologies of the syndrome, since most adrenal tumors cause low or undetectable ACTH levels [<2 pmol/L (10 pg/mL)]. Furthermore, ACTH-secreting pituitary macroadenomas and ACTH-producing nonendocrine tumors usually result in elevated ACTH levels. In the ectopic ACTH syndrome, ACTH levels may be elevated to >110 pmol/L (500 pg/mL), and in most patients the level is >40 pmol/L (200 pg/mL). In Cushing's syndrome as the result of a microadenoma or pituitary-hypothalamic dysfunction, ACTH levels range from 6 to 30 pmol/L (30 to 150 pg/mL) [normal, <14 pmol/L (<60 pg/mL)], with half of values falling in the normal range. However, the main problem with the use of ACTH levels in the differential diagnosis of Cushing's syndrome is that ACTH levels may be similar in individuals with hypothalamic-pituitary dysfunction, pituitary microadenomas, ectopic CRH production, and ectopic ACTH production (especially carcinoid tumors) (Table 5-4).

A useful step to distinguish patients with an ACTH-secreting pituitary microadenoma or hypothalamic-pituitary dysfunction from those with other forms of Cushing's syndrome is to determine the response of cortisol output to administration of high-dose dexamethasone (2 mg every 6 h for 2 days). An alternative 8-mg, overnight high-dose dexamethasone test has been developed; however, this test has a lower sensitivity and specificity than the standard test. When the diagnosis of Cushing's syndrome is clear-cut on the basis of baseline urinary and plasma assays, the high-dose dexamethasone suppression test may be used without performing the preliminary low-dose suppression test. The high-dose suppression test provides close to 100% specificity if the criterion used is suppression of urinary free cortisol by >90%. Occasionally, in individuals with bilateral nodular hyperplasia and/or ectopic CRH production, steroid output also is suppressed. Failure of low- and high-dose dexamethasone administration to suppress cortisol production (Table 5-4) can occur in patients with adrenal hyperplasia secondary to an ACTH-secreting pituitary macroadenoma or an ACTH-producing tumor of nonendocrine origin and in those with adrenal neoplasms.

Because of these difficulties, several additional tests have been advocated, such as the metyrapone and CRH infusion tests. The rationale underlying these tests is that steroid hypersecretion by an adrenal tumor or the ectopic production of ACTH will suppress the hypothalamic-pituitary axis so that inhibition of pituitary ACTH release can be demonstrated by either test. Thus, most patients with pituitary-hypothalamic dysfunction and/or a microadenoma have an increase in steroid or ACTH secretion in response to metyrapone or CRH administration, whereas most patients with ectopic ACTH-producing tumors do not. Most pituitary macroadenomas also respond to CRH, but their response to metyrapone is variable. However, false-positive and false-negative CRH tests can occur in patients with ectopic ACTH and pituitary tumors.

The main diagnostic dilemma in Cushing's syndrome is to distinguish those instances due to microadenomas of the pituitary from those due to ectopic sources (e.g., carcinoids or pheochromocytoma) that produce CRH and/or ACTH. The clinical manifestations are similar unless the ectopic tumor produces other symptoms, such as diarrhea and flushing from a carcinoid tumor or episodic hypertension from a pheochromocytoma. Sometimes, one can distinguish between ectopic and pituitary ACTH production by using metyrapone or CRH tests, as noted above. In these situations, computed tomography (CT) of the pituitary gland is usually normal. Magnetic resonance imaging (MRI) with the enhancing agent gadolinium may be better than CT for this purpose but demonstrates pituitary microadenomas in only half of patients with Cushing's disease. Because microadenomas can be detected in up to 10 to 20% of individuals without known pituitary disease, a positive imaging study does not prove that the pituitary is the source of ACTH excess. In those with negative imaging studies, selective petrosal sinus venous sampling for ACTH is now used in many referral centers. ACTH levels are measured at baseline and 2, 5, and 10 min after ovine CRH (1 μ/kg IV) injections. Peak petrosal:peripheral ACTH ratios of >3 confirm the presence of a pituitary ACTH-secreting tumor. In centers where petrosal sinus sampling is performed frequently, it has proved highly sensitive for distinguishing pituitary and nonpituitary sources of ACTH excess. However, the catheterization procedure is technically difficult, and complications have occurred.

The diagnosis of a *cortisol-producing adrenal adenoma* is suggested by low ACTH and disproportionate elevations in baseline urine free cortisol levels with only modest changes in urinary 17-ketosteroids or plasma DHEA sulfate. Adrenal androgen secretion is usually reduced in these patients owing to the cortisol-induced suppression of ACTH and subsequent involution of the androgen-producing zona reticularis.

The diagnosis of *adrenal carcinoma* is suggested by a palpable abdominal mass and by markedly elevated baseline values of both urine 17-ketosteroids and plasma DHEA sulfate. Plasma and urine cortisol levels are variably elevated. Adrenal carcinoma is usually resistant to both ACTH stimulation and dexamethasone suppression. Elevated adrenal androgen secretion often leads to virilization in the female. Estrogen-producing adrenocortical carcinoma usually presents with gynecomastia in men and dysfunctional uterine bleeding in women. These adrenal tumors secrete increased amounts of androstenedione, which is converted peripherally to the estrogens estrone and estradiol. Adrenal carcinomas that produce Cushing's syndrome are often associated with elevated levels of the intermediates of steroid biosynthesis (especially 11-deoxycortisol), suggesting inefficient conversion of the intermediates to the final product. This feature also accounts for the characteristic increase in 17-ketosteroids. Approximately 20% of adrenal carcinomas are not associated with endocrine syndromes and are presumed to be nonfunctioning or to produce biologically inactive steroid precursors. In addition, the excessive production of steroids is not always clinically evident (e.g., androgens in adult men).

Differential Diagnosis

Pseudo-Cushing's Syndrome Problems in diagnosis include patients with obesity, chronic alcoholism, depression, and acute illness of any type. Extreme *obesity* is uncommon in Cushing's syndrome; furthermore, with exogenous obesity, the adiposity is generalized, not truncal. On adrenocortical testing, abnormalities in patients with exogenous obesity are usually modest. Basal urine steroid excretion levels in obese patients also are either normal or slightly elevated, and the diurnal pattern in blood and urine levels is normal. Patients with *chronic alcoholism* and those with *depression* share similar abnormalities in steroid output: modestly elevated urine cortisol, blunted circadian rhythm of cortisol levels, and resistance to suppression using the overnight dexamethasone test. In contrast to alcoholic subjects, depressed patients do not have signs and symptoms of Cushing's syndrome. Following discontinuation of alcohol and/or improvement in the emotional status, results of steroid testing usually return to normal. One or more of three tests have been used to differentiate mild Cushing's syndrome and pseudo-Cushing's syndrome. The serum cortisol level following the standard 2-day low-dose dexamethasone test has very high sensitivity and specificity. Although the CRH test alone is less useful, in combination with the low-dose dexamethasone test, there is nearly complete discrimination between these two conditions. Finally, a midnight cortisol level obtained in awake patients may have similar predictive value as the low-dose dexamethasone test if a cut-off of 210 nmol/L (7.5 μg/dL) is used. Patients with *acute illness* often have abnormal results on laboratory tests and fail to exhibit pituitary-adrenal suppression in response to dexamethasone, since major stress (such as pain or fever) interrupts the normal regulation of ACTH secretion. *Iatrogenic Cushing's syndrome,* induced by the administration of glucocorticoids or other steroids such as megestrol that bind to the glucocorticoid receptor, is indistinguishable by physical findings from endogenous adrenocortical hyperfunction. The distinction can be made, however, by measuring blood or urine cortisol levels in a basal state; in the iatrogenic syndrome these levels are low secondary to suppression of the pituitary-adrenal axis. The severity of iatrogenic Cushing's syndrome is related to the total steroid dose, the biologic half-life of the steroid, and the duration of therapy. Also, individuals taking afternoon and evening doses of glucocorticoids develop Cushing's syndrome more readily and with a smaller total daily dose than do patients taking morning doses only.

Radiologic Evaluation for Cushing's Syndrome

The preferred radiologic study for visualizing the adrenals is a CT scan of the abdomen (**Fig. 5-8**). CT is of value both for localizing adrenal tumors and for diagnosing bilateral hyperplasia. All patients believed to have hypersecretion of pituitary ACTH should have

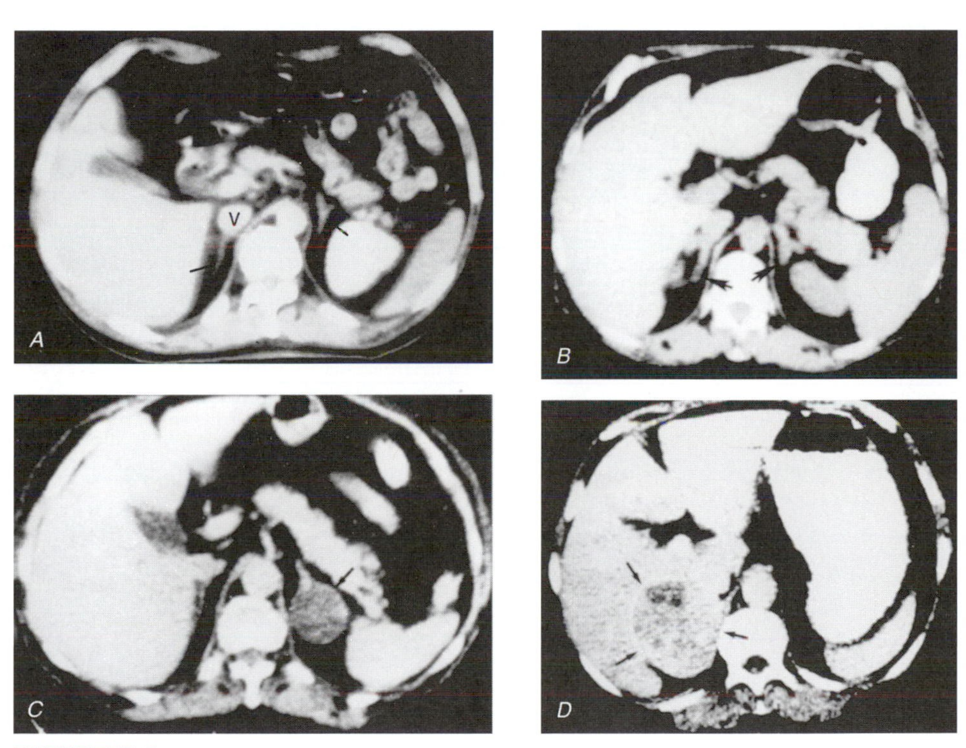

FIGURE 5-8

Computed tomography (CT) is the preferred method for visualizing the adrenal glands (*arrows*). ***A***. The normal right adrenal gland is adjacent to the inferior vena cava (V) where it emerges from the liver. Approximately 90% of right adrenal glands appear as linear structures extending posteriorly from the inferior vena cava into the space between the right lobe of the liver and the crus of the diaphragm. The normal left adrenal gland is lateral to the left crus of the diaphragm and below the stomach. Most left adrenal glands are shaped like an inverted V or Y. ***B***. Adrenal CT scan of a patient with ectopic ACTH production. Both adrenal glands (*arrows*) are enlarged (compare with *A*). In contrast, only 50% of patients with bilateral adrenal hyperplasia secondary to pituitary ACTH hypersecretion show enlargement of the adrenals when imaged by CT scan. ***C***. CT scan of a patient with Cushing's syndrome with biochemical evidence only of cortisol overproduction. The left adrenal has been replaced by a racquet-shaped 2-cm tumor (*arrow*). Attenuation of the tumor is low because of its high lipid content. ***D***. CT scan in a patient with Cushing's syndrome and biochemical evidence of an adrenal carcinoma. In contrast to the tumor in *C*, the right-sided mass in this patient is large and has a heterogeneous appearance—usual characteristics of an adrenal carcinoma.

a pituitary MRI scan with gadolinium contrast. Even with this technique, small microadenomas may be undetectable; alternatively, false-positive masses due to cysts or nonsecretory lesions of the normal pituitary may be imaged. In patients with ectopic ACTH production, high-resolution chest CT is a useful first step.

Evaluation of Asymptomatic Adrenal Masses

With abdominal CT scanning, many incidental adrenal masses (so-called incidentalomas) are discovered. This is not surprising, since 10 to 20% of subjects at autopsy have adrenocortical adenomas. The first step in evaluating such patients is to determine whether the tumor is functioning by means of appropriate screening tests, e.g., measurement of 24-h urine catecholamines and metabolites and serum potassium and assessment of adrenal cortical function by dexamethasone-suppression testing. However, 90% of incidentalomas are nonfunctioning. If an extraadrenal malignancy is present, there is a 30 to 50% chance that the adrenal tumor is a metastasis. If the primary tumor is being treated and there are no other metastases, it is prudent to obtain a fine-needle aspirate of the adrenal mass to establish the diagnosis. In the absence of a known malignancy the next step is unclear. The probability of adrenal carcinoma is <0.01%, the vast majority of adrenal masses being benign adenomas. Features suggestive of malignancy include large size (a size > 4 to 6 cm suggests carcinoma); irregular margins; and inhomogeneity, soft tissue calcifications visible on CT (Fig. 5-8), and findings characteristic of malignancy on a chemical-shift MRI image. If surgery is not performed, a repeat CT scan should be obtained in 3 to 6 months. Fine-needle aspiration is not useful to distinguish between benign and malignant primary adrenal tumors.

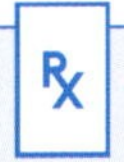

TREATMENT FOR ADRENAL NEOPLASM

When an adenoma or carcinoma is diagnosed, adrenal exploration is performed with excision of the tumor. Adenomas may be resected using laparoscopic techniques. Because of the possibility of atrophy of the contralateral adrenal, the patient is treated pre- and postoperatively as if for total adrenalectomy, even when a unilateral lesion is suspected, the routine being similar to that for an Addisonian patient undergoing elective surgery (see **Table 5-8**).

Despite operative intervention, most patients with adrenal carcinoma die within 3 years of diagnosis. Metastases occur most often to liver and lung. The principal drug for the treatment of adrenocortical carcinoma is mitotane (*o,p'*-DDD), an isomer of the insecticide DDT. This drug suppresses cortisol production and decreases plasma and urine steroid levels. Although its cytotoxic action is relatively selective for the glucocorticoid-secreting zone of the adrenal cortex, the zona glomerulosa also may be inhibited. Because mitotane also alters the extraadrenal metabolism of cortisol, plasma and urinary cortisol levels must be assessed to titrate the effect. The drug is usually given in divided doses three to four times a day, with the dose increased gradually to tolerability (usually <6 g daily). At higher doses, almost all patients experience side effects, which may be gastrointestinal (anorexia, diarrhea, vomiting) or neuromuscular (lethargy, somnolence, dizziness). All patients treated with mitotane should receive long-term glucocorticoid maintenance therapy, and, in some, mineralocorticoid replacement is appropriate. In approximately one-third of patients, both tumor and metastases regress, but long-term survival is not altered. In many patients, mitotane only inhibits steroidogenesis and does not cause regression of tumor metastases. Osseous metastases are usually refractory to the drug and should be treated with radiation therapy. Mitotane can also be given as adjunctive therapy after surgical resection of an adrenal carcinoma, although there is no evidence that this improves survival. Because of the absence of a long-term benefit with mitotane, alternative chemotherapeutic approaches based on platinum therapy have been used. However, there are no data presently available indicating a prolongation of life.

Bilateral hyperplasia

Patients with hyperplasia usually have a relative or absolute increase in ACTH levels. Since therapy would logically be directed at reducing ACTH levels, the ideal primary treatment for ACTH- or CRH-producing tumors, whether pituitary or ectopic, is surgical removal. Occasionally (particularly with ectopic ACTH production) surgical excision is not possible because the disease is far advanced. In this situation, "medical" or surgical adrenalectomy may correct the hypercortisolism.

Controversy exists as to the proper treatment for bilateral adrenal hyperplasia when the source of the ACTH overproduction is not apparent. In some centers, these patients (especially those who suppress after the administration of a high-dose dexamethasone test) undergo surgical exploration of the pituitary via a transsphenoidal approach in the expectation that a microadenoma will be found (Chap. 2). However, in most circumstances selective petrosal sinus venous sampling is recommended, and the patient is referred to an appropriate center if the procedure is not available locally. If a microadenoma is not found at the time of exploration, total hypophysectomy may be needed. Complications of transsphenoidal surgery include cerebrospinal fluid rhinorrhea, diabetes insipidus, panhypopituitarism, and optic or cranial nerve injuries.

In other centers, total adrenalectomy is the treatment of choice. The cure rate with this procedure is close to 100%. The adverse effects include the certain need for lifelong mineralocorticoid and glucocorticoid replacement and a 10 to 20% probability of a pituitary tumor developing over the next 10 years (Nelson's syndrome; Chap. 2). It is uncertain whether these tumors arise de novo or if they were present prior to adrenalectomy but were too small to be detected. Periodic radiologic evaluation of the pituitary gland by MRI as well as serial ACTH measurements should be performed in all individuals after bilateral adrenalectomy for Cushing's disease. Such pituitary tumors may become locally invasive and impinge on the optic chiasm or extend into the cavernous or sphenoid sinuses.

Except in children, pituitary irradiation is rarely used as primary treatment, being reserved rather for postoperative tumor recurrences. In some centers, high levels of gamma radiation can be focused on the desired site with less scattering to surrounding tissues by using stereotactic techniques. Side effects of radiation include ocular motor palsy and hypopituitarism. There is a long lag time between treatment and remission, and the remission rate is usually <50%.

Finally, in occasional patients in whom a surgical approach is not feasible, "medical" adrenalectomy may be indicated (**Table 5-5**). Inhibition of steroidogenesis may also be indicated in severely cushingoid subjects prior to surgical intervention. Chemical adrenalectomy may be accomplished by the administration of the inhibitor of steroidogenesis ketoconazole (600 to 1200 mg/d). In addition, mitotane (2 or 3 g/d) and/or the blockers of steroid synthesis aminoglutethimide (1 g/d) and metyrapone (2 or 3 g/d) may be effective either alone or in combination. Mitotane is slow to take effect (weeks). Mifepristone, a competitive inhibitor of the binding of glucocorticoid to its receptor, may be a treatment option. Adrenal insufficiency is a risk with all these agents, and replacement steroids may be required.

ALDOSTERONISM

Aldosteronism is a syndrome associated with hypersecretion of the mineralocorticoid aldosterone. In *primary* aldosteronism the cause for the excessive aldosterone production resides within the adrenal gland; in *secondary* aldosteronism the stimulus is extraadrenal.

Primary Aldosteronism

In the original descriptions of excessive and inappropriate aldosterone production, the disease was the result of an *aldosterone-producing adrenal adenoma* (Conn's syndrome). Most cases involve a unilateral adenoma, which is usually small and may occur on either side.

TABLE 5-5

TREATMENT MODALITIES FOR PATIENTS WITH ADRENAL HYPERPLASIA SECONDARY TO PITUITARY ACTH HYPERSECRETION
Treatments to reduce pituitary ACTH production
Transsphenoidal resection of microadenoma
Radiation therapy
Treatments to reduce or eliminate adrenocortical cortisol secretion
Bilateral adrenalectomy
Medical adrenalectomy (metyrapone, mitotane, aminoglutethimide, ketoconazole)[a]

[a]Not curative but effective as long as chronically administered in selected patients.
Note: ACTH, adrenocorticotropic hormone.

Rarely, primary aldosteronism is due to an adrenal carcinoma. Aldosteronism is twice as common in women as in men, usually occurs between the ages of 30 and 50, and is present in ~1% of unselected hypertensive patients. However, the prevalence may be as high as 5%, depending on the criteria and study population. In many patients with clinical and biochemical features of primary aldosteronism, a solitary adenoma is not found at surgery. Instead, these patients have *bilateral cortical nodular hyperplasia.* In the literature, this disease is also termed *idiopathic hyperaldosteronism,* and/or *nodular hyperplasia.* The cause is unknown.

Signs and Symptoms Hypersecretion of aldosterone increases the renal distal tubular exchange of intratubular sodium for secreted potassium and hydrogen ions, with progressive depletion of body potassium and development of hypokalemia. Most patients have diastolic hypertension, which may be very severe, and headaches. The hypertension is probably due to the increased sodium reabsorption and extracellular volume expansion. *Potassium depletion* is responsible for the muscle weakness and fatigue and is due to the effect of potassium depletion on the muscle cell membrane. The polyuria results from impairment of urinary concentrating ability and is often associated with polydipsia. However, some individuals with mild disease, particularly the bilateral hyperplasia type, may have normal potassium levels and therefore have no symptoms associated with hypokalemia.

Electrocardiographic and roentgenographic signs of left ventricular enlargement are, in part, secondary to the hypertension. However, the left ventricular hypertrophy is disproportionate to the level of blood pressure when compared to individuals with essential hypertension, and regression of the hypertrophy occurs even if blood pressure is not reduced after removal of an aldosteronoma. Electrocardiographic signs of potassium depletion include prominent U waves, cardiac arrhythmias, and premature contractions. In the absence of associated congestive heart failure, renal disease, or preexisting abnormalities (such as thrombophlebitis), edema is characteristically absent. However, structural damage to the cerebral circulation, retinal vasculature, and kidney occurs more frequently than would be predicted based on the level and duration of the hypertension. Proteinuria may occur in as many as 50% of patients with primary aldosteronism, and renal failure occurs in up to 15%. Thus, it is probable that excess aldosterone production induces cardiovascular damage independent of its effect on blood pressure.

Laboratory Findings Laboratory findings depend on both the duration and the severity of potassium depletion. An overnight concentration test often reveals impaired ability to concentrate the urine, probably secondary to the hypokalemia. Urine pH is neutral to alkaline because of excessive secretion of ammonium and bicarbonate ions to compensate for the metabolic alkalosis.

Hypokalemia may be severe (<3 mmol/L) and reflects body potassium depletion, usually >300 mmol. In mild forms of primary aldosteronism, potassium levels may be normal. *Hypernatremia* is infrequent but may be caused by sodium retention, concomitant water loss from polyuria, and resetting of the osmostat. Metabolic alkalosis and elevation of serum bicarbonate are caused by hydrogen ion loss into the urine and migration into potassium-depleted cells. The alkalosis is perpetuated by potassium deficiency, which increases the capacity of the proximal convoluted tubule to reabsorb filtered bicarbonate. If hypokalemia is severe, serum magnesium levels are also reduced.

Diagnosis The diagnosis is suggested by persistent hypokalemia in a nonedematous patient with a normal sodium intake who is not receiving potassium-wasting diuretics (furosemide, ethacrynic acid, thiazides). If hypokalemia occurs in a hypertensive patient taking a potassium-wasting diuretic, the diuretic should be discontinued and the patient should be given potassium supplements. After 1 to 2 weeks, the potassium level should be remeasured, and if hypokalemia persists, the patient should be evaluated for a mineralocorticoid excess syndrome (**Fig. 5-9**).

The criteria for the diagnosis of primary aldosteronism are (1) diastolic hypertension without edema, (2) hyposecretion of renin (as judged by low plasma renin activity levels) that fails to increase appropriately during volume depletion (upright posture, sodium depletion), and (3) hypersecretion of aldosterone that does not suppress appropriately in response to volume expansion.

Patients with primary aldosteronism characteristically *do not have edema,* since they exhibit an "escape" phenomenon from the sodium-retaining aspects of mineralocorticoids. Rarely, pretibial edema is present in patients with associated nephropathy and azotemia.

The estimation of plasma renin activity is of limited value in separating patients with primary aldosteronism from those with hypertension of other causes. Although failure of plasma renin activity to rise normally during volume-depletion maneuvers is a criterion for a diagnosis of primary aldosteronism, suppressed renin activity also occurs in ~25% of patients with essential hypertension.

Although a renin measurement alone lacks specificity, the ratio of serum aldosterone to plasma renin activity is a very useful screening test. A high ratio (>30), when aldosterone is expressed as ng/dL and plasma renin activity as ng/mL per hour, strongly suggests autonomy of aldosterone secretion. Aldosterone levels need to be >500 pmol/L (>15 ng/dL) when salt intake is not restricted. In some centers, the aldosterone/plasma renin activity ratio is used as a primary screen test in all normokalemic, difficult-to-control hypertensive patients, in addition to those with hypokalemia. Ultimately, it is necessary to demonstrate a lack of aldosterone suppression to diagnose primary aldosteronism (Fig. 5-9). The autonomy exhibited in these patients refers only to the resistance to suppression of secretion during volume expansion; aldosterone can and does respond in a normal or above-normal fashion to the stimulus of potassium loading or ACTH infusion.

Once hyposecretion of renin and failure of aldosterone secretion suppression are demonstrated, aldosterone-producing adenomas should be localized by abdominal CT scan, using a high-resolution scanner as many aldosteronomas are <1 cm in size. If the CT scan is negative, percutaneous transfemoral bilateral adrenal vein catheterization with adrenal vein sampling may demonstrate a two- to threefold increase in plasma aldosterone concentration on the involved side. In cases of hyperaldosteronism secondary to cortical nodular hyperplasia, no lateralization is found. It is important for samples to be obtained simultaneously if possible and for cortisol levels to be measured to ensure that false localization does not reflect dilution or an ACTH- or stress-induced rise in aldosterone levels. In a patient with an adenoma, the aldosterone/cortisol ratio lateralizes to the side of the lesion.

Differential Diagnosis Patients with hypertension and hypokalemia may have either primary or secondary hyperaldosteronism (**Fig. 5-10**). A useful maneuver to distinguish between these conditions is the measurement of plasma renin activity. Secondary hyperaldosteronism in patients with accelerated hypertension is due to elevated plasma renin levels; in contrast, patients with primary aldosteronism have suppressed plasma renin levels. Indeed, in patients with a serum potassium concentration of <2.5 mmol/L, a high ratio of plasma aldosterone to plasma renin activity in a random sample is usually sufficient to establish the diagnosis of primary aldosteronism without additional testing. Ectopic ACTH production also should be considered in patients with hypertension and severe hypokalemia.

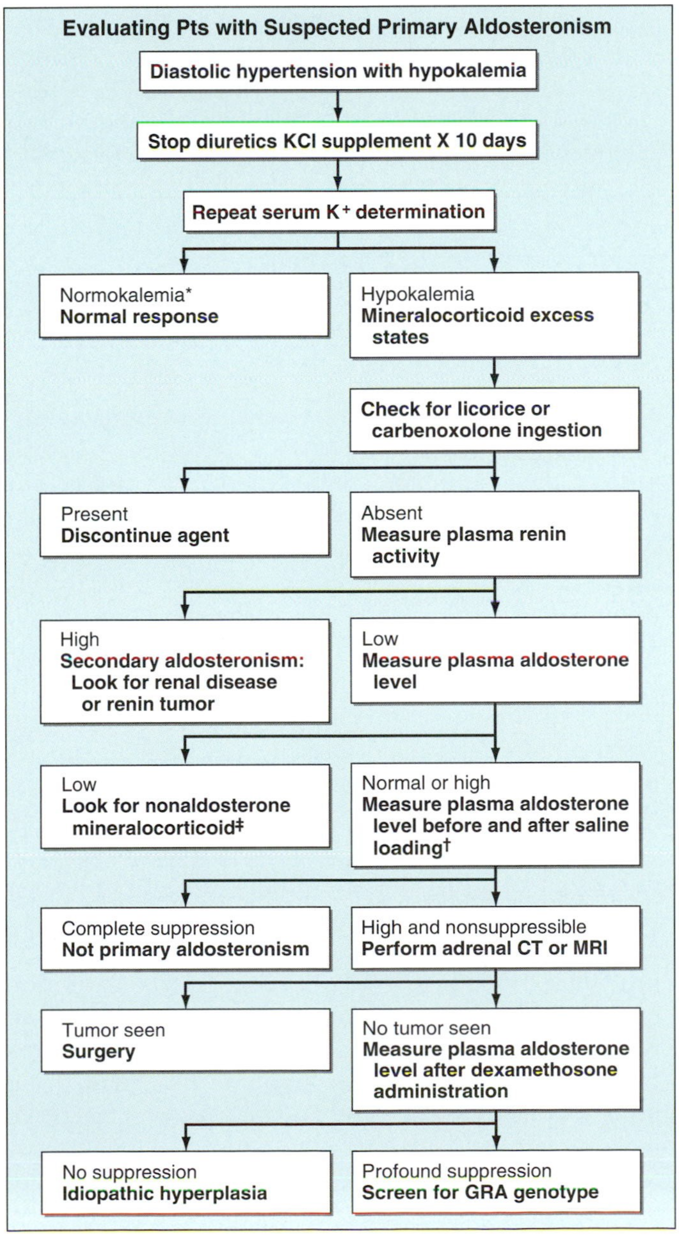

Evaluating Pts with Suspected Primary Aldosteronism

Diastolic hypertension with hypokalemia
→ Stop diuretics KCl supplement X 10 days
→ Repeat serum K^+ determination
- Normokalemia* — Normal response
- Hypokalemia — Mineralocorticoid excess states
→ Check for licorice or carbenoxolone ingestion
- Present — Discontinue agent
- Absent — Measure plasma renin activity
- High — Secondary aldosteronism: Look for renal disease or renin tumor
- Low — Measure plasma aldosterone level
- Low — Look for nonaldosterone mineralocorticoid‡
- Normal or high — Measure plasma aldosterone level before and after saline loading†
- Complete suppression — Not primary aldosteronism
- High and nonsuppressible — Perform adrenal CT or MRI
- Tumor seen — Surgery
- No tumor seen — Measure plasma aldosterone level after dexamethosone administration
- No suppression — Idiopathic hyperplasia
- Profound suppression — Screen for GRA genotype

FIGURE 5-9

Diagnostic flowchart for evaluating patients with suspected primary aldosteronism. *Serum K^+ may be normal in some patients with hyperaldosteronism who are taking potassium-sparing diuretics (spironolactone, triamterene) or who have a low sodium intake and a high potassium intake. †This step should not be taken if hypertension is severe (diastolic pressure > 115 mmHg) or if cardiac failure is present. Also, serum potassium levels should be corrected before the infusion of saline solution. Alternative methods that produce comparable suppression of aldosterone secretion include oral sodium loading (200 mmol/d) and the administration of fludrocortisone, 0.2 mg bid, for 3 days. For example, Liddle syndrome, apparent mineralocorticoid excess syndrome, or a deoxycorticosterone-secreting tumor. GRA, glucocorticoid-remediable aldosteronism; CT, computed tomography; MRI, magnetic resonance imaging.

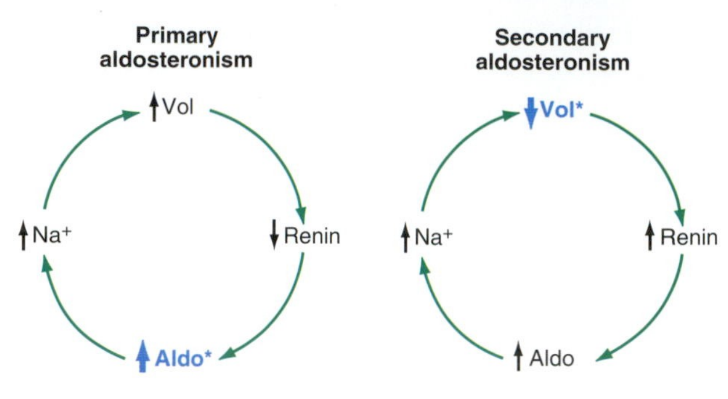

FIGURE 5-10
Responses of the renin-aldosterone volume control loop in primary versus secondary aldosteronism.

Primary aldosteronism must also be distinguished from other *hypermineralocorticoid states.* Nonaldosterone mineralocorticoid states will have suppressed plasma renin activity but low aldosterone levels. The most common problem is to distinguish between hyperaldosteronism due to an adenoma and that due to idiopathic bilateral nodular hyperplasia. This distinction is important because hypertension associated with idiopathic hyperplasia does not usually benefit from bilateral adrenalectomy, whereas hypertension associated with aldosterone-producing tumors is usually improved or cured by removal of the adenoma. Although patients with idiopathic bilateral nodular hyperplasia tend to have less severe hypokalemia, lower aldosterone secretion, and higher plasma renin activity than do patients with primary aldosteronism, differentiation is impossible solely on clinical and/or biochemical grounds. An anomalous postural decrease in plasma aldosterone and elevated plasma 18-hydroxycorticosterone levels are present in most patients with a unilateral lesion. However, these tests are also of limited diagnostic value in the individual patient, because some adenoma patients have an increase in plasma aldosterone with upright posture, so-called renin-responsive aldosteronoma. A definitive diagnosis is best made by radiographic studies, including bilateral adrenal vein catheterization, as noted above.

In a few instances, hypertensive patients with hypokalemic alkalosis have adenomas that secrete deoxycorticosterone. Such patients have reduced plasma renin activity levels, but aldosterone levels are either normal or reduced, suggesting the diagnosis of mineralocorticoid excess due to a hormone other than aldosterone. Several inherited disorders have clinical features similar to those of primary aldosteronism (see below).

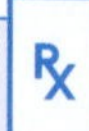

TREATMENT FOR PRIMARY ALDOSTERONISM

Primary aldosteronism due to an adenoma is usually treated by surgical excision of the adenoma. Where possible a laparoscopic approach is favored. However, dietary sodium restriction and the administration of an aldosterone antagonist—e.g., spironolactone—are effective in many cases. Hypertension and hypokalemia are usually controlled by doses of 25 to 100 mg spironolactone every 8 h. In some patients medical management has been successful for years, but chronic therapy in men is usually limited by side effects of spironolactone such as gynecomastia, decreased libido, and impotence.

When idiopathic bilateral hyperplasia is suspected, surgery is indicated only when significant, symptomatic hypokalemia cannot be controlled with medical therapy, i.e., by spironolactone, triamterene, or amiloride. Hypertension associated with idiopathic hyperplasia is usually not benefited by bilateral adrenalectomy.

Secondary Aldosteronism

Secondary aldosteronism refers to an appropriately increased production of aldosterone in response to activation of the renin-angiotensin system (Fig. 5-10). The production rate of aldosterone is often higher in patients with secondary aldosteronism than in those with primary aldosteronism. Secondary aldosteronism usually occurs in association with the accelerated phase of hypertension or on the basis of an underlying edema disorder. Secondary aldosteronism in pregnancy is a normal physiologic response to estrogen-induced increases in circulating levels of renin substrate and plasma renin activity and to the anti-aldosterone actions of progestogens.

Secondary aldosteronism in hypertensive states is due either to a primary overproduction of renin (primary reninism) or to an overproduction of renin secondary to a decrease in renal blood flow and/or perfusion pressure (Fig. 5-10). Secondary hypersecretion of renin can be due to a narrowing of one or both of the major renal arteries by atherosclerosis or by fibromuscular hyperplasia. Overproduction of renin from both kidneys also occurs in severe arteriolar nephrosclerosis (malignant hypertension) or with profound renal vasoconstriction (the accelerated phase of hypertension). The secondary aldosteronism is characterized by hypokalemic alkalosis, moderate to severe increases in plasma renin activity, and moderate to marked increases in aldosterone levels.

Secondary aldosteronism with hypertension can also be caused by rare renin-producing tumors (primary reninism). In these patients, the biochemical characteristics are of renal vascular hypertension, but the primary defect is renin secretion by a juxtaglomerular cell tumor. The diagnosis can be made by demonstration of normal renal vasculature and/or demonstration of a space-occupying lesion in the kidney by radiographic techniques and documentation of a unilateral increase in renal vein renin activity. Rarely, these tumors arise in tissues such as the ovary.

Secondary aldosteronism is present in many forms of *edema*. The rate of aldosterone secretion is usually increased in patients with edema caused by either cirrhosis or the nephrotic syndrome. In congestive heart failure, elevated aldosterone secretion varies depending on the severity of cardiac failure. The stimulus for aldosterone release in these conditions appears to be *arterial hypovolemia* and/or hypotension. Thiazides and furosemide often exaggerate secondary aldosteronism via volume depletion; hypokalemia and, on occasion, alkalosis can then become prominent features. On occasion secondary hyperaldosteronism occurs without edema or hypertension (Bartter and Gitelman syndromes, see below).

Aldosterone and Cardiovascular Damage

Although many studies have investigated the role of angiotensin II in mediating cardiovascular damage, additional evidence indicates that aldosterone has an important role that is independent of angiotensin II. Patients with primary aldosteronism (in which angiotensin II levels are usually very low) have a higher incidence of left ventricular hypertrophy (LVH), albuminuria, and stroke than do patients with essential hypertension. Experimental animal models mimicking secondary aldosteronism (angiotensin infusion) or primary aldosteronism (aldosterone infusion) reveal a common pathophysiologic sequence. Within the first few days there is activation of proinflammatory molecules with a histologic picture of perivascular macrophage infiltrate and inflammation, followed by cellular death, fibrosis, and ventricular hypertrophy. These events are prevented if an aldosterone receptor antagonist is used or if adrenalectomy is performed initially. The same pathophysiologic sequence is seen in animals with average aldosterone levels and cardiovascular damage, i.e., diabetes mellitus, or genetic hypertensive rats. Importantly, the level of sodium intake is a critical co-factor. If salt intake is severely restricted, no damage occurs even though the aldosterone levels are markedly elevated. Thus, it is not the level of aldosterone per se that is responsible for the damage, but its level relative to the volume or sodium status of the individual.

Four clinical studies support these experimental results. In the RALES trial, patients with class II/IV heart failure were randomized to standard care or a low dose of the mineralocorticoid receptor antagonist spironolactone. There was a 30% reduction in all-cause mortality and cardiovascular mortality and hospitalizations after 36 months. Two studies in hypertensive subjects addressed the question of the relative importance of a reduction of angiotensin II formation versus blockade of the MR in mediating cardiovascular damage. Subjects were randomized to eplerenone (an MR antagonist), enalapril (an ACE inhibitor), or both agents. In the first study the subjects had LVH, with the endpoint being a reduction in LVH. In the second, the subjects had diabetes mellitus and proteinuria, with the endpoint being a reduction in proteinuria. In both studies all three treatment arms substantially reduced the primary endpoint; however, the most potent effect occurred in the combination arms of the studies. In the monotherapy LVH arms, the reduction in LVH was similar, while in the proteinuria study, eplerenone produced a greater reduction than did enalapril. The final study was the EPHESUS trial, where individuals who developed congestive heart failure after an acute myocardial infarction were randomized to standard-of-care treatment with or without a small dose of eplerenone. Eplerenone administration produced a significantly greater reduction in mortality (15 to 17%) and in cardiovascular-related hospitalizations than the placebo arm. Thus, these four clinical studies provide strong support to the hypothesis that MR blockade has a significant added advantage over standard-of-care therapy in reducing cardiovascular mortality and surrogate endpoints.

SYNDROMES OF ADRENAL ANDROGEN EXCESS

Adrenal androgen excess results from excess production of DHEA and androstenedione, which are converted to testosterone in extraglandular tissues; elevated testosterone levels account for most of the virilization. Adrenal androgen excess may be associated with the secretion of greater or smaller amounts of other adrenal hormones and may, therefore, present as "pure" syndromes of virilization or as "mixed" syndromes associated with excessive glucocorticoids and Cushing's syndrome. For further discussion of hirsutism and virilization, see Chap. 12.

HYPOFUNCTION OF THE ADRENAL CORTEX

Cases of adrenal insufficiency can be divided into two general categories: (1) those associated with primary inability of the adrenal to elaborate sufficient quantities of hormone, and (2) those associated with a secondary failure due to inadequate ACTH formation or release (**Table 5-6**).

PRIMARY ADRENOCORTICAL DEFICIENCY (ADDISON'S DISEASE)

The original description of Addison's disease—"general languor and debility, feebleness of the heart's action, irritability of the stomach, and a peculiar change of the color of the skin"—summarizes the dominant clinical features. Advanced cases are usually easy to diagnose, but recognition of the early phases can be a real challenge.

Incidence

Acquired forms of primary insufficiency are relatively rare, may occur at any age, and affect both sexes equally. Because of the common therapeutic use of steroids, secondary adrenal insufficiency is relatively common.

Etiology and Pathogenesis

Addison's disease results from progressive destruction of the adrenals, which must involve >90% of the glands before adrenal insufficiency appears. The adrenal is a frequent site for chronic granulomatous diseases, predominantly tuberculosis but also histoplasmosis, coccidioidomycosis, and cryptococcosis. In early series, tuberculosis was responsible for 70 to 90% of cases, but the most frequent cause now is *idiopathic* atrophy, and an autoimmune mechanism is probably responsible. Rarely, other lesions are encountered, such as adrenoleukodystrophy, bilateral hemorrhage, tumor metastases, HIV, cytomegalovirus (CMV), amyloidosis, adrenomyeloneuropathy, familial adrenal insufficiency, or sarcoidosis.

Although half of patients with idiopathic atrophy have circulating adrenal antibodies, autoimmune destruction is probably secondary to cytotoxic T lymphocytes. Specific adrenal antigens to which autoantibodies may be directed include 21-hydroxylase (CYP21A2) and side chain cleavage enzyme, but the significance of these antibodies in the pathogenesis of adrenal insufficiency is unknown. Some antibodies cause adrenal insufficiency by blocking the binding of ACTH to its receptors. Some patients also have antibodies to thyroid, parathyroid, and/or gonadal tissue (Chap. 21). There is also an increased incidence of chronic lymphocytic thyroiditis, premature ovarian

TABLE 5-6

CLASSIFICATION OF ADRENAL INSUFFICIENCY
PRIMARY ADRENAL INSUFFICIENCY
Anatomic destruction of gland (chronic or acute)
"Idiopathic" atrophy (autoimmune, adrenoleukodystrophy)
Surgical removal
Infection (tuberculous, fungal, viral—especially in AIDS patients)
Hemorrhage
Invasion: metastatic
Metabolic failure in hormone production
Congenital adrenal hyperplasia
Enzyme inhibitors (metyrapone, ketoconazole, aminoglutethimide)
Cytotoxic agents (mitotane)
ACTH-blocking antibodies
Mutation in ACTH receptor gene
Adrenal hypoplasia congenita
SECONDARY ADRENAL INSUFFICIENCY
Hypopituitarism due to hypothalamic-pituitary disease
Suppression of hypothalamic-pituitary axis
By exogenous steroid
By endogenous steroid from tumor

Note: ACTH, adrenocorticotropic hormone.

failure, type 1 diabetes mellitus, and hypo- or hyperthyroidism. The presence of two or more of these autoimmune endocrine disorders in the same person defines the polyglandular autoimmune syndrome type II. Additional features include pernicious anemia, vitiligo, alopecia, nontropical sprue, and myasthenia gravis. Within families, multiple generations are affected by one or more of the above diseases. Type II polyglandular syndrome is the result of a mutant gene on chromosome 6 and is associated with the HLA alleles B8 and DR3.

The combination of parathyroid and adrenal insufficiency and chronic mucocutaneous candidiasis constitutes type I polyglandular autoimmune syndrome. Other autoimmune diseases in this disorder include pernicious anemia, chronic active hepatitis, alopecia, primary hypothyroidism, and premature gonadal failure. There is no HLA association; this syndrome is inherited as an autosomal recessive trait. It is caused by mutations in the *a*utoimmune *p*oly*e*ndocrinopathy *c*andidiasis *e*ctodermal *d*ystrophy (APECED) gene located on chromosome 21q22.3. The gene encodes a transcription factor thought to be involved in lymphocyte function. The type I syndrome usually presents during childhood, whereas the type II syndrome is usually manifested in adulthood.

Clinical suspicion of adrenal insufficiency should be high in patients with AIDS. CMV regularly involves the adrenal glands (so-called CMV necrotizing adrenalitis), and involvement with *Mycobacterium avium-intracellulare, Cryptococcus,* and Kaposi's sarcoma has been reported. Adrenal insufficiency in AIDS patients may not be manifest, but tests of adrenal reserve frequently give abnormal results. When interpreting tests of adrenocortical function, it is important to remember that medications such as rifampin, phenytoin, ketoconazole, megestrol, and opiates may cause or potentiate adrenal insufficiency. Adrenal hemorrhage and infarction occur in patients on anticoagulants and in those with circulating anticoagulants and hypercoagulable states, such as the antiphospholipid syndrome.

There are several rare genetic causes of adrenal insufficiency that present primarily in infancy and childhood (see below).

Clinical Signs and Symptoms

Adrenocortical insufficiency caused by gradual adrenal destruction is characterized by an insidious onset of fatigability, weakness, anorexia, nausea and vomiting, weight loss, cutaneous and mucosal pigmentation, hypotension, and occasionally hypoglycemia (**Table 5-7**). Depending on the duration and degree of adrenal hypofunction, the manifestations vary from mild chronic fatigue to fulminating shock associated with acute destruction of the glands, as described by Waterhouse and Friderichsen.

TABLE 5-7

FREQUENCY OF SYMPTOMS AND SIGNS IN ADRENAL INSUFFICIENCY

SIGN OR SYMPTOM	PERCENT OF PATIENTS
Weakness	99
Pigmentation of skin	98
Weight loss	97
Anorexia, nausea, and vomiting	90
Hypotension (<110/70)	87
Pigmentation of mucous membranes	82
Abdominal pain	34
Salt craving	22
Diarrhea	20
Constipation	19
Syncope	16
Vitiligo	9

Asthenia is the cardinal symptom. Early it may be sporadic, usually most evident at times of stress; as adrenal function becomes more impaired, the patient is continuously fatigued, and bed rest is necessary.

Hyperpigmentation may be striking or absent. It commonly appears as a diffuse brown, tan, or bronze darkening of parts such as the elbows or creases of the hand and of areas that normally are pigmented such as the areolae about the nipples. Bluish-black patches may appear on the mucous membranes. Some patients develop dark freckles, and irregular areas of vitiligo may paradoxically be present. As an early sign, tanning following sun exposure may be persistent.

Arterial hypotension with postural accentuation is frequent, and blood pressure may be in the range of 80/50 mmHg or less.

Abnormalities of gastrointestinal function are often the presenting complaint. Symptoms vary from mild anorexia with weight loss to fulminating nausea, vomiting, diarrhea, and ill-defined abdominal pain, which may be so severe as to be confused with an acute abdomen. Patients may have personality changes, usually consisting of excessive irritability and restlessness. Enhancement of the sensory modalities of taste, olfaction, and hearing is reversible with therapy. Axillary and pubic hair may be decreased in women due to loss of adrenal androgens.

Laboratory Findings

In the early phase of gradual adrenal destruction, there may be no demonstrable abnormalities in the routine laboratory parameters, but adrenal reserve is decreased—that is, while basal steroid output may be normal, a subnormal increase occurs after stress. Adrenal stimulation with ACTH uncovers abnormalities in this stage of the disease, eliciting a subnormal increase of cortisol levels or no increase at all. In more advanced stages of adrenal destruction, serum sodium, chloride, and bicarbonate levels are reduced, and the serum potassium level is elevated. The hyponatremia is due both to loss of sodium into the urine (due to aldosterone deficiency) and to movement into the intracellular compartment. This extravascular sodium loss depletes extracellular fluid volume and accentuates hypotension. Elevated plasma vasopressin and angiotensin II levels may contribute to the hyponatremia by impairing free water clearance. Hyperkalemia is due to a combination of aldosterone deficiency, impaired glomerular filtration, and acidosis. Basal levels of cortisol and aldosterone are subnormal and fail to increase following ACTH administration. Mild to moderate hypercalcemia occurs in 10 to 20% of patients for unclear reasons. The electrocardiogram may show nonspecific changes, and the electroencephalogram exhibits a generalized reduction and slowing. There may be a normocytic anemia, a relative lymphocytosis, and a moderate eosinophilia.

Diagnosis

The diagnosis of adrenal insufficiency should be made only with ACTH stimulation testing to assess adrenal reserve capacity for steroid production (see above for ACTH test protocols). In brief, the best screening test is the cortisol response 60 min after 250 μg of cosyntropin given intramuscularly or intravenously. Cortisol levels should exceed 495 nmol/L (18 μg/dL). If the response is abnormal, then primary and secondary adrenal insufficiency can be distinguished by measuring aldosterone levels from the same blood samples. In secondary, but not primary, adrenal insufficiency the aldosterone increment will be normal [$\geq$150 pmol/L (5 ng/dL)]. Furthermore, in primary adrenal insufficiency, plasma ACTH and associated peptides (β-LPT) are elevated because of loss of the usual cortisol-hypothalamic-pituitary feedback relationship, whereas in secondary adrenal insufficiency, plasma ACTH values are low or "inappropriately" normal (**Fig. 5-11**).

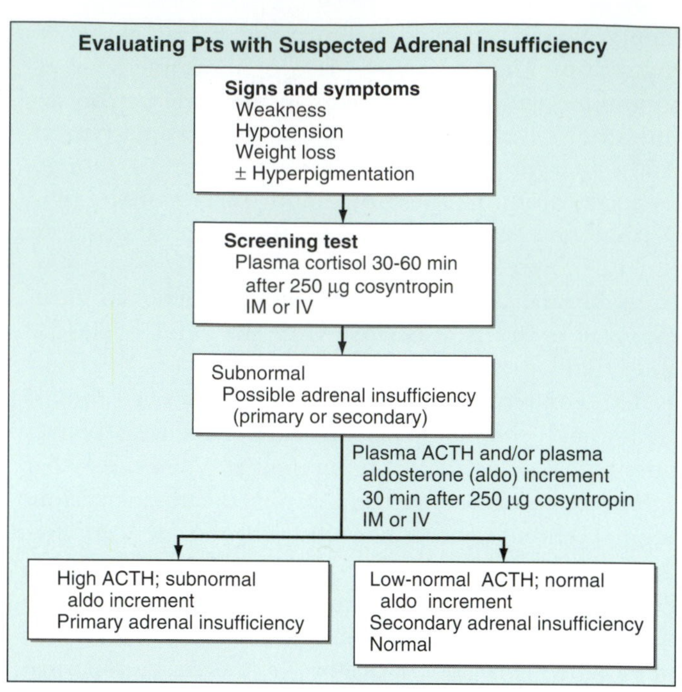

FIGURE 5-11

Diagnostic flowchart for evaluating patients with suspected adrenal insufficiency. Plasma adrenocorticotropic hormone (ACTH) levels are low in secondary adrenal insufficiency. In adrenal insufficiency secondary to pituitary tumors or idiopathic panhypopituitarism, other pituitary hormone deficiencies are present. On the other hand, ACTH deficiency may be isolated, as seen following prolonged use of exogenous glucocorticoids. Because the isolated blood levels obtained in these screening tests may not be definitive, the diagnosis may need to be confirmed by a continuous 24-h ACTH infusion. Normal subjects and patients with secondary adrenal insufficiency may be distinguished by insulin tolerance or metyrapone testing.

Differential Diagnosis

Because weakness and fatigue are common, diagnosis of early adrenocortical insufficiency may be difficult. However, the combination of mild gastrointestinal distress, weight loss, anorexia, and a suggestion of increased pigmentation makes it mandatory to perform ACTH stimulation testing to rule out adrenal insufficiency, particularly before steroid treatment is begun. Weight loss is useful in evaluating the significance of weakness and malaise. Facial pigmentation may be a problem, but a *recent* and progressive *increase* in pigmentation is usually reported by the patient with gradual adrenal destruction. Hyperpigmentation is usually absent when adrenal destruction is rapid, as in bilateral adrenal hemorrhage. The fact that hyperpigmentation occurs with other diseases may also present a problem, but the appearance and distribution of pigment in adrenal insufficiency are usually characteristic. When doubt exists, measurement of ACTH levels and testing of adrenal reserve with the infusion of ACTH provide clear-cut differentiation.

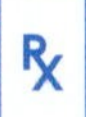

TREATMENT FOR PRIMARY ADRENAL INSUFFICIENCY

All patients with adrenal insufficiency should receive specific hormone replacement. These patients require careful education about the disease. Replacement therapy should correct both glucocorticoid and mineralocorticoid deficiencies. Hydrocortisone (cortisol) is the mainstay of treatment. The dose for most adults (depending on size) is 20 to 30 mg/d. Patients are advised to take glucocorticoids with meals or, if that is impractical, with milk or an antacid, because the drugs may increase gastric acidity and exert direct toxic effects on the gastric mucosa. To simulate the normal diurnal adrenal rhythm, two-thirds of the dose is taken in the morning, and the remaining one-third is taken in the late afternoon. Some patients exhibit insomnia, irritability, and mental excitement after initiation of therapy; in these, the dosage should be reduced. Other situations that may necessitate smaller doses are hypertension and diabetes mellitus. Obese individuals and those on anticonvulsive medications may require increased dosages. Measurements of plasma ACTH or cortisol or of urine cortisol levels do not appear to be useful in determining optimal glucocorticoid dosages.

Since the replacement dosage of hydrocortisone does not replace the mineralocorticoid component of the adrenal hormones, mineralocorticoid supplementation is usually needed. This is accomplished by the administration of 0.05 to 0.1 mg fludrocortisone per day by mouth. Patients should also be instructed to maintain an ample intake of sodium (3 to 4 g/d).

The adequacy of mineralocorticoid therapy can be assessed by measurement of blood pressure and serum electrolytes. Blood pressure should be normal and without postural changes; serum sodium, potassium, creatinine, and urea nitrogen levels should also be normal. Measurement of plasma renin levels also may be useful in titrating the dose.

In female patients with adrenal insufficiency, androgen levels also are low. Thus, some physicians believe that daily replacement with 25 to 50 mg of DHEA orally may improve quality of life and bone mineral density.

Complications of glucocorticoid therapy, with the exception of gastritis, are *rare* at the dosages recommended for treatment of adrenal insufficiency. Complications of mineralocorticoid therapy include hypokalemia, hypertension, cardiac enlargement, and even congestive heart failure due to sodium retention. Periodic measurements of body weight, serum potassium level, and blood pressure are useful. All patients with adrenal insufficiency should carry medical identification, should be instructed in the parenteral self-administration of steroids, and should be registered with a medical alerting system.

Special Therapeutic Problems

During periods of intercurrent illness, especially in the setting of fever, the dose of hydrocortisone should be doubled. With severe illness it should be increased to 75 to 150 mg/d. When oral administration is not possible, parenteral routes should be employed. Likewise, before surgery or dental extractions, supplemental glucocorticoids should be administered. Patients should also be advised to increase the dose of fludrocortisone and to add salt to their otherwise normal diet during periods of strenuous exercise with sweating, during extremely hot weather, and with gastrointestinal upsets such as diarrhea. A simple strategy is to supplement the diet one to three times daily with salty broth (1 cup of beef or chicken bouillon contains 35 mmol of sodium). For a representative program of steroid therapy for the patient with adrenal insufficiency who is undergoing major surgery, see **Table 5-8**. This schedule is designed so that on the day of surgery it will mimic the output of cortisol in normal individuals undergoing prolonged major stress (10 mg/h, 250 to 300 mg/d). Thereafter, if the patient is improving and is afebrile, the dose of hydrocortisone is tapered by 20 to 30% daily. Mineralocorticoid administration is unnecessary at hydrocortisone doses >100 mg/d because of the mineralocorticoid effects of hydrocortisone at such dosages.

SECONDARY ADRENOCORTICAL INSUFFICIENCY

ACTH deficiency causes *secondary* adrenocortical insufficiency; it may be a selective deficiency, as is seen following prolonged administration of excess glucocorticoids, or it may occur in association with deficiencies of

TABLE 5-8

STEROID THERAPY SCHEDULE FOR A PATIENT WITH ADRENAL INSUFFICIENCY UNDERGOING SURGERY[a]

	HYDROCORTISONE INFUSION, CONTINUOUS, MG/H		HYDROCORTISONE (ORALLY)		FLUDROCORTISONE (ORALLY), 8 A.M.
			8 A.M.	4 P.M.	
Routine daily medication			20	10	0.1
Day before operation			20	10	0.1
Day of operation	10				
Day 1	5–7.5				
Day 2	2.5–5				
Day 3	2.5–5	*or*	40	20	0.1
Day 4	2.5–5	*or*	40	20	0.1
Day 5			40	20	0.1
Day 6			20	20	0.1
Day 7			20	10	0.1

[a]All steroid doses are given in milligrams. An alternative approach is to give 100 mg hydrocortisone as an intravenous bolus injection every 8 h on the day of the operation (see text).

multiple pituitary hormones (panhypopituitarism) (Chap. 2). Patients with secondary adrenocortical hypofunction have many symptoms and signs in common with those having primary disease but are *not hyperpigmented,* since ACTH and related peptide levels are low. In fact, plasma ACTH levels distinguish between primary and secondary adrenal insufficiency, since they are elevated in the former and decreased to absent in the latter. Patients with total pituitary insufficiency have manifestations of multiple hormone deficiencies. An additional feature distinguishing primary adrenocortical insufficiency is the *near-normal level of aldosterone secretion* seen in pituitary and/or isolated ACTH deficiencies (Fig. 5-11). Patients with pituitary insufficiency may have hyponatremia, which can be dilutional or secondary to a subnormal increase in aldosterone secretion in response to severe sodium restriction. However, severe *dehydration, hyponatremia,* and *hyperkalemia* are characteristic of severe mineralocorticoid insufficiency and favor a diagnosis of primary adrenocortical insufficiency.

Patients receiving long-term steroid therapy, despite physical findings of Cushing's syndrome, may develop adrenal insufficiency because of prolonged pituitary-hypothalamic suppression and adrenal atrophy secondary to the loss of endogenous ACTH. These patients have two deficits, a loss of adrenal responsiveness to ACTH and a failure of pituitary ACTH release. They are characterized by low blood cortisol and ACTH levels, a low baseline rate of steroid excretion, and abnormal ACTH and metyrapone responses. Most patients with steroid-induced adrenal insufficiency eventually recover normal HPA responsiveness, but recovery time varies from days to months. The rapid ACTH test provides a convenient assessment of recovery of HPA function. Because the plasma cortisol concentrations after injection of cosyntropin and during insulin-induced hypoglycemia are usually similar, the rapid ACTH test assesses the integrated HPA function (see "Tests of Pituitary-Adrenal Responsiveness," above). Some investigators suggest using the low-dose (1 μg) ACTH test for suspected secondary ACTH deficiency. Additional tests to assess pituitary ACTH reserve include the standard metyrapone and insulin-induced hypoglycemia tests.

Glucocorticoid therapy in patients with secondary adrenocortical insufficiency does not differ from that for the primary disorder. Mineralocorticoid therapy is usually not necessary, as aldosterone secretion is preserved.

ACUTE ADRENOCORTICAL INSUFFICIENCY

Acute adrenocortical insufficiency may result from several processes. On the one hand, *adrenal crisis* may be a rapid and overwhelming intensification of chronic adrenal insufficiency, usually precipitated by sepsis or surgical stress. Alternatively, acute hemorrhagic destruction of both adrenal glands can occur in previously well individuals. In children, this event is usually associated with septicemia with *Pseudomonas* or meningococcemia (Waterhouse-Friderichsen syndrome). In adults, anticoagulant therapy or a coagulation disorder may result in bilateral adrenal hemorrhage. Occasionally, bilateral adrenal hemorrhage in the newborn results from birth trauma. Hemorrhage has been observed during pregnancy, following idiopathic adrenal vein thrombosis, and as a complication of venography (e.g., infarction of an adenoma). The third and most frequent cause of acute insufficiency is the rapid withdrawal of steroids from patients with adrenal atrophy owing to chronic steroid administration. Acute adrenocortical insufficiency may also occur in patients with congenital adrenal hyperplasia or those with decreased adrenocortical reserve when they are given drugs capable of inhibiting steroid synthesis (mitotane, ketoconazole) or of increasing steroid metabolism (phenytoin, rifampin).

Adrenal Crisis

The long-term survival of patients with adrenocortical insufficiency depends largely on the prevention and treatment of adrenal crisis. Consequently, the occurrence of infection, trauma (including surgery), gastrointestinal upsets, or other stresses necessitates an immediate increase in hormone. In untreated patients, preexisting symptoms are intensified. Nausea, vomiting, and abdominal pain may become intractable. Fever may be severe or absent. Lethargy deepens into somnolence, and hypovolemic vascular collapse ensues. In contrast, patients previously maintained on chronic glucocorticoid therapy may not exhibit dehydration or hypotension until they are in a preterminal state, since mineralocorticoid secretion is usually preserved. In all patients in crisis, a precipitating cause should be sought.

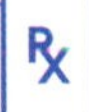

TREATMENT FOR SECONDARY AND ACUTE ADRENAL INSUFFICIENCY

Treatment is directed primarily toward repletion of circulating glucocorticoids and replacement of the sodium and water deficits. Hence an intravenous infusion of 5% glucose in normal saline solution should be started with a bolus intravenous infusion of 100 mg hydrocortisone followed by a continuous infusion of hydrocortisone at a rate of 10 mg/h. An alternative approach is to administer a 100-mg bolus of hydrocortisone intravenously every 6 h. However, only continuous infusion maintains the plasma cortisol constantly at stress levels [>830 nmol/L (30 μg/dL)]. Effective treatment of hypotension requires glucocorticoid replacement and repletion of sodium and water deficits. If the crisis was preceded by prolonged nausea, vomiting, and dehydration, several liters of saline solution may be required in the first few hours. Vasoconstrictive agents (such as dopamine) may be indicated in extreme conditions as adjuncts to volume replacement. With large doses of steroid, i.e., 100 to 200 mg hydrocortisone, the patient receives a maximal mineralocorticoid effect, and supplementary mineralocorticoid is superfluous. Following improvement, the steroid dosage is tapered over the next few days to maintenance levels, and mineralocorticoid therapy is reinstituted if needed (Table 5-8).

ADRENAL CORTICAL INSUFFICIENCY IN ACUTELY ILL PATIENTS

The physiology of the HPA axis is dramatically altered during critical illnesses such as trauma, surgery, sepsis, and shock. In such situations cortisol levels rise four- to sixfold, diurnal variation is abolished, and the unbound fractions of cortisol rise in the circulation and in target tissues. Inadequate cortisol production during critical illness can result in hypotension, reduced systemic vascular resistance, shock, and death.

A major area of controversy in presumably normal individuals is the correlation of clinical outcomes with the cortisol levels measured during critical illness. Subnormal cortisol production during acute severe illness has been termed "functional" or "relative" adrenal insufficiency. Conceptually, the elevated cortisol levels that are observed are viewed as insufficient to control the inflammatory response and maintain blood pressure. If such patients can be identified, treatment with supplementary cortisol could be beneficial.

A level of cortisol in a critically ill patient below which replacement glucocorticoids may improve prognosis is not firmly established, although many have accepted a level of ≤441 nmol/L (15 μg/dL). On the other hand, a random cortisol >938 nmol/L (34 μg/dL) in the setting of critical illness is unlikely to be associated with relative adrenal insufficiency. In patients who have random cortisol levels between 441 and 938 nmol/L (15 and 34 μg/dL), a cosyntropin stimulation test may identify patients with diminished adrenal reserve [increment <255 nmol/L (9 μg/dL)] who may benefit from supplementary cortisol treatment. If the diagnosis of relative or functional adrenal insufficiency is considered in an acutely ill, hypotensive patient, treatment with supplementary cortisol should be initiated promptly following the measurement of a random cortisol level and/or performing a cosyntropin stimulation test. Supplemental cortisol may be particularly beneficial in patients with septic shock where glucocorticoids have been reported to reduce mortality and the duration of vasopressor therapy. Such patients should be treated with 50 to 75 mg of intravenous hydrocortisone every 6 h as bolus treatment or the same amount as a continuous infusion. Treatment can be terminated if the cortisol levels obtained at the outset are normal. On the other hand, those patients with abnormal testing should be treated for 1 week and then tapered. In surviving patients, adrenal function should be reevaluated after resolution of the critical illness.

HYPOALDOSTERONISM

Isolated aldosterone deficiency accompanied by normal cortisol production occurs in association with hyporeninism, as an inherited biosynthetic defect, postoperatively following removal of aldosterone-secreting adenomas, during protracted heparin administration, in pretectal disease of the nervous system, and in severe postural hypotension.

The feature common to all forms of hypoaldosteronism is the inability to increase aldosterone secretion appropriately in response to salt restriction. Most patients have unexplained hyperkalemia, which is often exacerbated by restriction of dietary sodium intake. In severe cases, urine sodium wastage occurs at a normal salt intake, whereas in milder forms, excessive loss of urine sodium occurs only with salt restriction.

Most cases of isolated hypoaldosteronism occur in patients with a deficiency in renin production (so-called hyporeninemic hypoaldosteronism), most commonly in adults with diabetes mellitus and mild renal failure and in whom hyperkalemia and metabolic acidosis are out of proportion to the degree of renal impairment. Plasma renin levels fail to rise normally following sodium restriction and postural changes. The pathogenesis is uncertain. Possibilities include renal disease (the most likely), autonomic neuropathy, extracellular fluid volume expansion, and defective conversion of renin precursors to active renin. Aldosterone levels also fail to rise normally after salt restriction and volume contraction; this effect is probably related to the hyporeninism, since biosynthetic defects in aldosterone secretion usually cannot be demonstrated. In these patients, aldosterone secretion increases promptly after ACTH stimulation, but it is uncertain whether the magnitude of the response is normal. On the other hand, the level of aldosterone appears to be subnormal in relationship to the hyperkalemia.

Hypoaldosteronism can also be associated with high renin levels and low or elevated levels of aldosterone (see below). Severely ill patients may also have hyperreninemic hypoaldosteronism; such patients have a high mortality rate (80%). Hyperkalemia is not present. Possible explanations for the hypoaldosteronism include adrenal necrosis (uncommon) or a shift in steroidogenesis from mineralocorticoids to glucocorticoids, possibly related to prolonged ACTH stimulation.

Before the diagnosis of isolated hypoaldosteronism is considered for a patient with hyperkalemia, "pseudohyperkalemia" (e.g., hemolysis, thrombocytosis) should be excluded by measuring the *plasma* potassium level. The next step is to demonstrate a normal cortisol response to ACTH stimulation. Then, the response of renin and aldosterone levels to stimulation (upright posture, sodium restriction) should be measured. Low renin and aldosterone levels establish the diagnosis of hyporeninemic hypoaldosteronism. A combination of high renin levels and low aldosterone levels is consistent with an aldosterone biosynthetic defect or a selective unresponsiveness to angiotensin II. Finally, there is a condition that clinically and biochemically mimics hypoaldosteronism with elevated renin levels. However, the aldosterone levels are not low but high—so-called pseudohypoaldosteronism. This inherited condition is caused by a mutation in the epithelial sodium channel (see below).

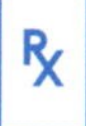

TREATMENT FOR HYPOALDOSTERONISM

The treatment is to replace the mineralocorticoid deficiency. For practical purposes, the oral administration of 0.05 to 0.15 mg fludrocortisone daily should restore electrolyte balance if salt intake is adequate (e.g., 150 to 200 mmol/d). However, patients with hyporeninemic hypoaldosteronism may require higher doses of mineralocorticoid to correct hyperkalemia. This need poses a potential risk in patients with hypertension, mild renal insufficiency, or congestive heart failure. An alternative approach is to reduce salt intake and to administer furosemide, which can ameliorate acidosis and hyperkalemia. Occasionally, a combination of these two approaches is efficacious.

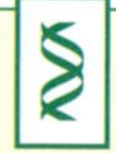

GENETIC CONSIDERATIONS

Glucocorticoid Diseases

CONGENITAL ADRENAL HYPERPLASIA

Congenital adrenal hyperplasia (CAH) is the consequence of recessive mutations that cause one of several distinct enzymatic defects (see below). Because cortisol is the principal adrenal steroid regulating ACTH elaboration and because ACTH stimulates adrenal growth and function, a block in cortisol synthesis may result in the enhanced secretion of adrenal androgens and/or mineralocorticoids depending on the site of the enzyme block. In severe congenital virilizing hyperplasia, the adrenal output of cortisol may be so compromised as to cause adrenal deficiency despite adrenal hyperplasia.

CAH is the most common adrenal disorder of infancy and childhood (Chap. 7). Partial enzyme deficiencies can be expressed after adolescence, predominantly in women with hirsutism and oligomenorrhea but minimal virilization. Late-onset adrenal hyperplasia may account for 5 to 25% of cases of hirsutism and oligomenorrhea in women, depending on the population.

Etiology Enzymatic defects have been described in 21-hydroxylase (CYP21A2), 17α-hydroxylase/17,20-lyase (CYP17), 11β-hydroxylase (CYP11B1), and (3β-HSD2) (Fig. 5-2). Although the genes encoding these enzymes have been cloned, the diagnosis of specific enzyme deficiencies with genetic techniques is not practical because of the large number of different deletions and missense mutations. CYP21A2 deficiency is closely linked to the HLA-B locus of chromosome 6 so that HLA typing and/or DNA polymorphism can be used to detect the heterozygous carriers and to diagnose affected individuals in some families (Chap. 2, in *Harrison's Rheumatology*). The clinical expression in the different disorders is variable, ranging from virilization of the female (CYP2/A2) to feminization of the male (3β-HSD2) (Chap. 7).

Adrenal virilization in the female at birth is associated with ambiguous external genitalia (*female pseudohermaphroditism*). Virilization begins after the fifth month of intrauterine development. At birth there may be enlargement of the clitoris, partial or complete fusion of the labia, and sometimes a urogenital sinus in the female. If the labial fusion is nearly complete, the female infant has external genitalia resembling a penis with hypospadias. In the *postnatal* period, CAH is associated with virilization in the female and isosexual precocity in the male. The excessive androgen levels result in accelerated growth, so that bone age exceeds chronologic age. Because epiphyseal closure occurs early, growth stops, but truncal development continues, the characteristic appearance being a short child with a well-developed trunk.

The most common form of CAH (95% of cases) is a result of impairment of CYP21A2. In addition to cortisol deficiency, aldosterone secretion is decreased in approximately one-third of the patients. Thus, with CYP21A2 deficiency, adrenal virilization occurs with or without a salt-losing tendency due to aldosterone deficiency (Fig. 5-2).

CYP11B1 deficiency causes a "hypertensive" variant of CAH. Hypertension and hypokalemia occur because of the impaired conversion of 11-deoxycorticosterone to corticosterone, resulting in the accumulation of 11-deoxycorticosterone, a potent mineralocorticoid. The degree of hypertension is variable. Steroid precursors are shunted into the androgen pathway.

CYP17 deficiency is characterized by hypogonadism, hypokalemia, and hypertension. This rare disorder causes decreased production of cortisol and shunting of precursors into the mineralocorticoid pathway with hypokalemic alkalosis, hypertension, and suppressed plasma renin activity. Usually, 11-deoxycorticosterone production is elevated. Because CYP17 hydroxylation is required for biosynthesis of both adrenal androgens and gonadal testosterone and estrogen, this defect is associated with sexual immaturity, high urinary gonadotropin levels, and low urinary 17-ketosteroid excretion. Female patients have primary amenorrhea and lack of development of secondary sexual characteristics. Because of deficient androgen production, male patients have either ambiguous external genitalia or a female phenotype (*male pseudohermaphroditism*). Exogenous glucocorticoids can correct the hypertensive syndrome, and treatment with appropriate gonadal steroids results in sexual maturation.

With 3β-HSD2 deficiency, conversion of pregnenolone to progesterone is impaired, so that the synthesis of both cortisol and aldosterone is blocked, with shunting into the adrenal androgen pathway via 17α-hydroxypregnenolone and DHEA. Because DHEA is a weak androgen, and because this enzyme deficiency is also present in the gonad, the genitalia of the male fetus may be incompletely virilized or feminized. Conversely, in the female, overproduction of DHEA may produce partial virilization.

Diagnosis The diagnosis of CAH should be considered in infants having episodes of acute adrenal insufficiency or salt wasting or hypertension. The diagnosis is further suggested by the finding of hypertrophy of the clitoris, fused labia, or a urogenital sinus in the female or of isosexual precocity in the male. In infants and children with a CYP21A2 defect, increased urine 17-ketosteroid excretion and increased plasma DHEA sulfate levels are typically associated with an increase in the blood levels of 17-hydroxyprogesterone and the excretion of its urinary metabolite pregnanetriol. Demonstration of elevated levels of 17-hydroxyprogesterone in amniotic fluid at 14 to 16 weeks of gestation allows prenatal detection of affected female infants.

The diagnosis of a *salt-losing form* of CAH due to defects in CYP21A2 is suggested by episodes of acute adrenal insufficiency with hyponatremia, hyperkalemia, dehydration, and vomiting. These infants and children often crave salt and have laboratory findings indicating deficits in both cortisol and aldosterone secretion.

With the *hypertensive form* of CAH due to CYP11B1 deficiency, 11-deoxycorticosterone and 11-deoxycortisol accumulate. The diagnosis is confirmed by demonstrating increased levels of 11-deoxycortisol in the blood or increased amounts of tetrahydro-11-deoxycortisol in the urine. Elevation of 17-hydroxyprogesterone levels does not imply a coexisting CYP21A2 deficiency.

Very high levels of urine DHEA with low levels of pregnanetriol and of cortisol metabolites in urine are characteristic of children with 3β-HSD2 deficiency. Marked salt-wasting may also occur.

Adults with *late-onset adrenal hyperplasia* (partial deficiency of CYP21A2, CYP11B1, or 3β-HSD2) are characterized by normal or moderately elevated levels of urinary 17-ketosteroids and plasma DHEA sulfate. A high basal level of a precursor of cortisol biosynthesis (such as 17-hydroxyprogesterone, 17-hydroxypregnenolone, or 11-deoxycortisol), or elevation of such a precursor after ACTH stimulation, confirms the diagnosis of a partial deficiency. Measurement of steroid precursors 60 min after bolus administration of ACTH is usually sufficient. Adrenal androgen output is easily suppressed by the standard low-dose (2 mg) dexamethasone test.

℞ TREATMENT FOR CAH

Therapy in CAH patients consists of daily administration of glucocorticoids to suppress pituitary ACTH secretion. Because of its low cost and intermediate half-life, prednisone is the drug of choice except in infants, in whom hydrocortisone is usually used. In adults with late-onset adrenal hyperplasia, the smallest single bedtime dose of a long- or intermediate-acting glucocorticoid that suppresses pituitary ACTH secretion should be administered. The amount of steroid required by children with CAH is approximately 1 to 1.5 times the normal cortisol production rate of 27 to 35 μmol (10 to 13 mg) of cortisol per square meter of body surface per day and is given in divided doses two or three times per day. The dosage schedule is governed by repetitive analysis of the urinary 17-ketosteroids, plasma DHEA sulfate, and/or precursors of cortisol biosynthesis. Skeletal growth and maturation also must be monitored closely, as overtreatment with glucocorticoid replacement therapy retards linear growth.

RECEPTOR MUTATIONS

Isolated glucocorticoid deficiency is a rare autosomal recessive disease secondary to a mutation in the ACTH receptor. Usually mineralocorticoid function is normal. Adrenal insufficiency is manifest within the first 2 years of life as hyperpigmentation, convulsions, and/or frequent episodes of hypoglycemia. In some patients the adrenal insufficiency is associated with achalasia and alacrima–Allgrove's, or triple A, syndrome. However, in some triple A syndrome patients, no mutation in the ACTH receptor has been identified, suggesting that a distinct genetic abnormality causes this syndrome. *Adrenal hypoplasia congenita* is a rare X-linked disorder caused by a mutation in the *DAX1* gene. This gene encodes an orphan nuclear receptor that plays an important role in the development of the adrenal cortex and also the hypothalamic-pituitary-gonadal axis. Thus, patients present with signs and symptoms secondary to deficiencies of all three major adrenal steroids–cortisol, aldosterone, and adrenal androgens–as well as gonadotropin deficiency. Finally a rare cause of hypercortisolism without cushingoid stigmata is *primary cortisol resistance* due to mutations in the glucocorticoid receptor. The resistance is incomplete because patients do not exhibit signs of adrenal insufficiency.

MISCELLANEOUS CONDITIONS

Adrenoleukodystrophy causes severe demyelination and early death in children, and adrenomyeloneuropathy is associated with a mixed motor and sensory neuropathy with spastic paraplegia in adults; both disorders are associated with elevated circulating levels of very long chain fatty acids and cause adrenal insufficiency. Autosomal recessive mutations in the *st*eroidogenic *a*cute *r*egulatory (STAR) protein gene cause congenital lipoid adrenal hyperplasia

(Chap. 7), which is characterized by adrenal insufficiency and defective gonadal steroidogenesis. Because STAR mediates cholesterol transport into the mitochondrion, mutations in the protein cause massive lipid accumulation in steroidogenic cells, ultimately leading to cell toxicity.

MINERALOCORTICOID DISEASES

Some forms of CAH have a mineralocorticoid component (see above). Others are caused by a mutation in other enzymes or ion channels important in mediating or mimicking aldosterone's action.

Hypermineralocorticoidism

Low Plasma Renin Activity Rarely, hypermineralocorticoidism is due to a defect in cortisol biosynthesis, specifically 11- or 17-hydroxylation. ACTH levels are increased, with a resultant increase in the production of the mineralocorticoid 11-deoxycorticosterone. Hypertension and hypokalemia can be corrected by glucocorticoid administration. The definitive diagnosis is made by demonstrating an elevation of precursors of cortisol biosynthesis in the blood or urine or by direct demonstration of the genetic defect.

Glucocorticoid administration can also ameliorate hypertension or produce normotension even though a hydroxylase deficiency cannot be identified (Fig. 5-9). These patients have normal to slightly elevated aldosterone levels that do not suppress in response to saline but do suppress in response to 2 days of dexamethasone (2 mg/d). The condition is inherited as an autosomal dominant trait and is termed *glucocorticoid-remediable aldosteronism* (GRA). This entity is secondary to a chimeric gene duplication whereby the 11-β hydroxylase gene promoter (which is under the control of ACTH) is fused to the aldosterone synthase coding sequence. Thus, aldosterone synthase activity is ectopically expressed in the zona fasciculata and is regulated by ACTH, in a fashion similar to the regulation of cortisol secretion. Screening for this defect is best performed by assessing the presence or absence of the chimeric gene. Because the abnormal gene may be present in the absence of hypokalemia, its frequency as a cause of hypertension is unknown. Individuals with suppressed plasma renin levels and juvenile-onset hypertension or a history of early-onset hypertension in first-degree relatives should be screened for this disorder. Early hemorrhagic stroke also occurs in GRA-affected individuals.

GRA documented by genetic analysis may be treated with glucocorticoid administration or antimineralocorticoids, i.e., spironolactone, triamterene, or amiloride. Glucocorticoids should be used only in small doses to avoid inducing iatrogenic Cushing's syndrome. A combination approach is often necessary.

High Plasma Renin Activity *Bartter syndrome* is characterized by severe hyperaldosteronism (hypokalemic alkalosis) with moderate to marked increases in renin activity and hypercalciuria, but normal blood pressure and no edema; this disorder usually begins in childhood. Renal biopsy shows juxtaglomerular hyperplasia. Bartter syndrome is caused by a mutation in the renal Na-K-2Cl co-transporter gene. The pathogenesis involves a defect in the renal conservation of sodium or chloride. The renal loss of sodium is thought to stimulate renin secretion and aldosterone production. Hyperaldosteronism produces potassium depletion, and hypokalemia further elevates prostaglandin production and plasma renin activity. In some cases, the hypokalemia may be potentiated by a defect in renal conservation of potassium.

Gitelman syndrome is an autosomal recessive trait characterized by renal salt wasting and as a result, as in Bartter syndrome, activation of the renin-angiotensin-aldosterone system. As a consequence affected individuals have low blood pressure, low serum potassium, low serum magnesium, and high serum bicarbonate. In contrast to Bartter syndrome, urinary calcium excretion is reduced. Gitelman syndrome results from loss-of-function mutations of the renal thiazide-sensitive Na-Cl co-transporter.

Increased Mineralocorticoid Action

Liddle syndrome is a rare autosomal dominant disorder that mimics hyperaldosteronism. The defect is in the genes encoding the β or η subunits of the epithelial sodium channel. Both renin and aldosterone levels are low, owing to the constitutively activated sodium channel and the resulting excess sodium reabsorption in the renal tubule.

A rare autosomal recessive cause of hypokalemia and hypertension is 11β-HSD II deficiency, in which cortisol cannot be converted to cortisone and hence binds to the MR and acts as a mineralocorticoid. This condition, also termed *apparent mineralocorticoid excess syndrome,* is caused by a defect in the gene encoding the renal isoform of this enzyme, 11β-HSD II. Patients can be identified either by documenting an increased ratio of cortisol to cortisone in the urine or by genetic analysis. Patients with the 11β-HSD deficiency syndrome can be treated with small doses of dexamethasone, which suppresses ACTH and endogenous cortisol production but binds less well to the mineralocorticoid receptor than does cortisol.

The ingestion of candies or chewing tobacco containing certain forms of licorice produces a syndrome that mimics primary aldosteronism. The component of such agents that causes sodium retention is glycyrrhizinic acid, which inhibits 11β-HSD II and hence

TABLE 5-9

A CHECKLIST FOR USE PRIOR TO THE ADMINISTRATION OF GLUCOCORTICOIDS IN PHARMACOLOGIC DOSES

Presence of tuberculosis or other chronic infection (chest x-ray, tuberculin test)
Evidence of glucose intolerance or history of gestational diabetes mellitus
Evidence of preexisting osteoporosis (bone density assessment in organ transplant recipients or postmenopausal patients)
History of peptic ulcer, gastritis, or esophagitis (stool guaiac test)
Evidence of hypertension or cardiovascular disease
History of psychological disorders

allows cortisol to act as a mineralocorticoid. The diagnosis is established or excluded by a careful history.

Decreased Mineralocorticoid Production or Action

In patients with a deficiency in aldosterone biosynthesis, the transformation of corticosterone into aldosterone is impaired, owing to a mutation in the aldosterone synthase (CYP11B2) gene. These patients have low to absent aldosterone secretion, elevated plasma renin levels, and elevated levels of the intermediates of aldosterone biosynthesis (corticosterone and 18-hydroxycorticosterone).

Pseudohypoaldosteronism type I (PHA-I) is an autosomal recessive disorder that is seen in the neonatal period and is characterized by salt wasting, hypotension, hyperkalemia, and high renin and aldosterone levels. In contrast to the gain-of-function mutations in the epithelial sodium channel in Liddle syndrome, mutations in PHA-I result in loss of epithelial sodium channel function.

PHARMACOLOGIC CLINICAL USES OF ADRENAL STEROIDS

The widespread use of glucocorticoids emphasizes the need for a thorough understanding of the metabolic effects of these agents. Before adrenal hormone therapy is instituted, the expected gains should be weighed against undesirable effects. Several important questions should be addressed before initiating therapy. First, how serious is the disorder (the more serious, the greater the likelihood that the risk/benefit ratio will be positive)? Second, how long will therapy be required (the longer the therapy, the greater the risk of adverse side effects)? Third, does the individual have preexisting conditions that glucocorticoids may exacerbate (**Table 5-9**)? If so, then a careful risk/benefit assessment is required to ensure that the ratio is favorable given the increased likelihood of harm by steroids in these patients. Supplementary measures to minimize undesirable metabolic effects are shown in **Table 5-10**. Fourth, which preparation is best?

TABLE 5-10

SUPPLEMENTARY MEASURES TO MINIMIZE UNDESIRABLE METABOLIC EFFECTS OF GLUCOCORTICOIDS

Monitor caloric intake to prevent weight gain.
Restrict sodium intake to prevent edema and minimize hypertension and potassium loss.
Provide supplementary potassium if necessary.
Provide antacid, H_2 receptor antagonist, and/or H^+, K^+-ATPase inhibitor therapy.
Institute alternate-day steroid schedule if possible. Patients receiving steroid therapy over a prolonged period should be protected by an appropriate increase in hormone level during periods of acute stress.
  A rule of thumb is to *double* the maintenance dose.
Minimize osteopenia by
  Administering gonadal hormone replacement therapy: 0.625–1.25 mg conjugated estrogens given cyclically with progesterone, unless the uterus is absent; testosterone replacement for hypogonadal men
Ensuring high calcium intake (should be approximately 1200 mg/d)
Administering supplemental vitamin D if blood levels of calciferol or 1,25 $(OH)_2$ vitamin D are reduced
Administering bisphosphonate prophylactically, orally or parenterally, in high-risk patients

THERAPEUTIC CONSIDERATIONS

The following considerations should be taken into account in deciding which steroid preparation to use:

1. *The biologic half-life.* The rationale behind alternate-day therapy is to decrease the metabolic effects of the steroids for a significant part of each 48-h period while still producing a pharmacologic effect durable enough to be effective. Too long a half-life would defeat the first purpose, and too short a half-life would defeat the second. In general, the more potent the steroid, the longer its biologic half-life.
2. *The mineralocorticoid effects of the steroid.* Most synthetic steroids have less mineralocorticoid effect than hydrocortisone (**Table 5-11**).
3. *The biologically active form of the steroid.* Cortisone and prednisone have to be converted to biologically active metabolites before anti-inflammatory effects can occur. Because of this, in a condition for which steroids are known to be effective and when an adequate dose has been given without response, one should consider substituting hydrocortisone or prednisolone for cortisone or prednisone.
4. *The cost of the medication.* This is a serious consideration if chronic administration is planned. Prednisone is the least expensive of available steroid preparations.
5. *The type of formulation.* Topical steroids have the distinct advantage over oral steroids in reducing the likelihood of systemic side effects. In addition, some inhaled steroids have been designed to minimize side effects by increasing their hepatic inactivation if they are swallowed (Chap. 236 in HPIM, 16e). However, all topical steroids can be absorbed into the systemic circulation.

ALTERNATE-DAY STEROID THERAPY

The most effective way to minimize the cushingoid effects of glucocorticoids is to administer the total 48-h dose as a *single* dose of *intermediate-acting steroid* in the morning, *every other day.* If symptoms of the underlying disorder can be controlled by this technique, it offers distinct advantages. Three considerations deserve mention: (1) The alternate-day schedule may be approached through transition schedules that allow the patient to adjust gradually; (2) supplementary nonsteroid medications may be needed on the "off" day to minimize symptoms of the underlying disorder; and (3) many symptoms that occur during the off day (e.g., fatigue, joint pain, muscle stiffness or tenderness, and fever) may represent relative adrenal insufficiency rather than exacerbation of the underlying disease.

TABLE 5-11

GLUCOCORTICOID PREPARATIONS

	ESTIMATED POTENCY[b]	
COMMONLY USED NAME[a]	GLUCOCORTICOID	MINERALOCORTICOID
Short-Acting		
Hydrocortisone	1	1
Cortisone	0.8	0.8
Intermediate-Acting		
Prednisone	4	0.25
Prednisolone	4	0.25
Methylprednisolone	5	<0.01
Triamcinolone	5	<0.01
Long-Acting		
Paramethasone	10	<0.01
Betamethasone	25	<0.01
Dexamethasone	30–40	<0.01

[a]The steroids are divided into three groups according to the duration of biologic activity. Short-acting preparations have a biologic half-life <12 h; long-acting, >48 h; and intermediate, between 12 and 36 h. Triamcinolone has the longest half-life of the intermediate-acting preparations.

[b]Relative milligram comparisons with hydrocortisone, setting the glucocorticoid and mineralocorticoid properties of hydrocortisone as 1. Sodium retention is insignificant for commonly employed doses of methylprednisolone, triamcinolone, paramethasone, betamethasone, and dexamethasone.

The alternate-day approach capitalizes on the fact that cortisol secretion and plasma levels normally are highest in the early morning and lowest in the evening. The normal pattern is mimicked by administering an intermediate-acting steroid in the morning (7 to 8 A.M.) (Table 5-11).

Initially, the steroid regimen often requires daily or more frequent doses of steroid to achieve the desired anti-inflammatory or immunity-suppressing action. *Only after this desired effect is achieved is an attempt made to switch to an alternate-day program.* A number of schedules can be used for transferring from a daily to an alternate-day program. The key points to be considered are flexibility in arranging a program and the use of supportive measures on the off day. One may attempt a gradual transition to the alternate-day schedule rather than an abrupt changeover. One approach is to keep the steroid dose constant on one day and gradually reduce it on the alternate day. Alternatively, the steroid dose can be increased on one day and reduced on the alternate day. In any case, it is important to anticipate that some increase in pain or discomfort may occur in the 36 to 48 h following the last dose.

WITHDRAWAL OF GLUCOCORTICOIDS FOLLOWING LONG-TERM USE

It is possible to reduce a daily steroid dose gradually and eventually to discontinue it, but under most circumstances withdrawal of steroids should be initiated by first implementing an alternate-day schedule. Patients who have been on an alternate-day program for a month or more experience less difficulty during termination regimens. The dosage is gradually reduced and finally discontinued after a replacement dosage has been reached (e.g., 5 to 7.5 mg prednisone). Complications rarely ensue unless undue stress is experienced, and patients should understand that for ≥1 year after withdrawal from long-term high-dose steroid therapy, supplementary hormone should be given in the event of a serious infection, operation, or injury. A useful strategy in patients with symptoms of adrenal insufficiency on a tapering regimen is to measure plasma cortisol levels prior to the steroid dose. A level <140 nmol/L (5 μg/dL) indicates suppression of the pituitary-adrenal axis and implies that a more cautious tapering of steroids is indicated.

In patients on high-dose daily steroid therapy, it is advised to reduce dosage to ~20 mg prednisone daily as a single morning dose before beginning the transition to alternate-day therapy. If a patient cannot tolerate an alternate-day program, consideration should be given to the possibility that the patient has developed primary adrenal insufficiency.

FURTHER READINGS

ARNALDI G et al: Diagnosis and complications of Cushing's syndrome: A consensus statement. J Clin Endocrinol Metab 88:5593, 2003

This consensus statement was developed by 50 endocrinologists with specific expertise in the management of Cushing's syndrome. In particular, it emphasizes the importance of managing the complications of Cushing's syndrome.

BARZON L et al: Risk factors and long-term follow-up of adrenal incidentalomas. J Clin Endocrinol Metab 84:520, 1999

BLACK HR: Evolving role of aldosterone blockers alone and in combination with angiotensin-converting enzyme inhibitors or angiotensin II receptor blockers in hypertension management: A review of mechanistic and clinical data. Am Heart J 147:564, 2004

CONLIN PR et al: Disorders of the renin-angiotensin-aldosterone system, in *Renal and Electrolyte Disorders,* 6th ed, RW Schrier (ed). Boston, Little, Brown, 2003, pp 303–340

COOPER MS et al: Current concepts: Corticosteroid insufficiency in acutely ill patients. N Engl J Med 348: 727, 2003

DORIN RI et al: Diagnosis of adrenal insufficiency. Ann Intern Med 139:194, 2003

This article summarizes the results of multiple studies involving the use of the cosyntropin stimulation test in primary and secondary adrenal insufficiency. The author concludes that both the low-dose (1 μg) and high-dose (250 μg) cosyntropin tests perform well in the diagnosis of primary adrenal insufficiency but lack sensitivity for reliable diagnosis of secondary adrenal insufficiency.

HAMRAHIAN AH et al: Clinical utility of noncontrast computed tomography attenuation value (hounsfield units) to differentiate adrenal adenomas/hyperplasias from nonadenomas: Cleveland Clinic experience. J Clin Endocrinol Metab 90:871, 2005

This study supports the idea that the combination of noncontrast CT and tumor size can predict whether an incidentaloma is likely to be benign or malignant.

KALTSAS GA et al: A critical analysis of the value of simultaneous inferior petrosal sinus sampling in Cushing's disease and the occult ectopic adrenocorticotropin syndrome. J Clin Endocrinol Metab 84:487, 1999

Keating GM et al: Eplerenone: A review of its use in left ventricular systolic dysfunction and heart failure after acute myocardial infarction. Drugs 64:2689, 2004

Eplerenone is a selective aldosterone blocker. This review summarizes the results of several large clinical trials indicating that the addition of eplerenone to standard medical therapy is an important new strategy for further improving mortality and morbidity in post-MI patients with LV systolic dysfunction and heart failure.

Mansmann G et al: The clinically inaparent adrenal mass: Update in diagnosis and management. Endocr Rev 25:309, 2004

Martinez DV et al: Cardiac damage prevention by eplerenone: Comparison with low sodium diet or potassium loading. Hypertension 39:614, 2002

Metherell LA et al: Mutations in MRAP, encoding a new interacting partner of the ACTH receptor, cause familial glucocorticoid deficiency type 2. Nat Genet 37:166, 2005

Based on linkage analyses in an inbred family, this report localizes a gene on chromosome 21q22.1 (with high levels of expression in the adrenal cortex) that encodes a single transmembrane-domain protein referred to as melanocortin 2 receptor accessory protein (MRAP). The identification of mutations in MRAP as a cause of familial glucocorticoid deficiency type-2 (FGD-2) and the molecular characterization of its interaction with MC2R define an important new mechanism underlying resistance to ACTH. Given the ubiquitous nature of G protein-coupled receptors in endocrine organs, it is possible that similar mechanisms may cause or contribute to states of hormone resistance in other receptor systems.

Mulatero P et al: Diagnosis of primary aldosteronism: From screening to subtype differentiation. Trends Endocrinol Metab 16:114, 2005

Newell-Price J et al: Diagnosis and management of Cushing's syndrome. Lancet 353:2087, 1999

Pitt B et al: Eplerenone, a selective aldosterone blocker, in patients with left ventricular dysfunction after myocardial infarction. N Engl J Med 348:1309, 2003

Young WF: Minireview: Primary aldosteronism–changing concepts in diagnosis and treatment. Endocrinology 144:2208, 2003

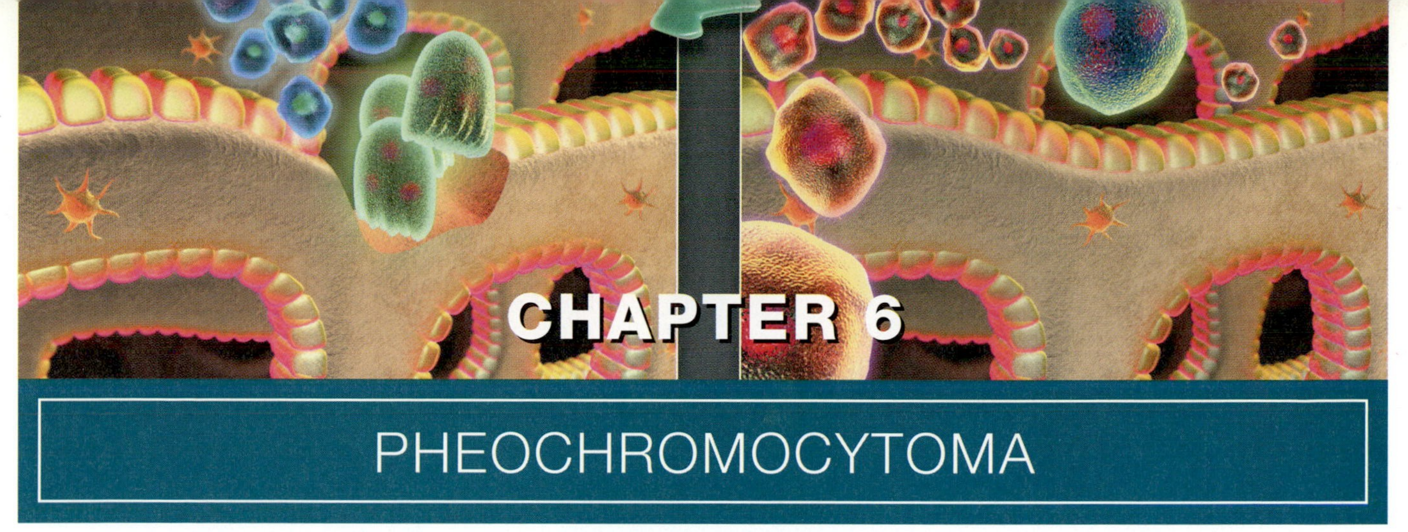

PHEOCHROMOCYTOMA

Lewis Landsberg
James B. Young

Pheochromocytomas produce, store, and secrete catecholamines. They are usually derived from the adrenal medulla but may develop from chromaffin cells in or about sympathetic ganglia (extraadrenal pheochromocytomas or paragangliomas). Related tumors that secrete catecholamines and produce similar clinical syndromes include chemodectomas derived from the carotid body and ganglioneuromas derived from the postganglionic sympathetic neurons.

The clinical features are due predominantly to the release of catecholamines and, to a lesser extent, to the secretion of other substances. Hypertension is the most common sign, and hypertensive paroxysms or crises, often spectacular and alarming, occur in over half the cases.

Pheochromocytoma occurs in approximately 0.1% of the hypertensive population but is, nevertheless, an important correctable cause of high blood pressure. Indeed, it is usually curable if diagnosed and treated, but it may be fatal if undiagnosed or mistreated. Postmortem series indicate that most pheochromocytomas are unsuspected clinically, even when the tumor is related to the fatal outcome.

PATHOLOGY

LOCATION AND MORPHOLOGY

In adults, approximately 80% of pheochromocytomas are unilateral and solitary, 10% are bilateral, and 10% are extraadrenal. In children, a fourth of tumors are bilateral, and an additional fourth are extraadrenal. Solitary lesions inexplicably favor the right side. Although pheochromocytomas may grow to large size (>3 kg), most weigh <100 g and are <10 cm in diameter. Pheochromocytomas are highly vascular.

The tumors are made up of large, polyhedral, pleomorphic chromaffin cells. Fewer than 10% of these tumors are malignant. As with several other endocrine tumors, malignancy cannot be determined from the histologic appearance; tumors that contain large numbers of aneuploid or tetraploid cells, as determined by flow cytometry, are more likely to recur. Local invasion of surrounding tissues or distant metastases indicate malignancy.

EXTRAADRENAL PHEOCHROMOCYTOMAS

Extraadrenal pheochromocytomas usually weigh 20 to 40 g and are <5 cm in diameter. Most are located within the abdomen in association with the celiac, superior mesenteric, and inferior mesenteric ganglia. Approximately 10% are in the thorax, 1% are within the urinary bladder, and <3% are in the neck, usually in association with the sympathetic ganglia or the extracranial branches of the ninth or tenth cranial nerves.

CATECHOLAMINE SYNTHESIS, STORAGE, AND RELEASE

Pheochromocytomas synthesize and store catecholamines by processes resembling those of the normal adrenal medulla. Little is known about the mechanisms of catecholamine release from pheochromocytomas, but changes in blood flow and necrosis within the tumor may be the cause in some instances. These tumors are not innervated, and catecholamine release does not result from neural stimulation. Pheochromocytomas also store and secrete a variety of peptides, including endogenous opioids, adrenomedullin, endothelin, erythropoietin, parathyroid hormone-related protein, neuropeptide Y, and chromagranin A. These peptides contribute to the clinical manifestations in selected cases, as noted below.

Epinephrine, Norepinephrine, and Dopamine

Most pheochromocytomas produce both norepinephrine and epinephrine, and the percentage of norepinephrine is usually greater than in the normal adrenal. Most extraadrenal pheochromocytomas secrete norepinephrine exclusively. Rarely, pheochromocytomas produce epinephrine alone, particularly in association with multiple endocrine neoplasia (MEN). Although epinephrine-producing tumors may cause a preponderance of metabolic and beta-receptor effects, in general the major catecholamine secreted cannot be predicted from the clinical presentation. Increased production of dopamine and homovanillic acid (HVA) is uncommon with benign lesions but may occur with malignant pheochromocytoma.

FAMILIAL PHEOCHROMOCYTOMA

Pheochromocytoma may be inherited as an autosomal dominant trait either alone or in combination with other abnormalities such as MEN type 2A (Sipple's syndrome) or type 2B (mucosal neuroma syndrome) (Chap. 21), von Hippel–Lindau's (VHL) retinal cerebellar hemangioblastomatosis, or von Recklinghausen's neurofibromatosis (type 1) and in association with paragangliomas of the neck. Recent evidence suggests that 25% of patients with pheochromocytoma may have an inherited form of the disease. Features that suggest familial disease include bilaterality, multicentricity (within the adrenal and at diverse sites), and age of onset <30 years.

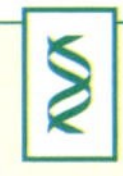

GENETIC CONSIDERATIONS

MEN 2

The MEN 2A and 2B syndromes are associated with abnormalities in the *RET* protooncogene located in the pericentromeric region of chromosome 10 (Chap. 21). These mutations result in the constitutive activation of the receptor tyrosine kinase, causing adrenal medullary chromaffin cell and thyroid parafollicular C cell hyperplasia and rendering the cells susceptible to malignant transformation. The *RET* mutations are located in the extracellular domain in MEN 2A and in the intracellular portion of the receptor in families with the MEN 2B syndrome. Mutations at specific sites in the *RET* protooncogene are highly predictive of pheochromocytoma. Pheochromocytomas in MEN 2 are multicentric and bilateral but not extraadrenal. Individuals at risk for MEN 2A and 2B should be screened periodically for pheochromocytoma by assay of a 24-h urine sample for catecholamines, including measurement of epinephrine. Pheochromocytoma should be excluded or removed before thyroid or parathyroid surgery.

VHL

In the VHL syndrome, mutation of one copy of the VHL tumor-suppressor gene is associated with the development of tumors characteristic of the syndrome, including pheochromocytomas. Loss of function of the VHL tumor-suppressor gene promotes tumor formation by mechanisms that are incompletely understood but may involve alterations in mRNA transcript elongation. In the VHL syndrome, the frequency of pheochromocytoma varies considerably but may be as high as 60% in some kindreds. As in the MEN 2 syndromes, certain VHL mutations are highly associated with the development of pheochromocytoma. Of further interest is the recent finding that the VHL mutation has been identified in some kindreds with familial pheochromocytoma as the sole manifestation without other clinical evidence of the VHL syndrome. Missense mutations, as opposed to deletions, insertions, or nonsense mutations, appear to be more commonly associated with pheochromocytoma, which may be adrenal, extraadrenal, or multifocal. A high incidence of germ-line VHL mutations in patients with thoracic extraadrenal pheochromocytomas also has been reported.

Familial Paraganglioma Syndromes

Mutations in the genes encoding succinate dehydrogenase subunit B (SDHB) and subunit D (SDHD) may occur in kindreds with inherited paraganglioma, usually located in the head or neck (glomus tumors) or carotid body. Paraganglioma in these syndromes is distinct from extraadrenal pheochromocytomas, which are also commonly referred to as *paragangliomas.* Adrenal or extraadrenal pheochromocytomas are often inherited in association with these paragangliomas.

Neurofibromatosis Type I

Mutations in the *NF-I* gene predispose to the development of pheochromocytoma, although the association is not very common. It has been estimated that 1% of patients with pheochromocytoma have an *NF-I* mutation. Pheochromocytomas may occur in patients with minor clinical manifestations of neurofibromatosis such as a few café au lait spots, vertebral abnormalities, or kyphoscoliosis.

Nonsyndromic Familial Pheochromocytoma

Patients presenting with a solitary adrenal pheochromocytoma, negative family history, and no evidence of associated disease may still have an inherited form of the disease. This is most common with the *SDHB* and *SDHD* mutations but also occurs with alterations in the *VHL* gene.

Screening for Genetic Disease

Genetic screening for the *RET* mutation is available and of established utility in the evaluation of families for the MEN 2 syndromes. Genetic tests for the *SDH, NF-I,* and *VHL* mutations are not yet generally available. Screening in these kindreds therefore is dependent on a vigorous search for the associated diseases and a complete evaluation of family history.

CLINICAL FEATURES

Pheochromocytoma occurs at all ages but is most common in young to midadult life. Some series show a slight female preponderance. Most patients come to medical attention as a result of hypertensive crisis, paroxysmal symptoms suggestive of seizure disorder or anxiety attacks, or hypertension that responds poorly to conventional treatment. Less commonly, unexplained hypotension or shock in association with surgery or trauma will suggest the diagnosis. Aberrant reactions to medications such as opioids or tricyclic antidepressants may bring the patient to clinical attention. In most patients the hypertension is associated with other symptoms, such as headaches, excessive sweating, and/or palpitations.

HYPERTENSION

Hypertension is the most common manifestation. In approximately 60% of cases the hypertension is sustained, although significant blood pressure lability is usually present, and half of patients with sustained hypertension have distinct crises or paroxysms. The other 40% have blood pressure elevations only during an attack. The hypertension is often severe, occasionally malignant, and may be resistant to treatment with standard antihypertensive drugs.

Paroxysms or Crises

The paroxysm or crisis occurs in over half of patients. In an individual patient, the symptoms are often similar with each attack. The paroxysms may be frequent or sporadic, occurring at intervals as long as weeks or months. With time, the paroxysms usually increase in frequency, duration, and severity.

The attack usually has a sudden onset. It may last from a few minutes to several hours or longer. Headache, profuse sweating, palpitations, and apprehension, often with a sense of impending doom, are common. Pain in the chest or abdomen may be associated with nausea and vomiting. Either pallor or flushing may occur during the attack. The blood pressure is elevated, often to alarming levels, and the elevation is usually accompanied by tachycardia.

The paroxysm may be precipitated by any activity that displaces the abdominal contents. In some cases a particular stimulus may induce an attack in a characteristic fashion, but in others no clearly defined precipitating event can be found. Although anxiety may accompany the attacks, mental or psychological stress does not usually provoke a crisis.

OTHER DISTINCTIVE CLINICAL FEATURES

Symptoms and signs of an increased metabolic rate, such as profuse sweating and mild to moderate weight loss, are common. Orthostatic hypotension is a consequence of diminished plasma volume and blunted sympathetic reflexes. Both these factors predispose the patient with unsuspected pheochromocytoma to hypotension or shock during surgery or trauma. Secretion of the hypotensive peptide adrenomedullin may contribute to the hypotension in some patients.

Cardiac Manifestations

Sinus tachycardia, sinus bradycardia, supraventricular arrhythmias, and ventricular premature contractions have all been noted. Angina and acute myocardial infarction may occur even in the absence of coronary artery disease. A catecholamine-induced increase in myocardial oxygen consumption and, perhaps, coronary spasm may play a role in these ischemic events. Electrocardiographic changes, including nonspecific ST-T wave changes, prominent U waves, left ventricular strain patterns, and right and left bundle branch blocks may be present in the absence of demonstrable ischemia or infarction. Cardiomyopathy, either congestive with myocarditis and myocardial fibrosis or hypertrophic with concentric or asymmetric hypertrophy, may be associated with heart failure and cardiac arrhythmias. Multiorgan system failure with noncardiogenic pulmonary edema may be the presenting manifestation. Elevated levels of amylase originating from damaged pulmonary endothelium and abdominal pain may suggest acute pancreatitis, although serum lipase levels are normal.

Carbohydrate Intolerance

Over half of patients have impaired carbohydrate tolerance due to suppression of insulin and stimulation of hepatic glucose output. The impaired glucose tolerance may require treatment with insulin and disappears after removal of the tumor.

Hematocrit

An elevated hematocrit may be secondary to diminished plasma volume. Rarely, production of erythropoietin by the tumor may cause a true erythrocytosis.

Other Manifestations

Hypercalcemia has been attributed to the ectopic secretion of parathyroid hormone–related protein. Fever and an elevated erythrocyte sedimentation rate have been reported in association with the production of interleukin 6. Elevated temperature more commonly reflects catecholamine-mediated increases in metabolic rate and diminished heat dissipation secondary to vasoconstriction. Polyuria is an occasional finding, and rhabdomyolysis with myoglobinuric renal failure may result from extreme vasoconstriction with muscle ischemia. Ectopic production of adrenocorticotropic hormone and vasoactive intestinal peptide have been documented in association with the characteristic manifestations of inappropriate secretion of these hormones (Chap. 1).

Pheochromocytoma of the Urinary Bladder

Pheochromocytoma in the wall of the urinary bladder may result in typical paroxysms in relation to micturition. The location in the bladder wall is responsible for the occurrence of symptoms while the tumors are quite small, and, consequently, catecholamine excretion may be normal or minimally elevated. Hematuria is present in over half of patients, and the tumor can often be visualized at cystoscopy.

ADVERSE DRUG INTERACTIONS

Severe and occasionally fatal paroxysms have been induced by opiates, histamine, adrenocorticotropin, saralasin, and glucagon. These agents appear to release catecholamines directly from the tumor. Indirect-acting sympathomimetic amines, including methyldopa (when administered intravenously), may increase blood pressure by releasing catecholamines from the augmented stores within nerve endings. Drugs that block neuronal uptake of catecholamines, such as tricyclic antidepressants, may enhance the physiologic effects of circulating catecholamines. Indeed, all medications should be considered carefully and administered cautiously in patients with known or suspected pheochromocytoma.

DIAGNOSIS

The diagnosis is established by the demonstration of increased production of catecholamines or catecholamine metabolites. The diagnosis can usually be made by the analysis of a single 24-h urine sample, provided the patient is hypertensive or symptomatic at the time of collection.

BIOCHEMICAL TESTS

The assays employed include those for vanillylmandelic acid (VMA), the metanephrines, and unconjugated or "free" catecholamines. The VMA assay is both less sensitive and less specific than assays of metanephrines or catecholamines. Accuracy of diagnosis is improved when two of three determinations are employed. The following considerations apply to all the urinary tests: (1) Despite claims for the adequacy of determinations made on random urine samples, analysis of a full 24-h urine sample is preferable. Creatinine also should be determined to assess the adequacy of collection. (2) Where possible, the collection should be made when the patient is at rest, on no medication, and without recent exposure to radiographic contrast media. When it is not practical to discontinue all medications, drugs known specifically to interfere with these assays (as noted below) should be avoided. (3) The urine should be acidified and refrigerated during and after collection. (4) With high-quality assays, dietary restrictions are minimal and should be specified by the laboratory performing the analyses. (5) Although most patients with pheochromocytoma excrete increased amounts of catecholamines and catecholamine metabolites at all times, the yield is increased in patients with paroxysmal hypertension if a 24-h urine collection is initiated during a crisis.

Free Catecholamines

The upper limit of normal for total urinary catecholamines is between 590 and 885 nmol (100 and 150 μg) per 24 h. In most patients with pheochromocytoma, values >1480 nmol (250 μg) per day are obtained. Measurement of epinephrine is often of value, since increased epinephrine excretion [>275 nmol (50 μg) per 24 h] is usually due to an adrenal lesion and may be the only abnormality in cases associated with MEN 2. False-positive increases in catecholamine excretion result from exogenous catecholamines and related drugs such as methyldopa, levodopa, labetalol, and sympathomimetic amines, which may elevate catecholamine excretion for up to 2 weeks. Endogenous catecholamines from stimulation of the sympathoadrenal system may also increase urinary catecholamine excretion. Relevant clinical situations that cause such increases include hypoglycemia, strenuous exertion, central nervous system disease with increased intracranial pressure, severe hypoxia, and clonidine withdrawal.

Metanephrines and VMA

In most laboratories, the upper limit of normal is 7 μmol (1.3 mg) of total metanephrines and 35 μmol (7.0 mg) of VMA excretion per 24 h. In most patients with pheochromocytoma, the increase in these urinary metabolites is considerable, often to more than three times the normal range. Metanephrine excretion is increased by exogenous and endogenous catecholamines and by treatment with monoamine oxidase inhibitors; propranolol may cause a spurious increase in metanephrine excretion, since a propranolol metabolite interferes in the commonly used spectrophotometric assay. VMA is less affected by endogenous and exogenous catecholamines but is spuriously increased by a variety of drugs, including carbidopa. VMA excretion is decreased by monoamine oxidase inhibitors.

Plasma Catecholamines

Measurement of plasma catecholamines has a limited application. The care required in obtaining basal levels and the satisfactory results with urinary determinations make measurement of plasma catecholamines unnecessary in most cases. Plasma catecholamine levels are affected by the same drugs and physiologic perturbations that increase urinary catecholamine excretion. In addition, α- and β-adrenergic receptor blocking agents may elevate plasma catecholamines by impairing clearance.

When the clinical features suggest pheochromocytoma and the urinary assay results are borderline, measurement of plasma catecholamines may be worthwhile. Markedly elevated basal levels of total catecholamines support the diagnosis, although approximately one-third of patients with pheochromocytoma have normal or slightly elevated basal values. The usefulness of plasma catecholamine determinations may be increased by agents that suppress sympathetic nervous system activity. Clonidine and ganglionic blocking agents reduce plasma catecholamine levels in normal subjects and in patients with essential hypertension. These drugs have little effect on catecholamine levels in patients with pheochromocytoma. In patients with elevated or borderline basal catecholamine values, failure to suppress plasma or urinary levels with clonidine supports the diagnosis of pheochromocytoma.

Plasma Metanephrines

Measurement of free (unconjugated) total plasma metanephrines, fractionated into normetanephrine and metanephrine, is a highly sensitive technique for the diagnosis of pheochromocytoma. Questions of specificity, particularly among the elderly, as well as the availability of high-quality assays need to be addressed before plasma metanephrines replace the 24-h urinary measurement of free catecholamines and metanephrines as the screening test of choice.

PHARMACOLOGIC TESTS

Reliable methods for the measurement of catecholamines and catecholamine metabolites in urine have rendered obsolete both the provocative and adrenolytic tests, which are nonspecific and entail considerable risk. A modified version of the adrenolytic test may be of some use, however, as a therapeutic trial in a patient in hypertensive crisis with features suggestive of pheochromocytoma. A positive response to phentolamine (5-mg bolus following a test dose of 0.5 mg) is a reduction in blood pressure of at least 35/25 mmHg after 2 min that persists for 10 to 15 min. The pharmacologic response is never diagnostic, and biochemical confirmation is essential. Provocative tests in normotensive patients are potentially dangerous and rarely indicated. However, a glucagon provocative test may be of use in patients with paroxysmal hypertension and nondiagnostic basal catecholamine levels. Glucagon has a negligible effect on blood pressure or plasma catecholamine levels in normal or hypertensive subjects. In patients with pheochromocytoma, on the other hand, glucagon may increase both blood pressure and circulating catecholamine levels. The elevation in plasma catecatcholamine concentration, moreover, may occur without a blood pressure response. It must be emphasized, however, that life-threatening pressor crises have occurred after administration of glucagon to patients with pheochromocytoma, so the test should never be performed casually. Careful continuous monitoring of the blood pressure is required, intravenous access must be adequate, and phentolamine must be at hand to terminate the test if a significant pressor reaction ensues.

DIFFERENTIAL DIAGNOSIS

Since the manifestations of pheochromocytoma can be protean, the diagnosis must be considered and excluded in many patients with suggestive clinical features. In patients with essential hypertension and "hyperadrenergic" features such as tachycardia, sweating, and increased cardiac output, and in patients with anxiety attacks associated with blood pressure elevations, analysis of a 24-h urine collection is usually decisive in excluding the diagnosis. Repeated determinations on urine collected during attacks may be necessary, however, before the diagnosis can be excluded with certainty. Pressor crises associated with clonidine withdrawal and the use of cocaine or monoamine oxidase inhibitors may mimic the paroxysms of pheochromocytoma. Factitious crises may be produced by self-administration of sympathomimetic amines in psychiatrically disturbed patients.

Intracranial lesions, particularly posterior fossa tumors or subarachnoid hemorrhage, may cause hypertension and increased excretion of catecholamines or catecholamine metabolites. While this is most common in patients with an obvious neurologic catastrophe, the possibility of subarachnoid or intracranial hemorrhage secondary to pheochromocytoma should be considered. Diencephalic or autonomic epilepsy may be associated with paroxysmal spells, hypertension, and increased plasma catecholamine levels. This rare entity may be difficult to distinguish from pheochromocytoma, but an aura, an abnormal electroencephalogram, and a beneficial response to anticonvulsant medications will often suggest this diagnosis.

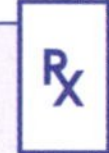

TREATMENT FOR PHEOCHROMOCYTOMA

Preoperative Management

The induction of stable α-adrenergic blockade provides the foundation for successful surgical treatment. Once the diagnosis is established, the patient should be placed on phenoxybenzamine to induce a long-lasting, noncompetitive α-receptor blockade. The usual initial dose is 10 mg every 12 h, with increments of 10 to 20 mg added every few days until the blood pressure is controlled and the paroxysms disappear. Because of the long duration of action, the therapeutic effects are cumulative, and the optimal dose must be achieved gradually with careful monitoring of supine and upright blood pressures. Most patients require between 40 and 80 mg phenoxybenzamine per day, although $\geq$200 mg may be necessary. Phenoxybenzamine should be administered for at least 10 to 14 days prior to surgery. Over this time, the combination of α-receptor blockade and a liberal salt intake will restore the contracted plasma volume to normal. Before adequate α-adrenergic blockade with phenoxybenzamine is achieved, paroxysms may be treated with oral prazosin or intravenous phentolamine. Selective α_1 antagonists have been employed for preoperative preparation, but their role in preparative management should be limited to the treatment of individual paroxysms. They may be useful as antihypertensive agents in patients with suspected pheochromocytoma while workup is in progress, since they are usually better tolerated than phenoxybenzamine and will prevent serious pressor crises if pheochromocytoma is present. Nitroprusside, calcium channel blocking agents, and possibly angiotensin-converting enzyme inhibitors reduce blood pressure in patients with pheochromocytoma. Nitroprusside may also be useful in the treatment of pressor crises.

β-Adrenergic receptor blocking agents should be given only after alpha blockade has been induced, since administration of such agents by themselves may cause a paradoxical increase in blood pressure by antagonizing beta-mediated vasodilation in skeletal muscle. Beta blockade is usually initiated when tachycardia develops during the induction of α-adrenergic blockade. Low doses often suffice, and a reasonable starting dose is 10 mg propranolol three to four times per day, increased as needed to control the pulse rate. Beta blockade is effective for catecholamine-induced arrhythmias, particularly those potentiated by anesthetic agents.

Preoperative Localization of the Tumor

Once pheochromocytoma is diagnosed, localization should be undertaken while the patient is being prepared for surgery. Computed tomography (CT) or magnetic resonance imaging (MRI) of the adrenals is usually successful in identifying intraadrenal lesions. Extraadrenal tumors within the chest can frequently be identified by conventional chest films or CT. MRI or positron emission tomography (PET) scanning with ^{18}F dopa is useful in identifying extraadrenal tumors. Abdominal aortography (once α-adrenergic blockade is complete) or venous sampling at different levels of the inferior and superior vena cava in search of catecholamine gradients has been useful in the past but are rarely necessary now. An additional localization technique involves a radionuclide scintiscan after administration of the radiopharmaceutical [^{131}I]metaiodobenzylguanidine (MIBG). This agent is concentrated by the amine uptake process and produces an external scintigraphic image at the site of the tumor. This type of scanning may be useful in characterizing lesions discovered by CT when biochemical confirmation is indeterminate but is less useful for localizing extraadrenal pheochromocytomas than MRI or PET. Percutaneous fine-needle aspiration of chromaffin tumors is contraindicated; indeed, pheochromocytoma should be considered before adrenal lesions are aspirated.

Surgery

Surgical treatment of pheochromocytoma is best performed in centers with experience in the preoperative, anesthetic, and intraoperative management of pheochromocytoma. Surgical mortality is <2 or 3%. Extensive experience with the laparoscopic approach over the past decade has demonstrated that in experienced hands pheochromocytoma can be safely and efficiently removed by this technique.

Monitoring during the surgical procedure should include continuous recording of arterial pressure and central venous pressure as well as electrocardiography; in the presence of cardiac disease or if congestive failure has been present, pulmonary capillary wedge pressure should be monitored. Adequate fluid replacement is crucial. Intraoperative hypotension responds better to volume replacement than to vasoconstrictors. Hypertension and cardiac arrhythmias are most likely during induction of anesthesia, intubation, and manipulation of the tumor. Intravenous phentolamine is usually sufficient to control the blood pressure, but nitroprusside may be required. Propranolol may be given in the treatment of tachycardia or ventricular ectopy.

PHEOCHROMOCYTOMA IN PREGNANCY

Spontaneous labor and vaginal delivery in unprepared patients are usually disastrous for mother and fetus. In early pregnancy, the patient should be prepared with phenoxybenzamine, and the tumor should be removed as soon as the diagnosis is confirmed. The pregnancy need not be terminated, but the operative procedure itself may result in spontaneous abortion. In the third trimester, treatment with adrenergic blocking agents should be undertaken; when the fetus is of sufficient size, cesarean section may be followed by extirpation of the tumor. Although the safety of adrenergic blocking drugs in pregnancy is not established, these agents have been administered in several cases without obvious adverse effect. Antepartum diagnosis and treatment lowers the maternal death rate to that approaching nonpregnant pheochromocytoma patients; fetal death rate, however, remains elevated.

UNRESECTABLE AND MALIGNANT TUMORS

In cases of metastatic or locally invasive tumor in patients with intercurrent illness that precludes surgery, long-term medical management is required. When the manifestations cannot be adequately controlled by adrenergic blocking agents, the concomitant administration of metyrosine may be required. This agent inhibits tyrosine hydroxylase, diminishes catecholamine production by the tumor, and often simplifies chronic management. Malignant pheochromocytoma frequently recurs in the retroperitoneum, and it metastasizes most commonly to bone and lung. Although these malignant tumors are resistant to radiotherapy, combination chemotherapy is occasionally of some benefit. Use of ^{131}I-MIBG has had limited success in the treatment of malignant pheochromocytoma, due to poor uptake of the radioligand.

PROGNOSIS AND FOLLOW-UP

The 5-year survival rate after surgery is usually >95%; the recurrence rate is <10%. After successful surgery, catecholamine excretion returns to normal in about 2 weeks and should be measured to ensure complete tumor removal. Catecholamine excretion should be assessed at the reappearance of suggestive symptoms or yearly if the patient remains asymptomatic. For malignant pheochromocytoma, the 5-year survival rate is usually <50%, although long-term survival is occasionally noted.

Complete removal cures the hypertension in approximately three-fourths of patients. In the remainder, hypertension recurs but is usually well controlled by standard antihypertensive agents. In this group, either underlying essential hypertension or irreversible vascular damage induced by catecholamines may cause the persistence of the hypertension.

FURTHER READINGS

BRYANT J et al: Pheochromocytoma: The expanding genetic differential diagnosis. J Natl Cancer Inst 95:1196, 2003

DANNENBERG H et al: Molecular genetic alterations in adrenal and extra-adrenal pheochromocytomas and paragangliomas. Endocr Pathol 14:329, 2003

Genetic predisposition to pheochromocytomas and paragangliomas includes von Hippel-Lindau disease (VHL), multiple endocrine neoplasia type 2 (MEN2), three familial paraganglioma (PGL) syndromes (PGL1, PGL3, PGL4), and neurofibromatosis type 1 (NF1). This review summarizes our current understanding of the molecular pathogenesis of pheochromocytoma and paraganglioma.

EISENHOFER G et al: Catecholamine metabolism: A contemporary view with implications for physiology and medicine. Pharmacol Rev 56:331, 2004

——— et al: Biochemical diagnosis of pheochromocytoma: How to distinguish true- from false-positive test results. J Clin Endocrinol Metab 88:2656, 2003

ILIAS I et al: Current approaches and recommended algorithm for the diagnostic localization of pheochromocytoma. J Clin Endocrinol Metab 89:479, 2004

After the biochemical diagnosis of pheochromocytoma, it is important to localize the tumor and evaluate the possibility of multicentric disease. This review focuses on a wide array of imaging techniques, including functional studies, that are used to localize pheochromocytomas.

LENDERS JW et al: Biochemical diagnosis of pheochromocytoma: Which test is best? JAMA 287:1427, 2002

NEUMANN HP et al: Germ-line mutations in nonsyndromic pheochromocytoma. N Engl J Med 346:1459, 2002

This study evaluated 271 patients who presented with nonsyndromic pheochromocytoma. Almost one-fourth of patients with apparently sporadic pheochromocytoma were found to be carriers of mutations in the RET, VHL, SDHD, or SDHB genes. While it remains to be seen if such a high prevalence is seen in other populations, this study provides important information about the molecular pathogenesis of pheochromocytoma and paraganglioma.

SAWKA AM et al: A comparison of biochemical tests for pheochromocytoma: Measurement of fractionated plasma metanephrines compared with the combination of 24-hour urinary metanephrines and catecholamines. J Clin Endocrinol Metab 88:553, 2003

This study, based on a retrospective review of patients evaluated at the Mayo Clinic, concludes that measurements of 24-h urinary total metanephrines and catecholamines yield fewer false-positive results in low-risk patients, but fractionated plasma metanephrine measurements are more effective for the diagnosis of high-risk patients with familial endocrine syndromes.

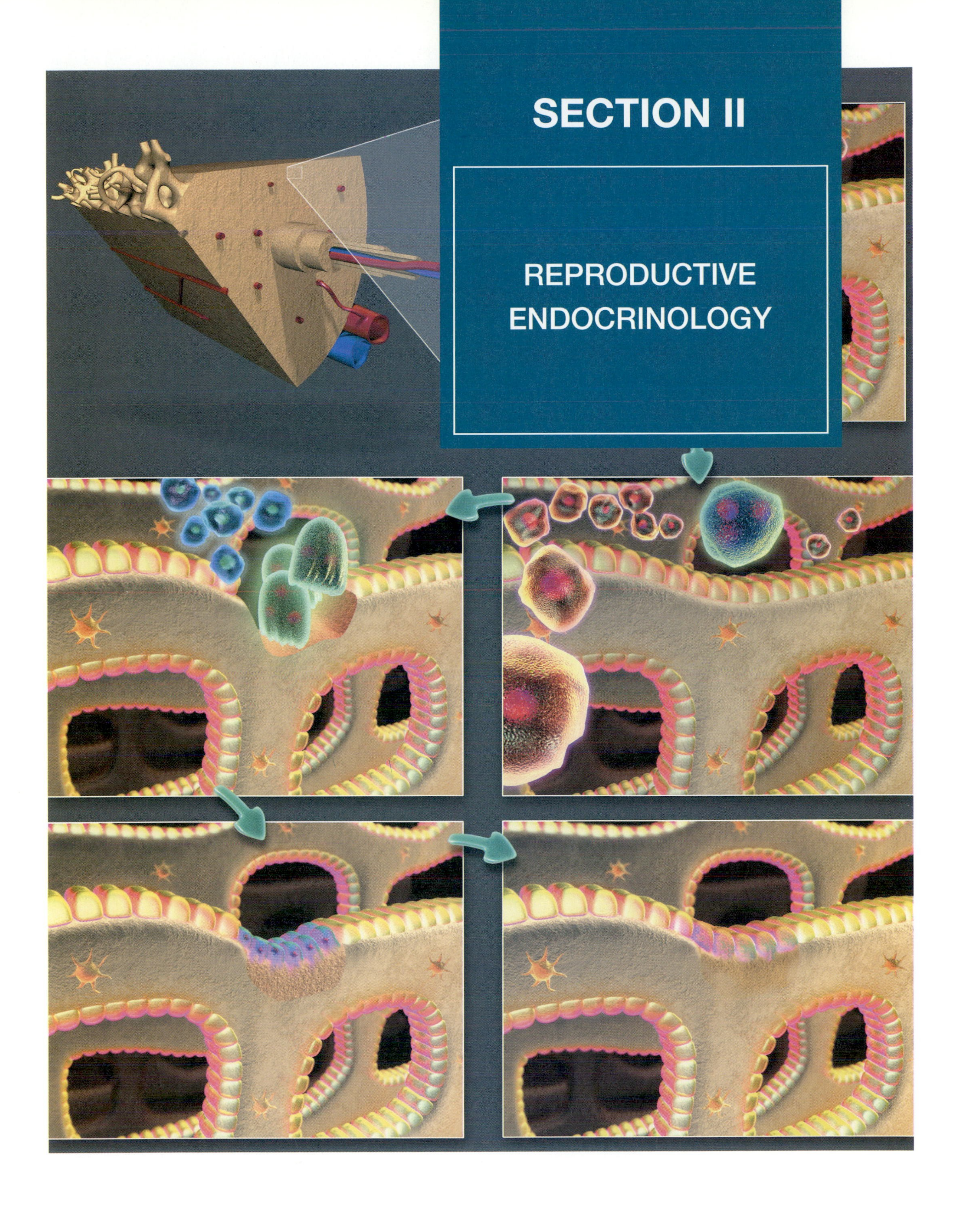

SECTION II

REPRODUCTIVE ENDOCRINOLOGY

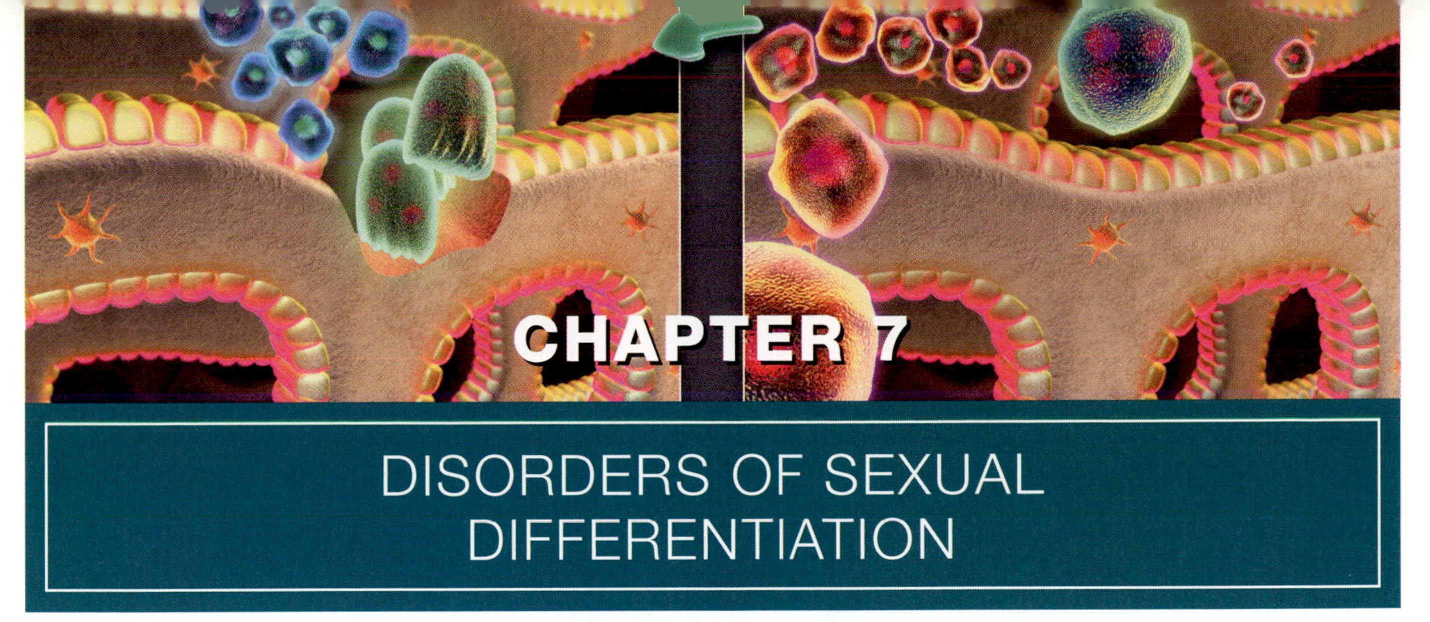

DISORDERS OF SEXUAL DIFFERENTIATION

John C. Achermann
J. Larry Jameson

Sexual differentiation begins in utero, but continues into young adulthood with the achievement of sexual maturity and reproductive capability. Sexual differentiation can be divided into three major components: chromosomal sex, gonadal sex, and phenotypic sex (**Fig. 7-1**). Abnormalities at each of these stages can result in disorders of sexual development. The child born with ambiguous genitalia requires urgent pediatric assessment, as some causes, such as congenital adrenal hyperplasia (CAH), are associated with potentially life-threatening adrenal crises. Early gender assignment and clear communication with parents about the diagnosis, prognosis, and treatment are essential. Disorders of sexual differentiation can also manifest later in life due to subtler forms of gonadal dysfunction [e.g., Klinefelter syndrome (KS)] and are often diagnosed by internists. There are many psychological, reproductive, and metabolic consequences associated with disorders of sexual differentiation; some of these patients avoid interactions with healthcare providers, and special effort is necessary to optimize long-term surgical, medical, and psychological management.

NORMAL SEXUAL DIFFERENTIATION

Chromosomal sex describes the sex chromosome complement (46,XY male; 46,XX female) that is established at the time of fertilization. The presence of a normal Y chromosome determines that testis development will occur, even in the presence of multiple X chromosomes (e.g., 47,XXY or 48,XXXY). The loss of an X chromosome impairs gonad development (45,X or 46,XY/45,X). Fetuses with no X material (45,Y) are not viable.

Gonadal sex refers to the assignment of gonadal tissue as testis or ovary. The embryonic gonad is bipotential, and can develop (at about 40 days gestation) into either a testis or ovary, depending on which genes are expressed. Ovarian development appears to be a constitutive pathway and occurs in the absence of specific genes that dictate testis determination and development (**Fig. 7-2**). Testis development is initiated by expression of the Y chromosome gene *SRY* (sex-determining region on the Y chromosome), which encodes an HMG box transcription factor. *SRY* is transiently expressed in cells destined to become Sertoli cells and serves as a pivotal switch to establish the testis lineage. Mutation of *SRY* prevents testis development in chromosomal 46,XY males, whereas translocation of *SRY* in 46,XX females is sufficient to induce testis development and a male phenotype. Other genes are necessary to continue testis development. *SOX9* (*SRY*-related HMG-box gene 9) is strikingly upregulated in the developing male gonad but is turned off in the female gonad. Transgenic expression of *SOX9* is sufficient to initiate testis formation in mice, and mutations that disrupt *SOX9* impair testis development. *WT1* (Wilms' tumor-related gene 1) is involved in renal and gonadal development. In the testis, *WT1* acts early in the genetic pathway and regulates the transcription of several genes including *SF1, DAX1,* and *AMH* (encoding *MIS,* müllerian-inhibiting substance).

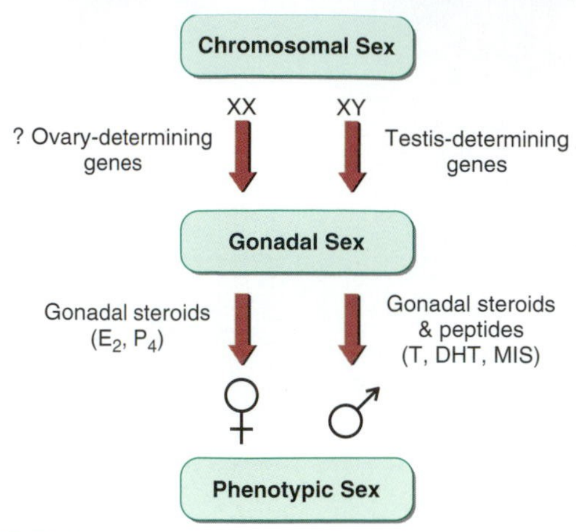

FIGURE 7-1
Sexual differentiation can be divided into three major components: chromosomal sex, gonadal sex, and phenotypic sex. T, testosterone; DHT, dihydrotestosterone; MIS, müllerian-inhibiting substance; E_2, estradiol; P_4, progesterone.

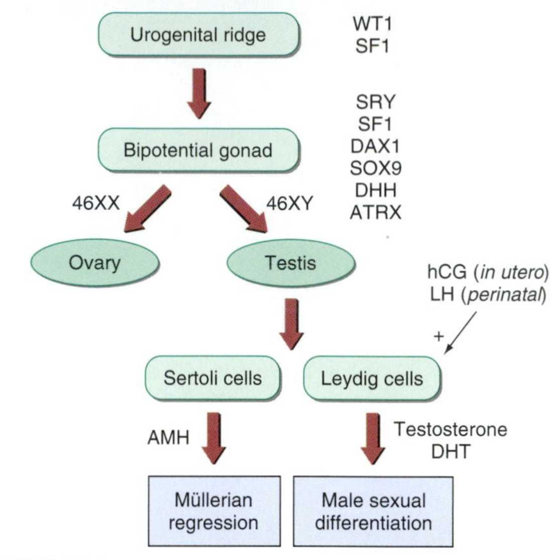

FIGURE 7-2
The genetic regulation of testis development. *WT1,* Wilms' tumor-related gene 1; *SF1,* steroidogenic factor 1; *SRY,* sex-related gene on the Y chromosome; *SOX9,* SRY-related HMG-box gene 9; *DHH,* desert hedgehog; *ATRX,* (α-thalassemia, mental retardation on the X); *DAX1,* dosage sensitive sex-reversal, adrenal hypoplasia congenita on the X chromosome, gene 1; AMH, anti-müllerian hormone (müllerian-inhibiting substance); DHT, dihydrotestosterone.

SF1 (steroidogenic factor 1) encodes a nuclear receptor and is required for adrenal and gonadal development (both testis and ovary). It functions in cooperation with other transcription factors to regulate a large array of adrenal and gonadal genes, including many genes involved in steroidogenesis. The early expression pattern of *SF1* in the gonad parallels that of another orphan nuclear receptor, *DAX1* (dosage-sensitive sex-reversal, adrenal hypoplasia congenita on the X chromosome, gene 1). In contrast to *SOX9, DAX1* is downregulated as the testis develops. Duplication of *DAX1* impairs testis development, possibly by antagonizing the function of SRY and SF1. Deletions or mutations of *DAX1,* on the other hand, lead to disordered formation of testis cords, revealing the exquisite sensitivity of the male sex-determining pathway to gene dosage effects. In addition to those mentioned above, human and murine mutations indicate that at least 10 other genes also are involved in gonadal differentiation and development as well as final positioning of the gonads.

It is unclear whether analogous "ovarian-determining genes" exist, or whether ovarian development only requires the absence of testis-determining genes. However, germ cells play a key role in supporting ovarian development and produce factors that inhibit the formation of testicular elements. This contrasts with the testis, which develops and undergoes steroidogenesis in the absence of germ cells. Once the ovary has formed, expression of a variety of specific genes is required for normal follicular development [e.g., follicle-stimulating hormone (FSH) receptor, *GDF9]*. Steroidogenesis in the ovary requires the development of follicles containing granulosa cells and theca cells surrounding the oocytes (Chap. 10). Thus, there is minimal ovarian steroidogenesis until gonadotropins are produced at puberty.

Phenotypic sex refers to the structures of the external and internal genitalia, and secondary sex characteristics. The male phenotype requires the secretion of anti-müllerian hormone (AMH, müllerian-inhibiting substance) from Sertoli cells and testosterone from testicular Leydig cells. AMH is a member of the transforming growth factor *β* (TGF-*β*) family and acts through specific receptors to cause regression of the müllerian structures (52 to 70 days gestation). At approximately 60 to 140 days gestation, testosterone supports the development of wolffian structures, including the epididymides, vasa deferentia, and seminal vesicles. Testosterone is also the precursor for dihydrotestosterone (DHT), a potent androgen that promotes development of the external genitalia, including the penis and scrotum (65 to 100 days, and beyond) (**Fig. 7-3**). The urogenital sinus develops into the prostate and prostatic urethra in the male and into the urethra and lower portion of the vagina in the female. The genital tubercle becomes the glans penis in the male and the clitoris in the female. The urogenital swellings form the scrotum or the labia majora, and the urethral folds fuse to form the shaft of the penis and the male urethra or the labia minora. In the female, wolffian ducts regress and the müllerian ducts form the fallopian tubes, uterus, and upper segment of the vagina. A normal female phenotype will develop in the absence of the gonad, but estrogen is needed for maturation of the uterus and breast at puberty.

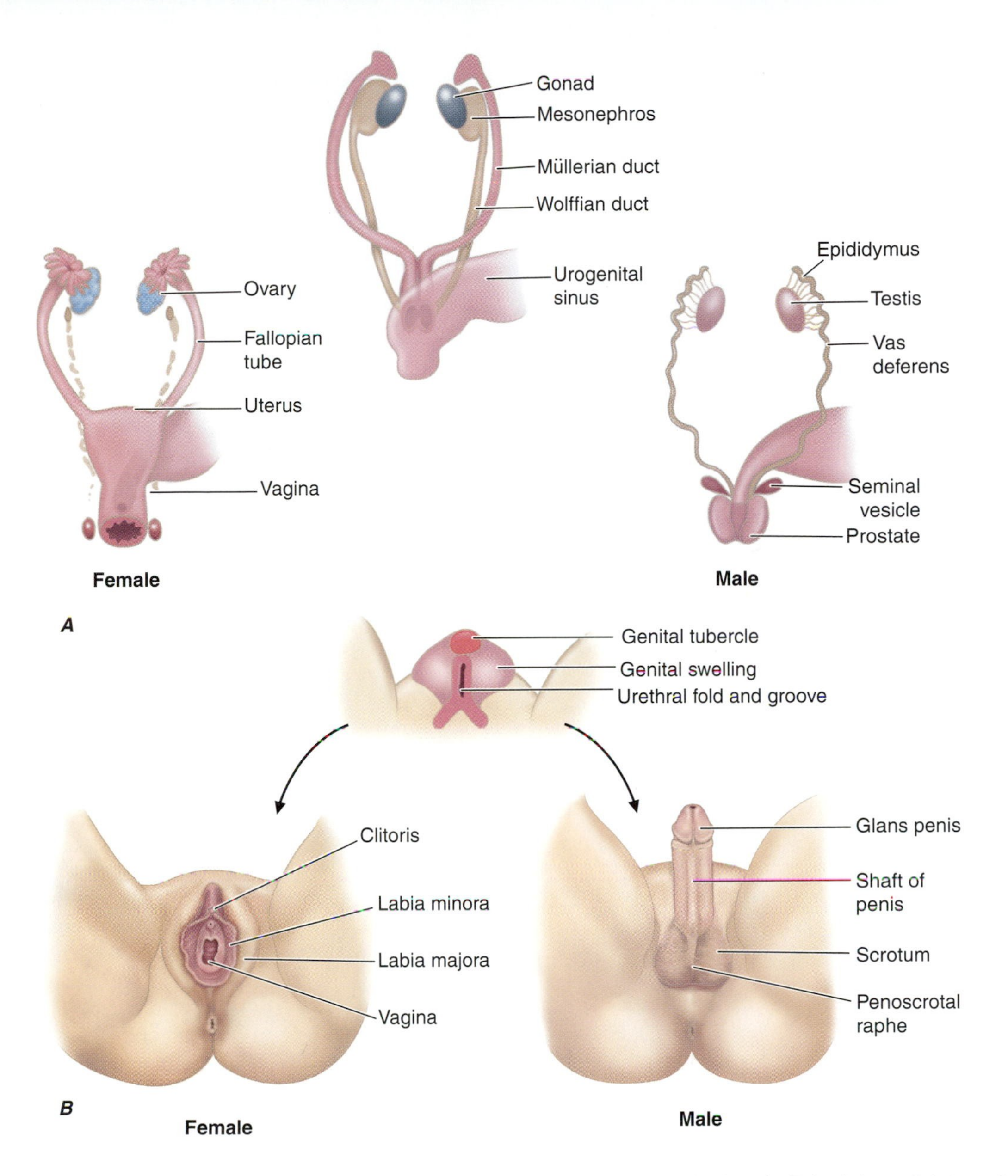

FIGURE 7-3

Normal sexual differentiation. ***A.*** Internal urogenital tract. ***B.*** External genitalia. [After JD Wilson, JE Griffin, in E Braunwald et al (eds): *Harrison's Principles of Internal Medicine,* 15th ed. New York, McGraw-Hill, 2001.]

DISORDERS OF CHROMOSOMAL SEX

Disorders of chromosomal sex result from abnormalities in the number or structure of the X or Y chromosomes (**Table 7-1**).

KLINEFELTER SYNDROME (47,XXY AND MOSAIC VARIANTS)

Pathophysiology

The classic form of Klinefelter syndrome (KS) (47,XXY) occurs following meiotic nondisjunction of the sex chromosomes during gametogenesis (40% during spermatogenesis, 60% during oogenesis). Mosaic forms of KS (46,XY/47,XXY) are thought to result from chromosomal mitotic nondisjunction within the zygote, and occur in at least 10% of individuals with this condition. Other chromosomal variants of KS (e.g., 48,XXYY; 48,XXXY) have been reported but are less common.

Clinical Features

KS is characterized by small testes, infertility, gynecomastia, eunuchoid proportions, and poor virilization in phenotypic males. It has an incidence of 1 in 500 to 1000 men. In severe cases, individuals present prepubertally with small testes, or with impaired androgenization and gynecomastia

TABLE 7-1

CLINICAL FEATURES OF THE DISORDERS OF CHROMOSOMAL SEX

DISORDER	COMMON CHROMOSOMAL COMPLEMENT	GONAD	GENITALIA		BREAST DEVELOPMENT	CLINICAL FEATURES
			EXTERNAL	INTERNAL		
Klinefelter syndrome	47, XXY or 46, XY/47, XXY	Hyalinized testes	Male	Male	Gynecomastia	Small testes, azoospermia, decreased facial and axillary hair, decreased libido, tall stature & increased leg length, decreased penile length, increased risk of breast tumors, learning diffficulties, obesity, varicose veins
Turner syndrome	45, X or 46, XX/45, X	Streak gonad or immature ovary	Female	Hypoplastic female	Immature female	Infancy: lymphedema, web neck, shield chest, low set hair line, cardiac defects and coarctation of the aorta, urinary tract malformations & horseshoe kidney Childhood: short stature, cubitus valgus, short neck, short 4th metacarpals, hypoplastic nails, microganthia, scoliosis, otitis media & sensorineural hearing loss, ptosis & amblyopia, multiple nevi & keloid formation, autoimmune thyroid disease, visuo-spatial learning difficulties Adulthood: pubertal failure & primary amenorrhea, hypertension, obesity, dyslipidemia, impaired glucose tolerance & insulin resistance, cardiovascular disease, aortic root dilatation, osteoporosis, inflammatory bowel disease, chronic hepatic dysfunction, increased risk of colon cancer, hearing loss
Mixed gonadal dysgenesis	46, XY/45, X	Testis or streak gonad	Variable—usually ambiguous	Variable	Usually male	Short stature, increased risk of gonadal tumors, some Turner syndrome features
True hermaphroditism	46, XY/46, XX	Testis & ovary or ovotestis	Variable—usually ambiguous	Variable	Gynecomastia	Increased risk of gonadal tumors

at the time of puberty. Developmental delay and learning disabilities may be a feature. Later in life, eunuchoid features or infertility lead to the diagnosis. Testes are small and firm [median length 2.5 cm (4 mL volume); almost always <3.5 cm (12 mL)], and typically seem inappropriately small for the degree of androgenization. Biopsies are not usually necessary but reveal seminiferous tubule hyalinization and azoospermia. Other clinical features of KS are listed in Table 7-1. Plasma concentrations of FSH and luteinizing hormone (LH) are increased in most patients with 47,XXY (90 and 80%, respectively) and plasma testosterone is decreased (50–75%), reflecting primary gonadal failure. Estradiol is often increased because of chronic Leydig cell stimulation by LH and because of aromatization of androstenedione by adipose tissue; the increased ratio of estradiol/testosterone results in gynecomastia. Patients with mosaic forms of KS have less severe clinical features, larger testes, and sometimes achieve fertility.

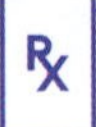

TREATMENT FOR KLINEFELTER SYNDROME

Disfiguring gynecomastia should be treated by surgical reduction. Androgen supplementation (Chap. 8) improves virilization, libido, energy, and bone mineralization in underandrogenized men, but may worsen gynecomastia. Fertility has been achieved using in vitro fertilization in men with oligospermia, or with intracytoplasmic sperm injection when spermatids can be recovered from testicular biopsy. However, the risk of transmission of this chromosomal abnormality needs to be considered, and preimplantation screening may be desired.

TURNER SYNDROME (GONADAL DYSGENESIS) (45,X AND MOSAIC VARIANTS)

Pathophysiology

Approximately one-half of individuals with Turner syndrome (TS) have a 45,X karyotype, one-fourth have 46,XX/45,X mosaicism, and the remainder have structural abnormalities of the X chromosome such as X fragments, isochromosomes, or rings. The clinical features of TS result from haploinsufficiency of multiple X chromosomal genes (e.g., Short Stature Homeobox, *SHOX*). However, imprinted genes may also be affected when the inherited X has different parental origins.

Clinical Features

TS is characterized by bilateral streak gonads, primary amenorrhea, short stature, and multiple congenital anomalies in phenotypic females. It affects approximately 1 in 2500 women and is diagnosed at different ages depending on the dominant clinical features (Table 7-1). Prenatally, a diagnosis of TS is usually made incidentally after chorionic villous sampling or amniocentesis for unrelated reasons, such as advanced maternal age. Prenatal ultrasound findings include increased nuchal translucency and reduced fetal growth. The postnatal diagnosis of TS should be considered in female neonates or infants with lymphedema, nuchal folds, low hairline, or left-sided cardiac defects, and in girls with unexplained growth failure or pubertal delay. Although limited spontaneous pubertal development occurs in up to 30% of girls with TS (10%, 45,X; 30–40%, 45,X/46,XY), and approximately 2% reach menarche, the vast majority of women with TS develop complete ovarian failure. This diagnosis should be considered, therefore, in all women who present with primary or secondary amenorrhea and elevated gonadotropin levels.

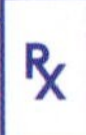

TREATMENT FOR TURNER SYNDROME

The management of girls and women with TS requires a multidisciplinary approach because of the number of potentially involved organ systems. Detailed cardiac and renal evaluation should be performed at the time of diagnosis. Individuals with congenital heart defects (CHD) (30%) (bicuspid aortic valve, 30 to 50%; coarctation of the aorta, 30%; aortic root dilatation, 5%) require long-term follow-up by an experienced cardiologist, antibiotic prophylaxis for dental or surgical procedures, and serial imaging of aortic root dimensions, as progressive aortic root dilatation can occur. Individuals found to have congenital renal and urinary tract malformations (30%) are at risk for urinary tract infections, hypertension, and nephrocalcinosis. Hypertension can occur independent of cardiac and renal malformations and should be monitored and treated as in other patients with essential hypertension. Clitoral enlargement or other evidence of virilization suggests the presence of covert, translocated Y chromosomal material and is associated with increased risk of gonadoblastoma, apparently the consequence of Y chromosomal genes distinct from *SRY*. Regular assessment of thyroid function, weight, dentition, hearing, speech, vision, and educational issues should be performed during childhood, and counseling about long-term growth and fertility issues should be provided. Patient support groups are active throughout the world.

The treatment of short stature in children with TS remains a challenge, as untreated final height rarely exceeds 150 cm. High-dose recombinant growth hormone stimulates growth rate in children with TS and may be used alone or in combination with low doses of the nonaromatizable anabolic steroid oxandrolone (up to 0.05 mg/kg per d) in the older child (>8 years). However, final height increments are often modest (5–10 cm), and individualization of treatment regimens to response may be beneficial. Girls with evidence of gonadal failure require estrogen replacement to induce breast and uterine development, to support growth, and to maintain bone mineralization. Low-dose estrogen therapy (approximately one-sixth of the adult dose, 2 to 5 μg/d ethinylestradiol) is initiated between 12 to 14 years of age and increased gradually to induce feminization over a 2- to 3-year period. Progestins are later added to regulate withdrawal bleeds, and some women with TS have now achieved successful pregnancy after ovum donation and in vitro fertilization. Long-term follow-up of women with TS involves careful surveillance of sex hormone replacement and reproductive function, bone mineralization, cardiac function and aortic root dimensions, blood pressure, weight and glucose tolerance, hepatic and lipid profiles, thyroid function, and hearing.

MIXED GONADAL DYSGENESIS (46,XY/45,X)

Mixed gonadal dysgenesis typically results from 46,XY/45,X mosaicism. The phenotype of patients with this condition varies considerably, depending on the proportion and distribution of 46,XY cells. Although some patients have a predominantly female phenotype with somatic features of TS, streak gonads, and müllerian structures, other 46,XY/45,X individuals have a male phenotype and testes, and the diagnosis is made incidentally after amniocentesis or during investigation of infertility. In practice, most children who present to clinicians have ambiguous genitalia and variable somatic features. A female sex-of-rearing is often chosen (60%) if phallic development is poor, uterine structures are present, and if height potential is limited. However, gonadectomy is indicated to prevent further androgen secretion and to prevent development of gonadoblastoma (up to 25%). Individuals raised as males may require reconstructive surgery for hypospadias and removal of streak gonads. Scrotal testes can be preserved but need regular examination for tumor development. Biopsy for carcinoma in situ is recommended in adolescence, and testosterone supplementation may be required for virilization in puberty.

TRUE HERMAPHRODITISM (46,XY/46,XX)

True hermaphroditism (TH) occurs when both an ovary and testis are found (or when an ovotestis is found) in one individual. For unclear reasons, gonadal asymmetry most often occurs with a testis on the right and an ovary on the left. True hermaphroditism due to 46,XY/46,XX mosaicism is rare and has a variable phenotype depending on the proportion of each cell line.

DISORDERS OF GONADAL AND PHENOTYPIC SEX

The clinical features of patients with disorders of gonadal and phenotypic sex are divided into the undervirilization of 46,XY males or inappropriate virilization of 46,XX females. These disorders comprise a spectrum of phenotypes ranging from complete "sex-reversal" (e.g., 46,XY phenotypic females or 46,XX males) to ambiguous genitalia.

UNDERVIRILIZED MALES (46,XY) (MALE PSEUDOHERMAPHRODITISM)

Undervirilization of the male (46,XY) reflects defects in androgen production or action. It can result from disorders of testis development, defects of androgen synthesis, or resistance to testosterone and DHT (**Table 7-2**).

DISORDERS OF TESTIS DEVELOPMENT

Testicular Dysgenesis Patients with *pure gonadal dysgenesis* have streak gonads, müllerian structures (due to insufficient MIS secretion), and a complete absence of virilization. Patients with *dysgenetic testes* produce enough MIS to regress the uterus and, sometimes, sufficient testosterone for partial virilization. Gonadal dysgenesis can result from mutations or deletions of testis-promoting genes (*WT1, SF1, SRY, SOX9, DAX1, DHH, ATRX, ARX*; also *DMRT,* and *SOX8* loci) or overexpression of factors that impair testis development when excessive (*WNT4, DAX1*) (**Table 7-3**). Associated clinical features may be present, reflecting additional functional roles for these genes. For example, renal dysfunction occurs in patients with specific *WT1* mutations (Denys-Drash and Frasier syndromes), primary adrenal failure occurs with *SF1* mutations, and severe cartilage abnormalities (campomelic dysplasia) are the predominant clinical feature of *SOX9* mutations. Dysgenetic testes should be removed to prevent malig-

TABLE 7-2

DISORDERS CAUSING UNDERVIRILIZATION IN KARYOTYPIC MALES (46, XY)
Disorders of testis development
True hermaphroditism (46, XY)
Gonadal dysgenesis
Absent testis syndrome
Disorders of androgen synthesis
LH receptor mutations
Smith-Lemli-Opitz syndrome
Steroidogenic acute regulatory protein mutations
Cholesterol side chain cleavage (*CYP 11A1*) deficiency
3β-Hydroxysteroid dehydrogenase 2 (*HSD3B2*) deficiency
17α-Hydroxylase/17,20-lyase(*CYP17*) deficiency
17β-Hydroxysteroid dehydrogenase 3 (*HSD17B3*) deficiency
5α-Reductase 2 deficiency (*SRD5A2*)
Aromatase overexpression
Disorders of androgen action
Androgen Insensitivity Syndrome
Androgen receptor cofactor defects
Other disorders of male reproductive tract
Persistent müllerian duct syndrome
Isolated hypospadias
Cryptorchidism

TABLE 7-3

GENETIC CAUSES OF UNDERVIRILIZATION OF KARYOTYPIC MALES (46, XY)

GENE	INHERITANCE	GONAD	UTERUS	EXTERNAL GENITALIA	ASSOCIATED FEATURES
		DISORDERS OF TESTIS DEVELOPMENT			
WT1	AD	Dysgenetic testis	+/−	Female or ambiguous	Wilms' tumor, renal abnormalities, gonadal tumors (WAGR, Denys-Drash & Frasier syndromes)
SF1	AR/AD	Dysgenetic testis	+	Female or ambiguous	Primary adrenal failure
SRY	Y	Dysgenetic testis or ovary	+/−	Female or ambiguous	
SOX9	AD	Dysgenetic testis or ovary	+/−	Female or ambiguous	Campomelic dysplasia
DHH	AR	Testis/streak	+	Female	Minifascicular neuropathy
ATRX	X	Dysgenetic testis	−	Female or ambiguous	α-Thalassemia, developmental delay
ARX	X	Dysgenetic testis	−	Male or ambiguous	Mental retardation; X-linked lissencephaly
DAX1	dupXp21	Dysgenetic testis or ovary	+/−	Female or ambiguous	
WNT4	dup1p35	Dysgenetic testis	+	Ambiguous	
		DISORDERS OF ANDROGEN SYNTHESIS			
LHR	AR	Testis	−	Female, ambiguous or micropenis	Leydig cell hypoplasia
DHCR7	AR	Testis	−	Variable	Smith-Lemli-Opitz syndrome: coarse facies, second-third toe syndactyly, failure to thrive, developmental delay, cardiac & visceral abnormalities
STAR	AR	Testis	−	Female	Congenital lipoid adrenal hyperplasia (primary adrenal failure)
CYP11A1	AR	Testis	−	Ambiguous	Congenital lipoid adrenal hyperplasia (primary adrenal failure)
HSD3B2	AR	Testis	−	Ambiguous	CAH, primary adrenal failure, partial virilization due to ↑ DHEA
CYP17	AR	Testis	−	Female or ambiguous	CAH, hypertension due to ↑ corticosterone & 11-deoxycorticosterone
HSD17B3	AR	Testis	−	Female or ambiguous	Partial virilization at puberty, ↑ androstenedione:testosterone ratio
SRD5A2	AR	Testis	−	Ambiguous	Partial virilization at puberty, ↑ testosterone: dihydrotestosterone ratio.
		DISORDERS OF ANDROGEN ACTION			
Androgen receptor	X	Testis	−	Female, ambiguous, micropenis or normal male	Phenotypic spectrum from complete androgen insensitivity syndrome (female external genitalia) and partial androgen insensitivity (ambiguous) to normal male genitalia and infertility

Note: AR, autosomal recessive; AD, autosomal dominant; *WT1,* Wilms' tumor-related gene 1; WAGR, Wilms' tumor, aniridia, genitourinary anomalies, and mental retardation; *SF1,* steroidogenic factor 1; *SRY,* sex-related gene on the Y chromosome; *SOX9, SRY*-related HMG-box gene 9; *DHH,* desert hedgehog; *ATRX,* (α-thalassemia, mental retardation on the X); *ARX,* aristaless related homeobox, X-linked; *DAX1,* dosage sensitive sex-reversal, adrenal hypoplasia congenita on the X chromosome, gene 1; *WNT4,* wingless-type mouse mammary tumor virus integration site, 4; *LHR,* LH receptor; *DHCR7,* sterol 7δ reductase; *STAR,* steroidogenic acute regulatory protein; *CYP11A1,* P450 cholesterol side-chain cleavage; *HSD3B2,* 3β-hydroxysteroid dehydrogenase type 2; *CYP17,* 17α-hydroxylase and 17,20-lyase; *HSD17B3,* 17β-hydroxysteroid dehydrogenase type 3; *CYP19,* aromatase; *SRD5A2,* 5α-reductase type 2.

nancy, and estrogens can be used to induce secondary sex characteristics in 46,XY individuals raised as females. *Absent (vanishing) testis syndrome* reflects regression of the testis during development. The etiology is unknown but the absence of müllerian structures indicates adequate secretion of MIS in utero. Early testicular regression causes impaired virilization. Individuals raised as female should receive estrogen replacement at puberty. More frequently, late regression results in an otherwise normal male with anorchia. These individuals can be offered testicular prostheses and should receive androgen replacement in adolescence.

Disorders of Androgen Synthesis

Defects in the pathway that regulates androgen synthesis (**Fig. 7-4**) cause undervirilization of the male fetus (Table 7-3). Müllerian regression is unaffected because Sertoli cell function is preserved.

LH Receptor Mutations in the LH receptor cause Leydig cell hypoplasia and androgen deficiency. Defects of LH receptor synthesis or function preclude hCG (human chorionic gonadotropin) stimulation of Leydig cells in utero, as well as LH stimulation of Leydig cells late in gestation and during the neonatal period. As a result, testosterone and DHT synthesis are insufficient for normal virilization of the internal and external genitalia, causing a spectrum of phenotypes that range from complete undervirilization to micropenis, depending on the severity of the mutation.

Congenital Adrenal Hyperplasia (CAH) Mutations in the genes that regulate cholesterol uptake and

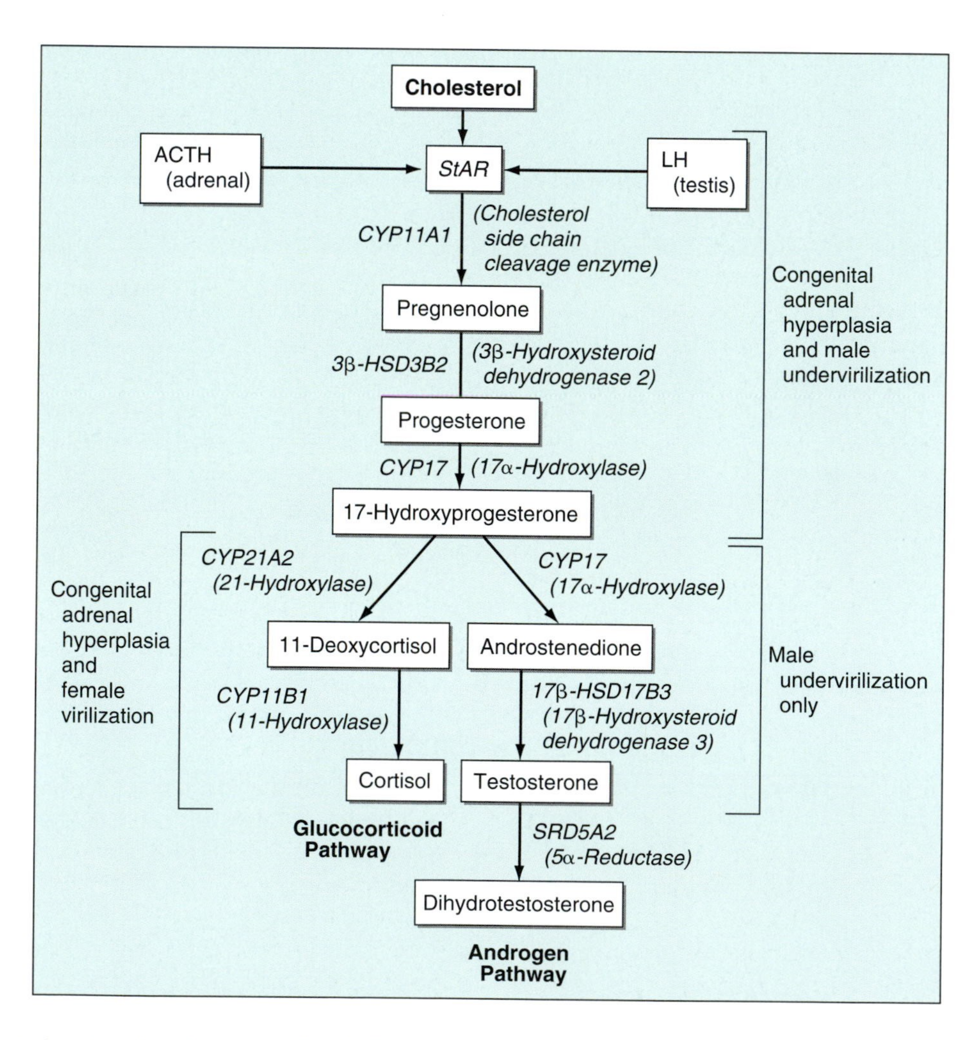

FIGURE 7-4

Pathways of glucocorticoid and androgen synthesis. Defects in *CYP21A2* and *CYP11B1* shunt steroid precursors into the androgen pathway and cause virilization of 46,XX females. Testosterone and dihydrotestosterone are synthesized in the testicular Leydig cells. Defects in enzymes involved in androgen synthesis result in undervirilization of 46,XY males. StAR, steroidogenic acute regulatory protein. [After JD Wilson, JE Griffin, in E Braunwald et al (eds): *Harrison's Principles of Internal Medicine,* 15th ed. New York, McGraw-Hill, 2001.]

modification [*steroidogenic acute regulatory protein (StAR), CYP11a*] affect both adrenal and gonadal steroidogenesis, and result in *congenital lipoid adrenal hyperplasia* (Chap. 5). Defects in *3β-hydroxysteroid dehydrogenase type 2* (*HSD3B2*) also cause adrenal insufficiency, but the accumulation of dehydroepiandrosterone (DHEA) has a mild virilizing effect. Patients with congenital adrenal hyperplasia due to *17α*-hydroxylase (CYP17) *deficiency* have variable undervirilization and develop hypertension due to the potent salt-retaining effects of corticosterone and 11-deoxycorticosterone. Some mutations in *CYP17* selectively impair 17,20 lyase activity, without altering 17α-hydroxylase activity, leading to undervirilization without mineralocorticoid excess and hypertension.

Sex-Steroid Pathway Enzymes Defects in *17β-hydroxysteroid dehydrogenase* type 3 *(HSD17B3)* and *5α-reductase type 2* (*SRD5A2*) interfere with the synthesis of testosterone and DHT, respectively (Fig. 7-4). These conditions are characterized by minimal masculinization in childhood, but some phallic development can occur during adolescence due to the action of other enzyme isoforms. Individuals with *5α-reductase type* 2 deficiency have normal wolffian structures and do not develop breast tissue. In some cultures, these individuals change gender role behavior from female to male at puberty, because the increase in testosterone induces muscle mass and other virilizing features. DHT cream can improve prepubertal phallic growth in patients raised as male. Individuals raised as female require gonadectomy, cosmetic surgery, and estrogen replacement.

Disorders of Androgen Action

Androgen Insensitivity Syndrome Mutations in the androgen receptor (AR) cause resistance to androgen (testosterone, DHT) action or the *androgen insensitivity syndrome (AIS)*. AIS is a spectrum of disorders that affects at least 1 in 100,000 chromosomal males. Because the androgen receptor is X-linked, only males are affected and maternal carriers are phenotypically normal. XY individuals with *complete AIS (testicular feminization syndrome)* have a female phenotype, normal breast development, a short vagina but no uterus (because MIS production is normal), scanty pubic and axillary hair, and female psychosexual orientation. Gonadotropins and testosterone levels can be low, normal, or elevated, depending on the degree of androgen resistance and the contribution of estradiol to feedback inhibition of the hypothalamic-pituitary gonadal axis. Most patients present with inguinal herniae (containing testes) in childhood or with primary amenorrhea in adulthood. Gonadectomy is usually performed, as there is a low risk of malignancy, and estrogen replacement is prescribed. Surgical reconstruction or mechanical dilatation of the vagina permits sexual intercourse. *Partial AIS (Reifenstein syndrome)* results from less severe AR mutations. Patients often present in infancy with perineoscrotal hypospadias and small cryptorchid testes, and with gynecomastia at the time of puberty. Those individuals raised as males require hypospadias repair in childhood and breast reduction in adolescence. Supplemental androgens rarely improve virilization significantly, as endogenous androgens are already increased. More severely undervirilized patients present with clitoral enlargement and labial fusion, and may be raised as females. The surgical and psychosexual management of both these groups of patients is complex and requires active involvement of the parents and the patient during the appropriate stages of development. *Azoospermia* and male-factor infertility have also been described in association with mild loss of function mutations in the androgen receptor. Trinucleotide (CAG) repeat expansion, from a mean of 22 repeats to greater than 40 repeats, within a highly polymorphic region of the androgen receptor is associated with spinal and bulbar muscular atrophy (also known as Kennedy disease). These patients may show evidence of partial androgen insensitivity in adolescence or adulthood (e.g., gynecomastia).

OTHER DISORDERS AFFECTING MALES (46,XY)

Persistent Müllerian Duct syndrome is the presence of a uterus in an otherwise normal male. This condition can result from mutations in AMH or its receptor (AMHR2). The uterus may be removed, but damage to vasa deferentia must be avoided. *Isolated hypospadias* occurs in approximately 1 in 200 males and is treated by surgical repair. Most cases are idiopathic, although evidence of penoscrotal hypospadias and bilateral cryptorchidism require investigation for an underlying genetic disorder (e.g., defect in testosterone action). *Cryptorchidism* (unilateral) affects up to 3% of boys at birth. Orchidopexy should be considered if the testis has not descended by early childhood. Bilateral cryptorchidism occurs less frequently, and should raise suspicion of gonadotropin deficiency or disorders of sexual development. A subset of patients with cryptorchidism have mutations in the insulin-like 3 (*INSL3*) gene or its receptor LGR8 (also known as *GREAT*), which mediates normal testicular descent.

VIRILIZED FEMALES (46,XX) (FEMALE PSEUDOHERMAPHRODITISM)

Inappropriate virilization of females can occur when the gonad (ovary) contains androgen-secreting testic-

TABLE 7-4

DISORDERS CAUSING VIRILIZATION IN KARYOTYPIC FEMALES (46,XX)

Ovarian transdifferentiation
- True hermaphroditism (46, XX)
- XX male

Increased androgen synthesis
- 3β-Hydroxysteroid dehydrogenase 2 (*HSD3B2*) deficiency
- 21-Hydroxylase (*CYP21A2*) deficiency
- 11β-Hydroxylase (*CYP11B1*) deficiency
- Aromatase (*CYP19*) deficiency
- Glucocorticoid receptor mutations

Increased androgen exposure
- Maternal virilizing tumors (e.g., luteomas of pregnancy)
- Androgenic drugs
- Nonvirilizing disorders of the female reproductive tract
- Ovarian dysgenesis
- Mülleriun agenesis
- Vaginal agenesis

ular material, or after increased androgen exposure (**Table 7-4**).

Gonadal Transdifferentiation

Testicular tissue can develop in 46,XX true hermaphrodites, and in 46,XX males with a translocation of *SRY* or duplication of *SOX9* (**Table 7-5**).

Increased Androgen Exposure

21-Hydroxylase Deficiency The *classic form* of 21-hydroxylase deficiency has an incidence of between 1 in 5000 and 15,000 and is the most frequent cause of virilization in chromosomal 46,XX females (**Table 7-5**; Chap. 5). Affected individuals are homozygous or compound heterozygous for severe mutations in the enzyme 21-hydroxylase (*CYP21A2*). This mutation causes a block in adrenal glucocorticoid and mineralocorticoid synthesis, increasing 17-hydroxyprogesterone and shunting steroid precursors into the androgen synthesis pathway (Fig. 7-4). Glucocorticoid insufficiency causes a compensatory elevation of adrenocorticotropin (ACTH), resulting in adrenal hyperplasia and additional synthesis of steroid precursors

TABLE 7-5

GENETIC CAUSES OF VIRILIZATION OF KARYOTYPIC FEMALES (46, XX)

GENE	INHERITANCE	GONAD	UTERUS	EXTERNAL GENITALIA	ASSOCIATED FEATURES
			OVARIAN TRANSDIFFERENTIATION		
SRY	translocation	Testis or ovotestis	–	Male or ambiguous	
SOX9	dup17q24	Unknown	–	Male or ambiguous	
			INCREASED ANDROGEN SYNTHESIS		
HSD3B2	AR	Ovary	+	Ambiguous	CAH, primary adrenal failure, partial virilization due to ↑ DHEA
CYP21A2	AR	Ovary	+	Ambiguous	CAH, phenotypic spectrum from severe salt-losing forms associated with adrenal failure to simple virilizing forms with compensated adrenal function, ↑ 17-hydroxyprogesterone
CYP11B1	AR	Ovary	+	Ambiguous	CAH, hypertension due to ↑ 11-deoxycortisol & 11-deoxycorticosterone
CYP19	AR	Ovary	+	Ambiguous	Maternal virilization during pregnancy, absent breast development at puberty
Glucocorticoid receptor	AR	Ovary	+	Ambiguous	↑ ACTH, 17-hydroxyprogesterone and cortisol; failure of dexamethasone suppression

Note: AR, autosomal recessive; *SRY,* sex-related gene on the Y chromosome; *SOX9,* SRY-related HMG-box gene 9; CAH, congenital adrenal hyperplasia; *HSD3B2,* 3β-hydroxysteroid dehydrogenase type 2; *CYP21A2,* 21-hydroxylase; *CYP11B1,* 11β-hydroxylase; *CYP19,* aromatase; ACTH, adrenocorticotropin.

proximal to the enzymatic block. Increased androgen synthesis *in utero* causes virilization of the female fetus. Ambiguous genitalia are seen at birth, with varying degrees of clitoral enlargement and labial fusion. Infants with the *salt-wasting* form of 21-hydroxylase deficiency develop primary adrenal failure in the first few weeks of life. Thus, a diagnosis of 21-hydroxylase deficiency should be considered in any baby with ambiguous genitalia; a salt-wasting crisis is a potentially life-threatening event. Males with this syndrome have no genital abnormalities at birth but are equally susceptible to adrenal insufficiency and salt-losing crises. If untreated, males undergo premature virilization (pseudopuberty) because of increased androgen levels during childhood. Females with the *classic simple virilizing* form of this disorder also present with genital ambiguity, but do not develop salt loss.

The diagnosis of classic 21-hydroxylase deficiency is made by neonatal screening tests for increased 17-hydroxyprogesterone in some centers. In most cases, 17-hydroxyprogesterone is markedly increased. In adults, ACTH stimulation (0.25 mg cosyntropin IV) with assays for 17-hydroxyprogesterone at 0 and 30 min can be useful for detecting nonclassic 21-hydroxylase deficiency and heterozygotes (Chap. 5).

Rx

TREATMENT FOR FEMALE PSEUDOHERMAPHRODITISM

Glucocorticoids must be given to correct the cortisol insufficiency and to suppress ACTH stimulation, thereby preventing further virilization, rapid skeletal maturation, and the development of polycystic ovaries. Typically, hydrocortisone (10 to 20 mg/m^2 per day in divided doses) is used with a goal of suppressing 17-hydroxyprogesterone to <1000 ng/dL. It is difficult, however, to fully suppress androgen production without using excessive glucocorticoid treatment, which can impair growth and predispose to obesity. Older adolescents and adults are often treated with dexamethasone at night to provide more complete ACTH suppression. In very severe cases, adrenalectomy has been advocated but incurs the risks of major surgery and total adrenal insufficiency. Salt-wasting conditions are treated with mineralocorticoid replacement. Infants usually need salt supplements up to the first year of life. Plasma renin activity and electrolytes are used to monitor mineralocorticoid replacement. Newer therapeutic approaches, such as antiandrogens and aromatase inhibitors (to block premature epiphyseal closure) are under evaluation. Parents and patients should be aware of the need for increased doses of steroids during sickness, and patients should carry medic alert systems.

Girls with significant virilization usually undergo clitoral reduction (maintaining the glans and nerve supply) and vaginal reconstruction, but the optimal timing of these procedures is the subject of debate. Surgical revision or regular vaginal dilatation may be needed in adolescence or adulthood, and long-term psychological support and psychosexual counseling may be appropriate.

Prenatal treatment of 21-hydroxylase deficiency by the administration of dexamethasone to mothers has been shown to reduce the degree of virilization in affected female fetuses. However, treatment on the mother and child must be started before 9 weeks gestation and ideally before 6–7 weeks; long-term effects are still under evaluation.

Other Causes Increased androgen synthesis can also occur in CAH due to defects in *11β-hydroxylase (CYP11B1)* and *3β-hydroxysteroid dehydrogenase type 2 (HSD3B2)*, and with mutations in the genes encoding *aromatase (CYP19)* and the glucocorticoid receptor. Increased androgen exposure *in utero* can occur with maternal virilizing tumors and with ingestion of androgenic compounds.

OTHER DISORDERS AFFECTING FEMALES (46,XX)

Congenital absence of the vagina occurs in association with *müllerian agenesis* or *hypoplasia* as part of the Mayer-Rokitansky-Kuster-Hauser syndrome. This diagnosis should be considered in otherwise phenotypically normal females with primary amenorrhea. Rarer associated features include renal (agenesis) and cervical spinal abnormalities.

ACKNOWLEDGMENTS

We are grateful to JD Wilson and JE Griffin, the authors of *Disorders of Sexual Differentiation* in the 15th edition of *Harrison's*, for contributions to this chapter.

FURTHER READINGS

Achermann JC et al: Genetic causes of human reproductive disease. J Clin Endocrinol Metab 87:2447, 2002

A review of genetic causes of reproductive disorders that affect the hypothalamic-pituitary-gonadal axis.

BOUVATTIER C et al: Postnatal changes of T, LH and FSH in 46,XY infants with mutations in the AR gene. J Clin Endocrinol Metab 87:29, 2002

During early infancy, LH and testosterone increase in males before falling and remaining suppressed until the time of puberty. This paper examines changes in LH and testosterone in XY infants with androgen receptor mutations. Unexpectedly, they show that the postnatal T and LH surge is absent in those with complete androgen insensitivity syndrome, suggesting that the postnatal T rise requires the receptivity of the hypothalamic-pituitary axis to testosterone.

FOREST MG: Recent advances in the diagnosis and management of congenital adrenal hyperplasia due to 21-hydroxylase deficiency. Hum Reprod Update 10:469, 2004

Congenital adrenal hyperplasia is among the most common causes of intersex disorders. Advances in early biochemical and genetic testing allow earlier diagnosis and treatment intervention.

JOSSO N: The undervirilized male child: Endocrine aspects. BJU Int 93(Suppl 3):3, 2004

LANFRANCO F et al: Klinefelter's syndrome. Lancet 364:273, 2004

This article reviews the epidemiology of Klinefelter's syndrome and its phenotypic variability. It reviews androgen replacement and the controversy related to using intracytoplasmic sperm injection (ICSI) to treat infertility in these patients.

MACLAUGHLIN DT et al: Sex determination and differentiation. N Engl J Med 350:367, 2004

An outstanding review of the genetic pathways that orchestrate sex determination with a focus on steps associated with human disease.

PARK SY et al: Minireview: Transcriptional regulation of gonadal development and differentiation. Endocrinology 146:1035, 2005

SYBERT VP et al: Turner's syndrome. N Engl J Med 351:1227, 2004

A summary of the spectrum of clinical manifestations of XO gonadal dysgenesis and management strategies at various stages of life from infancy through adulthood.

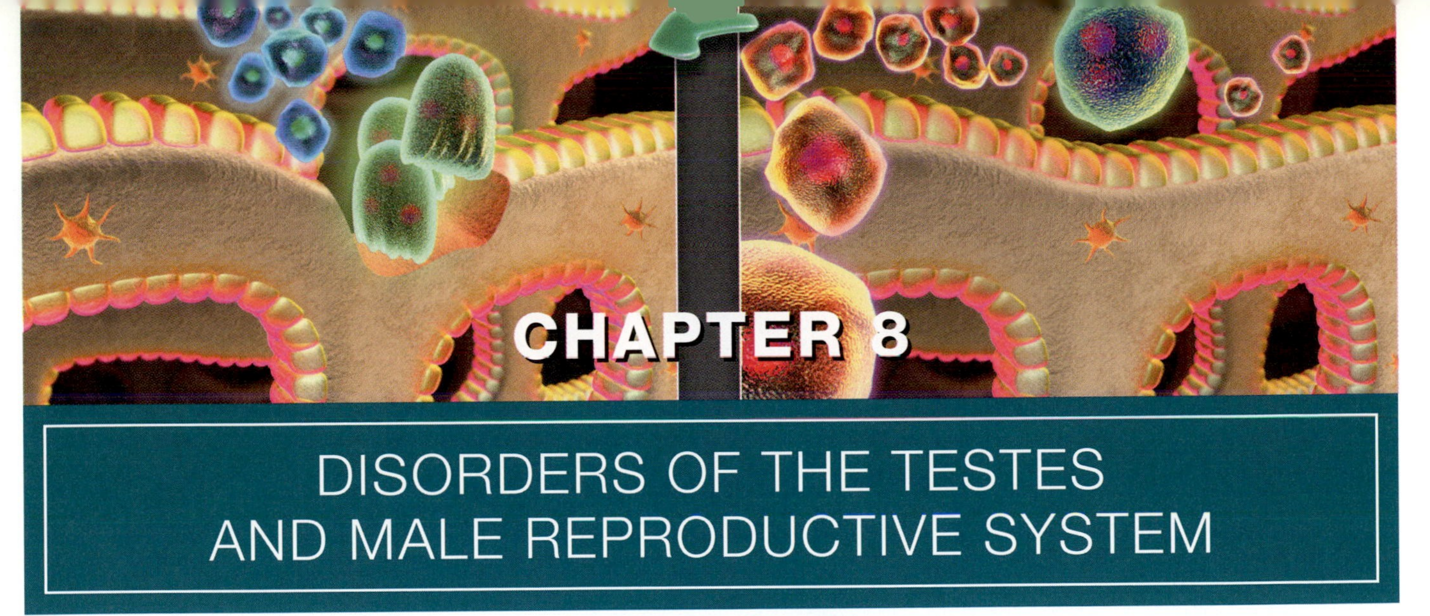

DISORDERS OF THE TESTES AND MALE REPRODUCTIVE SYSTEM

Shalendar Bhasin
J. Larry Jameson

The male reproductive system regulates sexual differentiation, virilization, and the hormonal changes that accompany puberty, ultimately leading to spermatogenesis and fertility. Under the control of the pituitary hormones—luteinizing hormone (LH) and follicle-stimulating hormone (FSH)—the Leydig cells of the testes produce testosterone and germ cells are nurtured by Sertoli cells to divide, differentiate, and mature into sperm. During embryonic development, testosterone and dihydrotestosterone (DHT) induce the wolffian duct and virilization of the external genitalia. During puberty, testosterone promotes somatic growth and the development of secondary sexual characteristics. In the adult, testosterone is necessary for spermatogenesis and stimulation of libido and normal sexual function. This chapter focuses on the physiology of the testes and disorders associated with decreased androgen production, which may be caused by gonadotropin deficiency or by primary testis dysfunction. A variety of testosterone formulations now allow more physiologic androgen replacement. Infertility occurs in ~5% of men and is increasingly amenable to treatment by hormone replacement or by using sperm transfer techniques (Chap. 15). For further discussion of sexual dysfunction, see Chap. 14.

DEVELOPMENT AND STRUCTURE OF THE TESTIS

The fetal testis develops from the undifferentiated gonad after expression of a genetic cascade that is initiated by the SRY (*s*ex-*r*elated gene on the *Y* chromosome) (Chap. 7). SRY induces differentiation of Sertoli cells, which surround germ cells, and together with peritubular myoid cells form testis cords that will later develop into seminiferous tubules. Fetal Leydig cells and endothelial cells migrate into the gonad from the adjacent mesonephros but may also arise from interstitial cells that reside between testis cords. Leydig cells produce testosterone, which supports the growth and differentiation of wolffian duct structures that develop into the epididymus, vas deferens, and seminal vesicles. Testosterone is also converted to DHT (see below), which induces formation of the prostate and the external male genitalia including the penis, urethra, and scrotum. Testicular descent through the inguinal canal is controlled in part by Leydig cell production of insulin-like factor 3 (INSL3), which acts via a receptor termed *Great* (*G* protein–coupled *re*ceptor *a*ffecting *t*estis descent). Sertoli cells produce müllerian inhibiting substance (MIS), which causes regression of the müllerian structures including the fallopian tube, uterus, and upper segment of the vagina.

NORMAL MALE PUBERTAL DEVELOPMENT

Although puberty commonly refers to the maturation of the reproductive axis and the development of secondary sex characteristics, it involves a coordinated response of multiple hormonal systems including the adrenal gland and the growth hormone (GH) axis (**Fig. 8-1**). The development of secondary sexual characteristics is initiated by *adrenarche,* which usually occurs between 6 and 8 years of age when the adrenal gland begins to produce greater amounts of androgens from the zona reticularis, the principal site of dehydroepiandrosterone (DHEA) production. The sexual maturation process is greatly accelerated by the activation of the hypothalamic-pituitary axis and the production of gonadotropin-releasing hormone (GnRH). The so-called GnRH pulse generator in the hypothalamus is active during fetal life and early infancy but is quiescent until the early stages of puberty, when the sensitivity to steroid inhibition is gradually lost, causing reactivation of GnRH secretion. Leptin, a hormone produced by adipose cells, may play a permissive role in this process, as leptin-deficient individuals fail to enter puberty (Chap. 16). Early puberty is characterized by nocturnal surges of LH and FSH. Growth of the testes is usually the first sign of puberty, reflecting an increase in seminiferous tubule volume. Increasing levels of testosterone deepen the voice and increase muscle growth. Conversion of testosterone to DHT leads to growth of the external genitalia and pubic hair. DHT also stimulates prostate and facial hair growth and initiates recession of the temporal hairline. The growth spurt occurs at a testicular volume of about 10 to 12 mL. GH increases early in puberty and is stimulated in part by the rise in gonadal steroids. GH increases the level of insulin-like growth factor 1 (IGF-1), which enhances linear bone growth. The prolonged pubertal exposure to gonadal steroids (mainly estradiol) ultimately causes epiphyseal closure and limits further bone growth.

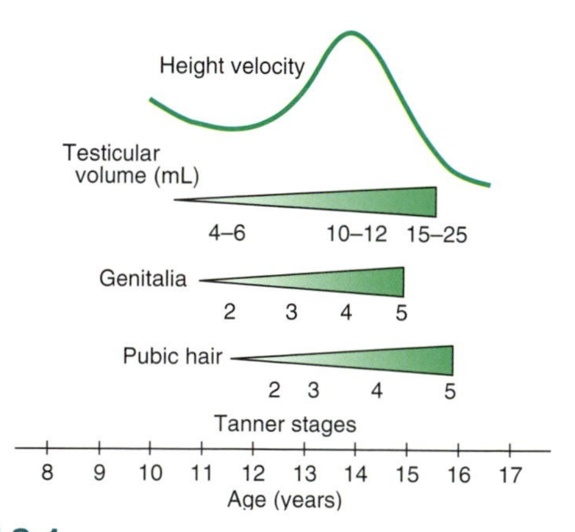

FIGURE 8-1

Pubertal events in males. Sexual maturity ratings for genitalia and pubic hair are divided into five stages. (*From WA Marshall, JM Tanner: Variations in the pattern of pubertal changes in boys. Arch Dis Child 45:13, 1970.*)

REGULATION OF TESTICULAR FUNCTION

REGULATION OF THE HYPOTHALAMIC-PITUITARY-TESTIS AXIS IN ADULT MAN

Hypothalamic GnRH regulates the production of the pituitary gonadotropins, LH and FSH (**Fig. 8-2**). GnRH is released in discrete pulses approximately every 2 h, resulting in corresponding pulses of LH and FSH. These dynamic hormone pulses account in part for the wide variations in LH and testosterone, even within the same individual. LH acts primarily on the Leydig cell to stimulate testosterone synthesis. The regulatory control of androgen synthesis is mediated by testosterone and estrogen feedback on both the hypothalamus and the pituitary. FSH acts on the Sertoli cell to regulate spermatogenesis and the production of Sertoli products such as inhibin B, which acts to selectively suppress pituitary FSH. Despite these somewhat distinct Leydig and Sertoli cell–regulated pathways, testis function is integrated at several levels: GnRH regulates both gonadotropins; spermatogenesis requires high levels of testosterone; and there are numerous paracrine interactions between Leydig and Sertoli cells that are necessary for normal testis function.

THE LEYDIG CELL: ANDROGEN SYNTHESIS

LH binds to its seven-transmembrane, G protein–coupled receptor to activate the cyclic AMP pathway. Stimulation of the LH receptor induces *st*eroid *a*cute *r*egulatory (StAR) protein, along with several steroidogenic enzymes involved in androgen synthesis. LH receptor mutations cause Leydig cell hypoplasia or agenesis, underscoring the importance of this pathway for Leydig cell development

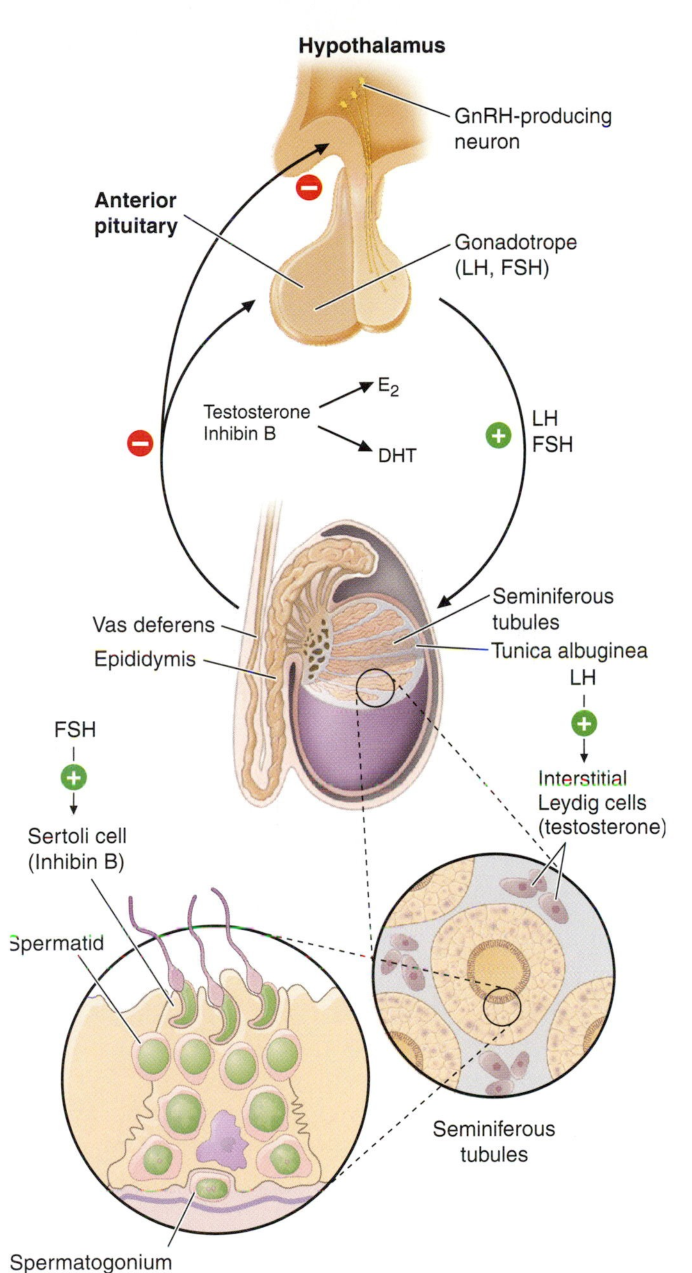

FIGURE 8-2
Human pituitary gonadotropin axis, structure of testis, seminiferous tubule. DHT, dihydrotestosterone; E_2, 17β estradiol.

and function. The rate-limiting process in testosterone synthesis is the delivery of cholesterol by the StAR protein to the inner mitochondrial membrane. Peripheral benzodiazepine receptor, a mitochondrial cholesterol-binding protein, is also an acute regulator of Leydig cell steroidogenesis. The five major enzymatic steps involved in testosterone synthesis are summarized in **Fig. 8-3**. After cholesterol transport into the mitochondrion, side chain cleavage by CYP11A1 to form pregnenolone is a limiting enzymatic step. The 17α-hydroxylase and the 17,20-lyase reactions are catalyzed by a single enzyme, CYP17; posttranslational modification (phosphorylation) of this enzyme and the presence of specific enzyme cofactors confer 17,20-lyase activity selectively in the testis and zona reticularis of the adrenal gland. Testosterone can be converted to the more potent DHT by 5α-reductase, or it can be aromatized to estradiol by CYP19 (aromatase).

Testosterone Transport and Metabolism

In males, 95% of circulating testosterone is derived from testicular secretion (3 to 10 mg/d). Direct secretion of testosterone by the adrenal and the peripheral conversion of androstenedione to testosterone collectively account for another 0.5 mg/d of testosterone. Only a small amount of DHT (70 μg/d) is secreted directly by the testis; most circulating DHT is derived from peripheral conversion of testosterone.

Circulating testosterone is bound to two plasma proteins: sex hormone–binding globulin (SHBG) and

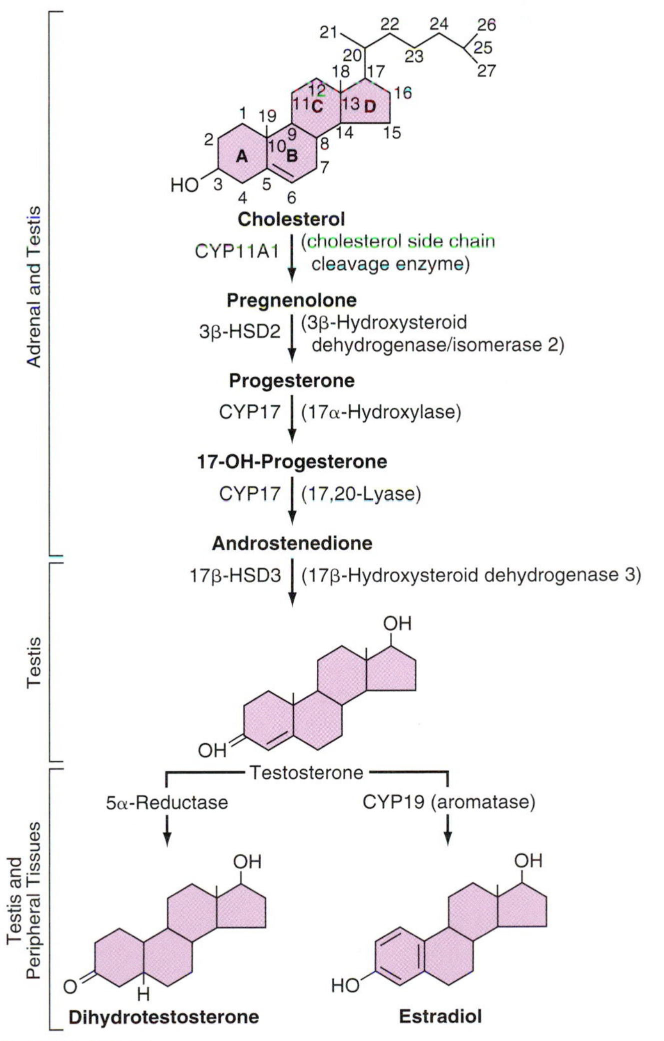

FIGURE 8-3
The biochemical pathway in the conversion of 27-carbon sterol cholesterol to androgens and estrogens.

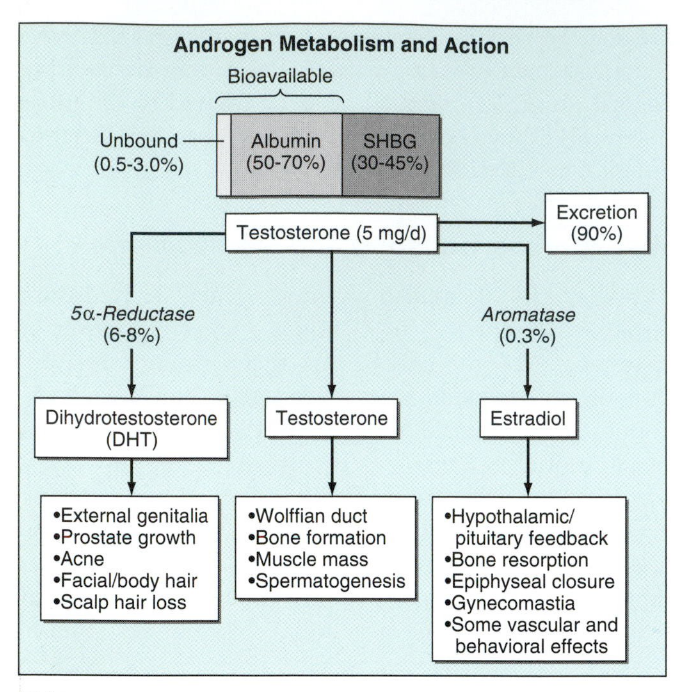

FIGURE 8-4

Androgen metabolism and actions. SHBG, sex hormone-binding globulin.

albumin (**Fig. 8-4**). SHBG binds testosterone with much greater affinity than albumin. Only 0.5 to 3% of testosterone is unbound. According to the "free hormone" hypothesis, only the unbound fraction is biologically active; however, albumin-bound hormone dissociates readily in the capillaries and may be bioavailable. SHBG concentrations are decreased by androgens, obesity, insulin, and nephrotic syndrome. Conversely, estrogen administration, hyperthyroidism, many chronic inflammatory illnesses, and aging are associated with high SHBG concentrations.

Testosterone is metabolized predominantly in the liver, although some degradation occurs in peripheral tissues, particularly the prostate and the skin. In the liver, testosterone is converted by a series of enzymatic steps into androsterone, etiocholanolone, DHT, and 3-α-androstanediol. These compounds undergo glucuronidation or sulfation before being excreted by the kidneys.

Mechanism of Androgen Action

The androgen receptor (AR) is homologous to other nuclear receptor proteins including the receptors for estrogen, glucocorticoids, and progesterone (Chap. 1). The AR is encoded by a gene on the long arm of the X chromosome and has a molecular mass of about 110 kDa. A polymorphic region in the amino terminus of the receptor, which contains a variable number of glutamine repeats, modifies the transcriptional activity of the receptor. The AR protein is distributed in both the cytoplasm and the nucleus. Androgen binding to the AR causes it to translocate into the nucleus where it binds to DNA or other transcription factors already bound to DNA. The ligand also induces conformational changes that allow the recruitment and assembly of tissue-specific cofactors. Thus, the AR is a ligand-regulated transcription factor. Some androgen effects may be mediated by nongenomic AR signal transduction pathways. Testosterone binds to AR with half the affinity of DHT. The DHT-AR complex also has greater thermostability, and a slower dissociation rate, than the testosterone-AR complex. However, the molecular basis for selective testosterone versus DHT actions remains incompletely explained.

THE SEMINIFEROUS TUBULES: SPERMATOGENESIS

The seminiferous tubules are convoluted, closed loops with both ends emptying into the rete testis, a network of progressively larger efferent ducts that ultimately form the epididymis (Fig. 8-2). The seminiferous tubules total about 600 m in length and constitute about two-thirds of testis volume. The walls of the tubules are formed by polarized Sertoli cells that are apposed to peritubular myoid cells. Tight junctions between Sertoli cells create a blood-testis barrier. Germ cells constitute the majority of the seminiferous epithelium (~60%) and are intimately embedded within the cytoplasmic extensions of the Sertoli cells, which function as "nurse cells." Germ cells progress through characteristic morphologic stages of spermiogenesis, requiring ~24 days. A pool of type A spermatogonia serve as stem cells capable of self-renewal. Primary spermatocytes are derived from type B spermatogonia and undergo meiosis before progressing to spermatids that mature and are ultimately released from Sertoli cells as mature spermatozoa. Peristaltic-type action by peritubular myoid cells transports sperm into the efferent ducts. The normal adult testes produce >100 million sperm per day.

Naturally occurring mutations in the *FSHβ* gene and in the FSH receptor confirm an important, but not essential, role for this pathway in spermatogenesis. Females with these mutations are hypogonadal and infertile because ovarian follicles do not mature; males exhibit variable degrees of reduced spermatogenesis, presumably because of impaired Sertoli cell function. Because Sertoli cells produce inhibin B, an inhibitor of FSH, seminiferous tubule damage (e.g., by radiation) causes a selective increase of FSH. Androgens reach very high concentrations locally in the testis and are essential for spermatogenesis. Several cytokines and growth factors are also involved in the regulation of spermatogenesis by paracrine and autocrine mechanisms. A number of knockout mouse models exhibit impaired germ cell development or spermatogenesis, presaging possible mutations associated with male infertility. In humans, microdeletions of several Y chromosome azoospermia factor (*AZF*) genes (e.g., RNA-binding motif, *RBM;* deleted in azoospermia, *DAZ*) are associated with oligospermia or azoospermia.

CLINICAL AND LABORATORY EVALUATION OF MALE REPRODUCTIVE FUNCTION

HISTORY AND PHYSICAL EXAMINATION

The history should focus on developmental stages such as puberty and growth spurts, as well as androgen-dependent events such as early morning erections, frequency and intensity of sexual thoughts, and frequency of masturbation or intercourse. Although libido and the overall frequency of sexual acts is decreased in androgen-deficient men, young hypogonadal men may achieve erections in response to visual erotic stimuli. Men with acquired androgen deficiency often report decreased energy and increased irritability.

The physical examination should focus on secondary sex characteristics such as hair growth, possible gynecomastia, testicular volume, prostate, and height and body proportions. Eunuchoidal proportions are defined as an arm span >2 cm greater than height and suggest that androgen deficiency occurred before epiphyseal fusion. Hair growth in the face, axilla, chest, and pubic regions is androgen-dependent; however, changes may not be noticeable unless androgen deficiency is severe and prolonged. Ethnicity also influences the intensity of hair growth (Chap. 12). Testicular volume is best measured by using a Prader orchidometer. Testes range from 3.5 to 5.5 cm in length, which corresponds to a volume of 12 to 25 mL. Advanced age does not influence testicular size, although the consistency becomes less firm. Asian men generally have smaller testes than western Europeans, independent of differences in body size. Because of its possible role in infertility, the presence of varicocele should be sought by palpation while the patient is standing; it is more common on the left side. Patients with Klinefelter syndrome have markedly reduced testicular volumes (1 to 2 mL). In congenital hypogonadotropic hypogonadism, testicular volumes provide a good index for the degree of gonadotropin deficiency and the likelihood of response to therapy.

GONADOTROPIN AND INHIBIN MEASUREMENTS

LH and FSH are measured using two-site immunoradiometric, immunofluorometric, or chemiluminescent assays, which have very low cross-reactivity with other pituitary glycoprotein hormones and human chorionic gonadotropin (hCG) and have sufficient sensitivity to measure the low levels present in patients with hypogonadotropic hypogonadism. In men with a low testosterone level, an LH level can distinguish hypergonadotropic (high LH) versus hypogonadotropic (low or inappropriately normal LH) hypogonadism. An elevated LH level indicates a primary defect at the testicular level, whereas a low or inappropriately normal LH level suggests a defect at the hypothalamic-pituitary level. LH pulses occur about every 1 to 3 h in normal men. Thus, gonadotropin levels fluctuate, and samples should be pooled or repeated when results are equivocal. FSH is less pulsatile than LH because it has a longer half-life. Increased FSH suggests damage to the seminiferous tubules. Inhibin B, a Sertoli cell product that suppresses FSH, is reduced with seminiferous tubule damage. Inhibin B is a dimer with α-β_B subunits and is measured by two-site immunoassays.

GnRH Stimulation Testing

The GnRH test is performed by measuring LH and FSH concentrations at baseline and at 30 and 60 min after intravenous administration of 100 μg of GnRH. A minimally acceptable response is a twofold LH increase and a 50% FSH increase. In the prepubertal period or with severe GnRH deficiency, the gonadotrope may not respond to a single bolus of GnRH because it has not been primed by endogenous hypothalamic GnRH; in these patients, GnRH responsiveness may be restored by chronic, pulsatile GnRH administration. With the availability of sensitive and specific LH assays, GnRH stimulation testing is used rarely except to evaluate gonadotrope function in patients who have undergone pituitary surgery or have a space-occupying lesion in the hypothalamic-pituitary region.

TESTOSTERONE ASSAYS

Total Testosterone

Total testosterone includes both unbound and protein-bound testosterone and is measured by radioimmunoassays or immunometric assays. A single random sample provides a good approximation of the average testosterone concentration with the realization that testosterone levels fluctuate in response to pulsatile LH. Testosterone is generally lower in the late afternoon and is reduced by acute illness. The testosterone concentration in healthy young men ranges from 300 to 1000 ng/dL in most laboratories. Alterations in SHBG levels due to aging, obesity, some types of medications, or chronic illness, or on a congenital basis, can affect total testosterone levels.

Measurement of Free Testosterone Levels

Most circulating testosterone is bound to SHBG and to albumin; only 0.5 to 3% of circulating testosterone is unbound or "free." Free testosterone concentrations can be calculated from algorithms based on total testosterone and SHBG concentrations. The free fraction is best measured by equilibrium dialysis. Tracer analogue methods are relatively inexpensive and convenient but they are less reliable because changes in SHBG affect the results. Bioavailable testosterone refers to unbound testosterone plus testosterone that is loosely bound to albumin; it can be estimated by the ammonium sulfate precipitation method.

hCG Stimulation Test

The hCG stimulation test is performed by administering a single injection of 1500 to 4000 IU of hCG intramuscularly and measuring testosterone levels at baseline and 24, 48, 72, and 120 h after hCG injection. An alternative regimen involves three injections of 1500 units of hCG on successive days, and measuring testosterone levels 24 h after the last dose. An acceptable response to hCG is a doubling of the testosterone concentration in adult men. In prepubertal boys, an increase in testosterone to >150 ng/dL indicates the presence of testicular tissue. No response may indicate an absence of testicular tissue or marked impairment of Leydig cell function. Measurement of MIS, a Sertoli cell product, is also used to detect the presence of testes in prepubertal boys with cryptorchidism.

SEMEN ANALYSIS

Semen analysis is the most important step in the evaluation of male infertility (Chap. 15). Samples are collected by masturbation following a period of abstinence for 2 to 3 days. Semen volumes and sperm concentrations vary considerably among fertile men, and several samples may be needed before concluding that the results are abnormal. Analysis should be performed within an hour of collection. The normal ejaculate volume is 2 to 6 mL and contains sperm counts of >20 million/mL, with a motility of >50% and >15% normal morphology. Some men with low sperm counts are nevertheless fertile. A variety of tests for sperm function can be performed in specialized laboratories, but these add relatively little to the treatment options.

TESTICULAR BIOPSY

Testicular biopsy is useful in some patients with oligospermia or azoospermia, as an aid in diagnosis and indication for the feasibility of treatment. Using local anesthesia, fine-needle aspiration biopsy is performed to aspirate tissue for histology. Alternatively, open biopsies can be performed under local or general anesthesia when more tissue is required. A normal biopsy in an azoospermic man with a normal FSH level suggests obstruction of the vas deferens, which may be correctable surgically. Biopsies are also used to harvest sperm for intracytoplasmic sperm injection (ICSI) and to classify disorders such as hypospermatogenesis (all stages present but in reduced numbers), germ cell arrest (usually at primary spermatocyte stage), and Sertoli cell–only syndrome (absent germ cells) or hyalinization (sclerosis with absent cellular elements).

DISORDERS OF SEXUAL DIFFERENTIATION

See Chap. 7.

DISORDERS OF PUBERTY

PRECOCIOUS PUBERTY

Puberty in boys before age 9 is considered precocious. *Isosexual precocity* refers to premature sexual development consistent with phenotypic sex and includes features such as the development of facial hair and phallic growth. Isosexual precocity is divided into gonadotropin-dependent and gonadotropin-independent causes of androgen excess (**Table 8-1**). *Heterosexual precocity* refers to the premature development of feminizing features in boys, such as breast development.

Gonadotropin-Dependent Precocious Puberty

This disorder is also called *central precocious puberty* (CPP) and is less common in boys than in girls. It is caused by premature activation of the GnRH pulse generator, sometimes because of central nervous system (CNS) lesions such as hypothalamic hamartomas, but it is often idiopathic. CPP is characterized by gonadotropin levels that are inappropriately elevated for age. Because pituitary priming has occurred, GnRH elicits LH and FSH responses typical of those seen in puberty or in adults. Magnetic resonance imaging (MRI) should be performed to exclude a mass, structural defect, or infectious or inflammatory process.

Gonadotropin-Independent Precocious Puberty

This group of disorders includes hCG-secreting tumors; congenital adrenal hyperplasia; sex steroid–producing tumors of the testis, adrenal, and ovary; accidental or deliberate exogenous sex steroid administration; hypothyroidism; and activating mutations of the LH recep-

TABLE 8-1

CAUSES OF PRECOCIOUS OR DELAYED PUBERTY IN BOYS

- **I. Precocious puberty**
  - A. Gonadotropin-dependent
    1. Idiopathic
    2. Hypothalamic hamartoma or other lesions
    3. CNS tumor or inflammatory state
  - B. Gonadotropin-independent
    1. Congenital adrenal hyperplasia
    2. hCG-secreting tumor
    3. McCune-Albright syndrome
    4. Activating LH receptor mutation
    5. Exogenous androgens
- **II. Delayed puberty**
  - A. Constitutional delay of growth and puberty
  - B. Systemic disorders
    1. Chronic disease
    2. Malnutrition
    3. Anorexia nervosa
  - C. CNS tumors and their treatment (radiotherapy and surgery)
  - D. Hypothalamic-pituitary causes of pubertal failure (low gonadotropins)
    1. Congenital disorders (Table 8-2)
       - a. Hypothalamic syndromes (e.g., Prader-Willi)
       - b. Idiopathic hypogonadotropic hypogonadism
       - c. Kallmann syndrome
       - d. GnRH receptor mutations
       - e. Adrenal hypoplasia congenital
       - f. PROPI mutations
       - g. Other mutations affecting pituitary development/function
    2. Acquired disorders
       - a. Pituitary tumors
       - b. Hyperprolactinemia
  - E. Gonadal causes of pubertal failure (elevated gonadotropins)
    1. Klinefelter syndrome
    2. Bilateral undescended testes or anorchia
    3. Orchitis
    4. Chemotherapy or radiotherapy
  - F. Androgen insensitivity

Note: CNS, central nervous system; hCG, human chronic gonadotropin; LH, luteinizing hormone; GnRH, gonadotropin-releasing hormone.

tor or $G_s\alpha$ subunit. In these cases, androgens from the testis or the adrenal are increased but gonadotropins are low.

Familial Male-Limited Precocious Puberty This is transmitted in an autosomal dominant manner. It is caused by activating mutations in the LH receptor, leading to constitutive stimulation of the cyclic AMP pathway and testosterone production. The disorder is also called *testotoxicosis*. Clinical features include premature virilization in boys, growth acceleration in early childhood, and advanced bone age followed by premature epiphyseal fusion. Testosterone is elevated and LH is suppressed. Treatment options include inhibitors of testosterone synthesis (e.g., ketoconazole), androgen receptor antagonists (e.g., flutamide), and aromatase inhibitors (e.g., anastrozole).

McCune-Albright Syndrome This is a sporadic disorder caused by somatic (postzygotic) activating mutations in the $G_s\alpha$ subunit that links G protein–coupled receptors to intracellular signaling pathways (Chap. 26). The mutations impair the guanosine triphosphatase activity of the $G_s\alpha$ protein, leading to constitutive activation of adenylyl cyclase. Like activating LH receptor mutations, this stimulates testosterone production and causes gonadotropin-independent precocious puberty. In addition to sexual precocity, affected individuals may have autonomy in the adrenals, pituitary, and thyroid glands. Café au lait spots are characteristic skin lesions that reflect the onset of the somatic mutations in melanocytes during embryonic development. Polyostotic fibrous dysplasia is caused by activation of the parathyroid hormone receptor pathway in bone. Treatment is similar to that in patients with activating LH receptor mutations. Bisphosphonates have been used to treat bone lesions.

Congenital Adrenal Hyperplasia Boys with congenital adrenal hyperplasia (CAH) who are not well controlled with glucocorticoid suppression of adrenocorticotropic hormone (ACTH) can develop premature virilization because of excessive androgen production by the adrenal gland (Chaps. 5 and 7). LH is low and the testes are small. Rarely, adrenal rests may develop within the testis because of chronic ACTH stimulation.

Heterosexual Sexual Precocity

Breast enlargement in prepubertal boys can result from familial aromatase excess, estrogen-producing tumors in the adrenal gland, Sertoli cell tumors in the testis, marijuana smoking, or estrogen use. Occasionally, germ cell tumors that secrete hCG can be associated with breast enlargement due to excessive stimulation of estrogen production (see "Gynecomastia," below).

APPROACH TO THE PATIENT WITH PRECOCIOUS PUBERTY

After verification of precocious development, serum LH and FSH levels should be measured to determine whether gonadotropins are increased in relation to chronologic age (gonadotropin-dependent) or whether sex steroid secretion is occurring independent of LH and FSH (gonadotropin-independent). In children with gonadotropin-dependent precocious puberty, CNS lesions should be excluded by history, neurologic examination, and MRI scan of the head. If organic causes are not found, one is left with the diagnosis of idiopathic central precocity. Patients with high testosterone but suppressed LH concentrations have gonadotropin-independent sexual precocity; in these patients, DHEA sulfate (DHEAS) and 17α-hydroxyprogesterone should be measured. High levels of testosterone and 17α-hydroxyprogesterone suggest the possibility of CAH due to 21α-hydroxylase or 11β-hydroxylase deficiency. If testosterone and DHEAS are elevated, adrenal tumors should be excluded by obtaining a computed tomography (CT) scan of the adrenal glands. Patients with elevated testosterone but without increased 17α-hydroxyprogesterone or DHEAS should undergo careful evaluation of the testis by palpation and ultrasound to exclude a Leydig cell neoplasm. Activating mutations of the LH receptor should be considered in children with gonadotropin-independent precocious puberty in whom CAH, androgen abuse, and adrenal and testicular neoplasms have been excluded.

℞ TREATMENT FOR PRECOCIOUS PUBERTY

In patients with a known cause (e.g., a CNS lesion or a testicular tumor), therapy should be directed toward the underlying disorder. In patients with idiopathic CPP, long-acting GnRH analogues can be used to suppress gonadotropins and decrease testosterone, halt early pubertal development, delay accelerated bone maturation, and prevent early epiphyseal closure. The treatment is most effective for increasing final adult height if it is initiated before age 6. Puberty resumes after discontinuation of the GnRH analogue. Counseling is an important aspect of the overall treatment strategy. In children with gonadotropin-independent precocious puberty, inhibitors of steroidogenesis, such as ketoconazole, and AR antagonists have been used empirically without data from clinical trials.

DELAYED PUBERTY

Puberty is delayed in boys if it has not ensued by age 14, an age that is 2 to 2.5 standard deviations above the mean for healthy children. Delayed puberty is more common in boys than in girls. There are four main categories of delayed puberty: (1) constitutional delay of growth and puberty (~60% of cases); (2) functional hypogonadotropic hypogonadism caused by systemic illness or malnutrition (~20% of cases); (3) hypogonadotropic hypogonadism caused by genetic or acquired defects in the hypothalamic-pituitary region (~10% of cases); and (4) hypergonadotropic hypogonadism secondary to primary gonadal failure (~15% of cases) (Table 8-1). Functional hypogonadotropic hypogonadism is more common in girls than in boys. Permanent causes of hypogonadotropic or hypergonadotropic hypogonadism are identified in <25% of boys with delayed puberty.

APPROACH TO THE PATIENT WITH DELAYED PUBERTY

Any history of systemic illness, eating disorders, excessive exercise, social and psychological problems, and abnormal patterns of linear growth during childhood should be verified. Boys with pubertal delay may have accompanying emotional and physical immaturity relative to their peers, which can be a source of anxiety. Physical examination should focus on height; arm span; weight; visual fields; and secondary sex characteristics including hair growth, testicular volume, phallic size, and scrotal reddening and thinning. Testicular size >2.5 cm generally indicates that the child has entered puberty.

The main diagnostic challenge is to distinguish those with constitutional delay, who will progress through puberty at a later age, from those with an underlying pathologic process. Constitutional delay should be suspected when there is a family history and when there are delayed bone age and short stature. Pituitary priming by pulsatile GnRH is required before LH and FSH are synthesized and secreted normally. Thus, blunted responses to exogenous GnRH can be seen in patients with constitutional delay, GnRH deficiency, or pituitary disorders (see "GnRH Stimulation Testing," above). On the other hand, low-normal basal gonadotropin levels or a normal response to exogenous GnRH is consistent with an early stage of puberty, which is often heralded by nocturnal GnRH secretion. Thus, constitutional delay is a diagnosis of exclusion that requires ongoing evaluation until the onset of puberty and the growth spurt.

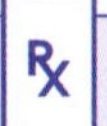

TREATMENT FOR DELAYED PUBERTY

If therapy is considered appropriate, it can begin with 25 to 50 mg testosterone enanthate or testosterone cypionate every 2 weeks, or by using a 2.5-mg testosterone patch or 25-mg testosterone gel. Because aromatization of testosterone to estrogen is obligatory for mediating androgen effects on epiphyseal fusion, concomitant treatment with aromatase inhibitors may allow attainment of greater final adult height. Testosterone treatment should be interrupted after 6 months to determine if endogenous LH and FSH secretion have ensued. Other causes of delayed puberty should be considered when there are associated clinical features or when boys do not enter puberty spontaneously after a year of observation or treatment.

Reassurance without hormonal treatment is appropriate for many individuals with presumed constitutional delay of puberty. However, the impact of delayed growth and pubertal progression on a child's social relationships and school performance is often underappreciated.

DISORDERS OF THE MALE REPRODUCTIVE AXIS DURING ADULTHOOD

HYPOGONADOTROPIC HYPOGONADISM

Because LH and FSH are trophic hormones for the testes, impaired secretion of these pituitary gonadotropins results in secondary hypogonadism, which is characterized by low testosterone in the setting of low LH and FSH. Those with the most severe deficiency have complete absence of pubertal development, sexual infantilism, and, in some cases, hypospadias and undescended testes. Patients with partial gonadotropin deficiency have delayed or arrested sexual development. The 24-h LH secretory profiles are heterogeneous in patients with hypogonadotropic hypogonadism, reflecting variable abnormalities of LH pulse frequency or amplitude. In severe cases, basal LH is low and there are no LH pulses. A smaller subset of patients has low-amplitude LH pulses or markedly reduced pulse frequency. Occasionally, only sleep-entrained LH pulses occur, reminiscent of the pattern seen in the early stages of puberty. Hypogonadotropic hypogonadism can be classified into congenital and acquired disorders. Congenital disorders most commonly involve GnRH deficiency, which leads to gonadotropin deficiency. Acquired disorders are much more common than congenital disorders and may result from a variety of sellar mass lesions or infiltrative diseases of the hypothalamus or pituitary.

Congenital Disorders Associated with Gonadotropin Deficiency

Most cases of congenital hypogonadotropic hypogonadism are idiopathic, despite extensive endocrine testing and imaging studies of the sellar region. Among known causes, familial hypogonadotropic hypogonadism can be transmitted as an X-linked (20%), autosomal recessive (30%), or autosomal dominant (50%) trait. Some individuals with idiopathic hypogonadotropic hypogonadism (IHH) have sporadic mutations in the same genes that cause inherited forms of the disorder. *Kallmann syndrome* is an X-linked disorder caused by mutations in the *KAL1* gene, which encodes anosmin, a protein that mediates the migration of neural progenitors of the olfactory bulb and GnRH-producing neurons. These individuals have GnRH deficiency and variable combinations of anosmia or hyposmia, renal defects, and neurologic abnormalities including mirror movements. Gonadotropin secretion and fertility can be restored by administration of pulsatile GnRH or by gonadotropin replacement. Mutations in the *FGFR1* gene cause an autosomal dominant form of hypogonadotropic hypogonadism that clinically resembles Kallmann syndrome. The *FGFR1* gene product may be the receptor for the *KAL1* gene product, anosmin, thereby explaining the similarity in clinical features. Other autosomal dominant causes remain unexplained. X-linked hypogonadotropic hypogonadism also occurs in adrenal hypoplasia congenita, a disorder caused by mutations in the *DAX1* gene, which encodes a nuclear receptor in the adrenal gland and reproductive axis. *Adrenal hypoplasia congenita* is characterized by absent development of the adult zone of the adrenal cortex, leading to neonatal adrenal insufficiency. Puberty usually does not occur or is arrested, reflecting variable degrees of gonadotropin deficiency. Although sexual differentiation is normal, some patients have testicular dysgenesis and impaired spermatogenesis despite gonadotropin replacement. *GnRH receptor mutations* account for ~40% of autosomal recessive and 10% of sporadic cases of hypogonadotropic hypogonadism. These patients have decreased LH response to exogenous GnRH. Some receptor mutations alter GnRH binding affinity, allowing apparently normal responses to pharmacologic doses of exogenous GnRH. Mutations in the G protein–coupled receptor GPR54 cause gonadotropin deficiency without anosmia. Patients retain responsiveness to exogenous GnRA, suggesting an abnormality in the neural pathways controlling GnRH release. Rarely, recessive mutations in the *LHβ* or *FSHβ* genes have been described in patients with selective

TABLE 8-2

CAUSES OF CONGENITAL HYPOGONADOTROPIC HYPOGONADISM

GENE	LOCUS	INHERITANCE	ASSOCIATED FEATURES
KAL1	Xp22	X-linked	Anosmia, renal agenesis, synkinesia, cleft lip/palate, oculomotor, visuospatial defects, gut malrotations
FGFR1	8p11-p12	AD	Anosmia, cleft lip/palate, synkinesia, syndactyly
LEP	7q31	AR	Obesity
LEPR	1p31	AR	Obesity
PC1	5q15-21	AR	Obesity, diabetes mellitus, ACTH deficiency
HESX1	3p21	AR	Septooptic dysplasia, CPHD
		AD	Isolated GH insufficiency
LHX3	9q35	AR	CPHD (ACTH spared), cervical spine rigidity
PROP1	5q35	AR	CPHD (ACTH usually spared)
GPR54	19p13	AR	None
GNRHR	4q21	AR	None
FSHβ	11p13	AR	↑ LH
LHβ	19q13	AR	↑ FSH
SFI (NR5A1)	9p33	AD/ AR	Primary adrenal failure, XY sex reversal
DAXI (NR0B1)	Xp21	X-linked	Primary adrenal failure impaired spermatogenesis

Abbreviations: ACTH, adrenocorticotropic hormone; AD, autosomal dominant; AR, autosomal recessive; CPHD, combined pituitary hormone deficiency; KAL1, Interval-1 gene; FGFR1, fibroblast growth factor receptor 1; LEP, leptin; LEPR, leptin receptor; PC1, prohormone convertase 1; HESX1, homeo box gene expressed in embryonic stem cells 1; LHX3, LIM homeobox gene 3; PROP1, Prophet of Pit 1; GPR54, G protein–coupled receptor 54, GNRHR, gonadotropin-releasing hormone receptor; FSHβ, follicle-stimulating hormone β-subunit; LHβ, luteinizing hormone β-subunit; SF1, steroidogenic factor 1; DAX1, dosage-sensitive sex-reversal, adrenal hypoplasia congenital, *X*-chromosome.

deficiencies of these gonadotropins. Deletions or mutations of the *GnRH* gene have not been found in patients with hypogonadotropic hypogonadism.

A number of homeodomain transcription factors are involved in the development and differentiation of the specialized hormone-producing cells within the pituitary gland (**Table 8-2**). Patients with mutations of *PROP1* have combined pituitary hormone deficiency that includes GH, prolactin (PRL), thyroid-stimulating hormone (TSH), LH, and FSH, but not ACTH. *LHX3* mutations cause combined pituitary hormone deficiency in association with cervical spine rigidity. *HESX1* mutations cause septooptic dysplasia and combined pituitary hormone deficiency.

Prader-Willi syndrome is characterized by obesity, hypotonic musculature, mental retardation, hypogonadism, short stature, and small hands and feet. Prader-Willi syndrome is a genomic imprinting disorder caused by deletions of the proximal portion of paternally derived chromosome 15q or by uniparental disomy of the maternal alleles. *Laurence-Moon syndrome* is an autosomal recessive disorder characterized by obesity, hypogonadism, mental retardation, polydactyly, and retinitis pigmentosa. Recessive mutations of leptin, or its receptor, cause severe obesity and pubertal arrest, apparently because of hypothalamic GnRH deficiency (Chap. 16).

Acquired Hypogonadotropic Disorders

Severe Illness, Stress, Malnutrition, and Exercise

These may cause reversible gonadotropin deficiency. Although gonadotropin deficiency and reproductive dysfunction are well documented in these conditions in women, men exhibit similar but less pronounced responses. Unlike women, most male runners and other endurance athletes have normal gonadotropin and sex steroid levels, despite low body fat and frequent intensive exercise. Testosterone levels fall at the onset of illness and recover during recuperation. The magnitude of gonadotropin suppression generally correlates with the severity of illness. Although hypogonadotropic hypogonadism is the most common cause of androgen deficiency in patients with acute illness, some have elevated levels of LH and FSH, which suggest primary gonadal dysfunction. The pathophysiology of reproductive dysfunction during acute illness is unknown but likely involves a combination of cytokine and/or glucocorticoid effects. There is a high frequency of low testosterone levels in patients with chronic illnesses such as HIV infection, end-stage renal disease, chronic obstructive lung disease, and many types of cancer and in patients receiving glucocorticoids. Some 20% of HIV-infected men with low testosterone levels have elevated LH and FSH levels; these patients presumably have primary testicular dysfunction. The remaining 80% have either normal or low LH and FSH levels; these men have a central hypothalamic-pituitary defect or a dual defect involving both the testis and the hypothalamic-pituitary centers. Muscle wasting is common in chronic diseases associated with hypogonadism, which also leads to debility, poor quality of life, and adverse outcome of disease. There is great interest in exploring strategies that can reverse androgen deficiency or attenuate the sarcopenia associated with chronic illness.

Men who are heavy users of marijuana have decreased testosterone secretion and sperm production. The mechanism of marijuana-induced hypogonadism is decreased GnRH secretion. Gynecomastia observed in marijuana users can also be caused by plant estrogens in crude preparations.

Obesity In men with mild to moderate obesity, SHBG levels decrease in proportion to the degree of obesity, resulting in lower total testosterone levels. However, free testosterone levels usually remain within the normal range. The decrease in SHBG levels is caused by increased circulating insulin, which inhibits SHBG production. Estradiol levels are higher in obese men compared with healthy, non-obese controls, because of aromatization of testosterone to estradiol in adipose tissue. Weight loss is associated with reversal of these abnormalities including an increase in total and free testosterone levels and a decrease in estradiol levels. A subset of massively obese men may have a defect in the hypothalamic-pituitary axis as suggested by low free testosterone in the absence of elevated gonadotropins.

Hyperprolactinemia (See also Chap. 2) Elevated PRL levels are associated with hypogonadotropic hypogonadism. PRL inhibits hypothalamic GnRH secretion either directly or through modulation of tuberoinfundibular dopaminergic pathways. A PRL-secreting tumor may also destroy the surrounding gonadotropes by invasion or compression of the pituitary stalk. Treatment with dopamine agonists reverses gonadotropin deficiency, although there may be a delay relative to PRL suppression.

Sellar Mass Lesions Neoplastic and nonneoplastic lesions in the hypothalamus or pituitary can directly or indirectly affect gonadotrope function. In adults, pituitary adenomas constitute the largest category of space-occupying lesions affecting gonadotropin and other pituitary hormone production. Pituitary adenomas that extend into the suprasellar region can impair GnRH secretion and mildly increase PRL secretion (usually <50 μg/L) because of impaired tonic inhibition by dopaminergic pathways. These tumors should be distinguished from prolactinomas, which typically secrete higher PRL levels. The presence of diabetes insipidus suggests the possibility of a craniopharyngioma, infiltrative disorder, or other hypothalamic lesions (Chap. 3).

Hemochromatosis (See also Chap. 336, in HPIM, 16e) Both the pituitary and testis can be affected by excessive iron deposition. However, the pituitary defect is the predominant lesion in most patients with hemochromatosis and hypogonadism. The diagnosis of hemochromatosis is suggested by the association of characteristic skin pigmentation, hepatic enlargement or dysfunction, diabetes mellitus, arthritis, cardiac conduction defects, and hypogonadism.

PRIMARY TESTICULAR CAUSES OF HYPOGONADISM

Common causes of primary testicular dysfunction include Klinefelter syndrome, uncorrected cryptorchidism, cancer chemotherapy, radiation to the testes, trauma, torsion, infectious orchitis, HIV infection, anorchia syndrome, and myotonic dystrophy. Primary testicular disorders may be associated with impaired spermatogenesis, decreased androgen production, or both. See Chap. 7 for disorders of testis development, androgen synthesis, and androgen action.

Klinefelter Syndrome (See also Chap. 7)

Klinefelter syndrome is the most common chromosomal disorder associated with testicular dysfunction and male infertility. It occurs in about 1 in 1000 live-born males. Azoospermia is the rule in men with Klinefelter syndrome who have the 47,XXY karyotype; however, men with mosaicism may have germ cells, especially at a younger age. Testicular histology shows hyalinization of seminiferous tubules and absence of spermatogenesis. Although their function is impaired, the number of Leydig cells appears to increase. Testosterone is decreased and estradiol is increased, leading to clinical features of undervirilization and gynecomastia.

Cryptorchidism

Cryptorchidism occurs when there is incomplete descent of the testis from the abdominal cavity into the scrotum. About 3% of full-term and 30% of premature male infants have at least one cryptorchid testis at birth, but descent is usually complete by the first few weeks of life. The incidence of cryptorchidism is <1% by 9 months of age. Cryptorchidism is associated with increased risk of malignancy and infertility. Unilateral cryptorchidism, even when corrected before puberty, is associated with decreased sperm counts, possibly reflecting unrecognized damage to the fully descended testis.

Acquired Testicular Defects

Viral orchitis may be caused by the mumps virus, echovirus, lymphocytic choriomeningitis virus, and group B arboviruses. Orchitis occurs in as many as one-fourth of adult men with mumps; the orchitis is unilateral in about two-thirds, and bilateral in the remainder. Orchitis usually develops a few days after the onset of parotitis but may precede it. The testis may return to normal size and function or undergo atrophy. Semen analysis returns to normal for three-fourths of men with unilateral involvement but normal for only one-third of men with bilateral orchitis. *Trauma,* including testicular torsion, can also cause secondary atrophy of the testes. The exposed position of the testes in the scrotum renders them susceptible to both thermal and physical trauma, particularly in men with hazardous occupations.

The testes are sensitive to *radiation damage.* Doses >200 mGy (20 rad) are associated with increased FSH and LH levels and damage to the spermatogonia. After ~800 mGy (80 rad), oligospermia or azoospermia develops, and higher doses may obliterate the germinal epithelium. Permanent androgen deficiency in adult men is uncommon after therapeutic radiation; however, most boys given direct testicular radiation therapy for acute lymphoblastic leukemia have permanently low testosterone levels. Sperm banking should be considered before patients undergo radiation treatment or chemotherapy.

Drugs interfere with testicular function by several mechanisms including inhibition of testosterone synthesis (e.g., ketoconazole), blockade of androgen action (e.g., spironolactone), increased estrogen (e.g., marijuana), or direct inhibition of spermatogenesis (e.g., chemotherapy). Cyclophosphamide causes azoospermia or extreme oligospermia within a few weeks after the initiation of therapy. In about half of patients, spermatogenesis returns within 3 years after cessation of therapy. Combination chemotherapy for acute leukemia, Hodgkin's disease, and other malignancies may impair Leydig cell function. Alcohol, when consumed in excess for prolonged periods, decreases testosterone, independent of liver disease or malnutrition. Elevated estradiol and decreased testosterone levels may occur in men taking digitalis.

The occupational and recreational history should be carefully evaluated in all men with infertility because of the toxic effects of many *chemical agents* on spermatogenesis. Known environmental hazards include microwaves and ultrasound and chemicals such as the nematocide dibromochloropropane, cadmium, and lead. In some populations, sperm density is said to have declined by as much as 40% in the past 50 years. Environmental estrogens or antiandrogens may be partly responsible.

Testicular failure also occurs as a part of *polyglandular autoimmune insufficiency* (Chap. 21). Sperm antibodies can cause isolated male infertility. In some instances, these antibodies are secondary phenomena resulting from duct obstruction or vasectomy. Granulomatous diseases can affect the testes, and testicular atrophy occurs in 10 to 20% of men with lepromatous leprosy because of direct tissue invasion by the mycobacteria. The tubules are involved initially, followed by endarteritis and destruction of Leydig cells.

Systemic disease can cause primary testis dysfunction in addition to suppressing gonadotropin production. In cirrhosis, a combined testicular and pituitary abnormality leads to decreased testosterone production independent of the direct toxic effects of ethanol. Impaired hepatic extraction of adrenal androstenedione leads to extraglandular conversion to estrone and estradiol, which partially suppresses LH. Testicular atrophy and gynecomastia are present in approximately one-half of men with cirrhosis. In chronic renal failure, androgen synthesis and sperm production decrease despite elevated gonadotropins. The elevated LH level is due to reduced clearance, but it does not restore normal testosterone production. About one-fourth of men with renal failure have hyperprolactinemia. Improvement in testosterone production with hemodialysis is incomplete, but successful renal transplantation may return testicular function to normal. Testicular atrophy is present in one-third of men with sickle cell anemia. The defect may be at either the testicular or the hypothalamic-pituitary level. Sperm density can decrease temporarily after acute febrile illness in the absence of a change in testosterone production. Infertility in men with celiac disease is associated with a hormonal pattern typical of androgen resistance, namely elevated testosterone and LH levels.

Neurologic diseases associated with altered testicular function include myotonic dystrophy, spinobulbar muscular atrophy, and paraplegia. In myotonic dystrophy, small testes may be associated with impairment of both spermatogenesis and Leydig cell function. Spinobulbar muscular atrophy is caused by an expansion of the glutamine repeat sequences in the amino-terminal region of the AR; this expansion impairs function of the AR, but it is unclear how the alteration is related to the neurologic manifestations. Men with spinobulbar muscular atrophy often have undervirilization and infertility as a late manifestation. Spinal cord lesions that cause paraplegia can lead to a temporary decrease in testosterone levels and may cause persistent defects in spermatogenesis; some patients retain the capacity for penile erection and ejaculation.

ANDROGEN INSENSITIVITY SYNDROMES

Mutations in the AR cause resistance to the action of testosterone and DHT. These X-linked mutations are associated with variable degrees of defective male phenotypic development and undervirilization (Chap. 7). Although not technically hormone insensitivity syndromes, two genetic disorders impair testosterone conversion to active sex steroids. Mutations in the *SRD5A2* gene, which encodes 5α-reductase type 2, prevent the conversion of testosterone to DHT, which is necessary for the normal development of the male external genitalia. Mutations in the *CYP19* gene, which encodes aromatase, prevent testosterone conversion to estradiol. Males with *CYP19* mutations have delayed epiphyseal fusion, tall stature, eunuchoidal proportions, and osteoporosis, consistent with evidence from an estrogen receptor–deficient individual that these testosterone actions are mediated indirectly via estrogen.

GYNECOMASTIA

Gynecomastia refers to enlargement of the male breast. It is caused by excess estrogen action and is usually the result of an increased estrogen/androgen ratio. True gynecomastia is associated with glandular breast tissue that is >4 cm in diameter and is often tender. Glandular tissue enlargement should be distinguished from excess adipose tissue; glandular tissue is firmer and contains fibrous-like cords. Gynecomastia occurs as a normal physiologic phenomenon in the newborn, during puberty, and with aging, but it can also result from pathologic conditions associated with androgen deficiency or estrogen excess. The prevalence of gynecomastia increases with age and body mass index (BMI), likely because of increased aromatase activity in adipose tissue. Medications that alter androgen metabolism or action may also cause gynecomastia. The relative risk of breast cancer is increased in men with gynecomastia, although the absolute risk is relatively small.

PATHOLOGIC GYNECOMASTIA

Any cause of *androgen deficiency* can lead to gynecomastia, reflecting an increased estrogen/androgen ratio, as estrogen synthesis still occurs by aromatization of residual adrenal and gonadal androgens. Gynecomastia is a characteristic feature of Klinefelter syndrome (Chap. 7). *Androgen insensitivity* disorders also cause gynecomastia. *Excess estrogen production* may be caused by tumors, including Sertoli cell tumors in isolation or in association with Peutz-Jeghers syndrome or Carney complex. Tumors that produce hCG, including some testicular tumors, stimulate Leydig cell estrogen synthesis. *Increased conversion of androgens to estrogens* can be a result of increased availability of substrate (androstenedione) for extraglandular estrogen formation (CAH, hyperthyroidism, and most feminizing adrenal tumors) or to diminished catabolism of androstenedione (liver disease) so that estrogen precursors are shunted to aromatase in peripheral sites. Obesity is associated with increased aromatization of androgen precursors to estrogens. Extraglandular aromatase activity can also be increased in tumors of the liver or adrenal gland or rarely as an inherited disorder. Several families with *increased peripheral aromatase activity* inherited as an autosomal or X-linked disorder have been described. *Drugs* can cause gynecomastia by acting directly as estrogenic substances (e.g., oral contraceptives, phytoestrogens, digitalis), inhibiting androgen synthesis (e.g., ketoconazole), or inhibiting action (e.g., spironolactone).

It is challenging to determine when to evaluate gynecomastia, since up to two-thirds of pubertal boys and half of hospitalized men have palpable glandular tissue (**Fig. 8-5**). In addition to the extent of gynecomastia, recent onset, rapid growth, tender tissue, and occurrence in a lean subject should prompt more extensive evaluation. This should include a careful drug history, measurement and examination of the testes, assessment of virilization, evaluation of liver function, and hormonal measurements including testosterone, estradiol, and androstenedione, LH, and hCG. If testes are small, a karyotype should be obtained to exclude Klinefelter syndrome. Despite this evaluation, the diagnosis is established in fewer than one-half of patients, probably because of subtle alterations of the estrogen/androgen ratio.

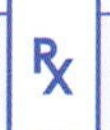

TREATMENT FOR GYNECOMASTIA

When the primary cause can be identified and corrected, breast enlargement usually subsides over several months. However, if gynecomastia is of long duration, surgery is the most effective therapy. Indications for surgery include severe psychological and/or cosmetic problems, continued growth or tenderness, or suspected malignancy. In patients who have painful gynecomastia and who are not candidates for other therapy, treatment with antiestrogens such as tamoxifen (20 mg/d)

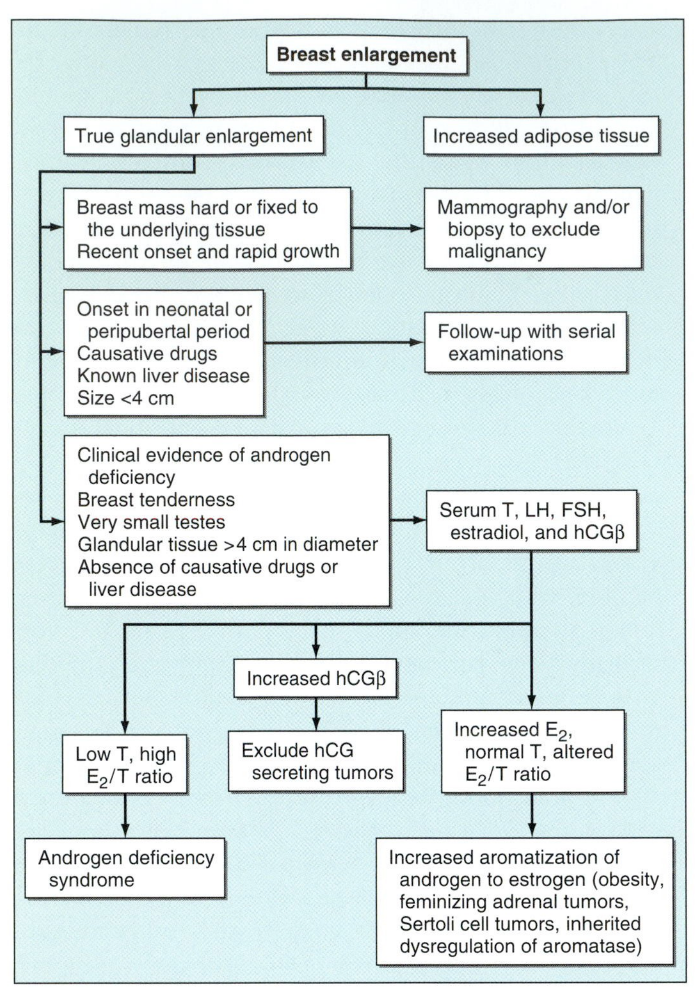

FIGURE 8-5

Evaluation of gynecomastia. E_2, 17β-estradiol; FSH, follicle-stimulating hormone; hCGβ, human chorionic gonadotropin β; LH, luteinizing hormone; T, testosterone.

reduces pain and breast tissue size in about two-thirds of patients. Aromatase inhibitors can be effective in the early proliferative phase of the disorder, although the experience is largely based on the use of testolactone, a relatively weak aromatase inhibitor; placebo-controlled trials with more potent aromatase inhibitors such as anastrozole, fadrozole, letrozole, or formestane are needed.

AGING-RELATED CHANGES IN MALE REPRODUCTIVE FUNCTION

A number of cross-sectional and longitudinal studies (e.g., The Baltimore Longitudinal Study of Aging and the Massachusetts Male Aging Study) have established that testosterone concentrations decrease with advancing age. This age-related decline starts in the third decade of life and progresses slowly; the rate of decline in testosterone concentrations is greater for men with chronic illness and for those taking medications than in healthy older men. Because SHBG concentrations are higher in older men than in younger men, free or bioavailable testosterone concentrations decline with aging to a greater extent than total testosterone concentrations. The age-related decline in testosterone is due to defects at all levels of the hypothalamic-pituitary-testicular axis: pulsatile GnRH secretion is attenuated, LH response to GnRH is reduced, and testicular response to LH is impaired. However, the gradual rise of LH with aging suggests that testis dysfunction is the main cause of declining androgen levels. The term *andropause* has been used to denote age-related decline in testosterone concentrations; this term is a misnomer because there is no discrete time when testosterone concentrations decline abruptly.

It is speculated that age-related decline in testosterone concentrations contributes to sexual dysfunction, loss of muscle mass and function, frailty, gain in fat mass, cognitive impairment, and loss of body hair. Initial studies of testosterone supplementation in older men with low or low normal testosterone levels have demonstrated a modest increase of fat-free mass and grip strength; a decrease in fat mass; an improved sense of well being, energy, visuo-spatial orientation, and verbal memory; and a modest increment in bone mineral density. However, the long-term risks of testosterone supplementation in older men remain largely unknown. In particular, physiologic testosterone replacement might increase the risk of prostate cancer or exacerbate cardiovascular disease. Population screening of all older men for low testosterone levels is not recommended, and testing should be restricted to men who have symptoms or physical features attributable to androgen deficiency. In men with documented androgen deficiency, testosterone replacement may be considered on an individualized basis and should be instituted after careful discussion of the risks and benefits (see "Testosterone Replacement," below).

Testicular morphology, semen production, and fertility are maintained up to a very old age in men. Although concern has been expressed about age-related increases in germ cell mutations and impairment of DNA repair mechanisms, the frequency of chromosomal aneuploidy or structural abnormalities does not increase in the sperm of older men. However, the incidence of autosomal dominant diseases, such as achondroplasia, polyposis coli, Marfan syndrome, and Apert syndrome, increases in the offspring of men who are advanced in age, consistent with transmission of sporadic missense mutations.

APPROACH TO THE PATIENT WITH AGING-RELATED CHANGES

Hypogonadism is often heralded by decreased sex drive, reduced frequency of sexual intercourse or inability to maintain erections, reduced beard growth, loss of muscle mass, decreased testicular size, and gynecomastia. Less than 10% of patients with erectile dysfunction alone have testosterone deficiency. Thus, it is useful to look for a constellation of symptoms and signs suggestive of androgen deficiency. Except when extreme, these clinical features may be difficult to distinguish from changes that occur with normal aging. Moreover, androgen deficiency may develop gradually. Population studies, such as the Massachusetts Male Aging Study, suggest that about 4% of men between the ages of 40 and 70 have testosterone levels <150 ng/dL. Thus, androgen deficiency is not uncommon. The challenges for the clinician are (1) to decide when to evaluate a man for possible androgen deficiency, (2) to assess when there is laboratory evidence for androgen deficiency and determine its cause, and (3) to decide when and how to treat patients with androgen deficiency.

When symptoms or clinical features suggest possible androgen deficiency, the laboratory evaluation is initiated by the measurement of total testosterone, preferably in the morning (**Fig. 8-6**). A total testosterone level <200 ng/dL, in association with symptoms, is evidence of testosterone deficiency. An early-morning testosterone level >350 ng/dL makes the diagnosis of androgen deficiency unlikely. In men with testosterone levels between 200 and 350 ng/dL, the total testosterone level should be repeated and a free testosterone level should be measured. In older men and in patients with other clinical states that are associated with alterations in SHBG levels, a direct measurement of free testosterone level by equilibrium dialysis can be useful in unmasking testosterone deficiency.

When androgen deficiency has been confirmed by low testosterone concentrations, LH should be measured to classify the patient as having hypergonadotropic (high LH) or hypogonadotropic (low or inappropriately normal LH) hypogonadism. An elevated LH level indicates that the defect is at the testicular level. Common causes of primary testicular failure include Klinefelter syndrome, HIV infection, uncorrected cryptorchidism, cancer chemotherapeutic agents, radiation, surgical orchiectomy, or prior infectious orchitis. Unless causes of primary testicular failure are known, a karyotype should be performed in men with low testosterone and elevated LH to exclude Klinefelter syndrome. Men who have a low testosterone but "inappropriately normal" or low LH levels have hypogonadotropic hypogonadism; their defect resides at the hypothalamic-pituitary level. Common causes of acquired hypogonadotropic hypogonadism include space-occupying lesions of the sella, hyperprolactinemia, chronic illness, hemochromatosis, excessive exercise, and substance abuse. Measurement of PRL and MRI scan of the hypothalamic-pituitary region can help exclude the presence of a space-occupying lesion. Patients in whom known causes of hypogonadotropic hypogonadism have been excluded are classified as having IHH. It is not unusual for congenital causes of hypogonadotropic hypogonadism, such as Kallmann syndrome, to be diagnosed in young adults.

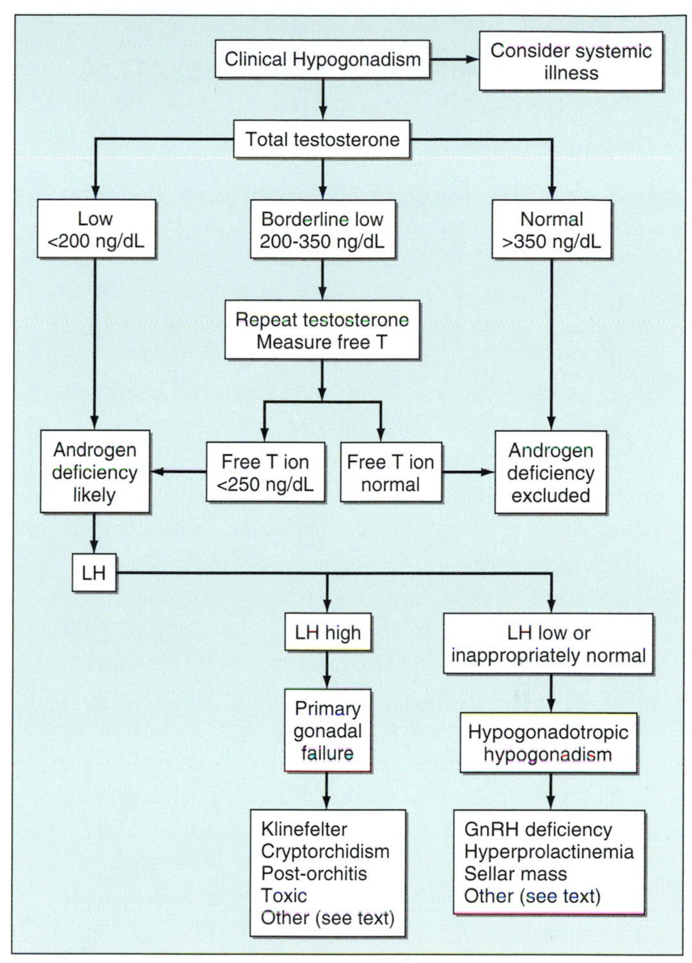

FIGURE 8-6

Evaluation of hypogonadism. GnRH, gonadotropin-releasing hormone; LH, luteinizing hormone; T, testosterone.

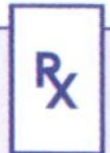

TREATMENT FOR AGING-RELATED CHANGES

Gonadotropins

Gonadotropin therapy is used to establish or restore fertility in patients with gonadotropin deficiency of any cause. Several gonadotropin preparations are available. Human menopausal gonadotropin (hMG) (purified from the urine of postmenopausal women) contains 75 IU FSH and 75 IU LH per vial. hCG (purified from the urine of pregnant women) has little FSH activity and resembles LH in its ability to stimulate testosterone production by Leydig cells. Recombinant hCG is now available. Because of the expense of hMG, treatment is usually begun with hCG alone, and hMG is added later to promote the FSH-dependent stages of spermatid development. Recombinant human FSH (hFSH) is now available and is indistinguishable from purified urinary hFSH in its biologic activity and pharmacokinetics in vitro and in vivo, although the mature β subunit of recombinant hFSH has seven fewer amino acids. Recombinant hFSH is available in ampules containing 75 IU (~7.5 μg FSH), which accounts for >99% of protein content. Once spermatogenesis is restored using combined FSH and LH therapy, hCG alone is often sufficient to maintain spermatogenesis.

Although a variety of treatment regimens are used, 1500 to 2000 IU of hCG administered intramuscularly three times weekly is a reasonable starting dose. Testosterone levels should be measured 6 to 8 weeks later, and 48 to 72 h after the hCG injection; the hCG dose should be adjusted to achieve testosterone levels in the mid-normal range. Sperm counts should be monitored on a monthly basis. It may take several months for spermatogenesis to be restored; therefore, it is important to forewarn patients about the potential length and expense of the treatment and to provide conservative estimates of success rates. If testosterone levels are in the mid-normal range but the sperm concentrations are low after 6 months of therapy with hCG alone, FSH should be added. This can be done by using hMG, highly purified urinary hFSH, or recombinant hFSH. The selection of FSH dose is empirical. A common practice is to start with the addition of 75 IU FSH three times each week in conjunction with the hCG injections. If sperm densities are still low after 3 months of combined treatment, the FSH dose should be increased to 150 IU. Occasionally, it may take ≥18 to 24 months for spermatogenesis to be restored.

The two best predictors of success using gonadotropin therapy in hypogonadotropic men are testicular volume at presentation and time of onset. In general, men with testicular volumes >8 mL have better response rates than those who have testicular volumes <4 mL. Patients who became hypogonadotropic after puberty experience higher success rates than those who have never undergone pubertal changes. Spermatogenesis can usually be reinitiated by hCG alone, with high rates of success for men with postpubertal onset of hypogonadotropism. The presence of a primary testicular abnormality, such as cryptorchidism, will attenuate testicular response to gonadotropin therapy. Prior androgen therapy does not affect subsequent response to gonadotropin therapy.

GnRH

In patients with documented GnRH deficiency, both pubertal development and spermatogenesis can be successfully induced by pulsatile administration of low doses of GnRH. This response requires normal pituitary and testicular function. Therapy usually begins with an initial dose of 25 ng/kg per pulse administered subcutaneously every 2 h by a portable infusion pump. Testosterone, LH, and FSH levels should be monitored. The dose of GnRH is increased until testosterone levels reach the mid-normal range. Doses ranging from 25 to 200 ng/kg may be required to induce virilization. Once pubertal changes have been initiated, the dose of GnRH can often be reduced. Increased sperm counts and testicular volume have been reported in >70% of treated men, and improvements in sexual function and virilization can be induced in >90% of patients. Cutaneous infections occur but are infrequent and minor. Carrying a portable infusion device can be cumbersome, and follow-up of these patients requires physician supervision and laboratory monitoring. Some patients with IHH have cryptorchidism; men with this additional testicular defect may not respond to GnRH or gonadotropin therapy.

Comparative studies of gonadotropin therapy and pulsatile GnRH administration demonstrate that these two therapies are similar in terms of the time to first appearance of sperm or pregnancy rates; both approaches are equally effective in inducing spermatogenesis in men with hypogonadotropic hypogonadism caused by GnRH deficiency. However, most patients find intermittent gonadotropin injections preferable to wearing a continuous infusion pump.

Testosterone Replacement

Androgen therapy is indicated to restore testosterone levels to normal to correct features of androgen deficiency. Testosterone replacement improves libido and overall sexual activity; increases energy, lean muscle mass, and bone density; and provides the patient a better sense of well-being. The benefits of testosterone replacement therapy have been proven only in men who have documented androgen deficiency, as demonstrated by testosterone levels that are well below the lower limit of normal (<250 ng/dL).

Testosterone is available in a variety of formulations with distinct pharmacokinetics (**Table 8-3**). Testosterone serves as a prohormone and is converted to 17β-estradiol by aromatase and to 5α-dihydrotestosterone by 5α-reductase. Therefore, when evaluating testosterone formulations, it is important to consider whether the formulation being used can achieve physiologic estradiol and DHT concentrations, in addition to normal testosterone concentrations. Although testosterone concentrations at the lower end of the normal male range can restore sexual function, it is not clear whether low-normal testosterone levels can maintain bone mineral density and muscle mass. The current recommendation is to restore testosterone levels to the mid-normal range.

ORAL DERIVATIVES OF TESTOSTERONE

Testosterone is well absorbed after oral administration but quickly degrades during the first pass through the liver. Therefore, it is not possible to achieve sustained blood levels of testosterone after oral administration of crystalline testosterone. 17α-alkylated derivatives of testosterone (e.g., 17α-methyl testosterone, oxandrolone, fluoxymesterone) are relatively resistant to hepatic degradation and can be administered orally; however, because of the potential for hepatotoxicity, including cholestatic jaundice, peliosis, and hepatoma, these formulations should not be used for testosterone replacement. Hereditary angioedema due to C1 esterase deficiency is the only exception to this general recommendation; in this condition, oral 17α-alkylated androgens are useful because they stimulate hepatic synthesis of the C1 esterase inhibitor.

INJECTABLE FORMS OF TESTOSTERONE

The esterification of testosterone at the 17β-hydroxy position makes the molecule hydrophobic and extends its duration of action. The slow release of testosterone ester from an oily depot in the muscle accounts for its extended duration of action. The longer the side chain, the greater the hydrophobicity of the ester and longer the duration of action. Thus, testosterone enanthate and cypionate with longer side chains have longer duration of action than testosterone propionate. Within 24 h after intramuscular administration of 200 mg testosterone enanthate or cypionate, testosterone levels rise into the high-normal or supraphysiologic range and then gradually decline into the hypogonadal range over the next 2 weeks. A bimonthly regimen of testosterone enanthate or cypionate therefore results in peaks and troughs in testosterone levels that are accompanied by changes in a patient's mood, sexual desire, and energy level. The kinetics of testosterone enanthate and cypionate are similar. Estradiol and DHT levels are normal if testosterone replacement is physiologic.

TRANSDERMAL TESTOSTERONE

Three transdermal testosterone patches are commercially available: a scrotal testosterone patch (Testoderm) and two nongenital patches (Androderm and Testoderm TTS). The scrotal transdermal testosterone patch, when applied daily to the scrotal skin, produces mid-normal testosterone levels in hypogonadal men 4 to 8 h after application followed by a gradual decrease in testosterone levels over the next 24 h. Estradiol levels are normal but DHT levels are increased due to the conversion of testosterone to DHT by the high amounts of 5α-reductase in scrotal skin. There was initial concern that exposure to high DHT levels might have deleterious effects on the prostate; however, long-term follow-up of men treated with the scrotal patch has not revealed an unexpected increase in prostate problems.

With nongenital testosterone patches, testosterone, DHT, and estradiol levels are in the mid-normal range 4 to 12 h after application. Sexual function and a sense of well-being are restored in androgen-deficient men treated with the nongenital patch. One 5-mg patch may not be sufficient to increase testosterone into the mid-normal male range in all hypogonadal men; some patients may need daily administration of two 5-mg patches to achieve

TABLE 8-3

CLINICAL PHARMACOLOGY OF TESTOSTERONE FORMULATIONS

FORMULATION	REGIMEN	PHARMACOKINETICS	DHT AND ESTRADIOL	ADVANTAGES	DISADVANTAGES
Testosterone enanthate or cypionate	100 mg IM weekly or 200 mg IM every 2 weeks	After a single IM injection, testosterone levels rise into the supraphysiologic range and then decline gradually into the hypogonadal range by the end of the dosing interval	DHT and estradiol levels rise in proportion to the increase in testosterone levels; T:DHT and T:EF_2 ratios do not change	Corrects symptoms of androgen deficiency Relatively inexpensive, if self-administered. Flexibility of dosing	Requires IM injection. Peaks and valleys in testosterone levels
Scrotal testosterone patch	One scrotal patch designed to deliver 6 mg over 24 h applied daily	Normalizes testosterone levels in many but not all androgen-deficient men	Estradiol levels are in the physiologic male range, but DHT levels rise into the supraphysiologic range	Corrects symptoms of androgen deficiency	To promote optimum adherence of the patch, scrotal skin needs to be shaved High DHT levels
Nongenital transdermal system	One or two patches, designed to deliver 5–10 mg testosterone over 24 h applied daily on nonpressure areas	Restores testosterone, DHT, and estradiol levels into the physiologic male range	T:DHT and T:estradiol levels are in the physiologic male range	Ease of application, corrects symptoms of androgen deficiency, and mimics the normal diurnal rhythm of testosterone secretion. Lesser increase in hemoglobin than injectable esters	Testosterone levels in some androgen-deficient men may be in the low-normal range; these men may need application of two patches daily Skin irritation at the application site in some patients
Testosterone gel	Testosterone gel containing 50 to 100 mg testosterone should be applied daily	Restores testosterone and estradiol levels into the physiologic male range	DHT levels and T:DHT ratios are lower in hypogonadal men treated with the testosterone gel than in healthy eugonadal men	Corrects symptoms of androgen deficiency, provides flexibility of dosing, ease of applications, good skin tolerability	Potential of transfer to a female partner or child by direct skin-to-skin contact; moderately high DHT levels
17 α-methy1 testosterone	Orally active, 17α-alkylated compound that should not be used because of potential for liver toxicity	Orally active			Clinical responses variable; potential for liver toxicity; should not be used for treatment of androgen deficiency
Buccal adhesive tetosterone	An adhesive, 10-mg tablet applied to buccal mucosa twice daily	Absorbed through buccal mucosa	Serum T and DHT in the normal male range	Ease of application	Limited experience no evidence of liver toxicity, effects of food and brushing unclear

Note: DHT, dihydrotestosterone; T, testosterone, E_2, 17β-estradiol.
Source: Adapted from: American College of Physicians/American Society of Internal Medicine Disease Management Module on Male Hypogonadism.

the targeted testosterone concentrations. The transdermal systems are more expensive than testosterone esters. The use of nongenital patches may be associated with skin irritation in some individuals.

TESTOSTERONE GEL

Two testosterone gels (Androgel and Testim) are available in 2.5- and 5-g unit doses that nominally deliver 25 and 50 mg of testosterone to the application site. Initial pharmacokinetic studies have demonstrated that 50-, 75-, and 100-mg doses applied daily to the skin can maintain total and free testosterone concentrations in the mid- to high-normal range in hypogonadal men. Total and free testosterone concentrations are uniform throughout the 24-h period. The current recommendations are to begin with a 50-mg dose and adjust the dose based on testosterone levels. The advantages of the testosterone gel are in its ease of application, its invisibility after application, and its flexibility of dosing. A major concern is the potential for inadvertent transfer of the gel to a sexual partner or to children who may come in close contact with the patient. The ratio of DHT to testosterone concentrations is higher in men treated with the testosterone gel.

A buccal adhesive testosterone tablet, which adheres to the buccal mucosa and releases testosterone as it is slowly dissolved, has been approved. After twice daily application of 10 to 20 mg tablets, serum testosterone levels are maintained within the normal male range in a majority of treated hypogonadal men. The adverse effects include buccal ulceration in a few subjects. The clinical experience with this formulation is limited, and the effects of food and brushing on absorption have not been studied in detail.

TESTOSTERONE FORMULATIONS NOT AVAILABLE IN THE UNITED STATES

Testosterone undecanoate, when administered orally in oleic acid, is absorbed preferentially through the lymphatics into the systemic circulation and is spared the first-pass degradation in the liver. Doses of 40 to 80 mg orally, two or three times daily, are typically used. However, the clinical responses are variable and suboptimal. DHT-to-testosterone ratios are higher in hypogonadal men treated with oral testosterone undecanoate, as compared with eugonadal men.

Implants of crystalline testosterone can be inserted in the subcutaneous tissue by means of a trocar through a small skin incision. Testosterone is released by surface erosion of the implant and absorbed into the systemic circulation. Four to six 200-mg implants can maintain testosterone in the mid- to high-normal range for up to 6 months. Potential drawbacks include incising the skin for insertion and removal, and spontaneous extrusions and fibrosis at the site of the implant.

NOVEL ANDROGEN FORMULATIONS

A number of androgen formulations with better pharmacokinetics or more selective activity profiles are under development. A biodegradable testosterone microsphere formulation provides physiologic testosterone levels for 10 to 11 weeks. Two long-acting esters, testosterone buciclate and testosterone undecanoate, when injected intramuscularly, can maintain circulating testosterone concentrations in the male range for 7 to 12 weeks. Initial clinical trials have demonstrated the feasibility of administering testosterone by the sublingual or buccal routes. 7α-methyl-19-nortestosterone is an androgen that cannot be 5α-reduced; therefore, compared to testosterone, it has relatively greater agonist activity in muscle and gonadotropin suppression but lesser activity on the prostate.

Analogous to the selective estrogen receptor modulators, such as raloxifene, it may be possible to develop selective androgen receptor modulators (SARMs) that exert the desired physiologic effects on muscle, bone, or sexual function but without adversely affecting the prostate and the cardiovascular system.

PHARMACOLOGIC USES OF ANDROGENS

In addition to hypogonadism, androgens have been used to treat a variety of disorders with the hope that anabolic actions of the agents (e.g., increase in nitrogen retention and muscle mass, increased hemoglobin) would outweigh any deleterious (e.g., virilization) actions of the drugs. The most common nonreplacement uses of androgen have been attempts to improve nitrogen balance in catabolic states (e.g., AIDS), self-administration by athletes to increase muscle mass and/or athletic performance, attempts to enhance erythropoiesis in refractory anemias (including the anemia of renal failure), treatment of hereditary angioedema and endometriosis, and management of growth retardation of various etiologies. Most of the expected benefits in these disorders have not been realized. The modest pharmacologic doses of androgens have little physiologic effect in men when superimposed on normal testicular androgen; in women, the virilizing side effects of androgens are formidable.

The most pervasive form of androgen abuse is by male athletes with the expectation that it will improve muscle development and athletic performance. In controlled studies using modest pharmacologic doses (two to four times the usual replacement doses), these agents do not consistently improve performance. However, at the doses frequently taken by athletes (which sometimes exceed 10 times the replacement dose), androgens enhance nitrogen balance and muscle mass; since the drugs have multiple side effects at high doses, these benefits do not outweigh the risks associated with androgen abuse in men, while androgen use by female athletes is associated with disfiguring virilization. The only established indications for androgen therapy aside from male hypogonadism are in selected patients with anemia due to bone marrow failure (an indication largely supplanted by erythropoietin) or for hereditary angioedema.

RECOMMENDED REGIMENS FOR ANDROGEN REPLACEMENT

Testosterone esters are administered weekly at doses of 75 to 100 mg intramuscularly, or 150 to 200 mg every 2 weeks. One 6-mg scrotal patch should be applied daily after shaving the scrotal skin. One or two 5-mg nongenital testosterone patches can be applied daily over the skin of the back, thigh, or upper arm away from pressure areas. Testosterone gel is typically applied over a covered area of skin at a dose of 50 to 100 mg daily; patients should wash their hands after gel application.

ESTABLISHING EFFICACY OF TESTOSTERONE REPLACEMENT THERAPY

Because a clinically useful marker of androgen action is not available, restoration of testosterone levels into the mid-normal range remains the goal of therapy. Measurements of LH and FSH are not useful in assessing the adequacy of testosterone replacement. Testosterone should be measured 3 months after initiating therapy to assess adequacy of therapy. In patients who are treated with testosterone enanthate or cypionate, testosterone levels should be 350 to 600 ng/dL 1 week after the injection. If testosterone levels are outside this range, adjustments should be made to either the dose or the interval between injections. In men on transdermal patch or gel therapy, testosterone levels should be in the mid-normal range (500 to 800 ng/dL) 4 to 12 h after application. If testosterone levels are outside this range, the dose should be adjusted.

Restoration of sexual function, secondary sex characteristics, and energy level and one's sense of well-being are important objectives of testosterone replacement therapy. The patient should also be asked about sexual desire and activity, the presence of early morning erections, and whether he is able to achieve and maintain erections that are adequate for sexual intercourse. Some hypogonadal men continue to complain about sexual dysfunction even after testosterone replacement has been instituted; these patients may benefit from counseling. The hair growth in response to androgen replacement is variable and depends on ethnicity. Hypogonadal men with prepubertal onset of androgen deficiency who begin testosterone therapy in their late 20s or 30s may find it difficult to adjust to their newly found sexuality and may benefit from counseling. If the patient has a sexual partner, the partner should be included in counseling because of the dramatic physical and sexual changes that occur with androgen treatment.

CONTRAINDICATIONS FOR ANDROGEN ADMINISTRATION

Testosterone administration is contraindicated in men with a history of prostate cancer because androgens can promote tumor growth (**Table 8-4**). Testosterone should not be prescribed to men with severe symptoms of benign prostatic hypertrophy (AUA symptom score > 22), because even small increases in prostate volume may exacerbate obstructive symptoms. Testosterone replacement should not be administered to men with baseline hematocrit ≥52%. Testosterone can induce and exacerbate sleep apnea because of its neuromuscular effects on the upper airway.

MONITORING POTENTIAL ADVERSE EXPERIENCES

The clinical effectiveness and safety of testosterone replacement therapy should be evaluated 3 and 6 months after initiating testosterone therapy and annually thereafter.

Hemoglobin Levels Administration of testosterone to androgen-deficient men is typically associated with a 3 to 5% increase in hemoglobin levels. Clinically significant erythrocytosis is uncommon in young hypogonadal men but can occur in men who have sleep apnea, a significant smoking history, or chronic obstructive lung disease, or those who are older in age. The magnitude of hemoglobin increase during testosterone therapy appears related to the peak testosterone levels. Transdermal testosterone replacement may produce a smaller hemoglobin increase than testosterone esters.

Digital Examination of the Prostate and Serum PSA Levels Testosterone replacement therapy increases prostate volume to the size seen in age-matched controls but should not increase prostate volume beyond that expected for age. There is no evidence that testosterone replacement causes prostate cancer. However, androgen administration can exacerbate preexisting prostate cancer.

TABLE 8-4

CONTRAINDICATIONS FOR ANDROGEN REPLACEMENT

- The presence or history of prostate cancer
- Baseline PSA ≥4 ng/mL, or a palpable abnormality of the prostate without urologic evaluation to rule out prostate cancer
- Severe symptoms of lower urinary tract obstruction as indicated by IPSS or AUA symptom score of ≥22
- Baseline hematocrit >52%
- Severe sleep apnea
- Class IV congestive heart failure

Note: PSA, prostate-specific antigen, IPSS, International Prostate Symptom Score; AUA, American Urological Association.

Many older men harbor microscopic foci of cancer in their prostates. It is not known whether long-term testosterone administration will induce these microscopic foci to grow into clinically significant cancers.

Prostate-specific antigen (PSA) levels are lower in testosterone-deficient men and are restored to normal after testosterone replacement. There is considerable test-retest variability in PSA measurements; the average interassay coefficient of variation of PSA assays is 15%. The 95% confidence interval for the change in PSA values, measured 3 to 6 months apart, is 1.4 ng/mL. Increments in PSA levels after testosterone supplementation in androgen-deficient men are generally <0.5 ng/mL, and increments >1.0 ng/mL over a 3- to 6-month period are unusual. Nevertheless, administration of testosterone to men with baseline PSA levels between 2.5 and 4.0 ng/mL will cause PSA levels to exceed 4.0 ng/mL for some, and many of these men may undergo prostate biopsies. PSA velocity criteria can be used for patients who have sequential PSA measurements for >2 years; a change of >0.40 ng/mL per year merits closer urologic follow-up.

Cardiovascular Risk Assessment The long-term effects of testosterone supplementation on cardiovascular risk are unknown. Testosterone effects on lipids depend on the dose (physiologic or supraphysiologic), the route of administration (oral or parenteral), and the formulation (whether aromatizable or not). Physiologic testosterone replacement by an aromatizable androgen has a modest effect on high-density lipoprotein (HDL) or no effect at all. In middle-aged men with low testosterone levels, physiologic testosterone replacement has been shown to improve insulin sensitivity and reduce visceral obesity. In epidemiologic studies, testosterone concentrations are inversely related to waist-to-hip ratio and directly correlated with HDL cholesterol levels. These data suggest that physiologic testosterone concentrations are correlated with factors associated with reduced cardiovascular risk. However, no prospective studies have examined the effect of testosterone replacement on cardiovascular risk.

MALE SEXUAL DYSFUNCTION See Chap. 14.

MALE INFERTILITY See Chap. 15.

ACKNOWLEDGMENT

We are grateful to James E. Griffin and Jean D. Wilson, authors of Disorders of the Testes in the 15th edition of *Harrison's,* for contributions to this chapter.

FURTHER READINGS

De Martino MU et al: Dynamic testing in the evaluation of male gonadal function. J Endocrinol Invest 26:107, 2003

Because the pituitary is sensitive to GnRH priming and desensitization, testing the function of the hypothalamic-pituitary-gonadal axis can be challenging. This paper illustrates the normal and pathologic responses associated with GnRH and hCG stimulation tests.

Feldman HA et al: Age trends in the level of serum testosterone and other hormones in middle-aged men: Longitudinal results from the Massachusetts male aging study. J Clin Endocrinol Metab 87:589, 2002

Results from this longitudinal study of 1709 men suggest that chronic illness accelerates the age-related decline of testosterone levels.

Harman SM et al: Longitudinal effects of aging on serum total and free testosterone levels in healthy men. Baltimore Longitudinal Study of Aging. J Clin Endocrinol Metab 86:724, 2001

IOVANE A et al: New insights in the genetics of isolated hypogonadotropic hypogonadism. Eur J Endocrinol 151(Suppl 3):U83, 2004

A number of new genetic causes of hypogonadotropic hypogonadism, including mutations in the KAL1, FGFR1, and GPR54 genes, are reviewed.

LIU PY et al: Androgens and cardiovascular disease. Endocr Rev 24:313, 2003

RHODEN EL et al: Risks of testosterone-replacement therapy and recommendations for monitoring. N Engl J Med 350:482, 2004

A comprehensive review of indications and potential complications associated with testosterone replacement therapy.

SEDLMEYER IL, PALMERT MR: Delayed puberty: Analysis of a large case series from an academic center. J Clin Endocrinol Metab 87:1613, 2002

VALDES-SOCIN H et al: Hypogonadism in a patient with a mutation in the luteinizing hormone β-subunit gene. N Engl J Med 351:2619, 2004

SHOZU M et al: Estrogen excess associated with novel gain-of-function mutations affecting the aromatase gene. N Engl J Med 348:19, 2003

Aromatase converts androgens to estrogens. This report describes a novel mechanism for aromatase excess and gynecomastia.

WICKMAN S: A specific aromatase inhibitor and potential increase in adult height in boys with delayed puberty: A randomised controlled trial. Lancet 357:1743, 2001

This study shows that an aromatase inhibitor, letrozole, increases predicted height in boys with delayed puberty. These findings are consistent with the important role that estrogen plays in the closure of epiphyseal growth plates.

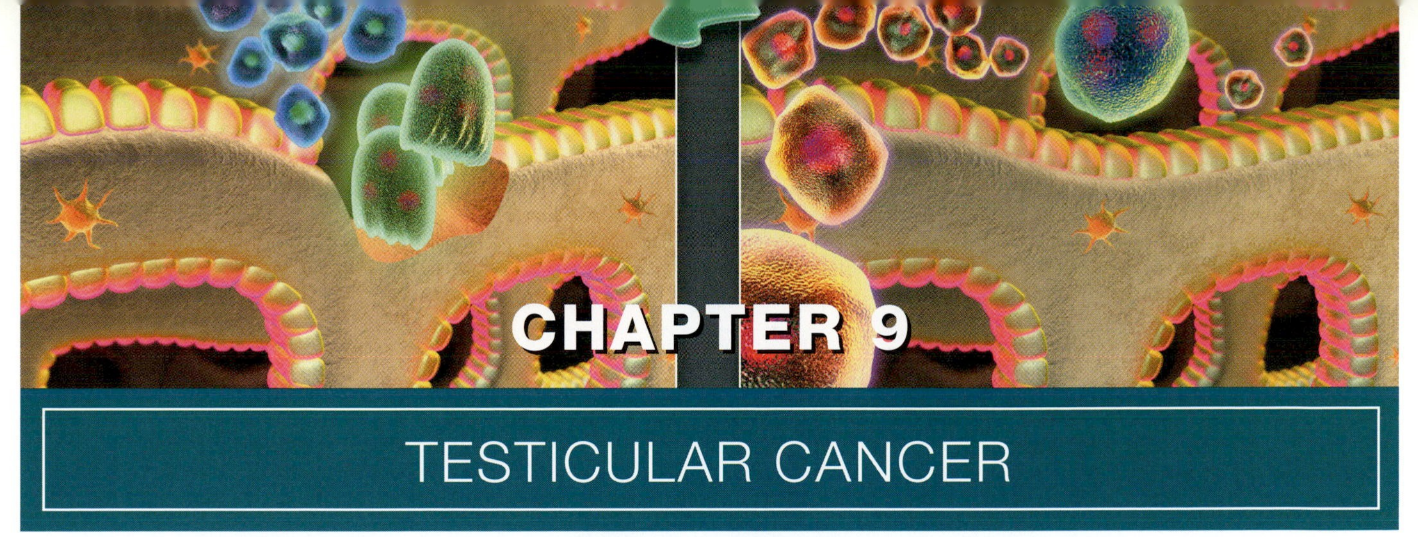

TESTICULAR CANCER

Robert J. Motzer
George J. Bosl

Primary germ cell tumors (GCTs) of the testis, arising by the malignant transformation of primordial germ cells, constitute 95% of all testicular neoplasms. Infrequently, GCTs arise from an extragonadal site, including the mediastinum, retroperitoneum, and, very rarely, the pineal gland. This disease is notable for the young age of the afflicted patients, the totipotent capacity for differentiation of the tumor cells, and its curability; about 95% of all newly diagnosed patients will be cured. Experience in the management of GCTs leads to improved outcome.

INCIDENCE AND EPIDEMIOLOGY

Nearly 9000 new cases of testicular GCT were diagnosed in the United States in 2004; the incidence of this malignancy has increased slowly over the past 40 years. The tumor occurs most frequently in men between the ages of 20 and 40. A testicular mass in a man ≥50 years should be regarded as a lymphoma until proved otherwise. GCT is at least four to five times more common in white than in African-American males, and a higher incidence has been observed in Scandinavia and New Zealand than in the United States.

ETIOLOGY AND GENETICS

Cryptorchidism is associated with a severalfold higher risk of GCT. Abdominal cryptorchid testes are at a higher risk than inguinal cryptorchid testes. Orchiopexy should be performed before puberty, if possible. Early orchiopexy reduces the risk of GCT and improves the ability to save the testis. An abdominal cryptorchid testis that cannot be brought into the scrotum should be removed. About 2% of men with GCTs of one testis will develop a primary tumor in the other testis. Testicular feminization syndromes increase the risk of testicular GCT, and Klinefelter syndrome is associated with mediastinal GCT.

An isochromosome of the short arm of chromosome 12 [i(12p)] is pathognomonic for GCT of all histologic types. Excess 12p copy number either in the form of i(12p) or as increased 12p on aberrantly banded marker chromosomes occurs in nearly all GCTs, but the gene(s) on 12p involved in the pathogenesis are not yet defined.

CLINICAL PRESENTATION

A painless testicular mass is pathognomonic for a testicular malignancy. More commonly, patients present with testicular discomfort or swelling suggestive of epididymitis and/or orchitis. In this circumstance, a trial of antibiotics is reasonable. However, if symptoms persist or a residual abnormality remains, then testicular ultrasound examination is indicated.

Ultrasound of the testis is indicated whenever a testicular malignancy is considered and for persistent or painful testicular swelling. If a testicular mass is detected, a radical inguinal orchiectomy should be performed. Because the testis develops from the gonadal ridge, its blood supply and lymphatic drainage originate in the abdomen and descend with the testis into the scrotum. An inguinal approach is taken to avoid breaching anatomical barriers and permitting additional pathways of spread.

Back pain from retroperitoneal metastases is common and must be distinguished from musculoskeletal pain. Dyspnea from pulmonary metastases occurs infrequently. Patients with increased serum levels of human chorionic gonadotropin (hCG) may present with

TABLE 9-1

GERM CELL TUMOR STAGING AND TREATMENT

		TREATMENT	
STAGE	EXTENT OF DISEASE	SEMINOMA	NONSEMINOMA
IA	Testis only, no vascular/ lymphatic invasion (T1)	Radiation therapy	RPLND or observation
IB	Testis only, with vascular/ lymphatic invasion (T2), or extension through tunica albuginea (T2), or involvement of spermatic cord (T3) of scrotum (T4)	Radiation therapy	RPLND
IIA	Nodes <2 cm	Radiation therapy	RPLND or chemotherapy often followed by RPLND
IIB	Nodes 2–5 cm	Radiation therapy	RPLND +/− adjuvant chemotherapy or chemotherapy followed by RPLND
IIC	Nodes >5 cm	Chemotherapy	Chemotherapy, often followed by RPLND
III	Distant metastases	Chemotherapy	Chemotherapy, often followed by surgery (biopsy or resection)

Note: RPLND, retroperitoneal lymph node dissection.

gynecomastia. A delay in diagnosis is associated with a more advanced stage and possibly worse survival.

The staging evaluation for GCT includes a determination of serum levels of α fetoprotein (AFP), hCG, and lactate dehydrogenase (LDH). After orchiectomy, a chest radiograph and a computed tomography (CT) scan of the abdomen and pelvis should be performed. A chest CT scan is required if pulmonary nodules or mediastinal or hilar disease is suspected. Stage I disease is limited to the testis, epididymis, or spermatic cord. Stage II disease is limited to retroperitoneal (regional) lymph nodes. Stage III disease is disease outside the retroperitoneum, involving supradiaphragmatic nodal sites or viscera. The staging may be "clinical"—defined solely by physical examination, blood marker evaluation, and radiographs—or "pathologic"—defined by an operative procedure.

The regional draining lymph nodes for the testis are in the retroperitoneum, and the vascular supply originates from the great vessels (for the right testis) or the renal vessels (for the left testis). As a result, the lymph nodes that are involved first by a right testicular tumor are the interaortocaval lymph nodes just below the renal vessels. For a left testicular tumor, the first involved lymph nodes are lateral to the aorta (para-aortic) and below the left renal vessels. In both cases, further nodal spread is inferior and contralateral and, less commonly, above the renal hilum. Lymphatic involvement can extend cephalad to the retrocrural, posterior mediastinal, and supraclavicular lymph nodes. Treatment is determined by tumor histology (seminoma versus nonseminoma) and clinical stage (**Table 9-1**).

PATHOLOGY

GCTs are divided into nonseminoma and seminoma subtypes. Nonseminomatous GCTs are most frequent in the third decade of life and can display the full spectrum of embryonic and adult cellular differentiation. This entity comprises four histologies: embryonal carcinoma, teratoma, choriocarcinoma, and endodermal sinus (yolk sac) tumor. Choriocarcinoma, consisting of both cytotrophoblasts and syncytiophoblasts, represents malignant trophoblastic differentiation and is invariably associated with secretion of hCG. Endodermal sinus tumor is the malignant counterpart of the fetal yolk sac and is associated with secretion of AFP. Pure embryonal carcinoma may secrete AFP or hCG, or both; this pattern is biochemical evidence of differentiation.

Teratoma is composed of somatic cell types derived from two or more germ layers (ectoderm, mesoderm, or endoderm). Each of these histologies may be present alone or in combination with others. Nonseminomatous GCTs tend to metastasize early to sites such as the retroperitoneal lymph nodes and lung parenchyma. One-third of patients present with disease limited to the testis (stage I), one-third with retroperitoneal metastases (stage II), and one-third with more extensive supradiaphragmatic nodal or visceral metastases (stage III).

Seminoma represents about 50% of all GCTs, has a median age in the fourth decade, and generally follows a more indolent clinical course. Most patients (70%) present with stage I disease, about 20% with stage II disease, and 10% with stage III disease; lung or other visceral metastases are rare. Radiation therapy is the treatment of choice in patients with stage I disease and stage II disease where the nodes are <5 cm in maximum diameter. When a tumor contains both seminoma and nonseminoma components, patient management is directed by the more aggressive nonseminoma component.

TUMOR MARKERS

Careful monitoring of the serum tumor markers AFP and hCG is essential in the management of patients with GCT, as these markers are important for diagnosis, as prognostic indicators, in monitoring treatment response, and in the detection of early relapse. Approximately 70% of patients presenting with disseminated nonseminomatous GCT have increased serum concentrations of AFP and/or hCG. While hCG concentrations may be increased in patients with either nonseminoma or seminoma histology, the AFP concentration is increased only in patients with nonseminoma. The presence of an increased AFP level in a patient whose tumor showed only seminoma indicates that an occult nonseminomatous component exists and the patient should be treated for nonseminomatous GCT. LDH levels are not as specific as AFP or hCG, but are increased in 50 to 60% patients with metastatic nonseminoma and in up to 80% of patients with advanced seminoma.

AFP, hCG, and LDH levels should be determined before and after orchiectomy. Increased serum AFP and hCG concentrations decay according to first-order kinetics; the half-life is 24 to 36 h for hCG and 5 to 7 days for AFP. AFP and hCG should be assayed serially during and after treatment. The reappearance of hCG and/or AFP or the failure of these markers to decline according to the predicted half-life is an indicator of persistent or recurrent tumor.

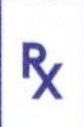

TREATMENT FOR TESTICULAR CANCER

STAGE I NONSEMINOMA

If, after an orchiectomy (for clinical stage I disease), radiographs and physical examination show no evidence of disease, and serum AFP and hCG concentrations are either normal or declining to normal according to the known half-life, patients may be managed by either a nerve-sparing retroperitoneal lymph node dissection (RPLND) or surveillance. The retroperitoneal lymph nodes are involved by GCT (pathologic stage II) in 20 to 50% of these patients. The choice of surveillance or RPLND is based on the pathology of the primary tumor. If the primary tumor shows no evidence for lymphatic or vascular invasion and is limited to the testis (T1), then either option is reasonable. If lymphatic or vascular invasion is present or the tumor extends into the tunica, spermatic cord, or scrotum (T2 through T4), then surveillance should not be offered. Either approach should cure >95% of patients.

A RPLND is the standard operation for removal of the regional lymph nodes of the testis (retroperitoneal nodes). The operation removes the lymph nodes ipsilateral to the primary site and the nodal groups adjacent to the primary landing zone. The standard (modified bilateral) RPLND removes all node-bearing tissue down to the bifurcation of the great vessels, including the ipsilateral iliac nodes. The major long-term effect of this operation is retrograde ejaculation and infertility. A nerve-sparing RPLND, usually accomplished by identification and dissection of individual nerve fibers, may avoid injury to the sympathetic nerves responsible for ejaculation. Normal ejaculation is preserved in ~90% of patients. Patients with pathologic stage I disease are observed, and only the <10% who relapse require additional therapy. If retroperitoneal nodes are found to be involved at RPLND, then a decision regarding adjuvant chemotherapy is made on the basis of the extent of retroperitoneal disease (see below).

Surveillance is an option in the management of clinical stage I disease when no vascular/lymphatic invasion is found (T1). Only 20 to 30% of patients have pathologic stage II disease, implying that most RPLNDs in this situation are not therapeutic. Although surveillance has not been compared to RPLND in a randomized trial, all large studies show that surveillance and RPLND lead to equivalent long-term survival rates. Patient compliance is essential if surveillance is to be successful. Patients must be carefully followed with periodic chest radiography, physical examination, CT scan of the abdomen, and serum tumor marker determinations. The median time to relapse is about 7 months, and late relapses (>2 years) are rare. The 70 to 80% of patients who do not relapse require no intervention after orchiectomy; treatment is reserved for those who do relapse. When the primary tumor is classified as T2 through T4 (extension beyond testis and epididymis or lymphatic/vascular invasion is identified), nerve-sparing RPLND is preferred. About 50% of these patients have pathologic stage II disease and are destined to relapse without the RPLND.

STAGE II NONSEMINOMA

Patients with limited, ipsilateral retroperitoneal adenopathy (nodes usually ≤3 cm in largest diameter) and normal levels of AFP and hCG generally undergo a modified bilateral RPLND as primary management. Increased levels of either AFP or hCG or both imply metastatic disease outside the retroperitoneum; chemotherapy is used in this setting. The local recurrence rate after a properly performed RPLND is very low. Depending on the extent of disease, the postoperative management options include either surveillance or two cycles of adjuvant chemotherapy. Surveillance is the preferred approach for patients with resected "low-volume" metastases (tumor nodes ≤2 cm in diameter *and* <6 nodes involved) because the probability of relapse is one-third or less. For those who relapse, risk-directed chemotherapy is indicated (see below). Because relapse occurs in ≥50% of patients with "high-volume" metastases (>6 nodes involved, *or* any involved node >2 cm in largest diameter, *or* extranodal tumor extension), two cycles of adjuvant chemotherapy should be considered, as it results in cure in ≥98% of patients. Regimens consisting of etoposide (100 mg/m^2 daily on days 1 through 5) plus cisplatin (20 mg/m^2 daily on days 1 through 5) with or without bleomycin (30 U per day on days 2, 9, and 16) given at 3-week intervals are effective and well tolerated.

STAGES I AND II SEMINOMA

Inguinal orchiectomy followed by retroperitoneal radiation therapy cures ~98% of patients with stage I seminoma. The dose of radiation therapy (2500 to 3000 cGy) is low and well tolerated, and the in-field recurrence rate is negligible. About 2% of patients relapse with supradiaphragmatic or systemic disease. Surveillance has been proposed as an option, and studies have shown that about 15% of patients relapse. The median time to relapse is 12 to 15 months, and late relapses (>5 years) may be more frequent than with nonseminoma. The relapse is usually treated with chemotherapy. Surveillance for clinical stage I seminoma is generally not recommended.

Nonbulky retroperitoneal disease (stage IIA and IIB) is also treated with radiation therapy. Prophylactic supradiaphragmatic fields are not used. Relapses in the anterior mediastinum are unusual. Approximately 90% of patients achieve relapse-free survival with retroperitoneal masses <5 cm in diameter. Because at least one-third of patients with bulkier disease relapse, initial chemotherapy is preferred for stage IIC disease.

CHEMOTHERAPY FOR ADVANCED GCT

Regardless of histology, patients with stage IIC and stage III GCT are treated with chemotherapy. Combination chemotherapy programs based on cisplatin at doses of 100 mg/m^2 plus etoposide at doses of 500 mg/m^2 per cycle cure 70 to 80% of such patients, with or without bleomycin, depending on risk stratification (see below). A complete response (the complete disappearance of all clinical evidence of tumor on physical examination and radiography plus normal serum levels of AFP and hCG for ≥1 month) occurs after chemotherapy alone in ~60% of patients, and another 10 to 20% become disease-free with surgical resection of residual masses containing viable GCT. Lower doses of cisplatin result in inferior survival rates.

The toxicity of four cycles of the cisplatin/bleomycin/etoposide (BEP) regimen is substantial. Nausea, vomiting, and hair loss occur in most patients, although nausea and vomiting have been markedly ameliorated by modern antiemetic regimens. Myelosuppression is frequent, and symptomatic bleomycin pulmonary toxicity occurs in ~5% of patients. Treatment-induced mortality due to neutropenia with septicemia or bleomycin-induced pulmonary failure occurs in 1 to 3% of patients. Dose reductions for myelosuppression are rarely indicated. Long-term permanent toxicities include nephrotoxicity (reduced glomerular filtration and persistent magnesium wasting), ototoxicity, and peripheral neuropathy. When bleomycin is administered by weekly bolus injection, Raynaud's phenomenon appears in 5 to 10% of patients. Other evidence of small blood vessel damage is seen less often, including transient ischemic attacks and myocardial infarction.

RISK-DIRECTED CHEMOTHERAPY

Because not all patients are cured and treatment may cause significant toxicities, patients are stratified into "good-risk" and "poor-risk" groups according to pretreatment clinical features. For good-risk patients, the goal is to achieve maximum efficacy with minimal toxicity. For poor-risk patients, the goal is to identify more effective therapy with tolerable toxicity.

The International Germ Cell Cancer Consensus Group (IGCCCG) developed criteria to assign patients to three risk groups (good, intermediate, poor) (**Table 9-2**). The marker cut-offs have been incorporated into the revised TNM staging of GCT. Hence, TNM stage groupings are now based on both anatomy (site and extent of disease) and biology (marker status and histology). Seminoma is either good or intermediate risk based on the absence or presence of nonpulmonary visceral metastases. No poor-risk category exists for seminoma. Marker levels play no role in defining risk for seminoma. Nonseminomas have good-, intermediate-, and poor-risk categories based on the site of the primary tumor, the presence or absence of nonpulmonary visceral metastases, and marker levels.

For ~90% of patients with good-risk GCTs, four cycles of etoposide plus cisplatin (EP) or three cycles of BEP produce durable complete responses, with minimal acute and chronic toxicity. Pulmonary toxicity is absent when bleomycin is not used and is rare when therapy is limited to 9 weeks; myelosuppression with neutropenic fever is less frequent; and the treatment mortality rate is negligible. About 75% of intermediate-risk patients and 45% of poor-risk patients achieve durable complete remission with four cycles of BEP, and no regimen has proved superior. More effective therapy is needed.

POSTCHEMOTHERAPY SURGERY

Resection of residual metastases after the completion of chemotherapy is an integral part of therapy. If the initial histology is nonseminoma and the marker values have normalized, all sites of residual disease should be resected. In general, residual retroperitoneal disease requires a modified bilateral RPLND. Thoracotomy (unilateral or bilateral) and neck dissection are less frequently required to remove residual mediastinal, pulmonary parenchymal, or cervical nodal disease. Viable tumor (semi-

TABLE 9-2

IGCCCG RISK CLASSIFICATION FOR ADVANCED GERM CELL TUMORS

RISK	NONSEMINOMA	SEMINOMA
Good	Gonadal or retroperitoneal primary site Absent nonpulmonary visceral metastases AFP <1000 ng/mL. Beta-hCG < 5000 mIU/mL LDH< 1.5 × upper limit or normal (ULN)	Any primary site Absent nonpulmonary visceral metastases Any LDH, hCG
Intermediate	Gonadal or retroperitoneal primary site Absent nonpulmonary visceral metastases AFP 1000–10,000 ng/mL Beta-hCG 5000–50,000 mIU/mL LDH 1.5–10 × ULN	Any primary site Presence of nonpulmonary visceral metastases Any LDH, hCG
Poor	Mediastinal primary site Presence of nonpulmonary visceral metastases AFP ≥10,000 ng/ML Beta-hCG > 50,000 mIU/mL LDH >10 × ULN	No patients classified as poor prognosis

Note: AFP, α fetoprotein; hCG, human chorionic gonadotropin; LDH, lactate dehydrogenase.
Source: International Germ Cell Cancer Consensus Group: International Germ Cell Consensus Classification: A prognostic factor-based staging system for metastatic germ cell cancers. J Clin Oncol 15:594, 1997. Reprinted with permission from the American Society of Clinical Oncology.

noma, embryonal carcinoma, yolk sac tumor, or choriocarcinoma) will be present in 15%, mature teratoma in 40%, and necrotic debris and fibrosis in 45% of resected specimens. The frequency of teratoma or viable disease is highest in residual mediastinal tumors. If necrotic debris or mature teratoma is present, no further chemotherapy is necessary. If viable tumor is present but is completely excised, two additional cycles of chemotherapy are given.

If the initial histology is pure seminoma, mature teratoma is rarely present, and the most frequent finding is necrotic debris. For residual retroperitoneal disease, a complete RPLND is technically difficult owing to extensive postchemotherapy fibrosis. Observation is recommended when no radiographic abnormality exists or a residual mass $<$3 cm is present. Controversy exists over what to do when the residual mass exceeds 3 cm in diameter. About 25% of such masses contain viable GCT. Some investigators prefer excision or biopsy, but radiation therapy and surveillance are alternatives.

SALVAGE CHEMOTHERAPY

Of patients with advanced GCT, 20 to 30% fail to achieve a durable complete response to first-line chemotherapy. A combination of cisplatin, ifosfamide, and vinblastine (VeIP) will cure about 25% of patients as a second-line therapy. Substitution of paclitaxel for vinblastine may be more effective in this setting. Patients are more likely to achieve a durable complete response if they had a testicular primary tumor and relapsed from a prior complete remission to first-line cisplatin-containing chemotherapy. In contrast, if the patient failed to achieve a complete response or has a primary mediastinal nonseminoma, then standard-dose salvage therapy is rarely beneficial. Treatment options for such patients include dose-intensive treatment, experimental therapies, and surgical resection.

Chemotherapy consisting of dose-intensive, high-dose carboplatin ($\geq$1500 mg/m^2) plus etoposide ($\geq$1200 mg/m^2), with or without cyclophosphamide or ifosfamide, with peripheral blood stem cell support induces a complete response in 25 to 40% of patients who have progressed after ifosfamide-containing salvage chemotherapy. About one-half of the complete responses will be durable. High-dose therapy is the treatment of choice and standard of care for this patient population. Paclitaxel is also active in previously treated patients and shows promise in high-dose combination programs. Cure is still possible in some relapsed patients.

EXTRAGONADAL GCT AND MIDLINE CARCINOMA OF UNCERTAIN HISTOGENESIS

The prognosis and management of patients with extragonadal GCTs depends on the tumor histology and site of origin. All patients with a diagnosis of extragonadal GCT should have a testicular ultrasound examination. Nearly all patients with retroperitoneal or mediastinal seminoma achieve a durable complete response to BEP or EP. The clinical features of patients with primary retroperitoneal nonseminoma GCT are similar to those of patients with a primary of testis origin, and careful evaluation will find evidence of a primary testicular GCT in about two-thirds of cases. In contrast, a primary mediastinal nonseminomatous GCT is associated with a poor prognosis; one-third of patients are cured with standard therapy (four cycles of BEP). Patients with newly diagnosed mediastinal nonseminoma are considered to have poor-risk disease and should be considered for clinical trials testing regimens of possibly greater efficacy. In addition, mediastinal nonseminoma is associated with hematologic disorders, including acute myelogenous leukemia, myelodysplastic syndrome, and essential thrombocytosis unrelated to previous chemotherapy. These hematologic disorders are very refractory to treatment. Nonseminoma of any primary site may change into other malignant histologies such as embryonal rhabdomyosarcoma or adenocarcinoma. This is called malignant transformation. i(12p) has been identified in the transformed cell type, indicating GCT clonal origin.

A group of patients with poorly differentiated tumors of unknown histogenesis, midline in distribution, and not associated with secretion of AFP or hCG has been described; a few (10 to 20%) are cured by standard cisplatin-containing chemotherapy. i(12p) is present in ~25% of such tumors (the fraction that are cisplatin-responsive), confirming their origin from primitive germ cells. This finding is also predictive of the response to cisplatin-based chemotherapy and resulting long-term survival. These tumors are heterogeneous; neuroepithelial tumors and lymphoma also may present in this fashion.

FERTILITY

Infertility is an important consequence of the treatment of GCTs. Preexisting infertility or impaired fertility is often present. Azoospermia and/or oligospermia are present at diagnosis in at least 50% of patients with testicular GCTs. Ejaculatory dysfunction is associated with RPLND, and germ cell damage may result from cisplatin-containing chemotherapy. Nerve-sparing techniques to preserve the retroperitoneal sympathetic nerves have made retrograde ejaculation less likely in the subgroups of patients who are candidates for this operation. Spermatogenesis does recur in some patients after chemotherapy. However, because of the significant risk of impaired reproductive capacity, semen analysis and cryopreservation of sperm in a sperm bank should be recommended to all patients before treatment.

FURTHER READINGS

HONECKER F et al: New insights into the pathology and molecular biology of human germ cell tumors. World J Urol 22:15, 2004

Germ cell tumors manifest many similarities to early germ cell development, most likely related to their cell of origin. This article highlights the diagnostic value of OCT3/4, a transcription factor and marker for pluripotency, as well as chromosomal aberrations that have prognostic value.

KONDAGUNTA GV, MOTZER R: Adjuvant chemotherapy for stage II nonseminomatous germ cell tumors. Semin Urol 20:239, 2002

LUTKE HOLZIK MF et al: Genetic predisposition to testicular germ-cell tumours. Lancet Oncol 5:363, 2004

Genome-wide screens have provided evidence of a testicular germ cell tumor susceptibility gene on chromosome Xq27 (TGCT1) that might also predispose to cryptorchism. Insight into inheritance of TGCT might lead to the identification of individuals at increased risk of developing the disorder.

MACVICAR GR et al: Testicular cancer. Curr Opin Oncol 16:253, 2004

OOSTERHUIS JW et al: Testicular germ-cell tumours in a broader perspective. Nat Rev Cancer 5:210, 2005

This review proposes that different types of germ cell tumors can be divided into five entities, in which the developmental potential is determined by the maturation stage and imprinting status of the originating germ cell.

RYAN CJ, BAJORIN DF: Chemotherapy for good-risk germ-cell tumors. Semin Urol Oncol 20:244, 2002

SCHMOLL HJ ET AL: European consensus on diagnosis and treatment of germ cell cancer: A report of the European Germ Cell Cancer Consensus Group (EGCCCG). Ann Oncol 15:1377, 2004

ULBRIGHT TM: Germ cell tumors of the gonads: A selective review emphasizing problems in differential diagnosis, newly appreciated, and controversial issues. Mod Pathol 18(Suppl 2):S61, 2005

A detailed summary of pathologic features and classification of different types of germ cell tumors.

VAENA DA et al: Long-term survival after high-dose salvage chemotherapy for germ cell malignancies with adverse prognostic variables. J Clin Oncol 21:4100, 2003

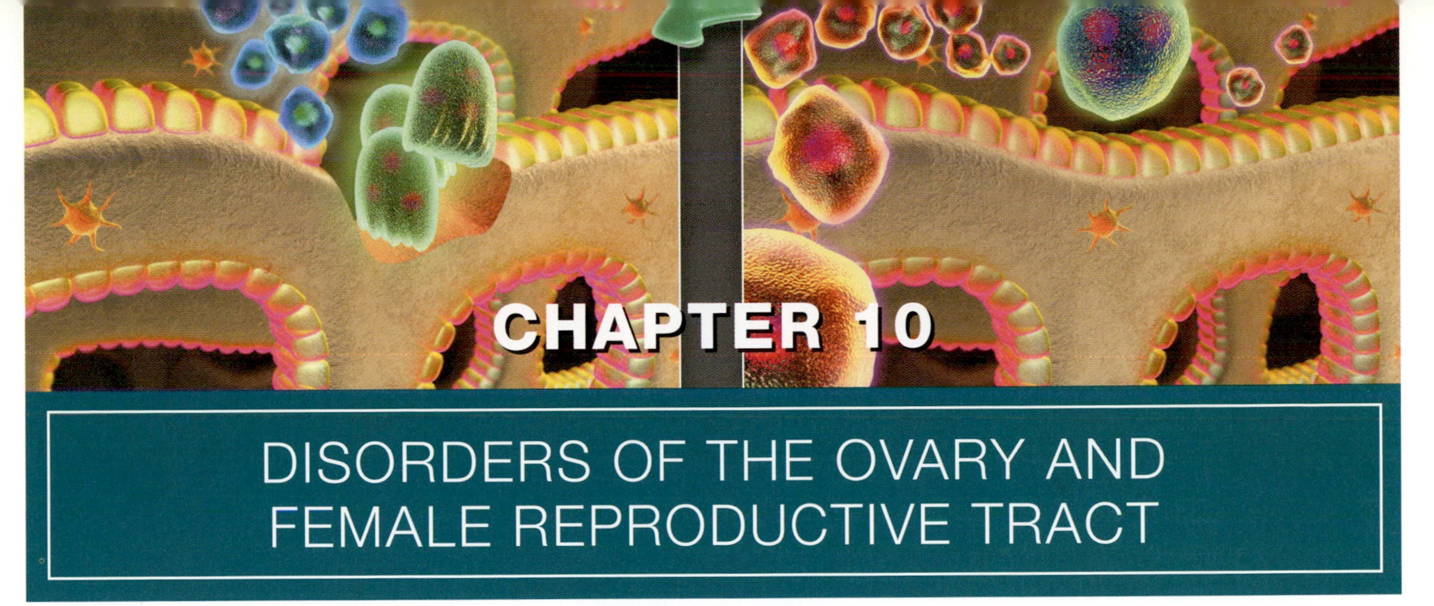

DISORDERS OF THE OVARY AND FEMALE REPRODUCTIVE TRACT

Bruce R. Carr
Karen D. Bradshaw

Normal female reproduction requires the integrated action of the central nervous system, the pituitary gland, and the ovary to orchestrate the monthly cycle of ovarian follicle development and the release of ova. The hormonal changes associated with the menstrual cycle prepare the uterus for implantation if fertilization occurs. After menopause, these cycles cease, and there is a marked reduction in sex steroid levels, leading to physiologic changes. Disorders of the female reproductive system may be developmental, structural, or hormonal in etiology. The reproductive tract is also susceptible to sexually transmitted diseases, which may cause active or chronic infections and predispose to infertility and neoplasia. Gynecologic malignancies, particularly of the ovary, uterus, and cervix, are relatively common. Although many women receive specialized care from obstetrician-gynecologists, a good understanding of the female reproductive system and its disorders is essential for comprehensive healthcare by internists and family practitioners.

DEVELOPMENT, STRUCTURE, AND FUNCTION OF THE OVARY

EMBRYOLOGY

The primordial germ cells migrate to the genital ridge adjacent to the mesonephric kidney by the fifth week of gestation and undergo mitotic division. The gonads exist in an undifferentiated state until the seventh week of fetal life, at which time the primitive ovary can be distinguished from the testis (Chap. 7). From the fifth month of fetal life, the primordial follicle consists of the primary oocyte arrested in meiosis, a single surrounding layer of granulosa cells, and a basement membrane that separates the primordial follicle from surrounding stromal (interstitial) tissues. The ovary contains a finite number of germ cells, the number peaking at about 7 million oogonia by the fifth to sixth month of gestation. Subsequently, the germ cells decrease in number through a process of atresia so that approximately 1 million remain at birth, 400,000 are present at menarche, and only a few remain at menopause.

PUBERTAL MATURATION

The final maturation of ovarian follicles commences during puberty. The two major hormones that regulate follicular development are the pituitary gonadotropins—follicle-stimulating hormone (FSH) and luteinizing hormone (LH) (**Fig. 10-1**). In the neonate, concomitant

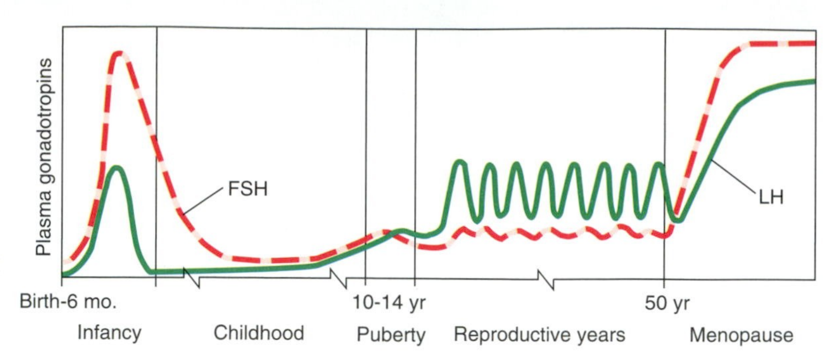

FIGURE 10-1
Pattern of gonadotropin secretion during different stages of life in women. FSH, follicle-stimulating hormone; LH, luteinizing hormone.

with the decrease in estrogen and progesterone levels caused by separation from the placenta, there is a rebound increase in gonadotropin secretion for the first few months of life. With continued maturation of the hypothalamic-pituitary system, the hypothalamic-pituitary axis (the so-called gonadostat) becomes exquisitely sensitive to negative feedback by low levels of circulating steroid hormones, and plasma gonadotropins again decrease. As the time of puberty nears, a decrease in the sensitivity of the gonadostat allows for increased secretion of FSH and LH, possibly secondary to increased episodic or pulsatile secretion of gonadotropin-releasing hormone (GnRH) by the hypothalamus (Chap. 2). The increase in estrogen secretion exerts a positive feedback, which leads to an exaggeration of the pulsatile release of LH and eventually to menarche and ovulation, after which plasma gonadotropin concentrations reach adult values but vary across the menstrual cycle. After the menopause, plasma gonadotropin levels rise; then plateau 5 to 10 years after menopause and remain fairly constant until the eighth to ninth decade of life, when the levels may fall. Although ovarian function is regulated primarily by LH and FSH, the ovary is a source of protein hormones and growth factors such as inhibin and activin that play an important role in ovarian function and regulation. The production of inhibin by the mature ovary accounts, in part, for the selective reduction in FSH that is seen during the reproductive years (Fig. 10-1).

At age 10 to 11, the first secondary sexual characteristics begin to appear in girls-namely, development of the breast buds (*thelarche*), followed by the development of pubic hair (*pubarche*), and later by the development of axillary hair (*adrenarche*). The growth of pubic and axillary hair is believed to be initiated by adrenal androgens, the levels of which begin to rise at approximately 6 to 8 years of age. A growth spurt ensues, and peak growth rate is attained by age 12.

The culmination of puberty is the onset of predictable, cyclic menses. The average time between the beginning of breast development and the onset of menses (*menarche*) is 2 years. During the first few years after menarche, menstrual cycles are often irregular and unpredictable due to anovulation. The age of menarche is variable and is influenced by socioeconomic and genetic factors and by general health. In the United States, the mean age of menarche is believed to have decreased at a rate of 3 to 4 months per decade over the past 100 years and is now approximately 12 years of age, a change believed to be due to improved nutrition. Leptin levels have been correlated with the onset of the pubertal process. A critical combination of total body weight and percent body fat is associated with development of hypothalamic insensitivity to feedback by steroids that leads to increased secretion of gonadotropins and finally to menarche. Obese girls have earlier menarche than girls with normal body weight. In contrast, active participation in sports or ballet, malnutrition, and chronic debilitating disease can delay menarche.

MATURE OVARY

Morphology

The anatomic components and function of the adult ovary are illustrated schematically in **Fig. 10-2.** Under the influence of gonadotropins, a group of primary follicles are recruited, and by day 6 to 8 of the menstrual cycle, one follicle becomes mature or "dominant," a process characterized by accelerated growth of granulosa cells and enlargement of the fluid-filled antrum. The follicles not destined to ovulate undergo degeneration, similar to the atresia that occurs during embryogenesis. Just prior to ovulation, meiosis resumes in the ovum of the dominant follicle, and the first meiotic division results in formation of the first polar body. The antrum rapidly enlarges (up to 10 to 25 mm in size), follicular fluid increases in amount, and the follicular surface thins and forms a conical stigma. Ovulation from the dominant follicle occurs 16 to 23 h after the LH peak and 24 to 38 h after the onset of the LH surge when the follicular wall ruptures in the area of the stigma. The ovum is then expelled together with a mass of surrounding granulosa cells called *cumulus cells.* The rupture is believed to result from the action of hydrolytic enzymes on the surface of the follicle, possibly under the control of prostaglandins.

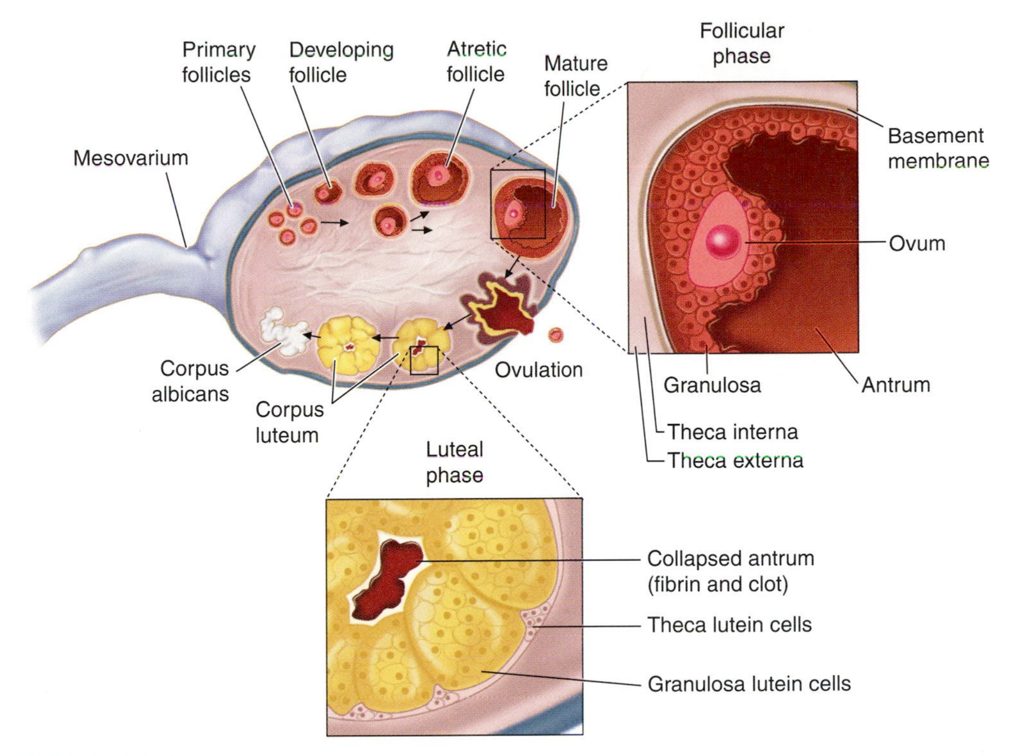

FIGURE 10-2
Developmental changes in the adult ovary during a complete 28-day cycle.

The second meiotic division occurs after the egg is fertilized by a sperm, and the second polar body is then extruded. The formation of the *corpus luteum* begins in the retained remnant of the ovulated follicle; the remaining granulosa and theca cells increase in size and accumulate lipids and a yellow pigment, lutein, to become "luteinized." After a period of 14 ± 2 days (the functional life of the corpus luteum), the corpus luteum begins to atrophy, to be replaced in time by a fibrous scar, the *corpus albicans*. The factors that limit the life span of the human corpus luteum are not known, but if pregnancy occurs, the corpus luteum persists under the influence of placental chorionic gonadotropin, and progesterone is produced by the corpus luteum for the support of pregnancy.

Hormone Formation

Steroid Hormones Like other steroid hormones, ovarian steroids are derived from cholesterol (**Fig. 10-3**). The ovary can synthesize cholesterol de novo and can also utilize cholesterol obtained from circulating lipoproteins as substrate for steroid hormone formation. Virtually all ovarian cells are believed to possess the complete complement of enzymes required for the synthesis of estradiol from cholesterol (Fig. 10-3); however, different cell types in the ovary contain different amounts of these enzymes so that the main steroids produced vary in different compartments. For example, the corpus luteum forms mainly progesterone and 17-hydroxyprogesterone, whereas theca and stromal cells convert cholesterol to androstenedione and testosterone. Granulosa cells are particularly rich in the aromatase enzyme responsible for estrogen synthesis and utilize as substrates for this process androgens synthesized in the adjacent theca cells.

LH acts primarily to regulate the early steps in steroid hormone biosynthesis, namely, the transport of cholesterol into the mitochondria by steroidogenic acute regulatory (StAR) protein and its conversion to pregnenolone. FSH acts mainly to regulate the final process by which androgens are aromatized to estrogens. As a consequence, LH enhances substrate flow and the formation of androgens and/or progesterone in the absence of FSH, whereas FSH action is impeded in the absence of LH because of diminished substrate for aromatization.

Estrogens The principal estrogen secreted by the ovary and the most potent estrogen is estradiol. Estrone is also produced by the ovary, but most estrone is formed by extraglandular conversion of androstenedione in peripheral tissues. Estriol (16-hydroxyestradiol), the main estrogen in urine, arises from the 16-hydroxylation of estrone and estradiol. Catechol estrogens are formed by hydroxylation of estrogens at the C-2 or C-4 position and may act

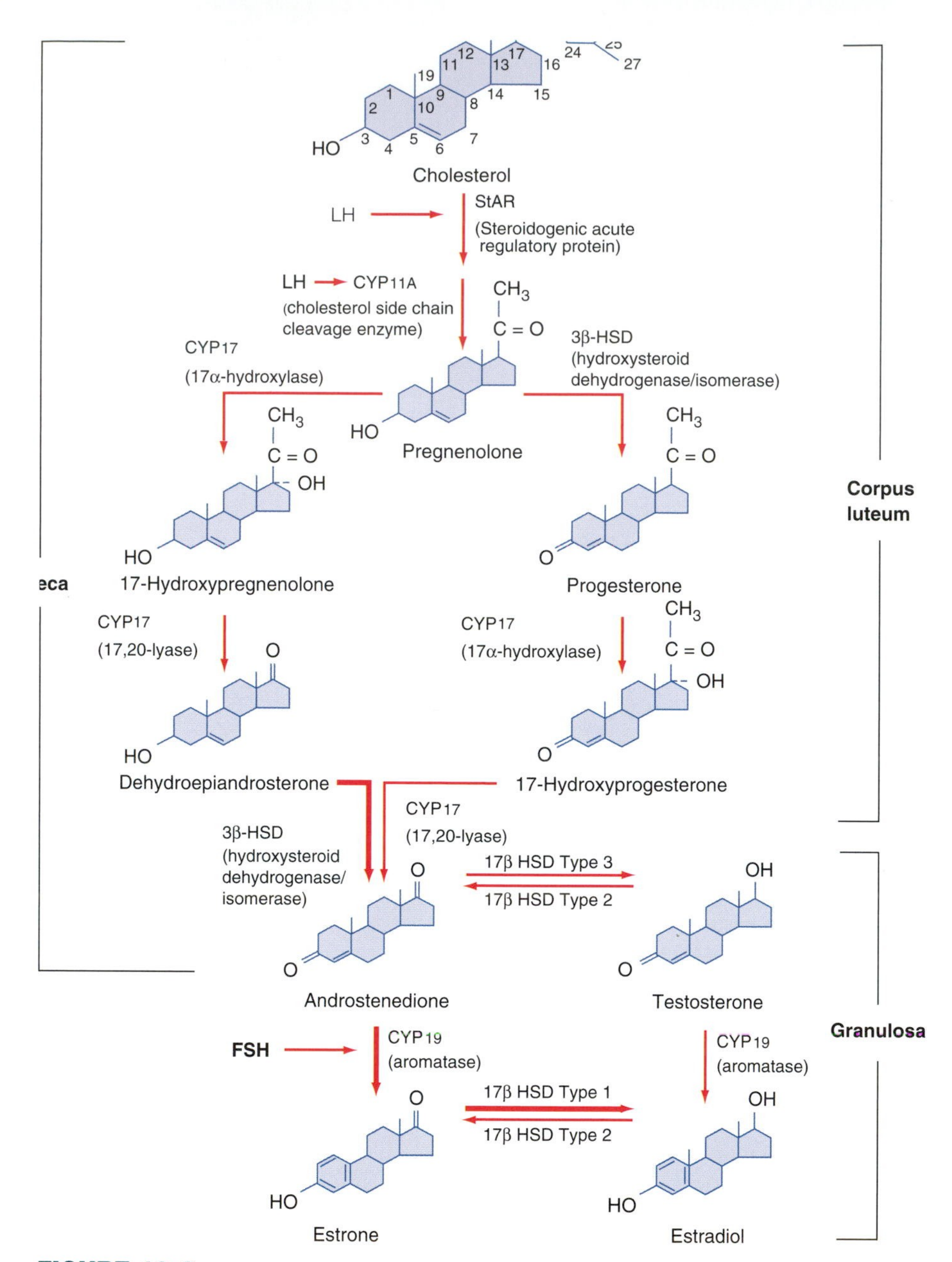

FIGURE 10-3

The principal pathway of steroid hormone biosynthesis in the ovary. The major enzyme complements for the corpus luteum, stroma, and granulosa cells are shown by the brackets; as a consequence, these cells produce predominantly progesterone and 17-OH progesterone, androgen, and estrogen, respectively. The major sites of action of luteinizing hormone (LH) and follicle-stimulating hormone (FSH) in mediating this pathway are shown in the horizontal arrows. The thin arrow emphasizes that the metabolism of 17-hydroxyprogesterone is limited in the human ovary. 17β HSD, 17β-hydroxysteroid dehydrogenase.

as the intracellular mediators of some estrogen action. Estrogens promote development of the secondary sexual characteristics in women and cause uterine growth, thickening of the vaginal mucosa, thinning of the cervical mucus, and development of the ductule system of the breasts. Estrogens also alter lipid profiles and exert effects on the vascular endothelilum. The classic mechanism of estrogen action in target tissues is similar to that for other steroid hormones and involves binding to a nuclear steroid receptor—either estrogen receptor (ER)α or ERβ—and enhancement of the transcription of various target genes (Chap. 1). There is growing evidence that

ERs also act through nonclassic mechanisms to alter signal transduction, independent of receptor binding to DNA. ERs have specific tissue site expression and bind various estrogens with different affinities, thereby conferring selective actions. The relatively promiscuous binding of synthetic and environmental estrogens by the ER has allowed the development of selective estrogen receptor modulators (SERMs), such as tamoxifen and raloxifene.

Progesterone Progesterone is the principal hormone secreted by the corpus luteum and is responsible for progestational effects, i.e., induction of secretory activity in the endometrium of the estrogen-primed uterus in preparation for implantation of the fertilized egg. Progesterone also induces a decidual reaction in endometrium. Other effects include inhibition of uterine contractions, an increase in the viscosity of cervical mucus, glandular development of the breasts, and an increase in basal body temperature (thermogenic effect).

Androgens The ovary synthesizes a variety of 19-carbon steroids, including dehydroepiandrosterone, androstenedione, testosterone, and dihydrotestosterone, principally in stromal and thecal cells. The major ovarian 19-carbon steroid is androstenedione (Fig. 10-3), part of which is secreted into the plasma and part of which is converted to estrogen in granulosa cells or to testosterone in the interstitium. Androstenedione can also be converted to testosterone and estrogens in peripheral tissues. Only testosterone and dihydrotestosterone are true androgens that interact with the androgen receptor and induce virilizing signs in women (Chap. 12).

Other Hormones *Inhibin* is secreted in two forms (A and B) by the follicle and inhibits the release of FSH by the hypothalamic-pituitary unit. *Activin* is also secreted by the follicle and may enhance FSH secretion as well as having local effects on ovarian steroidogenesis. *Follistatin* is an activin-binding protein that attenuates the actions of activin and other members of the transforming growth factor β (TGF-β) family.

Some ovarian hormones play an uncertain role in human physiology. *Relaxin,* a polypeptide hormone produced by the human corpus luteum and by the decidua, causes softening of the cervix and loosening of the symphysis pubis in preparation for parturition in animals. *Oxytocin, vasopressin,* and other hypothalamic and pituitary hormones are also present in granulosa and/or luteal cells, but their function in these cells is unknown. Granulosa cells secrete *oocyte maturation inhibitor* (OMI), a factor that prevents premature ovulation. In addition, in the gonads of both sexes a *meiosis-inducing substance* triggers the onset of meiosis, an event that occurs earlier in ovarian than in testicular development. Local growth factors [including insulin-like growth factors (IGFs) 1 and 2 and TGF-α and -β] may also influence steroid secretion by the ovary.

The Normal Menstrual Cycle

The menstrual cycle is divided into a follicular or proliferative phase and a luteal, or secretory, phase (**Fig. 10-4**). The secretion of FSH and LH is fundamentally under negative feedback control by ovarian steroids (particularly estradiol) and by inhibin (which selectively suppresses FSH), but the response of gonadotropins to different levels of estradiol varies. FSH secretion is inhibited progressively as estrogen levels increase—typical negative feedback. In contrast, LH secretion is suppressed maximally by sustained low levels of estrogen and is enhanced by a rising level of estradiol—positive feedback. Feedback of estrogen involves both the hypothalamus and pituitary. Negative feedback suppresses GnRH and inhibits gonadotropin production. Positive feedback is associated with an increased frequency of GnRH secretion and enhanced pituitary sensitivity to GnRH.

The length of the menstrual cycle is defined as the time from the onset of one menstrual bleeding episode to onset of the next. In women of reproductive age, the cycle averages 28 $\pm$ 3 days and the mean duration of flow is 4 $\pm$ 2 days. Longer menstrual cycles (usually characterized by anovulation) occur at menarche and near the onset of menopause. At the end of a cycle, plasma levels of estrogen and progesterone fall and circulating levels of FSH increase. Under the influence of FSH, follicular recruitment results in development of the follicle that will be dominant during the next cycle.

After the onset of menses, follicular development continues, but FSH levels decrease. Approximately 8 to 10 days prior to the midcycle LH surge, plasma estradiol levels begin to rise as the result of estradiol formation by the granulosa cells of the dominant follicle. During the second half of the follicular phase, LH levels also begin to rise (owing to positive feedback). Just before ovulation, estradiol secretion reaches a peak and then falls. Immediately thereafter, a further rise in the plasma level of LH mediates the final maturation of the follicle, followed by follicular rupture and ovulation 16 to 23 h after the LH peak. The rise in LH is accompanied by a smaller increase in the level of plasma FSH, the physiologic significance of which is unclear. The plasma progesterone level also begins to rise just prior to midcycle and facilitates the positive feedback action of estradiol on LH secretion.

At the onset of the luteal phase, plasma gonadotropins decrease and plasma progesterone increases. A secondary rise in estrogens causes further gonadotropin suppression.

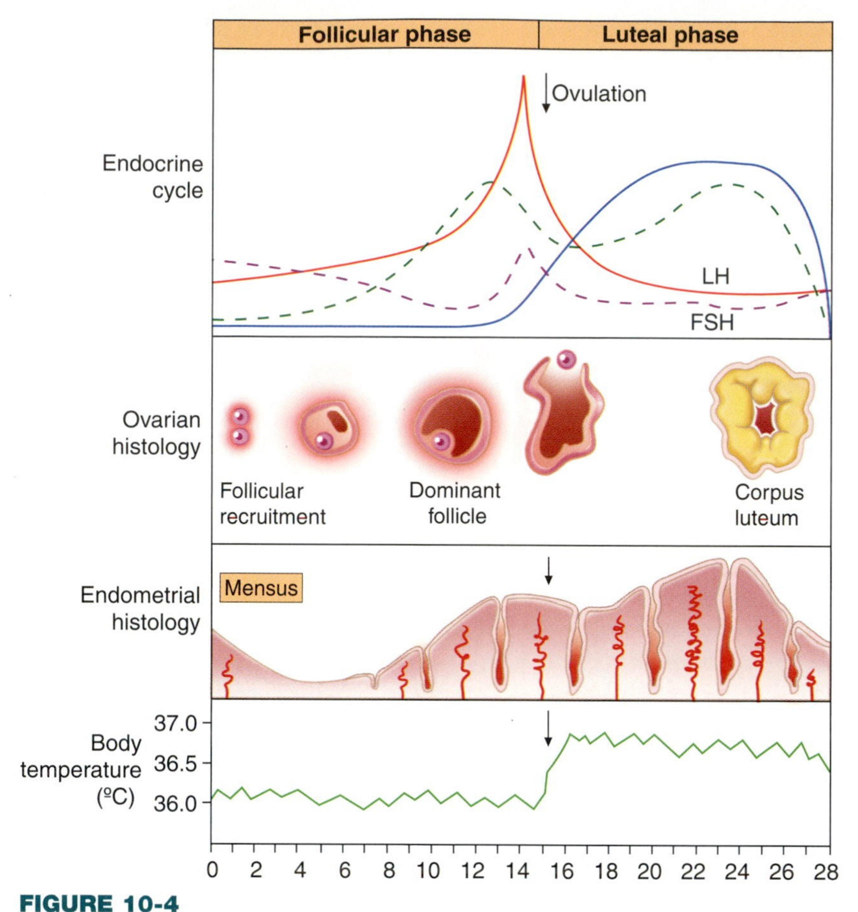

FIGURE 10-4

The hormonal, ovarian, endometrial, and basal body temperature changes and relationships throughout the normal menstrual cycle.

Near the end of the luteal phase, progesterone and estrogen levels fall, and FSH levels begin to rise to initiate the development of the next follicle (usually in the contralateral ovary) and the next menstrual cycle. Inhibin A levels are low in the follicular phase but reach a peak in the luteal phase. Inhibin B levels, in contrast, are increased in the follicular phase and low in the luteal phase.

The endometrium lining the uterine cavity undergoes marked alterations in response to the changing plasma levels of ovarian hormones (Fig. 10-4). Concurrent with the decrease in plasma estrogen and progesterone and the decline of corpus luteum function in the late luteal phase, intense vasospasm occurs in the spiral arterioles supplying blood to the endometrium, causing ischemic necrosis, endometrial desquamation, and bleeding. This vasospasm is caused by locally synthesized prostaglandins. The onset of bleeding marks the first day of the menstrual cycle. By the fourth to fifth day, the endometrium is thin. During the proliferative phase, glandular growth of the endometrium is mediated by estrogen. After ovulation, increased progesterone levels lead to further thickening of the endometrium, but the rapid growth slows. The endometrium then enters the secretory phase, characterized by tortuosity of the glands, curling of the spiral arterioles, and glandular secretion. As corpus luteum function begins to wane in the absence of conception, the sequence of events leading to menstruation is again set into action.

Biphasic changes in basal body temperature are characteristic of the ovulatory cycle and are mediated by alterations in progesterone levels (Fig. 10-4). An increase in basal body temperature by 0.3° to 0.5°C begins after ovulation, persists during the luteal phase, and returns to the normal baseline (36.2° to 36.4°C) after the onset of the subsequent menses.

MENOPAUSE

The *menopause* is defined as the final episode of menstrual bleeding in women. Menopause is the consequence of exhaustion of ovarian follicles, a process that begins during fetal development. The median age of women at the time of cessation of menstrual bleeding is 50 to 51 years. Preceding the menopause, the pattern of menstrual cycles is variable, but the interval between menses usually becomes shorter, as follicular recruitment is hastened by increases in FSH. Day 3 FSH and 17β-estradiol (E_2) levels are often elevated. Ovulatory cycles continue for some period of time, then anovulation becomes common.

The ovaries of postmenopausal women are small and wrinkled, and the residual cells are predominantly stromal. Estrogen and androgen levels in plasma are reduced but not absent. Before the menopause, plasma androstenedione is derived almost equally from the adrenals and the ovaries; after menopause, the ovarian contribution ceases so that the plasma levels of androstenedione fall by 50%. However, the menopausal ovary continues to secrete testosterone, presumably formed in stromal cells. After menopause, extraglandular estrogen formation is the major pathway for estrogen synthesis. Because adipose tissue is a major site of extraglandular estrogen production, peripheral estrogen formation may actually be enhanced in obese postmenopausal women. The predominant estrogen formed is estrone rather than estradiol. For discussion of the management of menopause, see Chap. 11.

LABORATORY AND CLINICAL ASSESSMENT OF HORMONAL STATUS

The hormonal status of women can usually be assessed by history and physical examination. In general, the presence of secondary sexual characteristics such as normal female breast development indicates adequate estrogen secretion in the past, and the presence of regular, predictable, cyclic menses implies that ovulation and the production of gonadotropins, estrogen, progesterone, and androgens are adequate and that the outflow tract is intact. Such a history may be more valuable than laboratory tests in evaluating ovarian hormone status. However, laboratory tests provide valuable ancillary information in the evaluation of women with endocrine dysfunction or infertility (Chap. 15).

PITUITARY GONADOTROPINS

Plasma gonadotropins are assessed by immunoassay. Because both FSH and LH are secreted in a pulsatile manner, the results obtained from a single serum sample may be difficult to interpret. Moreover, the values vary widely during the menstrual cycle, particularly at the time of the midcycle gonadotropin surge. Consequently, plasma gonadotropin measurements are of greatest use in evaluating women with suspected ovarian failure and in supporting the diagnosis of polycystic ovarian syndrome (PCOS) or hypogonadotropic hypogonadism. FSH levels that are persistently >40 IU/L are diagnostic of ovarian failure, and an LH value <0.8 IU/L suggests hypogonadotropic hypogonadism. In practice, however, gonadotropin values may be equivocal and must be interpreted in the context of other historic, physical, and laboratory findings.

OVARIAN HORMONES

Estrogen

The presence of normal secondary sexual characteristics implies that estrogen production was adequate in the past. The current estrogen status can be estimated by pelvic examination. The presence of a moist, rugated vagina with copious, clear, thin cervical mucus that can be stretched and that exhibits arborization or ferning when spread on a slide is strong evidence of adequate estrogen production. Cytologic demonstration of mature vaginal epithelial cells and abundant cornified squamous epithelial cells with pyknotic nuclei confirms the presence of adequate estrogen levels.

The progesterone-withdrawal test provides a functional assessment of the endometrium, outflow tract, and estrogen status. If menses appear within a week to 10 days after the end of a trial of medroxyprogesterone acetate (10 mg by mouth once or twice a day for 5 days) or after a single intramuscular injection of progesterone (100 mg), then prior estrogen priming was adequate to allow withdrawal bleeding.

Owing to its variable level in plasma during the normal cycle and the difficulty of estimating the day of the cycle in women with abnormal cycles, the measurement of estrogen levels in plasma or urine is of little use in the routine assessment of estrogen status. Measurement of plasma estradiol is useful during attempts to induce ovulation with gonadotropins to prevent the development of the ovarian hyperstimulation syndrome and is used along with ultrasound assessment to monitor follicular growth in women during in vitro fertilization.

Progesterone

Cyclic, predictable menses also imply that adequate progesterone is secreted during the luteal phase of the menstrual cycle. Assessment of progesterone is useful to detect ovulation and to evaluate the adequacy of the luteal phase in infertile women. Several functional assays of progesterone can be used. The least expensive and most useful is the daily measurement of basal body temperature throughout a cycle. Owing to the thermogenic properties of progesterone, a normal biphasic monthly curve showing a temperature elevation lasting for approximately 2 weeks after ovulation is a valid indication of progesterone secretion during the luteal phase (Fig. 10-4). The presence of viscous cervical mucus that does not stretch or fern and of predominantly intermediate cells on vaginal cytology or demonstration of a secretory epithelium in an endometrial biopsy during the luteal phase on days 20 to 22 of the cycle provides additional assessment of progesterone secretion. In addition, plasma progesterone can be measured to assess the function of the corpus luteum; a level > 10 μmol/L (>3 ng/mL) suggests successful ovulation and adequate corpus luteum function.

Androgen

Under normal conditions, the ovary secretes androstenedione, testosterone, and dehydroepiandrosterone. In conditions of androgen excess, hirsutism and/or virilization are common. The evaluation of androgen excess is discussed in Chap. 12.

DIAGNOSIS OF PREGNANCY

Pregnancy is usually recognized on the basis of history and physical examination. That is, a woman with previously cyclic, predictable menses develops amenorrhea accompanied by breast tenderness, malaise, lassitude, and nausea, and on physical examination the uterus is soft and enlarged.

Human chorionic gonadotropin (hCG) is secreted by the trophoblastic cells of the placenta into the maternal plasma and excreted in the urine. Plasma or urine assays of hCG make it possible to detect pregnancies 8 to 10 days after ovulation, before the first missed menstrual period and long before pregnancy can be diagnosed by clinical assessments. Sensitive and specific hCG-based pregnancy tests are now available for patients to use at home.

DISORDERS OF OVARIAN FUNCTION

PREPUBERTAL YEARS

Puberty is said to be *precocious* if breast budding begins before age 8 or if menarche occurs before age 9. Those disorders in which the developing sexual characteristics are appropriate for the genetic and gonadal sex—i.e., feminization in girls or virilization in boys—are termed *isosexual precocity,* whereas *heterosexual precocity* occurs when sexual characteristics are not in accord with the genetic sex, namely, virilization in girls or feminization in boys. Pubertal disorders of boys are described in Chap. 8.

Isosexual Precocious Puberty

Isosexual precocious puberty in girls can be divided into three major categories (**Table 10-1**).

True Precocious Puberty True precocious puberty (gonadotropin-dependent) is characterized by an early but otherwise normal sequence of pubertal development, including increased secretion of gonadotropins and ovulatory menstrual cycles. Constitutional or idiopathic precocious puberty accounts for 90% of cases. The disorder is more common in girls than boys. No cause for the premature maturation of the central nervous system–hypothalamic–pituitary axis can be identified, and the diagnosis is confirmed by finding an adult pattern of LH and FSH release on a GnRH stimulation test. Premature appearance of secondary sexual characteristics and of ovulatory cycles with the accompanying risk of fertility may cause significant emotional disturbance. Therefore, prompt initiation of therapy is imperative. GnRH analogues suppress gonadotropins and inhibit estrogen synthesis, thereby blocking precocious puberty; they may also prevent premature closure of the epiphyses and the resulting short stature.

About 10% of cases are due to organic brain diseases, including brain tumors (hypothalamic gliomas, astrocytomas, ependymomas, germinomas, and hamartomas), encephalitis, meningitis, hydrocephalus, head injury, tuberous sclerosis, and neurofibromatosis. It is essential to distinguish this group of patients from those with the idiopathic disorder, and patients whose disorder is designated as idiopathic occasionally prove to have such tu-

TABLE 10-1

DIFFERENTIAL DIAGNOSIS OF SEXUAL PRECOCITY

- **I. Isosexual precocity**
  - A. True precocious puberty
    1. Constitutional
    2. Organic brain disease
    3. Congenital adrenal hyperplasia
  - B. Precocious pseudopuberty
    1. Ovarian tumors
    2. Adrenal tumors
    3. McCune-Albright syndrome
    4. Hypothyroidism
    5. Russell-Silver syndrome
    6. Estrogen-containing medications
  - C. Incomplete sexual precocity
    1. Premature thelarche
    2. Premature adrenarche
    3. Premature pubarche
- **II. Heterosexual precocity**
  - A. Ovarian tumors
  - B. Adrenal tumors
  - C. Congenital adrenal hyperplasia

mors. Most patients with organic lesions serious enough to cause precocious puberty have obvious neurologic signs and symptoms. Evaluation of all patients with precocious puberty should include, at a minimum, computed tomography (CT) or magnetic resonance imaging (MRI) of the brain. The success of treatment depends on the nature of the lesion, but surgical and radiation treatment of well-localized tumors is occasionally successful.

A rare cause of isosexual precocity is congenital adrenal hyperplasia due to 21-hydroxylase deficiency in girls when treatment has been delayed until 4 to 8 years of age (Chap. 5). After initiation of glucocorticoid replacement, such individuals may undergo isosexual precocious puberty.

Precocious Pseudopuberty Precocious pseudopuberty (gonadotropin-independent) occurs when girls undergo feminization as a consequence of enhanced estrogen formation but do not ovulate or develop cyclic menses. Ovarian cysts or tumors that secrete estrogen (granulosa-theca cell tumors) are the most frequent cause of precocious pseudopuberty. Granulosa-theca cell tumors associated with intestinal polyps and pigmentation of the mucous membranes occur in the Peutz-Jeghers syndrome. Other ovarian tumors that secrete estrogens (or androgens that can be converted to estrogens at extraglandular sites) include dysgerminomas, teratomas, cystadenomas, and ovarian carcinomas (Chap. 13). Ovarian tumors can usually be detected by rectoabdominal examination or by ultrasound, CT, MRI, and/or laparoscopy. Ovarian teratomas and choriocarcinomas and other carcinomas that secrete hCG do not cause precocious puberty in girls unless they also secrete estrogen (hCG or LH in the absence of FSH does not induce ovarian estrogen production). Rarely, feminizing tumors of the adrenal cause isosexual precocious puberty by direct formation of estrogens or by secretion of weak androgens, which are converted to estrogens in extraglandular tissues. The *McCune-Albright syndrome* (polyostotic fibrous dysplasia) is due to an activating mutation in the G protein, $G_{s\alpha}$, that occurs during embryogenesis, leading to a mosaic pattern of expression in various tissues. It is characterized by café au lait spots, cystic fibrous dysplasia of bones, and sexual precocity. In the ovary, the $G_{s\alpha}$ mutation mimics the action of FSH, leading to autonomous follicle development and estrogen formation. Occasionally, this disorder leads to true precocious puberty. *Primary hypothyroidism* is occasionally associated with enhanced secretion of FSH, inducing ovarian estrogen secretion. High levels of thyroid-stimulating hormone (TSH) caused by hypothyroidism also may stimulate the FSH receptor. The *Russell-Silver syndrome,* or congenital asymmetry, is associated with short stature and precocious feminization. *Estrogen-containing medications,* including use of estrogen-containing creams for diaper rash or the ingestion of meat from estrogen-treated animals or poultry or of any estrogen by mouth, can cause this disorder.

Incomplete Isosexual Precocity This term is used to describe the premature development of a single pubertal event and encompasses several entities. Breast budding before age 7 (*premature thelarche*) without other evidence of estrogen secretion and without premature bone maturation is believed to be due to a transient increase in estrogen secretion or to increased sensitivity to the small amounts of circulating estrogens formed before puberty. Usually, the disorder is self-limited and resolves spontaneously. Occasionally, axillary hair and/or pubic hair (*premature adrenarche* and *premature pubarche*) appear without any other secondary sexual development. The phenomenon is associated with adrenal androgen secretion in the range of normal puberty and can be distinguished from syndromes of virilization by the absence of clitoromegaly. It requires no treatment, and patients enter puberty at about the average time.

Heterosexual Precocity

Virilization in a prepubertal female is usually due to congenital adrenal hyperplasia or to androgen secretion by an ovarian or adrenal tumor. The manifestations of virilization are described in Chap. 12. Virilization in girls with congenital adrenal hyperplasia usually occurs in a background of variable sexual ambiguity (Chap. 7).

Evaluation of Sexual Precocity

The evaluation of sexual precocity involves a careful history and physical examination, including rectoabdominal examination, abdominal sonography, determination of bone age, and GnRH stimulation test, and measurement of thyroid hormones, TSH, and gonadotropins (and androgen or estrogen levels when appropriate). MRI and/or CT scans should be obtained if a neurologic disorder is suspected and no evidence of an ovarian or adrenal tumor is found.

REPRODUCTIVE YEARS

Disorders of the Menstrual Cycle

Abnormal Uterine Bleeding Between menarche and the menopause, almost every woman experiences one or more episodes of abnormal uterine bleeding, here defined as any bleeding pattern that differs in frequency, duration, or amount from the pattern observed during a normal menstrual cycle. In normal women, the average menstrual cycle is 28 ± 3 days, the mean duration of menstrual flow is 4 ± 2 days, and the average blood loss is 35 to 80 mL. A variety of descriptive terms (such as *menorrhagia, metrorrhagia,* and *menometrorrhagia*) have been used to characterize patterns of abnormal uterine bleeding. A more logical approach is to divide abnormal uterine bleeding into those patterns associated with ovulatory cycles and those associated with anovulatory cycles.

Ovulatory Cycles Normal menstrual bleeding with ovulatory cycles is spontaneous, regular, cyclic, and predictable and is frequently associated with discomfort (*dysmenorrhea*). Deviations from this pattern associated with cycles that are still regular and predictable are most often due to organic disease of the outflow tract. For example, regular but prolonged and excessive bleeding episodes unassociated with bleeding dyscrasias (hypermenorrhea or menorrhagia) can result from abnormalities of the uterus such as submucous leiomyomas, adenomyosis, or endometrial polyps. Regular, cyclic, predictable menstruation characterized by spotting or light bleeding is termed *hypomenorrhea* and is due to obstruction of the outflow tract as from intrauterine synechiae or scarring of the cervix. Intermenstrual bleeding between episodes of regular, ovulatory menstruation is also often due to cervical or endometrial lesions. An exception to the association between organic disease and abnormal uterine bleeding is the occurrence of regular menstruation more frequently than 21 days apart (*polymenorrhea*). Such cycles may be a normal variant.

Anovulatory Cycles Dysfunctional uterine bleeding refers to bleeding that is unpredictable with respect to amount, onset, and duration and is usually painless. This disorder is not due to abnormalities of the uterus but rather to chronic anovulation and occurs when there is interruption of the normal sequence of follicular and luteal phases under the influence of a dominant follicle and its resulting corpus luteum. As discussed above, uterine bleeding in ovulatory cycles occurs because of progesterone withdrawal and requires that the endometrium first be primed with estrogen. (When castrates or postmenopausal women are given progesterone, withdrawal bleeding usually does not occur.)

Dysfunctional uterine bleeding can occur in women who have a transient disruption of the synchronous hypothalamic-pituitary-ovarian patterns necessary for ovulatory cycles, most often at the extremes of the reproductive life—in the early menarche and in the perimenopausal period—but also after temporary stress or intercurrent illness.

Primary dysfunctional uterine bleeding can result from three disorders.

1. ***Estrogen withdrawal bleeding*** occurs when estrogen is given to a castrated or postmenopausal woman and then withdrawn. As in other types of dysfunctional uterine bleeding, this form of menstrual bleeding is usually painless.
2. ***Estrogen breakthrough bleeding*** occurs when there is continuous estrogen stimulation of the endometrium not interrupted by cyclic progesterone secretion and withdrawal. This is the most common type of dysfunctional uterine bleeding and is usually due to anovulation associated with chronic acyclic estrogen production, as in women with PCOS. Such women may have histories of irregular, unpredictable menses; oligomenorrhea; or amenorrhea (see below). Alternatively, estrogen breakthrough bleeding can occur in hypogonadal women given estrogens chronically rather than intermittently and in women with estrogen-secreting tumors of the ovary. Estrogen breakthrough bleeding may be profuse and is unpredictable with respect to duration, amount of flow, and time of occurrence. The endometrium is typically thin because its repair between episodes of bleeding is incomplete.
3. ***Progesterone breakthrough bleeding*** occurs in the presence of abnormally high ratios of progesterone to estrogen, i.e., in women using continuous low-dose oral contraceptives.

The approach to a patient with dysfunctional uterine bleeding begins with a careful history of menstrual patterns and prior hormonal therapy. Since not all urogenital tract bleeding is from the uterus, rectal, bladder, and vaginal or cervical sources must be excluded by physical examination. If the bleeding is from the uterus, a pregnancy-related disorder such as abortion or ectopic pregnancy must be ruled out.

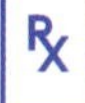

TREATMENT FOR DYSFUNCTIONAL UTERINE BLEEDING

Once the diagnosis of dysfunctional uterine bleeding is established, a rational approach to management is as follows: During a first episode of dysfunctional bleeding, it is reasonable to observe the patient without intervention, provided the bleeding is not copious and no evidence of bleeding dyscrasia is present. If bleeding is moderately severe, control can be achieved with relatively high dose estrogen oral contraceptives for 3 weeks. Alternatively, a regimen of three or four low-dose oral contraceptive pills per day for 1 week followed by tapering to the usual dosage for up to 3 weeks is also effective. If uterine bleeding is more severe, hospitalization, bed rest, and intramuscular injections of estradiol valerate (10 mg) and hydroxyprogesterone caproate (500 mg) or intravenous or intramuscular conjugated estrogens (25 mg) usually control the bleeding. After initial treatment, iron replacement should be instituted, and recurrence can be prevented by cyclic oral contraceptives for 2 to 3 months (or more if pregnancy is not desired). Alternatively, menses can be induced every 2 to 3 months with medroxyprogesterone acetate, 10 mg taken orally once or twice a day for 10 days. If hormone therapy fails to control uterine bleeding, an endometrial biopsy, hysteroscopy, or dilatation and curettage may be required for diagnosis and therapy. Indeed, uterine sampling should be performed prior to hormone therapy in women at risk for endometrial cancer (e.g., in women who are approaching the age of menopause or who are massively obese); endometrial cancer is rare in ovulatory women of reproductive age.

Amenorrhea An acceptable definition of amenorrhea is failure of menarche by age 15, irrespective of the presence or absence of secondary sexual characteristics, or the absence of menstruation for 6 months in a woman with previous periodic menses. However, women who do not fulfill these criteria should be evaluated if (1) the patient and/or her family are greatly concerned, (2) no breast development has occurred by age 13, or (3) any sexual ambiguity or virilization is present. Amenorrhea is commonly categorized as either primary (the woman has never menstruated) or secondary (when menstruation has been present for a variable period of time in the past and has ceased). However, some disorders can cause either primary or secondary amenorrhea. For example, most women with gonadal dysgenesis have primary amenorrhea, but some have a few follicles and ovulate for short periods so that pregnancy occurs rarely. Furthermore, patients with chronic anovulation (PCOS) usually have secondary amenorrhea but on occasion have primary amenorrhea. For these reasons, categorization of amenorrhea into primary and secondary types is less helpful than a classification based on the underlying physiologic derangements: (1) anatomical defects, (2) ovarian failure, and (3) chronic anovulation with or without estrogen present.

Anatomical Defects Anatomical or structural defects of the genital tract can preclude menstrual bleeding. Starting from the caudal end of the female genital tract, labial fusion is often associated with disorders of sexual development, particularly female pseudohermaphroditism (congenital adrenal hyperplasia or exposure to maternal androgens in utero; Chap. 7). Congenital defects of the vagina, imperforate hymen, and transverse vaginal septae can also cause amenorrhea. These women frequently have accumulation of menstrual blood behind the obstruction and may have cyclic, predictable episodes of abdominal pain.

More severe müllerian anomalies include müllerian agenesis (the Mayer-Rokitansky-Küster-Hauser syndrome), second in frequency only to gonadal dysgenesis as a cause of primary amenorrhea. It can be caused by mutations in the genes encoding anti-müllerian hormone (AMH) or its receptor (AMHR). Women with this syndrome have a 46,XX karyotype, female secondary sex characteristics, and normal ovarian function, including cyclic ovulation, but have absence or hypoplasia of the vagina. The uterus usually consists of only rudimentary bicornuate cords, but if the uterus contains endometrium, cyclic abdominal pain and accumulation of blood may occur, as in other forms of outlet obstruction. One-third of women with this syndrome have abnormalities of the urogenital tract, and one-tenth have skeletal anomalies, usually involving the spine. The major diagnostic problem is distinguishing müllerian agenesis from complete androgen insensitivity syndrome, in which 46,XY genetic males with testes differentiate as phenotypic women but with a blind vaginal pouch and no uterus (Chap. 7). Androgen insensitivity can be diagnosed by demonstrating a male level of serum testosterone and a 46,XY karyotype, whereas demonstration of a 46,XX karyotype, the biphasic basal body temperature curve characteristic of ovulation, and elevated levels of progesterone during the luteal phase establish the diagnosis of müllerian agenesis.

Other abnormalities of the uterus that cause amenorrhea include obstruction due to scarring or stenosis of the cervix, often as a result of surgery, electrocautery, laser therapy, or cryosurgery. Such destruction of the endometrium (Asherman's syndrome) usually follows vigorous curettage for postpartum hemorrhage or after therapeutic abortion complicated by infection. This diagnosis is confirmed by hysterosalpingography or by direct visual examination of the endometrial scarring or synechiae using a hysteroscope.

Treatment of disorders of the outflow tract is surgical.

Ovarian Failure Primary ovarian failure is associated with elevated plasma gonadotropin levels and can result from several causes. The most frequent cause is *gonadal* *dysgenesis,* in which the germ cells are absent and the ovary is replaced by a fibrous streak (Chap. 7). A 45,X karyotype is found in about half of women with this disorder, and most have somatic defects, including short stature, webbed neck, shield chest, and cardiovascular defects, collectively termed the *Turner phenotype.* The remainder of women with X chromosome abnormalities have chromosomal mosaicism with or without associated structural abnormalities of the X. Approximately 90% of women with gonadal dysgenesis due to partial or complete deletion of the X never have menstrual bleeding, and the remaining 10% have sufficient follicles to experience menses and, rarely, fertility; the menstrual and reproductive lives of such individuals are invariably brief.

One-tenth of individuals identified as having bilateral streak gonads have a normal 46,XX or 46,XY karyotype and are said to have *pure gonadal dysgenesis.* These individuals have either normal or above-average stature, owing to failure of estrogen-mediated epiphyseal closure in the presence of a normal chromosomal constitution. Pure gonadal dysgenesis does not constitute a phenotypic or chromosomally homogeneous disorder.

Other causes of ovarian failure and amenorrhea include deficiency of the *CYP17* gene that encodes 17α-hydroxylase and 17,20-lyase activities, premature ovarian failure, the resistant-ovary syndrome, and ovarian failure secondary to chemotherapy or radiation therapy for malignancy. *17α-Hydroxylase deficiency* is a rare, autosomal recessive disorder characterized by primary amenorrhea, sexual infantilism, and hypertension, the latter due to increased production of desoxycorticosterone (DOC); women with *17,20-lyase deficiency* have primary amenorrhea and sexual infantilism with normal blood pressure. The diagnosis of *premature ovarian failure* or *premature menopause* applies to women who cease menstruating before age 40. The ovaries in such women are similar to those of postmenopausal women, containing few or no follicles as the result of accelerated follicular atresia. Premature ovarian failure due to ovarian antibodies may be one component of polyglandular failure, together with adrenal insufficiency, hypothyroidism, and other autoimmune disorders (Chap. 21). A rare form of ovarian failure is the *resistant-ovary syndrome,* in which the ovaries contain many follicles that are arrested in development prior to the antral stage, possibly because of resistance to the action of FSH in the ovary. A subset of these individuals have mutations in FSH or its receptor. To differentiate this disorder from the 46,XX variety of pure gonadal dysgenesis, which is also associated with sexual immaturity, it is necessary to perform ovarian biopsy or genetic testing. Women with ovarian failure who desire pregnancy have been treated with hormone replacement and transfer of donor embryos to the uterine cavity or fallopian tubes.

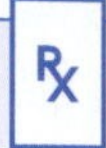

TREATMENT FOR AMENORRHEA

In women with decreased estrogen production, whether due to ovarian dysfunction or to hypogonadotropic hypogonadism, treatment with cyclic estrogens should be instituted to induce the development and maintenance of female secondary sexual characteristics and to prevent osteoporosis. The most commonly used medications are conjugated estrogens (0.625 to 1.25 mg/d by mouth) together with medroxyprogesterone acetate (2.5 mg/d or 5 to 10 mg during the last several days of monthly estrogen treatment to prevent development of endometrial hyperplasia). Alternatively, oral contraceptives may be given to premenopausal-age women (Chap. 15). Abnormal bleeding in women receiving estrogen replacement mandates histologic evaluation of the endometrium.

Chronic Anovulation At least 80% or more of gynecologic endocrine disorders result from chronic anovulation. Women with chronic anovulation fail to ovulate spontaneously but may ovulate with appropriate therapy. The ovaries of such women do not secrete estrogen in a normal cyclic pattern. It is clinically useful to differentiate those women who produce enough estrogen to have withdrawal bleeding after progestogen therapy from those who do not; the latter often have hypothalamic-pituitary dysfunction.

Chronic Anovulation with Estrogen Present This disorder is most commonly caused by *polycystic ovarian syndrome (PCOS),* which is characterized by infertility, hirsutism, obesity, insulin resistance, and amenorrhea or oligomenorrhea. When spontaneous uterine bleeding occurs in women with PCOS, it is unpredictable as to time of onset, duration, and amount; on occasion the bleeding can be severe.

PCOS, as originally described by Stein and Leventhal, was characterized by enlarged, polycystic ovaries, but it is now known to be associated with a variety of pathologic findings in the ovaries, only some of which result in enlargement and none of which are pathognomonic. The most common finding is a white, smooth, sclerotic ovary with a thickened capsule, multiple follicular cysts in various stages of atresia, a hyperplastic theca and stroma, and rare or absent corpora albicans. Other ovaries have hyperthecosis in which the ovarian stroma is hyperplastic and may contain lipid-laden luteal cells. Thus, the diagnosis of PCOS is a clinical one, based on the coexistence of chronic anovulation and varying degrees of androgen excess. The fundamental defect that causes PCOS is unknown, and it is likely to have several distinct causes.

In most women with PCOS, menarche occurs at the expected time, but oligomenorrhea ensues after a variable period. Signs of androgen excess (hirsutism) usually become evident soon after menarche. One scenario suggests that this disorder originates as an exaggerated adrenarche in obese girls (**Fig. 10-5**). The combination of elevated levels of adrenal androgens and obesity leads to increased formation of extraglandular estrogen. This estrogen exerts a positive feedback on LH secretion and negative feedback on FSH secretion, resulting in a ratio of LH to FSH levels in plasma that is characteristically greater than 2. The increased LH levels can then lead to hyperplasia of the ovarian stroma and theca cells and increased androgen production, which in turn provides more substrate for peripheral aromatization and perpetuates the chronic anovulation. In the advanced stage of the disorder, the ovary is the major site of androgen production, but the adrenal may continue to secrete excess androgen as well. Ovarian follicles from women with PCOS have low aromatase activity, but normal aromatase can be induced by treatment with FSH. An association exists between PCOS/hyperthecosis, virilization, acanthosis nigricans, and insulin resistance; in the ovary, insulin may interact via the insulin-like growth factor receptors to enhance androgen synthesis in insulin-resistant states. Women with PCOS have an increased incidence of impaired glucose tolerance and type 2 diabetes mellitus.

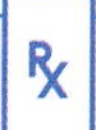

TREATMENT FOR PCOS

Treatment for PCOS is directed toward interrupting the self-perpetuating cycle and can be accomplished in several ways, such as by decreasing ovarian androgen secretion (by wedge resection or the use of oral contraceptive agents), decreasing peripheral estrogen formation (by weight reduction), or enhancing FSH secretion [by administration of clomiphene, human menopausal gonadotropin (hMG), GnRH (gonadorelin) by portable infusion pump, or purified FSH (urofollitropin)]. The choice of therapy depends on the clinical findings and the needs of the patient. An attempt at weight reduction is appropriate in all who are obese. If the woman is not hirsute and does not desire pregnancy, periodic withdrawal menses can be induced with medroxyprogesterone acetate 10 days per month; such treatment prevents the development of endometrial hyperplasia. If the woman is hirsute and does not desire pregnancy, the ovarian (and possibly the adrenal)

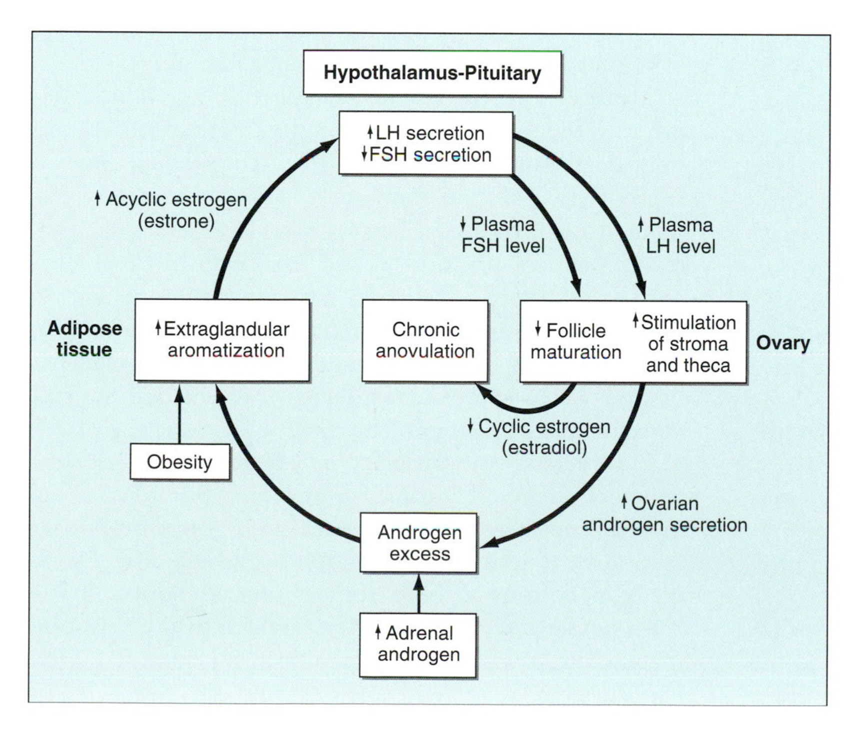

FIGURE 10-5
Proposed mechanism for the initiation and perpetuation of chronic anovulation in polycystic ovarian syndrome (PCOS). This cycle may be entered or initiated via adrenal androgen excess or obesity, both of which result in enhanced extraglandular formation of estrogens. The therapy of PCOS involves interruption of the cycle at any of several steps. *[From SSC Yen et al (eds), Reproductive Endocrinology. Philadelphia, Saunders, 1999; and from U Goebelmann, in Reproductive Endocrinology, Infertility, and Contraception, 2d ed, DR Mishell Jr, V Davajan (eds), Philadelphia, Davis, 1986.]*

component of androgen production can be suppressed with combined estrogen-progestogen oral contraceptive agents. Combined oral contraceptives are also indicated if prolonged or excessive menstrual bleeding is present. Once androgen excess is controlled, treatment of previously existing hair growth by shaving, depilatories, or electrolysis may be indicated (Chap. 12). If pregnancy is desired, ovulation must be induced. Insulin-sensitizing drugs, such as metformin and the thiazolidinediones, improve fertility in women with PCOS. Clomiphene promotes ovulation in three-fourths of cases, or ovulation can be induced with hMG, urofollitropin, or gonadorelin (Chap. 15). Pretreatment with GnRH analogues prior to use of hMG, urofollitropin, or gonadorelin may improve the rates of ovulation and pregnancy. Women with PCOS are at increased risk of ovarian hyperstimulation after treatment with gonadotropins. They also experience increased rates of spontaneous abortion. An alternative therapy is ovarian drilling by laser or cautery performed at laparoscopy when hormonal therapy is not effective; however, the procedure is associated with a high incidence of ovarian adhesions.

Chronic anovulation with estrogen present may also occur with tumors of the ovary. These include granulosa-theca cell tumors, Brenner tumors, cystic teratomas, mucous cystadenomas, and Krukenberg tumors (Chap. 13). Such tumors can either secrete excess estrogen themselves or produce androgens that are aromatized in extraglandular sites. Chronic anovulation and the clinical features of PCOS result. Occasionally, areas of the ovary not involved with tumors show the characteristic histologic changes of PCOS. Other causes of chronic anovulation with estrogen present include adrenal production of excess androgen (usually adult-onset adrenal hyperplasia due to partial 21-hydroxylase deficiency) and hypothyroidism.

Chronic Anovulation with Estrogen Absent Women with chronic anovulation who have low or absent estrogen production and do not experience withdrawal bleeding after progestogen treatment usually have hypogonadotropic hypogonadism due to disease of either the pituitary or the central nervous system.

Isolated hypogonadotropic hypogonadism associated with defects of smell (olfactory bulb defects) is known as the *Kallmann syndrome* (Chap. 2), which is due to a single gene defect in the X-linked *KAL* gene. Affected women are sexually infantile and have a defect in the synthesis and/or release of GnRH. Hypothalamic lesions that impair GnRH production and cause hypogonadotropic hypogonadism include craniopharyngioma, germinoma (pinealoma), glioma, Hand-Schüller-Christian disease, teratomas, endodermal-sinus tumors, tuberculosis, sarcoidosis, and metastatic tumors that cause suppression or destruction of the hypothalamus. Central nervous system trauma and irradiation can also cause hypothalamic amenorrhea and deficiencies in secretion of growth hormone, adrenocorticotropic hormone (ACTH), vasopressin, and thyroid hormone. Rare, autosomal recessive defects in the GnRH receptor have also been described.

More commonly, gonadotropin deficiency leading to chronic anovulation is believed to arise from functional disorders of the hypothalamus or higher centers. A history of a stressful event in a young woman is frequent. Gonadotropin and estrogen levels are in the low to low-normal range as compared with normal women in the early follicular phase of the cycle. In addition, rigorous exercise, such as jogging or ballet, and diets that result in excessive weight loss may lead to chronic anovulation, particularly in girls with a history of prior menstrual irregularity. The amenorrhea in these women does not appear to be a result of weight loss alone but a combination of a decrease in body fat and chronic stress. An extreme form of weight loss with chronic anovulation occurs in anorexia nervosa. In anorexia nervosa amenorrhea can precede, follow, or coincide with weight loss.

In addition, chronic debilitating diseases such as end-stage kidney disease, malignancy, inflammatory bowel disease, and malabsorption can lead to hypogonadotropic hypogonadism via a hypothalamic mechanism.

Treatment of chronic anovulation due to hypothalamic disorders includes ameliorating the stressful situation, decreasing exercise, and correcting weight loss, as appropriate. These women are susceptible to the development of osteoporosis; estrogen replacement therapy is recommended to induce and maintain normal secondary sexual characteristics and prevent bone loss in those who do not desire pregnancy, and gonadotropin or gonadorelin therapy is indicated when pregnancy is desired. When appropriate, therapy is directed at the primary disease of the hypothalamus.

Disorders of the pituitary can lead to the estrogen-deficient form of chronic anovulation by at least two mechanisms—direct interference with gonadotropin secretion by lesions that either obliterate or interfere with the gonadotrope cells (chromophobe adenomas, Sheehan's syndrome) or inhibition of gonadotropin secretion in association with excess prolactin (prolactinoma). *Pituitary tumors* may secrete no hormone, one hormone, or more than one hormone (Chap. 2). Prolactin levels are elevated in 50 to 70% of patients with pituitary tumors, either because of prolactin secretion by the tumor itself (in the case of prolactinomas) or because the tumor mass interferes with the normal hypothalamic inhibition of prolactin secretion.

Prolactin excess associated with low levels of LH and FSH constitutes a specific subtype of hypogonadotropic hypogonadism. One-tenth or more of amenorrheic women have increased levels of prolactin, and more than half of women with both galactorrhea and amenorrhea have elevated prolactin levels. The amenorrhea is most often associated with decreased or absent estrogen production, but prolactin-secreting tumors on occasion are associated with normal ovulatory menses or chronic anovulation with estrogen present. In the latter half of pregnancy, prolactin-secreting pituitary tumors may expand, leading to headaches, compression of the optic chiasm, bitemporal hemianopia, and blindness. Therefore, before inducing ovulation for the purposes of achieving pregnancy, it is mandatory to exclude the presence of a pituitary tumor. The evaluation, differential diagnosis, and management of hyperprolactinemia are described in Chap. 2.

Large pituitary tumors such as null cell adenomas—whether or not hyperprolactinemia is present—are likely to be associated with deficiency of hormones in addition to gonadotropins (Chap. 2).

Craniopharyngiomas, which are thought to arise from remnants of Rathke's pouch, occur most frequently in the second decade of life and often extend into the suprasellar region. Many of these tumors calcify and can be diagnosed by conventional skull film or CT. Patients often present with sexual infantilism, delayed puberty, and amenorrhea due to gonadotropin deficiency; secretion of TSH, ACTH, growth hormone, and vasopressin also may be impaired.

Panhypopituitarism can be caused by mutations in transcription factors (Pit-1; Prop-1) involved in pituitary gland development, result from surgical or radiation treatment of pituitary adenomas, or develop after postpartum hemorrhage (Sheehan's syndrome) (Chap. 2). **Table 10-2** outlines the incidence and mode of single gene mutations associated with reproductive dysfunction in women.

Evaluation of Amenorrhea A general scheme for the evaluation of women with amenorrhea is given in **Fig. 10-6.** On physical examination, attention should be given to three features: (1) the degree of maturation of the breasts, pubic and axillary hair, and external genitalia; (2) the current estrogen status; and (3) the presence or absence of a uterus. Pregnancy should be excluded in all women with amenorrhea; it is prudent to perform a suitable pregnancy screening test even when the history and physical examination are not suggestive. Once that is done, the cause of amenorrhea can frequently be diagnosed clinically. For example, Asherman's syndrome is suggested by a history of curettage in a woman who previously menstruated; in women with primary amenorrhea and sexual infantilism, the essential differential diagnosis is between gonadal dysgenesis and hypopituitarism; and the diagnosis of gonadal dysgenesis (Turner's syndrome) or of anatomical defects of the outflow tract (müllerian agenesis, testicular feminization, and cervical stenosis) is frequently suggested on the basis of physical findings. When a specific cause is suspected, it is appropriate to proceed directly to confirm the diagnosis (obtaining a chromosomal karyotype or measure-

TABLE 10-2

INCIDENCE AND MODE OF TRANSMISSION OF SINGLE-GENE MUTATIONS ASSOCIATED WITH REPRODUCTIVE DYSFUNCTION IN WOMEN

PHENOTYPE	GENE	INCIDENCE	MODE OF TRANSMISSION
Kallmann's syndrome	*KAL*	1 in 50,000	X-linked
Gonadotropin-releasing hormone resistance	*GNRHR*	Rare	Autosomal recessive
Isolated follicle-stimulating hormone deficiency	*FSHB*	Rare	Autosomal recessive
Hypergonadotropic hypogonadal ovarian failure	*FSHR*	1 in 8300 (Finland)	Autosomal recessive
Luteinizing hormone resistance	*LHR*	Rare	Autosomal recessive
Congenital lipoid adrenal hyperplasia	*STAR*	Rare	Autosomal recessive
Galactosemia	*GALT*	1 in 187,000	Autosomal recessive
McCune-Albright syndrome	*GNASI*	Rare	Dominant postzygotic mutation
Aromatase deficiency	*CYP19*	Rare	Autosomal recessive
3β-Hydroxysteroid dehydrogenase type II deficiency	*HSD3B2*	Rare	Autosomal recessive
17α-Hydroxylase deficiency	*CYP17*	Rare	Autosomal recessive

Source: From EY Adashi, JD Hennbold: Single-gene mutations resulting in reproductive dysfunction in women. N Engl J Med 340:709, 1999.

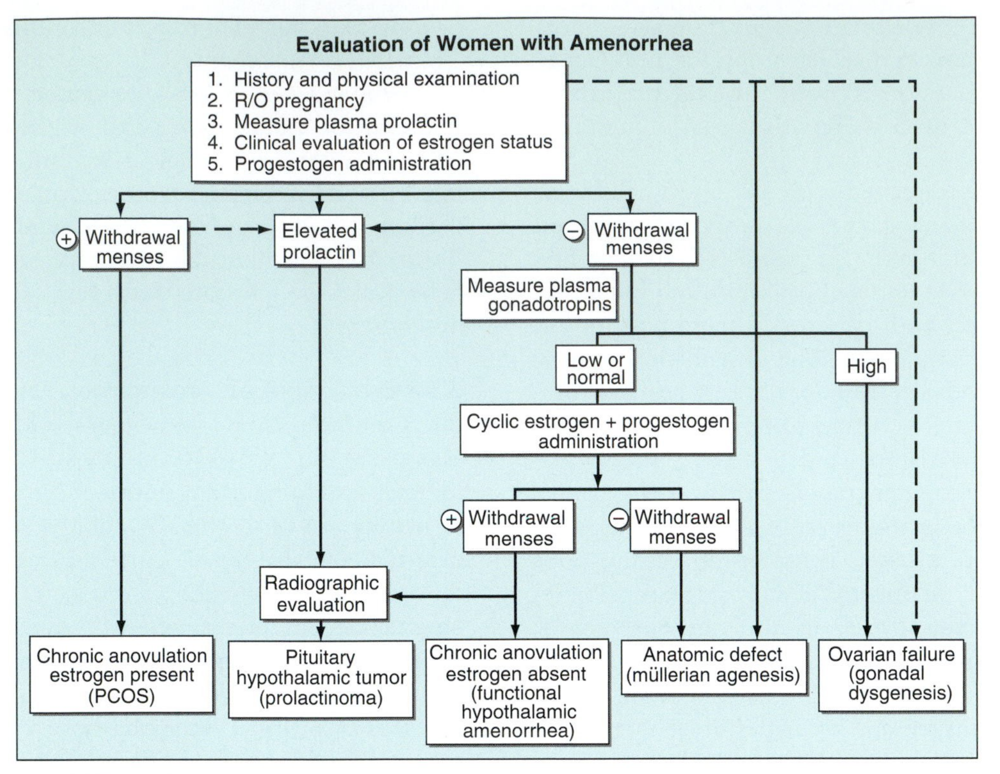

FIGURE 10-6

Flow diagram for the evaluation of women with amenorrhea. The most common diagnosis for each category is shown in parentheses. The dotted lines indicate that in some instances a correct diagnosis can be reached on the basis of history and physical examination alone. PCOS, polycystic ovarian syndrome.

ment of plasma gonadotropins). It is also useful to measure serum prolactin and FSH levels during the initial evaluation.

Estrogen status is evaluated by determining if the vaginal mucosa is moist and rugated and if the cervical mucus can be stretched and shown to fern upon drying. If these criteria are indeterminate, a progestational challenge is indicated, most often the administration of 10 mg medroxyprogesterone acetate by mouth once or twice daily for 5 days or 100 mg progesterone in oil intramuscularly. (It should be emphasized that progestogen should never be administered until pregnancy is excluded.) If estrogen levels are adequate (and the outflow tract is intact), menstrual bleeding should occur within 1 week of ending the progestogen treatment. If withdrawal bleeding occurs, the diagnosis is chronic anovulation with estrogen present, usually caused by PCOS.

If no withdrawal bleeding or only minimal vaginal spotting occurs, the nature of the subsequent workup depends on the results of the initial prolactin assay. If plasma prolactin is elevated, or if galactorrhea is present, radiography of the pituitary should be undertaken. When the plasma prolactin level is normal in an anovulatory woman with estrogen absent and with elevated FSH levels, the diagnosis is ovarian failure. If the gonadotropins are in the low or normal range, the diagnosis is either hypothalamic-pituitary disorder or an anatomical defect of the outflow tract. As indicated previously, the diagnosis of outflow tract disorder is usually suspected or established on the basis of the history and physical findings. When the physical findings are not clear-cut, it is useful to administer cyclic estrogen plus progestogen (1.25 mg oral conjugated estrogens per day for 3 weeks, with 10 mg medroxyprogesterone acetate added for the last 7 to 10 days of estrogen treatment), followed by 10 days of observation. If no bleeding occurs, the diagnosis of Asherman's syndrome or another anatomical defect of the outflow tract is confirmed by hysterosalpingography or hysteroscopy. If withdrawal bleeding occurs following the estrogen-progestogen combination, the diagnosis of chronic anovulation with estrogen absent (functional hypothalamic amenorrhea) is suggested. Radiologic evaluations of the pituitary-hypothalamic areas may be indicated in the latter cases—irrespective of the prolactin level—because of the risk of overlooking a pituitary-hypothalamic tumor and because the diagnosis of functional hypothalamic amenorrhea is one of exclusion.

Infertility

Infertility, the failure to become pregnant after 1 year of unprotected intercourse, affects approximately 10 to 15% of couples and is a common reason for seeking gynecologic assistance. Male factors account for at least 25% of infertility problems (Chap. 8). In women, failure of ovulation accounts for 40% of cases; pelvic factors, such as tubal disease or endometriosis, account for half. In 10 to 20% of infertile women no etiology is found. The evaluation and management of infertility are discussed in Chap. 15.

Pregnancy

The possibility of pregnancy should be considered in all women of reproductive age who are evaluated for medical illness or considered for surgery. Procedures such as x-ray exposure, drugs, and anesthetics may be harmful to the developing fetus, and a variety of medical problems may worsen during pregnancy, including hypertension; diseases of the heart, lungs, kidney, and liver; and metabolic and endocrine disorders. Abnormal vaginal bleeding or amenorrhea during the reproductive years should prompt consideration of a complication of pregnancy, such as incomplete abortion, ectopic pregnancy, or trophoblastic disease (hydatidiform mole or choriocarcinoma). Women who present with these complications of pregnancy often have histories of abdominal pain and vaginal bleeding and may have evidence of intra-abdominal hemorrhage.

Choriocarcinoma is a particular problem because of its protean manifestations. Half of these malignancies follow pregnancies complicated by hydatidiform mole, and the remainder occur after spontaneous abortion, ectopic pregnancy, or normal deliveries. Patients may present with intra-abdominal bleeding due to rupture of the uterus, liver, or ovary, with pulmonary manifestations (cough, hemoptysis, pleuritic pain, dyspnea, and respiratory failure) or gastrointestinal symptoms, usually chronic blood loss or melena. In addition, patients can present with cerebral metastases or renal involvement. The diagnosis can be established by demonstrating an elevated level of the β subunit of hCG in plasma. Treatment and cure are possible with chemotherapeutic agents (dactinomycin and/or methotrexate).

OTHER DISORDERS OF THE FEMALE REPRODUCTIVE TRACT

VULVA

Most disorders of the vulva are a result of sexually transmitted diseases, most commonly syphilis (painless chancre), condylomata acuminata (venereal warts), and herpes vulvitis. All other lesions of the vulva, particularly in older women, must be biopsied. Early biopsy of cancer of the vulva is mandatory, because when it becomes symptomatic (pruritus and bleeding), it has often progressed to an advanced stage.

VAGINA

Infections of the vagina usually present as vaginal discharge and pruritus. The most frequent organisms are *Trichomonas, Candida albicans,* and *Gardnerella vaginalis*. The diagnosis is made by microscopic examination of the discharge, and appropriate therapy can be instituted using vaginal or oral antibiotics.

Abnormalities of the vagina and cervix in female offspring of women given diethylstilbestrol during pregnancy include adenosis of the vagina and structural abnormalities of the vagina, cervix, and uterus; the risk of developing a rare vaginal cancer (adenocarcinoma, clear cell type) is increased (2 per 10,000 exposed women). Periodic examination of women at risk should begin at age 12 to 14, and reexamination should be done after any episode of abnormal bleeding.

CERVIX

Preinvasive lesions of the cervix (also known as *cervical intraepithelial neoplasia*) and invasive carcinoma of the cervix can be detected reliably by obtaining a Papanicolaou (Pap) smear.

Evaluation of the Pap Smear

The incidence of invasive cervical cancer has declined as a result of Pap smear screening. In the United States, approximately 2 to 3 million abnormal Pap smears are found each year. Most represent low-grade lesions but require appropriate follow-up. The follow-up of abnormal Pap smears requires an understanding of the Bethesda system for evaluating such smears (see below) and of the limitations of cytologic screening systems. Further evaluation may require repeat cytologic examination, colposcopy, or both.

Current Screening Recommendations

Risk factors for cervical neoplasia include a history of multiple sexual partners, coitus beginning at an early age, a history of infection with human papilloma virus (HPV), infection with HIV or another immunosuppressed state, and a history of cancer of the lower genital tract. Cervical cancer screening is recommended annually beginning at 18 years of age or when the woman becomes sexually active, if earlier than age 18. Less frequent screening is sufficient when three consecutive, negative, satisfactory annual Pap smears have been obtained or if the woman is in a low-risk category. There is no upper age limit for screening, because the prevalence of invasive cancer shows a linear increase with age, most of these cancers being diagnosed after age 50. Even after hysterectomy, annual screening should be performed if there is a history of abnormal Pap smears or other lower genital tract neoplasia.

The Bethesda System of Cytologic Examination

Pap smears are evaluated in regard to the adequacy of the specimen (satisfactory for evaluation, satisfactory but limited, or unsatisfactory for evaluation because of a stated reason), the general diagnosis (normal or abnormal), and a descriptive diagnosis if the smear is abnormal. The descriptive diagnoses include benign cellular changes, reactive cellular changes, and epithelial cell abnormalities, the latter including (1) atypical squamous cells of undetermined significance (ASCUS); (2) low-grade squamous intraepithelial lesion (LSIL), which is further categorized to include HPV infection, cervical intraepithelial neoplasia (CIN 1), and high-grade squamous intraepithelial lesion (HSIL), which is itself subdivided into CIN 2 and CIN 3); and (3) squamous cell carcinoma.

Guidelines for the Management of Women with Abnormal Pap Smears

For ASCUS smears that are unqualified or suggest a reactive process, a repeat smear should be obtained every 4 to 6 months for 2 years until three consecutive negative smears have been obtained. For ASCUS smears that are unqualified but have severe inflammation, any specific cause should be treated, and the smear should be repeated in 2 to 3 months; because invasive carcinoma can be obscured by severe inflammation, clinical evaluation is mandatory. For postmenopausal women not using hormone replacement, a course of topical estrogen should be applied before the test is repeated. For LSIL smears, the Pap test is repeated every 4 to 6 months for 2 years until three consecutive negative smears have been obtained; treatment of HPV is of no established benefit, and there is a high rate of regression of LSIL, so that in compliant, low-risk individuals, the outcome is usually favorable. If LSIL is persistent, colposcopy with directed biopsy is performed, and endocervical curettage is undertaken if a specific diagnosis is made by biopsy. Cervical cone biopsy or loop electrosurgical excision procedures are performed for higher-grade lesions such as HSIL. If cervical cancer is diagnosed by biopsy, clinical staging is performed, and the patient is treated with radiation therapy or surgery.

UTERUS

Only 40% of cases of endometrial adenocarcinoma are detected by Pap smear. In women at high risk for endometrial carcinoma (because of obesity, a history of chronic anovulatory cycles, diabetes mellitus, hypertension, or unopposed estrogen treatment), yearly endometrial sampling should be performed. Measurement of endometrial thickness by sonography can indicate which patients are at risk for endometrial pathology. Endometrial thickness <5 mm is rarely associated with either hyperplasia or cancer. Low-dose oral estrogen therapy rarely causes breakthrough or withdrawal bleeding in postmenopausal women. Therefore, irrespective of whether the patient is using estrogen therapy, the occurrence of postmenopausal bleeding makes it mandatory to obtain a tissue diagnosis by either endometrial sampling or curettage to exclude endometrial cancer.

One of the most common disorders of the uterus and the most frequent tumor of women (one of four women affected) is the uterine leiomyoma, or fibroid tumor. Three-fourths of women with leiomyoma are asymptomatic, and the diagnosis is made on routine pelvic examination. When the tumor is associated with excessive menstrual blood loss, is large or fast-growing, or causes significant pelvic pain (see below), the preferred treatment is hysterectomy if there is no desire for further childbearing. Embolism of the vascular supply to the tumor may be possible. In young women, myomectomy is sometimes indicated when infertility or repeated fetal wastage is a manifestation or where future childbearing is desired.

FALLOPIAN TUBES AND OVARIES

Pelvic Inflammatory Disease (PID)

This is a common disorder of the fallopian tubes and usually becomes symptomatic after a menstrual period; symptoms include fever, chills, abdominal pain, and vaginal discharge, and pelvic tenderness on physical examination is common. The initiating organism most often is *Chlamydia trachomatis* or *Neisseria gonorrhoeae,* but tuboovarian abscess and sterility are probably caused by mixed aerobic and anaerobic superinfections and require wide-spectrum antibiotic treatment.

Endometriosis

This is a benign disorder characterized by the presence and proliferation of endometrial tissue (stroma and glands) outside the endometrial cavity. The clinical manifestations are variable. Endometriosis occurs most commonly between the ages of 30 and 40 and is found incidentally at the time of surgery in approximately one-fifth of all gynecologic operations. The fertility rate is reduced in affected women. The disorder usually involves the posterior cul-de-sac or the ovaries and it occasionally involves distant sites (lung, umbilicus). The major symptom is pelvic pain, characteristically dysmenorrhea (see below). However, the frequency and severity of symptoms correlate poorly with the extent of disease. Other manifestations include dyspareunia, pain with defecation, and infertility. The characteristic physical findings are multiple tender nodules palpable along the uterosacral ligament at the time of rectal-vaginal examination, a posteriorly fixed uterus, or enlarged, cystic ovaries. The diagnosis can be confirmed only by direct visualization, usually at diagnostic laparoscopy. Treatment depends on the degree of involvement and the desires of the patient and includes observation for mild disease with no associated infertility or pain, hormonal suppressive therapy, conservative surgery by laparoscopy or laparotomy if fertility is desired, or removal of the uterus, tubes, and ovaries in severe disease. Endometriosis is rare after the menopause.

Any adnexal mass that persists for more than 6 weeks or is larger than 6 cm must be evaluated. Although ovarian cysts and neoplasms are the most common pelvic adnexal masses, tumors of the fallopian tubes, uterus, gastrointestinal tract, or urinary tract also should be considered. Sonography or radiographic evaluation is often helpful in identifying the nature of the adnexal mass prior to surgical exploration. For a discussion of ovarian tumors, see Chap. 13.

EVALUATION OF PELVIC PAIN

The evaluation of pelvic pain requires a careful history and pelvic examination. This often leads to the correct diagnosis and institution of appropriate treatment. Pelvic pain may originate in the pelvis or be referred from another region of the body. A pelvic source is suggested by the history (e.g., dysmenorrhea and dyspareunia) and physical findings, but a high index of suspicion must be entertained for extrapelvic disorders that refer to the pelvis, such as appendicitis, diverticulitis, cholecystitis, intestinal obstruction, and urinary tract infections. If the pain is severe and the diagnosis is unclear, the workup should follow that outlined for the acute abdomen.

"PHYSIOLOGIC" PELVIC PAIN

Pain Associated with Ovulation ("Mittelschmerz")

Many women experience low abdominal discomfort with ovulation, typically a dull aching pain at midcycle in one lower quadrant lasting from minutes to hours. It is rarely severe or incapacitating. The pain may result from peritoneal irritation by follicular fluid released into the peritoneal cavity at ovulation. The onset of discomfort at midcycle, and short duration of pain, suggest this diagnosis.

Premenstrual or Menstrual Pain

In normal ovulatory women, somatic symptoms during the few days prior to menses may be insignificant or disabling. Such symptoms include edema, breast engorgement, and abdominal bloating or discomfort. A symptom complex of cyclic irritability, depression, and lethargy is known as *premenstrual syndrome,* which appears to be caused by changes in gonadal steroid levels. Although there is no consensus about therapy, randomized, controlled trials suggest improvement in some women with the daily use of serotonin-reuptake inhibitors.

Severe or incapacitating uterine cramping during ovulatory menses and in the absence of demonstrable disorders of the pelvis is termed *primary dysmenorrhea.* Primary dysmenorrhea is caused by prostaglandin-induced uterine ischemia and is treated with nonsteroidal anti-inflammatory drugs and/or oral contraceptive agents.

PELVIC PAIN DUE TO ORGANIC CAUSES

Severe dysmenorrhea associated with disease of the pelvis is termed *secondary dysmenorrhea.* Organic causes of pelvic pain can be classified as (1) uterine, (2) adnexal, (3) vulvar or vaginal, and (4) pregnancy-associated.

Uterine Pain

Pain of uterine etiology is often chronic and continuous and increases in intensity during menstruation and intercourse. Causes include leiomyomas of the uterus (particularly submucous and degenerating leiomyomas), adenomyosis, and cervical stenosis. Infections of the uterus associated with intrauterine manipulation following dilatation and curettage or with the insertion of intrauterine devices also can cause pelvic pain. Pelvic pain due to endometrial or cervical cancer is usually a late manifestation.

Adnexal Pain

The most common cause of pain in the adnexae (fallopian tubes and ovaries) is infection. Acute salpingo-oophoritis presents as low abdominal pain, fever, and chills and begins a few days after a menstrual period. Chronic PID results from either a single episode or multiple episodes of infection and may present as infertility associated with chronic pelvic pain that increases in intensity with menses and intercourse. On physical examination, cervical motion tenderness, adnexal tenderness, and adnexal thickening and/or masses may be present. PID may become a surgical emergency if peritonitis results from rupture of a tuboovarian abscess. Ovarian cysts or neoplasms may cause pelvic pain that becomes more severe with torsion or rupture of the mass, and ectopic pregnancy must be considered in the differential diagnosis. If there is a question of an adnexal mass or if the patient is so obese as to preclude a thorough pelvic examination, abdominal or vaginal ultrasound may be useful. Endometriosis involving fallopian tubes, ovaries, or peritoneum may cause both chronic low abdominal pain and infertility; the magnitude of tissue involvement does not always correlate with the severity of symptoms. Endometriosis pain typically increases with menstruation and, if the posterior ligaments of the uterus are involved, with intercourse.

Vulvar or Vaginal Pain

Pain in these areas is most often due to infectious vaginitis and is characteristically associated with vaginal discharge and pruritus. Herpetic vulvitis, other dermatologic conditions of the vulva, condyloma acumination, and cysts or abscesses of Bartholin's glands also may cause vulvar pain.

Pregnancy-Associated Disorders

Pregnancy must be considered in the differential diagnosis of pelvic pain during the reproductive years. Threatened abortion or incomplete abortion often presents with uterine cramping, bleeding, or passage of tissue following a period of amenorrhea. Ectopic pregnancy may be insidious in presentation or result in abrupt intraperitoneal hemorrhage and maternal death. A culdocentesis may be indicated if a ruptured ectopic pregnancy is suspected. Serial hCG measurements may help in establishing a diagnosis of tubal pregnancy and are useful in determining if an intrauterine pregnancy is viable.

FURTHER READINGS

ALBERS JR et al: Abnormal uterine bleeding. Am Fam Physician 69:1915, 2004

This review provides practical approaches to managing abnormal uterine bleeding in women at different stages of reproductive life.

AZZIZ R et al: Androgen excess in women: experience with over 1000 consecutive patients. J Clin Endocrinol Metab 89:453, 2004

In this large study of consecutive patients presenting with clinically evident androgen excess, specific identifiable disorders (NCAH, CAH, HAIRAN syndrome, and androgen-secreting neoplasms) were observed in approximately 7% of subjects, whereas functional androgen excess, principally PCOS, was observed in the remainder. Hirsutism, menstrual dysfunction, or acne, but not alopecia, improved in the majority of patients treated with a combination suppressive therapy.

BUKULMEZ O et al: Assessment of ovarian reserve. Curr Opin Obstet Gynecol 16:231, 2004

This review highlights challenges in using hormonal measures of hormonal reserve, such as follicular phase FSH and inhibin B, or the clomiphene stimulation test, in populations with different causes of infertility.

DAVISON SL et al: Androgen levels in adult females: Changes with age, menopause, and oophorectomy. J Clin Endocrinol Metab 90:3847, 2005

This large study of 1423 healthy Australian women, ages 18 to 75, provides normative data for androgen concentrations. The study shows a gradual decrease in androgens, although the degree to which this decline reflects aging ovarian function versus a decline in adrenal precursor steroids remains unknown.

HALL JE: Neuroendocrine physiology of the early and late menopause. Endocrinol Metab Clin North Am 33:637, 2004

The progressive loss of ovarian follicles with normal aging is accompanied by an initial decrease in inhibin B and a concomitant increase in follicle-stimulating hormone. Studies in postmenopausal women suggest that there are also age-related changes in the neuroendocrine axis that are independent of the changing ovarian hormonal milieu.

HEWITT GD: Acute and chronic pelvic pain in female adolescents. Med Clin North Am 84:1009, 2000

PALMERT MR et al: Screening for abnormal glucose tolerance in adolescents with polycystic ovary syndrome. J Clin Endocrinol Metab 87:1017, 2002

◪ PALOMBA S et al: Prospective parallel randomized, double-blind, double-dummy controlled clinical trial comparing clomiphene citrate and metformin as the first-line treatment for ovulation induction in nonobese anovulatory women with polycystic ovary syndrome. J Clin Endocrinol Metab 90:4068, 2005

This study suggests that metformin may be more effective than clomiphene in the treatment of infertility in anovulatory women with PCOS.

◪ SCHMIDT D et al: The murine winged-helix transcription factor Foxl2 is required for granulosa cell differentiation and ovary maintenance. Development 131:933, 2004

Human blepharophimosis/ptosis/epicanthus inversus syndrome (BPES) type I is an autosomal dominant disorder associated with premature ovarian failure (POF) caused by mutations in FOXL2, *a winged-helix/forkhead domain transcription factor. Using targeted mutagenesis in mice, this report shows that the* Foxl2 *gene is essential for granulosa cell differentiation and ovary maintenance. In the absence of functional granulosa cells, oocytes undergo atresia and progressive follicular depletion.*

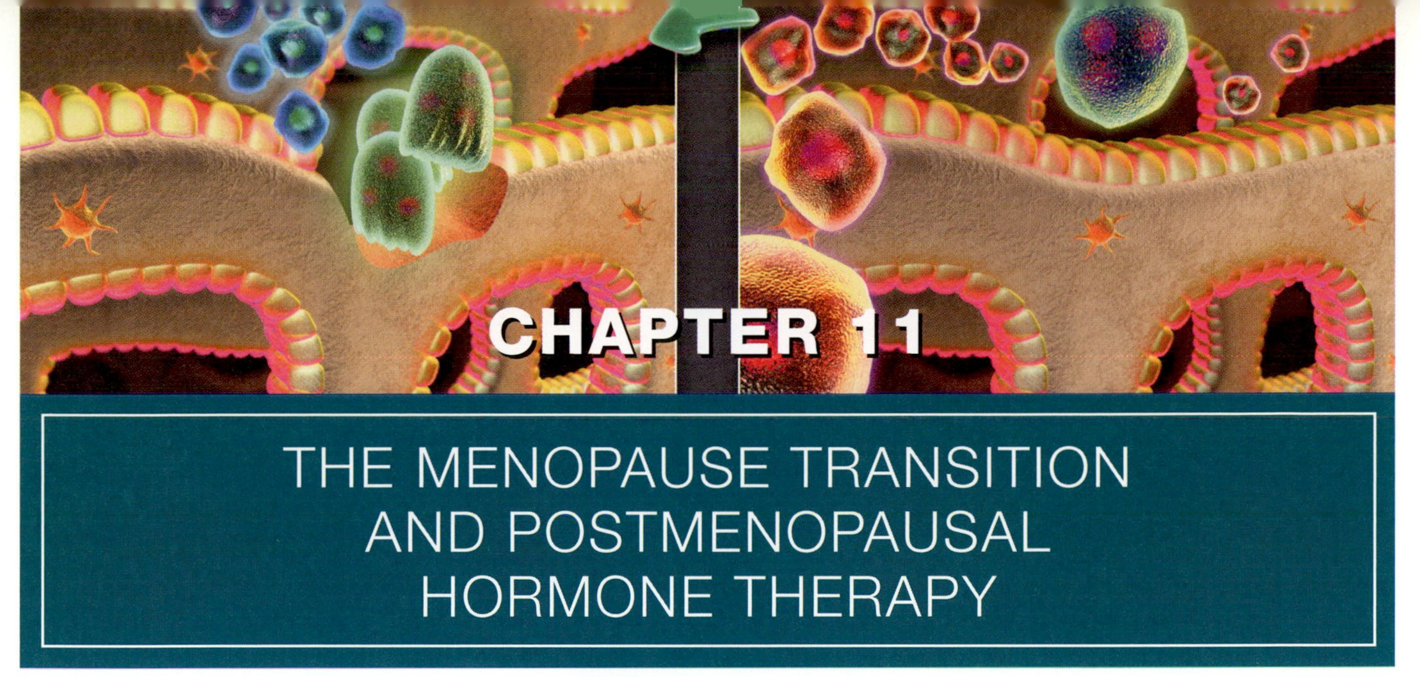

THE MENOPAUSE TRANSITION AND POSTMENOPAUSAL HORMONE THERAPY

JoAnn E. Manson
Shari S. Bassuk

Menopause is the permanent cessation of menstruation due to loss of ovarian follicular function. It is diagnosed retrospectively after 12 months of amenorrhea. The average age at menopause is 51 years among U.S. women. *Perimenopause* refers to the time period preceding menopause, when fertility wanes and menstrual cycle irregularity increases, until the first year after cessation of menses. The onset of perimenopause precedes the final menses by 2 to 8 years, with a mean duration of 4 years. Smoking accelerates the menopausal transition by 2 years.

Although the peri- and postmenopausal periods share many symptoms, the physiology and clinical management of the two periods differ. Low-dose oral contraceptives have become a therapeutic mainstay in perimenopause, whereas postmenopausal hormone therapy (HT) has been a common method of symptom alleviation after menstruation ceases.

PERIMENOPAUSE

PHYSIOLOGY

Ovarian mass and fertility decline sharply after age 35 and even more precipitously during perimenopause; depletion of primary follicles, a process that begins before birth, occurs steadily until menopause (Chap. 10). In perimenopause, intermenstrual intervals shorten significantly (typically by 3 days) due to an accelerated follicular phase. Follicle-stimulating hormone (FSH) levels rise, due to altered folliculogenesis and reduced inhibin secretion. In contrast to the consistently high FSH and low estradiol levels seen in menopause, perimenopause is characterized by "irregularly irregular" hormone levels. The propensity for anovulatory cycles can produce a hyperestrogenic, hypoprogestagenic environment that may account for the increased incidence of endometrial hyperplasia or carcinoma, uterine polyps, and leiomyoma observed among women of perimenopausal age. Mean serum levels of selected ovarian and pituitary hormones during the menopausal transition are shown in **Fig. 11-1**. With transition into menopause, estradiol levels fall markedly, whereas estrone levels are relatively preserved, reflecting peripheral aromatization of adrenal and ovarian androgens. FSH levels increase more than those of luteinizing hormone (LH), presumably because of the loss of inhibin, as well as estrogen feedback.

DIAGNOSTIC TESTS

Because of their extreme intraindividual variability, FSH and estradiol levels are imperfect diagnostic indicators of perimenopause in menstruating women. However, a low FSH in the early follicular phase (days 2 to 5) of the menstrual cycle is inconsistent with a diagnosis of perimenopause. FSH measurement can also aid in assessing fertility; levels of <20 mIU/mL, 20 to <30 mIU/mL, and ≥30 mIU/mL measured on day 3 of the cycle indicate a good, fair, and poor likelihood of achieving pregnancy, respectively.

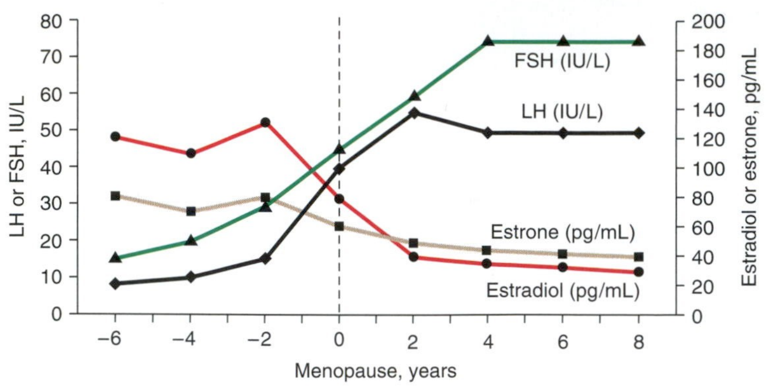

FIGURE 11-1

Mean serum levels of ovarian and pituitary hormones during the menopausal transition. FSH, follicle-stimulating hormone; LH, luteinizing hormone. *(From JL Shifren, I Schiff: The aging ovary. J Women's Health Gend-Based Med 9:S–3, 2000, with permission.)*

SYMPTOMS

Anovulatory cycles may be associated with irregular bleeding. Some perimenopausal women experience classic postmenopausal symptoms such as hot flashes and night sweats, insomnia, vaginal dryness, mood swings, or depression. In one U.S. study, nearly 60% of women reported hot flashes in the 2 years before their final menses. Symptom intensity, duration, and frequency are highly variable.

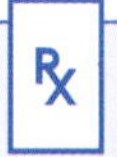

TREATMENT IN PERIMENOPAUSE

For women with irregular or heavy menses or hormonally related symptoms that impair quality of life, low-dose combined oral contraceptives are a staple of therapy. Static doses of estrogen and progestin (e.g., 20 μg of ethinyl estradiol and 1 mg of norethindrone acetate daily for 21 days each month) can eliminate vasomotor symptoms and restore regular cyclicity. Oral contraceptives provide other benefits, including protection against ovarian and endometrial cancers and increased bone density, although it is not clear whether use during perimenopause decreases fracture risk later in life. Moreover, the contraceptive benefit is important, given that the unintentional pregnancy rate among women in their forties rivals that of adolescents. Contraindications to oral contraceptive use include cigarette smoking, liver disease, a history of thromboembolism or cardiovascular disease, breast cancer, or unexplained vaginal bleeding. Progestin-only formulations (e.g., 0.35 mg norethindrone daily) or medroxyprogesterone (Depo-Provera) injections (e.g., 150 mg intramuscularly every 3 months) may provide an alternative for the treatment of perimenopausal menorrhagia in women who smoke or have cardiovascular risk factors. Although progestins neither regularize cycles nor reduce the number of bleeding days, they reduce the volume of menstrual flow.

Nonhormonal strategies to reduce menstrual flow include use of nonsteroidal anti-inflammatory agents such as mefenamic acid (initial dose of 500 mg at start of menses, then 250 mg qid for 2 to 3 days) or, when medical approaches fail, endometrial ablation. It should be noted that menorrhagia requires an evaluation to rule out uterine disorders. Transvaginal ultrasound with saline enhancement is useful for detecting leiomyomata or polyps, and endometrial aspiration can identify hyperplastic changes.

TRANSITION TO MENOPAUSE

For sexually active women using contraceptive hormones to alleviate perimenopausal symptoms, the question of when and if to switch to HT must be individualized. Estrogen and progestin doses in HT are lower than those in oral contraceptives and have not been documented to prevent pregnancy. Although a 1-year absence of spontaneous menses reliably indicates ovulation cessation, it is not possible to assess the natural menstrual pattern while a woman is taking an oral contraceptive. Women willing to switch to a barrier method of contraception should do so; if menses occur spontaneously, oral contraceptive use can be resumed. The average age of final menses among relatives can serve as a guide for when to initiate this process, which can be repeated yearly until menopause has occurred.

MENOPAUSE AND POSTMENOPAUSAL HORMONE THERAPY

One of the most complex health care decisions facing women is whether to use postmenopausal hormone therapy(HT). HT, once prescribed primarily to relieve vasomotor symptoms, has been promoted as a strategy to forestall various disorders that accelerate after menopause, including osteoporosis and cardiovascular disease. More than 30% of postmenopausal women in the United States currently use HT. This widespread use is unwarranted given the paucity of conclusive data, until very recently, on the health consequences of such therapy. Although many women rely on their health care providers for a definitive answer to the question of whether to use postmenopausal hormones, balancing the benefits and risks for an individual patient is challenging.

Although observational studies suggest that HT prevents cardiovascular and other chronic diseases, the apparent benefits may result at least in part from differences between women who opt to take postmenopausal hormones and women who do not. Those choosing HT tend to be healthier, have greater access to medical care, are more compliant with prescribed treatments, and maintain a more health-promoting lifestyle. Randomized trials, which eliminate these confounding factors, have not consistently confirmed the benefits found in observational studies. Indeed, one arm of the largest trial of HT to date, the Women's Health Initiative (WHI), which examined more than 16,000 postmenopausal women for an average of 5.2 years, was stopped early because of an overall unfavorable risk-benefit ratio associated with estrogen-progestin therapy.

The following summary offers a decision-making guide based on a synthesis of currently available evidence. The decision is divided into one of short- (<5 years) or long-term (≥5 years) use of HT. Prevention of cardiovascular disease is eliminated from the equation due to lack of evidence for such benefits in recent randomized clinical trials.

BENEFITS AND RISKS OF POSTMENOPAUSAL HORMONE THERAPY (Table 11-1)

DEFINITE BENEFITS

Symptoms Of Menopause

Compelling evidence, including data from randomized clinical trials, indicates that estrogen therapy is highly effective for controlling vasomotor and genitourinary symptoms. Alternative approaches, including the use of antidepressants (such as venlafaxine, 75 to 150 mg/d), clonidine (0.1 to 0.2 mg/d), or vitamin E (400 to 800 IU/d) or the consumption of soy-based products or other phytoestrogens, also may alleviate vasomotor symptoms, although they are less effective than HT. For genitourinary symptoms, the efficacy of vaginal estrogen is similar to that of oral or transdermal estrogen.

Osteoporosis (see also Chap. 25)

Bone Density By reducing bone turnover and resorption rates, estrogen slows the aging-related bone loss experienced by most postmenopausal women. More than 50 randomized trials have demonstrated that postmenopausal estrogen therapy, with or without a progestin, rapidly increases bone mineral density at the spine by 4 to 6% and at the hip by 2 to 3%, and maintains those increases during treatment.

Fractures Data from observational studies indicate a 50 to 80% lower risk of vertebral fracture and a 25 to 30% lower risk of hip, wrist, and other peripheral fractures among current estrogen users; addition of a progestin does not appear to modify this benefit. Discontinuation of estrogen therapy leads to a diminution of protection. In the WHI, 5 to 6 years of either combined estrogen-progestin or estrogen-only therapy was associated with a 30 to 40% reduction in hip fracture and 20 to 30% fewer total fractures among a population unselected for osteoporosis. Bisphosphonates (such as alendronate, 10 mg/d or 70 mg once per week or risedronate, 5 mg/d or 35 mg once a week) and raloxifene (60 mg/d), a selective estrogen receptor modulator (SERM), have each been shown in randomized trials to increase bone mass density and to decrease fracture rates. These agents, unlike estrogen, do not appear to have adverse effects on the endometrium or breast. Increased physical activity and adequate calcium (1000 to 1500 mg/d in two to three divided doses) and vitamin D (400 to 800 IU/d) intakes also may reduce the risk of osteoporosis-related fractures.

DEFINITE RISKS

Endometrial Cancer

A combined analysis of 30 observational studies found a tripling of risk of endometrial cancer among short-term (1 to 5 years) users of unopposed estrogen and a nearly tenfold increased risk among users for 10 or more years. These findings are supported by results from the randomized Postmenopausal Estrogen/Progestin Interventions (PEPI) trial, in which 24% of women assigned to unopposed estrogen for 3 years developed atypical endometrial hyperplasia, a premalignant lesion, compared with only 1% of women assigned to placebo. Use of a progestin, which opposes the effects of estrogen on the endometrium, eliminates these risks.

Venous Thromboembolism

A recent meta-analysis of 12 studies—8 case-control, 1 cohort, and 3 randomized trials—found that current

TABLE 11-1

BENEFITS AND RISKS OF POSTMENOPAUSAL HORMONE THERAPY (HT)

VARIABLE	EFFECT	BENEFIT OR RISK		SOURCES OF EVIDENCE
		RELATIVE	ABSOLUTE	
DEFINITE BENEFITS				
Symptoms of menopause (vasomotor, genitourinary)	Definite improvement	>70 to 80% decrease		Observational studies and randomized trials
Osteoporosis	Definite increase in bone mineral density and decrease in fracture risk	2–5% increase in bone density; 25–50% decrease in risk of fractures	WHI: 50 fewer hip fractures (100 vs. 150) per 100,000 woman-years	Observational studies and randomize trials, including WHI
DEFINITE RISKS				
Endometrial cancer	Definite increase in risk with use of unopposed[a] estrogen; no increase with use of estrogen plus progestin	8-to 10-fold increased risk with use of unopposed estrogen for ≥10 yr; no excess risk with estrogen-progestin therapy	46 excess cases (52 vs. 6) per 100,000 woman-years of unopposed estrogen use (≥ 10 years of use); no excess with estrogen-progestin therapy	Observational studies and randomized trials
Venous thromboembolism	Definite increase in risk	≥2-fold increase	Secondary prevention: 390 excess cases per 100,000 woman-years	Randomized trial (HERS)
			Primary prevention: 180 excess cases per 100,000 woman-years	Observational studies and randomized trial (WHI)
Breast cancer	Increase in risk with long-term use (≥5 yr)	1.35-fold overall increase with HT use ≥5 yr	10–30 excess cases per 10,000 women using HT for 5 yr; 30–90 excess cases after 10 yr of use; 50–200 excess cases after 15 yr of use	Observational data (meta-analysis of 51 studies)
		25–30% increase with 5.2 yr of estrogen-progestin therapy; no increase with estrogen-only	WHI: 80 excess cases (300 vs. 380) per 100,000 woman-years of estrogen-progestin therapy	Randomized trials (WHI, HERS)
PROBABLE OR UNCERTAIN RISKS AND BENEFITS				
Cardiovascular disease				
Primary prevention	Probable increase in risk	WHI: 29% increase in CHD with estrogen-progestin: no apparent increase or decrease with estrogen-only	WHI: 70 excess cases (370 vs. 300) of CHD per 100,000 woman- years with estrogen-progestin	Observational studies suggest a 35–50% decrease in risk, while randomized trials show no effect or a harmful effect; most studies have assessed conjugated equine estrogen alone or in combination with medroxyprogesterone acetate
		40% increase in stroke with either estrogen-progestin or estrogen-only	80 excess cases (290 vs. 210) of stroke per 100,000 woman-years	

(Continued)

TABLE 11-1 *(Continued)*

BENEFITS AND RISKS OF POSTMENOPAUSAL HORMONE THERAPY (HT)

VARIABLE	EFFECT	BENEFIT OR RISK: RELATIVE	BENEFIT OR RISK: ABSOLUTE	SOURCE OF EVIDENCE
Secondary prevention	Probable early increase in risk	HERS: 50% increase in CHD in year 1; no overall effect over 4 years	Equal number of CHD cases over 4 years	Observational studies and randomized secondary prevention trials
Gallbladder disease	Probable increase in risk	1.4-fold increase	360 excess cases per 100,000 woman-years	Randomized trials (HERS)
Colorectal cancer	Probable decrease in risk	20–37% decrease with estrogen-progestin	24–60 fewer cases per 100,000 woman-years	Observational data, randomized trial (WHI)
Cognitive dysfunction	Unproven decrease in risk	Apparent increase in dementia after age 65	Uncertain	Inconsistent data from observational studies and randomized trials

[a]"Unopposed estrogen" refers to the use of estrogen without progestin.
Note: WHI, Women's Health Initiative; HERS, Hearth and Estrogen/progestin Replacement Study; CHD, coronary heart disease.

Source: Manson JE, Martin KA: Clinical practice: Postmenopausal hormone-replacement therapy. N Engl J Med 345:34, 2001.

estrogen use was associated with a doubling of risk for venous thromboembolism in postmenopausal women. Relative risks of thromboembolic events were even greater (2.7 to 5.1) in the three trials included in the meta-analysis. Results from the WHI indicate a twofold increase in risk of venous and pulmonary thromboembolism.

Breast Cancer

An increased risk of breast cancer has been found among current or recent estrogen users in observational studies; this risk is directly related to duration of use. In a meta-analysis of 51 case-control and cohort studies, short-term use (<5 years) of postmenopausal hormone therapy did not appreciably elevate breast cancer incidence, whereas long-term use (≥5 years) was associated with a 35% increase in risk. In contrast to findings for endometrial cancer, combined estrogen-progestin regimens appear to increase breast cancer risk more than estrogen alone. Data from randomized trials also indicate that HT raises breast cancer risk. In the WHI, women assigned to receive combination therapy for an average of 5.2 years were 26% more likely to develop breast cancer than women assigned to placebo, but estrogen-only therapy did not increase risk. In the Heart and Estrogen/progestin Replacement Study (HERS), 4 years of combination therapy was associated with a 27% increase in breast cancer risk. Although the latter finding was not statistically significant, the totality of evidence strongly implicates estrogen-progestin therapy in breast carcinogenesis.

PROBABLE OR UNCERTAIN RISKS AND BENEFITS

Coronary Heart Disease/Stroke

Until recently, HT had been enthusiastically recommended as a possible cardioprotective agent. In the past three decades, multiple observational studies suggested, in the aggregate, that estrogen use leads to a 35 to 50% reduction in coronary heart disease incidence among postmenopausal women. The biologic plausibility of such an association is supported by data from randomized trials demonstrating that exogenous estrogen lowers plasma low-density lipoprotein (LDL) cholesterol and raises high-density lipoprotein (HDL) cholesterol levels by 10 to 15%. Administration of estrogen also favorably affects lipoprotein(a) levels, LDL oxidation, endothelial vascular function, and fibrinogen and plasminogen activator inhibitor-1. However, estrogen therapy also has unfavorable effects on other biomarkers of cardiovascular risk; it boosts triglyceride levels; promotes coagulation via factor VII, prothrombin fragments 1 and 2, and fibrinopeptide A elevations; and raises levels of the inflammatory marker C-reactive protein.

Randomized trials of estrogen or combined estrogen-progestin in women with preexisting cardiovascular disease have not confirmed the benefits reported in observational studies. In HERS, a secondary prevention trial designed to test the efficacy and safety of estrogen-progestin therapy on clinical cardiovascular outcomes, the 4-year incidence of coronary mortality and nonfatal myocardial infarction was similar in the active treatment and placebo groups, and a 50% increase in risk of coronary events was noted during the first year of the study among participants assigned to the active treatment group. Although it is possible that progestin may mitigate estrogen's benefits, the Estrogen Replacement and Atherosclerosis (ERA) trial indicated that angiographically determined progression of coronary atherosclerosis was unaffected by either opposed or unopposed estrogen treatment. Moreover, the Papworth Hormone Replacement Therapy Atherosclerosis Study, a trial of transdermal estradiol with and without norethindrone, the Women's Estrogen for Stroke Trial (WEST), a trial of oral 17β-estradiol, and the EStrogen in the Prevention of ReInfarction Trial (ESPRIT), a trial of oral estradiol valerate, found no cardiovascular benefits of the regimens studied. Thus, in clinical trials, HT has not proved effective for the secondary prevention of cardiovascular disease in postmenopausal women.

Primary prevention trials also suggest an early increase in cardiovascular risk and absence of cardioprotection with postmenopausal HT. Results from the large-scale WHI suggest a deleterious cardiovascular effect of hormone therapy. Women assigned to 5 years of estrogen-progestin therapy were 29% more likely to develop coronary heart disease and 41% more likely to suffer a stroke than those assigned to placebo. In the estrogen-only arm of the WHI, a similar increase in stroke and no effect on CHD were observed. Further research is needed on clinical characteristics as well as on biomarkers that predict increases or decreases in cardiovascular risk associated with exogenous hormone therapy. Whether different doses, formulations, or routes of administration of hormone therapy will produce different cardiovascular effects remains uncertain.

Gallbladder Disease

Several large observational studies report a two- to threefold increased risk of gallstones or cholecystectomy among postmenopausal women taking estrogen. In HERS, women randomized to 4 years of estrogen-progestin therapy had a 38% greater risk of developing gallbladder disease than those assigned to placebo, a risk that climbed to 48% after 2.7 additional years of observational follow-up.

Colorectal Cancer

Observational studies have suggested that HT reduces risks of colon and rectal cancer, although the estimated magnitudes of the relative benefits ranged from 8 to 33% in various meta-analyses. In the WHI, the only trial to examine the issue, estrogen-progestin therapy was associated with a significant 37% reduction in colorectal cancer over a 5-year period; no benefit was seen with estrogen-only therapy.

Cognitive Decline and Dementia

A meta-analysis of 10 case-control and 2 cohort studies suggested that postmenopausal HT is associated with a 33% decreased risk of dementia. Subsequent randomized trials, however, failed to demonstrate any benefit of estrogen therapy on the progression of mild to moderate Alzheimer's disease and indicated a potential adverse effect of estrogen-progestin therapy on the incidence of dementia.

Ovarian Cancer and Other Disorders

On the basis of limited observational and randomized data, it has been hypothesized that HT increases the risk of ovarian cancer and reduces the risk of type 2 diabetes mellitus. These hypotheses require confirmation in additional clinical trials.

APPROACH TO THE POSTMENOPAUSAL PATIENT

The rational use of postmenopausal hormone therapy requires balancing the potential benefits and risks. **Figure 11-2** provides one approach to decision-making. The clinician should first determine whether the patient has an indication for initiating HT. Relief of menopausal symptoms and prevention of osteoporosis are the most valid reasons. The benefits and risks of such therapy should then be reviewed with the patient, giving more emphasis to absolute than to relative measures of effect, and pointing out uncertainties in clinical knowledge where relevant. Potential side effects—especially vaginal bleeding that may result from use of combined estrogen-progestin formulations recommended for women with an intact uterus—should be noted. The patient's own preference regarding therapy should be elicited and factored into the decision. Contraindications to HT should be assessed routinely and include unexplained vaginal bleeding, active liver disease, venous thromboembolism, or history of endometrial cancer (except stage 1 without deep invasion) or breast cancer. Relative contraindications include hypertriglyceridemia (>400 mg/dL) and active gallbladder disease (in such cases, transdermal estrogen is an option). Neither primary nor secondary prevention of heart disease should be viewed as an expected benefit of HT, and an increase in stroke and a small early increase in coronary artery disease risk should be considered. Nevertheless, such therapy may be

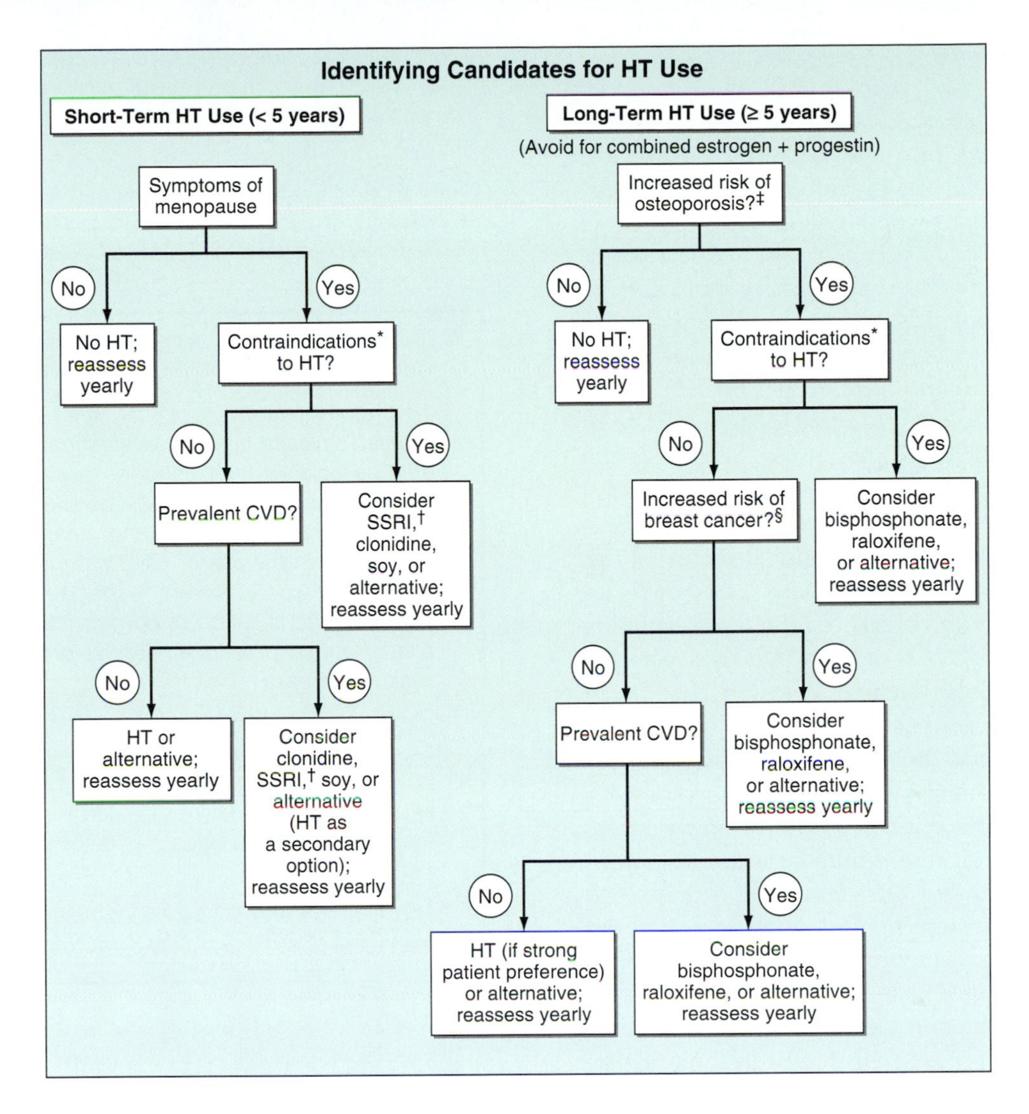

FIGURE 11-2

Flowchart for identifying appropriate candidates for short-term and long-term use of postmenopausal hormone therapy (HT). *Contraindications include unexplained vaginal bleeding, active liver disease, venous thromboembolism, or history of endometrial cancer (except stage 1 without deep invasion) or breast cancer. Relative contraindications include hypertriglyceridemia (>400 mg/dL) and active gallbladder disease (in such cases, transdermal estrogen is an option). †SSRI denotes selective serotonin reuptake inhibitor. ‡Increased risk of osteoporosis: documented osteopenia or osteoporosis, personal or family history of nontraumatic fracture, current smoking, or a body mass index <22 kg/m^2. §Increased risk of breast cancer: one or more first-degree relatives with breast cancer; susceptibility genes such as *BRCA1* or *BRCA2*; or a personal history of breast biopsy demonstrating atypia. CVD, cardiovascular disease. *(Manson JE, Martin KA: Clinical practice: Postmenopausal hormone-replacement therapy. N Engl J Med 345:34, 2001. Copyright © 2001 Massachusetts Medical Society. Used with permission.)*

appropriate, if the noncoronary benefits of treatment clearly outweigh risks. A woman who suffers an acute coronary event or stroke while on HT should stop therapy immediately.

Short-term use (<5 years) of HT is appropriate for relief of menopausal symptoms among women without contraindications to such use. However, such therapy should be avoided or considered only as a secondary option among women with preexisting heart disease or stroke due to their elevated baseline risk of future cardiovascular events. Women who have contraindications, or are opposed to HT, may derive benefit from the use of selective antidepressants, clonidine, or soy, and, for genitourinary symptoms, intravaginal estrogen creams or devices.

Long-term use (≥5 years) of HT is more problematic because a heightened risk of breast cancer must be factored into the decision. Reasonable candidates for such use include a small percentage of postmenopausal women and comprise those who have persistent severe vasomotor symptoms and/or have an increased risk of osteoporosis (e.g., those with osteopenia, a personal or family history of nontraumatic fracture, or a body mass index <22 kg/m^2), who also have no personal or family history of breast cancer in a first-degree relative or other contraindications, and who have a strong personal preference for therapy. Poor candidates are women with cardiovascular disease, those at low risk of osteoporosis, and those at increased risk of breast cancer (e.g., women who have a first-degree relative with breast cancer, susceptibility genes such as BRCA1 or BRCA2, or a personal history of cellular atypia detected by breast biopsy). Even in reasonable candidates, strategies to minimize dose and duration of use should be employed. For example, women using hormone replacement to relieve intense vasomotor symptoms in early postmenopause should consider discontinuing therapy before 5 years, resuming it only if vasomotor symptoms persist and/or an increased risk of osteoporosis is evident. In the latter situation, alternative therapies such as bisphosphonates or SERMs should be considered. Research on androgen-containing preparations has been limited, particularly in terms of long-term safety.

In addition to HT, control of symptoms and prevention of chronic disease can be accomplished by lifestyle choices, including smoking abstention, adequate physical activity, and a healthy diet. An expanding array of pharmacologic options—e.g., bisphosphonates or SERMs for osteoporosis, and cholesterol-lowering or antihypertensive agents for cardiovascular disease—also should reduce the widespread reliance on hormone use. However, short-term HT may still benefit some women.

FURTHER READINGS

Cushman M et al: Estrogen plus progestin and risk of venous thrombosis. JAMA 292:1573, 2004

Estrogen plus progestin doubles the risk of venous thrombosis. Estrogen plus progestin therapy increased the risks associated with age, overweight or obesity, and factor V Leiden.

Gabriel SR et al: Hormone replacement therapy for preventing cardiovascular disease in post-menopausal women. Cochrane Database Syst Rev CD002229, 2005

Grady D et al: Cardiovascular disease outcomes during 6.8 years of hormone therapy: Heart and Estrogen/progestin Replacement Study follow-up (HERS II). JAMA 288:49, 2002

Manson JE et al: Estrogen plus progestin and the risk of coronary heart disease. N Engl J Med 349:523, 2003

This study summarizes the final results from the Women's Health Initiative evaluating the risks and benefits associated with estrogen and progestin therapy after menopause. The study concludes that estrogen plus progestin does not confer cardiac protection and may increase the risk of CHD among generally healthy postmenopausal women, especially during the first year after the initiation of hormone use. This treatment should not be prescribed for the prevention of cardiovascular disease.

National Institutes of Health: National Institutes of Health State-of-the-Science Conference statement: Management of menopause-related symptoms. Ann Intern Med 142:1003, 2005

This is a comprehensive review, by an expert panel, of managing postmenopausal symptoms.

Nelson HD: Commonly used types of postmenopausal estrogen for treatment of hot flashes: Scientific review. JAMA 291:1610, 2004

Rossouw JE et al: Risks and benefits of estrogen plus progestin in healthy postmenopausal women. Principal results from the Women's Health Initiative randomized controlled trial. Writing Group for the Women's Health Initiative Investigators. JAMA 288:321, 2002

Wassertheil-Smoller S et al: Effect of estrogen plus progestin on stroke in postmenopausal women: The Women's Health Initiative: A randomized trial. JAMA 289:2673, 2003

This report demonstrates that estrogen plus progestin increases the risk of ischemic stroke in generally healthy postmenopausal women.

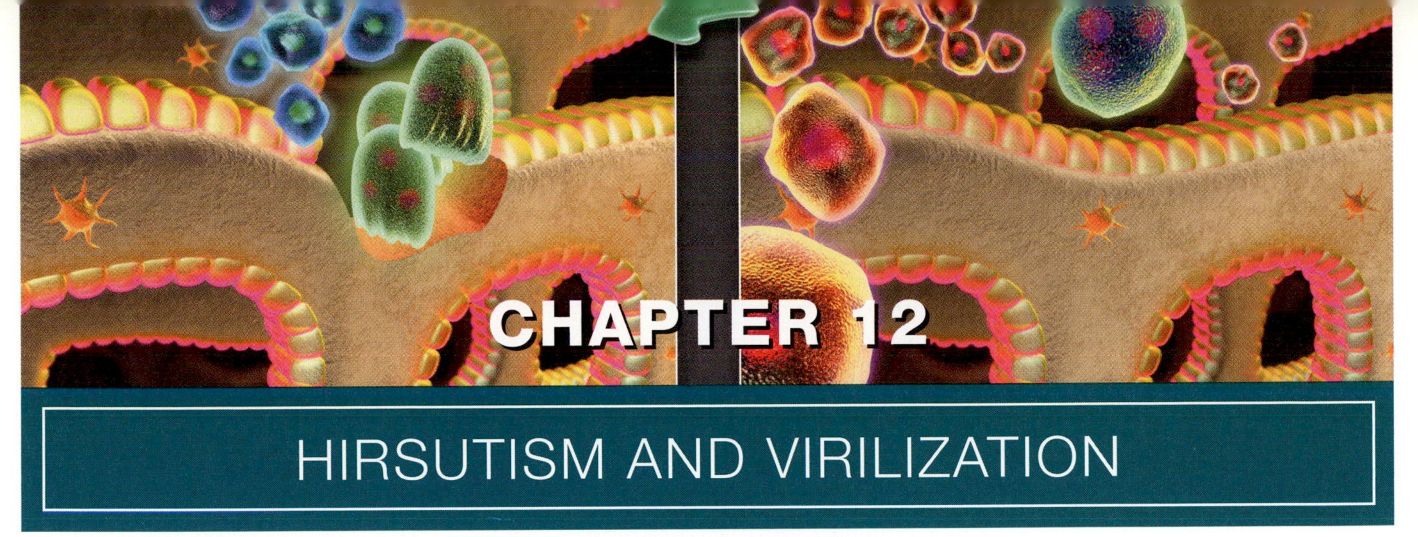

HIRSUTISM AND VIRILIZATION

David A. Ehrmann

Hirsutism, defined as excessive male-pattern hair growth, affects approximately 10% of women. If often represents a variation of normal hair growth, but rarely it is a harbinger of a serious underlying condition. Hirsutism is often idiopathic but may be caused by conditions associated with androgen excess, such as polycystic ovarian syndrome (PCOS) or congenital adrenal hyperplasia (CAH) (**Table 12-1**). Cutaneous manifestations commonly associated with hirsutism include acne and male-pattern balding (androgenic alopecia). *Virilization* refers to the state in which androgen levels are sufficiently high to cause additional signs and symptoms such as deepening of the voice, breast atrophy, increased muscle bulk, clitoromegaly, and increased libido; virilization is an ominous sign that suggests the possibility of an ovarian or adrenal neoplasm.

HAIR FOLLICLE GROWTH AND DIFFERENTIATION

Hair can be categorized as either *vellus* (fine, soft, and not pigmented) or *terminal* (long, coarse, and pigmented). The number of hair follicles does not change over an individual's lifetime, but the follicle size and type of hair can change in response to numerous factors, particularly androgens. Androgens are necessary for terminal hair and sebaceous gland development and mediate differentiation of pilosebaceous units (PSUs) into either a terminal hair follicle or a sebaceous gland. In the former case, androgens transform the vellus hair into a terminal hair; in the latter, the sebaceous component proliferates and the hair remains vellus.

There are three phases in the cycle of hair growth: (1) *anagen* (growth phase), (2) *catagen* (involution phase), and (3) *telogen* (rest phase). Depending on the body site, hormonal regulation may play an important role in the hair growth cycle. For example, the eyebrows, eyelashes, and vellus hairs are androgen-insensitive, whereas the axil-

TABLE 12-1

CAUSES OF HIRUSTISM
Gonadal hyperandrogenism
Ovarian hyperandrogenism
Polycystic ovary syndrome/functional ovarian hyperandrogenism
Ovarian steroidogenic blocks
Syndromes of extreme insulin resistance
Ovarian neoplasms
Adrenal hyperandrogenism
Premature adrenarche
Functional adrenal hyperandrogenism
Congenital adrenal hyperplasia (nonclassic and classic)
Abnormal cortisol action/metabolism
Adrenal neoplasms
Other endocrine disorders
Cushing's syndrome
Hyperprolactinemia
Acromegaly
Peripheral androgen overproduction
Obesity
Idiopathic
Pregnancy-related hyperandrogenism
Hyperreactio luteinalis
Thecoma of pregnancy
Drugs
Androgens
Oral contraceptives containing androgenic progestins
Minoxidil
Phenytoin
Diazoxide
Cyclosporine
True hermaphroditism

lary and pubic areas are sensitive to low levels of androgens. Hair growth on the face, chest, upper abdomen, and back requires greater levels of androgens and is therefore more characteristic of the pattern typically seen in males. Androgen excess in women leads to increased hair growth in most androgen-sensitive sites except in the scalp region, where hair loss occurs because androgens cause scalp hairs to spend less time in the anagen phase.

Although androgen excess underlies most cases of hirsutism, there is only a modest correlation between androgen levels and the quantity of hair growth. This is due to the fact that hair growth from the follicle also depends on local growth factors, and there is variability in end-organ sensitivity. Genetic factors and ethnic background also influence hair growth. In general, dark-haired individuals tend to be more hirsute than blonde or fair individuals. Asians and Native Americans have relatively sparse hair in regions sensitive to high androgen levels, whereas people of Mediterranean descent are more hirsute.

CLINICAL ASSESSMENT

Historic elements relevant to the assessment of hirsutism include the age of onset and rate of progression of hair growth and associated symptoms or signs (e.g., acne). Depending on the cause, excess hair growth is typically first noted during the second and third decades. The growth is usually slow but progressive. Sudden development and rapid progression of hirsutism suggests the possibility of an androgen-secreting neoplasm, in which case virilization may also be present.

The age of onset of menstrual cycles (menarche) and the pattern of the menstrual cycle should be ascertained; irregular cycles from the time of menarche onward are more likely to result from ovarian rather than adrenal androgen excess. Associated symptoms such as galactorrhea should prompt evaluation for hyperprolactinemia (Chap. 2) and possibly hypothyroidism (Chap. 4). Hypertension, striae, easy bruising, centripetal weight gain, and weakness suggest hypercortisolism (Cushing's syndrome; Chap. 5). Rarely, patients with growth hormone excess (i.e., acromegaly) will present with hirsutism. Use of medications such as phenytoin, minoxidil, or cyclosporine may be associated with androgen-independent causes of excess hair growth (i.e., hypertrichosis). A family history of infertility and/or hirsutism may indicate disorders such as nonclassic CAH (Chap. 5).

Physical examination should include measurement of height, weight, and calculation of body mass index (BMI). A BMI >25 kg/m^2 is indicative of excess weight for height, and values >30 kg/m^2 are often seen in association with hirsutism. Notation should be made of blood pressure, as adrenal causes may be associated with hypertension. Cutaneous signs sometimes associated with androgen excess and insulin resistance include acanthosis nigricans and skin tags.

An objective clinical assessment of hair distribution and quantity is central to the evaluation in any woman presenting with hirsutism. This assessment permits the distinction between hirsutism and hypertrichosis and provides a baseline reference point to gauge the response to treatment. A simple and commonly used method to grade hair growth is the modified scale of Ferriman and Gallwey (**Fig. 12-1**), where each of nine androgen-sensitive sites is graded from 0 to 4. Approximately 95% of Caucasian women have a score below 8 on this scale; thus, it is normal for most women to have some hair growth in androgen-sensitive sites. Scores above 8 suggest excess androgen-mediated hair growth, a finding that should be assessed further by hormonal evaluation (see below). In racial/ethnic groups that are less likely to manifest hirsutism (e.g., Asian women), additional cutaneous evidence of androgen excess should be sought, including pustular acne or thinning hair.

HORMONAL EVALUATION

Androgens are secreted by the ovaries and adrenal glands in response to their respective tropic hormones, luteinizing hormone (LH) and adrenocorticotropic hormone (ACTH). The principal circulating steroids involved in the etiology of hirsutism are testosterone, androstenedione, dehydroepiandrosterone (DHEA) and its sulfated form (DHEAS). The ovaries and adrenal glands normally contribute about equally to testosterone production. Approximately half of the total testosterone originates from direct glandular secretion, and the remainder is derived from the peripheral conversion of androstenedione and DHEA (Chap. 8).

Although it is the most important circulating androgen, testosterone is, in effect, the penultimate androgen in mediating hirsutism; it is converted to the more potent dihydrotestosterone (DHT) by the enzyme 5α-

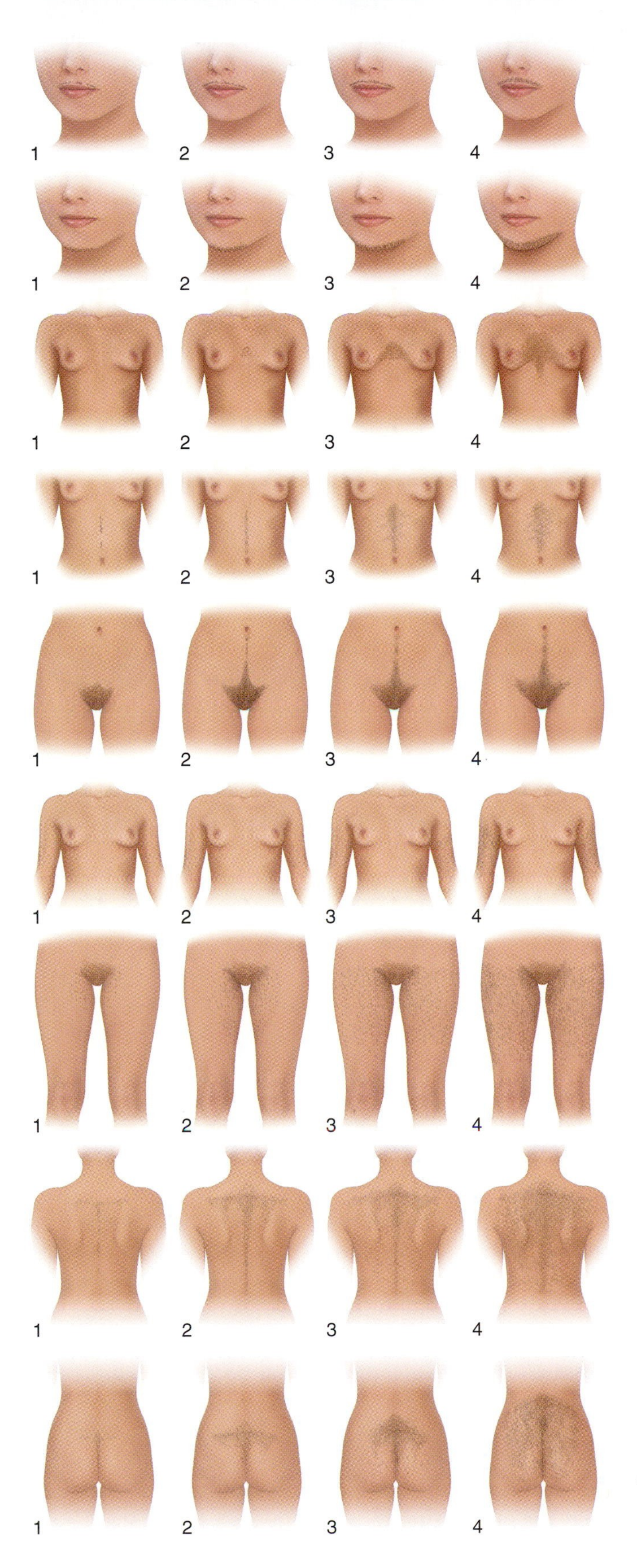

reductase, which is located in the PSU. DHT has a higher affinity for, and slower dissociation from, the androgen receptor. The local production of DHT allows it to serve as the primary mediator of androgen action at the level of the pilosebaceous unit. There are two isoenzymes of 5α-reductase: type 2 is found in the prostate gland and in hair follicles, whereas type 1 is found primarily in sebaceous glands.

One approach to testing for hyperandrogenemia is depicted in **Fig. 12-2.** In addition to measuring blood levels of testosterone and DHEAS, it is also important to measure the level of free (or unbound) testosterone. The fraction of testosterone that is not bound to its carrier protein, sex-hormone binding globulin (SHBG), is biologically available for conversion to DHT and for binding to androgen receptors. Hyperinsulinemia and/or androgen excess decrease hepatic production of SHBG, resulting in levels of total testosterone within the high-normal range, whereas the unbound hormone is more substantially elevated. Although there is a decline in ovarian testosterone production after menopause, ovarian estrogen production decreases to an even greater extent, and the concentration of SHBG is reduced. Consequently, there is an increase in the relative proportion of unbound testosterone, and it may exacerbate hirsutism after menopause.

Because adrenal androgens are readily suppressed by low doses of glucocorticoids, the dexamethasone androgen-suppression test may broadly distinguish ovarian from adrenal androgen overproduction. A blood sample is obtained before and after administering dexamethasone (0.5 mg orally every 6 h for 4 days). An adrenal source is suggested by suppression of unbound testosterone into the normal range; incomplete suppression suggests ovarian androgen excess.

A baseline plasma total testosterone level >12 nmol/L (>3.5 ng/mL) usually indicates a virilizing tumor,

FIGURE 12-1

Hirsutism scoring scale of Ferriman and Gallwey. The nine body areas possessing androgen-sensitive areas are graded from 0 (no terminal hair) to 4 (frankly virile) to obtain a total score. A normal hirsutism score is less than 8. [*Reproduced from DA Ehrmann et al: Hyperandrogenism, hirsutism, and polycystic ovarian syndrome, in LJ DeGroot et al (eds), Endocrinology, 4th ed. Philadelphia, Saunders, 2000; with permission.*]

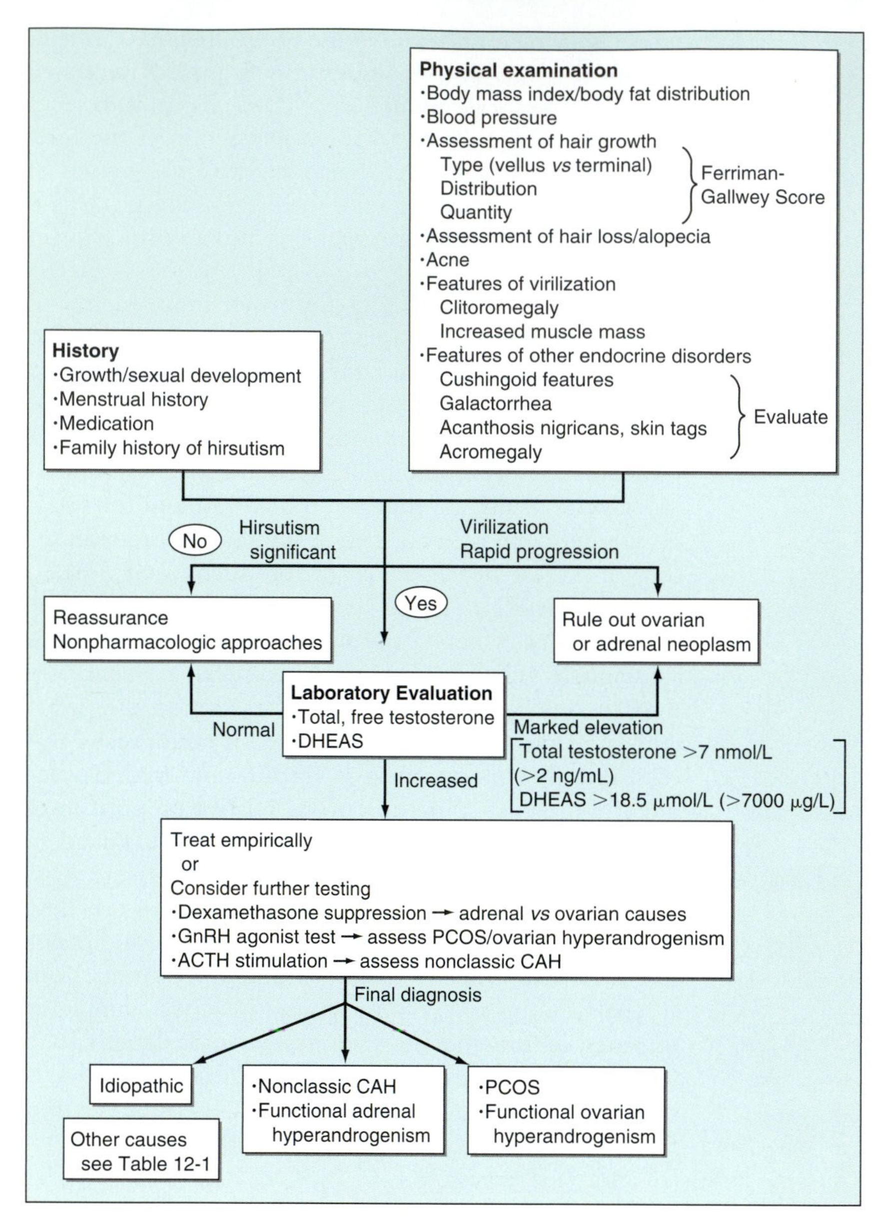

FIGURE 12-2

Algorithm for the evaluation and differential diagnosis of hirsutism. ACTH, adrenocorticotropic hormone; CAH, congenital adrenal hyperplasia; DHEAS, sulfated form of dehydroepiandrosterone; GnRH, gonadotropin-releasing hormone; PCOS, polycystic ovarian syndrome.

whereas a level >7 nmol/L (>2 ng/mL) is suggestive. A basal DHEAS level >18.5 μmol/L (>7000 μg/L) suggests an adrenal tumor. Although DHEAS has been proposed as a "marker" of predominant adrenal androgen excess, it is not unusual to find modest elevations in DHEAS among women with PCOS. Computed tomography (CT) or magnetic resonance imaging (MRI) should be used to localize an adrenal mass, and ultrasound will usually suffice to identify an ovarian mass, if clinical evaluation and hormonal levels suggest these possibilities.

PCOS is the most common cause of ovarian androgen excess (Chap. 10). However, the increased ratio of LH to follicle-stimulating hormone that is characteristic of carefully studied patients with PCOS is not seen in up to half of these women due to the pulsatility of gonadotropins. If performed, ultrasound shows enlarged ovaries and increased stroma in many women with PCOS. However, polycystic ovaries may also be found in women without clinical or laboratory features of PCOS. Therefore, polycystic ovaries are a relatively insensitive and nonspecific finding for the diagnosis of ovarian hyperandrogenism. Gonadotropin-releasing hormone agonist testing can be used to make a specific diagnosis of ovarian hyperandrogenism. A peak 17-hydroxyprogesterone level ≥7.8 nmol/L (≥2.6 μg/L), after the administration of 100 μg nafarelin (or 10 μg/kg leuprolide) subcutaneously, is virtually diagnostic of ovarian hyperandrogenism.

Nonclassic CAH is most commonly due to 21-hydroxylase deficiency but can also be caused by autosomal recessive defects in other steroidogenic enzymes necessary for adrenal corticosteroid synthesis (Chap. 5). Because of the enzyme defect, the adrenal gland cannot secrete glucocorticoids efficiently (especially cortisol). This results in diminished negative feedback inhibition of ACTH, leading to compensatory adrenal hyperplasia and the accumulation of steroid precursors that are subsequently converted to androgen.

Deficiency of 21-hydroxylase can be reliably excluded by determining a morning 17-hydroxyprogesterone level <6 nmol/L (<2 μg/L) (drawn in the follicular phase). Alternatively, 21-hydroxylase deficiency can be diagnosed by measurement of 17-hydroxyprogesterone 1 h after administration of 250 μg of synthetic ACTH (cosyntropin) intravenously.

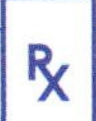

TREATMENT FOR HIRSUTISM

Treatment of hirsutism may be accomplished pharmacologically or by mechanical means of hair removal. Nonpharmacologic treatments should be considered in all patients, either as the only treatment or as an adjunct to drug therapy.

Nonpharmacologic treatments include (1) bleaching; (2) depilatory (removal from the skin surface) such as shaving and chemical treatments; or (3) epilatory (removal of the hair including the root) such as plucking, waxing, electrolysis, and laser therapy. Despite perceptions to the contrary, shaving does not increase the rate or density of hair growth. Chemical depilatory treatments may be useful for mild hirsutism that affects only limited skin areas, though they can cause skin irritation. Wax treatment removes hair temporarily but is uncomfortable. Electrolysis is effective for more permanent hair removal, particularly in the hands of a skilled electrologist. Laser phototherapy appears to be efficacious for hair removal. It delays hair regrowth and causes permanent hair removal in most patients. The long-term effects and complications associated with laser treatment are being evaluated.

Pharmacologic therapy is directed at interrupting one or more of the steps in the pathway of androgen synthesis and action: (1) suppression of adrenal and/or ovarian androgen production; (2) enhancement of androgen-binding to plasma-binding proteins, particularly SHBG; (3) impairment of the peripheral conversion of androgen precursors to active androgen; and (4) inhibition of androgen action at the target tissue level. Attenuation of hair growth is typically not evident until 4 to 6 months after initiation of medical treatment and, in most cases, leads to only a modest reduction in hair growth.

Combination estrogen-progestin therapy, in the form of an oral contraceptive, is usually the first-line endocrine treatment for hirsutism and acne, after cosmetic and dermatologic management. The estrogenic component of most oral contraceptives currently in use is either ethinyl estradiol or mestranol. The suppression of LH leads to reduced production of ovarian androgens. The reduced androgen levels also result in a dose-related increase in SHBG, thereby lowering the fraction of unbound plasma testosterone. Combination therapy has also been demonstrated to decrease DHEAS, perhaps by reducing ACTH levels. Estrogens also have a direct, dose-dependent suppressive effect on sebaceous cell function.

The choice of a specific oral contraceptive should be predicated on the progestational component, as progestins vary in their suppressive effect on SHBG levels and in their androgenic potential. Ethynodiol diacetate has relatively low androgenic potential, whereas progestins such as norgestrel and levonorgestrel are particularly androgenic, as judged from their attenuation of the estrogen-induced increase in SHBG. Norgestimate exemplifies the newer generation of progestins that are virtually nonandrogenic. Drospirenone, an analogue of spironolactone that has both antimineralocorticoid and antiandrogenic activities, has been approved for use as a progestational agent in combination with ethinyl estradiol. Its properties suggest that it should be the preferred choice for the treatment of hirsutism.

Oral contraceptives are contraindicated in women with a history of thromboembolic disease or in women with increased risk of breast or other estrogen-dependent cancers (Chap. 11). There is a relative contraindication to the use of oral contraceptives in smokers or in those with hypertension or a history of migraine headaches. In most trials, estrogen-progestin therapy alone improves the extent of acne by a maximum of 50 to 70%. The effect on hair growth may not be evident for 6 months, and the maximum effect may require 9 to 12 months owing to the length of the hair growth cycle. Improvements in hirsutism are typically in the range of 20%, but there may be an arrest of further progression of hair growth.

Adrenal androgens are more sensitive than cortisol to the suppressive effects of glucocorticoids. Therefore, glucocorticoids are the mainstay of treatment in patients with CAH. Although glucocorticoids have been reported to restore ovulatory function in some women with PCOS, this effect is highly variable. Because of side effects from excessive glucocorticoids, low doses should be used. Dexamethasone (0.2 to 0.5 mg) or prednisone (5 to 10 mg) should be taken at bedtime to achieve maximal suppression by inhibiting the nocturnal surge of ACTH.

Cyproterone acetate is the prototypic antiandrogen. It acts mainly by competitive inhibition of the binding of testosterone and DHT to the androgen receptor. In addition, it may act to enhance the metabolic clearance of testosterone by inducing hepatic enzymes. Although not available for use in the United States, cyproterone acetate is widely used in Canada, Mexico, and Europe. Cyproterone (50 to 100 mg) is given on days 1 to 15 and ethinyl estradiol (50 μg) is given on days 5 to 26 of the menstrual cycle. Side effects include irregular uterine bleeding, nausea, headache, fatigue, weight gain, and decreased libido.

Spironolactone, usually used as a mineralocorticoid antagonist, is also a weak antiandrogen. It is almost as effective as cyproterone acetate when used at high enough doses (100 to 200 mg daily). Patients should be monitored intermittently for hyperkalemia or hypotension, though these side effects are uncommon. Pregnancy should be avoided because of the risk of feminization of a male fetus. Spironolactone can also cause menstrual irregularity. It is often used in combination with an oral contraceptive, which suppresses ovarian androgen production and helps prevent pregnancy.

Flutamide is a potent nonsteroidal antiandrogen that is effective in treating hirsutism, but concerns about the induction of hepatocellular dysfunction have limited its use. Finasteride is a competitive inhibitor of 5α-reductase type 2. Beneficial effects on hirsutism have been reported, but the predominance of 5α-reductase type 1 in the PSU appears to account for its limited efficacy. Finasteride would also be expected to impair sexual differentiation in a male fetus, and it should not be used in women who may become pregnant.

Eflornithine cream (Vaniqa) has been approved as a novel treatment for unwanted facial hair in women, but long-term efficacy remains to be established. It can cause skin irritation under exaggerated conditions of use. Ultimately, the choice of any specific agent(s) must be tailored to the unique needs of the patient being treated. As noted previously, pharmacologic treatments for hirsutism should be used in conjunction with nonpharmacologic approaches. It is also helpful to review the pattern of female hair distribution in the normal population to dispel unrealistic expectations.

FURTHER READINGS

CARMINA E: Antiandrogens for the treatment of hirsutism. Expert Opin Investig Drugs 11:357, 2002

FALSETTI L et al: Management of hirsutism. Am J Clin Dermatol 1:89, 2000

HORDINSKY M et al: Hair loss and hirsutism in the elderly. Clin Geriatr Med 18:121, 2002

LACOMBE VG: Laser hair removal. Facial Plast Surg 20:85, 2004

A review of the physics of laser-skin interactions and guidelines for safe and effective clinical treatments. Four wavelengths of lasers and intense light sources have proven successful for a variety of skin types. Average rates of long-term hair reduction are between 70 and 90% after 6 months.

LANIGAN SW: Management of unwanted hair in females. Clin Exp Dermatol 26:644, 2001

SAHIN Y ET AL: Medical treatment regimens of hirsutism. Reprod Biomed Online 8:538, 2004

Review of various combinations of anti-androgens used in the management of hirsutism.

SANCHEZ LA et al: Laser hair reduction in the hirsute patient: A critical assessment. Hum Reprod Update 8:169, 2002

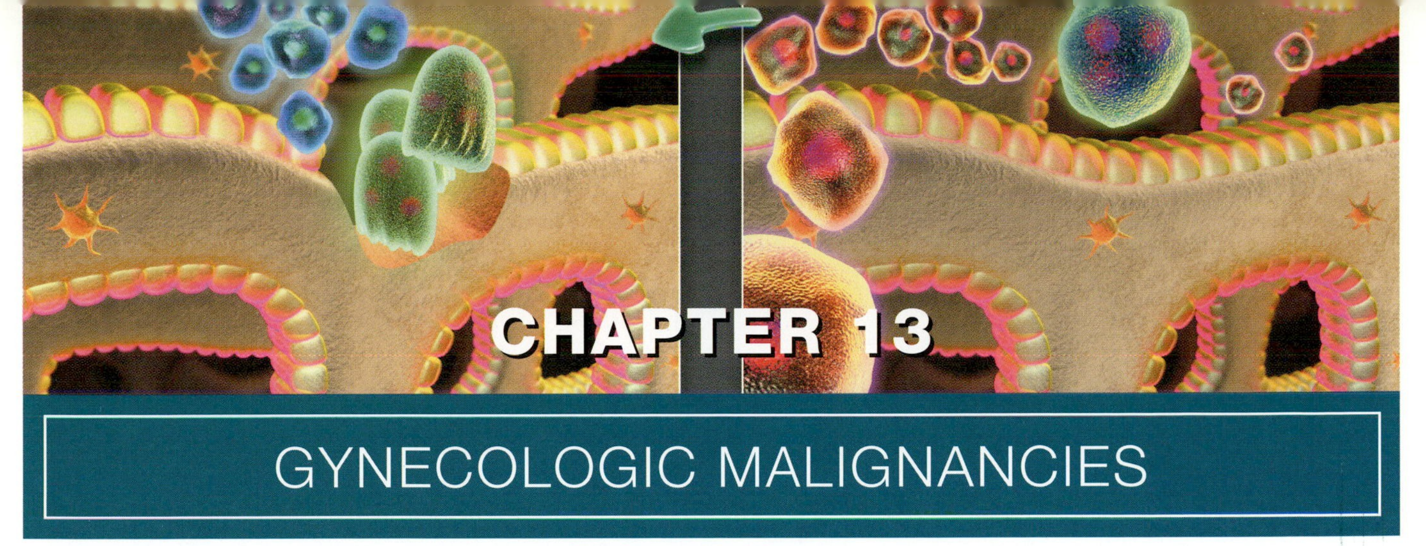

GYNECOLOGIC MALIGNANCIES

Robert C. Young

OVARIAN CANCER

Incidence and Epidemiology

Epithelial ovarian cancer is the leading cause of death from gynecologic cancer in the United States. In 2004, 25,580 new cases were diagnosed and 16,090 women died from ovarian cancer. The disease accounts for 5% of all cancer deaths in women in the United States; more women die of this disease than from cervix and endometrial cancer combined.

The age-specific incidence of the common epithelial type of ovarian cancer increases progressively and peaks in the eighth decade. Epithelial tumors, unlike germ cell and stromal tumors, are uncommon before the age of 40. Epidemiologic studies suggest higher incidences in industrialized nations and an association with disordered ovarian function, including infertility, nulliparity, frequent miscarriages, and use of ovulation-inducing drugs such as clomiphene. Each pregnancy reduces the ovarian cancer risk by about 10%, and breast-feeding and tubal ligation also appear to reduce the risk. Oral contraceptives reduce the risk of ovarian cancer in patients with a familial history of cancer and in the general population. Many of these risk-reduction factors support the "incessant ovulation" hypothesis for ovarian cancer etiology, which implies that an aberrant repair process of the surface epithelium is central to ovarian cancer development. Estrogen replacement after menopause does not appear to increase the risk of ovarian cancer, although one study showed a modest increase in risk with >11 years of use.

Familial cases account for about 5% of all ovarian cancer, and a family history of ovarian cancer is a major risk factor. Compared to a lifetime risk of 1.6% in the general population, women with one affected first-degree relative have a 5% risk. In families with two or more affected first-degree relatives, the risk may exceed 50%. Three types of autosomal dominant familial cancer are recognized: (1) site-specific, in which only ovarian cancer is seen; (2) families with cancer of the ovary and breast; and (3) the Lynch type II cancer family syndrome with nonpolyposis colorectal cancer, endometrial cancer, and ovarian cancer.

Etiology and Genetics

In women with hereditary breast/ovarian cancer, two susceptibility loci have been identified: *BRCA1,* located on chromosome 17q12-21, and *BRCA2,* on 13q12-13. Both are tumor-suppressor genes, and their protein products act as inhibitors of tumor growth. Both genes are large, and numerous mutations have been described; most are frameshift or nonsense mutations, and 86% produce truncated protein products. The implications of the many other mutations including many missense mutations are not known. The cumulative risk of ovarian cancer with critical mutations of *BRCA1* or −*2* is 25%, compared to the lifetime risk of 50% for breast cancer for similar mutations. Men in such families have an increased risk of prostate cancer.

Cytogenetic analysis of sporadic epithelial ovarian cancers generally reveals complex karyotypic rearrangements. Structural abnormalities frequently appear on chromosomes 1 and 11, and loss of heterozygosity is common on 3q, 6q, 11q, 13q, and 17. Abnormalities of oncogenes are frequently found in ovarian cancer and include c-*myc,* H-*ras,* K-*ras,* and *neu.*

Ovarian tumors (usually not epithelial) are sometimes components of complex genetic syndromes. Peutz-Jeghers syndrome (mucocutaneous pigmentation and intestinal polyps) is associated with ovarian sex cord stromal tumors and Sertoli cell tumors in men. Patients with gonadal dysgenesis (46XY genotype or mosaic for Y-containing cell lines) develop gonadoblastomas, and women with nevoid basal cell carcinomas have an increased risk of ovarian fibromas.

Clinical Presentation and Differential Diagnosis

Most patients with ovarian cancer are first diagnosed when the disease has already spread beyond the true pelvis. The occurrence of abdominal pain, bloating, and urinary symptoms usually indicates advanced disease. Localized ovarian cancer is generally asymptomatic. However, progressive enlargement of a localized ovarian tumor can produce urinary frequency or constipation, and rarely torsion of an ovarian mass causes acute abdominal pain or a surgical abdomen. In contrast to cervical or endometrial cancer, vaginal bleeding or discharge is rarely seen with early ovarian cancer. The diagnosis of early disease usually occurs with palpation of an asymptomatic adnexal mass during routine pelvic examination. However, most ovarian enlargements discovered this way, especially in premenopausal women, are benign functional cysts that characteristically resolve over one to three menstrual cycles. Adnexal masses in premenarchal or postmenopausal women are more likely to be pathologic. A solid, irregular, fixed pelvic mass is usually ovarian cancer. Other causes of adnexal masses include pedunculated uterine fibroids, endometriosis, benign ovarian neoplasms, and inflammatory lesions of the bowel.

Evaluation of patients with suspected ovarian cancer should include measurement of serum levels of the tumor marker CA-125. CA-125 determinants are glycoproteins with molecular masses from 220 to 1000 kDa, and a radioimmunoassay is used to determine circulating CA-125 antigen levels. Between 80 and 85% of patients with epithelial ovarian cancer have levels of CA-125 ≥ 35 U/mL. Other malignant tumors can also elevate CA-125 levels, including cancers of the endometrium, cervix, fallopian tubes, pancreas, breast, lung, and colon. Certain nonmalignant conditions that can produce moderate elevations of CA-125 levels include pregnancy, endometriosis, pelvic inflammatory disease, and uterine fibroids. About 1% of normal females have serum CA-125 levels >35 U/mL. However, in postmenopausal women with an asymptomatic pelvic mass and CA-125 levels ≥65 U/mL, the test has a sensitivity of 97% and a specificity of 78%.

Screening

In contrast to patients who present with advanced disease, patients with early ovarian cancers (stages I and II) are commonly curable with conventional therapy. Thus, effective screening procedures would improve the cure rate in this disease. Although pelvic examination can occasionally detect early disease, it is a relatively insensitive screening procedure. Transvaginal sonography is often useful, but significant false-positive results are noted, particularly in premenopausal women. In one study, 67 laparotomies were required to diagnose 1 primary ovarian cancer. Doppler flow imaging coupled with transvaginal ultrasound may improve accuracy and reduce the high rate of false positives.

CA-125 has been studied as a screening tool. Unfortunately, half of women with stages I and II ovarian cancer have CA-125 levels <65 U/mL. Attempts have been made to improve the sensitivity and specificity by combinations of procedures, commonly transvaginal ultrasound and CA-125 levels. In a screening study of 22,000 women, 42 had a positive screen and 11 had ovarian cancer (7 with advanced disease). In addition, eight women with a negative screen developed ovarian cancer. Thus, the false-positive rate would lead to a large number of unnecessary (i.e., negative) laparotomies if each positive screen resulted in a surgical exploration. The National Institutes of Health Consensus Conference recommended against screening for ovarian cancer among the general population without known risk factors for the disease. Although no evidence shows that screening saves lives, many physicians use annual pelvic examinations, transvaginal ultrasound, and CA-125 levels to screen women with a family history of ovarian cancer or breast/ovarian cancer syndromes.

In one study, proteomic spectra in the serum analyzed by an iterative searching algorithm were used to identify women with ovarian cancer. Preliminary studies have identified all 50 stage I patients with a sensitivity of 100%, a specificity of 95%, and a positive predictive value of 94%. The procedure can be automated, requires a pinprick of blood, and has many characteristics of an ideal screening test. However, difficulty in consistency of replicate samples, variation in spectroscopy equipment, and the tendency of the artificial intelligence algorithms to overfit the data makes conformation studies necessary before widespread application to screening is warranted.

Pathology

Common epithelial tumors comprise most (85%) of the ovarian neoplasms. These may be benign (50%), frankly malignant (33%), or tumors of low malignant potential (16%) (tumors of borderline malignancy). Epithelial tumors of low malignant potential have the cytologic features of malignancy but do not invade the ovarian stroma. More than 75% of borderline malignancies present in early stage and generally occur in younger women. They have a much better natural history than their malignant counterpart.

There are five major subtypes of common epithelial tumors: serous (50%), mucinous (25%), endometroid (15%), clear cell (5%), and Brenner tumors (1%), the latter derived from the urothelium. Benign common epithelial tumors are almost always serous or mucinous and develop in women ages 20 to 60. They are frequently large (20 to 30 cm), bilateral, and cystic.

Malignant epithelial tumors are usually seen in women over 40. They present as solid masses, with areas of necrosis and hemorrhage. Masses >10 to 15 cm have usually already spread into the intraabdominal space. Spread eventually results in intraabdominal carcinomatosis, which leads to bowel and renal obstruction and cachexia.

Although most ovarian tumors are epithelial, two other important ovarian tumor types exist—stromal and germ cell tumors. These tumors are distinct in their cell of origin but also have different clinical presentations and natural histories and are often managed differently (see below).

Metastasis to the ovary can occur from breast, colon, gastric, and pancreatic cancers, and the Krukenberg tumor was classically described as bilateral ovarian masses from metastatic mucin-secreting gastrointestinal cancers.

Staging and Prognostic Factors

Laparotomy is often the primary procedure used to establish the diagnosis. Less invasive studies useful in defining the extent of spread include chest x-rays, abdominal computed tomography scans, and abdominal and pelvic sonography. If the woman has specific gastrointestinal symptoms, a barium enema or gastrointestinal series can be performed. Symptoms of bladder or renal dysfunction can be evaluated by cystoscopy or intravenous pyelography.

A careful staging laparotomy will establish the stage and extent of disease and allow for the cytoreduction of tumor masses in patients with advanced disease. Proper laparotomy requires a vertical incision of sufficient length to ensure adequate examination of the abdominal contents. The presence, amount, and cytology of any ascites fluid should be noted. The primary tumor should be evaluated for rupture, excrescences, or dense adherence. Careful visual and manual inspection of the diaphragm and peritoneal surfaces is required. In addition to total abdominal hysterectomy and bilateral salpingo-oophorectomy, a partial omentectomy should be performed and the paracolic gutters inspected. Pelvic lymph nodes as well as para-aortic nodes in the region of the renal hilus should be biopsied. Since this surgical procedure defines stage, establishes prognosis, and determines the necessity for subsequent therapy, it should be performed by a surgeon with special expertise in ovarian cancer staging. Studies have shown that patients operated upon by gynecologic oncologists were properly staged 97% of the time, compared to 52% and 35% of cases staged by obstetricians/gynecologists and general surgeons, respectively. At the end of staging, 23% of women have stage I disease (cancer confined to the ovary or ovaries); 13% have stage II (disease confined to the true pelvis); 47% have stage III (disease spread into but confined to the abdomen); and 16% have stage IV disease (spread outside the pelvis and abdomen). The 5-year survival correlates with stage of disease: stage I—90%, stage II—70%, stage III—15 to 20%, and stage IV—1 to 5% (**Table 13-1**).

TABLE 13-1

STAGING AND SURVIVAL IN GYNECOLOGIC MALIGNANCIES

STAGE	OVARIAN	5-YEAR SURVIVAL, %	ENDOMETRIAL	5-YEAR SURVIVAL, %	CERVIX	5-YEAR SURVIVAL, %
0	—		—		Carcinoma in situ	100
I	Confined to ovary	90	Confined to corpus	89	Confined to uterus	85
II	Confined to pelvis	70	Involves corpus and cervix	80	Invades beyond uterus but not to pelvic wall	60
III	Intraabdominal spread	15–20	Extends outside the uterus but not outside the true pelvis	30	Extends to pelvic wall and/or lower third of vagina, or hydronephrosis	33
IV	Spread outside abdomen	1–5	Extends outside the true pelvis or involves the bladder or rectum	9	Invades mucosa of bladder or rectum or extends beyond the true pelvis	7

Prognosis in ovarian cancer is dependent not only upon stage but on the extent of residual disease and histologic grade. Patients presenting with advanced disease but left without significant residual disease after surgery have a median survival of 39 months, compared to 17 months for those with suboptimal tumor resection.

Prognosis of epithelial tumors is also highly influenced by histologic grade but less so by histologic type. Although grading systems differ among pathologists, all grading systems show a better prognosis for well- or moderately differentiated tumors and a poorer prognosis for poorly differentiated histologies. Typical 5-year survivals for patients with all stages of disease are: well-differentiated—88%, moderately differentiated—58%, poorly differentiated—27%.

The prognostic significance of pre- and postoperative CA-125 levels is uncertain. Serum levels generally reflect volume of disease, and high levels usually indicate unresectability and a poorer survival. Postoperative levels, if elevated, usually indicate residual disease. The rate of decline of CA-125 levels during initial therapy or the absolute level after one to three cycles of chemotherapy correlates with prognosis but is not sufficiently accurate to guide individual treatment decisions. Even when the CA-125 level falls to normal after surgery or chemotherapy, "second-look" laparotomy identifies residual disease in 60% of women.

Genetic and biologic factors may influence prognosis. Increased tumor levels of p53 are associated with a worse prognosis in advanced disease. Epidermal growth factor receptors in ovarian cancer are associated with a high risk of progression, but the increased expression of HER-2/neu has given conflicting prognostic results, and expression of Mdr-1 has not been of prognostic value. HER-2/neu is highly expressed in 20% of ovarian cancers, and responses have been seen to trastuzumab in this subset of patients.

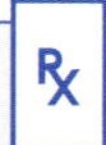

TREATMENT FOR OVARIAN CANCER

The selection of therapy for patients with epithelial ovarian cancer depends upon the stage, extent of residual tumor, and histologic grade. In general, patients are considered in three separate treatment groups: (1) those with early (stages I and II) ovarian cancer and microscopic or no residual disease; (2) patients with advanced (stage III) disease but minimal residual tumor (<1 cm) after initial surgery; and (3) patients with bulky residual tumor and advanced (stage III or IV) disease.

Patients with stage I disease, no residual tumor, and well or moderately differentiated tumors need no adjuvant therapy after definitive surgery, and 5-year survival exceeds 95%. For all other patients with early disease and those stage I patients with poor prognosis histologic grade, adjuvant therapy is probably warranted, and single-agent cisplatin or platinum-containing drug combinations improve survival by 8% (82% vs 76%, $p = .08$).

For the patients with advanced (stage III) disease but with limited or no residual disease after definitive cytoreductive surgery (about half of all stage III patients), the primary therapy is platinum-based combination chemotherapy. Approximately 70% of women respond to initial combination chemotherapy, and 40 to 50% have a complete regression of disease. Only about half of these patients are free of disease if surgically restaged. Although a variety of combinations are active, a randomized prospective trial of paclitaxel and cisplatin compared to paclitaxel and carboplatin in patients with optimally resected advanced disease demonstrated equivalent results (median time to progression 20.7 months vs 19.4 months, median survival 57.4 months vs 48.7 months) but with significantly reduced toxicity using carboplatin. This regimen of paclitaxel, 175 mg/m^2 by 3-h infusion, and carboplatin, dosed to an AUC (area under the curve) of 7.5 is the treatment of choice for patients with previously untreated advanced-stage disease.

Patients with advanced disease (stages III and IV) and bulky residual tumor are generally treated with a paclitaxel-platinum combination regimen as well and, while the overall prognosis is poorer, 5-year survival may reach 10 to 15%.

Historically, patients who had an excellent initial response to chemotherapy and no clinical evidence of disease have had a second-look laparotomy. For patients with stage I ovarian cancer or for germ cell tumors, the operation rarely detects residual tumor and has been largely abandoned. Even for those with stages II and III epithelial tumors, the second-look surgical procedure itself does not prolong overall survival. Its routine use cannot be recommended. Maintenance therapy (12 cycles of paclitaxel every 28 days) may extend progression-free survival among patients who achieve a complete response; an effect on overall survival has not yet been shown.

Patients with advanced disease whose disease recurs after initial treatment are usually not curable but may benefit significantly from limited surgery to relieve intestinal obstruction, localized radiation therapy to relieve pressure or pain from mass lesions or metastasis, or palliative chemotherapy. The selection of chemotherapy for palliation depends upon the initial regimen and evidence of drug resistance. Patients who have a complete regression of disease that lasts ≥6 months often respond to reinduction with the same agents. Patients relapsing within the first 6 months of initial therapy rarely do. Chemotherapeutic agents with >15% response rates in patients relapsing after initial combination chemotherapy include gemcitabine, topotecan, liposomal doxorubicin, and vinorelbine. Intraperitoneal chemotherapy (usually cisplatin) may be used if a small residual volume (<1 cm^3) of tumor exists. Progestational agents and antiestrogens produce responses in 5 to 15% of patients and have minimal side effects.

Patients with tumor of low malignant potential, even with advanced-stage disease, have longer survivals when managed with surgery alone. The added value of radiation and chemotherapy has not been shown.

OVARIAN GERM CELL TUMORS

Fewer than 5% of all ovarian tumors are germ cell in origin. They include teratoma, dysgerminoma, endodermal sinus tumor, and embryonal carcinoma. Germ cell tumors of the ovary generally occur in younger women (75% of ovarian malignancies in women <30), display an unusually aggressive natural history, and are commonly cured with less extensive nonsterilizing surgery and chemotherapy. Women cured of these malignancies are able to conceive and have normal children.

These neoplasms can be divided into three major groups: (1) benign tumors (usually dermoid cysts); (2) malignant tumors that arise from dermoid cysts; and (3) primitive malignant germ cell tumors including dysgerminoma, yolk sac tumors, immature teratomas, embryonal carcinomas, and choriocarcinoma.

Dermoid cysts are teratomatous cysts usually lined by epidermis and skin appendages. They often contain hair, and calcified bone or teeth can sometimes be seen on conventional pelvic x-ray. They are almost always curable by surgical resection. Approximately 1% of these tumors have malignant elements, usually squamous cell carcinoma.

Malignant germ cell tumors are usually large (median—16 cm). Bilateral disease is rare except in dysgerminoma (10 to 15% bilaterality). Abdominal or pelvic pain in young women is the usual presenting symptom. Serum human chorionic gonadotropin (β-hCG) and α fetoprotein levels are useful in the diagnosis and management of these patients. Before the advent of chemotherapy, extensive surgery was routine, but it has now been replaced by careful evaluation of extent of spread followed by resection of bulky disease and preservation of one ovary, uterus, and cervix, if feasible. This allows many affected women to preserve fertility. After surgical staging, 60 to 75% of women have stage I disease and 25 to 30% have stage III disease. Stages II and IV are infrequent.

Most of the malignant germ cell tumors are managed with chemotherapy after surgery. Regimens used in testicular cancer such as PVB (cisplatin, vinblastine, bleomycin) and BEP (bleomycin, 30 units IV weekly; etoposide, 100 mg/m^2 days 1 to 5; and cisplatin, 20 mg/m^2 days 1 to 5), with three or four courses given at 21-day intervals, have produced 95% long-term survival in patients with stages I to III disease. This regimen is the treatment of choice for all malignant germ cell tumors except grade I, stage I immature teratoma, where surgery alone is adequate, and perhaps early-stage dysgerminoma, where surgery and radiation therapy are used.

Dysgerminoma is the ovarian counterpart of testicular seminoma. The tumor is very sensitive to radiation therapy. The 5-year disease-free survival is 100% in early-stage patients and 61% in stage III disease. Unfortunately, the use of radiation therapy makes many patients infertile. BEP chemotherapy is equally or more effective and does not cause infertility. In incompletely resected patients with dysgerminoma, the 2-year disease-free survival is 95% and infertility is not observed. Combination chemotherapy (BEP) has replaced postoperative radiation therapy as the treatment of choice in women with ovarian dysgerminoma.

OVARIAN STROMAL TUMORS

Stromal tumors make up <10% of ovarian tumors. They are named for the stromal tissue involved: granulosa, theca, Sertoli, Leydig, and collagen-producing stromal cells. The granulosa and theca cell stromal cell tumors occur most frequently in the first three decades of life. Granulosa cell tumors frequently produce estrogen and cause menstrual abnormalities, bleeding, and precocious puberty. Endometrial carcinoma can be seen in 5% of these women, perhaps related to the persistent hyperestrogenism. Sertoli and Leydig cell tumors, when functional, produce androgens with resultant virilization or hirsutism. Some 75% of these stromal cell tumors present in stage I and can be cured with total abdominal hysterectomy and bilateral salpingo-oophorectomy. Stromal tumors generally grow slowly, and recurrences can occur 5 to 10 years after initial surgery. Neither radiation therapy nor chemotherapy have been documented to be consistently effective, and surgical management remains the primary treatment.

CARCINOMA OF THE FALLOPIAN TUBE

The fallopian tube is the least common site of cancer in the female genital tract, although its epithelial surface far exceeds that of the ovary, where epithelial cancer is 20 times more common. Approximately 300 new cases occur yearly; 90% are papillary serous adenocarcinomas, with the remainder being mixed mesodermal, endometroid, and transitional cell tumors. *BRCA1* and *−2* mutations are found in 7% of cases. The gross and microscopic characteristics and the spread of the tumor are similar to those of ovarian cancer but can be distinguished if the tumor arises from the endosalpinx where the tubal epithelium shows a transition between benign and malignant, and the ovaries and endometrium are normal or minimally involved. The differential diagnosis includes primary or metastatic ovarian cancer, chronic salpingitis, tuberculous salpingitis, salpingitis isthmica nodosa, and cautery artifact.

Unlike patients with ovarian cancer, patients often present with early symptoms, usually postmenopausal vaginal bleeding, pain, and leukorrhea. Surgical staging is similar to that used for ovarian cancer, and prognosis is related to stage and extent of residual disease. Patients with stages I and II disease are generally treated with surgery alone or with surgery and pelvic radiation therapy, although radiation therapy does not clearly improve 5-year survival (5-year survival stage I: 74 versus 75%, stage II: 43 versus 48%). Patients with stages III and IV disease are treated with the same chemotherapy regimens used in advanced ovarian carcinoma, and 5-year survival is similar (stage III—20%, stage IV—5%).

UTERINE CANCER

Carcinoma of the endometrium is the most common female pelvic malignancy. Approximately 40,300 new cases are diagnosed yearly, although in most (75%), tumor is confined to the uterine corpus at diagnosis and therefore most can be cured. The 7000 deaths yearly make uterine cancer only the eighth leading cause of cancer death in females. It is primarily a disease of postmenopausal women, although 25% of cases occur in women <age 50 and 5% <age 40. The disease is common in Eastern Europe and the United States and uncommon in Asia.

Phenotypic characteristics and risk factors common in patients with endometrial cancer include obesity, altered menstruation, low fertility index, late menopause, anovulation, and postmenopausal bleeding. Exposure to unopposed estrogen from either endogenous or exogenous sources may play a central etiologic role. Women taking tamoxifen for breast cancer treatment or prevention have a twofold increased risk.

Endometrial carcinoma occurs most often in the sixth and seventh decades of life. Symptoms often include abnormal vaginal discharge (90%); abnormal bleeding (80%), which is usually postmenopausal; and leukorrhea (10%). Evaluation of such patients should include a history and physical and pelvic examinations followed by an endometrial biopsy or a fractional dilation and curettage. Outpatient procedures such as endometrial biopsy or aspiration curettage can be used but are definitive only when positive.

Between 75 and 80% of all endometrial carcinomas are adenocarcinomas, and the prognosis depends upon stage, histologic grade, and extent of myometrial invasion. Grade I tumors are highly differentiated adenocarcinomas, grade II contain some solid areas, and grade III tumors are largely solid or undifferentiated. Adenocarcinoma with squamous differentiation is seen in 10% of patients; the most differentiated form is known as *adenoacanthoma,* and the poorly differentiated form is called *adenosquamous carcinoma.* Other less common pathologies include mucinous carcinoma (5%) and papillary serous carcinoma (<10%). This latter type has a natural history similar to ovarian carcinoma and should be managed as an ovarian cancer. Rarer histologies include secretory (2%), ciliated, clear cell, and undifferentiated carcinomas.

The staging of endometrial cancer requires surgery to establish the extent of disease and the depth of myometrial invasion. Peritoneal fluid should be sampled; the abdomen and pelvis explored; and pelvic and para-aortic lymphadenectomy performed depending upon the histology, grade, and depth of invasion in the uterine specimen on frozen section. After evaluation and staging, 74% of patients are stage I, 13% are stage II, 9% are stage III, and 3% are stage IV. Five-year survival by stage is as follows: stage I—89%, stage II—80%, stage III—30%, and stage IV—9% (Table 13-1).

Patients with uncomplicated endometrial carcinoma are effectively managed with total abdominal hysterectomy and bilateral salpingo-oophorectomy. Pre- or postoperative irradiation has been used, and although vaginal cuff recurrence is reduced, survival is not altered. In women with poor histologic grade, deep myometrial invasion, or extensive involvement of the lower uterine segment or cervix, intracavitary or external beam irradiation is warranted.

About 15% of women have endometrial carcinoma with extension to the cervix only (stage II), and management depends upon the extent of cervical invasion. Superficial cervical invasion can be managed like stage I disease, but extensive cervical invasion requires radical hysterectomy or preoperative radiotherapy followed by extrafascial hysterectomy. Once disease is outside the uterus but still confined to the true pelvis (stage III), management generally includes surgery and irradiation. Patients who have involvement only of the ovary or fallopian tubes generally do well with such therapy (5-year survivals of 80%). Other stage III patients with disease extending beyond the adnexa or those with serous carcinomas of the endometrium have a significantly poorer prognosis (5-year survival of 15%).

Patients with stage IV disease (outside the abdomen or invading the bladder or rectum) are treated palliatively with irradiation, surgery, and/or progestational agents. Progestational agents produce responses in about 25% of patients. Well-differentiated tumors respond most frequently, and response can be correlated with the level of progesterone receptor expression in the tumor. The commonly used progestational agents hydroxyprogesterone (Dilalutin), megastrol (Megace), and deoxyprogesterone (Provera) all produce similar response rates, and the antiestrogen tamoxifen (Nolvadex) produces responses in 10 to 25% of patients in a salvage setting.

Chemotherapy is not very successful in advanced endometrial carcinoma. The most active single agents with consistent response rates of ≥20% include cisplatin, carboplatin, doxorubicin, epirubicin, and paclitaxel. Combinations of drugs with or without progestational agents have generally produced response rates similar to single agents.

CERVIX CANCER

Carcinoma of the cervix was once the most common cause of cancer death in women, but over the past 30 years, the mortality rate has decreased by 50% due to widespread screening with the Pap smear. In 2004, ~10,500 new cases of invasive cervix cancer occurred, and >50,000 cases of carcinoma in situ were detected. There were 3900 deaths from the disease, and of those patients, ~85% had never had a Pap smear. It remains the major gynecologic cancer in underdeveloped countries. It is more common in lower socioeconomic groups, in women with early initial sexual activity and/or multiple sexual partners, and in smokers. Venereal transmission of human papilloma virus (HPV) has an important etiologic role. Over 66 types of HPVs have been isolated, and many are associated with genital warts. Those types associated with cervical carcinoma are 16, 18, 31, 45, and 51 to 53. These, along with many other types, are also associated with cervical intraepithelial neoplasia (CIN). The protein product of HPV-16, the E7 protein, binds and inactivates the tumor-suppressor gene Rb, and the E6 protein of HPV-18 has sequence homology to the SV40 large T antigen and has the capacity to bind and inactivate the tumor-suppressor gene p53. E6 and E7 are both necessary and sufficient to cause cell transformation in vitro. These binding and inactivation events may explain the carcinogenic effects of the viruses.

Vaccination against pathologic HPV appears quite promising as a cervix cancer prevention strategy. The administration of HPV-16 vaccine in a double-blind study of 2392 women completely prevented infection with the virus, and no cases of HPV-16-related CIN were seen in vaccinated women. Although this vaccine is promising, polyvalent vaccines incorporating the known pathologic HPV virus types may ultimately be required.

Uncomplicated HPV lower genital tract infection and condylomatous atypia of the cervix can progress to CIN. This lesion precedes invasive cervical carcinoma and is classified as low-grade squamous intraepithelial lesion (SIL), high-grade SIL, and carcinoma in situ. Carcinoma in situ demonstrates cytologic evidence of neoplasia without invasion through the basement membrane, can persist unchanged for 10 to 20 years, but eventually progresses to invasive carcinoma.

The Pap smear is 90 to 95% accurate in detecting early lesions such as CIN but is less sensitive in detecting cancer when frankly invasive cancer or fungating masses are present. Inflammation, necrosis, and hemorrhage may produce false-positive smears, and colposcopic-directed biopsy is required when any lesion is visible on the cervix, regardless of Pap smear findings. The American Cancer Society recommends that women after onset of sexual activity, or >age 20, have two consecutive yearly smears. If negative, smears should be repeated every 3 years. The American College of Obstetrics and Gynecology recommends yearly Pap smears with routine annual pelvic and breast examinations. The Pap smear can be reported as normal (includes benign, reactive, or reparative changes); atypical squamous cells of undetermined significance (ASCUS) or cannot exclude high-grade SIL (ASC-H); low- or high-grade CIN; or frankly malignant. Women with ASCUS, ASC-H, or low-grade CIN should have repeat smears in 3 to 6 months and be tested for HPV. Women with high-grade CIN or frankly malignant Pap smears should have colposcopic-directed cervical biopsy. Colposcopy is a technique using a binocular microscope and 3% acetic acid applied to the cervix in which abnormal areas appear white and can be biopsied directly. Cone biopsy is still required when endocervical tumor is suspected, colposcopy is inadequate, the biopsy shows microinvasive carcinoma, or when a discrepancy is noted between the Pap smear and the colposcopic findings. Cone biopsy alone is therapeutic for CIN in many patients, although a less radical electrocautery excision may be sufficient.

Approximately 80% of invasive cervix cancers are squamous cell tumors, 10 to 15% are adenocarcinomas, 2 to 5% are adenosquamous with epithelial and glandular structures, and 1 to 2% are clear cell mesonephric tumors.

Patients with cervix cancer generally present with abnormal bleeding or postcoital spotting that may increase to intermenstrual or prominent menstrual bleeding. Yellowish vaginal discharge, lumbosacral back pain, and urinary symptoms can also be seen.

The staging of cervical carcinoma is clinical and generally completed with a pelvic examination under anesthesia with cystoscopy and proctoscopy. Chest x-rays, intravenous pyelograms, and computed tomography are generally required, and magnetic resonance imaging (MRI) may be used to assess extracervical extension. Stage 0 is carcinoma in situ, stage I is disease confined to the cervix, stage II disease invades beyond the cervix but not to the pelvic wall or lower third of the vagina, stage III disease extends to the pelvic wall or lower third of the vagina or causes hydronephrosis, stage IV is present when the tumor invades the mucosa of bladder or rectum or extends beyond the true pelvis. Five-year survivals are as follows: stage I—85%, stage II—60%, stage III—33%, and stage IV—7% (Table 13-1).

Carcinoma in situ (stage 0) can be managed successfully by cone biopsy or by abdominal hysterectomy. For stage I disease, results appear equivalent for either radical hysterectomy or radiation therapy. Patients with stages II to IV disease are primarily managed with radical radiation therapy or combined modality therapy. Retroperitoneal lymphadenectomy has no proven therapeutic role. Pelvic exenterations, although uncommon, are performed for centrally recurrent or persistent disease. Reconstruction of the vagina, bladder, and rectum can often be done following this operation.

In women with locally advanced disease (stages IIB to IVA), platinum-based chemotherapy given concomitantly with radiation therapy improves survival compared to radiation therapy alone. Cisplatin, 75 mg/m^2 over 4 h, followed by 5-fluorouracil (5-FU), 4 g given by 96-h infusion on days 1 to 5 of radiation therapy, is a common regimen. Two additional cycles of chemotherapy are given at 3-week intervals. Concurrent chemoradiotherapy reduced the risk of recurrence by 30 to 50% across a wide spectrum of stages and presentations and is the treatment of choice in stages IIB to IV cervix cancer.

Chemotherapy has been used in patients with unresectable advanced disease or recurrent disease. Active agents with ≥20% response rates include cisplatin, 5-FU, ifosfamide, and irinotecan. No combination of agents has proved better than single agents. Intraarterial chemotherapy has been studied, either pre- or postoperatively, but is associated with substantial local toxicity and response rates of 20%.

GESTATIONAL TROPHOBLASTIC NEOPLASIA

Gestational trophoblastic diseases are a group of interrelated diseases that form a spectrum from benign hydatidiform mole to trophoblastic malignancy (placental-site trophoblastic tumor and choriocarcinoma). Malignant forms account for <1% of female gynecologic malignancies and can be cured with appropriate chemotherapy. Deaths from this disease have become rare in the United States.

Epidemiology

The incidence is about 1 per 1500 pregnancies in the United States and is nearly tenfold higher in Asia. Maternal age >45 years is a risk factor for hydatidiform mole. A prior history of molar pregnancy is also a risk factor. Choriocarcinoma occurs in ~1 in 25,000 pregnancies or 1 in 20,000 live births. Prior history of hydatidiform mole is a risk factor for choriocarcinoma. A woman with a molar pregnancy is 1000 times more likely to develop choriocarcinoma than a woman with a prior normal-term pregnancy.

Pathology and Etiology

The trophoblastic neoplasms have been divided by morphology into complete or partial hydatidiform mole, invasive mole, placental-site trophoblastomas, and choriocarcinomas. Hydatidiform moles contain clusters of villi with hydropic changes, hyperplasia of the trophoblast, and the absence of fetal vessels. Invasive moles differ only by invasion into the uterine myometrium. Placental-site trophoblastic tumors are predominantly made up of cytotrophoblast cells arising from the placental implantation site. Choriocarcinomas consist of anaplastic trophoblastic tissue with both cytotrophoblastic and syncytiotrophoblastic elements and no identifiable villi.

Complete moles result from uniparental disomy in which loss of the maternal genes (23 autosomes plus X) occurs by unknown mechanisms and is followed by duplication of the paternal haploid genome (23 autosomes plus X). Uncommonly (5%), moles result from dispermic fertilization of an empty egg, resulting in either 46XY or 46XX genotype. Partial moles result from dispermic fertilization of an egg with retention of the maternal haploid set of chromosomes, resulting in diandric triploidy.

Clinical Presentation

Molar pregnancies are generally associated with first-trimester bleeding, ectopic pregnancies, or threatened abortions. The uterus is inappropriately large for the length of gestation, and β-hCG levels are higher than expected.

Fetal parts and heart sounds are not present. The diagnosis is generally made by the passage of grapelike clusters from the uterus, but ultrasound demonstration of the hydropic mole can be diagnostic. Patients suspected of a molar pregnancy require a chest film, careful pelvic examinations, and weekly serial monitoring of β-hCG levels.

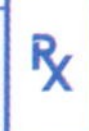

TREATMENT FOR GESTATIONAL TROPHOBLASTIC NEOPLASIA

Patients with hydatidiform moles require suction curettage coupled with postevacuation monitoring of β-hCG levels. In most women (80%), the β-hCG titer progressively declines within 8 to 10 days of evacuation (serum half-life is 24 to 36 h). Patients should be monitored on a monthly basis and should not become pregnant for at least a year. Patients found to have invasive mole at curettage are generally treated with hysterectomy and chemotherapy. Approximately half of patients with choriocarcinoma develop the malignancy after a molar pregnancy, and the other half develop the malignancy after abortion, ectopic pregnancy, or occasionally after a normal full-term pregnancy.

Chemotherapy is generally used for gestational trophoblastic neoplasia and is often used in hydatidiform mole if β-hCG levels rise or plateau or if metastases develop. Patients with invasive mole or choriocarcinoma require chemotherapy. Several regimens are effective, including methotrexate at 30 mg/m^2 intramuscularly on a weekly basis until β-hCG titers are normal. However, methotrexate (1 mg/kg) every other day for 4 days followed by leukovorin (0.1 mg/kg) intravenously 24 h after methotrexate is associated with a cure rate of ≥90% and low toxicity. Intermittent courses are continued until the β-hCG titer becomes undetectable for 3 consecutive weeks, and then patients are monitored monthly for a year.

Patients with high-risk tumors (high β-hCG levels, disease presenting ≥4 months after antecedent pregnancy, brain or liver metastasis, or failure of single-agent methotrexate) are initially treated with combination chemotherapy. EMA-CO (a cyclic non-cross-resistant combination of etoposide, methotrexate, and dactinomycin alternating with cyclophosphamide and vincristine); cisplatin, bleomycin, and vinblastine; and cisplatin, etoposide, and bleomycin are effective regimens. EMA-CO is now the regimen of choice for patients with high-risk disease because of excellent survival rates (>80%) and less toxicity. The use of etoposide carries a 1.5% lifetime risk of acute myeloid leukemia (16-fold relative risk). Because of this problem, etoposide-containing regimens should be reserved for patients with high-risk features. Patients with brain or liver metastases are usually treated with local irradiation to metastatic sites in conjunction with chemotherapy. Long-term studies of patients cured of trophoblastic disease have not demonstrated an increased risk of maternal complications or fetal abnormalities with subsequent pregnancies.

FURTHER READINGS

CANNISTRA SA: Cancer of the ovary. N Engl J Med 351:2519, 2004

A thorough review of the clinical features and management of ovarian cancer, including women with genetic predisposition. The article also highlights advances in chemotherapy that have resulted in improved survival and in more effective treatment of relapsed disease.

KOUTSKY LA: A controlled trial of a human papilloma virus type 16 vaccine. N Engl J Med 347:1645, 2002

Approximately 20% of adults become infected with human papillomavirus type 16 (HPV-16). This trial demonstrates that an HPV-16 vaccine reduced the incidence of both HPV-16 infection and HPV-16-related cervical intraepithelial neoplasia.

MARKMAN M et al: Phase III randomized trial of 12 versus 3 months of maintenance paclitaxel in patients with advanced ovarian cancer after complete response to platinum and paclitaxel-based chemotherapy: A Southwest Oncology Group and Gynecologic Oncology Group Trial. J Clin Oncol 21:2460, 2003

NELSON HD ET AL: Genetic risk assessment and *BRCA* mutation testing for breast and ovarian cancer susceptibility: Systematic evidence review for the U.S. Preventive Services Task Force. Ann Intern Med 143:362, 2005

POSADAS EM ET AL: Proteomics and ovarian cancer: Implications for diagnosis and treatment: A critical review of the recent literature. Curr Opin Oncol 16:478, 2004

Mass spectral blood and tissue analysis are being explored to identify potential diagnostic biomarkers of ovarian cancer. These methods will require validation in clinical trials but provide novel approaches for earlier detection of ovarian cancer.

SOLOMON D et al: The 2001 Bethesda System. JAMA 287:2114, 2002

STEHMAN FB et al: Innovations in the treatment of invasive cervical cancer. Cancer 98:2052, 2003

WRIGHT JD, MUTCH DG: Treatment of high-risk gestational trophoblastic tumors. Clin Obstet Gynecol 46:593, 2003

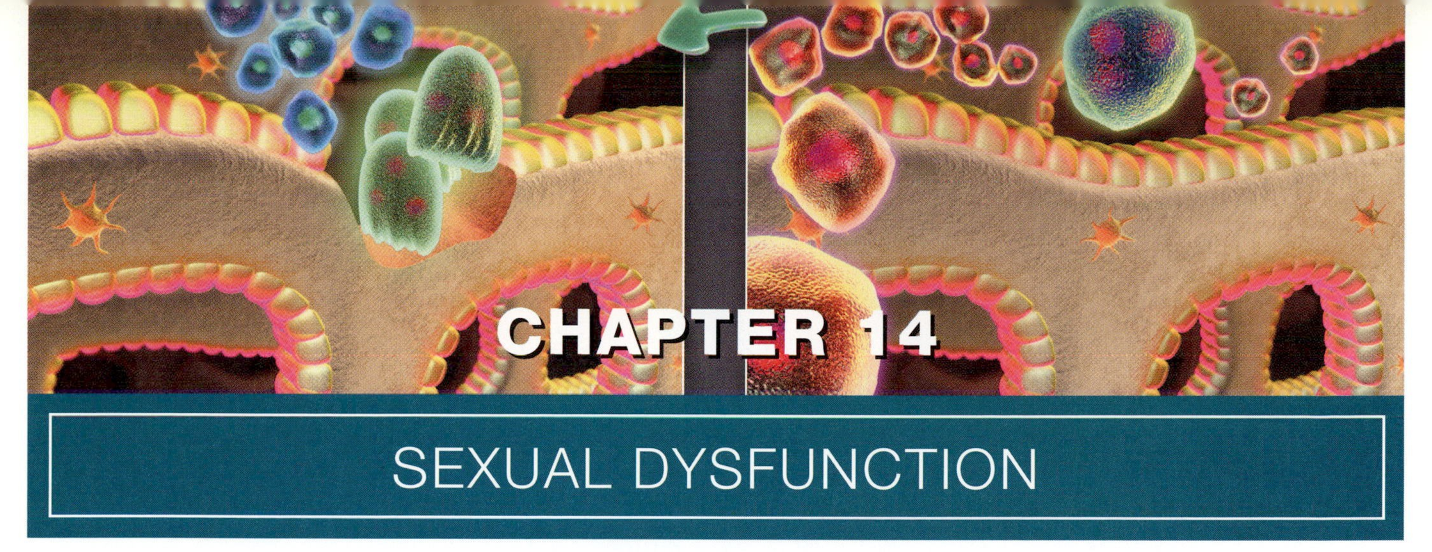

SEXUAL DYSFUNCTION

Kevin T. McVary

Male sexual dysfunction affects 10 to 25% of middle-aged and elderly men. Female sexual dysfunction occurs with a similar frequency. Demographic changes, the popularity of newer treatments, and greater awareness of sexual dysfunction by patients and society have led to increased diagnosis and associated health care expenditures for the management of this common disorder. Because many patients are reluctant to initiate discussion of their sex lives, the physician should address this topic directly to elicit a history of sexual dysfunction.

PHYSIOLOGY OF MALE SEXUAL RESPONSE

Normal male sexual function requires (1) an intact libido, (2) the ability to achieve and maintain penile erection, (3) ejaculation, and (4) detumescence. *Libido* refers to sexual desire and is influenced by a variety of visual, olfactory, tactile, auditory, imaginative, and hormonal stimuli. Sex steroids, particularly testosterone, act to increase libido. Libido can be diminished by hormonal or psychiatric disorders or by medications.

Penile tumescence leading to erection depends on the increased flow of blood into the lacunar network after complete relaxation of the arteries and corporal smooth muscle. The microarchitecture of the corpora is composed of a mass of smooth muscle (trabecula) which contains a network of endothelial-lined vessels (lacunar spaces). Subsequent compression of the trabecular smooth muscle against the fibroelastic tunica albuginea causes a passive closure of the emissary veins and accumulation of blood in the corpora. In the presence of a full erection and a competent valve mechanism, the corpora become noncompressible cylinders from which blood does not escape.

The central nervous system exerts an important influence by either stimulating or antagonizing spinal pathways that mediate erectile function and ejaculation. The erectile response is mediated by a combination of central (psychogenic) and peripheral (reflexogenic) innervation. Sensory nerves that originate from receptors in the penile skin and glans converge to form the dorsal nerve of the penis, which travels to the S2-S4 dorsal root ganglia via the pudendal nerve. Parasympathetic nerve fibers to the penis arise from neurons in the intermediolateral columns of S2-S4 sacral spinal segments. Sympathetic innervation originates from the T-11 to the L-2 spinal segments and descends through the hypogastric plexus.

Neural input to smooth muscle tone is crucial to the initiation and maintenance of an erection. There is also an intricate interaction between the corporal smooth muscle cell and its overlying endothelial cell lining (**Fig. 14-1***A*). Nitric oxide, which induces vascular relaxation, promotes erection and is opposed by endothelin-1 (ET-1), which mediates vascular contraction. Nitric oxide is synthesized from L-arginine by nitric oxide synthase (NOS) and is released from the nonadrenergic, noncholinergic (NANC) autonomic nerve supply to act postjunctionally on smooth muscle cells. Nitric oxide increases the production of cyclic 3′,5′-guanosine monophosphate (cyclic GMP), which induces relaxation of the smooth muscle (Fig. 14-1*B*). Cyclic GMP is gradually broken down by phosphodiesterase type 5 (PDE-5). Inhibitors of PDE-5, such as the oral medication sildenafil, maintain erections by reducing the breakdown of cyclic GMP. However, if

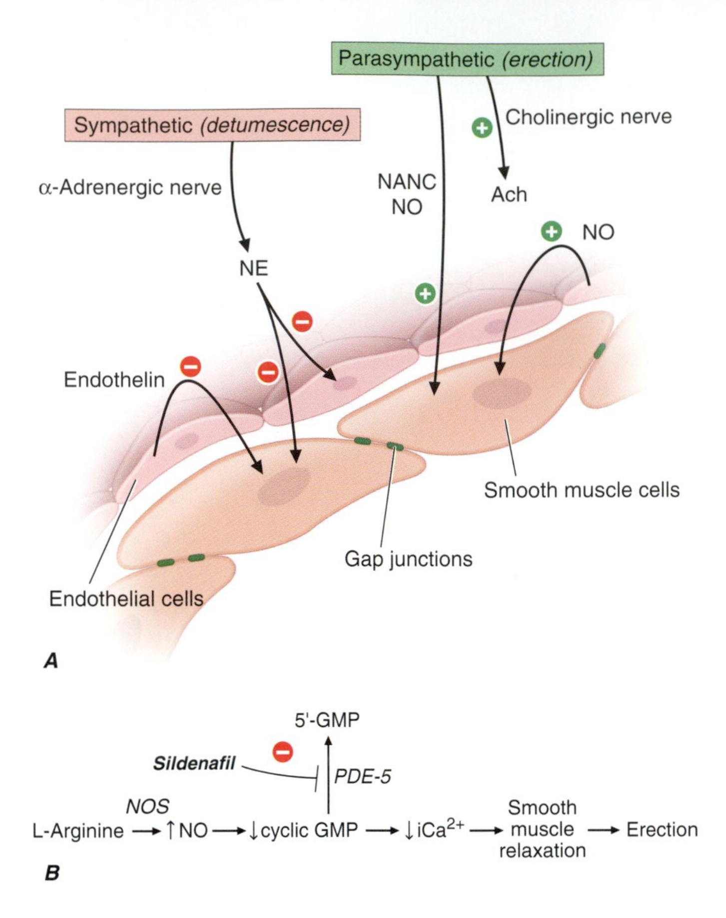

FIGURE 14-1

Pathways that control erection and detumescence. ***A***. Erection is mediated by cholinergic parasympathetic pathways, and nonadrenergic, noncholinergic (NANC) pathways, which release nitric oxide (NO). Endothelial cells also release NO, which induces vascular smooth muscle cell relaxation, allowing enhanced blood flow, and leading to erection. Detumescence is mediated by sympathetic pathways that release norepinephrine and stimulate α-adrenergic pathways, leading to contraction of vascular smooth muscle cells. Endothelin, released from endothelial cells, also induces contraction. ***B***. Biochemical pathways of NO synthesis and action. Sildenafil enhances erectile function by inhibiting phosphodiesterase type 5 (PDE-5), thereby maintaining high levels of cyclic 3′,5′-guanosine monophosphate (cyclic GMP). NOS, nitric oxide synthase; iCa^{2+}, intracellular calcium.

nitric oxide is not produced at some level, the addition of PDE-5 inhibitor is not effective, as the drug facilitates but does not initiate the initial enzyme cascade. In addition to nitric oxide, vasoactive prostaglandins (PGE_1, $PGF_{2\alpha}$) are synthesized within the cavernosal tissue and increase cyclic GMP levels, also leading to relaxation of cavernosal smooth muscle cells.

Ejaculation is stimulated by the sympathetic nervous system, which results in contraction of the epididymis, vas deferens, seminal vesicles, and prostate, causing seminal fluid to enter the urethra. Seminal fluid emission is followed by rhythmic contractions of the bulbocavernosus and ischiocavernosus muscles, leading to ejaculation. *Premature ejaculation* is usually related to anxiety or a learned behavior and is amenable to behavioral therapy or treatment with medications such as selective serotonin reuptake inhibitors (SSRIs). *Retrograde ejaculation* results when the internal urethral sphincter does not close, and it may occur in men with diabetes or after surgery involving the bladder neck.

Detumescence is mediated by released norepinephrine from the sympathetic nerves, release of endothelin from the vascular surface, and contraction of smooth muscle induced by activation of postsynaptic α-adrenergic receptors. These events increase venous outflow and restore the flaccid state. Venous leak can cause premature detumescence and is thought to be caused by insufficient relaxation of the corporal smooth muscle rather than a specific anatomical defect. *Priapism* refers to a persistent and painful erection and may be associated with sickle cell anemia, hypercoagulable states, spinal cord injury, or injection of vasodilator agents into the penis.

ERECTILE DYSFUNCTION

EPIDEMIOLOGY

Erectile dysfunction (ED) is not considered a normal part of the aging process. Nonetheless, it is associated with certain physiologic and psychological changes related to age. In the Massachusetts Male Aging Study (MMAS), a community-based survey of men between the ages of 40 and 70, 52% of responders reported some degree of ED. Complete ED occurred in 10% of respondents, moderate ED occurred in 25%, and minimal ED in 17%. The incidence of moderate or severe ED more than doubled between the ages of 40 and 70. In the National Health and Social Life Survey (NHSLS), which was a nationally representative sample of men and women age 18 to 59 years, 10% of men reported being unable to maintain an erection (corresponding to the proportion of men in the MMAS reporting severe ED). Incidence was highest among men in the 50 to 59 age group (21%) and among men who were poor (14%), divorced (14%), and less educated (13%).

The incidence of ED is also higher among men with certain medical disorders such as diabetes mellitus, heart disease, hypertension, and decreased high-density lipoprotein levels. Smoking is a significant risk factor in the development of ED. Medications used to treat diabetes or cardiovascular disease are additional risk factors (see below). There is a higher incidence of ED among men who have undergone radiation or surgery for prostate cancer and in those with a lower spinal cord injury. Psychological causes of ED include depression, anger, or stress from unemployment or other causes.

PATHOPHYSIOLOGY

ED may result from three basic mechanisms: (1) failure to initiate (psychogenic, endocrinologic, or neurogenic), (2) failure to fill (arteriogenic), or (3) failure to store (veno-occlusive dysfunction) adequate blood volume within the lacunar network. These categories are not mutually exclusive, and multiple factors contribute to ED in many patients. For example, diminished filling pressure can lead secondarily to venous leak. Psychogenic factor frequently coexist with other etiologic factors and should be considered in all cases. Diabetic, atherosclerotic, and drug-related causes account for >80% of cases of ED in older men.

Vasculogenic

The most frequent organic cause of ED is a disturbance of blood flow to and from the penis. Atherosclerotic or traumatic arterial disease can decrease flow to the lacunar spaces, resulting in decreased rigidity and an increased time to full erection. Excessive outflow through the veins, despite adequate inflow, may also contribute to ED. This situation may be due to insufficient relaxation of trabecular smooth muscle and may occur in anxious individuals with excessive adrenergic tone or in those with damaged parasympathetic outflow. Structural alterations to the fibroelastic components of the corpora may cause a loss of compliance and an inability to compress the tunical veins. This condition may result from aging, increased cross-linking of collagen fibers induced by nonenzymatic glycosylation, hypoxia, or altered synthesis of collagen associated with hypercholesterolemia.

Neurogenic

Disorders that affect the sacral spinal cord or the autonomic fibers to the penis preclude nervous system relaxation of penile smooth muscle, thus leading to ED. In patients with spinal cord injury, the degree of ED depends on the completeness and level of the lesion. Patients with incomplete lesions or injuries to the upper part of the spinal cord are more likely to retain erectile capabilities than those with complete lesions or injuries to the lower part. Although 75% of patients with spinal cord injuries have some erectile capability, only 25% have erections sufficient for penetration. Other neurologic disorders commonly associated with ED include multiple sclerosis and peripheral neuropathy. The latter is often due to either diabetes or alcoholism. Pelvic surgery may cause ED through disruption of the autonomic nerve supply.

Endocrinologic

Androgens increase libido, but their exact role in erectile function remains unclear. Individuals with castrate levels of testosterone can achieve erections from visual or sexual stimuli. Nonetheless, normal levels of testosterone appear to be important for erectile function, particularly in older males. Androgen replacement therapy can improve depressed erectile function when it is secondary to hypogonadism; it is not useful for ED when endogenous testosterone levels are normal. Increased prolactin may decrease libido by suppressing gonadotropin-releasing hormone (GnRH), and it also leads to decreased testosterone levels. Treatment of hyperprolactinemia with dopamine agonists can restore libido and testosterone.

Diabetic

ED occurs in 35 to 75% of men with diabetes mellitus. Pathologic mechanisms are primarily related to diabetes-associated vascular and neurologic complications. Diabetic macrovascular complications are mainly related to age, whereas microvascular complications correlate with the duration of diabetes and the degree of glycemic control (Chap. 17). Individuals with diabetes also have reduced amounts of nitric oxide synthase in both endothelial and neural tissues.

Psychogenic

Two mechanisms contribute to the inhibition of erections in psychogenic ED. First, psychogenic stimuli to the sacral cord may inhibit reflexogenic responses, thereby blocking activation of vasodilator outflow to the penis. Second, excess sympathetic stimulation in an anxious man may increase penile smooth muscle tone. The most common causes of psychogenic ED are performance anxiety, depression, relationship conflict, loss of attraction, sexual inhibition, conflicts over sexual preference, sexual abuse in childhood, and fear of pregnancy or sexually transmitted disease. Almost all patients with ED, even when it has a clear-cut organic basis, develop a psychogenic component as a reaction to ED.

Medication-Related

Medication-induced ED (**Table 14-1**) is estimated to occur in 25% of men seen in general medical outpatient

TABLE 14-1

DRUGS ASSOCIATED WITH ERECTILE DYSFUNCTION

CLASSIFICATION	DRUGS
Diuretics	Thiazides Spironolactone
Antihypertensives	Calcium channel blockers Methyldopa Clonidine Reserpine β-Blockers Guanethidine
Cardiac/anti-hyperlipidemics	Digoxin Gemfibrozil Clofibrate
Antidepressants	Selective serotonin reuptake inhibitors Tricyclic antidepressants Lithium Monoamine oxidase inhibitors
Tranquilizers	Butyrophenones Phenothiazines
H_2 antagonists	Ranitidine Cimetidine
Hormones	Progesterone Estrogens Glucocorticoids GnRH agonists 5α-Reductase inhibitors Cyproterone acetate
Cytotoxic agents	Cyclophosphamide Methotrexate Roferon-A
Anticholinergics	Disopyramide Anticonvulsants
Recreational	Ethanol Cocaine Marijuana

clinics. Among the antihypertensive agents, the thiazide diuretics and beta blockers have been implicated most frequently. Calcium channel blockers and angiotensin-converting enzyme inhibitors are less frequently cited. These drugs may act directly at the corporal level (e.g., calcium channel blockers) or indirectly by reducing pelvic blood pressure, which is important in the development of penile rigidity. α-Adrenergic blockers are less likely to cause ED. Estrogens, GnRH agonists, H_2 antagonists, and spironolactone cause ED by suppressing gonadotropin production or by blocking androgen action. Antidepressant and antipsychotic agents—particularly neuroleptics, tricyclics, and SSRIs—are associated with erectile, ejaculatory, orgasmic, and sexual desire difficulties.

Although many medications can cause ED, patients frequently have concomitant risk factors that confound the clinical picture. If there is a strong association between the institution of a drug and the onset of ED, alternative medications should be considered. Otherwise, it is often practical to treat the ED without attempting multiple changes in medications, as it may be difficult to establish a causal role for the drug.

CLINICAL EVALUATION

A good physician-patient relationship helps to unravel the possible causes of ED, many of which require discussion of personal and sometimes embarrassing topics. For this reason, a primary care provider is often ideally suited to initiate the evaluation. A complete medical and sexual history should be taken in an effort to assess whether the cause of ED is organic, psychogenic, or

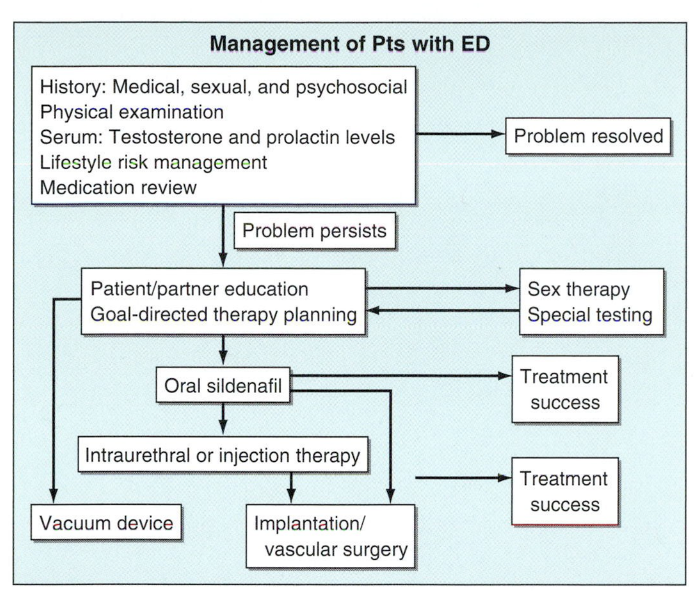

FIGURE 14-2
Algorithm for the evaluation and management of patients with ED.

multifactorial (**Fig. 14-2**). Initial questions should focus on the onset of symptoms, the presence and duration of partial erections, and the progression of ED. A history of nocturnal or early morning erections is useful for distinguishing physiologic from psychogenic ED. Nocturnal erections occur during rapid eye movement (REM) sleep and require intact neurologic and circulatory systems. Organic causes of ED are generally characterized by a gradual and persistent change in rigidity or the inability to sustain nocturnal, coital, or self-stimulated erections. The patient should also be questioned about the presence of penile curvature or pain with coitus. It is also important to address libido, as decreased sexual drive and ED are sometimes the earliest signs of endocrine abnormalities (e.g., increased prolactin, decreased testosterone levels). It is useful to ask whether the problem is confined to coitus with one or other partners; ED arises not uncommonly in association with new or extramarital sexual relationships. Situational ED, as opposed to consistent ED, suggests psychogenic causes. Ejaculation is much less commonly affected than erection, but questions should be asked about whether ejaculation is normal, premature, delayed, or absent. Relevant risk factors should be identified, such as diabetes mellitus, coronary artery disease, lipid disorders, hypertension, peripheral vascular disease, smoking, alcoholism, and endocrine or neurologic disorders. The patient's surgical history should be explored with an emphasis on bowel, bladder, prostate, or vascular procedures. A complete drug history is also important. Social changes that may precipitate ED are also crucial to the evaluation, including health worries, spousal death, divorce, relationship difficulties, and financial concerns.

The physical examination is an essential element in the assessment of ED. Signs of hypertension as well as evidence of thyroid, hepatic, hematologic, cardiovascular, or renal diseases should be sought. An assessment should be made of the endocrine and vascular systems, the external genitalia, and the prostate gland. The penis should be carefully palpated along the corpora to detect fibrotic plaques. Reduced testicular size and loss of secondary sexual characteristics are suggestive of hypogonadism. Neurologic examination should include assessment of anal sphincter tone, the bulbocavernosus reflex, and testing for peripheral neuropathy.

Although hyperprolactinemia is uncommon, a serum prolactin level should be measured, as decreased libido and/or erectile dysfunction may be the presenting symptoms of a prolactinoma or other mass lesions of the sella (Chap. 2). The serum testosterone level should be measured and, if low, gonadotropins should be measured to determine whether hypogonadism is primary (testicular) or secondary (hypothalamic-pituitary) in origin (Chap. 8). Serum chemistries, complete blood count, and lipid profiles may be of value, if not performed recently, as they can yield evidence of anemia, diabetes, hyperlipidemia, or other systemic diseases associated with ED. Determination of serum prostate-specific antigen (PSA) should be conducted according to recommended clinical guidelines.

Additional diagnostic testing is rarely necessary in the evaluation of ED. However, in selected patients, specialized testing may provide insight into pathologic mechanisms of ED and aid in the selection of treatment options. Optional specialized testing includes: (1) studies of nocturnal penile tumescence and rigidity, (2) vascular testing (in-office injection of vasoactive substances, penile Doppler ultrasound, penile angiography, dynamic infusion cavernosography/cavernosometry), (3) neurologic testing (biothesiometry-graded vibratory perception; somatosensory evoked potentials), and (4) psychological diagnostic tests. The information potentially gained from these procedures must be balanced against their invasiveness and cost.

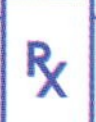

TREATMENT FOR ERECTILE DYSFUNCTION

Patient Education

Patient and partner education are essential in the treatment of ED. In goal-directed therapy, education facilitates understanding of the disease, results of the tests, and selection of treatment. Discussion of treatment options helps to clarify how treatment is best offered, and to stratify first- and second-line therapies. Patients with high-risk life-style issues, such as smoking, alcohol abuse, or recreational drug use, should be counseled on the role these factors play in the development of ED.

Oral Agents

Sildenafil, vardenafil, and tadalafil have been approved for the treatment of ED. They exhibit similar efficacy but tadalafil has a longer duration of action. Sildenafil is representative of this class of drugs. It has markedly improved the management of ED because it is effective for the treatment of a broad range of causes of ED, including psychogenic, diabetic, vasculogenic, post-radical prostatectomy (nerve-sparing procedures), and spinal cord injury. Sildenafil is a selective and potent inhibitor of PDE-5, the predominant phosphodiesterase isoform found in the penis. It is administered in doses of 25, 50, or 100 mg and enhances erections after sexual stimulation. The onset of action is ~60 to 90 min. Reduced initial doses should be considered for patients who are elderly, have renal insufficiency, or are taking medications that inhibit the CYP3A4 metabolic pathway in the liver (e.g., erythromycin, cimetidine, ketoconazole, and, possibly, itraconazole and mibefradil), as they may increase the serum concentration of sildenafil. The drug does not affect ejaculation, orgasm, or sexual drive. Side effects associated with sildenafil include headaches (19%), facial flushing (9%), dyspepsia (6%) and nasal congestion (4%). Approximately 7% of men may experience transient altered color vision (blue halo effect). Sildenafil is contraindicated in men receiving nitrate therapy for cardiovascular disease, including agents delivered by oral, sublingual, transnasal, or topical routes. These agents can potentiate its hypotensive effect and may result in profound shock. Likewise, amyl/butyl nitrates "poppers" may have a fatal synergistic effect on blood pressure. Sildenafil should also be avoided in patients with congestive heart failure and cardiomyopathy because of the risk of vascular collapse. Because sexual activity leads to an increase in physiologic expenditure [5 to 6 metabolic equivalents (METS)], physicians have been advised to exercise caution in prescribing any drug for sexual activity to those with active coronary disease, heart failure, borderline hypotension, hypovolemia, and to those on complex antihypertensive regimens.

Androgen Therapy

Testosterone replacement is used to treat both primary and secondary causes of hypogonadism (Chap. 8). Androgen supplementation in the setting of normal testosterone is rarely efficacious and is discouraged. Methods of androgen replacement include parenteral administration of long-acting testosterone esters (enanthate and cypionate), oral preparations (17 α-alkylated derivatives), and transdermal patches and gels (Chap. 8). The long-acting 17 β-hydroxy esters of testosterone are the safest, most cost-effective, and practical preparations available. The administration of 200 to 300 mg intramuscularly every 2 to 3 weeks provides a practical option but is far from an ideal physiologic replacement. Oral androgen preparations have the potential for hepatotoxicity and should be avoided. Transdermal delivery of testosterone using patches or gels more closely mimics physiologic testosterone levels, but it is unclear whether this translates into improved sexual function. Testosterone therapy is contraindicated in men with androgen-sensitive cancers and may be inappropriate for men with bladder neck obstruction. It is generally advisable to measure PSA before giving androgen. Hepatic function should be tested before and during testosterone therapy.

Vacuum Constriction Devices

Vacuum constriction devices (VCD) are a well-established, noninvasive therapy. They are a reasonable treatment alternative for select patients who cannot take sildenafil or do not desire other interventions. VCD draw venous blood into the penis and use a constriction ring to restrict venous return and maintain tumescence. Adverse events with VCD include pain, numbness, bruising, and altered ejaculation. Additionally, many patients complain that the devices are cumbersome and that the induced erections have a nonphysiologic appearance.

Intraurethral Alprostadil

If a patient fails to respond to oral agents, a reasonable next choice is intraurethral or self-injection of vasoactive substances. Intraurethral prostaglandin E_1 (alprostadil), in the form of a semisolid pellet (doses of 125 to 1000 μg), is delivered with an applicator. Approximately 65% of men receiving intraurethral alprostadil respond with an erection when tested in the office, but only 50% of those achieve successful coitus at home. Intraurethral insertion is associated with a markedly reduced incidence of priapism in comparison to intracavernosal injection.

Intracavernosal Self-Injection

Injection of synthetic formulations of alprostadil is effective in 70 to 80% of patients with ED, but discontinuation rates are high because of the invasive nature of administration. Doses range between 1 and 40 μg. Injection therapy is contraindicated in men with a history of hypersensitivity to the drug and in men at risk for priapism (hypercoagulable states, sickle cell disease). Side effects include local adverse events, prolonged erections, pain, and fibrosis with chronic use. Various combinations of alprostadil, phentolamine, and/or papaverine are sometimes used.

Surgery

A less frequently used form of therapy for ED involves the surgical implantation of a semi-rigid or inflatable penile prosthesis. These surgical treatments are invasive, associated with potential complications, and generally reserved for treatment of refractory ED. Despite their high cost and invasiveness, penile prostheses are associated with high rates of patient satisfaction.

Sex Therapy

A course of sex therapy may be useful for addressing specific interpersonal factors that may affect sexual functioning. Sex therapy generally consists of in-session discussion and at-home exercises specific to the person and the relationship. It is preferable if therapy includes both partners, provided the patient is involved in an ongoing relationship.

FEMALE SEXUAL DYSFUNCTION

Female sexual dysfunction (FSD) has traditionally included disorders of desire, arousal, pain, and muted orgasm. The associated risk factors for FSD are similar to those in males: cardiovascular disease, endocrine disorders, hypertension, neurologic disorders, and smoking (**Table 14-2**).

EPIDEMIOLOGY

Epidemiologic data are limited but the available estimates suggest that as many as 43% of women complain of at least one sexual problem. Despite the recent interest in organic causes of FSD, desire and arousal phase disorders (including lubrication complaints) remain the most common presenting problems when surveyed in a community-based population.

PHYSIOLOGY OF THE FEMALE SEXUAL RESPONSE

Although there are the obvious anatomical differences as well as variation in the density of vascular and neural beds in males and females, the primary effectors of sexual response are strikingly similar. Intact sensation is

TABLE 14-2

RISK FACTORS FOR FEMALE SEXUAL DYSFUNCTION
Neurologic disease: stroke, spinal cord injury, Parkinsonism
Trauma, genital surgery, radiation
Endocrinopathies: diabetes, hyperprolactinemia
Liver and/or renal failure
Cardiovascular disease
Psychological factors and interpersonal relationship disorders: sexual abuse, life stressors
Medications
Antiandrogens: Cimetidine, spironolactone
Antidepressants, Alcohol, hypnotics, sedatives
Antiestrogens or GnRH antagonists
Antihistamines, sympathomimetic amines
Antihypertensives: Diuretics, calcium channel blockers
Alkylating agents
Anticholinergies

important for arousal. Thus, reduced levels of sexual functioning are more common in women with peripheral neuropathies (e.g., diabetes). Vaginal lubrication is a transudate of serum that results from the increased pelvic blood flow associated with arousal. Vascular insufficiency from a variety of causes may compromise adequate lubrication and result in dyspareunia. Similar to the male response, cavernosal and arteriole smooth muscle relaxation occur via increased NOS activity and produce engorgement in the clitoris and surrounding vestibule. Orgasm requires an intact sympathetic outflow tract; hence, orgasmic disorders are common in female patients with spinal cord injuries.

CLINICAL EVALUATION

The evaluation of FSD previously occurred mainly in a psychosocial context. However, inconsistencies between diagnostic categories based on only psychosocial considerations, and the emerging recognition of organic etiologies, have led to a new classification of FSD. This diagnostic scheme is based on four components that are not mutually exclusive:

1. *Hypoactive sexual desire*—the persistent or recurrent lack of sexual thoughts and/or receptivity to sexual activity, which causes personal distress. Hypoactive sexual desire may result from endocrine failure or may be associated with psychological or emotional disorders.
2. *Sexual arousal disorder*—the persistent or recurrent inability to attain or maintain sexual excitement, which causes personal distress.
3. *Orgasmic disorder*—the persistent or recurrent loss of orgasmic potential after sufficient sexual stimulation and arousal, which causes personal distress.
4. *Sexual pain disorder*—persistent or recurrent genital pain associated with noncoital sexual stimulation, which causes personal distress.

This newer classification emphasizes "personal distress" as a requirement for dysfunction and provides clinicians an organized framework for evaluation prior to or in conjunction with more traditional counseling methods.

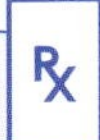

TREATMENT FOR FSD

Patient Education

Patient and partner education are essential in the treatment of FSD. Educating the couple about normal anatomy and physiologic responses is often necessary. Physiologic changes associated with aging and/or disease should be explained. Maximizing physical health and avoiding life-styles (e.g., smoking, alcohol abuse) and medications likely to produce FSD are prudent (Table 14-2).

Hormonal Therapy

In postmenopausal women, estrogen replacement therapy may be helpful in treating vaginal atrophy, decreasing coital pain, and improving clitoral sensitivity (Chap. 11). Estrogen replacement in the form of local cream is the preferred method, as it avoids systemic side effects. Androgen levels in women decline substantially before menopause. However, low levels of testosterone or dehydroepiandrosterone (DHEA) are not effective predictors of a positive therapeutic outcome with androgen therapy. The widespread use of exogenous androgens is not supported by the literature except in select circumstances (premature ovarian failure or menopausal states) and in secondary arousal disorders.

Oral Agents

The efficacy of PDE-5 inhibitors in FDS has been a marked disappointment given the proposed role of nitric oxide–dependent physiology in the normal female sexual response. The use of sildenafil for FSD should be discouraged pending proof that it is effective.

Clitoral Vacuum Device

In patients with arousal and orgasmic difficulties, the option of using a clitoral vacuum device may be explored. This handheld battery-operated device has a small soft plastic cup that applies a vacuum over the stimulated clitoris. This causes increased cavernosal blood flow, engorgement, and vaginal lubrication.

FURTHER READINGS

Araujo AB et al: Changes in sexual function in middle-aged and older men: Longitudinal data from the Massachusetts Male Aging Study. J Am Geriatr Soc 52:1502, 2004

Androgen deficiency was assessed in 1087 men from the Massachusetts Male Aging Study. Based on these incidence data (12.3 per 1000 person-years), this study estimates ~481,000 new cases of androgen deficiency per year in U.S. men 40–69 years old.

■ BRAUNSTEIN GD ET AL: Safety and efficacy of a testosterone patch for the treatment of hypoactive sexual desire disorder in surgically menopausal women. Arch Intern Med 165:1582, 2005

This study found that a 300-μg/d testosterone patch increased sexual desire and frequency of satisfying sexual activity in women who developed hypoactive sexual desire disorder after surgical menopause. Although there is increasing evidence for the efficacy of testosterone patches after surgical menopause, inappropriate or long-term use of testosterone carries the risk of masculinization and possibly more serious side effects.

■ DAVIS SR et al: Circulating androgen levels and self-reported sexual function in women. JAMA 294:91, 2005

This study of over 1000 women found that circulating androgen levels did not correlate with self-reported sexual function.

■ DOGGRELL SA: Comparison of clinical trials with sildenafi, vardenafil, and tadalafil in erectile dysfunction. Expert Opin Pharmacother 6:75, 2005

This review summarizes the efficacy and side effects of various phosphodiesterase inhibitors used to treat erectile dysfunction. While the efficacy of the three drugs is similar, vardenafil does not affect color perception and tadalafil has a longer duration of action.

KLONER RA: Cardiovascular effect of the three phosphodiesterase-5 inhibitors approved for the treatment of erectile dysfunction. Circulation 110:3149, 2004.

KOVALEVSKY G: Female sexual dysfunction and use of hormone therapy in postmenopausal women. Semin Reprod Med 23:180, 2005

LESSER J: Sexual dysfunction in the older woman: Complex medical, psychiatric illnesses should be considered in evaluation and management. Geriatrics 60:18, 2005

MCVARY KT et al: Smoking and erectile dysfunction: Evidence based analysis. J Urol 166:1624, 2001

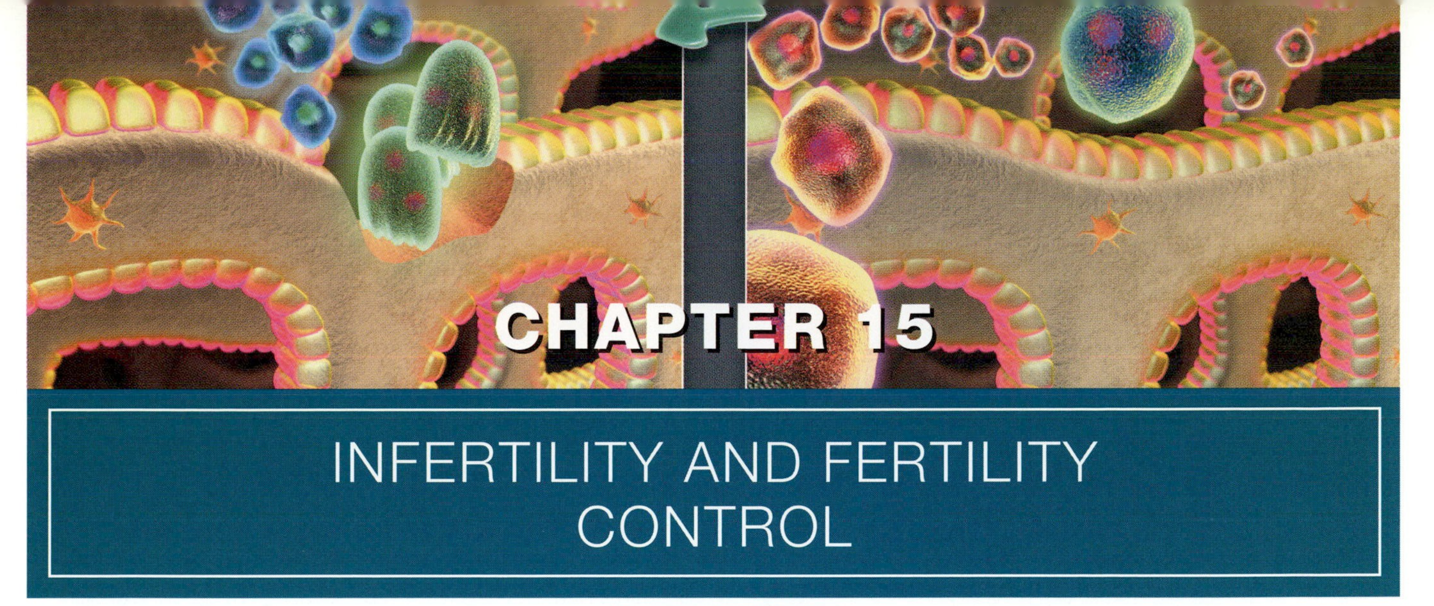

INFERTILITY AND FERTILITY CONTROL

Janet E. Hall

The concept of reproductive choice is now firmly entrenched in developed countries and has dramatically altered reproductive behavior. The availability of effective contraceptive methods prevents unintended pregnancies and has important economic and social implications. Infertility, on the other hand, can be accompanied by substantial stress and disappointment. Fortunately, the ability to diagnose and to treat various causes of infertility now provides an array of effective new approaches to this condition.

INFERTILITY

DEFINITION AND PREVALENCE

Infertility is defined as the inability to conceive after 12 months of unprotected sexual intercourse. In a study of 5574 English and American women who ultimately conceived, pregnancy occurred in 50% within 3 months, 72% within 6 months, and 85% within 12 months. These findings are consistent with predictions based on *fecundability*, the probability of achieving pregnancy in one menstrual cycle (approximately 20 to 25% in healthy young couples). Assuming a fecundability of 0.25, 98% of couples should conceive within 13 months. Based on this definition, the National Survey of Family Growth reports a 14% rate of infertility in the United States in married women aged 15 to 44. The infertility rate has remained relatively stable over the past 30 years, although the proportion of couples without children has risen, reflecting a trend to delay childbearing. This trend has important implications because of an age-related decrease in fecundability, which begins at age 35 and is exacerbated after age 40.

CAUSES OF INFERTILITY

The spectrum of infertility ranges from reduced conception rates or the need for medical intervention to irreversible causes of infertility (*sterility*). Infertility can be attributed primarily to male factors in 25%, female factors in 58%, and is unexplained in about 17% of couples (**Fig. 15-1**). Not uncommonly, both male and female factors contribute to infertility.

APPROACH TO THE PATIENT WITH INFERTILITY

Initial Evaluation

In all couples presenting with infertility, the initial evaluation includes discussion of the appropriate timing of intercourse and discussion of modifiable risk factors such as smoking, alcohol, caffeine, and obesity. A description of the range of investigations that may be required and a brief description of infertility treatment options, including adoption, should be reviewed. Initial investigations are focused on determining whether the primary cause of the infertility is male, female, or both. These investigations include a semen analysis in the male, confirmation of ovulation in the female,

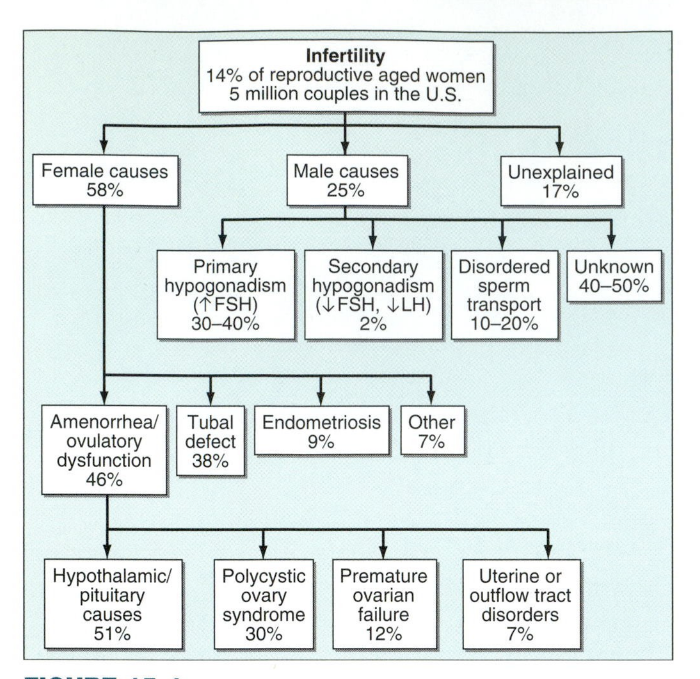

FIGURE 15-1

Causes of infertility. FSH, follicle-stimulating hormone; LH, luteinizing hormone.

and, in the majority of situations, documentation of tubal patency in the female. Although frequently used in the past, recent studies have not supported the efficacy of postcoital testing of sperm interaction with cervical mucus as a routine component of initial testing. Strategies for further evaluation are described below and in Chaps. 8 and 10. In some cases, after an extensive evaluation has excluded identifiable male or female causes of infertility, the disorder is classified as unexplained infertility.

Psychological Aspects of Infertility

Infertility is invariably associated with psychological stress. In addition to the diagnostic and therapeutic procedures, stress may result from repeated cycles of hope and loss associated with each new procedure or cycle of treatment that does not result in the birth of a child. These feelings are often combined with a sense of isolation from friends and family. Counseling and stress-management techniques should be introduced early in the evaluation of infertility. When extreme, stress can contribute to infertility; for example, stress may impair hypothalamic control of ovulation. Infertility and its treatment do not appear to be associated with long-term psychological sequelae.

Female Causes

Abnormalities in menstrual function constitute the most common cause of female infertility. These disorders, which include ovulatory dysfunction and abnormalities of the uterus or outflow tract, may present as amenorrhea (absence of menses) or as irregular or short menstrual cycles. A careful history and physical examination and a limited number of laboratory tests will help to determine whether the abnormality is (1) hypothalamic or pituitary [low follicle-stimulating hormone (FSH), luteinizing hormone (LH), and estradiol with or without an increase in prolactin], (2) polycystic ovarian syndrome (PCOS; irregular cycles and hyperandrogenism in the absence of other causes of androgen excess), (3) ovarian (low estradiol with increased FSH), or (4) uterine or outflow tract abnormality. The frequency of these diagnoses depends on whether the amenorrhea is primary or occurs after normal puberty and menarche (Fig. 15-1). The approach to further evaluation of these disorders is described in detail in Chap. 10.

OVULATORY DYSFUNCTION

In women with a history of regular menstrual cycles, *evidence of ovulation* should be sought by using urinary ovulation predictor kits (they reflect the preovulatory gonadotropin surge but do not confirm ovulation), basal body temperature charts, or a mid-luteal phase progesterone level. The mid-luteal phase progesterone increase (usually >3 ng/mL) confirms ovulation and corpus luteum function and is responsible for the rise in basal body temperature [>0.3°C (>0.6°F) for 10 days]. An endometrial biopsy to exclude luteal phase insufficiency is no longer considered an essential part of the infertility workup for most patients. Even in the presence of ovulatory cycles, evaluation of *ovarian reserve* is recommended for women over 35 by measurement of FSH on day 3 of the cycle or in response to clomiphene, an estrogen antagonist (see below). An FSH level <10 IU/mL on cycle day 3 predicts adequate ovarian oocyte reserve. Inhibin B, an ovarian hormone that selectively suppresses FSH, is not of additional benefit in assessment of ovarian reserve.

TUBAL DISEASE

Tubal disease may result from pelvic inflammatory disease (PID), appendicitis, endometriosis, pelvic adhesions, tubal surgery, and previous use of an intrauterine device (IUD). However, a specific cause is not identified in up to 50% of patients with documented tubal factor infertility. Because of the high prevalence of tubal disease, evaluation of tubal patency by hysterosalpingogram or laparoscopy should occur early in the majority of couples with infertility. Subclinical infection with *Chlamydia trachomatis* may be an underdiagnosed cause of tubal infertility and requires the treatment of both partners.

ENDOMETRIOSIS

Endometriosis is defined as the presence of endometrial glands or stroma outside the endometrial cavity and uterine musculature. Its presence is suggested by a history of dyspareunia (painful intercourse), worsening dysmenorrhea that often begins before menses, or by a thickened rectovaginal septum or deviation of the cervix on pelvic examination. The pathogenesis of the infertility associated with endometriosis is unclear but may involve cytokine effects on the normal endometrium as well as adhesions. Endometriosis is often clinically silent, however, and can only be excluded definitively by laparoscopy.

Male Causes

Known causes of male infertility include primary testicular dysfunction, disorders of sperm transport, and hypothalamic-pituitary disease resulting in secondary hypogonadism. However, the etiology is not ascertained in up to half of men with suspected male factor infertility (Fig. 15-1). The key initial diagnostic test is a *semen analysis*. Although 95% confidence limits can be used to define normal semen parameters, data relating sperm counts to fecundability are more useful. Such studies suggest that normal fertility is associated with sperm counts of >48 million/mL, with a motility of >63%, with >12% exhibiting normal morphology, whereas subfertility is seen with sperm counts of <13 million/mL, motility of <32%, and <9% normal morphology. Abnormalities of spermatogenesis may have a genetic component. Y chromosome microdeletions and *POLG* variants are increasingly recognized as a cause of *azoospermia* (absence of sperm) or *oligospermia* (low sperm count). Y chromosome microdeletions have also been identified in a subset of men with elevated FSH levels and idiopathic infertility. Testosterone levels should be measured if the sperm count is low on repeated examination or if there is clinical evidence of hypogonadism. A low testosterone level may result from *primary gonadal deficiency*; in this condition, levels of LH and FSH will be elevated. Less commonly, low testosterone and decreased spermatogenesis result from hypothalamic or pituitary disease, in which case the LH and FSH levels will be low (Chap. 8).

Acquired disorders of the testes are often associated with impaired spermatogenesis with relatively preserved Leydig cell function; thus, testosterone levels may be normal. Such abnormalities include viral orchitis (especially mumps) and other infectious causes such as tuberculosis or sexually transmitted diseases (STDs), chemotherapy (especially the alkylating agents cyclophosphamide and chlorambucil), ionizing radiation, and drugs that may impair fertility directly or through inhibition of testicular androgen production or action. Anabolic androgen abuse should be considered in a well-androgenized man with low gonadotropins and testosterone but a suppressed sperm count. Prolonged elevation of testicular temperature may impair spermatogenesis, e.g., cryptorchidism, after an acute febrile illness or in association with varicocele. A potential role for environmental toxins as a cause of impaired spermatogenesis has been suggested based on an apparent decrease in sperm counts over the past several decades, but a direct cause-and-effect relationship has not been established.

SECONDARY HYPOGONADISM

Low gonadotropin levels, associated with low testosterone, may signal the presence of a pituitary macroadenoma or hypothalamic tumor (in both cases prolactin levels may be elevated; Chap. 2) or may be the first presentation of hemochromatosis or other systemic illness. Recent studies have identified several genetic causes of gonadotropin-releasing hormone (GnRH) deficiency (*KAL* and *DAX-1*), as well as mutations that lead to isolated gonadotropin deficiency (GnRH receptor, LHβ, FSHβ mutations) (Chap. 2).

DISORDERED SPERM TRANSPORT

Patients with low sperm counts and normal hormonal levels may be found to have obstructive abnormalities of the vas deferens or epididymus. The most common causes of vas deferens obstruction are previous vasectomy or accidental ligation during inguinal surgery. Congenital absence of the vas deferens can be diagnosed by a deficiency of fructose in the ejaculate and is often associated with an abnormality of the cystic fibrosis transmembrane regulator (*CFTR*) gene. Young's syndrome, characterized by inspissated secretions, can also preclude normal sperm transport.

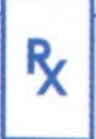

TREATMENT FOR INFERTILITY

The treatment of infertility should be tailored to the problems unique to each couple. In many situations, including unexplained infertility, mild to moderate endometriosis, and/or borderline semen parameters, a stepwise approach to infertility is optimal, beginning with low-risk interventions and moving to more invasive, higher risk interventions only if necessary. After determination of all infertility factors and their correction, if possible, this approach might include, in increasing order of complexity: (1) expectant management, (2) clomiphene citrate (see below) with or without intrauterine insemination (IUI), (3) gonadotropins with or without IUI, and (4) in vitro fertilization (IVF). The time used to complete the evaluation, correction, and expectant management can be longer in women <30, but this process should be advanced rapidly in women >35. In some situations, expectant management will not be appropriate.

Ovulatory Dysfunction

Treatment of ovulatory dysfunction should first be directed at identification of the etiology of the disorder to allow specific management when possible. Dopamine agonists, for example, may be indicated in patients with hyperprolactinemia (Chap. 2); life-style modification may be successful in women with low body weight or a history of intensive exercise.

Medications used for ovulation induction include clomiphene citrate, gonadotropins, and pulsatile GnRH. *Clomiphene citrate* is a nonsteroidal estrogen antagonist that increases FSH and LH levels by blocking estrogen negative feedback at the hypothalamus. The efficacy of clomiphene for ovulation induction is highly dependent on patient selection. It induces ovulation in 70 to 80% of women with PCOS and is the initial treatment of choice in these patients, particularly in conjunction with the use of insulin-sensitizing agents, such as metformin. Clomiphene citrate is less successful in patients with hypogonadotropic hypogonadism.

Gonadotropins are highly effective for ovulation induction in women with hypogonadotropic hypogonadism and PCOS and are used to induce multiple follicular recruitment in unexplained infertility and in older reproductive-aged women. Disadvantages include a significant risk of multiple gestation and the risk of ovarian hyperstimulation, but careful monitoring and a conservative approach to ovarian stimulation reduce these risks. Currently available gonadotropins include urinary preparations of LH and FSH, highly purified FSH, and recombinant FSH. Though FSH is the key component, the addition of some LH (or human chorionic gonadotropin) may improve results, particularly in hypogonadotropic patients.

Pulsatile GnRH is highly effective for restoring ovulation in patients with hypothalamic amenorrhea but is not widely available in the United States. Pregnancy rates are similar to those following the use of gonadotropins, but rates of multiple gestation are lower and there is virtually no risk of ovarian hyperstimulation.

None of these methods are effective in women with premature ovarian failure in whom donor oocyte or adoption are the methods of choice.

Tubal Disease

If hysterosalpingography suggests a tubal or uterine cavity abnormality, or if a patient is ≥35 at the time of initial evaluation, laparoscopy with tubal lavage is recommended, often with a hysteroscopy. Although tubal reconstruction may be attempted if tubal disease is identified, IVF is often used instead, as these patients are at increased risk of developing an ectopic pregnancy.

Endometriosis

Though 60% of women with minimal or mild endometriosis may conceive within 1 year without treatment, laparoscopic resection or ablation appears to improve conception rates. Medical management of advanced stages of endometriosis is widely used for symptom control but has not been shown to enhance fertility (Chap. 10). In moderate to severe endometriosis, conservative surgery is associated with pregnancy rates of 50 and 39% respectively, compared with rates of 25 and 5% with expectant management alone. In some patients, IVF may be the treatment of choice.

Male Factor Infertility

Treatment options for male factor infertility have expanded greatly in recent years. Secondary hypogonadism is highly amenable to treatment with pulsatile GnRH or gonadotropins (Chap. 8). In vitro techniques have provided new opportunities for patients with primary testicular failure and disorders of sperm transport. Choice of initial treatment options depends on sperm concentration and motility. Expectant management should be attempted initially in men with mild male factor infertility (sperm count of 15 to 20 × 10^6/mL and normal motility). Moderate male factor infertility (10 to 15 × 10^6/mL and 20 to 40% motility) should begin with IUI alone or in combination with treatment of the female partner with clomiphene or gonadotropins, but it may require IVF with or without intracytoplasmic sperm injection (ICSI). For men with a severe defect (sperm count of <10 × 10^6/mL, 10% motility), IVF with ICSI or donor sperm should be used.

Assisted Reproductive Technologies

The development of assisted reproductive technologies (ART) has dramatically altered the treatment of male and female infertility. IVF is indicated for patients with many causes of infertility that have not been successfully managed with more conservative approaches. IVF or ICSI is often the treatment of choice in couples with a significant male factor or tubal disease, whereas IVF using donor oocytes is used in patients with premature ovarian failure and in women of advanced reproductive age. Success rates depend on the age of the woman and the cause of the infertility and are generally 18 to 24% per cycle when initiated in women <40. In women >40, there is a marked decrease in both the number of oocytes retrieved and their ability to be fertilized. Though often effective, IVF is expensive and requires careful monitoring of ovulation induction and invasive techniques, including the aspiration of multiple follicles. IVF is associated with a significant risk of multiple gestation (31% twins, 6% triplets, and 0.2% higher order multiples).

CONTRACEPTION

Though various forms of contraception are widely available, ~30% of births in the United States are the result of unintended pregnancy. Teenage pregnancies continue to represent a serious public health problem in the United States, with >1 million unintended pregnancies each year—a significantly greater incidence than in other industrialized nations.

Contraceptive methods are widely used (**Table 15-1**). Only 15% of couples report having unprotected sexual intercourse in the past 3 months. A reversible form of contraception is used by >50% of couples. Sterilization (in either the male or female) has been employed as a permanent form of contraception by over a third of couples. Pregnancy termination is relatively safe when directed by health care professionals but is rarely the option of choice.

No single contraceptive method is ideal, although all are safer than carrying a pregnancy to term. The effectiveness of a given method of contraception is dependent on the efficacy of the method itself, compliance, and appropriate use. Knowledge of the advantages and disadvantages of each contraceptive is essential for counseling an individual about the methods that are safest and most consistent with his or her life-style. Discrepancies between theoretical and actual effectiveness emphasize the importance of patient education and compliance when considering various forms of contraception (Table 15-1).

BARRIER METHODS

Barrier contraceptives (such as condoms, diaphragms, and cervical caps) and spermicides are easily available, reversible, and have fewer side effects than hormonal methods. However, their effectiveness is highly dependent on compliance and proper use (Table 15-1). A major advantage of barrier contraceptives is the protection provided against STDs. Consistent use is associated with a decreased risk of gonorrhea, nongonococcal urethritis, and genital herpes, probably due in part to the concomitant use of spermicides. Condom use also reduces the transmission of HIV infection. Natural membrane condoms may be less effective than latex condoms, and petroleum-based lubricants can degrade condoms and decrease their efficacy for preventing HIV infection. A highly effective female condom, which also provides protection against STDs, was approved in 1994 but has not achieved widespread use.

STERILIZATION

Sterilization is the method of birth control most frequently chosen by fertile men and multiparous women >30 (Table 15-1). Sterilization prevents fertilization by surgical interruption of the fallopian tubes in women or the vas deferens in men. Although tubal ligation and vasectomy are potentially reversible, these procedures should be considered permanent and should not be undertaken without careful patient counseling.

Several methods of *tubal ligation* have been developed, all of which are highly effective with a 10-year cumulative pregnancy rate of 1.85 per 100 women. However, when pregnancy does occur, the risk of ectopic pregnancy may be as high as 30%. In addition to prevention of pregnancy, tubal ligation reduces the risk of ovarian cancer, possibly by limiting the upward migration of potential carcinogens.

Vasectomy is an outpatient surgical procedure that has little risk and is highly effective. The development of azoospermia may be delayed for 2 to 6 months, and other forms of contraception must be used until two sperm-free ejaculations provide proof of sterility.

TABLE 15-1

EFFECTIVENESS OF DIFFERENT FORMS OF CONTRACEPTION

METHOD OF CONTRACEPTION	THEORETICAL EFFECTIVENESS, %[a]	ACTUAL EFFECTIVENESS, %[a]	% CONTINUING USE AT 1 YEAR[b]	CONTRACEPTIVE METHODS USED BY U.S. WOMEN[c]
Barrier methods				
Condoms	98	88	63	20
Diaphragm	94	82	58	2
Cervical cap	94	82	50	<1
Spermicides	97	79	43	1
Sterilization				
Male	99.9	99.9	100	11
Female	99.8	99.6	100	28
Intrauterine device				1
Copper T380	99	97	78	
Progestasert	98	97	81	
Mirena	99.9	99.8		
Oral contraceptive pill			72	27
Combination	99.9	97		
Progestin only	99.5	97		
Long-acting progestins				
Depo-Provera	99.7	99.7	70	<1
Norplant	99.7	99.7	85	1

[a]Adapted from Trussel J et al, Obstet Gynecol 76:558, 1990.
[b]Adapted from Contraceptive Technology Update. Contraceptive Technology, Feb. 1996, vol 17, No 1, pp 13–24.
[c]Adapted from Piccinino LJ and Mosher WD, Fam Plan Perspective 30:4, 1998.

INTRAUTERINE DEVICES

IUDs inhibit pregnancy primarily through a spermicidal effect caused by a sterile inflammatory reaction produced by the presence of a foreign body in the uterine cavity (copper IUDs) or by the release of progestins (Progestasert, Mirena). IUDs provide a high level of efficacy in the absence of systemic metabolic effects, and ongoing motivation is not required to ensure efficacy once the device has been placed. However, only 1% of women in the United States use this method compared to a utilization rate of 15 to 30% in much of Europe and Canada. This relatively low utilization rate continues despite evidence that the newer devices are not associated with increased rates of pelvic infection and infertility, as occurred with earlier devices. Screening for STDs should be performed prior to insertion, and an IUD should not be used in women at high risk for development of STDs or in women at high risk for bacterial endocarditis.

HORMONAL METHODS

Oral Contraceptive Pills

Because of their ease of use and efficacy, oral contraceptive pills are the most widely used form of hormonal contraception. They act by suppressing ovulation, changing cervical mucus, and altering the endometrium. The current formulations are made from synthetic estrogens and progestins. The estrogen component of the pill consists of ethinyl estradiol or mestranol, which is metabolized to ethinyl estradiol. Multiple synthetic progestins are available. Norethindrone and its derivatives are used in many formulations. Low-dose norgestimate and the more recently developed progestins (desogestrel, gestodene, drospirenone) have a less androgenic profile; levonorgestrel appears to be the most androgenic of the progestins and should be avoided in patients with hyperandrogenic features. The three major formulations of oral contraceptives are: (1) fixed-dose estrogen-progestin combination, (2) phasic estrogen-progestin combination, and (3) progestin only. Combination formulations are administered daily for 3 weeks followed by a week of no medication during which menstrual bleeding generally occurs. Progestin-only pills are administered continuously. There has been recent interest in the development of extended oral contraceptives, reducing the number of episodes of withdrawal bleeding. An oral, trimonthly regimen is currently under investigation in the United States. Preliminary studies indicate that headache is reduced, although there is an early incidence of breakthrough bleeding.

TABLE 15-2

ORAL CONTRACEPTIVES: CONTRAINDICATIONS AND DISEASE RISK

I. Contraindications
- A. Absolute
  1. Previous thromboembolic event or stroke
  2. History of an estrogen-dependent tumor
  3. Active liver disease
  4. Pregnancy
  5. Undiagnosed abnormal uterine bleeding
  6. Hypertriglyceridemia
  7. Women over age 35 who smoke heavily (>15 cigarettes per day)
- B. Relative
  1. Hypertension
  2. Women receiving anticonvulsant drug therapy

II. Disease risks
- A. Increased
  1. Coronary heart disease—increased only in smokers >35; no relation to progestin type
  2. Hypertension—relative risk 1.8 (current users) and 1.2 (previous users)
  3. Venous thrombosis—relative risk ~4; markedly increased with factor V Leiden or prothrombin-gene mutations
  4. Stroke—increased only in combination with hypertension; unclear relation to migraine headache
  5. Cerebral vein thrombosis—relative risk ~13–15; synergistic with prothrombin-gene mutation
  6. Cervical cancer—relative risk 2–4
- B. Decreased
  1. Ovarian cancer—50% reduction in risk
  2. Endometrial cancer—40% reduction in risk
- C. No effect
  1. Breast cancer

Current doses of ethinyl estradiol range from 20 to 50 μg. However, indications for the 50-μg dose are rare, and the majority of formulations contain 35 μg of ethinyl estradiol. The reduced estrogen and progesterone content in the second- and third-generation pills has decreased both side effects and risks associated with oral contraceptive use (**Table 15-2**). At the currently used doses, patients must be cautioned not to miss pills due to the potential for ovulation. Side effects, including break-through bleeding, amenorrhea, breast tenderness, and weight gain, are often responsive to a change in formulation.

The microdose progestin-only minipill is less effective as a contraceptive, having a pregnancy rate of 2 to 7 per 100 women-years. However, it may be appropriate for women with cardiovascular disease or for women who cannot tolerate synthetic estrogens.

New Methods

A *weekly contraceptive patch* (Ortho Evra) is now available. It has similar efficacy to oral contraceptives and may be associated with less breakthrough bleeding. Approximately 2% of patches fail to adhere, and a similar percentage of women have skin reactions. Efficacy is lower in women >90 kg. A *monthly contraceptive injection* (Lunelle) is also available. This estrogen/progestin combination is highly effective, with a first-year failure rate of <0.2%, but it may be less effective in obese women. Its use is associated with bleeding irregularities that diminish over time. Fertility returns rapidly after discontinuation. A *monthly vaginal ring* (NuvaRing) is now approved for contraceptive use. It is highly effective, with a 12-month failure rate of 0.7%. The device is intended to be left in place during intercourse. If removed during intercourse, it must be reinserted within 3 h. Ovulation returns within the first recovery cycle after discontinuation.

Long-Term Contraceptives

Long-term progestin administration in the form of Depo-Provera and Norplant (Table 15-1) act primarily by inhibiting ovulation and causing changes in the endometrium and cervical mucus that result in decreased implantation and sperm transport. Depo-Provera requires an intramuscular injection and is effective for 3 months, but return of fertility after discontinuation may be delayed for up to 12 to 18 months. Norplant requires surgical insertion but is effective for up to 5 years afer insertion; fertility is possible shortly after its removal. Amenorrhea, irregular bleeding, and weight gain are the most common adverse effects associated with both injectable forms of contraception. A major advantage of the injectable progestin-based contraceptives is the apparent lack of increased arterial and venous thromboembolic events, but increased gallbladder disease and decreased bone density may result.

POSTCOITAL CONTRACEPTION

Postcoital contraceptive methods prevent implantation or cause regression of the corpus luteum and are highly efficacious if used appropriately. Unprotected intercourse without regard to the time of the month carries an 8% incidence of pregnancy, an incidence that can be reduced to 2% by the use of emergency contraceptives within 72 h of unprotected intercourse. Certain oral contraceptive pills can be used within 72 h of unprotected intercourse [Ovral (2 tablets, 12 h apart) and Lo/Ovral (4 tablets, 12 h apart)]. Preven (50 mg ethinyl estradiol and 0.25 mg levonorgestrel) and Plan B (0.75 mg levonorgestrel) are now approved for postcoital contraception. Side effects are common with these high doses of hormones and include nausea, vomiting, and breast soreness. Recent studies suggest that 600 mg mifepristone (RU486), a progesterone receptor antagonist, may be equally as effective or more effective than hormonal regimens, with fewer side effects.

MALE HORMONAL CONTRACEPTION

An effective and reversible male contraceptive has long been sought, and surveys indicate that a "male pill" would be acceptable to both men and women. Complete suppression of spermatogenesis is required for acceptable contraception but is not achieved reliably with testosterone alone. However, the combination of a long-acting testosterone preparation with a GnRH antagonist or a progestin such as norgestral, desonorgestrel, or norethisterone results in effective contraception, suggesting that a male contraceptive may be forthcoming.

FURTHER READINGS

ANDERSON RA et al: Male contraception. Endocr Rev 23:735, 2002

GRIFFIN DK ET AL: The genetic and cytogenetic basis of male infertility. Hum Fertil 8:19, 2005

GRIMES D et al: Steroid hormones for contraception in men. Cochrane Database Syst Rev:CD004316, 2004

This review concludes that no male hormonal contraceptive is currently ready for clinical use. Most studies to date have been relatively small, and the definition of oligospermia has been imprecise or inconsistent. Nonetheless, efforts to develop effective male contraceptives show gradual progress.

GUZIK DS et al: Sperm morphology, motility and concentration in fertile and infertile men. N Engl J Med 345:1388, 2001

KURODA-KAWAGUCHI T et al: The AZFc region of the Y chromosome features massive palindromes and uniform recurrent deletions in infertile men. Nat Genet 29:279, 2001

MARCHBANKS PA et al. Oral contraceptives and the risk of breast cancer. N Engl J Med 346:2025, 2002

MISHELL DR JR: State of the art in hormonal contraception: An overview. Am J Obstet Gynecol 190:S1, 2004

A review of advances in contraception including the introduction of new formulations of oral contraceptives, continued development of existing injectable and implantable delivery methods, and the development and approval of novel delivery systems of contraceptive steroids.

PETITTI DB: Clinical practice. Combination estrogen-progestin oral contraceptives. N Engl J Med 349:1443, 2003

VANDENBROUCKE JP et al: Oral contraceptives and the risk of venous thrombosis. N Engl J Med 344:1527, 2001

WANG C ET AL: Male hormonal contraception. Am J Obstet Gynecol 190:S60, 2004

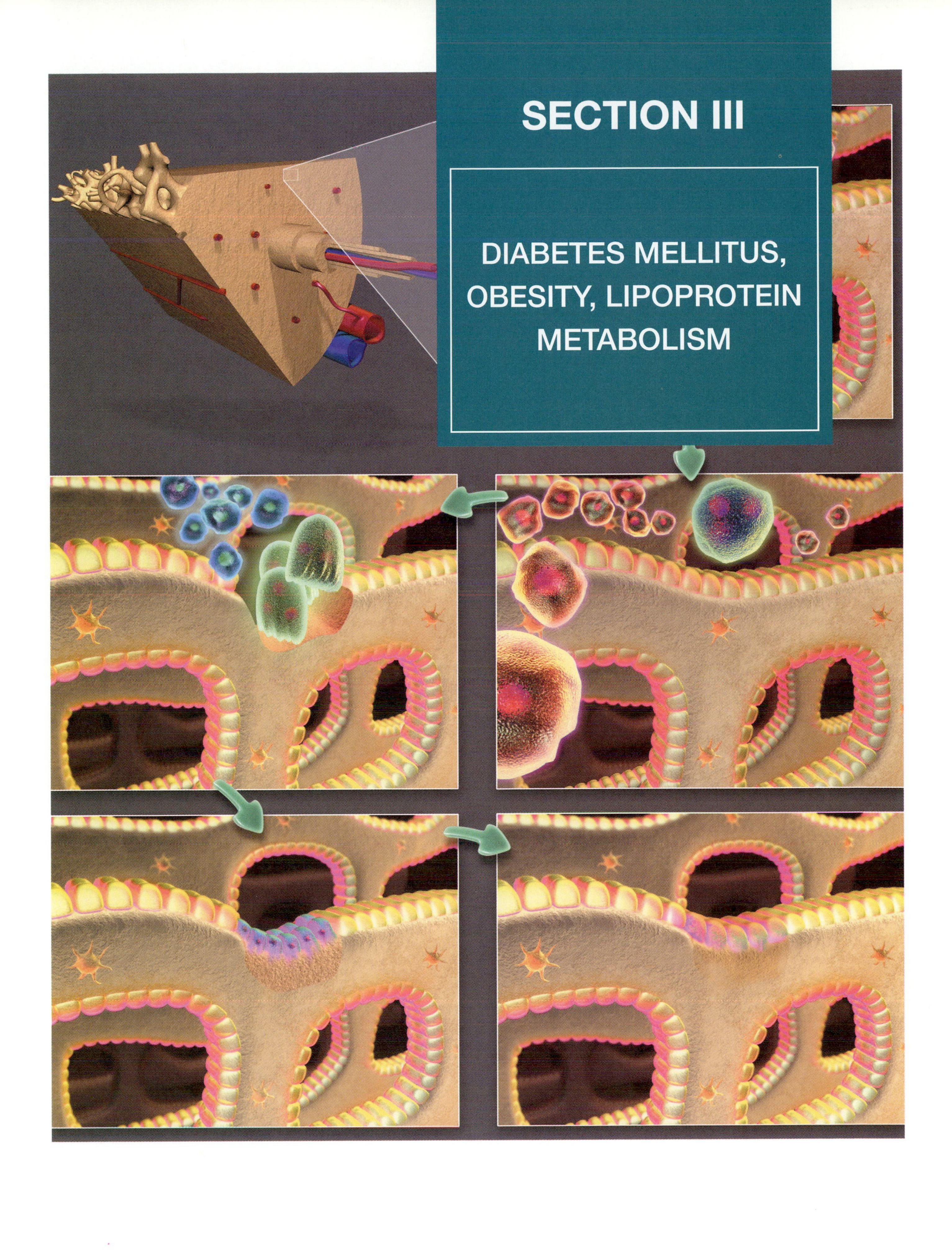

SECTION III

DIABETES MELLITUS, OBESITY, LIPOPROTEIN METABOLISM

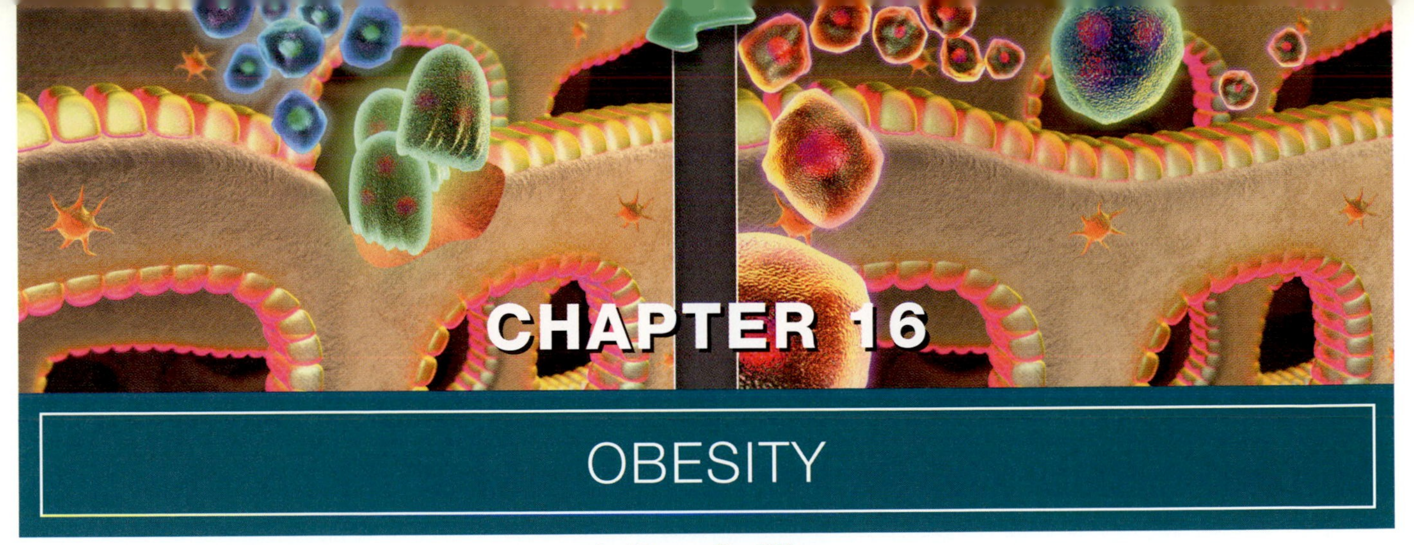

OBESITY

Jeffrey S. Flier
Eleftheria Maratos-Flier

In a world where food supplies are intermittent, the ability to store energy in excess of what is required for immediate use is essential for survival. Fat cells, residing within widely distributed adipose tissue depots, are adapted to store excess energy efficiently as triglyceride and, when needed, to release stored energy as free fatty acids for use at other sites. This physiologic system, orchestrated through endocrine and neural pathways, permits humans to survive starvation for as long as several months. However, in the presence of nutritional abundance and a sedentary life-style, and influenced importantly by genetic endowment, this system increases adipose energy stores and produces adverse health consequences.

DEFINITION AND MEASUREMENT

Obesity is a state of excess adipose tissue mass. Although often viewed as equivalent to increased body weight, this need not be the case—lean but very muscular individuals may be overweight by arbitrary standards without having increased adiposity. Body weights are distributed continuously in populations, so that a medically meaningful distinction between lean and obese is somewhat arbitrary. Obesity is therefore more effectively defined by assessing its linkage to morbidity or mortality.

Although not a direct measure of adiposity, the most widely used method to gauge obesity is the *body mass index* (BMI), which is equal to weight/height^2 (in kg/m^2) (**Fig. 16-1**). Other approaches to quantifying obesity include anthropometry (skin-fold thickness), densitometry (underwater weighing), computed tomography (CT) or magnetic resonance imaging (MRI), and electrical impedance. Using data from the Metropolitan Life Tables, BMIs for the midpoint of all heights and frames among both men and women range from 19 to 26 kg/m^2; at a similar BMI, women have more body fat than men. Based on unequivocal data of substantial morbidity, a BMI of 30 is most commonly used as a threshold for obesity in both men and women. Large-scale epidemiologic studies suggest that all-cause, metabolic, cancer, and cardiovascular morbidity begin to rise (albeit at a slow rate) when BMIs are $\geq$25, suggesting that the cut-off for obesity should be lowered. Some authorities use the term *overweight* (rather than obese) to describe individuals with BMIs between 25 and 30. A BMI between 25 and 30 should be viewed as medically significant and worthy of therapeutic intervention, especially in the presence of risk factors that are influenced by adiposity, such as hypertension and glucose intolerance.

The distribution of adipose tissue in different anatomical depots also has substantial implications for morbidity. Specifically, intraabdominal and abdominal

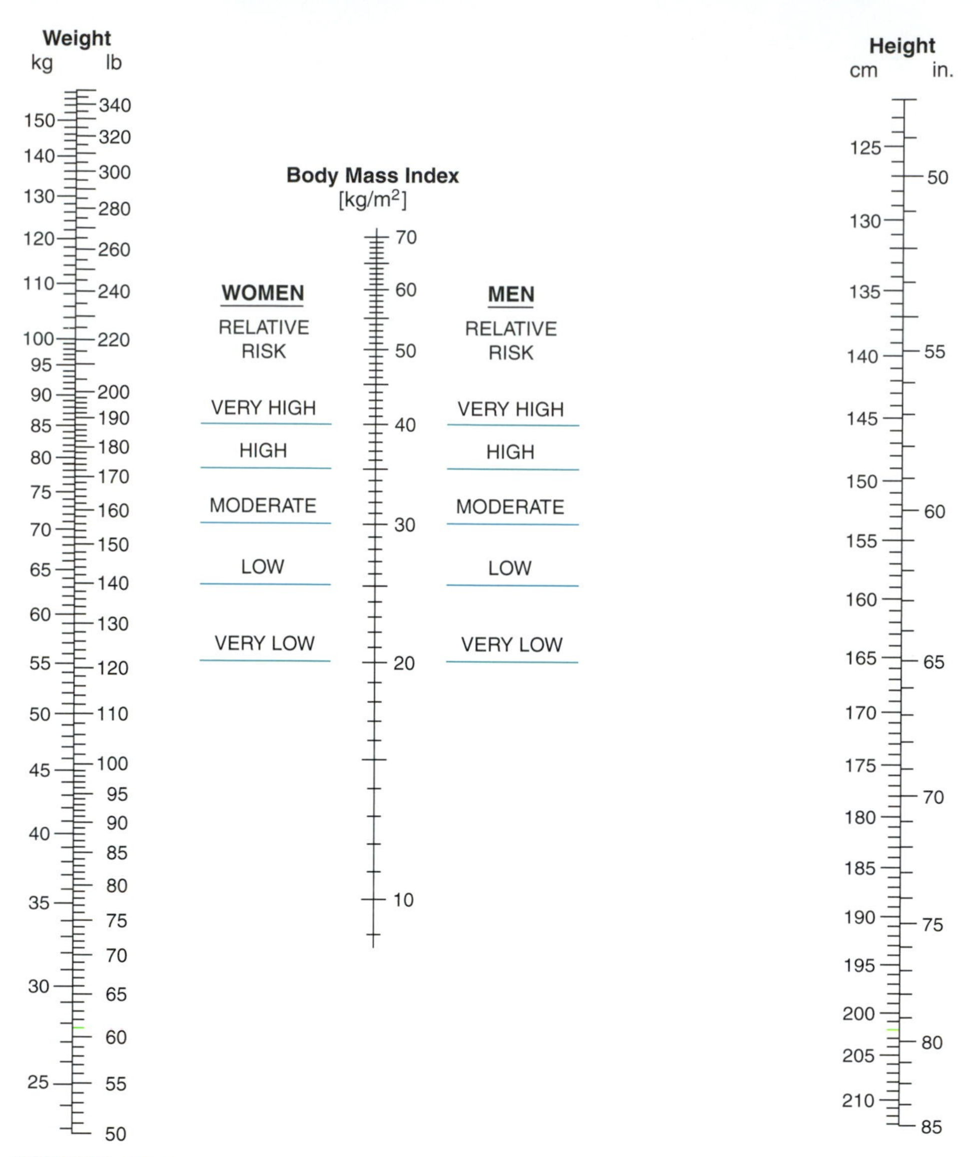

FIGURE 16-1

Nomogram for determining body mass index. To use this nomogram, place a ruler or other straight edge between the body weight (without clothes) in kilograms or pounds located on the left-hand line and the height (without shoes) in centimeters or inches located on the right-hand line. The body mass index is read from the middle of the scale and is in metric units. (*Copyright 1979, George A. Bray, M.D. Used with permission.*)

subcutaneous fat have more significance than subcutaneous fat present in the buttocks and lower extremities. This distinction is most easily made by determining the waist-to-hip ratio, with a ratio >0.9 in women and >1.0 in men being abnormal. Many of the most important complications of obesity, such as insulin resistance, diabetes, hypertension, hyperlipidemia, and hyperandrogenism in women, are linked more strongly to intraabdominal and/or upper body fat than to overall adiposity. The mechanism underlying this association is unknown but may relate to the fact that intraabdominal adipocytes are more lipolytically active than those from other depots. Release of free fatty acids into the portal circulation has adverse metabolic actions, especially on the liver.

PREVALENCE

Data from the National Health and Nutrition Examination Surveys (NHANES) show that the percent of the American adult population with obesity (BMI > 30) has increased from 14.5% (between 1976 and 1980) to 30.5% (between 1999 and 2000). As many as 64% of U.S. adults ≥20 years of age were overweight (defined as

BMI > 25) between the years of 1999 and 2000. Extreme obesity (BMI ≥ 40) has also increased and affects 4.7% of the population. The increasing prevalence of medically significant obesity raises great concern. Obesity is more common among women and in the poor; the prevalence in children is also rising at a worrisome rate.

PHYSIOLOGIC REGULATION OF ENERGY BALANCE

Substantial evidence suggests that body weight is regulated by both endocrine and neural components that ultimately influence the effector arms of energy intake and expenditure. This complex regulatory system is necessary because even small imbalances between energy intake and expenditure will ultimately have large effects on body weight. For example, a 0.3% positive imbalance over 30 years would result in a 9-kg (20-lb) weight gain. This exquisite regulation of energy balance cannot be monitored easily by calorie-counting in relation to physical activity. Rather, body weight regulation or dysregulation depends on a complex interplay of hormonal and neural signals. Alterations in stable weight by forced overfeeding or food deprivation induce physiologic changes that resist these perturbations: with weight loss, appetite increases and energy expenditure falls; with overfeeding, appetite falls and energy expenditure increases. This latter compensatory mechanism frequently fails, however, permitting obesity to develop when food is abundant and physical activity is limited. A major regulator of these adaptative responses is the adipocyte-derived hormone leptin, which acts through brain circuits (predominantly in the hypothalamus) to influence appetite, energy expenditure, and neuroendocrine function (see below).

Appetite is influenced by many factors that are integrated by the brain, most importantly within the hypothalamus (**Fig. 16-2**). Signals that impinge on the hypothalamic center include neural afferents, hormones, and metabolites. Vagal inputs are particularly important, bringing information from viscera, such as gut distention. Hormonal signals include leptin, insulin, cortisol, and gut peptides such as ghrelin, peptide YY (PYY), and cholecystokinin, which signal to the brain through direct action on hypothalamic control centers and/or via the vagus nerve. Metabolites, including glucose, can influence appetite, as seen by the effect of hypoglycemia to induce hunger; however, glucose is not normally a major regulator of appetite. These diverse hormonal, metabolic, and neural signals act by influencing the expression and release of various hypothalamic peptides [e.g., neuropeptide Y (NPY), Agouti-related peptide (AgRP), α melanocyte-stimulating hormone (α-MSH), and melanin-concentrating hormone (MCH)] that are

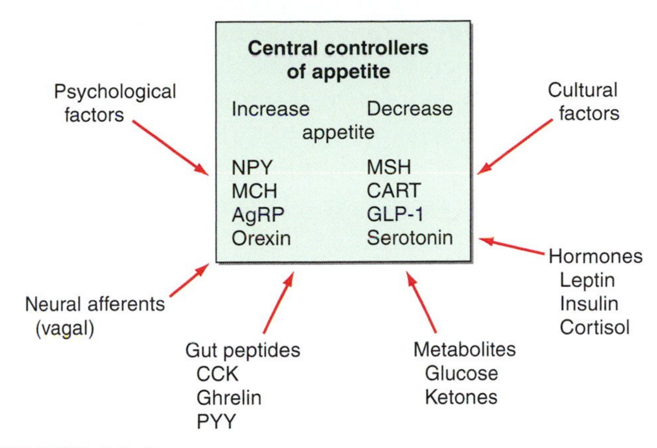

FIGURE 16-2

The factors that regulate appetite through effects on central neural circuits. Some factors that increase or decrease appetite are listed. NPY, neuropeptide Y; MCH, melanin-concentrating hormone; AgRP, Agouti-related peptide; MSH, melanocyte-stimulating hormone; CART, cocaine- and amphetamine-related transcript; GLP-1, glucagon-related peptide-1; CCK, cholecystokinin.

integrated with serotonergic, catecholaminergic, and opioid signaling pathways (see below). Psychological and cultural factors also appear to play a role in the final expression of appetite. Apart from rare syndromes involving leptin, its receptor, and the melanocortin system, specific defects in this complex appetite control network that influence common causes of obesity are not well understood.

Energy expenditure includes the following components:

(1) resting or basal metabolic rate;
(2) the energy cost of metabolizing and storing food;
(3) the thermic effect of exercise; and
(4) adaptive thermogenesis, which varies in response to chronic caloric intake (rising with increased intake).

Basal metabolic rate accounts for about 70% of daily energy expenditure, whereas active physical activity contributes 5 to 10%. Thus, a significant component of daily energy consumption is fixed.

Genetic models in mice indicate that mutations in certain genes (e.g., targeted deletion of the insulin receptor in adipose tissue) protect against obesity, apparently by increasing energy expenditure. Adaptive thermogenesis occurs in *brown adipose tissue* (BAT), which plays an important role in energy metabolism in many mammals. In contrast to white adipose tissue, which is used to store energy in the form of lipids, BAT expends stored energy as heat. A mitochondrial *uncoupling protein* (UCP-1) in BAT dissipates the hydrogen ion gradient in the oxidative respiration chain and releases energy as heat. The metabolic activity of BAT is increased by a central action of leptin, acting through the sympathetic nervous system, which heavily innervates this tissue. In rodents, BAT deficiency causes obesity and diabetes; stimulation of BAT with a specific adrenergic agonist (β_3 agonist) protects against diabetes and obesity. Although BAT exists in humans (especially neonates), its physiologic role is not yet established. Homologues of UCP-1 may mediate uncoupled mitochondrial respiration in other tissues.

THE ADIPOCYTE AND ADIPOSE TISSUE

Adipose tissue is composed of the lipid-storing adipose cell and a stromal/vascular compartment in which preadipocytes reside. Adipose mass increases by enlargement of adipose cells through lipid deposition, as well as by an increase in the number of adipocytes. The process by which adipose cells are derived from a mesenchymal preadipocyte involves an orchestrated series of differentiation steps mediated by a cascade of specific transcription factors. One of the key transcription factors is *peroxisome proliferator-activated receptor* γ (PPARγ), a nuclear receptor that binds the thiazoladinedione class of insulin-sensitizing drugs used in the treatment of type 2 diabetes (Chap. 17).

Although the adipocyte has generally been regarded as a storage depot for fat, it is also an endocrine cell that releases numerous molecules in a regulated fashion (**Fig. 16-3**). These include the energy balance regulating hormone leptin, cytokines such as tumor necrosis factor (TNF) α, complement factors such as factor D (also known as *adipsin*), prothrombotic agents such as plasminogen activator inhibitor I, and a component of the blood pressure regulating system, angiotensinogen. Adiponectin (or ACRP30) enhances insulin sensitivity and lipid oxidation, whereas resistin may induce insulin resistance. These factors, and others not yet identified, play a role in the physiology of lipid homeostasis, insulin sensitivity, blood pressure control, and coagulation and are likely to contribute to obesity-related pathologies.

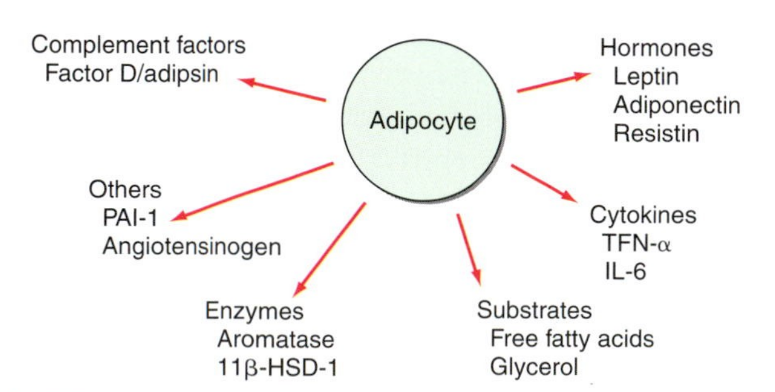

FIGURE 16-3

Factors released by the adipocyte that can affect peripheral tissues. PAI, plasminogen activator inhibitor; TNF, tumor necrosis factor.

ETIOLOGY OF OBESITY

Though the molecular pathways regulating energy balance are beginning to be illuminated, the causes of obesity remain elusive. In part, this reflects the fact that obesity is a heterogeneous group of disorders. At one level, the pathophysiology of obesity seems simple: a chronic excess of nutrient intake relative to the level of energy expenditure. However, due to the complexity of the neuroendocrine and metabolic systems that regulate energy intake, storage, and expenditure, it has been difficult to quantitate all the relevant parameters (e.g., food intake and energy expenditure) over time in human subjects.

ROLE OF GENES VERSUS ENVIRONMENT

Obesity is commonly seen in families, and the heredibility of body weight is similar to that for height. Inheritance is usually not Mendelian, however, and it is difficult to distinguish the role of genes and environmental factors. Adoptees usually resemble their biologic rather than adoptive parents with respect to obesity, providing strong support for genetic influences. Likewise, identical twins have very similar BMIs whether reared together or apart, and their BMIs are much more strongly correlated than those of dizygotic twins. These genetic effects appear to relate to both energy intake and expenditure.

Whatever the role of genes, it is clear that the environment plays a key role in obesity, as evidenced by the fact that famine prevents obesity in even the most obesity-prone individual. In addition, the recent increase in the prevalence of obesity in the United States is too rapid to be due to changes in the gene pool. Undoubtedly, genes influence the susceptibility to obesity when confronted with specific diets and availability of nutrition. Cultural factors are also important—these relate to both availability and composition of the diet and to changes in the level of physical activity. In industrial societies, obesity is more common among poor women, whereas in underdeveloped countries, wealthier women are more often obese. In children, obesity correlates to some degree with time spent watching television. High-fat diets may promote obesity, as may diets rich in simple (as opposed to complex) carbohydrates.

SPECIFIC GENETIC SYNDROMES

For many years obesity in rodents has been known to be caused by a number of distinct mutations distributed through the genome. Most of these single-gene mutations cause both hyperphagia and diminished energy expenditure, suggesting a link between these two parameters of energy homeostasis. Identification of the *ob* gene mutation in genetically obese (ob/ob) mice represented a major breakthrough in the field. The ob/ob mouse develops severe obesity, insulin resistance, and hyperphagia, as well as efficient metabolism (e.g., it gets fat even when given the same number of calories as lean littermates). The product of the *ob* gene is the peptide leptin, a name derived from the Greek root *leptos*, meaning thin. Leptin is secreted by adipose cells and acts primarily through the hypothalamus. Its level of production provides an index of adipose energy stores (**Fig. 16-4**). High leptin levels decrease food intake and increase energy expenditure. Another mouse mutant, db/db, which is resistant to leptin, has a mutation in the leptin receptor and develops a similar syndrome. The *OB* gene is present in humans and expressed in fat. Several families with morbid, early-onset obesity caused by inactivating mutations in either leptin or the leptin receptor have been described, thus demonstrating the biologic relevance of leptin in humans. The obesity in these individuals begins shortly after birth, is severe, and is accompanied by neuroendocrine abnormalities. The most prominent of these is hypogonadotropic hypogonadism, which is reversed by leptin replacement. Central hypothyroidism and growth retardation are seen in the mouse model, but their occurrence in leptin-deficient humans is less clear.

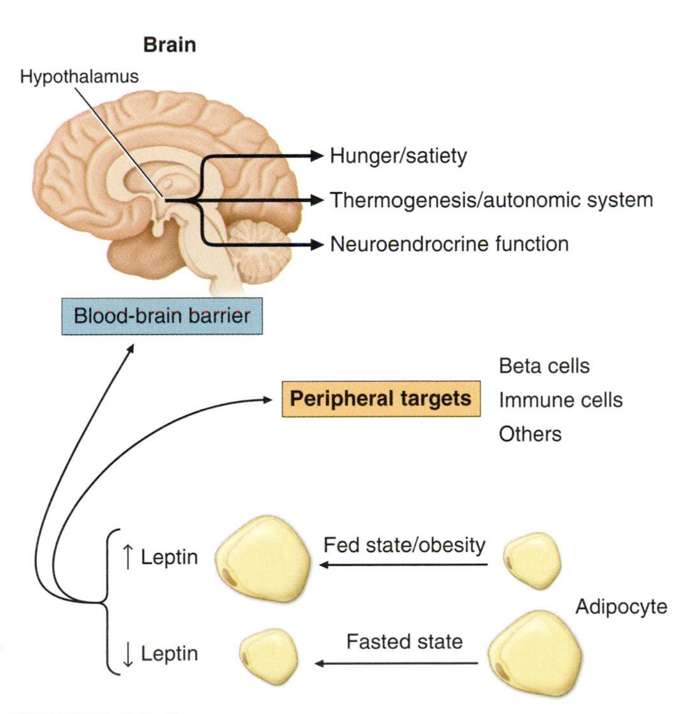

FIGURE 16-4

The physiologic system regulated by leptin. Rising or falling leptin levels act through the hypothalamus to influence appetite, energy expenditure, and neuroendocrine function and through peripheral sites to influence systems such as the immune system.

To date, there is no evidence to suggest that mutations or polymorphisms in the leptin or leptin receptor genes play a prominent role in common forms of obesity.

Mutations in several other genes cause severe obesity in humans (**Table 16-1**); each of these syndromes is rare. Mutations in the gene encoding proopiomelanocortin (POMC) cause severe obesity through failure to synthesize α-MSH, a key neuropeptide that inhibits appetite in the hypothalamus. The absence of POMC also causes secondary adrenal insufficiency due to absence of adrenocorticotropic hormone (ACTH), as well as pale skin and red hair due to absence of MSH. Proenzyme convertase 1 (PC-1) mutations are thought to cause obesity by preventing synthesis of α-MSH from its precursor peptide, POMC. α-MSH binds to the type 4 melanocortin receptor (MC4R), a key hypothalamic receptor that inhibits eating. Heterozygous mutations of this receptor appear to account for as much as 5% of severe obesity. These five genetic defects define a pathway through which leptin (by stimulating POMC and increasing MSH) restricts food intake and limits weight (**Fig. 16-5**).

In addition to these human obesity genes, studies in rodents reveal several other molecular candidates for hypothalamic mediators of human obesity or leanness. The *tub* gene encodes a hypothalamic peptide of unknown function; mutation of this gene causes late-onset obesity. The *fat* gene encodes carboxypeptidase E, a peptide-processing enzyme; mutation of this gene is thought to cause obesity by disrupting production of one or more neuropeptides. AgRP is coexpressed with NPY in arcuate nucleus neurons. AgRP antagonizes α-MSH action at MC4 receptors, and its overexpression induces obesity. In contrast, a mouse deficient in the peptide MCH, whose administration causes feeding, is lean.

A number of complex human syndromes with defined inheritance are associated with obesity (**Table 16-2**). Although specific genes are undefined at present, their identification will likely enhance our understanding of more common forms of human obesity. In the Prader-Willi syndrome, obesity coexists with short stature, mental retardation, hypogonadotropic hypogonadism, hypotonia, small hands and feet, fish-shaped mouth, and hyperphagia. Most patients have a chromosome 15 deletion. Laurence-Moon-Biedl syndrome is characterized by obesity, mental retardation, retinitis pigmentosa, polydactyly, and hypogonadotropic hypogonadism.

OTHER SPECIFIC SYNDROMES ASSOCIATED WITH OBESITY

Cushing's Syndrome

Although obese patients commonly have central obesity, hypertension, and glucose intolerance, they lack other

TABLE 16-1

SOME OBESITY GENES IN HUMANS AND MICE

GENE	GENE PRODUCT	MECHANISM OF OBESITY	IN HUMAN	IN RODENT
Lep (ob)	Leptin, a fat-derived hormone	Mutation prevents leptin from delivering satiety signal; brain perceives starvation	Yes	Yes
LepR (db)	Leptin receptor	Same as above	Yes	Yes
POMC	Proopiomelanocortin, a precursor of several hormones and neuropeptides	Mutation prevents synthesis of melanocyte-stimulating hormone (MSH), a satiety signal	Yes	Yes
MC4R	Type 4 receptor for MSH	Mutation prevents reception of satiety signal from MSH	Yes	Yes
AgRP	Agouti-related peptide, a neuropeptide expressed in the hypothalamus	Overexpression inhibits signal through MC4R	No	Yes
PC-1	Prohormone convertase 1, a processing enzyme	Mutation prevents synthesis of neuropeptide, probably MSH	Yes	No
Fat	Carboxypeptidase E, a processing enzyme	Same as above	No	Yes
Tab	Tub, a hypothalamic protein of unknown function	Hypothalamic dysfunction	No	Yes

specific stigmata of Cushing's syndrome (Chap. 5). Nonetheless, a potential diagnosis of Cushing's syndrome is often entertained. Cortisol production and urinary metabolites (17OH steroids) may be increased in simple obesity. Unlike in Cushing's syndrome, however, cortisol levels in blood and urine in the basal state and in response to corticotropin-releasing hormone (CRH) or ACTH are normal; the overnight 1-mg dexamethasone suppression test is normal in 90%, with the remainder being normal on a standard 2-day low-dose dexamethasone suppression test. Obesity may be associated with local reactivation of cortisol in fat by 11β hydroxysteroid dehydrogenase 1, an enzyme that converts cortisone to cortisol.

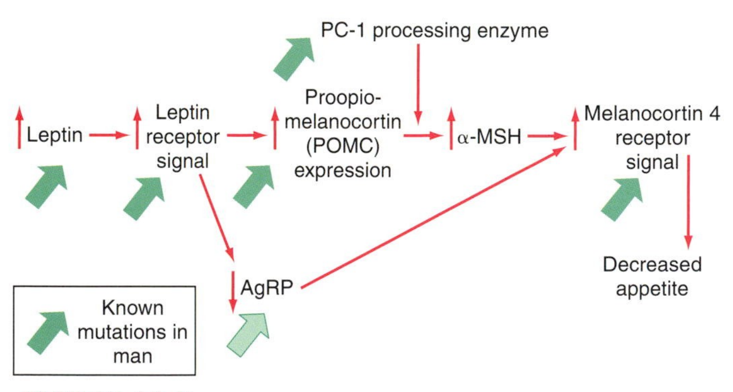

FIGURE 16-5

A central pathway through which leptin acts to regulate appetite and body weight. Leptin signals through proopiomelanocortin (POMC) neurons in the hypothalamus to induce increased production of α melanocyte-stimulating hormone (α-MSH), requiring the processing enzyme PC-1 (proenzyme convertase 1). α-MSH acts as an agonist on melanocortin-4 receptors to inhibit appetite, and the neuropeptide AgRp (Agouti-related peptide) acts as an antagonist of this receptor. Mutations that cause obesity in humans are indicated by the solid green arrows.

Hypothyroidism

The possibility of hypothyroidism should be considered, but it is an uncommon cause of obesity; hypothyroidism is easily ruled out by measuring thyroid-stimulating hormone (TSH). Much of the weight gain that occurs in hypothyroidism is due to myxedema (Chap. 4).

Insulinoma

Patients with insulinoma often gain weight as a result of overeating to avoid hypoglycemia symptoms (Chap. 19). The increased substrate plus high insulin levels promote energy storage in fat. This can be marked in some individuals but is modest in most.

Craniopharyngioma and Other Disorders Involving the Hypothalamus

Whether through tumors, trauma, or inflammation, hypothalamic dysfunction of systems controlling satiety, hunger, and energy expenditure can cause varying degrees of obesity (Chap. 2). It is uncommon to identify

TABLE 16-2

A COMPARISON OF SYNDROMES OF OBESITY—HYPOGONADISM AND MENTAL RETARDATION

	SYNDROME				
FEATURE	PRADER-WILLI	LAURENCE-MOON-BIEDL	AHLSTROM	COHEN	CARPENTER
Inheritance	Sporadic; two-thirds have defect	Autosomal recessive	Autosomal recessive	Probably autosomal recessive	Autosomal recessive
Stature	Short	Normal; infrequently short	Normal; infrequently short	Short or tall	Normal
Obesity	Generalized Moderate to severe Onset 1–3 yrs	Generalized Early onset, 1–2 yrs	Truncal Early onset, 2–5 yrs	Truncal Mid-childhood, age 5	Truncal, gluteal
Craniofacies	Narrow bifrontal diameter Almond-shaped eyes Strabismus V-shaped mouth High-arched palate	Not distinctive	Not distinctive	High nasal bridge Arched palate Open mouth Short philtrum	Acrocephaly Flat nasal bridge High-arched palate
Limbs	Small hands and feet Hypotonia	Polydactyly	No abnormalities	Hypotonia Narrow hands and feet	Polydactyly Syndactyly Genu valgum
Reproductive status	1° Hypogonadism	1° Hypogonadism	Hypogonadism in males but not in females	Normal gonadal function or hypogonadotrophic hypogonadism	2° Hypogonadism
Other features	Enamel hypoplasia Hyperphagia Temper tantrums Nasal speech			Dysplastic ears Delayed puberty	
Mental retardation	Mild to moderate		Normal intelligence	Mild	Slight

a discrete anatomical basis for these disorders. Subtle hypothalamic dysfunction is probably a more common cause of obesity than can be documented using currently available imaging techniques. Growth hormone (GH), which exerts lipolytic activity, is diminished in obesity and is increased with weight loss. Despite low GH levels, insulin-like growth factor (IGF) I (somatomedin) production is normal, suggesting that GH suppression is a compensatory response to increased nutritional supply.

PATHOGENESIS OF COMMON OBESITY

Obesity can result from increased energy intake, decreased energy expenditure, or a combination of the two. Thus, identifying the etiology of obesity should involve measurements of both parameters. However, it is nearly impossible to perform direct and accurate measurements of energy intake in free-living individuals. Obese people, in particular, often underreport intake. Measurements of chronic energy expenditure have only recently become available using doubly labeled water or metabolic chamber/rooms. In subjects at stable weight and body composition, energy intake equals expenditure. Consequently, these techniques allow determination of energy intake in free-living individuals. The level of energy expenditure differs in established obesity, during periods of weight gain or loss, and in the pre- or postobese state. Studies that fail to take note of this phenomenon are not easily interpreted.

There is increased interest in the concept of a body weight "set point." This idea is supported by physiologic mechanisms centered around a sensing system in adipose tissue that reflects fat stores and a receptor, or "adipostat," that is in the hypothalamic centers. When fat stores are depleted, the adipostat signal is low, and the hypothalamus responds by stimulating hunger and decreasing energy expenditure to conserve energy. Conversely, when fat stores are abundant, the signal is increased, and the hypothalamus responds by decreasing hunger and increasing energy expenditure. The recent discovery of the *ob* gene, and its product leptin, provides a molecular basis for this physiologic concept (see above).

WHAT IS THE STATUS OF FOOD INTAKE IN OBESITY? (DO THE OBESE EAT MORE THAN THE LEAN?)

This question has stimulated much debate, due in part to the methodologic difficulties inherent in determining food intake. Many obese individuals believe that they eat small quantities of food, and this claim has often been supported by the results of food intake questionnaires. However, it is now established that average energy expenditure increases as people get more obese, due primarily to the fact that metabolically active lean tissue mass increases with obesity. Given the laws of thermodynamics, the obese person must therefore eat more than the average lean person to maintain their increased weight. It may be the case, however, that a subset of individuals who are predisposed to obesity have the capacity to become obese initially without an absolute increase in caloric consumption.

WHAT IS THE STATE OF ENERGY EXPENDITURE IN OBESITY?

The average total daily energy expenditure is higher in obese than lean individuals when measured at stable weight. However, energy expenditure falls as weight is lost, due in part to loss of lean body mass and to decreased sympathetic nerve activity. When reduced to near-normal weight and maintained there for a while, (some) obese individuals have lower energy expenditure than (some) lean individuals. There is also a tendency for those who develop obesity as infants or children to have lower resting energy expenditure rates than those who remain lean.

The physiologic basis for variable rates of energy expenditure (at a given body weight and level of energy intake) is essentially unknown. A mutation in the human β_3 adrenergic receptor may be associated with increased risk of obesity and/or insulin resistance in certain (but not all) populations. Homologues of the BAT uncoupling protein, named UCP-2 and UCP-3, have been identified in both rodents and humans. UCP-2 is expressed widely, whereas UCP-3 is primarily expressed in skeletal muscle. These proteins may play a role in disordered energy balance.

One newly described component of thermogenesis, called *nonexercise activity thermogenesis* (NEAT), has been linked to obesity. It is the thermogenesis that accompanies physical activities other than volitional exercise, such as the activities of daily living, fidgeting, spontaneous muscle contraction, and maintaining posture. NEAT accounts for about two-thirds of the increased daily energy expenditure induced by overfeeding. The wide variation in fat storage seen in overfed individuals is predicted by the degree to which NEAT is induced. The molecular basis for NEAT and its regulation are unknown.

LEPTIN IN TYPICAL OBESITY

The vast majority of obese people have increased leptin levels but do not have mutations of either leptin or its receptor. They appear, therefore, to have a form of functional "leptin resistance." Data suggesting that some individuals produce less leptin per unit fat mass than others or have a form of relative leptin deficiency that predisposes to obesity are at present contradictory and unsettled. The mechanism for leptin resistance, and whether it can be overcome by raising leptin levels, is not yet established. Some data suggest that leptin may not effectively cross the blood-brain barrier as levels rise. It is also possible that leptin signaling inhibitors are involved in the leptin-resistant state.

PATHOLOGIC CONSEQUENCES OF OBESITY

Obesity has major adverse effects on health. Morbidly obese individuals (>200% ideal body weight) have as much as a twelvefold increase in mortality. Mortality rates rise as obesity increases, particularly when obesity is associated with increased intraabdominal fat (see above). It is also apparent that the degree to which obesity affects particular organ systems is influenced by susceptibility genes that vary in the population.

INSULIN RESISTANCE AND TYPE 2 DIABETES MELLITUS

Hyperinsulinemia and insulin resistance are pervasive features of obesity, increasing with weight gain and diminishing with weight loss. Insulin resistance is more strongly linked to intraabdominal fat than to fat in other depots. The molecular link between obesity and insulin resistance in tissues such as fat, muscle, and liver has been sought for many years. Major factors under investigation include: (1) insulin itself, by inducing receptor downregulation; (2) free fatty acids, known to be increased and capable of impairing insulin action; (3) intracellular lipid accumulation; and (4) various circulating peptides produced by adipocytes, including the cytokines TNF-α and interleukin (IL) 6, and the "adipokines" adiponectin and resistin, which are produced by adipocytes, have altered expression in obese adipocytes, and are capable of modifying insulin action. Despite nearly universal insulin resistance, most obese individuals do not develop diabetes, suggesting that the onset of diabetes requires an interaction between obesity-induced insulin resistance and other factors that predispose to diabetes, such as impaired insulin secretion (Chap. 17). Obesity, however, is a major risk factor for diabetes, and as many as 80% of patients with type 2 diabetes mellitus are obese. Weight loss and exercise, even of modest degree, are associated with increased insulin sensitivity and often improve glucose control in diabetes.

REPRODUCTIVE DISORDERS

Disorders that affect the reproductive axis are associated with obesity in both men and women. Male hypogonadism is associated with increased adipose tissue, often distributed in a pattern more typical of females. In men ≥160% ideal body weight, plasma testosterone and sex hormone–binding globulin (SHBG) are often reduced, and estrogen levels (derived from conversion of adrenal androgens in adipose tissue) are increased (Chap. 8). Gynecomastia may be seen. However, masculinization, libido, potency, and spermatogenesis are preserved in most of these individuals. Free testosterone may be decreased in morbidly obese men whose weight exceeds 200% ideal body weight.

Obesity has long been associated with menstrual abnormalities in women, particularly in women with upper body obesity (Chap. 10). Common findings are increased androgen production, decreased SHBG, and increased peripheral conversion of androgen to estrogen. Most obese women with oligomenorrhea have the polycystic ovarian syndrome (PCOS), with its associated anovulation and ovarian hyperandrogenism; 40% of women with PCOS are obese. Most nonobese women with PCOS are also insulin-resistant, suggesting that insulin resistance, hyperinsulinemia, or the combination of the two are causative or contribute to the ovarian pathophysiology in PCOS in both obese and lean individuals. In obese women with PCOS, weight loss or treatment with insulin-sensitizing drugs often restores normal menses. The increased conversion of androstenedione to estrogen, which occurs to a greater degree in women with lower body obesity, may contribute to the increased incidence of uterine cancer in postmenopausal women with obesity.

CARDIOVASCULAR DISEASE

The Framingham Study revealed that obesity was an independent risk factor for the 26-year incidence of cardiovascular disease in men and women [including coronary disease, stroke, and congestive heart failure (CHF)]. The waist/hip ratio may be the best predictor of these risks. When the additional effects of hypertension and glucose intolerance associated with obesity are included, the adverse impact of obesity is even more evident. The effect of obesity on cardiovascular mortality in women may be seen at BMIs as low as 25. Obesity, especially abdominal obesity, is associated with an atherogenic lipid profile, with increased low-density lipoprotein (LDL) cholesterol, very low density lipoprotein, and triglyceride, and decreased high-density lipoprotein cholesterol (Chap. 18). Obesity is also associated with hypertension. Measurement of blood pressure in the obese requires use of a larger cuff size to avoid artifactual increases. Obesity-induced hypertension is associated with increased peripheral resistance and cardiac output, increased sympathetic nervous system tone, increased salt sensitivity, and insulin-mediated salt retention; it is often responsive to modest weight loss.

PULMONARY DISEASE

Obesity may be associated with a number of pulmonary abnormalities. These include reduced chest wall compliance, increased work of breathing, increased minute ventilation due to increased metabolic rate, and decreased total lung capacity and functional residual capacity. Severe obesity may be associated with obstructive sleep apnea and the "obesity hypoventilation syndrome." Sleep apnea can be obstructive (most common), central, or mixed. Weight loss (10 to 20 kg) can bring substantial improvement, as can major weight loss following gastric bypass or restrictive surgery. Continuous positive airway pressure has been used with some success.

GALLSTONES

Obesity is associated with enhanced biliary secretion of cholesterol, supersaturation of bile, and a higher incidence of gallstones, particularly cholesterol gallstones. A person 50% above ideal body weight has about a sixfold increased incidence of symptomatic gallstones. Paradoxically, fasting increases supersaturation of bile by decreasing the phospholipid component. Fasting-induced cholecystitis is a complication of extreme diets.

CANCER

Obesity in males is associated with higher mortality from cancer, including cancer of the esophagus, colon, rectum, pancreas, liver, and prostate; obesity in females is associated with higher mortality from cancer of the gallbladder, bile ducts, breasts, endometrium, cervix, and ovaries. Some of the latter may be due to increased rates of conversion of androstenedione to estrone in adipose tissue of obese individuals. It was recently estimated that obesity accounts for 14% of cancer deaths in men, and 20% in women in the United States.

BONE, JOINT, AND CUTANEOUS DISEASE

Obesity is associated with an increased risk of osteoarthritis, no doubt partly due to the trauma of added weight bearing and joint malalignment. The prevalence of gout may also be increased. Among the skin problems associated with obesity is acanthosis nigricans, manifested by darkening and thickening of the skin folds on the neck, elbows, and dorsal interphalangeal spaces. Acanthosis reflects the severity of underlying insulin resistance and diminishes with weight loss. Friability of skin may be increased, especially in skin folds, enhancing the risk of fungal and yeast infections. Finally, venous stasis is increased in the obese.

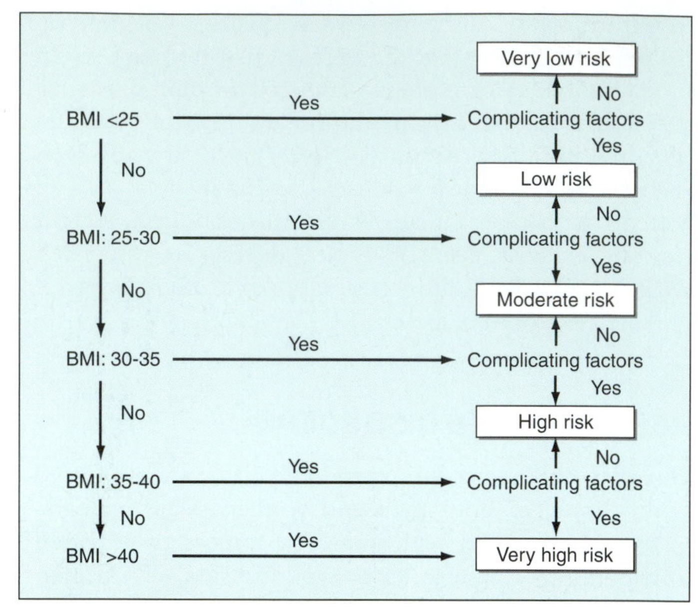

FIGURE 16-6
Risk classification algorithm. The patient is first placed into a category based on body mass index. The presence or absence of complicating factors determines the degree of health risk. Complicating factors include elevated abdominal-gluteal ratio (male: 1.0, female: 0.9), diabetes mellitus, hypertension, hyperlipidemia, male sex, and age ≤40. (*Copyright 1987, George A. Bray, MD. Used with permission.*)

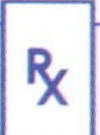

TREATMENT FOR OBESITY

Obesity is a chronic medical condition. Successful treatment, defined as the sustained attainment of normal body weight without producing unacceptable treatment-induced morbidity, is rarely achieved in clinical practice. Many approaches produce short-term weight loss, and this has clear benefits for associated morbidities such as hypertension and diabetes. Although enormous resources are expended in pursuit of obesity therapies, most patients are unsuccessful at achieving and sustaining weight loss over time.

Treatment goals should be guided by the health risks of obesity in any given individual (**Fig. 16-6**). The clinician should always consider the possibility that an individual has an identified cause of obesity, such as hypothyroidism, hypercortisolism, male hypogonadism, insulinoma, or central nervous system disease that affects hypothalamic function. Although they are infrequent causes of obesity, specific therapy may be available.

Behavior Modification

The principles of behavior modification provide the underpinnings for many current programs of weight reduction. Typically, the patient is requested to monitor and record the circumstances related to eating, and rewards are designed to modify maladaptive behaviors. Patients may benefit from counseling offered in a stable group setting for extended periods of time, including after weight loss.

Diet

Reduced caloric intake is the cornerstone of obesity treatment. The fundamental goal is the sustained reduction of energy intake below that of energy expenditure. The difficulty in achieving this goal has led to a wide array of suggested diets that vary in recommended calorie content (from total fasting to mild reductions), as well as specific food content and form (e.g., liquid vs. solid). There is no scientific evidence to validate the utility of specific "fad diets." The main diet regimens in use follow several general facts relevant to food intake and weight loss. First, a deficit of 7500 kcal will produce a weight loss of ~1 kg. Therefore, eating 100 kcal/d less for a year should cause a 5-kg weight loss, and a deficit of 1000 kcal/d should cause a loss of ~1 kg per week. The rate of weight loss on a given caloric intake is related to the rate of energy expenditure. Because obese individuals have a higher metabolic rate than lean individuals, and because men have a higher metabolic rate than women (due to their greater lean body mass), the rate of weight loss is greater among the more obese and among men (relative to women). With chronic caloric restriction, metabolic rate diminishes because of reduced lean body mass (along with much greater loss in fat mass) and possibly because of other adaptations. This fall in metabolic rate with food restriction slows the rate of weight loss on a constant diet. With total starvation or diets restricted to <600 kcal/d, initial weight loss over the first week results predominantly from natriuresis and the loss of fluids.

Very low energy diets (e.g., 400 to 600 kcal/d) may be appropriate for short-term treatment of obesity in selected patients. They are most commonly used for periods of 1 to 2 months to initiate more rapid weight loss, improve comorbidities, and provide patients with positive feedback. The liquid protein diets popularized in the 1970s were proved to be unsafe, causing >60 deaths. Life-threatening arrhythmias were documented in the clinical research setting, a consequence of both low-quality protein and deficiencies of vitamins, minerals, and trace elements. These types of diets have now been substantially modified. A very low energy diet consisting of 45 to 70 g high-quality protein, 30 to 50 g carbohydrate, and ~2 g fat per day, as well as supplements of vitamins, minerals, and trace elements, appears to be safe in selected patients under medical supervision. Patients should not be started on such diets unless they are >130% of their ideal body weight. Contraindications include pregnancy, cancer, recent myocardial infarction, cerebrovascular disease, hepatic disease, or untreated psychiatric disease. When used in patients with diabetes who are receiving insulin or oral agent therapy, close supervision is required and diabetic treatment will need to be adjusted. Whenever possible, exercise regimens and behavioral modification approaches should be used in conjunction with the diet.

Advantages of very low calorie diets are the greater rate of weight loss compared to less restrictive diets, as well as the possible beneficial effect of hunger suppression brought about by the production of ketones. In patients on such diets, blood pressure, blood glucose, cholesterol, and triglyceride levels fall, and pulmonary function and exercise tolerance improve. Sleep apnea may improve within a few weeks. Complications of these very low energy diets are usually minor and include fatigue, constipation or diarrhea, dry skin, hair loss, menstrual irregularities, orthostatic dizziness, and difficulty concentrating. Cholelithiasis and pancreatitis may occur when such diets are interrupted by binge eating; gallstones have been shown to develop in as many as 25% of patients while on the diet.

Low-calorie diets, >800 kcal/d, are applicable to most patients and have fewer restrictions than the very low calorie diets. Considerable controversy has attended the question of which diet composition is most appropriate for promoting weight loss. Though commonly recommended, benefits resulting from very low fat diets are modest at best. Nonetheless, the health effects of low-fat diets—apart from curbing obesity—may be important. A diet rich in fruits, vegetables, whole grains, and other low–glycemic index carbohydrates may promote weight loss and is preferable to low-fat diets in which large amounts of simple carbohydrates are substituted for fats. The latter may actually promote obesity. Some have advocated diets with protein replacement of simple carbohydrates in an effort to minimize insulin production. The efficacy of this strategy, aside from overall calorie reduction, is unknown. Recent data suggest that very low carbohydrate "Atkins" style diets are more effective for short-term weight loss when compared to standard caloric restriction. Weight loss on such diets is not associated with adverse effects on such indices as lipid profile, glycemic control, or blood pressure. However, these diets have not been shown to be more effective in maintaining weight loss, and the possible long-term consequences of maintaining a lower body weight at the expense of consuming more saturated fat are unknown.

An important aspect of diet therapy should include education aimed at preventing weight gain. Knowledge of the caloric and nutritional content of foods is generally poor. In the absence of studies demonstrating convincingly that one type of diet is more effective and safe than another, an emphasis on helping patients understand the caloric content of specific portions is a helpful aid to weight loss and weight maintenance in many individuals.

Exercise

Exercise is an important component of the overall approach to treating obesity. Increased energy expenditure is the most obvious mechanism for an effect of exercise. The impact of an exercise regimen as a sole therapy of obesity has been difficult to document. On the other hand, exercise appears to be a valuable means to sustain diet therapy (**Fig. 16-7**). Even if exercise had no such salutary

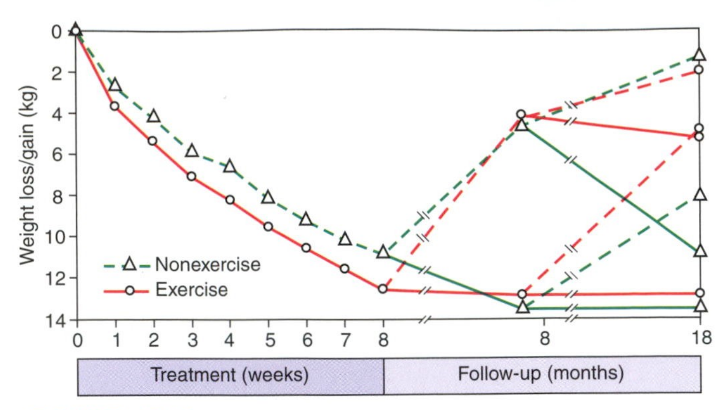

FIGURE 16-7

Weight loss and exercise. During the first 8 weeks, subjects were divided into two groups, one treated with diet and the other with diet plus exercise, with no difference in weight loss. Thereafter the subjects who exercised maintained better weight loss than those that did not. (*After KN Pavlou et al: Am J Clin Nutr 49:1115, 1989.*)

effect, it would be valuable in the obese individual for its effects on cardiovascular tone and blood pressure. Because many obese individuals have not engaged in exercise on a regular basis and may have cardiovascular risk factors, it should be introduced gradually and under medical supervision, especially in the most obese individuals.

Drugs

Despite modest short-term benefits from several agents, medication-induced weight loss is not a cure and is often associated with rebound weight gain after the cessation of drug use. Substantial side effects from several anti-obesity medications, and the potential for drug abuse, have combined to create a wariness about this approach. On the other hand, there is a great medical need for safe and effective therapies, so many possible compounds have been evaluated. On the basis of placebo-controlled trials, the U.S. Food and Drug Administration (FDA) approved several amphetamine-like agents for short-term use. Phentermine is an amphetamine-like drug with low addictive potential that showed modest efficacy (10 vs. 4.4 kg of weight loss over a 24-week period in a well-controlled study). This class of drugs is thought to act centrally by reducing appetite. The over-the-counter drug phenylpropanolamine HCl, had similar efficacy to prescription appetite suppressants in short-term studies but was withdrawn from the market in 2001 because of an association with cerebral hemorrhage. Drugs that promote serotonin release or inhibit serotonin reuptake, such as fenfluramine, have had modest efficacy as single agents. When fenfluramine was administered together with phentermine, as "fen-phen," the combination gained wide use for several years based on controlled trials that demonstrated modest but definite efficacy and reduction of comorbidities. However, the risk of primary pulmonary hypertension was increased up to 20-fold in association with this treatment. The FDA withdrew approval of the fen-phen combination in 1997 when reports demonstrated an association with right- and left-sided valvular heart disease. The histopathologic features of the valvular disease are similar to those seen in carcinoid syndrome and are thought to result from fenfluramine. The occurrence of this complication has been verified in multiple studies, and fenfluramine has been removed from the market.

Sibutramine is a central reuptake inhibitor of both norepinephrine and serotonin that was originally developed as an antidepressant. Using a once-daily dose over 24 weeks, it produced a 7% weight loss in a double-blind, placebo-controlled trial. It lowered cholesterol and triglyceride levels and exhibited similar clinical efficacy to fenfluramine. Sibutramine increases pulse by an average of 4 to 5 beats per minute and blood pressure by 1 to 3 mmHg, and this plus modest efficacy has limited its broad adoption. Orlistat is an inhibitor of intestinal lipase with no systemic availability that causes modest weight loss due to drug-induced fat malabsorption. A randomized, double-blind trial over 2 years revealed modest weight loss (8.7 kg for 120 mg orlistat versus 5.8 kg from diet alone) during the first year and better maintenance of weight loss in a second year compared to the placebo-treated group (3.2 kg regained vs. 5.6 kg regained for placebo). LDL cholesterol and insulin levels were also reduced. Gastrointestinal side effects include oily stools, flatulence, and fecal urgency and usually diminish as patients choose to limit fat intake to avoid the symptoms. Absorption of fat-soluble vitamins is decreased. In patients with obesity and type 2 diabetes mellitus, the antidiabetic medication metformin tends to decrease body weight. The mechanism appears to involve inhibition of appetite. Thyroid hormone has little place in the treatment of obesity, as the vast majority of obese individuals are euthyroid. It promotes loss of lean body mass and raises the risk of complications from the hyperthyroid state.

In the rare cases of leptin deficiency caused by mutations of the leptin gene, the administration of recombinant leptin is highly effective for regulating hunger and inducing loss of fat mass while preserving lean body mass. The response to leptin is limited or absent in common obesity, which is associated with hyperleptinemia and leptin resistance. New drugs are also being developed based on recent insights into central pathways that regulate body weight. These include antagonists for NPY receptors (subtypes Y1, Y5) and MCH receptors and agonists for melanocortin 4 receptors.

Surgery

Morbid obesity, commonly defined as a BMI >40, is estimated to increase mortality by as much as twelvefold in men between 25 and 34 years of age and sixfold between 35 and 45 years of age. Deaths from cardiovascular disease, diabetes, and accidents have been documented. In response to typically ineffective treatment using diet, exercise, and available drugs, surgical approaches are increasingly being employed. The potential benefits of surgery include major weight loss and improvement in hypertension, diabetes, sleep apnea, CHF, angina, hyperlipidemia, and venous disease. Several different approaches have been used, sometimes without adequate long-term assessment of efficacy and complications. Jejunoileal bypass surgery has been abandoned because of complications, which included electrolyte disturbances, nephrolithiasis, gallstones, gastric ulcers, arthritis, and hepatic dysfunction, with cirrhosis occurring in as many as 7% of patients. Two procedures in common use today are the vertical-banded gastroplasty and the Roux-en-Y gastric bypass (**Fig. 16-8**). The former is a purely restrictive procedure, while the latter combines restriction with slight malabsorption and may also reduce appetite via suppression of the gastric hormone ghrelin, which stimulates appetite. Gastric bypass is most often performed by laparotomy but may be performed laparascopically in some patients. A third procedure, laparascopic adjustable gastric banding, is widely used in Europe and Australia and is being introduced in the United States. This procedure may be viewed as "less drastic" than gastric bypass but appears capable of producing substantial weight loss, albeit with shorter periods of follow-up.

Following the National Institutes of Health Consensus Conference on Gastrointestinal Surgery for Severe Obesity in 1991, it was recommended that suitable patients be selected using the following criteria: (1) a BMI >35 with an associated comorbidity or a BMI >40; (2) repeated failures of other therapeutic approaches; (3) at eligible weight for 3 to 5 years; (4) capability of tolerating surgery; (5) absence of alcoholism, other addictions, or major psychopathology; and (6) prior clearance by a psychiatrist. It is recommended that an appropriately experienced surgeon work together with nutritionists and other support personnel; evaluation and follow-up programs should be monitored closely.

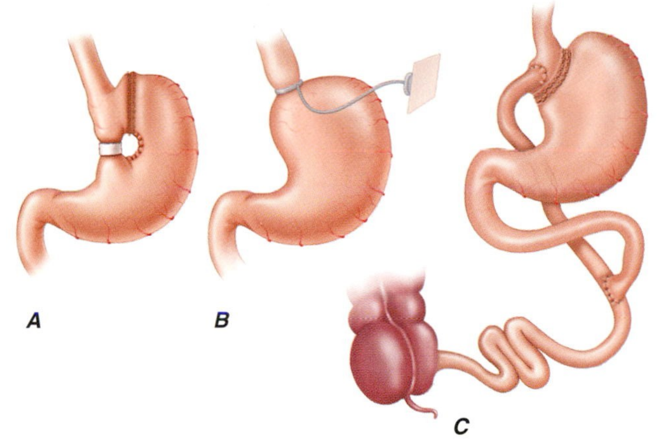

FIGURE 16-8
Examples of operative interventions used for surgical manipulation of the gastrointestinal tract. ***A.*** Vertical banded gastroplasty; ***B.*** adjustable gastric banding; ***C.*** Roux-en-Y gastric bypass.

ACKNOWLEDGMENT

The authors acknowledge the contributions of Dr. George A. Bray, who wrote this chapter in the 14th edition.

FURTHER READINGS

Branson R et al: Binge eating as a major phenotype of melanocortin 4 receptor gene mutations. N Engl J Med 348:1096, 2003

Buchwald H et al: Bariatric surgery: A systematic review and meta-analysis. JAMA 292: 1724, 2004

This report examined 136 previous studies to assess the impact of bariatric surgery on weight loss, operative mortality outcome, and obesity comorbidities (diabetes, hyperlipidemia, hypertension, and obstructive sleep apnea). The mean percentage of excess weight loss was 61% for all procedures. Opera-

tive mortality was 0.1% for the purely restrictive procedures, 0.5% for gastric bypass, and 1.1% for biliopancreatic diversion or duodenal switch. Diabetes was completely resolved in 77% of patients and resolved or improved in 86%. Hyperlipidemia improved in 70% or more of patients. Hypertension and obstructive sleep apnea also resolved most patients.

FAROOQI IS et al: Clinical spectrum of obesity and mutations in the melanocortin 4 receptor gene. N Engl J Med 348:1085, 2003

FLEGAL KM et al: Excess deaths associated with underweight, overweight, and obesity. JAMA 293: 1861, 2005

This study assessed the relative risks of mortality associated with different levels of BMI based on data from National Health and Nutrition Examination Survey (NHANES) results between 1971 and 2000. The results indicate that both underweight and obesity, particularly higher levels of obesity, were associated with increased mortality relative to the normal weight category.

HAFFNER S et al: Epidemic obesity and the metabolic syndrome. Circulation 108: 1541, 2003

LARSEN LH et al: Prevalence of mutations and functional analyses of melanocortin 4 receptor variants identified among 750 men with juvenile-onset obesity. J Clin Endocrinol Metab 90: 219, 2005

This study examined 750 Danish men with juvenile-onset obesity for mutations in MC4R. A total of 14 different mutations were identified, suggesting a carrier frequency of pathogenic mutations in the MC4R gene of 2.5% in a population-based study of obese men.

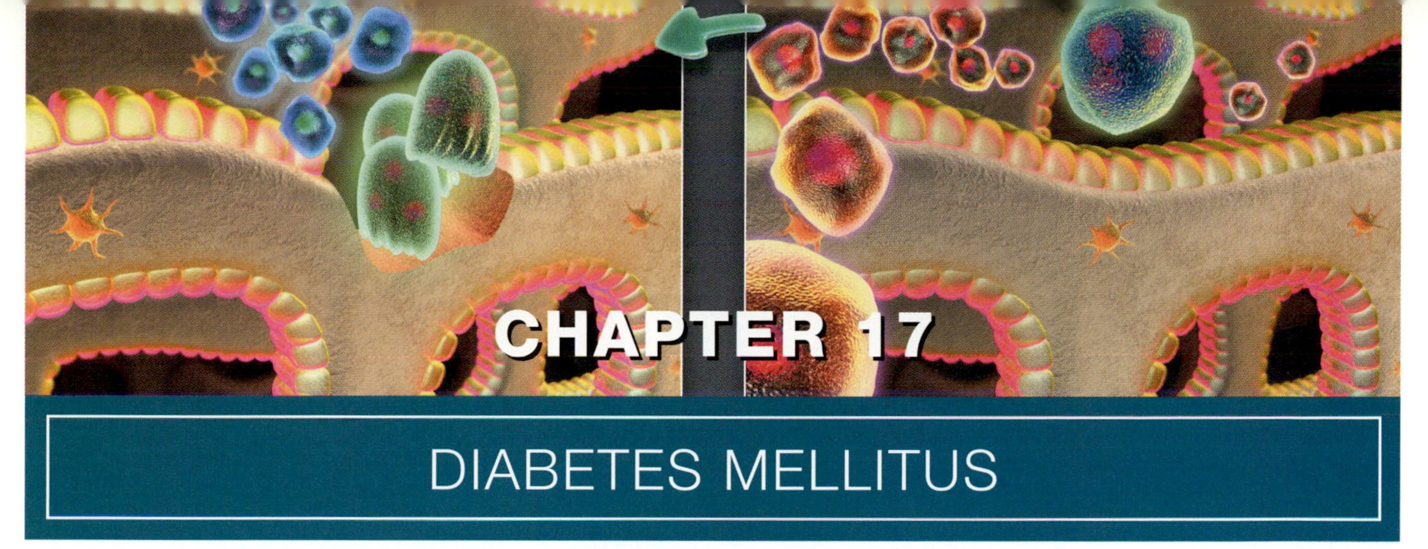

CHAPTER 17

DIABETES MELLITUS

Alvin C. Powers

Diabetes mellitus (DM) comprises a group of common metabolic disorders that share the phenotype of hyperglycemia. Several distinct types of DM exist and are caused by a complex interaction of genetics, environmental factors, and life-style choices. Depending on the etiology of the DM, factors contributing to hyperglycemia may include reduced insulin secretion, decreased glucose utilization, and increased glucose production. The metabolic dysregulation associated with DM causes secondary pathophysiologic changes in multiple organ systems that impose a tremendous burden on the individual with diabetes and on the health care system. In the United States, DM is the leading cause of end-stage renal disease (ESRD), nontraumatic lower extremity amputations, and adult blindness. With an increasing incidence worldwide, DM will be a leading cause of morbidity and mortality for the foreseeable future.

CLASSIFICATION

DM is classified on the basis of the pathogenic process that leads to hyperglycemia, as opposed to earlier criteria such as age of onset or type of therapy (**Fig. 17-1**). The two broad categories of DM are designated type 1 and type 2 (**Table 17-1**). Type 1A DM results from autoimmune beta cell destruction, which leads to insulin deficiency. Individuals with type 1B DM lack immunologic markers indicative of an autoimmune destructive process of the beta cells. However, they develop insulin deficiency by unknown mechanisms and are ketosis prone. Relatively few patients with type 1 DM are in the type 1B idiopathic category; many of these individuals are either African-American or Asian in heritage.

Type 2 DM is a heterogeneous group of disorders characterized by variable degrees of insulin resistance, impaired insulin secretion, and increased glucose production. Distinct genetic and metabolic defects in

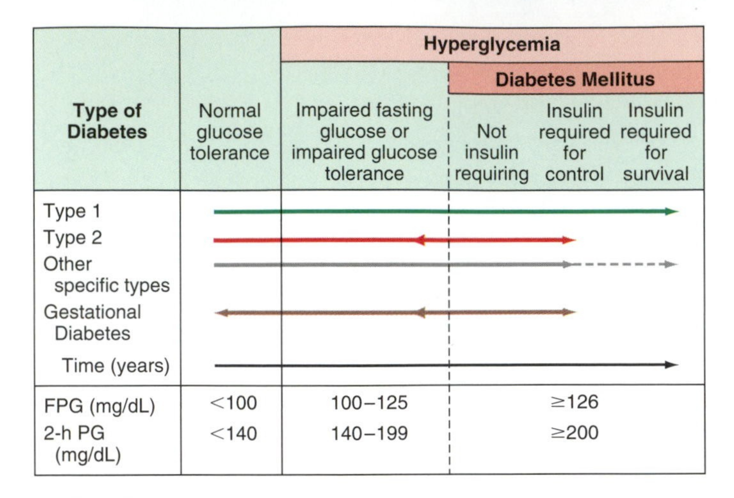

FIGURE 17-1

Spectrum of glucose homeostasis and diabetes mellitus (DM). The spectrum from normal glucose tolerance to diabetes in type 1 DM, type 2 DM, other specific types of diabetes, and gestational DM is shown from left to right. In most types of DM, the individual traverses from normal glucose tolerance to impaired glucose tolerance to overt diabetes. Arrows indicate that changes in glucose tolerance may be bi-directional in some types of diabetes. For example, individuals with type 2 DM may return to the impaired glucose tolerance category with weight loss; in gestational DM diabetes may revert to impaired glucose tolerance or even normal glucose tolerance after delivery. The fasting plasma glucose (FPG) and 2-h plasma glucose (PG), after a glucose challenge for the different categories of glucose tolerance, are shown at the lower part of the figure. These values do not apply to the diagnosis of gestational DM. Some types of DM may or may not require insulin for survival, hence the dotted line. (Conventional units are used in the figure.) *(Adapted from American Diabetes Association: Diagnosis and classification of diabetes mellitus. Diabetes Care 29 (suppl 1): S43, 2006.)*

insulin action and/or secretion give rise to the common phenotype of hyperglycemia in type 2 DM (see below). Distinct pathogenic processes in type 2 DM have important potential therapeutic implications, as pharmacologic agents that target specific metabolic derangements have become available. Type 2 DM is preceded by a period of abnormal glucose homeostasis classified as impaired fasting glucose (IFG) or impaired glucose tolerance (IGT).

Two features of the current classification of DM diverge from previous classifications. First, the terms *insulin-dependent diabetes mellitus* (IDDM) and *noninsulin-dependent diabetes mellitus* (NIDDM) are obsolete. Since many individuals with type 2 DM eventually require insulin treatment for control of glycemia, the use of the term NIDDM generated considerable confusion. A second difference is that age is not a criterion in the classification system. Although type 1 DM most commonly develops before the age of 30, an autoimmune beta cell destructive process can develop at any age. It is estimated that between 5 and 10% of individuals who develop DM after age 30 have type 1A DM. Likewise, type 2 DM more typically develops with increasing age, but it also occurs in children, particularly in obese adolescents.

TABLE 17-1

ETIOLOGIC CLASSIFICATION OF DIABETES MELLITUS

- **I. Type 1 diabetes** (β cell destruction, usually leading to absolute insulin deficiency)
  - A. Immune-mediated
  - B. Idiopathic
- **II. Type 2 diabetes** (may range from predominantly insulin resistance with relative insulin deficiency to a predominantly insulin secretory defect with insulin resistance)
- **III. Other specific types of diabetes**
  - A. Genetic defects of β cell function characterized by mutations in:
    1. Hepatocyte nuclear transcription factor (HNF) 4α (MODY 1)
    2. Glucokinase (MODY 2)
    3. HNF-1α (MODY 3)
    4. Insulin promoter factor (IPF) 1 (MODY 4)
    5. HNF-1β (MODY 5)
    6. NeuroD1 (MODY 6)
    7. Mitochondrial DNA
    8. Proinsulin or insulin conversion
  - B. Genetic defects in insulin action
    1. Type A insulin resistance
    2. Leprechaunism
    3. Rabson-Mendenhall syndrome
    4. Lipodystrophy syndromes
  - C. Diseases of the exocrine pancreas — pancreatitis, pancreatectomy, neoplasia, cystic fibrosis, hemochromatosis, fibrocalculous pancreatopathy
  - D. Endocrinopathies — acromegaly, Cushing's syndrome, glucagonoma, pheochromocytoma, hyperthyroidism, somatostatinoma, aldosteronoma
  - E. Drug- or chemical-induced — Vacor, pentamidine, nicotinic acid, glucocorticoids, thyroid hormone, diazoxide, β-adrenergic agonists, thiazides, phenytoin, α-interferon, protease inhibitors, clozapine, beta blockers
  - F. Infections — congenital rubella, cytomegalovirus, coxsackie
  - G. Uncommon forms of immune-mediated diabetes — "stiff-man" syndrome, anti-insulin receptor antibodies
  - H. Other genetic syndromes sometimes associated with diabetes — Down's syndrome, Klinefelter's syndrome, Turner's syndrome, Wolfram's syndrome, Friedreich's ataxia, Huntington's chorea, Laurence-Moon-Biedl syndrome, myotonic dystrophy, porphyria, Prader-Willi syndrome
- **VI. Gestational diabetes mellitus (GDM)**

Note: MODY, maturity onset of diabetes of the young.
Source: From American Diabetes Association: Diagnosis and classification of diabetes mellitus. Diabetes Care 29(suppl 1): S43–S48, 2006.

OTHER TYPES OF DM

Other etiologies for DM include specific genetic defects in insulin secretion or action, metabolic abnormalities that impair insulin secretion, mitochondrial abnormalities, and a host of conditions that impair glucose tolerance (Table 17-1). *Maturity onset diabetes of the young* (MODY) is a subtype of DM characterized by autosomal dominant inheritance, early onset of hyperglycemia, and impairment in insulin secretion (discussed below). Mutations in the insulin receptor cause a group of rare disorders characterized by severe insulin resistance.

DM can result from pancreatic exocrine disease when the majority of pancreatic islets (>80%) are destroyed. Hormones that antagonize the action of insulin can lead to DM. Thus, DM is often a feature of endocrinopathies, such as acromegaly and Cushing's disease. Viral infections have been implicated in pancreatic islet destruction, but are an extremely rare cause of DM. Congenital rubella greatly increases the risk for DM; however, most of these individuals also have immunologic markers indicative of autoimmune beta cell destruction.

GESTATIONAL DIABETES MELLITUS (GDM)

Glucose intolerance may develop during pregnancy. Insulin resistance related to the metabolic changes of late pregnancy increases insulin requirements and may lead to IGT. GDM occurs in ~4% of pregnancies in the United States; most women revert to normal glucose tolerance post-partum but have a substantial risk (30 to 60%) of developing DM later in life.

EPIDEMIOLOGY

The worldwide prevalence of DM has risen dramatically over the past two decades. Likewise, prevalence rates of IFG are also increasing. Although the prevalence of both type 1 and type 2 DM is increasing worldwide, the prevalence of type 2 DM is expected to rise more rapidly in the future because of increasing obesity and reduced activity levels. DM increases with aging. In 2000, the prevalence of DM was estimated to be 0.19% in persons <20 years old and 8.6% in those >20 years old. In individuals >65 years the prevalence of DM was 20.1%. The prevalence is similar in men and women throughout most age ranges but is slightly greater in men >60 years.

There is considerable geographic variation in the incidence of both type 1 and type 2 DM. Scandinavia has the highest incidence of type 1 DM (e.g., in Finland, the incidence is 35/100,000 per year). The Pacific Rim has a much lower rate (in Japan and China, the incidence is 1 to 3/100,000 per year) of type 1 DM; Northern Europe and the United States share an intermediate rate (8 to 17/100,000 per year). Much of the increased risk of type 1 DM is believed to reflect the frequency of high-risk HLA alleles among ethnic groups in different geographic locations. The prevalence of type 2 DM and its harbinger, IGT, is highest in certain Pacific islands, intermediate in countries such as India and the United States, and relatively low in Russia and China. This variability is likely due to genetic, behavioral, and environmental factors. DM prevalence also varies among different ethnic populations within a given country. In 2000, the prevalence of DM in the United States was 13% in African Americans, 10.2% in Hispanic Americans, 15.5% in Native Americans (American Indians and Alaska natives), and 7.8% in non-Hispanic whites. The onset of type 2 DM occurs, on average, at an earlier age in ethnic groups other than non-Hispanic whites.

DIAGNOSIS

The National Diabetes Data Group and World Health Organization have issued diagnostic criteria for DM (**Table 17-2**) based on the following premises: (1) the spectrum of fasting plasma glucose (FPG) and the response to an oral glucose load varies among normal individuals, and (2) DM is defined as the level of glycemia at which diabetes-specific complications occur rather than on deviations from a population-based mean. For example, the prevalence of retinopathy in Native Americans (Pima Indian population) begins to increase at a FPG > 6.4 mmol/L (116 mg/dL) (**Fig. 17-2**).

Glucose tolerance is classified into three categories based on the FPG: (1) FPG < 5.6 mmol/L (100 mg/dL) is considered normal; (2) FPG ≥ 5.6 mmol/L (100 mg/dL) but < 7.0 mmol/L (126 mg/dL) is defined

TABLE 17-2

CRITERIA FOR THE DIAGNOSIS OF DIABETES MELLITUS

- Symptoms of diabetes plus random blood glucose concentration ≥11.1 mmol/L (200 mg/dL)[a] *or*
- Fasting plasma glucose ≥7.0 mmol/L (126 mg/dL)[b] *or*
- Two-hour plasma glucose ≥11.1 mmol/L (200 mg/dL) during an oral glucose tolerance test[a]

[a]Random is defined as without regard to time since the last meal.
[b]Fasting is defined as no caloric intake for at least 8 h.
[c]The test should be performed using a glucose load containing the equivalent of 75 g anhydrous glucose dissolved in water; not recommended for routine clinical use.
Note: In the absence of unequivocal hyperglycemia and acute metabolic decompensation, these criteria should be confirmed by repeat testing on a different day.
Source: Adapted from American Diabetes Association: Diagnosis and classification of diabetes mellitus. Diabetes Care 29 (suppl 1): S43, 2006.

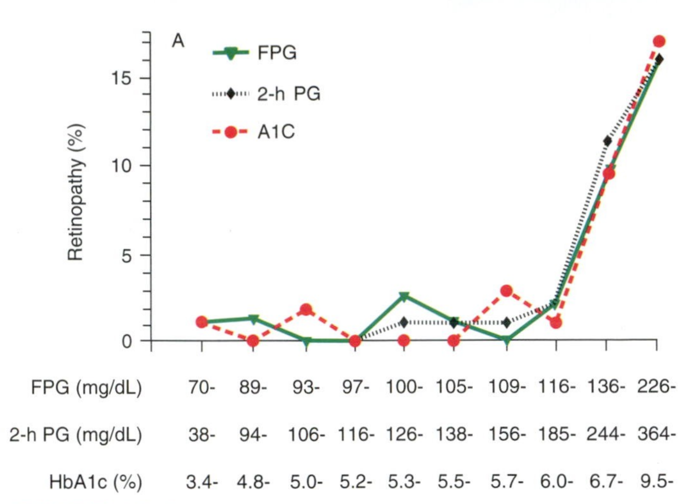

FIGURE 17-2

Relationship of diabetes-specific complication and glucose tolerance. This figure shows the incidence of retinopathy in Pima Indians as a function of the fasting plasma glucose (FPG), the 2-h plasma glucose after a 75-g oral glucose challenge (2-h PG), or glycated hemoglobin (A1C). Note that the incidence of retinopathy greatly increases at a fasting plasma glucose >116 mg/dL, or a 2-h plasma glucose of 185 mg/dL, or a A1C >6.0%. (Conventional units for blood glucose are used in the figure.) *Copyright 2002, American Diabetes Association. From Diabetes Care 25(Suppl 1): S5–S20, 2002. Reprinted with permission from The American Diabetes Association.*

as IFG; and (3) FPG ≥ 7.0 mmol/L (126 mg/dL) warrants the diagnosis of DM. IFG is comparable to IGT, which is defined as plasma glucose levels between 7.8 and 11.1 mmol/L (140 and 200 mg/dL) 2 h after a 75-g oral glucose load (Table 17-2). Individuals with IFG or IGT are at substantial risk for developing type 2 DM (40% risk over the next 5 years) and cardiovascular disease.

The revised criteria for the diagnosis of DM emphasize the FPG as a reliable and convenient test for diagnosing DM in asymptomatic individuals. A random plasma glucose concentration ≥ 11.1 mmol/L (200 mg/dL) accompanied by classic symptoms of DM (polyuria, polydipsia, weight loss) is sufficient for the diagnosis of DM (Table 17-2). Oral glucose tolerance testing, although still a valid mechanism for diagnosing DM, is not recommended as part of routine care.

Some investigators have advocated the hemoglobin A1c (A1C) as a diagnostic test for DM. Though there is a strong correlation between elevations in the plasma glucose and the A1C (discussed below), the relationship between the FPG and the A1C in individuals with normal glucose tolerance or mild glucose intolerance is less clear and thus the use of the A1C is not currently recommended for the diagnosis of diabetes.

The diagnosis of DM has profound implications for an individual from both a medical and financial standpoint. Thus, these diagnostic criteria must be satisfied before assigning the diagnosis of DM. Abnormalities on screening tests for diabetes should be repeated before making a definitive diagnosis of DM, unless acute metabolic derangements or a markedly elevated plasma glucose are present (Table 17-2). The revised criteria also allow for the diagnosis of DM to be withdrawn in situations where the FPG reverts to normal.

SCREENING

Widespread use of the FPG as a screening test for type 2 DM is recommended because: (1) a large number of individuals who meet the current criteria for DM are asymptomatic and unaware that they have the disorder, (2) epidemiologic studies suggest that type 2 DM may be present for up to a decade before diagnosis, (3) as many as 50% of individuals with type 2 DM have one or more diabetes-specific complications at the time of their diagnosis, and (4) treatment of type 2 DM may favorably alter the natural history of DM. The American Diabetes Association (ADA) recommends screening all individuals >45 years every 3 years and screening individuals with additional risk factors (**Table 17-3**) at an earlier age. In contrast to type 2 DM, a long asymptomatic period of hyperglycemia is rare prior to the diagnosis of type 1 DM. A number of immunologic markers for type 1 DM are becoming available (discussed below), but their routine use is discouraged pending the identification of clinically beneficial interventions for individuals at high risk for developing type 1 DM.

TABLE 17-3

RISK FACTORS FOR TYPE 2 DIABETES MELLITUS

- Family history of diabetes (i.e., parent or sibling with type 2 diabetes)
- Obesity (BMI ≥25 kg/m^2)
- Habitual physical inactivity
- Race/ethnicity (e.g., African American, Hispanic American, Native American, Asian American, Pacific Islander)
- Previously identified IFG or IGT
- History of GDM or delivery of baby >4kg (>9 1b)
- Hypertension (blood pressure ≥140/90 mmHg)
- HDL cholesterol level ≤35mg/dL (0.09 mmol/L) and/or a triglyceride level ≥250 mg/dL (2.82 mmol/L)
- Polycystic ovary syndrome or acanthosis nigricans
- History of vascular disease

Note: BMI, body mass index; IFG, impaired fasting glucose; IGT, impaired glucose tolerance; GDM, gestational diabetes mellitus; HDL, high-density lipoprotein.

Source: Adapted from American Diabetes Association: Standards of medical care in diabetes—2006. Diabetes Care 29(suppl 1): S4, 2006.

INSULIN BIOSYNTHESIS, SECRETION, AND ACTION

BIOSYNTHESIS

Insulin is produced in the beta cells of the pancreatic islets. It is initially synthesized as a single-chain 86-amino-acid precursor polypeptide, preproinsulin. Subsequent proteolytic processing removes the aminoterminal signal peptide, giving rise to proinsulin. Proinsulin is structurally related to insulin-like growth factors I and II, which bind weakly to the insulin receptor (Chap. 1). Cleavage of an internal 31-residue fragment from proinsulin generates the C peptide and the A (21 amino acids) and B (30 amino acids) chains of insulin, which are connected by disulfide bonds. The mature insulin molecule and C peptide are stored together and cosecreted from secretory granules in the beta cells. Because the C peptide is less susceptible than insulin to hepatic degradation, it is a useful marker of insulin secretion and allows discrimination of endogenous and exogenous sources of insulin in the evaluation of hypoglycemia (Chap. 19). Human insulin is now produced by recombinant DNA technology; structural alterations at one or more residues are useful for modifying its physical and pharmacologic characteristics (see below).

SECRETION

Glucose is the key regulator of insulin secretion by the pancreatic beta cell, although amino acids, ketones, various nutrients, gastrointestinal peptides, and neurotransmitters also influence insulin secretion. Glucose levels >3.9 mmol/L (70 mg/dL) stimulate insulin synthesis, primarily by enhancing protein translation and processing. Glucose stimulation of insulin secretion begins with its transport into the beta cell by the GLUT2 glucose transporter (**Fig. 17-3**). Glucose phosphorylation by glucokinase is the rate-limiting step that controls glucose-regulated insulin secretion. Further metabolism of glucose-6-phosphate via glycolysis generates ATP, which inhibits the activity of an ATP-sensitive K^+ channel. This channel consists of two separate proteins: one is the receptor for certain oral hypoglycemics (e.g., sulfonylureas, meglitinides); the other is an inwardly rectifying K^+ channel protein. Inhibition of this K^+ channel induces beta cell membrane depolarization, which opens voltage-dependent calcium channels (leading to an influx of calcium), and stimulates insulin secretion. Insulin secretory profiles reveal a pulsatile pattern of hormone release, with small secretory bursts occurring about every 10 min, superimposed upon greater amplitude oscillations of about 80 to 150 min. Meals or other major stimuli of insulin secretion induce large (four- to fivefold increase versus baseline) bursts of insulin secretion that usually last for 2 to 3 h before returning to baseline.

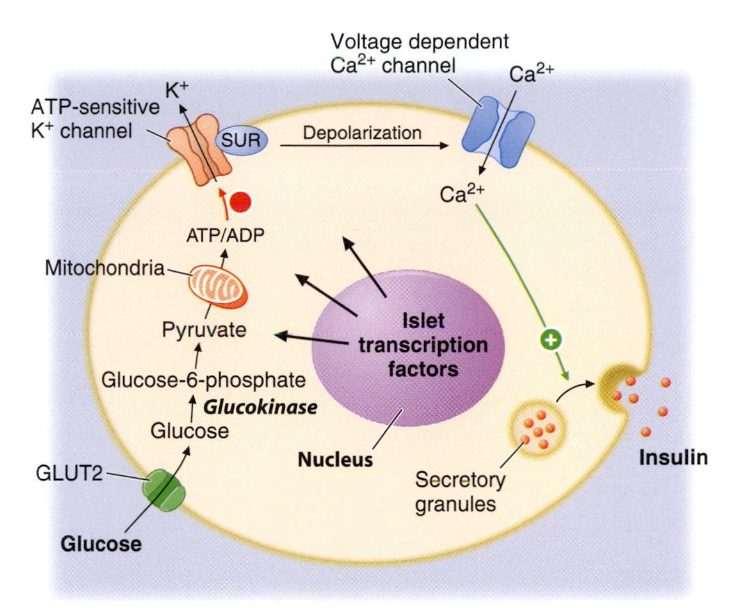

FIGURE 17-3

Diabetes and abnormalities in glucose-stimulated insulin secretion. Glucose and other nutrients regulate insulin secretion by the pancreatic beta cell. Glucose is transported by the GLUT2 glucose transporter; subsequent glucose metabolism by the beta cell alters ion channel activity, leading to insulin secretion. The SUR receptor is the binding site for drugs that act as insulin secretagogues. Mutations in the events or proteins underlined are a cause of maturity onset diabetes of the young (MODY) or other forms of diabetes. SUR, sulfonylurea receptor; ATP, adenosine triphosphate; ADP, adenosine diphosphate. *(Adapted from WL Lowe, in JL Jameson (ed): Principles of Molecular Medicine. Totowa, NJ, Humana, 1998.)*

Derangements in these normal secretory patterns are one of the earliest signs of beta cell dysfunction in DM.

ACTION

Once insulin is secreted into the portal venous system, ~50% is degraded by the liver. Unextracted insulin enters the systemic circulation where it binds to receptors in target sites. Insulin binding to its receptor stimulates intrinsic tyrosine kinase activity, leading to receptor autophosphorylation and the recruitment of intracellular signaling molecules, such as insulin receptor substrates (IRS) (**Fig. 17-4**). These and other adaptor proteins initiate a complex cascade of phosphorylation and dephosphorylation reactions, resulting in the widespread metabolic and mitogenic effects of insulin. As an example, activation of the phosphatidylinositol-3′-kinase (PI-3-kinase) pathway stimulates translocation of glucose transporters (e.g., GLUT4) to the cell surface, an event that is crucial for glucose uptake by skeletal muscle and fat. Activation of other insulin receptor signaling pathways induces glycogen synthesis, protein synthesis,

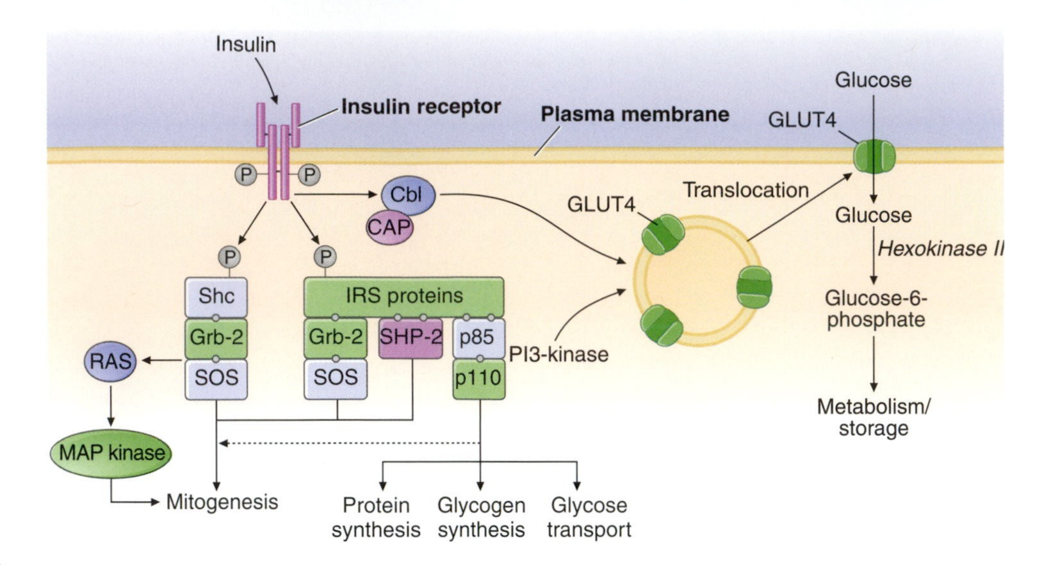

FIGURE 17-4

Insulin signal transduction pathway in skeletal muscle. The insulin receptor has intrinsic tyrosine kinase activity and interacts with insulin receptor substrates (IRS and Shc) proteins. A number of "docking" proteins bind to these cellular proteins and initiate the metabolic actions of insulin [GrB-2, SOS, SHP-2, p65, p110, and phosphatidylinositol-3′-kinase (PI-3-kinase)]. Insulin increases glucose transport through PI-3-kinase and the Cbl pathway, which promotes the translocation of intracellular vesicles containing GLUT4 glucose transporter to the plasma membrane. *(Adapted from WL Lowe, in Principles of Molecular Medicine, JL Jameson (ed). Totowa, NJ, Humana, 1998; A Virkamaki et al: J Clin Invest 103:931, 1999. For additional details see AR Saltiel and CR Kahn, Nature 414: 799, 2001.)*

lipogenesis, and regulation of various genes in insulin-responsive cells.

Glucose homeostasis reflects a precise balance between hepatic glucose production and peripheral glucose uptake and utilization. Insulin is the most important regulator of this metabolic equilibrium, but neural input, metabolic signals, and hormones (e.g., glucagon) result in integrated control of glucose supply and utilization (Chap. 19; see Fig. 19-1). In the fasting state, low insulin levels increase glucose production by promoting hepatic gluconeogenesis and glycogenolysis. Glucagon also stimulates glycogenolysis and gluconeogenesis by the liver and renal medulla. Low insulin levels decrease glycogen synthesis, reduce glucose uptake in insulin-sensitive tissues, and promote mobilization of stored precursors. Postprandially, the glucose load elicits a rise in insulin and fall in glucagon, leading to a reversal of these processes. The major portion of postprandial glucose is utilized by skeletal muscle, an effect of insulin-stimulated glucose uptake. Other tissues, most notably the brain, utilize glucose in an insulin-independent fashion.

PATHOGENESIS

TYPE 1 DM

Type 1A DM develops as a result of the synergistic effects of genetic, environmental, and immunologic factors that ultimately destroy the pancreatic beta cells. The temporal development of type 1A DM is shown schematically as a function of beta cell mass in **Fig. 17-5**. Individuals with a genetic susceptibility have normal beta cell mass at birth but begin to lose beta cells secondary to autoimmune destruction that occurs over months to years. This autoimmune process is thought to be triggered by an infectious or environmental stimulus and to be sustained by a beta cell–specific molecule. In the majority of individuals, immunologic markers appear after the triggering event but before diabetes becomes clinically overt. Beta cell mass then begins to decline, and insulin secretion becomes progressively impaired, although normal glucose tolerance is maintained. The rate of decline in beta cell mass varies widely among individuals, with some patients progressing rapidly to clinical diabetes and others evolving more slowly. Features of diabetes do not become evident until a majority of beta cells are destroyed (~80%). At this point, residual functional beta cells still exist but are insufficient in number to maintain glucose tolerance. The events that trigger the transition from glucose intolerance to frank diabetes are often associated with increased insulin requirements, as might occur during infections or puberty. After the initial clinical presentation of type 1A DM, a "honeymoon" phase may ensue during which time glycemic control is achieved with modest doses of insulin or, rarely, insulin is not needed.

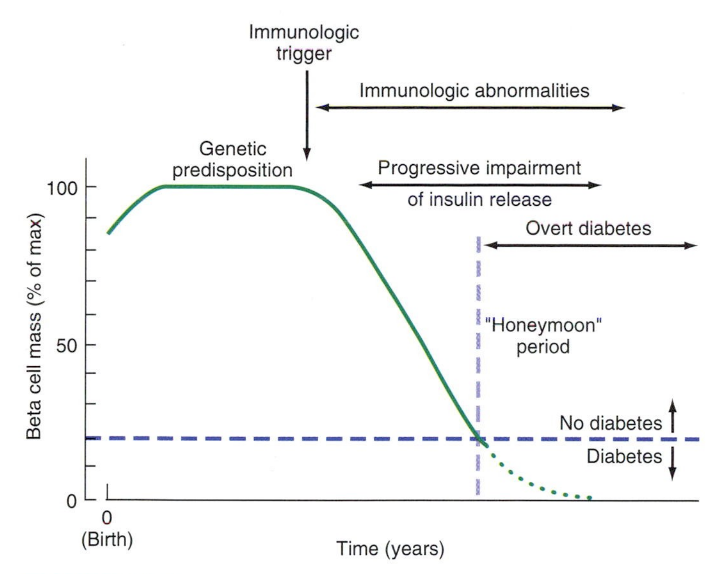

FIGURE 17-5

Temporal model for development of type 1 diabetes. Individuals with a genetic predisposition are exposed to an immunologic trigger that initiates an autoimmune process, resulting in a gradual decline in beta cell mass. The downward slope of the beta cell mass varies among individuals. This progressive impairment in insulin release results in diabetes when ~80% of the beta cell mass is destroyed. A "honeymoon" phase may be seen in the first 1 or 2 years after the onset of diabetes and is associated with reduced insulin requirements. *(Adapted from Medical Management of Type 1 Diabetes, 3d ed, JS Skyler (ed). Alexandria, VA, American Diabetes Association, 1998.)*

However, this fleeting phase of endogenous insulin production from residual beta cells disappears as the autoimmune process destroys the remaining beta cells, and the individual becomes completely insulin deficient.

Genetic susceptibility to type 1A DM involves multiple genes. The concordance of type 1A DM in identical twins ranges between 30 and 70%, indicating that additional modifying factors must be involved in determining whether diabetes develops. The major susceptibility gene for type 1A DM is located in the HLA region on chromosome 6. Polymorphisms in the HLA complex account for 40 to 50% of the genetic risk of developing type 1A DM. This region contains genes that encode the class II MHC molecules, which present antigen to helper T cells and thus are involved in initiating the immune response. The ability of class II MHC molecules to present antigen is dependent on the amino acid composition of their antigen-binding sites. Amino acid substitutions may influence the specificity of the immune response by altering the binding affinity of different antigens for class II molecules.

Most individuals with type 1A DM have the HLA DR3 and/or DR4 haplotype. Refinements in genotyping of HLA loci have shown that the haplotypes DQA1*0301, DQB1*0302, DQA1*501, and DQB1*0201 are most strongly associated with type 1A DM. These haplotypes are present in 40% of children with type 1A DM as compared to 2% of the normal U.S. population.

In addition to MHC class II associations, at least 17 different genetic loci contribute susceptibility to type 1A DM. For example, polymorphisms in the promoter region of the insulin gene account for ~10% of the predisposition to type 1A DM. Genes that confer protection against the development of the disease also exist. The haplotype DQA1*0102, DQB1*0602 is present in 20% of the U.S. population but is extremely rare in individuals with type 1A DM (<1%).

The risk of developing type 1A DM is increased tenfold in relatives of individuals with the disease. Nevertheless, most individuals with predisposing haplotypes do not develop diabetes. In addition, most individuals with type 1A DM do not have a first-degree relative with this disorder.

Autoimmune Factors

Although other islet cell types [alpha cells (glucagon-producing), delta cells (somatostatin-producing), or PP cells (pancreatic polypeptide–producing)] are functionally and embryologically similar to beta cells and express most of the same proteins as beta cells, they are inexplicably spared from the autoimmune process. Pathologically, the pancreatic islets are infiltrated with lymphocytes (in a process termed *insulitis*). After all beta cells are destroyed, the inflammatory process abates, the islets become atrophic, and immunologic markers disappear. Studies of the autoimmune process in humans and animal models of type 1A DM (NOD mouse and BB rat) have identified the following abnormalities in both the humoral and cellular arms of the immune system: (1) islet cell autoantibodies; (2) activated lymphocytes in the islets, peripancreatic lymph nodes, and systemic circulation; (3) T lymphocytes that proliferate when stimulated with islet proteins; and (4) release of cytokines within the insulitis. Beta cells seem to be particularly susceptible to the toxic effect of some cytokines [tumor necrosis factor α (TNF-α), interferon γ, and interleukin-1 (IL-1)]. The precise mechanisms of beta cell death are not known but may involve formation of nitric oxide metabolites, apoptosis, and direct CD8+ T cell cytotoxicity. Islet autoantibodies are not thought to be involved in the destructive process, as these antibodies do not generally react with the cell surface of islet cells and are not capable of transferring diabetes mellitus to animals.

Pancreatic islet molecules targeted by the autoimmune process include insulin, glutamic acid decarboxylase (GAD, the biosynthetic enzyme for the neurotransmitter GABA), ICA-512/IA-2 (homology with tyrosine phosphatases), and phogrin (insulin secretory granule protein). Other less clearly defined autoantigens include an islet ganglioside and carboxypeptidase H. With the exception of insulin, none of the autoantigens are beta cell specific, which raises the question of how the beta cells are selectively destroyed. Current theories favor initiation of an autoimmune process directed at one beta cell molecule, which then spreads to other islet molecules as the immune process destroys beta cells and creates a series of secondary autoantigens. The beta cells of individuals who develop type 1A DM do not differ from beta cells of normal individuals, since transplanted islets are destroyed by a recurrence of the autoimmune process of type 1A DM.

Immunologic Markers

Islet cell autoantibodies (ICAs) are a composite of several different antibodies directed at pancreatic islet molecules such as GAD, insulin, IA-2/ICA-512, and an islet ganglioside and serve as a marker of the autoimmune process of type 1A DM. Assays for autoantibodies to GAD-65 are commercially available. Testing for ICAs can be useful in classifying the type of DM as type IA and in identifying nondiabetic individuals at risk for developing type 1A DM. ICAs are present in the majority of individuals (>75%) diagnosed with new-onset type 1A DM, in a significant minority of individuals with newly diagnosed type 2 DM (5 to 10%), and occasionally in individuals with GDM (<5%). ICAs are present in 3 to 4% of first-degree relatives of individuals with type 1A DM. In combination with impaired insulin secretion after intravenous glucose tolerance testing, they predict a >50% risk of developing type 1A DM within 5 years. Without this impairment in insulin secretion, the presence of ICAs predicts a 5-year risk of <25%. Based on these data, the risk of a first-degree relative developing type 1A DM is relatively low. At present, the measurement of ICAs in nondiabetic individuals is a research tool because no treatments have been approved to prevent the occurrence or progression of type 1A DM.

Environmental Factors

Numerous environmental events have been proposed to trigger the autoimmune process in genetically susceptible individuals; however, none have been conclusively linked to diabetes. Identification of an environmental trigger has been difficult because the event may precede the onset of DM by several years (Fig. 17-5). Putative environmental triggers include viruses (coxsackie and rubella most prominently), bovine milk proteins, and nitrosourea compounds.

Prevention of Type 1A DM

A number of interventions have successfully delayed or prevented diabetes in animal models. Some interventions have targeted the immune system directly (immunosuppression, selective T cell subset deletion, induction of immunologic tolerance to islet proteins), whereas others have prevented islet cell death by blocking cytotoxic cytokines or increasing islet resistance to the destructive process. Though results in animal models are promising, these interventions have not been successful in preventing type 1A DM in humans. The Diabetes Prevention Trial—type 1 recently concluded that administering insulin to individuals at high risk for developing type 1A DM did not prevent type 1A DM.

TYPE 2 DM

Insulin resistance and abnormal insulin secretion are central to the development of type 2 DM. Although controversy remains regarding the primary defect, most studies support the view that insulin resistance precedes insulin secretory defects and that diabetes develops only if insulin secretion becomes inadequate.

Type 2 DM has a strong genetic component. Major genes that predispose to this disorder have yet to be identified, but it is clear that the disease is polygenic and multifactorial. Various genetic loci contribute to susceptibility, and environmental factors (such as nutrition and physical activity) further modulate phenotypic expression of the disease. The concordance of type 2 DM in identical twins is between 70 and 90%. Individuals with a parent with type 2 DM have an increased risk of diabetes; if both parents have type 2 DM, the risk approaches 40%. Insulin resistance, as demonstrated by reduced glucose utilization in skeletal muscle, is present in many nondiabetic, first-degree relatives of individuals with type 2 DM. However, definition of the genetic susceptibility remains a challenge because the genetic defect in insulin secretion or action may not manifest itself unless an environmental event or another genetic defect, such as obesity, is superimposed. Mutations in various molecules involved in insulin action (e.g., the insulin receptor and enzymes involved in glucose homeostasis) account for a very small fraction of type 2 DM. Likewise, genetic defects in proteins involved in insulin secretion have not been found in most individuals with type 2 DM. Genome-wide scanning for mutations or polymorphisms associated with type 2 DM is being used in an effort to identify genes associated with type 2 DM. The gene for the protease, calpain 10, is associated with type 2 DM in Hispanic and some other populations.

Pathophysiology

Type 2 DM is characterized by three pathophysiologic abnormalities: impaired insulin secretion, peripheral insulin resistance, and excessive hepatic glucose production. Obesity, particularly visceral or central (as evidenced by the hip-waist ratio), is very common in type 2 DM. Adipocytes secrete a number of biologic products (leptin, TFN-α, free fatty acids, resistin, and adiponectin) that modulate insulin secretion, insulin action, and body weight and may contribute to the insulin resistance. In the early stages of the disorder, glucose tolerance remains normal, despite insulin resistance, because the pancreatic beta cells compensate by increasing insulin output (**Fig. 17-6**). As insulin resistance and compensatory hyperinsulinemia progress, the pancreatic islets in certain individuals are unable to sustain the hyperinsulinemic state. IGT, characterized by elevations in postprandial glucose, then develops. A further decline in insulin secretion and an increase in hepatic glucose production lead to overt diabetes with fasting hyperglycemia. Ultimately, beta cell failure may ensue. Markers of inflammation such as IL-6 and C-reactive protein are often elevated in type 2 diabetes.

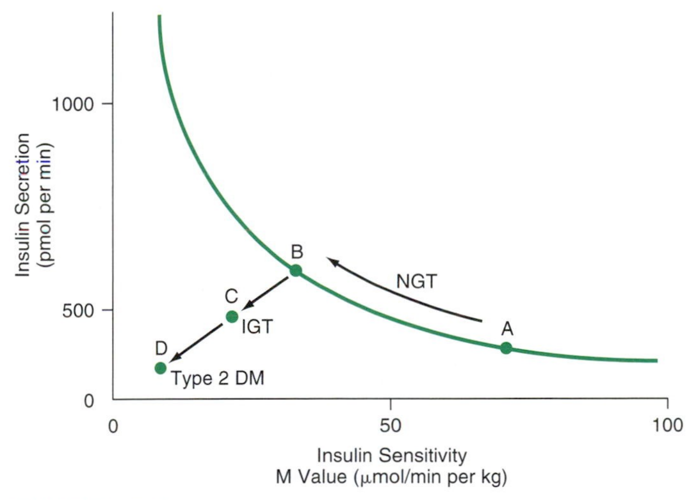

FIGURE 17-6

Metabolic changes during the development of type 2 diabetes mellitus (DM). Insulin secretion and insulin sensitivity are related, and as an individual becomes more insulin resistant (by moving from point A to point B), insulin secretion increases. A failure to compensate by increasing the insulin secretion results initially in impaired glucose tolerance (IGT; point C) and ultimately in type 2 DM (point D). *(Adapted from SE Kahn, J Clin Endocrinol Metab 86:4047, 2001; RN Bergman, M Ader, Trends Endocrinol Metab 11:351, 2000.)*

Metabolic Abnormalities

Insulin Resistance The decreased ability of insulin to act effectively on peripheral target tissues (especially muscle and liver) is a prominent feature of type 2 DM and results from a combination of genetic susceptibility and obesity. Insulin resistance is relative, however, since supernormal levels of circulating insulin will normalize the plasma glucose. Insulin dose-response curves exhibit a rightward shift, indicating reduced sensitivity, and a reduced maximal response, indicating an overall decrease in maximum glucose utilization (30 to 60% lower than normal individuals). Insulin resistance impairs glucose utilization by insulin-sensitive tissues and increases hepatic glucose output; both effects contribute to the hyperglycemia. Increased hepatic glucose output predominantly accounts for increased FPG levels, whereas decreased peripheral glucose usage results in postprandial hyperglycemia. In skeletal muscle, there is a greater impairment in nonoxidative glucose usage (glycogen formation) than in oxidative glucose metabolism through glycolysis. Glucose metabolism in insulin-independent tissues is not altered in type 2 DM.

The precise molecular mechanism of insulin resistance in type 2 DM has not been elucidated. Insulin receptor levels and tyrosine kinase activity in skeletal muscle are reduced, but these alterations are most likely secondary to hyperinsulinemia and are not a primary defect. Therefore, postreceptor defects are believed to play the predominant role in insulin resistance (Fig. 17-4). Polymorphisms in IRS-1 may be associated with glucose intolerance, raising the possibility that polymorphisms in various postreceptor molecules may combine to create an insulin-resistant state. The pathogenesis of insulin resistance is currently focused on a PI-3-kinase signaling defect, which reduces translocation of GLUT4 to the plasma membrane, among other abnormalities. Of note, not all insulin signal transduction pathways are resistant to the effects of insulin [e.g., those controlling cell growth and differentiation and using the mitogen-activated protein (MAP) kinase pathway; Fig. 17-4]. Consequently, hyperinsulinemia may increase the insulin action through these pathways, potentially accelerating diabetes-related conditions such as atherosclerosis.

Another emerging theory proposes that elevated levels of free fatty acids, a common feature of obesity, may contribute to the pathogenesis of type 2 DM. Free fatty acids can impair glucose utilization in skeletal muscle, promote glucose production by the liver, and impair beta cell function.

Impaired Insulin Secretion Insulin secretion and sensitivity are interrelated (Fig. 17-6). In type 2

DM, insulin secretion initially increases in response to insulin resistance to maintain normal glucose tolerance. Initially, the insulin secretory defect is mild and selectively involves glucose-stimulated insulin secretion. The response to other nonglucose secretagogues, such as arginine, is preserved. Eventually, the insulin secretory defect progresses to a state of grossly inadequate insulin secretion.

The reason(s) for the decline in insulin secretory capacity in type 2 DM is unclear. Despite the assumption that a second genetic defect—superimposed upon insulin resistance—leads to beta cell failure, intense genetic investigation has so far excluded mutations in islet candidate genes. Islet amyloid polypeptide or amylin is cosecreted by the beta cell and likely forms the amyloid fibrillar deposit found in the islets of individuals with long-standing type 2 DM. Whether such islet amyloid deposits are a primary or secondary event is not known. The metabolic environment of diabetes may also negatively impact islet function. For example, chronic hyperglycemia paradoxically impairs islet function ("glucose toxicity") and leads to a worsening of hyperglycemia. Improvement in glycemic control is often associated with improved islet function. In addition, elevation of free fatty acid levels ("lipotoxicity") and dietary fat may also worsen islet function.

Increased Hepatic Glucose Production In type 2 DM, insulin resistance in the liver reflects the failure of hyperinsulinemia to suppress gluconeogenesis, which results in fasting hyperglycemia and decreased glycogen storage by the liver in the postprandial state. Increased hepatic glucose production occurs early in the course of diabetes, though likely after the onset of insulin secretory abnormalities and insulin resistance in skeletal muscle.

Insulin Resistance Syndromes

The insulin resistance condition comprises a spectrum of disorders, with hyperglycemia representing one of the most readily diagnosed features. The *metabolic syndrome,* the *insulin resistance syndrome,* or *syndrome X* are terms used to describe a constellation of metabolic derangements that includes insulin resistance, hypertension, dyslipidemia [low high-density lipoprotein (HDL) and elevated triglycerides], central or visceral obesity, type 2 diabetes or IGT/IFG, and accelerated cardiovascular disease. This syndrome is very common. The Centers for Disease Control and Prevention (CDC) estimates that 20% of U.S. adults have this syndrome. Epidemiologic evidence supports hyperinsulinemia as a marker for coronary artery disease risk, though an etiologic role has not been demonstrated.

A number of relatively rare forms of severe insulin resistance include features of type 2 DM or IGT (Table 17-1). *Acanthosis nigricans* and signs of hyperandrogenism (hirsutism, acne, and oligomenorrhea in women) are also common physical features. Two distinct syndromes of severe insulin resistance have been described in adults: (1) type A, which affects young women and is characterized by severe hyperinsulinemia, obesity, and features of hyperandrogenism; and (2) type B, which affects middle-aged women and is characterized by severe hyperinsulinemia, features of hyperandrogenism, and autoimmune disorders. Individuals with the type A insulin resistance syndrome have an undefined defect in the insulin-signaling pathway; individuals with the type B insulin resistance syndrome have autoantibodies directed at the insulin receptor. These receptor autoantibodies may block insulin binding or may stimulate the insulin receptor, leading to intermittent hypoglycemia.

Polycystic ovary syndrome (PCOS) is a common disorder that affects premenopausal women and is characterized by chronic anovulation and hyperandrogenism (Chap. 10). Insulin resistance is seen in a significant subset of women with PCOS, and the disorder substantially increases the risk for type 2 DM, independent of the effects of obesity. Both metformin and the thiazolidinediones attenuate hyperinsulinemia, ameliorate hyperandrogenism, induce ovulation, and improve plasma lipids, but they are not approved for this indication.

Prevention

Type 2 DM is preceded by a period of IGT, and a number of life-style modifications and pharmacologic agents prevent or delay the onset of DM. The Diabetes Prevention Program (DPP) demonstrated that intensive changes in life-style (diet and exercise for 30 min/day five times/week) in individuals with IGT prevented or delayed the development of type 2 diabetes by 58% compared to placebo. This effect was seen in individuals regardless of age, sex, or ethnic group. In the same study, metformin prevented or delayed diabetes by 31% compared to placebo. The life-style intervention group lost 5 to 7% of their body weight during the 3 years of the study. Studies in Finnish and Chinese populations noted similar efficacy of diet and exercise in preventing or delaying type 2 DM; acarbose, metformin, and the thiazolidinediones prevent or delay type 2 DM, but are not approved for this purpose. When administered to nondiabetic individuals for other reasons (cardiac, cholesterol lowering, etc.), two pharmacologic agents (ramipril, pravastatin) reduced the number of new cases of diabetes. Individuals with a strong family history, those at high risk for developing DM, or those with IFG or IGT should be strongly encouraged to maintain a normal body mass index (BMI) and engage in regular physical activity.

GENETICALLY DEFINED, MONOGENIC FORMS OF DIABETES MELLITUS

Several monogenic forms of DM have been identified. Five different variants of MODY, caused by mutations in genes encoding islet cell transcription factors or glucokinase (Fig. 17-3), have been identified so far, and all are transmitted as autosomal dominant disorders (Table 17-1). MODY 2 is the result of mutations in the glucokinase gene that lead to mild-to-moderate hyperglycemia. Glucokinase catalyzes the formation of glucose-6-phosphate from glucose, a reaction that is important for glucose sensing by the beta cells and for glucose utilization by the liver. As a result of glucokinase mutations, higher glucose levels are required to elicit insulin secretory responses, thus altering the set point for insulin secretion. Homozygous mutations in glucokinase cause severe, neonatal diabetes. MODY 1, MODY 3, and MODY 5 are caused by mutations in the hepatocyte nuclear transcription factors (HNF) 4α, HNF-1α, and HNF-1β, respectively. As their names imply, these transcription factors are expressed in the liver but also in other tissues, including the pancreatic islets and kidney (as a result, patients may also have renal absorption abnormalities and renal cysts). The mechanisms by which such mutations lead to DM is not well understood, but it is likely that these factors affect islet development or the transcription of genes that are important in stimulating insulin secretion. MODY 1 and 3 begin with mild hyperglycemia, but progressive impairment of insulin secretion requires treatment with oral agents or insulin. MODY 4 is a rare variant caused by mutations in the insulin promoter factor (IPF) 1, which is a transcription factor that regulates pancreatic development and insulin gene transcription. Homozygous inactivating mutations cause pancreatic agenesis, whereas heterozygous mutations result in DM. Studies of populations with type 2 DM suggest that mutations in the glucokinase gene and various islet cell transcription factors are very rare in ordinary type 2 DM.

ACUTE COMPLICATIONS OF DM

Diabetic ketoacidosis (DKA) and hyperglycemic hyperosmolar state (HHS) are acute complications of diabetes. DKA was formerly considered a hallmark of type 1 DM, but it also occurs in individuals who lack immunologic features of type 1A DM and who can subsequently be treated with oral glucose-lowering agents (these individuals with type 2 DM are often of Hispanic or African-American descent). HHS is primarily seen in individuals with type 2 DM. Both disorders are associated with absolute or relative insulin deficiency, volume depletion, and acid-base abnormalities. DKA and HHS exist along a continuum of hyperglycemia, with or without ketosis. The metabolic similarities and differences in DKA and HHS are highlighted in **Table 17-4.** Both disorders are associated with potentially serious complications if not promptly diagnosed and treated.

TABLE 17-4

LABORATORY VALUES IN DIABETIC KETOACIDOSIS (DKA) AND HYPERGLYCEMIC HYPEROSMOLAR STATE (HHS) (REPRESENTATIVE RANGES AT PRESENTATION)

	DKA	HHS
Glucose,[a] μmol/L (mg/dL)	13.9 – 33.3 (250 – 600)	33.3–66.6 (600–1200)
Sodium, meq/L	125–135	135–145
Potassium,[a] meg/L	Normal to ↑[b]	Normal
Magnesium[a]	Normal[b]	Normal
Chloride[a]	Normal	Normal
Phosphate[a]	↓	Normal
Creatinine, μmol/L (mg/dL)	Slightly ↑	Moderately ↑
Osmolality (mOsm/mL)	300–320	330–380
Plasma ketones[a]	++++	+/−
Serum bicarbonate,[a] meq/L	<15 meq/L	Normal to slightly ↓
Arterial pH	6.8–7.3	>7.3
Arterial Pco_2,[a] mmHg	20–30	Normal
Anion gap[a] [Na − (Cl + HCO_3)], meq/L	↑	Normal to slightly ↑

[a]Large changes occur during treatment of DKA.
[b]Although plasma levels may be normal or high at presentation, total-body stores are usually depleted.

DIABETIC KETOACIDOSIS

Clinical Features

The symptoms and physical signs of DKA are listed in **Table 17-5** and usually develop over 24 hours. DKA may be the initial symptom complex that leads to a diagnosis of type 1 DM, but more frequently it occurs in individuals with established diabetes. Nausea and vomiting are often prominent, and their presence in an individual with diabetes warrants laboratory evaluation for DKA. Abdominal pain may be severe and can resemble acute pancreatitis or ruptured viscous. Hyperglycemia leads to glucosuria, volume depletion, and tachycardia. Hypotension can occur because of volume depletion in combination with peripheral vasodilation. Kussmaul respirations and a fruity odor on the patient's breath (secondary to metabolic acidosis and increased acetone) are classic signs of the disorder. Lethargy and central nervous system depression may evolve into coma with severe DKA but should also prompt evaluation for other reasons for altered mental status (infection, hypoxia, etc.). Cerebral edema, an extremely serious complication of DKA, is seen most frequently in children. Signs of infection, which may precipitate DKA, should be sought on physical examination, even in the absence of fever. Tissue ischemia (heart, brain) can also be a precipitating factor.

Pathophysiology

DKA results from relative or absolute insulin deficiency combined with counterregulatory hormone excess (glucagon, catecholamines, cortisol, and growth hormone). Both insulin deficiency and glucagon excess, in particular, are necessary for DKA to develop. The decreased ratio of insulin to glucagon promotes gluconeogenesis, glycogenolysis, and ketone body formation in the liver, as well as increases in substrate delivery from fat and muscle (free fatty acids, amino acids) to the liver.

The combination of insulin deficiency and hyperglycemia reduces the hepatic level of fructose-2,6-phosphate, which alters the activity of phosphofructokinase and fructose-1,6-bisphosphatase. Glucagon excess decreases the activity of pyruvate kinase, whereas insulin deficiency increases the activity of phosphoenolpyruvate carboxykinase. These changes shift the handling of pyruvate toward glucose synthesis and away from glycolysis. The increased levels of glucagon and catecholamines in the face of low insulin levels promote glycogenolysis. Insulin deficiency also reduces levels of the GLUT4 glucose transporter, which impairs glucose uptake into skeletal muscle and fat and reduces intracellular glucose metabolism (Fig. 17-4).

Ketosis results from a marked increase in free fatty acid release from adipocytes, with a resulting shift toward ketone body synthesis in the liver. Reduced insulin levels, in combination with elevations in catecholamines and growth hormone, increase lipolysis and the release of free fatty acids. Normally, these free fatty acids are converted to triglycerides or very low density lipoproteins (VLDL) in the liver. However, in DKA, hyperglucagonemia alters hepatic metabolism to favor ketone body formation, through activation of the enzyme carnitine palmitoyltransferase I. This enzyme is crucial for regulating fatty acid transport into the mitochondria, where beta oxidation and conversion to ketone bodies occur. At physiologic pH, ketone bodies exist as ketoacids, which are neutralized by bicarbonate. As bicarbonate stores are depleted, metabolic acidosis ensues. Increased lactic acid production also contributes to the acidosis. The increased free fatty acids increase triglyceride and VLDL production. VLDL clearance is also reduced because the activity of insulin-sensitive lipopro-

TABLE 17-5

MANIFESTATIONS OF DIABETIC KETOACIDOSIS

Symptoms	**Physical findings**
Nausea/vomiting	Tachycardia
Thirst/polyuria	Dry mucous membranes/reduced skin turgor
Abdominal pain	Dehydration/hypotension
Shortness of breath	Tachypnea/Kussmaul respirations/respiratory distress
Precipitating events	Abdominal tenderness (may resemble acute pancreatitis or surgical abdomen)
Inadequate insulin administration	Lethargy/obtundation/cerebral edema/possibly coma
Infection (pneumonia/UTI/gastroenteritis/sepsis)	
Infarction (cerebral, coronary, mesenteric, peripheral)	
Drugs (cocaine)	
Pregnancy	

Note: UTI, urinary tract infection.

tein lipase in muscle and fat is decreased. Hypertriglyceridemia may be severe enough to cause pancreatitis.

DKA is initiated by inadequate levels of plasma insulin (Table 17-5). Most commonly, DKA is precipitated by increased insulin requirements, as might occur during a concurrent illness. Failure to augment insulin therapy often compounds the problem. Occasionally, complete omission of insulin by the patient or health care team (in a hospitalized patient with type 1 DM) precipitates DKA. Patients using insulin infusion devices with short-acting insulin are at increased risk of DKA, since even a brief interruption in insulin delivery (e.g., mechanical malfunction) quickly leads to insulin deficiency.

Laboratory Abnormalities and Diagnosis

The timely diagnosis of DKA is crucial and allows for prompt initiation of therapy. DKA is characterized by hyperglycemia, ketosis, and metabolic acidosis (increased anion gap) along with a number of secondary metabolic derangements (Table 17-4). Occasionally, the serum glucose is only minimally elevated. Serum bicarbonate is frequently <10 mmol/L, and arterial pH ranges between 6.8 and 7.3, depending on the severity of the acidosis. Despite a total-body potassium deficit, the serum potassium at presentation may be mildly elevated, secondary to the acidosis. Total-body stores of sodium, chloride, phosphorous, and magnesium are also reduced in DKA but are not accurately reflected by their levels in the serum because of dehydration and hyperglycemia. Elevated blood urea nitrogen (BUN) and serum creatinine levels reflect intravascular volume depletion. Interference from acetoacetate may falsely elevate the serum creatinine measurement. Leukocytosis, hypertriglyceridemia, and hyperlipoproteinemia are commonly found as well. Hyperamylasemia may suggest a diagnosis of pancreatitis, especially when accompanied by abdominal pain. However, in DKA the amylase is usually of salivary origin and thus is not diagnostic of pancreatitis. Serum lipase should be obtained if pancreatitis is suspected.

The measured serum sodium is reduced as a consequence of the hyperglycemia [1.6 mmol/L (1.6 meq) reduction in serum sodium for each 5.6 mmol/L (100 mg/dL) rise in the serum glucose]. A normal serum sodium in the setting of DKA indicates a more profound water deficit. In "conventional" units, the calculated serum osmolality [2 × (serum sodium + serum potassium) + plasma glucose (mg/dL)/18 + BUN/2.8] is mildly to moderately elevated, though to a lesser degree than that found in HHS (see below).

In DKA, the ketone body, β-hydroxybutyrate, is synthesized at a threefold greater rate than acetoacetate; however, acetoacetate is preferentially detected by a commonly used ketosis detection reagent (nitroprusside). Serum ketones are present at significant levels (usually positive at serum dilution of ≥1:8). The nitroprusside tablet, or stick, is often used to detect urine ketones; certain medications such as captopril or penicillamine may cause false-positive reactions. Serum or plasma assays for β-hydroxybutyrate more accurately reflect the true ketone body level.

The metabolic derangements of DKA exist along a spectrum, beginning with mild acidosis with moderate hyperglycemia evolving into more severe findings. The degree of acidosis and hyperglycemia do not necessarily correlate closely since a variety of factors determine the level of hyperglycemia (oral intake, urinary glucose loss). Ketonemia is a consistent finding in DKA and distinguishes it from simple hyperglycemia. The differential diagnosis of DKA includes starvation ketosis, alcoholic ketoacidosis (bicarbonate > 15 meq/L) and other increased anion gap acidosis.

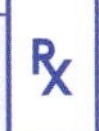

TREATMENT FOR DKA

The management of DKA is outlined in **Table 17-6.** After initiating intravenous fluid replacement and insulin therapy, the agent or event that precipitated the episode of DKA should be sought and aggressively treated. If the patient is vomiting or has altered mental status, a nasogastric tube should be inserted to prevent aspiration of gastric contents. Central to successful treatment of DKA is careful monitoring and frequent reassessment to ensure that the patient and the metabolic derangements are improving. A comprehensive flow sheet should record chronologic changes in vital signs, fluid intake and output, and laboratory values as a function of insulin administered.

After the initial bolus of normal saline, replacement of the sodium and free water deficit is carried out over the next 24 h (fluid deficit is often 3 to 5 L). When hemodynamic stability and adequate urine output are achieved, intravenous fluids should be switched to 0.45% saline at a rate of 200 to 300 mL/h, depending on the calculated volume deficit. The change to 0.45% saline helps to reduce the trend toward hyperchloremia later in the course of DKA. Alternatively, initial use of lactated Ringer's intravenous solution may reduce the hyperchloremia that commonly occurs with normal saline.

A bolus of intravenous (0.15 units/kg) or intramuscular (0.4 units/kg) regular insulin should be administered immediately (Table 17-6), and subsequent treatment should provide continuous and

TABLE 17-6

MANAGEMENT OF DIABETIC KETOACIDOSIS

1. Confirm diagnosis (↑ plasma glucose, positive serum ketones, metabolic acidosis).
2. Admit to hospital; intensive-care setting may be necessary for frequent monitoring or if pH < 7.00 or unconscious.
3. Assess: Serum electrolytes (K^+, Na^+, Mg^{2+}, C1$^-$, bicarbonate, phosphate)
   Acid-base status — pH, HCO_3^-, P_{co_2}, β-hydroxybutyrate
   Renal function (creatinine, urine output).
4. Replace fluids: 2–3 L of 0.9% saline over first 1–3 h (5–10 mL/kg per hour); subsequently, 0.45% saline at 150–300 mL/h; change to 5% glucose and 0.45% saline at 100–200 mL/h when plasma glucose reaches 250 mg/dL (14 mmol/L).
5. Administer regular insulin: IV (0.1 units/kg) or IM (0.4 units/kg), then 0.1 units/kg per hour by continuous IV infusion; increase 2- to 10-fold if no response by 2–4 h. If initial serum potassium <3.3 mmol/L (3.3 meq/L), do not administer insulin until the potassium is corrected to >3.3 mmol/L (3.3. meq/L).
6. Assess patient: What precipitated the episode (noncompliance, infection, trauma, infarction, cocaine)? Initiate appropriate workup for precipitating event (cultures, CXR, ECG).
7. Measure capillary glucose every 1–2 h; measure electrolytes (especially K^+, bicarbonate, phosphate) and anion gap every 4 h for first 24 h.
8. Monitor blood pressure, pulse, respirations, mental status, fluid intake and output every 1–4 h.
9. Replace K^+: 10 meq/h when plasma K^+ <5.5 meq/L, ECG normal, urine flow and normal creatinine documented; administer 40–80 meq/h when plasma K^+<3.5 meg/L or if bicarbonate is given.
10. Continue above until patient is stable, glucose goal is 150–250 mg/dL, and acidosis is resolved. Insulin infusion may be decreased to 0.05–0.1 units/kg per hour.
11. Administer intermediate or long-acting insulin as soon as patient is eating. Allow for overlap in insulin infusion and subcutaneous insulin injection.

Note: CXR, chest x-ray; ECG, electrocardiogram.
Source: Adapted from M Sperling, in *Therapy for Diabetes Mellitus and Related Disorders,* American Diabetes Association, Alexandria, VA, 1998; and AE Kitabchi et al: Diabetes Care 24:131, 2001.

adequate levels of circulating insulin. Intravenous administration is preferred (0.1 units/kg per hour), because it assures rapid distribution and allows adjustment of the infusion rate as the patient responds to therapy. Intravenous regular insulin should be continued until the acidosis resolves and the patient is metabolically stable. As the acidosis and insulin resistance associated with DKA resolve, the insulin infusion rate can be decreased (to 0.05 to 0.1 units/kg per hour). Intermediate or long-acting insulin, in combination with subcutaneous regular insulin, should be administered as soon as the patient resumes eating, as this facilitates transition to an outpatient insulin regimen and reduces length of hospital stay. It is crucial to continue the insulin infusion until adequate insulin levels are achieved by the subcutaneous route. Even relatively brief periods of inadequate insulin administration in this transition phase may result in DKA relapse.

Hyperglycemia usually improves at a rate of 4.2 to 5.6 mmol/L (75 to 100 mg/dL) per hour as a result of insulin-mediated glucose disposal, reduced hepatic glucose release, and rehydration. The latter reduces catecholamines, increases urinary glucose loss, and expands the intravascular volume. The decline in the plasma glucose within the first 1 to 2 h may be more rapid and is mostly related to volume expansion. When the plasma glucose reaches 13.9 mmol/L (250 mg/dL), glucose should be added to the 0.45% saline infusion to maintain the plasma glucose in the 11.1 to 13.9 mmol/L (200 to 250 mg/dL) range, and the insulin infusion should be continued. Ketoacidosis begins to resolve as insulin reduces lipolysis, increases peripheral ketone body use, suppresses hepatic ketone body formation, and promotes bicarbonate regeneration. However, the acidosis and ketosis resolve more slowly than hyperglycemia. As ketoacidosis improves, β-hydroxybutyrate is converted to acetoacetate. Ketone body levels may appear to increase if measured by laboratory assays that use the nitroprusside reaction, which only detects acetoacetate and acetone. The improvement in acidosis and anion gap, a result of bicarbonate regeneration and decline in ketone bodies, is reflected by a rise in the serum bicarbonate level and the arterial pH. Depending on the rise of serum chloride, the anion gap (but not bicarbonate) will normalize. A hyperchloremic acidosis [serum bicarbonate of 15 to 18 mmol/L (15 to 18 meq/L)] often follows successful treatment and gradually resolves as the kidneys regenerate bicarbonate and excretes chloride.

Potassium stores are depleted in DKA [estimated deficit 3 to 5 mmol/kg (3 to 5 meq/kg)]. During treatment with insulin and fluids, various factors contribute to the development of hypokalemia. These include insulin-mediated potassium transport into cells, resolution of the acidosis (which also promotes potassium entry into cells), and urinary loss of potassium salts of organic acids. Thus, potassium repletion should commence as soon as adequate urine output and a normal serum potassium are documented. If the initial serum potassium level is elevated, then potassium repletion should be delayed until the potassium falls into the normal range. Inclusion of 20 to 40 meq of potassium in each liter of intravenous fluid is reasonable, but additional potassium supplements may also be required. To reduce the amount of chloride administered, potassium phosphate or acetate can be substituted for the chloride salt. The goal is to maintain the serum potassium > 3.5 mmol/L (3.5 meq/L). If the initial serum potassium is <3.3 mmol/L (3.3 meq/L), do not administer insulin until the potassium is supplemented to >3.3 mmol/L (3.3 meq/L).

Despite a bicarbonate deficit, bicarbonate replacement is not usually necessary. In fact, theoretical arguments suggest that bicarbonate administration and rapid reversal of acidosis may impair cardiac function, reduce tissue oxygenation, and promote hypokalemia. The results of most clinical trials do not support the routine use of bicarbonate replacement, and one study in children found that bicarbonate use was associated with an increased risk of cerebral edema. However, in the presence of severe acidosis (arterial pH < 7.0 after initial hydration), the ADA advises bicarbonate [50 mmol/L (meq/L) of sodium bicarbonate in 200 mL of 0.45% saline over 1 h if pH = 6.9 to 7.0; or 100 mmol/L (meq/L) of sodium bicarbonate in 400 mL of 0.45% saline over 2 h if pH 7 < 6.9]. Hypophosphatemia may result from increased glucose usage, but randomized clinical trials have not demonstrated that phosphate replacement is beneficial in DKA. If the serum phosphate is <0.32 mmol/L (1.0 mg/dL), then phosphate supplement should be considered and the serum calcium monitored. Hypomagnesemia may develop during DKA therapy and may also require supplementation.

With appropriate therapy, the mortality of DKA is low (<5%) and is related more to the underlying or precipitating event, such as infection or myocardial infarction. The major nonmetabolic complication of DKA therapy is cerebral edema, which most often develops in children as DKA is resolving. The etiology and optimal therapy for cerebral edema are not well established, but overreplacement of free water should be avoided. Venous thrombosis, upper gastrointestinal bleeding, and acute respiratory distress syndrome occasionally complicate DKA.

Following treatment, the physician and patient should review the sequence of events that led to DKA to prevent future recurrences. Foremost is patient education about the symptoms of DKA, its precipitating factors, and the management of diabetes during a concurrent illness. During illness or when oral intake is compromised, patients should: (1) frequently measure the capillary blood glucose; (2) measure urinary ketones when the serum glucose > 16.5 mmol/L (300 mg/dL); (3) drink fluids to maintain hydration; (4) continue or increase insulin; and (5) seek medical attention if dehydration, persistent vomiting, or uncontrolled hyperglycemia develop. Using these strategies, early DKA can be prevented or detected and treated appropriately on an outpatient basis.

HYPERGLYCEMIC HYPEROSMOLAR STATE

Clinical Features

The prototypical patient with HHS is an elderly individual with type 2 DM, with a several week history of polyuria, weight loss, and diminished oral intake that culminates in mental confusion, lethargy, or coma. The physical examination reflects profound dehydration and hyperosmolality and reveals hypotension, tachycardia, and altered mental status. Notably absent are symptoms of nausea, vomiting, and abdominal pain and the Kussmaul respirations characteristic of DKA. HHS is often precipitated by a serious, concurrent illness such as myocardial infarction or stroke. Sepsis, pneumonia, and other serious infections are frequent precipitants and should be sought. In addition, a debilitating condition (prior stroke or dementia) or social situation that compromises water intake may contribute to the development of the disorder.

Pathophysiology

Relative insulin deficiency and inadequate fluid intake are the underlying causes of HHS. Insulin deficiency increases hepatic glucose production (through glycogenolysis and gluconeogenesis) and impairs glucose utilization in skeletal muscle (see above discussion of DKA). Hyperglycemia induces an osmotic diuresis that leads to intravascular volume depletion, which is exacerbated by inadequate fluid replacement. The absence of ketosis in HHS is not completely understood. Presumably, the insulin deficiency is only relative and less severe than in DKA. Lower levels of counterregulatory hormones and free fatty acids have been found in HHS than in DKA in some studies. It is also possible that the liver is less capable of ketone body synthesis or that the insulin/glucagon ratio does not favor ketogenesis.

Laboratory Abnormalities and Diagnosis

The laboratory features in HHS are summarized in Table 17-4. Most notable are the marked hyperglycemia [plasma glucose may be >55.5 mmol/L (1000 mg/dL)], hyperosmolality (>350 mosmol/L), and prerenal azotemia. The measured serum sodium may be normal or slightly low despite the marked hyperglycemia. The corrected serum sodium is usually increased [add 1.6 meq to measured sodium for each 5.6-mmol/L (100 mg/dL) rise in the serum glucose]. In contrast to DKA, acidosis and ketonemia are absent or mild. A small anion gap metabolic acidosis may be present secondary to increased lactic acid. Moderate ketonuria, if present, is secondary to starvation.

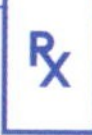

TREATMENT FOR HHS

Volume depletion and hyperglycemia are prominent features of both HHS and DKA. Consequently, therapy of these disorders shares several elements (Table 17-6). In both disorders, careful monitoring of the patient's fluid status, laboratory values, and insulin infusion rate is crucial. Underlying or precipitating problems should be aggressively sought and treated. In HHS, fluid losses and dehydration are usually more pronounced than in DKA due to the longer duration of the illness. The patient with HHS is usually older, more likely to have mental status changes, and more likely to have a life-threatening precipitating event with accompanying comorbidities. Even with proper treatment, HHS has a substantially higher mortality than DKA (up to 15% in some clinical series).

Fluid replacement should initially stabilize the hemodynamic status of the patient (1 to 3 L of 0.9% normal saline over the first 2 to 3 h). Because the fluid deficit in HHS is accumulated over a period of days to weeks, the rapidity of reversal of the hyperosmolar state must balance the need for free water repletion with the risk that too rapid a reversal may worsen neurologic function. If the serum sodium is >150 mmol/L (150 meq/L), 0.45% saline should be used. After hemodynamic stability is achieved, the intravenous fluid administration is directed at reversing the free water deficit using hypotonic fluids (0.45% saline initially then 5% dextrose in water, D_5W). The calculated free water deficit (which averages 9 to 10 L) should be reversed over the next 1 to 2 days (infusion rates of 200 to 300 mL/h of hypotonic solution). Potassium repletion is usually necessary and should be dictated by repeated measurements of the serum potassium. In patients taking diuretics, the potassium deficit can be quite large and may be accompanied by magnesium deficiency. Hypophosphatemia may occur during therapy and can be improved by using KPO_4 and beginning nutrition.

As in DKA, rehydration and volume expansion lower the plasma glucose initially, but insulin is also required. A reasonable regimen for HHS begins with an intravenous insulin bolus of 5 to 10 units followed by intravenous insulin at a constant infusion rate (3 to 7 units/h). As in DKA, glucose should be added to intravenous fluid when the plasma glucose falls to 13.9 mmol/L (250 mg/dL), and the insulin infusion rate should be decreased to 1 to 2 units/h. The insulin infusion should be continued until the patient has resumed eating and can be transferred to a subcutaneous insulin regimen. The patient should be discharged from the hospital on insulin, though some patients can later switch to oral glucose-lowering agents.

CHRONIC COMPLICATIONS OF DM

The chronic complications of DM affect many organ systems and are responsible for the majority of morbidity and mortality associated with the disease. Chronic complications can be divided into vascular and nonvascular complications (**Table 17-7**). The vascular complications of DM are further subdivided into microvascular (retinopathy, neuropathy, nephropathy) and macrovascular complications (coronary artery disease, peripheral arterial disease, cerebrovascular disease). Nonvascular complications include problems such as gastroparesis, infections, and skin changes. The risk of chronic complications increases as a function of the duration of hyperglycemia; they usually become apparent in the second decade of hyperglycemia. Since type 2 DM often has a long asymptomatic period of hyperglycemia, many individuals with type 2 DM have complications at the time of diagnosis.

The microvascular complications of both type 1 and type 2 DM result from chronic hyperglycemia. Large, randomized clinical trials of individuals with type 1 or type 2 DM have conclusively demonstrated that a reduction in chronic hyperglycemia prevents or delays retinopathy, neuropathy, and nephropathy. Other incompletely defined factors may modulate the development of complications. For example, despite long-standing DM, some individuals never develop nephropathy or retinopathy. Many of these patients have glycemic control that is indistinguishable from those who develop microvascular complications, suggesting that there is a genetic susceptibility for developing particular complications.

Evidence implicating a causative role for chronic hyperglycemia in the development of macrovascular complications is less conclusive. However, coronary heart disease events and mortality are two to four times greater in patients with type 2 DM. These events correlate with fasting and postprandial plasma glucose levels as well as with the A1C. Other factors (dyslipidemia and hypertension) also play important roles in macrovascular complications.

TABLE 17-7

CHRONIC COMPLICATIONS OF DIABETES MELLITUS

CHRONIC COMPLICATIONS OF DIABETES MELLITUS
Microvascular
Eye disease
Retinopathy (nonproliferative/proliferative)
Macular edema
Neuropathy
Sensory and motor (mono- and polyneuropathy)
Autonomic
Nephropathy
Macrovasular
Coronary artery disease
Peripheral vascular disease
Cerebrovascular disease
Other
Gastrointestinal (gastroparesis, diarrhea)
Genitourinary (uropathy/sexual dysfunction)
Dermatologic
Infectious
Cataracts
Glaucoma

MECHANISMS OF COMPLICATIONS

Although chronic hype rglycemia is an important etiologic factor leading to complications of DM, the mechanism(s) by which it leads to such diverse cellular and organ dysfunction is unknown. Four prominent theories, which are not mutually exclusive, have been proposed to explain how hyperglycemia might lead to the chronic complications of DM (**Fig. 17-7**).

One theory is that increased intracellular glucose leads to the formation of advanced glycosylation end products (AGEs) via the nonenzymatic glycosylation of intra- and extracellular proteins. Nonenzymatic glycosylation results from the interaction of glucose with amino groups on proteins. AGEs have been shown to cross-link proteins (e.g., collagen, extracellular matrix proteins), accelerate atherosclerosis, promote glomerular dysfunction, reduce nitric oxide synthesis, induce endothelial dysfunction, and alter extracellular matrix composition and structure. The serum level of AGEs correlates with the level of glycemia, and these products accumulate as glomerular filtration rate declines.

A second theory is based on the observation that hyperglycemia increases glucose metabolism via the sorbitol pathway. Intracellular glucose is predominantly metabolized by phosphorylation and subsequent glycolysis, but when increased, some glucose is converted to sorbitol by the enzyme aldose reductase. Increased sorbitol concentration alters redox potential, increases cellular osmolality, generates reactive oxygen species, and likely leads to other types of cellular dysfunction. However, testing of this theory in humans, using aldose reductase inhibitors, has not demonstrated significant beneficial effects on clinical endpoints of retinopathy, neuropathy, or nephropathy.

A third hypothesis proposes that hyperglycemia increases the formation of diacylglycerol leading to activation of protein kinase C (PKC). Among other actions, PKC alters the transcription of genes for fibronectin, type IV collagen, contractile proteins, and extracellular matrix proteins in endothelial cells and neurons.

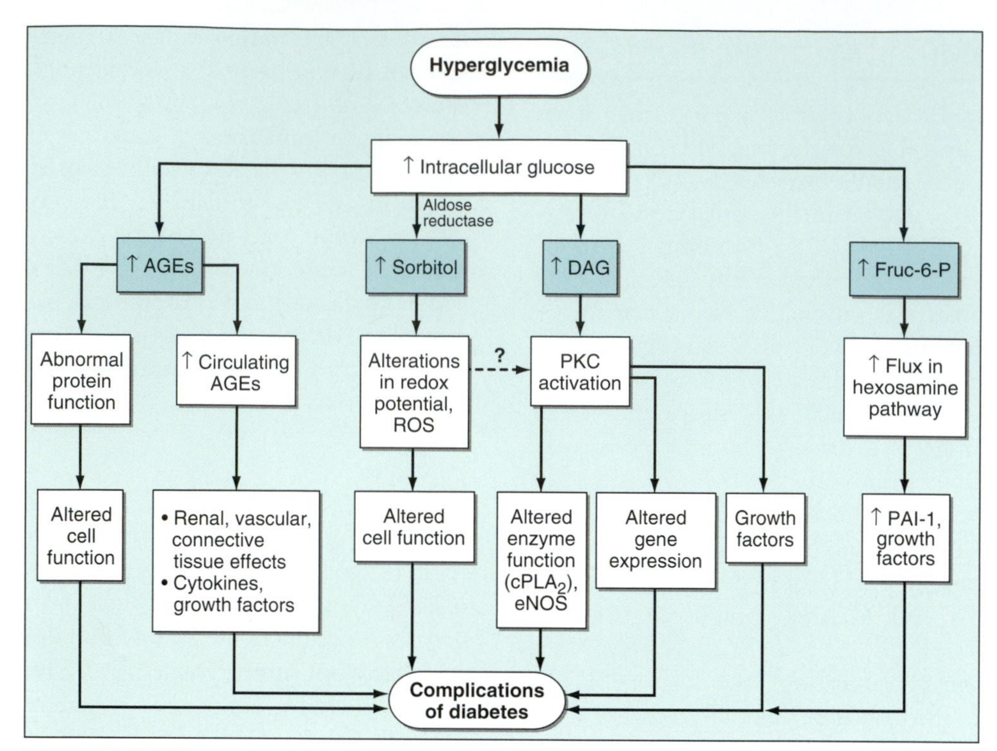

FIGURE 17-7

Possible molecular mechanisms of diabetes-related complications. AGEs, advanced glycation end products; PKC, protein kinase C; DAG, diacylglycerol; $cPLA_2$, phospholipase A_2; eNOS, endothelial nitric oxide synthase; ROS, reactive oxygen species; Fruc-6-P, fructose-6-phosphate; PAI-1, plasminogen activor inhibitor-1.

A fourth theory proposes that hyperglycemia increases the flux through the hexosamine pathway, which generates fructose-6-phosphate, a substrate for O-linked glycosylation and proteoglycan production. The hexosamine pathway may alter function by glycosylation of proteins such as endothelial nitric oxide synthase or by changes in gene expression of transforming growth factor β (TGF-β) or plasminogen activator inhibitor-1 (PAI-1).

Growth factors appear to play an important role in DM-related complications, and their production is increased by most of these proposed pathways. Vascular endothelial growth factor (VEGF) is increased locally in diabetic proliferative retinopathy and decreases after laser photocoagulation. TGF-β is increased in diabetic nephropathy and stimulates basement membrane production of collagen and fibronectin by mesangial cells. Other growth factors, such as platelet-derived growth factor, epidermal growth factor, insulin-like growth factor I, growth hormone, basic fibroblast growth factor, and even insulin, have been suggested to play a role in DM-related complications. A possible unifying mechanism is that hyperglycemia leads to increased production of reactive oxygen species or superoxide in the mitochondria; these compounds may activate all four of the pathways described above. Although hyperglycemia serves as the initial trigger for complications of diabetes, it is still unknown whether the same pathophysiologic processes are operative in all complications or whether some pathways predominate in certain organs.

GLYCEMIC CONTROL AND COMPLICATIONS

The Diabetes Control and Complications Trial (DCCT) provided definitive proof that reduction in chronic hyperglycemia can prevent many of the early complications of type 1 DM. This large multicenter clinical trial randomized over 1400 individuals with type 1 DM to either intensive or conventional diabetes management, and prospectively evaluated the development of retinopathy, nephropathy, and neuropathy. Individuals in the intensive diabetes management group received multiple administrations of insulin each day along with extensive educational, psychological, and medical support. Individuals in the conventional diabetes management group received twice-daily insulin injections and quarterly nutritional, educational, and clinical evaluation. The goal in the former group was normoglycemia; the goal in the latter group was prevention of symptoms of diabetes. Individuals in the intensive diabetes management group achieved a substantially lower hemoglobin A1C (7.3%) than individuals in the conventional diabetes management group (9.1%).

The DCCT demonstrated that improvement of glycemic control reduced nonproliferative and proliferative retinopathy (47% reduction), microalbuminuria (39% reduction), clinical nephropathy (54% reduction), and neuropathy (60% reduction). Improved glycemic control also slowed the progression of early diabetic complications. There was a nonsignificant trend in reduction of macrovascular events. The results of the DCCT predicted that individuals in the intensive diabetes management group would gain 7.7 additional years of vision, 5.8 additional years free from ESRD, and 5.6 years free from lower extremity amputations. If all complications of DM were combined, individuals in the intensive diabetes management group would experience 15.3 more years of life without significant microvascular or neurologic complications of DM, compared to individuals who received standard therapy. This translates into an additional 5.1 years of life expectancy for individuals in the intensive diabetes management group. The benefit of the improved glycemic control during the DCCT persisted even after the study concluded and glycemic control worsened.

The benefits of an improvement in glycemic control occurred over the entire range of A1C values (**Fig. 17-8**), suggesting that at any A1C level, an improvement in glycemic control is beneficial. Therefore, there is no threshold beneath which the A1C can be reduced and the complications of DM prevented. The clinical implication of this finding is that the goal of therapy is to achieve an A1C level as close to normal as possible, without subjecting the patient to excessive risk of hypoglycemia.

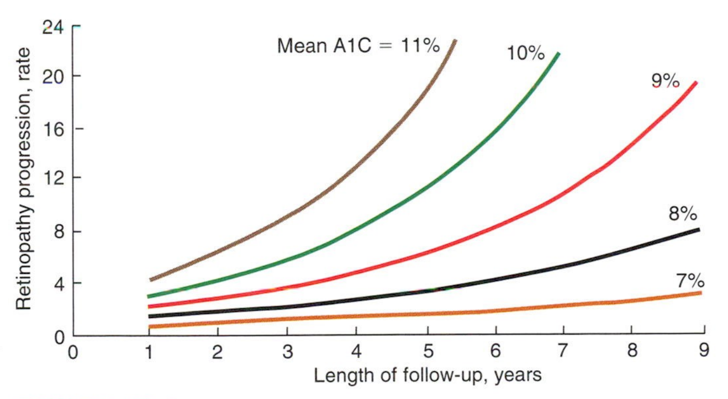

FIGURE 17-8

Relationship of glycemic control and diabetes duration to diabetic retinopathy. The progression of retinopathy in individuals in the Diabetes Control and Complications Trial is graphed as a function of the length of follow-up with different curves for different A1C values. *(Adapted from The Diabetes Control and Complications Trial Research Group, Diabetes 44:968, 1995. Copyright © 1995 American Diabetes Association. Reprinted with permission.)*

The United Kingdom Prospective Diabetes Study (UKPDS) studied the course of >5000 individuals with type 2 DM for >10 years. This study utilized multiple treatment regimens and monitored the effect of intensive glycemic control and risk factor treatment on the development of diabetic complications. Newly diagnosed individuals with type 2 DM were randomized to (1) intensive management using various combinations of insulin, a sulfonylurea, or metformin; or (2) conventional therapy using dietary modification and pharmacotherapy with the goal of symptom prevention. In addition, individuals were randomly assigned to different antihypertensive regimens. Individuals in the intensive treatment arm achieved an A1C of 7.0%, compared to a 7.9% A1C in the standard treatment group. The UKPDS demonstrated that each percentage point reduction in A1C was associated with a 35% reduction in microvascular complications. As in the DCCT, there was a continuous relationship between glycemic control and development of complications. Improved glycemic control did not conclusively reduce (nor worsen) cardiovascular mortality but was associated with improvement with lipoprotein risk profiles, such as reduced triglycerides and increased HDL.

One of the major findings of the UKPDS was that strict blood pressure control significantly reduced both macro- and microvascular complications. In fact, the beneficial effects of blood pressure control were greater than the beneficial effects of glycemic control. Lowering blood pressure to moderate goals (144/82 mmHg) reduced the risk of DM-related death, stroke, microvascular end points, retinopathy, and heart failure (risk reductions between 32 and 56%). Despite concerns that insulin therapy is associated with weight gain and may worsen underlying insulin resistance and hyperinsulinemia, most available data support strict glycemic control in individuals with type 2 DM.

Similar reductions in the risks of retinopathy and nephropathy were also seen in a small trial of lean Japanese individuals with type 2 DM randomized to either intensive glycemic control or standard therapy with insulin (Kumamoto study). These results demonstrate the effectiveness of improved glycemic control in individuals of different ethnicity, and, presumably a different etiology of DM (i.e., phenotypically different from those in the DCCT and UKPDS).

The findings of the DCCT, UKPDS, and Kumamoto study support the idea that chronic hyperglycemia plays a causative role in the pathogenesis of diabetic microvascular complications. These landmark studies prove the value of metabolic control and emphasize the importance of (1) intensive glycemic control in all forms of DM, and (2) early diagnosis and strict blood pressure control in type 2 DM.

OPHTHALMOLOGIC COMPLICATIONS OF DIABETES MELLITUS

DM is the leading cause of blindness between the ages of 20 and 74 in the United States. The gravity of this problem is highlighted by the finding that individuals with DM are 25 times more likely to become legally blind than individuals without DM. Blindness is primarily the result of progressive diabetic retinopathy and clinically significant macular edema. Diabetic retinopathy is classified into two stages: nonproliferative and proliferative. *Nonproliferative diabetic retinopathy* usually appears late in the first decade or early in the second decade of the disease and is marked by retinal vascular microaneurysms, blot hemorrhages, and cotton wool spots (**Fig. 17-9**). Mild nonproliferative retinopathy progresses to more extensive disease, characterized by changes in venous vessel caliber, intraretinal microvascular abnormalities, and more numerous microaneurysms and hemorrhages. The pathophysiologic mechanisms invoked in nonproliferative retinopathy include loss of retinal pericytes, increased retinal vascular permeability, alterations in retinal blood flow, and abnormal retinal microvasculature, all of which lead to retinal ischemia.

The appearance of neovascularization in response to retinal hypoxia is the hallmark of *proliferative diabetic retinopathy*. These newly formed vessels appear near the optic nerve and/or macula and rupture easily, leading to vitreous hemorrhage, fibrosis, and ultimately retinal detachment. Not all individuals with nonproliferative retinopathy develop proliferative retinopathy, but the more severe the nonproliferative disease, the greater the chance of evolution to proliferative retinopathy within 5 years. This creates an important opportunity for early detection and treatment of diabetic retinopathy. *Clinically significant macular edema* can occur when only nonproliferative retinopathy is present. Fluorescein angiography is useful to detect macular edema, which is associated with a 25% chance of moderate visual loss over the next 3 years.

Duration of DM and degree of glycemic control are the best predictors of the development of retinopathy; hypertension is also a risk factor. Nonproliferative retinopathy is found in almost all individuals who have had DM for >20 years (25% incidence with 5 years, and 80% incidence with 15 years of type 1 DM). Although there is genetic susceptibility for retinopathy, it confers less influence than either the duration of DM or the degree of glycemic control.

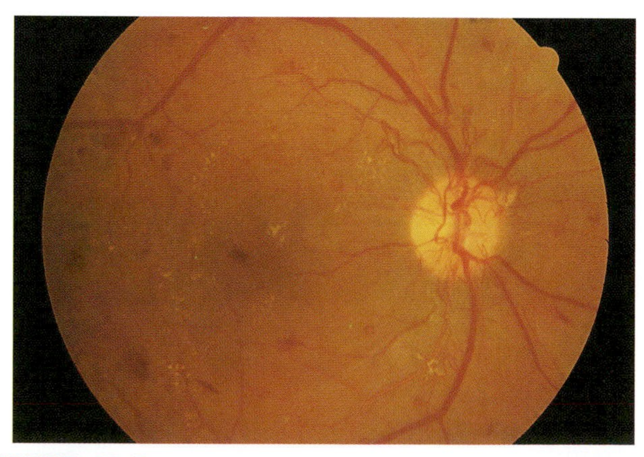

FIGURE 17-9

Diabetic retinopathy results in scattered hemorrhages and yellow exudates. This patient has neovascular vessels proliferating from the optic disc, requiring urgent pan retinal laser photocoagulation.

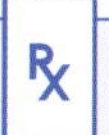

TREATMENT FOR DIABETIC RETINOPATHY

The most effective therapy for diabetic retinopathy is prevention. Intensive glycemic and blood pressure control will delay the development or slow the progression of retinopathy in individuals with either type 1 or type 2 DM. Paradoxically, during the first 6 to 12 months of improved glycemic control, established diabetic retinopathy may transiently worsen. Fortunately, this progression is temporary, and in the long term, improved glycemic control is associated with less diabetic retinopathy. Individuals with known retinopathy are candidates for prophylactic photocoagulation when initiating intensive therapy. Once advanced retinopathy is present, improved glycemic control imparts less benefit, though adequate ophthalmologic care can prevent most blindness.

Regular, comprehensive eye examinations are essential for all individuals with DM. Most diabetic eye disease can be successfully treated if detected early. Routine, nondilated eye examinations by the primary care provider or diabetes specialist are *inadequate* to detect diabetic eye disease, which requires an ophthalmologist for optimal care of these disorders. Laser photocoagulation is very successful in preserving vision. Proliferative retinopathy is usually treated with panretinal laser photocoagulation, whereas macular edema is treated with focal laser photocoagulation. Although exercise has not been conclusively shown to worsen proliferative diabetic retinopathy, most ophthalmologists advise individuals with advanced diabetic eye disease to limit physical activities associated with repeated Valsalva maneuvers. Aspirin therapy (650 mg/d) does not appear to influence the natural history of diabetic retinopathy, but studies of other antiplatelet agents are under way.

RENAL COMPLICATIONS OF DIABETES MELLITUS

Diabetic nephropathy is the leading cause of ESRD in the United States and a leading cause of DM-related morbidity and mortality. Proteinuria in individuals with DM is associated with markedly reduced survival and increased risk of cardiovascular disease. Individuals with diabetic nephropathy almost always have diabetic retinopathy.

Like other microvascular complications, the pathogenesis of diabetic nephropathy is related to chronic hyperglycemia (Fig. 17-7). The mechanisms by which chronic hyperglycemia leads to ESRD, though incompletely defined, involve the effects of soluble factors (growth factors, angiotensin II, endothelin, AGEs), hemodynamic alterations in the renal microcirculation (glomerular hyperfiltration or hyperperfusion, increased glomerular capillary pressure), and structural changes in the glomerulus (increased extracellular matrix, basement membrane thickening, mesangial expansion, fibrosis). Some of these effects may be mediated through angiotensin II receptors. Smoking accelerates the decline in renal function.

The natural history of diabetic nephropathy is characterized by a fairly predictable sequence of events that was initially defined for individuals with type 1 DM but appears to be similar in type 2 DM (**Fig. 17-10**). Glomerular hyperperfusion and renal hypertrophy occur in the first years after the onset of DM and cause an increase of the glomerular filtration rate (GFR). During the first 5 years of DM, thickening of the glomerular basement membrane, glomerular hypertrophy, and mesangial volume expansion occur as the GFR returns to normal. After 5 to 10 years of type 1 DM, ~40% of individuals begin to excrete small amounts of albumin in the urine. *Microalbuminuria* is defined as 30 to 300 mg/d in a 24-h collection or 30 to 300 μg/mg creatinine in a spot collection (preferred method). The appearance of microalbuminuria (incipient nephropathy) in type 1 DM is an important predictor of progression to overt proteinuria (>300 mg/d) or overt nephropathy. Blood pressure may rise slightly at this point but usually remains in the normal range. Once overt proteinuria is present, there is a steady decline in GFR, and ~50% of individuals reach ESRD in 7 to 10 years. The early pathologic changes and albumin excretion abnormalities are reversible with normalization of plasma glucose. However, once overt nephropathy develops, the pathologic changes are likely irreversible.

The nephropathy that develops in type 2 DM differs from that of type 1 DM in the following respects: (1) microalbuminuria or overt nephropathy may be present when type 2 DM is diagnosed, reflecting its long asymptomatic period; (2) hypertension more commonly accompanies microalbuminuria or overt nephropathy in type 2 DM; and (3) microalbuminuria may be less predictive of diabetic nephropathy and progression to overt nephropathy in type 2 DM. Finally, it should be noted that albuminuria in type 2 DM may be secondary to factors unrelated to DM, such as hypertension, congestive heart failure, prostate disease, or infection. Diabetic nephropathy and ESRD secondary to this develop more commonly in African Americans, Native Americans, and Hispanic individuals than in Caucasians with type 2 DM.

Type IV renal tubular acidosis (hyporeninemic hypoaldosteronism) also occurs in type 1 or 2 DM. These individuals develop a propensity to hyperkalemia, which may be exacerbated by medications [especially angiotensin-converting enzyme (ACE) inhibitors and angiotensin receptor blockers (ARBs)]. Patients with DM

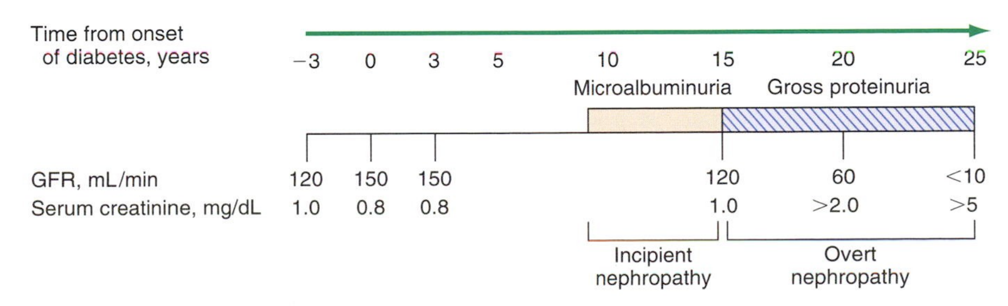

FIGURE 17-10

Time course of development of diabetic nephropathy. The relationship of time from onset of diabetes, the glomerular filtration rate (GFR), and the serum creatinine are shown. *(Adapted from RA DeFronzo, in Therapy for Diabetes Mellitus and Related Disorders, American Diabetes Association, Alexandria, VA, 1998.)*

are predisposed to radiocontrast-induced nephrotoxicity. Risk factors for radiocontrast-induced nephrotoxicity are preexisting nephropathy and volume depletion. Individuals with DM undergoing radiographic procedures with contrast dye should be well hydrated before and after dye exposure, and the serum creatinine should be monitored for several days following the procedure. Treatment with acetylcysteine (600 mg bid) on the day before and the day of the dye study appears to protect high-risk patients [creatinine, >212 μmol/L (>2.4 mg/dL)] from radiocontrast-induced nephrotoxicity.

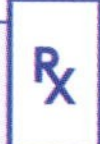

TREATMENT FOR DIABETIC NEPROPATHY

The optimal therapy for diabetic nephropathy is prevention. As part of comprehensive diabetes care, microalbuminuria should be detected at an early stage when effective therapies can be instituted. The recommended strategy for detecting microalbuminuria is outlined in **Fig. 17-11.** Interventions effective in slowing progression from microalbuminuria to overt nephropathy include: (1) near normalization of glycemia, (2) strict blood pressure control, and (3) administration of ACE inhibitors or ARBs, and (4) treatment of dyslipidemia.

Improved glycemic control reduces the rate at which microalbuminuria appears and progresses in type 1 and type 2 DM. However, once overt nephropathy exists, it is unclear whether improved glycemic control will slow progression of renal disease. During the phase of declining renal function, insulin requirements may fall as the kidney is a site of insulin degradation. Furthermore, glucose-lowering medications (sulfonylureas and metformin) are contraindicated in advanced renal insufficiency.

Many individuals with type 1 or type 2 DM develop hypertension. Numerous studies in both type 1 and type 2 DM demonstrate the effectiveness of strict blood pressure control in reducing albumin excretion and slowing the decline in renal function. Blood pressure should be maintained at <130/80 mmHg in diabetic individuals without proteinuria. A slightly lower blood pressure (125/75) should be considered for individuals with microalbuminuria or overt nephropathy (see "Hypertension," below).

ACE inhibitors and ARBs reduce the progression of overt nephropathy in individuals with type 1 or type 2 DM and should be prescribed in individuals with type 1 or type 2 DM and microalbuminuria. After 2 to 3 months of therapy, measurement of proteinuria should be repeated and the drug dose increased until either the albuminuria disappears or the maximum dose is reached. If an ACE inhibitor has an unacceptable side-effect profile (hyperkalemia, cough, and renal insufficiency), ARBs can be used as alternatives. If use of either of these types of agents is not possible, then calcium channel blockers (non-dihydropyridine class) can be used. However, their efficacy in slowing the fall in the GFR is not proven. Blood pressure control with any agent is extremely important, but a drug-specific benefit in diabetic nephropathy, independent of blood pressure control, has been shown only for ACE inhibitors in type 1 DM and ARBs in type 2 DM.

A consensus panel of the ADA suggests modest restriction of protein intake in diabetic individuals with microalbuminuria (0.8 g/kg per day) or overt nephropathy (<0.8 g/kg per day, which is the adult Recommended Daily Allowance, or about 10% of the daily caloric intake). Conclusive proof of the efficacy of protein restriction is lacking.

Nephrology consultation should be considered after the diagnosis of early incipient nephropathy. Once overt nephropathy ensues, the likelihood of ESRD is very high. As compared to nondiabetic individuals, hemodialysis in patients with DM is associated with more frequent complications, such

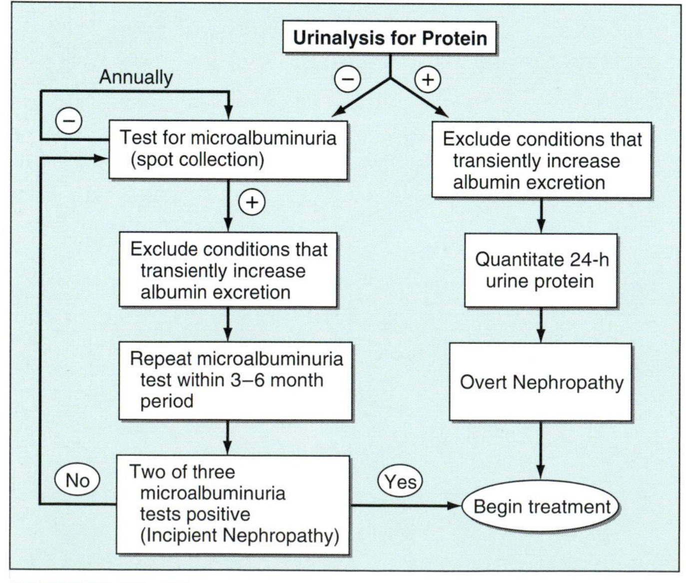

FIGURE 17-11
Screening for microalbuminuria. *(Adapted from RA DeFronzo, in Therapy for Diabetes Mellitus and Related Disorders, American Diabetes Association, Alexandria, VA, 1998.)*

as hypotension (due to autonomic neuropathy or loss of reflex tachycardia), more difficult vascular access, and accelerated progression of retinopathy. Survival after the onset of ESRD is shorter in the diabetic population compared to nondiabetics with similar clinical features. Atherosclerosis is the leading cause of death in diabetic individuals on dialysis, and hyperlipidemia should be treated aggressively. Renal transplantation from a living-related donor is the preferred therapy but requires chronic immunosuppression. Combined pancreas-kidney transplant offers the promise of normoglycemia but requires substantial expertise.

NEUROPATHY AND DIABETES MELLITUS

Diabetic neuropathy occurs in ~50% of individuals with long-standing type 1 and type 2 DM. It may manifest as polyneuropathy, mononeuropathy, and/or autonomic neuropathy. As with other complications of DM, the development of neuropathy correlates with the duration of diabetes and glycemic control; both myelinated and unmyelinated nerve fibers are lost. Because the clinical features of diabetic neuropathy are similar to those of other neuropathies, the diagnosis of *diabetic neuropathy* should be made only after other possible etiologies are excluded.

Polyneuropathy/Mononeuropathy

The most common form of diabetic neuropathy is distal symmetric *polyneuropathy.* It most frequently presents with distal sensory loss. Hyperesthesia, paresthesia, and dysesthesia also occur. Any combination of these symptoms may develop as neuropathy progresses. Symptoms include a sensation of numbness, tingling, sharpness, or burning that begins in the feet and spreads proximally. Neuropathic pain develops in some of these individuals, occasionally preceded by improvement in their glycemic control. Pain typically involves the lower extremities, is usually present at rest, and worsens at night. Both an acute (lasting <12 months) and a chronic form of painful diabetic neuropathy have been described. As diabetic neuropathy progresses, the pain subsides and eventually disappears, but a sensory deficit in the lower extremities persists. Physical examination reveals sensory loss, loss of ankle reflexes, and abnormal position sense.

Diabetic polyradiculopathy is a syndrome characterized by severe disabling pain in the distribution of one or more nerve roots. It may be accompanied by motor weakness. Intercostal or truncal radiculopathy causes pain over the thorax or abdomen. Involvement of the lumbar plexus or femoral nerve may cause pain in the thigh or hip and may be associated with muscle weakness in the hip flexors or extensors (diabetic amyotrophy). Fortunately, diabetic polyradiculopathies are usually self-limited and resolve over 6 to 12 months.

Mononeuropathy (dysfunction of isolated cranial or peripheral nerves) is less common than polyneuropathy in DM and presents with pain and motor weakness in the distribution of a single nerve. A vascular etiology has been suggested, but the pathogenesis is unknown. Involvement of the third cranial nerve is most common and is heralded by diplopia. Physical examination reveals ptosis and ophthalmoplegia with normal pupillary constriction to light. Sometimes cranial nerves IV, VI, or VII (Bell's palsy) are affected. Peripheral mononeuropathies or simultaneous involvement of more than one nerve (mononeuropathy multiplex) may also occur.

Autonomic Neuropathy

Individuals with long-standing type 1 or 2 DM may develop signs of autonomic dysfunction involving the cholinergic, noradrenergic, and peptidergic (peptides such as pancreatic polypeptide, substance P, etc.) systems. DM-related autonomic neuropathy can involve multiple systems, including the cardiovascular, gastrointestinal, genitourinary, sudomotor, and metabolic systems. Autonomic neuropathies affecting the cardiovascular system cause a resting tachycardia and orthostatic hypotension. Reports of sudden death have also been attributed to autonomic neuropathy. Gastroparesis and bladder-emptying abnormalities are often caused by the autonomic neuropathy seen in DM (discussed below). Hyperhidrosis of the upper extremities and anhidrosis of the lower extremities result from sympathetic nervous system dysfunction. Anhidrosis of the feet can promote dry skin with cracking, which increases the risk of foot ulcers. Autonomic neuropathy may reduce counterregulatory hormone release, leading to an inability to sense hypoglycemia appropriately (*hypoglycemia unawareness*; Chap. 19), thereby subjecting the patient to the risk of severe hypoglycemia and complicating efforts to improve glycemic control.

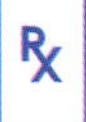

TREATMENT FOR DIABETIC NEUROPATHY

Treatment for diabetic neuropathy is less than satisfactory. Improved glycemic control should be pursued and will improve nerve conduction velocity, but the symptoms of diabetic neuropathy may not necessarily improve. Efforts to improve glycemic control may be confounded by autonomic neuropathy and hypoglycemia unawareness. Avoidance of neurotoxins (alcohol), supplementation with vitamins for possible deficiencies (B_{12}, B_6, folate, and symptomatic treatment are the mainstays of therapy. Aldose reductase inhibitors do not offer significant symptomatic relief. Loss of sensation in the foot places the patient at risk for ulceration and its sequelae; consequently, prevention of such problems is of paramount importance. Since the pain of acute diabetic neuropathy may resolve over the first year, analgesics may be discontinued as progressive neuronal damage from DM occurs. Chronic, painful diabetic neuropathy is difficult to treat but may respond to tricyclic antidepressants (amitriptyline, desipramine, nortriptyline), gabapentin, nonsteroidal anti-inflammatory agents (avoid in renal dysfunction), and other agents (mexilitine, phenytoin, carbamazepine, capsaicin cream). Referral to a pain management center may be necessary.

Therapy of orthostatic hypotension secondary to autonomic neuropathy is challenging. A variety of agents have limited success (fludrocortisone, midodrine, clonidine, octreotide, and yohimbine) but each has significant side effects. Nonpharmacologic maneuvers (adequate salt intake, avoidance of dehydration and diuretics, and lower extremity support hose) may offer some benefit.

GASTROINTESTINAL/GENITOURINARY DYSFUNCTION

Long-standing type 1 and 2 DM may affect the motility and function of gastrointestinal (GI) and genitourinary systems. The most prominent GI symptoms are delayed gastric emptying (gastroparesis) and altered small- and large-bowel motility (constipation or diarrhea). *Gastroparesis* may present with symptoms of anorexia, nausea, vomiting, early satiety, and abdominal bloating. Nuclear medicine scintigraphy after ingestion of a radiolabeled meal is the best study to document delayed gastric emptying, but noninvasive "breath tests" following ingestion of a radiolabeled meal are under development. Though parasympathetic dysfunction secondary to chronic hyperglycemia is important in the development of gastroparesis, hyperglycemia itself also impairs gastric emptying. Nocturnal diarrhea, alternating with constipation, is a common feature of DM-related GI autonomic neuropathy. In type 1 DM, these symptoms should also prompt evaluation for celiac sprue because of its increased frequency. Esophageal dysfunction in long-standing DM is common but usually asymptomatic.

Diabetic autonomic neuropathy may lead to genitourinary dysfunction including cystopathy, erectile dysfunction, and female sexual dysfunction (reduced sexual desire, dyspareunia, reduced vaginal lubrication). Symptoms of diabetic cystopathy begin with an inability to sense a full bladder and a failure to void completely. As bladder contractility worsens, bladder capacity and the post-void residual increase, leading to symptoms of urinary hesitancy, decreased voiding frequency, incontinence, and recurrent urinary tract infections. Diagnostic evaluation includes cystometry and urodynamic studies.

Erectile dysfunction and retrograde ejaculation are very common in DM and may be one of the earliest signs of diabetic neuropathy (Chap. 14). Erectile dysfunction, which increases in frequency with the age of the patient and the duration of diabetes, may occur in the absence of other signs of diabetic autonomic neuropathy.

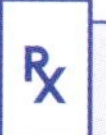

TREATMENT FOR GASTROINTESTINAL/ GENITOURINARY DYSFUNCTION

Current treatments for these complications of DM are inadequate. Improved glycemic control should be a primary goal, as some aspects (neuropathy, gastric function) may improve. Smaller, more frequent meals that are easier to digest (liquid) and low in fat and fiber may minimize symptoms of gastroparesis. Cisapride (10 to 20 mg before each meal) is probably the most effective medication but has been removed from use in the United States except under special circumstances. Other agents with some efficacy include dopamine agonists (metoclopramide, 5 to 10 mg, and domperidone, 10 to 20 mg, before each meal) and bethanechol (10 to 20 mg before each meal). Erythromycin interacts with the motilin receptor and may promote gastric emptying. Diabetic diarrhea in the absence of bacterial overgrowth is treated symptomatically with loperamide but may respond to clonidine at higher doses (0.6 mg tid) or octreotide (50 to 75 μg tid subcutaneously). Treatment of bacterial overgrowth with antibiotics is sometimes useful.

Diabetic cystopathy should be treated with timed voiding or self-catherization. Medications (bethanechol) are inconsistently effective. The drug of choice for erectile dysfunction is sildenafil, but the efficacy in individuals with DM is slightly lower than in the nondiabetic population (Chap. 14). Sexual dysfunction in women may be improved with use of vaginal lubricants, treatment of vaginal infections, and systemic or local estrogen replacement.

CARDIOVASCULAR MORBIDITY AND MORTALITY

Cardiovascular disease is increased in individuals with type 1 or type 2 DM. The Framingham Heart Study revealed a marked increase in peripheral arterial disease, congestive heart failure, coronary artery disease, myocardial infarction (MI), and sudden death (risk increase from one- to fivefold) in DM. The American Heart Association recently designated DM as a major risk factor for cardiovascular disease (same category as smoking, hypertension, and hyperlipidemia). Type 2 diabetes patients without a prior MI have a similar risk for coronary artery–related events as nondiabetic individuals who have had a prior myocardial infarction. Because of the extremely high prevalence of underlying cardiovascular disease in individuals with diabetes (especially in type 2 DM), evidence of atherosclerotic vascular disease should be sought in an individual with diabetes who has symptoms suggestive of cardiac ischemia, peripheral or carotid arterial disease, a resting electrocardiogram indicative of prior infarction, plans to initiate an exercise program, proteinuria, or two other cardiac risk factors (ADA recommendations). The absence of chest pain ("silent ischemia") is common in individuals with diabetes, and a thorough cardiac evaluation is indicated in individuals undergoing major surgical procedures. The prognosis for individuals with diabetes who have coronary artery disease or myocardial infarction is worse than for nondiabetics. Coronary artery disease is more likely to involve multiple vessels in individuals with DM.

The increase in cardiovascular morbidity and mortality appears to relate to the synergism of hyperglycemia with other cardiovascular risk factors. For example, after controlling for all known cardiovascular risk factors, type 2 DM increases the cardiovascular death rate twofold in men and fourfold in women. Risk factors for macrovascular disease in diabetic individuals include dyslipidemia, hypertension, obesity, reduced physical activity, and cigarette smoking. Additional risk factors specific to the diabetic population include microalbuminuria, gross proteinuria, an elevation of serum creatinine, and abnormal platelet function. Insulin resistance, as reflected by elevated serum insulin levels, is associated with an increased risk of cardiovascular complications in individuals with and without DM. Individuals with insulin resistance and type 2 DM have elevated levels of plasminogen activator inhibitors (especially PAI-1) and fibrinogen, which enhances the coagulation process and impairs fibrinolysis, thus favoring the development of thrombosis. Diabetes is also associated with endothelial, vascular smooth muscle, and platelet dysfunction.

Proof that improved glycemic control reduces cardiovascular complications in DM is lacking; in fact, it is possible that macrovascular complications may be unaffected or even worsened by such therapy. Concerns about the atherogenic potential of insulin remain, since in nondiabetic individuals, higher serum insulin levels (indicative of insulin resistance) are associated with a greater risk of cardiovascular morbidity and mortality. In the DCCT, the number of cardiovascular events did not differ between the standard and intensively treated groups. However, the duration of DM in these individuals was relatively short, and the total number of events was very low. An improvement in the lipid profile of individuals in the intensive group [lower total and low-density lipoprotein (LDL) cholesterol, lower triglycerides] suggested that intensive therapy may reduce the risk of cardiovascular morbidity and mortality associated with DM. In the UKPDS, improved glycemic control did not conclusively reduce cardiovascular mortality. Importantly, treatment with insulin and the sulfonylureas did not appear to increase the risk of cardiovascular disease in individuals with type 2 DM, refuting prior claims about the atherogenic potential of these agents.

In addition to coronary artery disease, cerebrovascular disease is increased in individuals with DM (threefold increase in stroke). Individuals with DM have an increased incidence of congestive heart failure (diabetic cardiomyopathy). The etiology of this abnormality is probably multifactorial and includes factors such as myocardial ischemia from atherosclerosis, hypertension, and myocardial cell dysfunction secondary to chronic hyperglycemia.

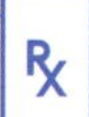

TREATMENT FOR CARDIOVASCULAR DISEASE

In general, the treatment for coronary disease is no different in the diabetic individual. Revascularization procedures for coronary artery disease, including percutaneous coronary interventions (PCI) and coronary artery bypass grafting (CABG), are less efficacious in the diabetic individual. Initial success rates of PCI in diabetic individuals are similar to those in the nondiabetic population, but diabetic patients have higher rates of restenosis and lower long-term patency and survival rates. The use of stents and a GPIIb/IIIa platelet inhibitor has improved the outcome in diabetic patients. Perioperative mortality from CABG is not altered in DM, but both short- and long-term survival are reduced. Recent trials indicate that diabetic individuals with multivessel coronary artery disease or recent Q-wave MI have better long-term survival with CABG than PCI.

The ADA has emphasized the importance of glycemic control and aggressive cardiovascular risk modification in all individuals with DM. Past trepidation about using beta blockers in individuals who have diabetes should not prevent use of these agents since they clearly benefit diabetic patients after MI. ACE inhibitors may also be particularly beneficial and should be considered in individuals with type 2 DM and other risk factors (smoking, dyslipidemia, history of cardiovascular disease, microalbuminuria).

Antiplatelet therapy reduces cardiovascular events in individuals with DM who have coronary artery disease. Current recommendations by the ADA include the use of aspirin for secondary prevention of coronary events. Although data demonstrating efficacy in primary prevention of coronary events in DM are lacking, antiplatelet therapy should be strongly considered, especially in diabetic individuals with other coronary risk factors such as hypertension, smoking, or dyslipidemia. The aspirin dose (81 to 325 mg) is the same as that in nondiabetic individuals. Aspirin therapy does not have detrimental effects on renal function or hypertension, nor does it influence the course of diabetic retinopathy.

Cardiovascular Risk Factors

DYSLIPIDEMIA

Individuals with DM may have several forms of dyslipidemia (Chap. 18). Because of the additive cardiovascular risk of hyperglycemia and hyperlipidemia, lipid abnormalities should be aggressively detected and treated as part of comprehensive diabetes care (**Fig. 17-12**). The most common pattern of dyslipidemia is hypertriglyc-

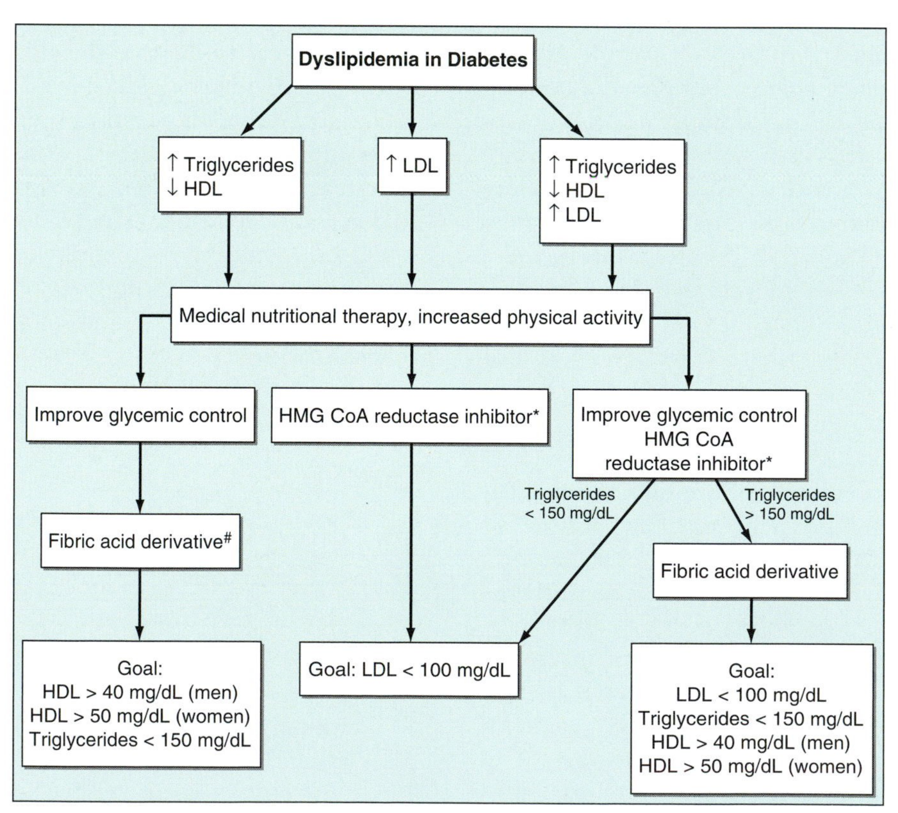

FIGURE 17-12

Dyslipidemia management in diabetes. *Second line treatment: fibric acid derivative or bile acid–binding resin. #Alternative treatment: high dose HMG CoA reductase inhibitor. The level of HDL in women should be 10 mg/dL higher. LDL, low-density lipoprotein; HDL, high-density lipoprotein.

eridemia and reduced HDL cholesterol levels. DM itself does not increase levels of LDL, but the small dense LDL particles found in type 2 DM are more atherogenic because they are more easily glycated and susceptible to oxidation. According to guidelines of the ADA and the American Heart Association, the target lipid values in diabetic individuals without cardiovascular disease should be: LDL < 2.6 mmol/L (100 mg/dL); HDL > 1.1 mmol/L (40 mg/dL) in men and >1.38 mmol/L (50 mg/dL) in women; and triglycerides < 1.7 mmol/L (150 mg/dL). The National Cholesterol Education Program Adult Treatment Panel III also recommends lowering the LDL to < 2.6 mmol/L (100 mg/dL) in diabetics. This is because the incidence of MI in type 2 DM is the same as that in patients without diabetes who have had a prior MI.

Almost all studies of diabetic dyslipidemia have been performed in individuals with type 2 DM because of the greater frequency of dyslipidemia in this form of diabetes. Interventional studies have shown that the beneficial effects of LDL reduction are similar in the diabetic and nondiabetic populations. Large prospective trials of primary and secondary intervention for coronary heart disease have included some individuals with type 2 DM, and subset analyses have consistently found that reductions in LDL reduce cardiovascular events and morbidity in individuals with DM. Most clinical trials used HMG CoA reductase inhibitors, although a fibric acid derivative has also shown to be beneficial. No prospective studies have addressed similar questions in individuals with type 1 DM.

Based on the guidelines provided by the ADA and the American Heart Association, the order of priorities in the treatment of hyperlipidemia is: (1) lower the LDL cholesterol, (2) raise the HDL cholesterol, and (3) decrease the triglycerides. A treatment strategy depends on the pattern of lipoprotein abnormalities (Fig. 17-11). Initial therapy for all forms of dyslipidemia should include dietary changes, as well as the same life-style modifications recommended in the nondiabetic population (smoking cessation, control of blood pressure, weight loss, increased physical activity). The dietary recommendations for individuals with DM are similar to those advocated by the National Cholesterol Education Program (Chap. 18) and include an increase in monounsaturated fat and carbohydrates and a reduction in saturated fats and cholesterol. Though viewed as important, the response to dietary alterations is often modest [<0.6-mmol/L (<25-mg/dL) reduction in the LDL]. Improvement in glycemic control will lower triglycerides and have a modest beneficial effect on raising HDL. HMG CoA reductase inhibitors are the agents of choice for lowering the LDL. Recent data suggest that all individuals >40 years with diabetes and total cholesterol >135 mg/dL may benefit from an HMG CoA reductase inhibitor. Fibric acid derivatives have some efficacy and should be considered when the HDL is low. Combination therapy with an HMG CoA reductase inhibitor and fibric acid derivative may be useful but increases the possibility of myositis. Nicotinic acid effectively raises HDL, but in high doses (>2 g/d) may worsen glycemic control and increase insulin resistance. Bile acid–binding resins should not be used if hypertriglyceridemia is present.

HYPERTENSION

Hypertension can accelerate other complications of DM, particularly cardiovascular disease and nephropathy. Hypertension therapy should first emphasize life-style modifications such as weight loss, exercise, stress management, and sodium restriction. Antihypertensive agents should be selected based on the advantages and disadvantages of the therapeutic agent in the context of an individual patient's risk factor profile. DM-related considerations include the following:

1. ACE inhibitors are either glucose- and lipid-neutral or glucose- and lipid-beneficial and thus positively impact the cardiovascular risk profile. For example, captopril improves insulin resistance, reduces LDL slightly, and increases HDL slightly. α-Adrenergic blockers slightly improve insulin resistance and positively impact the lipid profile, whereas beta blockers and thiazide diuretics can increase insulin resistance and negatively impact the lipid profile. Calcium channel blockers, central adrenergic antagonists, and vasodilators are lipid- and glucose-neutral.
2. Beta blockers may slightly increase the risk of developing type 2 DM. Although often questioned because of the potential masking of hypoglycemic symptoms, beta blockers are safe in most patients with diabetes and reduce car-

diovascular events. In one study of nondiabetic individuals, the ACE inhibitor ramipril reduced the risk of developing type 2 DM.

3. Sympathetic inhibitors and α-adrenergic blockers may worsen orthostatic hypotension in the diabetic individual with autonomic neuropathy.
4. Equivalent reduction in blood pressure by different classes of agents may not translate into equivalent protection from cardiovascular and renal endpoints. Thiazides, beta blockers, ACE inhibitors, and ARBs positively impact cardiovascular endpoints (MI or stroke). The cardiovascular protective effect of calcium channel blockers, central adrenergic antagonists, and α-adrenergic blockers is either controversial or not known. ACE inhibitors (in types 1 and 2 DM) and ARBs (in type 2 DM) slow the progression of diabetic renal disease; the effect of other classes of agents on diabetic nephropathy is not known.
5. Non-dihydropyridine calcium channel blockers (verapamil and diltiazem), rather than dihydropyridine agents (amlodipine and nifedipine), are preferred in diabetics.

If microalbuminuria or overt albuminuria is present, the optimal antihypertensive agent is an ACE inhibitor (in types 1 and 2 DM) or an ARB (in type 2 DM). Most prefer ARBs over ACE inhibitors in type 2 DM with hypertension and microalbuminuria. If albumin excretion is normal, then an ACE inhibitor is usually prescribed initially. A low-dose thiazide diuretic, beta blockers, or an ARB may also be used as the initial agent. Non-dihydropyridine calcium channel blockers, α-adrenergic blockers, and central adrenergic antagonists should be considered as additional or second-line agents. Since hypertension is often difficult to control with a single agent (especially in type 2 DM), multiple antihypertensive agents are usually required when blood pressure goals (<130/80 mmHg) are not achieved. Because of the high prevalence of atherosclerotic disease in individuals with DM, the possibility of renovascular hypertension should be considered when the blood pressure is not readily controlled.

LOWER EXTREMITY COMPLICATIONS

DM is the leading cause of nontraumatic lower extremity amputation in the United States. Foot ulcers and infections are also a major source of morbidity in individuals with DM. The reasons for the increased incidence of these disorders in DM involve the interaction of several pathogenic factors: neuropathy, abnormal foot biomechanics, peripheral arterial disease, and poor wound healing. The peripheral sensory neuropathy interferes with normal protective mechanisms and allows the patient to sustain major or repeated minor trauma to the foot, often without knowledge of the injury. Disordered proprioception causes abnormal weight bearing while walking and subsequent formation of callus or ulceration. Motor and sensory neuropathy lead to abnormal foot muscle mechanics and to structural changes in the foot (hammer toe, claw toe deformity, prominent metatarsal heads, Charcot joint). Autonomic neuropathy results in anhidrosis and altered superficial blood flow in the foot, which promote drying of the skin and fissure formation. Peripheral arterial disease and poor wound healing impede resolution of minor breaks in the skin, allowing them to enlarge and to become infected.

Approximately 15% of individuals with DM develop a foot ulcer, and a significant subset will ultimately undergo amputation (14 to 24% risk with that ulcer or subsequent ulceration). Risk factors for foot ulcers or amputation include: male sex, diabetes >10 years' duration, peripheral neuropathy, abnormal structure of foot (bony abnormalities, callus, thickened nails), peripheral arterial disease, smoking, history of previous ulcer or amputation, and poor glycemic control.

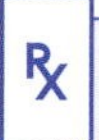

TREATMENT FOR LOWER EXTREMITY COMPLICATIONS

The optimal therapy for foot ulcers and amputations is prevention through identification of high-risk patients, education of the patient, and institution of measures to prevent ulceration. High-risk patients should be identified during the routine foot examination performed on all patients with DM (see "Ongoing Aspects of Comprehensive Diabetes Care," below). Patient education should emphasize: (1) careful selection of footwear, (2) daily inspection of the feet to detect early signs of poor-fitting footwear or minor trauma, (3) daily foot hygiene to keep the skin clean and moist, (4) avoidance of self-treatment of foot abnormalities and high-risk behavior (e.g., walking barefoot), and (5) prompt consultation with a health care provider if an abnormality arises. Patients at high risk for ulceration or amputation may benefit from evaluation by a foot care specialist. Interventions directed at risk factor modification include orthotic shoes and devices, callus management, nail care, and prophylactic measures to reduce increased skin pressure from abnormal bony architecture. Attention to other risk factors for vascular disease (smoking, dyslipidemia, hypertension) and improved glycemic control are also important.

Despite preventive measures, foot ulceration and infection are common and represent a potentially serious problem. Due to the multifactorial pathogenesis of lower extremity ulcers, management of these lesions is multidisciplinary and often demands expertise in orthopedics, vascular surgery, endocrinology, podiatry, and infectious diseases. The plantar surface of the foot is the most common site of ulceration. Ulcers may be primarily neuropathic (no accompanying infection) or may have surrounding cellulitis or osteomyelitis. Cellulitis without ulceration is also frequent and should be treated with antibiotics that provide broad-spectrum coverage, including anaerobes (see below).

An infected ulcer is a clinical diagnosis, since superficial culture of any ulceration will likely find multiple possible bacterial pathogens. The infection surrounding the foot ulcer is often the result of multiple organisms (gram-positive and -negative organisms and anaerobes), and gas gangrene may develop in the absence of clostridial infection. Cultures taken from the debrided ulcer base or from purulent drainage are most helpful. Wound depth should be determined by inspection and probing with a blunt-tipped sterile instrument. Plain radiographs of the foot should be performed to assess the possibility of osteomyelitis in chronic ulcers that have not responded to therapy. Nuclear medicine bone scans may be helpful, but overlying subcutaneous infection is often difficult to distinguish from osteomyelitis. Indium-labeled white cell studies are more useful in determining if the infection involves bony structures or only soft tissue, but they are technically demanding. Magnetic resonance imaging of the foot may be the most specific modality, although distinguishing bony destruction due to osteomyelitis from destruction secondary to Charcot arthropathy is difficult. If surgical debridement is necessary, bone biopsy and culture may provide the answer.

Osteomyelitis is best treated by a combination of prolonged antibiotics (IV then oral) and possibly debridement of infected bone. The possible contribution of vascular insufficiency should be considered in all patients. Noninvasive blood-flow studies are often unreliable in DM, and angiography may be required, recognizing the risk of contrast-induced nephrotoxicity. Peripheral arterial bypass procedures are often effective in promoting wound healing and in decreasing the need for amputation of the ischemic limb.

A growing number of possible treatments for diabetic foot ulcers exist, but they have yet to demonstrate clear efficacy in prospective, controlled trials. A recent consensus statement from the ADA identified six interventions with demonstrated efficacy in diabetic foot wounds: (1) off-loading, (2) debridement, (3) wound dressings, (4) appropriate use of antibiotics, (5) revascularization, and (6) limited amputation. Off-loading is the complete avoidance of weight bearing on the ulcer, which removes the mechanical trauma that retards wound healing. Bed rest and a variety of orthotic devices or contact casting limit weight bearing on wounds or pressure points. Surgical debridement is important and effective, but clear efficacy of other modalities for wound cleaning (enzymes, soaking, whirlpools) is lacking. Dressings promote wound healing by creating a moist environment and protecting the wound. Antiseptic agents and topical antibiotics should be avoided. Referral for physical therapy, orthotic evaluation, and rehabilitation may be useful once the infection is controlled.

Mild or non-limb-threatening infections can be treated with oral antibiotics (cephalosporin, clindamycin, amoxicillin/clavulanate, and fluoroquinolones), surgical debridement of necrotic tissue, local wound care (avoidance of weight bearing over the ulcer), and close surveillance for progression of infection. More severe ulcers may require intravenous antibiotics as well as bed rest and local wound care. Urgent surgical debridement may be required. Intravenous antibiotics should provide broad-spectrum coverage directed toward *Staphylococcus aureus,* streptococci, gram-negative aerobes, and anaerobic bacteria. Initial antimicrobial regimens include cefotetan, ampicillin/sulbactam, or the combination of clindamycin and a fluoroquinolone. Severe infections, or infections that do not improve after 48 h of antibiotic therapy, require expansion of antimicrobial therapy to treat methicillin-resistant *S. aureus* (e.g., vancomycin) and *Pseudomonas aeruginosa.* If the infection surrounding the ulcer is not improving with intravenous antibiotics, reassessment of antibiotic coverage and reconsideration of the need for surgical debridement or revascularization are indicated. With clinical improvement, oral antibiotics and local wound care can be continued on an outpatient basis with close follow-up.

New information about wound biology has led to a number of new technologies (e.g., living skin equivalents and growth factors such as basic fibroblast growth factor) that may prove useful. Recombinant platelet-derived growth factor has some benefit and complements the therapies of off-loading, debridement, and antibiotics. Hyperbaric oxygen has been used, but rigorous proof of efficacy is lacking.

INFECTIONS

Individuals with DM have a greater frequency and severity of infection. The reasons for this include incompletely defined abnormalities in cell-mediated immunity and phagocyte function associated with hyperglycemia, as well as diminished vascularization. Hyperglycemia aids the colonization and growth of a variety of organisms (*Candida* and other fungal species). Many common infections are more frequent and severe in the diabetic population, whereas several rare infections are seen almost exclusively in the diabetic population. Examples of this latter category includes rhinocerebral mucormycosis, emphysematous infections of the gall bladder and urinary tract, and "malignant" or invasive otitis externa. Invasive otitis externa is usually secondary to *P. aeruginosa* infection in the soft tissue surrounding the external auditory canal, usually begins with pain and discharge, and may rapidly progress to osteomyelitis and meningitis. These infections should be sought, in particular, in patients presenting with HHS.

Pneumonia, urinary tract infections, and skin and soft tissue infections are all more common in the diabetic population. In general, the organisms that cause pulmonary infections are similar to those found in the nondiabetic population; however, gram-negative organisms, *S. aureus,* and *Mycobacterium tuberculosis* are more frequent pathogens. Urinary tract infections (either lower tract or pyelonephritis) are the result of common bacterial agents such as *Escherichia coli,* though several yeast species (*Candida* and *Torulopsis glabrata*) are commonly observed. Complications of urinary tract infections include emphysematous pyelonephritis and emphysematous cystitis. Bacteriuria occurs frequently in individuals with diabetic cystopathy. Susceptibility to furunculosis, superficial candidal infections, and vulvovaginitis are increased. Poor glycemic control is a common denominator in individuals with these infections. Diabetic individuals have an increased rate of colonization of *S. aureus* in the skin folds and nares. Diabetic patients also have a greater risk of postoperative wound infections. Strict glycemic control reduces postoperative infections in diabetic individuals undergoing CABG and should be the goal in all diabetic patients with an infection.

DERMATOLOGIC MANIFESTATIONS

The most common skin manifestations of DM are protracted wound healing and skin ulcerations. Diabetic dermopathy, sometimes termed *pigmented pretibial papules,* or "diabetic skin spots," begins as an erythematous area and evolves into an area of circular hyperpigmentation. These lesions result from minor mechanical trauma in the pretibial region and are more common in elderly men with DM. Bullous diseases (shallow ulcerations or erosions in the pretibial region) are also seen. *Necrobiosis lipoidica diabeticorum* is a rare disorder of DM that predominantly affects young women with type 1 DM, neuropathy, and retinopathy. It usually begins in the pretibial region as an erythematous plaque or papules that gradually enlarge, darken, and develop irregular margins, with atrophic centers and central ulceration. They may be painful. *Acanthosis nigricans* (hyperpigmented velvety plaques seen on the neck, axilla, or extensor surfaces) is sometimes a feature of severe insulin resistance and accompanying diabetes. Generalized or localized *granuloma annulare* (erythematous plaques on the extremities or trunk) and *scleredema* (areas of skin thickening on the back or neck at the site of previous superficial infections) are more common in the diabetic population. *Lipoatrophy* and *lipohypertrophy* can occur at insulin injection sites but are unusual with the use of human insulin. Xerosis and pruritus are common and are relieved by skin moisturizers.

APPROACH TO THE PATIENT WITH DM

DM and its complications produce a wide range of symptoms and signs; those secondary to acute hyperglycemia may occur at any stage of the disease, whereas those related to chronic complications begin to appear during the second decade of hyperglycemia. Individuals with previously undetected type 2 DM may present with chronic complications of DM at the time of diagnosis. The history and physical examination should assess for symptoms or signs of acute hyperglycemia and should screen for the chronic complications and conditions associated with DM.

History

A complete medical history should be obtained with special emphasis on DM-relevant aspects such as weight, family history of DM and its complications, risk factors for cardiovascular disease, exercise, smoking, and ethanol use. Symptoms of hyperglycemia include polyuria, polydipsia, weight loss, fatigue, weakness, blurry vision, frequent superficial infections (vaginitis, fungal skin infections), and slow healing of skin lesions after minor trauma. Metabolic derangements relate mostly to hyperglycemia (osmotic diuresis, reduced glucose entry into muscle) and to the catabolic state of the patient (urinary loss of glucose and calories, muscle breakdown due to protein degradation and decreased protein synthesis). Blurred vision results from changes in the water content of the lens and resolves as the hyperglycemia is controlled.

In a patient with established DM, the initial assessment should also include special emphasis on prior diabetes care, including the type of therapy, prior hemoglobin A1C levels, self-monitoring blood glucose results, frequency of hypoglycemia, presence of DM-specific complications, and assessment of the patient's knowledge about diabetes. The chronic complications may afflict several organ systems, and an individual patient may exhibit some, all, or none of the symptoms related to the complications of DM (see above). In addition, the presence of DM-related comorbidities should be sought (cardiovascular disease, hypertension, dyslipidemia).

Physical Examination

In addition to a complete physical examination, special attention should be given to DM-relevant aspects such as weight or BMI, retinal examination, orthostatic blood pressure, foot examination, peripheral pulses, and insulin injection sites. Blood pressure > 130/80 mmHg is considered hypertension in individuals with diabetes. Careful examination of the lower extremities should seek evidence of peripheral neuropathy, calluses, superficial fungal infections, nail disease, and foot deformities (such as hammer or claw toes and Charcot foot) in order to identify sites of potential skin ulceration. Vibratory sensation (128-MHz tuning fork at the base of the great toe) and the ability to sense touch with a monofilament (5.07, 10-g monofilament) are useful to detect moderately advanced diabetic neuropathy. Since periodontal disease is more frequent in DM, the teeth and gums should also be examined.

Classification of DM in an Individual Patient

The etiology of diabetes in an individual with new-onset disease can usually be assigned on the basis of clinical criteria. Individuals with type 1 DM tend to have the following characteristics: (1) onset of disease prior to age 30; (2) lean body habitus; (3) requirement of insulin as the initial therapy; (4) propensity to develop ketoacidosis; and (5) an increased risk of other autoimmune disorders such as autoimmune thyroid disease, adrenal insufficiency, pernicious anemia, and vitiligo. In contrast, individuals with type 2 DM often exhibit the following features: (1) develop diabetes after the age of 30; (2) are usually obese (80% are obese, but elderly individuals may be lean); (3) may not require insulin therapy initially; and (4) may have associated conditions such as insulin resistance, hypertension, cardiovascular disease, dyslipidemia, or PCOS. In type 2 DM, insulin resistance is often associated with abdominal obesity (as opposed to hip and thigh obesity) and hypertriglyceridemia. Although most individuals diagnosed with type 2 DM are older, the age of diagnosis is declining in some ethnic groups, and there is a marked increase among overweight children and adolescents. Some individuals with phenotypic type 2 DM present with DKA but lack autoimmune markers and may be later treated with oral glucose-lowering agents rather than insulin. On the other hand, some individuals (5 to 10%) with the phenotypic appearance of type 2 DM do not have absolute insulin deficiency but have autoimmune markers (ICA, GAD autoantibodies) suggestive of type 1A DM (termed *autoimmune diabetes not requiring insulin at diagnosis* or *latent autoimmune diabetes of the adult*). Such individuals are much more likely to require insulin treatment within 5 years. Thus, despite the revised classification of DM, it remains difficult to categorize some patients unequivocally. Individuals who deviate from the clinical profile of type 1 and type 2 DM, or who have other associated defects such as deafness, pancreatic exocrine disease, and other endocrine disorders, should be classified accordingly (Table 17-1).

Laboratory Assessment

The laboratory assessment should first determine whether the patient meets the diagnostic criteria for DM (Table 17-2) and then assess the degree of glycemic control (A1C, discussed below). In addition to the standard laboratory evaluation, the patient should be screened for DM-associated conditions (e.g., microalbuminuria, dyslipidemia, thyroid dysfunction). Individuals at high risk for cardiovascular disease should be screened for asymptomatic coronary artery disease by appropriate cardiac stress testing, when indicated.

The classification of the type of DM may be facilitated by laboratory assessments. Serum insulin or C-peptide measurements do not always distinguish type 1 from type 2 DM, but a low C-peptide level confirms a patient's need for insulin. Many individuals with new-onset type 1 DM retain some C-peptide production. Measurement of islet cell antibodies at the time of diabetes onset may be useful if the type of DM is not clear based on the characteristics described above.

LONG-TERM TREATMENT

OVERALL PRINCIPLES

The goals of therapy for type 1 or type 2 DM are to: (1) eliminate symptoms related to hyperglycemia, (2) reduce or eliminate the long-term microvascular and macrovascular complications of DM, and (3) allow the patient to achieve as normal a life-style as possible. To reach these goals, the physician should identify a target level of glycemic control for each patient, provide the patient with the educational and pharmacologic resources necessary to reach this level, and monitor/treat DM-related complications. Symptoms of diabetes usually resolve when the plasma glucose is <11.1 mmol/L (200 mg/dL), and thus most DM treatment focuses on achieving the second and third goals.

The care of an individual with either type 1 or type 2 DM requires a multidisciplinary team. Central to the success of this team are the patient's participation, input, and enthusiasm, all of which are essential for optimal diabetes management. Members of the health care team include the primary care provider and/or the endocrinologist or diabetologist, a certified diabetes educator, and a nutritionist. In addition, when the complications of DM arise, subspecialists (including neurologists, nephrologists, vascular surgeons, cardiologists, ophthalmologists, and podiatrists) with experience in DM-related complications are essential.

A number of names are sometimes applied to different approaches to diabetes care, such as intensive insulin therapy, intensive glycemic control, and "tight control." The current chapter, however, will use the term *comprehensive diabetes care* to emphasize the fact that optimal diabetes therapy involves more than plasma glucose management. Though glycemic control is central to optimal diabetes therapy, comprehensive diabetes care of both type 1 and type 2 DM should also detect and manage DM-specific complications and modify risk factors for DM-associated diseases. In addition to the physical aspects of DM, social, family, financial, cultural, and employment-related issues may impact diabetes care.

PATIENT EDUCATION ABOUT DM, NUTRITION, AND EXERCISE

The patient with type 1 or type 2 DM should receive education about nutrition, exercise, care of diabetes during illness, and medications to lower the plasma glucose. Along with improved compliance, patient education allows individuals with DM to assume greater responsibility for their care. Patient education should be viewed as a continuing process with regular visits for reinforcement; it should *not* be a process that is completed after one or two visits to a nurse educator or nutritionist.

Diabetes Education

The diabetes educator is a health care professional (nurse, dietician, or pharmacist) with specialized patient education skills who is certified in diabetes education (e.g., American Association of Diabetes Educators). Education topics important for optimal diabetes care include self-monitoring of blood glucose; urine ketone monitoring (type 1 DM); insulin administration; guidelines for diabetes management during illnesses; management of hypoglycemia; foot and skin care; diabetes management before, during, and after exercise; and risk factor–modifying activities.

Nutrition

Medical nutrition therapy (MNT) is a term used by the ADA to describe the optimal coordination of caloric intake with other aspects of diabetes therapy (insulin, exercise, weight loss). Historically, nutrition education imposed restrictive, complicated regimens on the patient. Current practices have greatly changed, though many patients and health care providers still view the diabetic diet as monolithic and static. For example, MNT now includes foods with sucrose and seeks to modify other risk factors such as hyperlipidemia and hypertension rather than focusing exclusively on weight loss in individuals with type 2 DM. Like other aspects of DM therapy, MNT must be adjusted to meet the goals of the individual patient. Furthermore, MNT education is an important component of comprehensive diabetes care and should be reinforced by regular patient education. In general, the components of optimal MNT are similar for individuals with type 1 or type 2 DM (**Table 17-8**).

TABLE 17-8

NUTRITIONAL RECOMMENDATIONS FOR ALL PERSONS WITH DIABETES

- Protein to provide ~15 – 20% of kcal/d (~10% for those with nephropathy)
- Saturated fat to provide <10% of kcal/d (<7% for those with elevated LDL)
- Polyunsaturated fat to provide ~10% of kcal; avoid trans-unsaturated fatty acids
- 60–70% of calories to be divided between carbohydrate and monounsaturated fat, based on medical needs and personal tolerance; glycemic index of food not as important
- Use of caloric sweeteners, including sucrose, is acceptable.
- Fiber (20–35 g/d) and sodium (≤3000 mg/d) levels as recommended for the general healthy population
- Cholesterol intake ≤300 mg/d
- The same precautions regarding alcohol use in the general population also apply in individuals with diabetes. Alcohol may increase risk for hypoglycemia and therefore should be taken with food.

Note: LDL, low-density lipoprotein.
Source: Adapted from R Farkas-Hirsch, *Intensive Diabetes Management,* Alexandria, VA, American Diabetes Association, 1998; and American Diabetes Association: Diabetes Care 25:SI, 2002.

The goal of MNT in the individual with type 1 DM is to coordinate and match the caloric intake, both temporally and quantitatively, with the appropriate amount of insulin. MNT in type 1 DM and self-monitoring of blood glucose must be integrated to define the optimal insulin regimen. MNT must be flexible enough to allow for exercise, and the insulin regimen must allow for deviations in caloric intake. An important component of MNT in type 1 DM is to minimize the weight gain often associated with intensive diabetes management.

The goals of MNT in type 2 DM are slightly different and address the greatly increased prevalence of cardiovascular risk factors (hypertension, dyslipidemia, obesity) and disease in this population. The majority of these individuals are obese, and weight loss is strongly encouraged and should remain an important goal. Medical treatment of obesity is a rapidly evolving area and is discussed in Chap. 16. Hypocaloric diets and modest weight loss often result in rapid and dramatic glucose lowering in individuals with new-onset type 2 DM. Nevertheless, numerous studies document that long-term weight loss is uncommon. Current MNT for type 2 DM should emphasize modest caloric reduction, reduced fat intake, increased physical activity, and reduction of hyperlipidemia and hypertension. Increased consumption of soluble, dietary fiber may improve glycemic control in individuals with type 2 DM.

Exercise

Exercise has multiple positive benefits including cardiovascular risk reduction, reduced blood pressure, maintenance of muscle mass, reduction in body fat, and weight loss. For individuals with type 1 or type 2 DM, exercise is also useful for lowering plasma glucose (during and following exercise) and increasing insulin sensitivity.

Despite its benefits, exercise presents challenges for individuals with DM because they lack the normal glucoregulatory mechanisms (insulin falls and glucagon rises during exercise). Skeletal muscle is a major site for metabolic fuel consumption in the resting state, and the increased muscle activity during vigorous, aerobic exercise greatly increases fuel requirements. Individuals with type 1 DM are prone to either hyperglycemia or hypoglycemia during exercise, depending on the preexercise plasma glucose, the circulating insulin level, and the level of exercise-induced catecholamines. If the insulin level is too low, the rise in catecholamines may increase the plasma glucose excessively, promote ketone body formation, and possibly lead to ketoacidosis. Conversely, if the circulating insulin level is excessive, this relative hyperinsulinemia may reduce hepatic glucose production (decreased glycogenolysis, decreased gluconeogenesis) and increase glucose entry into muscle, leading to hypoglycemia.

To avoid exercise-related hyper- or hypoglycemia, individuals with type 1 DM should: (1) monitor blood glucose before, during, and after exercise; (2) delay exercise if blood glucose is >14 mmol/L (250 mg/dL), <5.5 mmol/L (100 mg/dL), or if ketones are present; (3) monitor glucose during exercise and ingest carbohydrate to prevent hypoglycemia; (4) decrease insulin doses (based on previous experience) before exercise and inject insulin into a nonexercising area; and (5) learn individual glucose responses to different types of exercise and increase food intake for up to 24 h after exercise, depending on intensity and duration of exercise. In individuals with type 2 DM, exercise-related hypoglycemia is less common but can occur in individuals taking either insulin or sulfonylureas.

Because asymptomatic cardiovascular disease appears at a younger age in both type 1 and type 2 DM, formal exercise tolerance testing may be warranted in diabetic individuals with any of the following: age >35 years, diabetes duration >15 years (type 1 DM) or >10 years (type 2 DM), microvascular complications of DM (retinopathy, microalbuminuria, or nephropathy), peripheral arterial disease, other risk factors of coronary artery disease, or autonomic neuropathy. Untreated proliferative retinopathy is a relative contraindication to vigorous exercise, as this may lead to vitreous hemorrhage or retinal detachment.

MONITORING THE LEVEL OF GLYCEMIC CONTROL

Optimal monitoring of glycemic control involves plasma glucose measurements by the patient and an assessment of long-term control by the physician (measurement of hemoglobin A1C and review of the patient's self-measurements of plasma glucose). These measurements are complementary: the patient's measurements provide a picture of short-term glycemic control, whereas the A1C reflects average glycemic control over the previous 2 to 3 months.

Self-Monitoring of Blood Glucose

Self-monitoring of blood glucose (SMBG) is the standard of care in diabetes management and allows the patient to monitor his or her blood glucose at any time. In SMBG, a small drop of blood and an easily detectable enzymatic reaction allow measurement of the capillary plasma glucose. A number of devices accurately measure glucose in blood obtained from the fingertip; alternative testing sites (e.g., forearm) are less reliable. By combining glucose measurements with diet history, medication changes, and exercise history, the physician and patient can improve the treatment program.

The frequency of SMBG measurements must be individualized and adapted to address the goals of diabetes care. Individuals with type 1 DM should routinely measure their plasma glucose four to eight times per day to estimate and select mealtime boluses of short-acting insulin and to modify long-acting insulin doses. Most individuals with type 2 DM require less frequent monitoring, though the optimal frequency of SMBG has not been clearly defined. Individuals with type 2 DM who are on oral medications should utilize SMBG as a means of assessing the efficacy of their medication and the impact of diet. Since plasma glucose levels fluctuate less in these individuals, one to two SMBG measurements per day (or fewer) may be sufficient. Individuals with type 2 DM who are on insulin should utilize SMBG more frequently than those on oral agents. Urine glucose testing does not provide an accurate assessment of glycemic control.

Two devices for continuous blood glucose monitoring have been recently approved by the U.S. Food and Drug Administration (FDA). The Glucowatch uses iontophoresis to assess glucose in interstitial fluid, whereas the Minimed device uses an indwelling subcutaneous catheter to monitor interstitial fluid glucose. Both devices utilize immobilized glucose oxidase to generate electrons in response to changing glucose levels. Though clinical experience with these devices is limited, they perform well in clinical trials and appear to provide useful short-term information about the patterns of glucose changes as well as an enhanced ability to detect hypoglycemic episodes. These devices are not yet used routinely in diabetes management.

Ketones are an indicator of early diabetic ketoacidosis and should be measured in individuals with type 1 DM when the plasma glucose is consistently >16.7 mmol/L (300 mg/dL); during a concurrent illness; or with symptoms such as nausea, vomiting, or abdominal pain. Blood measurement of β-hydroxybutyrate is preferred over urine testing with nitroprusside-based assays that measure only acetoacetate and acetone.

Assessment of Long-Term Glycemic Control

Measurement of glycated hemoglobin is the standard method for assessing long-term glycemic control. When plasma glucose is consistently elevated, there is an increase in nonenzymatic glycation of hemoglobin; this alteration reflects the glycemic history over the previous 2 to 3 months, since erythrocytes have an average life span of 120 days. There are numerous laboratory methods for measuring the various forms of glycated hemoglobin, and these have significant interassay variations. Since glycated hemoglobin measurements are usually compared to prior measurements, it is essential for the assay results to be comparable. Depending on the assay methodology, hemoglobinopathies, anemias, and uremia may interfere with the A1C result.

Glycated hemoglobin or A1C should be measured in all individuals with DM during their initial evaluation and as part of their comprehensive diabetes care. As the primary predictor of long-term complications of DM, the A1C should mirror, to a certain extent, the short-term measurements of SMBG. These two measurements are complementary in that recent intercurrent illnesses may impact the SMBG measurements but not the A1C. Likewise, postprandial and nocturnal hyperglycemia may not be detected by the SMBG of fasting and preprandial capillary plasma glucose but will be reflected in the A1C. In standardized assays, the A1C approximates the following mean plasma glucose values: an A1C of 6% is 7.5 mmol/L (135 mg/dL), 7% is 9.5 mmol/L (170 mg/dL), 8% is 11.5 mmol/L (205 mg/dL), etc. [A 1% rise in the A1C translates into a 2.0-mmol/L (35 mg/dL) increase in the mean glucose.] In patients achieving their glycemic goal, the ADA recommends measurement of the A1C twice per year. More frequent testing (every 3 months) is warranted when glycemic control is inadequate, when therapy has changed, or in most patients with type 1 DM. The degree of glycation of other proteins, such as albumin, has been used as an alternative indicator of glycemic control when the A1C is inaccurate (hemolytic anemia, hemoglobinopathies). The fructosamine assay (measuring glycated albumin) reflects the glycemic status over the prior 2 weeks. Current consensus statements do not favor the use of alternative assays of glycemic control, as there are no studies to indicate whether such assays accurately predict the complications of DM.

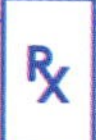

TREATMENT FOR DM COMPLICATIONS

ESTABLISHMENT OF A TARGET LEVEL OF GLYCEMIC CONTROL

Because the complications of DM are related to glycemic control, normoglycemia or near normoglycemia is the desired, but often elusive, goal for most patients. However, normalization of the plasma glucose for long periods of time is extremely difficult, as demonstrated by the DCCT. Regardless of the level of hyperglycemia, improvement in glycemic control will lower the risk of diabetes complications (Fig. 17-8).

The target for glycemic control (as reflected by the A1C) must be individualized, and the goals of therapy should be developed in consultation with the patient after considering a number of medical, social, and life-style issues. Some important factors to consider include the patient's age, ability to understand and implement a complex treatment regimen, presence and severity of complications of diabetes, ability to recognize hypoglycemic symptoms, presence of other medical conditions or treatments that might alter the response to therapy, life-style and occupation (e.g., possible consequences of experiencing hypoglycemia on the job), and level of support available from family and friends.

The ADA has established suggested glycemic goals based on the premise that glycemic control predicts development of DM-related complications. In general, the target A1C should be <7.0% (**Table 17-9**). Other consensus groups (such as the Veterans Administration) have suggested A1C goals that take into account the patient's life expectancy at the time of diagnosis and the presence of microvascular complications. Such recommendations strive to balance the financial and personal costs of glycemic therapy with anticipated benefits (reduced health care costs, reduced morbidity). One limitation to this approach is that the onset of hyperglycemia in type 2 DM is difficult to ascertain and likely predates the diagnosis.

TYPE 1 DIABETES MELLITUS

GENERAL ASPECTS

The ADA recommendations for fasting and bedtime glycemic goals and A1C targets are summarized in Table 17-9. The goal is to design and implement insulin regimens that mimic physiologic insulin secretion. Because individuals with type 1 DM lack endogenous insulin production, administration of basal, exogenous insulin is essential for regulating glycogen breakdown, gluconeogenesis, lipolysis, and ketogenesis. Likewise, insulin replacement for meals should be appropriate for the carbohydrate intake and promote normal glucose utilization and storage.

TABLE 17-9

IDEAL GOALS FOR GLYCEMIC CONTROL[a]

INDEX	GOAL
Preprandial plasma glucose, mmol/L (mg/dL)	5.0–7.2 (90–130)
Peak postprandial plasma glucose, mmol/L (mg/dL)	<10 (<180)
A1C, %	<7

[a]Plasma glucose values are 10–15% higher than whole blood values. The upper limit of the A1C reference range is 6.0% (mean 5.0%, with a standard deviation of 0.5%). These goals must be individualized for each patient and must consider the patient's age and other medical conditions.

Note: A1C, hemoglobin A1c.

Source: Adapted from American Diabetes Association: Standards of Medical Care in Diabetes—2006. Diabetes Care (suppl 1): S4, 2006.

INTENSIVE MANAGEMENT

Intensive diabetes management has the goal of achieving euglycemia or near-normal glycemia. This approach requires multiple resources including thorough and continuing patient education, comprehensive recording of plasma glucose measurements and nutrition intake by the patient, and a variable insulin regimen that matches glucose intake and insulin dose. Insulin regimens usually include multiple-component insulin regimens, multiple daily injections (MDI), or insulin infusion devices (each discussed below).

The benefits of intensive diabetes management and improved glycemic control include a reduction in the microvascular complications of DM and a possible delay or reduction in the macrovascular complications of DM. From a psychological standpoint, the patient experiences greater control over his or her diabetes and often notes an improved sense of well-being, greater flexibility in the timing and content of meals, and the capability to alter insulin dosing with exercise. In addition, intensive diabetes management in pregnancy reduces the risk of fetal malformations and morbidity. Intensive diabetes management is strongly encouraged in newly diagnosed patients with type 1 DM because it may prolong the period of C-peptide production, which may result in better glycemic control and a reduced risk of serious hypoglycemia.

Although intensive management confers impressive benefits, it is also accompanied by significant personal and financial costs and is therefore not appropriate for all individuals. Circumstances in which intensive diabetes management should be strongly considered are listed in **Table 17-10.**

TABLE 17-10

INDICATIONS FOR INTENSIVE DIABETES MANAGEMENT
• Otherwise healthy adults with either type 1 or type 2 diabetes (selected adolescents and older children)
• Purposeful, therapeutic attempt to avoid or lessen microvascular complications
• All pregnant women with diabetes; all women with diabetes who are planning pregnancy
• Management of labile diabetes
• Availability of health care professionals with appropriate expertise
• Patients who have had kidney transplantation for diabetic nephropathy

Source: Adapted from R Farkas-Hirsch: *Intensive Diabetes Management*, Alexandria, VA American Diabetes Association, 1998.

INSULIN PREPARATIONS

Current insulin preparations are generated by recombinant DNA technology and consist of the amino acid sequence of human insulin or variations thereof. Animal insulin (beef or pork) is no longer used. Human insulin has been formulated with distinctive pharmacokinetics to mimic physiologic insulin secretion (**Table 17-11**). In the United States, all insulin is formulated as U-100 (100 units/mL), whereas in some other countries it is available in other units (e.g., U-40 = 40 units/mL). One short-acting insulin formulation, lispro, is an insulin analogue in which the 28th and 29th amino acids (lysine and proline) on the insulin B chain have been reversed by recombinant DNA technology. Insulin aspart is another genetically modified insulin analogue with very similar properties to lispro. These insulin analogues have full biologic activity but less tendency toward subcutaneous aggregation, resulting in more rapid absorption and onset of action and a shorter duration of action. These characteristics are particularly advantageous for allowing entrainment of insulin injection and action to rising plasma glucose levels following meals. The shorter duration of action also appears to be associated with a decreased number of hypoglycemic episodes, primarily because the delay of lispro action corresponds to the decline in plasma glucose after a meal. Insulin glargine is a long-acting biosynthetic human insulin that differs from normal insulin in that asparagine is replaced by glycine at amino acid 21, and two arginine residues are added to the C-terminus of the B chain. Compared to NPH insulin, the onset of insulin glargine action is later, the duration of action is longer (~24 h), and there is no pronounced peak. A lower incidence of hypoglycemia, especially at night, has been reported with insulin glargine when compared to NPH insulin. Additional insulin analogues are currently under development.

Basal insulin requirements are provided by intermediate (NPH insulin or lente insulin) or long-acting (ultralente insulin or insulin glargine) insulin formulations. These are usually combined with short-acting insulin in an attempt to mimic physiologic insulin release with meals. Although mixing of intermediate and short-acting insulin formulations is common practice, this mixing

TABLE 17-11

PHARMACOKINETICS OF INSULIN PREPARATIONS

PREPARATION	TIME OF ACTION		
	ONSET, H	PEAK, H	EFFECTIVE DURATION, H
Short-acting			
Lispro	<0.25	0.5 – 1.5	3–4
Insulin aspart	<0.25	0.5–1.5	3–4
Regular	0.5–1.0	2–3	3–6
Intermediate-acting			
NPH	2–4	6–10	10–16
Lente	3–4	6–12	12–18
Long-acting			
Ultralente	6–10	10–16	18–20
Glargine	4	—[a]	24
Combinations			
75/25–75% protamine lispro, 25% lispro	0.5–1	Dual	10–14
70/30–70% NPH, 30% regular	0.5–1	Dual	10–16
50/50–50% NPH, 50% regular	0.5–1	Dual	10–16

[a]Glargine has minimal peak activity.

Source: Adapted from JS Skyler, *Therapy for Diabetes Mellitus and Related Disorders,* American Diabetes Association, Alexandria, VA, 1998.

may alter the insulin absorption profile (especially the short-acting insulins). For example, the absorption of regular insulin is delayed when mixed for even short periods of time (<5 min) with lente or ultralente insulin, but not when mixed with NPH insulin. Lispro absorption is delayed by mixing with NPH but not ultralente. Insulin glargine should not be mixed with other insulins and is not stable at room temperature. The miscibility of human regular and NPH insulin allows for the production of combination insulins that contain 70% NPH and 30% regular (70/30) or equal mixtures of NPH and regular (50/50). These combinations of insulin are more convenient for the patient but prevent adjustment of only one component of the insulin formulation. The alteration in insulin absorption when the patient mixes different insulin formulation should not discourage the patient from mixing insulin. However, the following guidelines should be followed: (1) mix the different insulin formulations in the syringe immediately before injection (inject within 2 min after mixing); (2) do not store insulin as a mixture; and (3) follow the same routine in terms of insulin mixing and administration to standardize the physiologic response to injected insulin. Several insulin formulations are available as insulin "pens," which may be more convenient for some patients.

INSULIN REGIMENS

Representations of the various insulin regimens that may be utilized in type 1 DM are illustrated in **Fig. 17-13.** Although the insulin profiles are depicted as "smooth," symmetric curves, there is considerable patient-to-patient variation in the peak and duration. In all regimens, intermediate- or long-acting insulins (NPH, lente, ultralente, or glargine insulin) supply basal insulin, whereas regular, insulin aspart, or lispro insulin provides prandial insulin. Lispro and insulin aspart should be injected just before or just after a meal; regular insulin is given 30 to 45 min prior to a meal.

A shortcoming of current insulin regimens is that injected insulin immediately enters the systemic circulation, whereas endogenous insulin is secreted into the portal venous system. Thus, exogenous insulin administration exposes the liver to subphysiologic insulin levels. No insulin regimen reproduces the precise insulin secretory pattern of the pancreatic islet. However, the most physiologic regimens entail more frequent insulin injections, greater reliance on short-acting insulin, and more frequent capillary plasma glucose measurements. In general, individuals with type 1 DM require 0.5 to

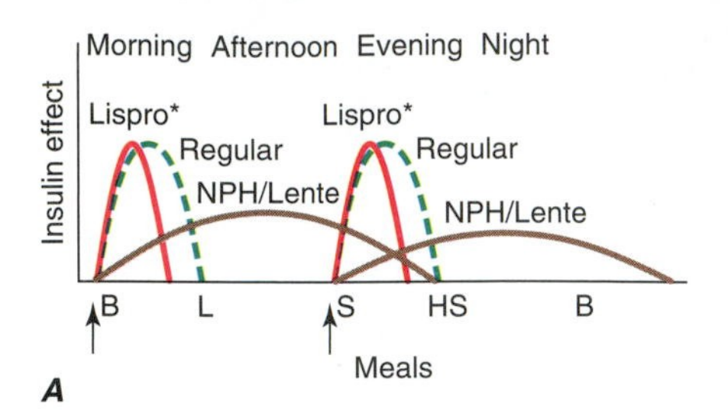

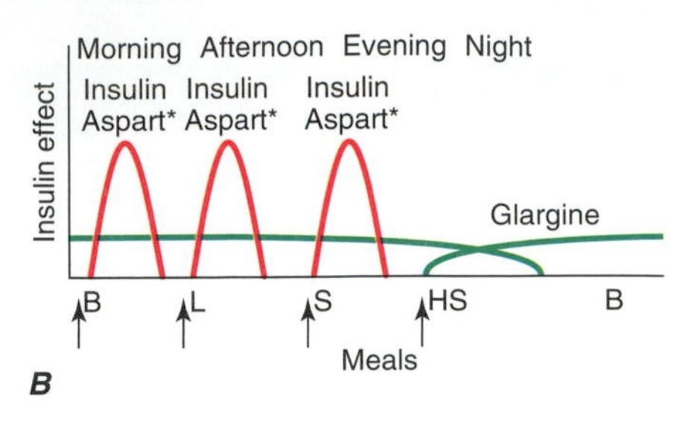

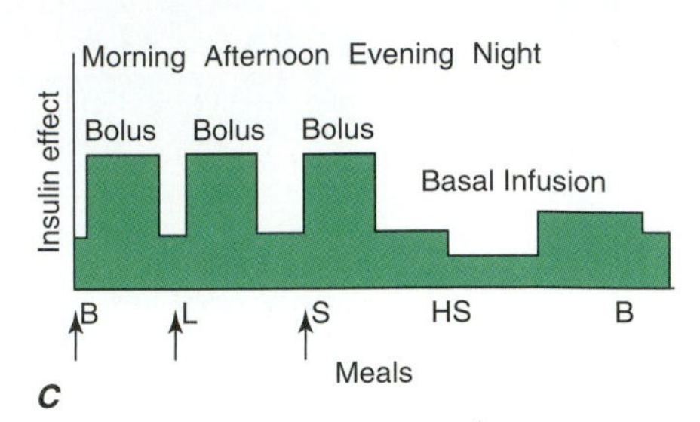

FIGURE 17-13

Representative insulin regimens for the treatment of diabetes. For each panel, the *y*-axis shows the amount of insulin effect and the *x*-axis shows the time of day. B, breakfast; L, lunch; S, supper; HS, bedtime; CSII, continuous subcutaneous insulin infusion. *Either lispro or insulin aspart can be used. The time of insulin injection is shown with a vertical arrow. The type of insulin is noted above each insulin curve. ***A***. The injection of two shots of intermediate-acting insulin (NPH or lente) and short-acting insulin (lispro, insulin aspart, or regular). Only one formulation of short-acting insulin is used. ***B***: A multiple-component insulin regimen consisting of one shot of glargine at bedtime to provide basal insulin coverage and three shots of lispro or insulin aspart to provide glycemic coverage for each meal. ***C***: Insulin administration by insulin infusion device is shown with the basal insulin and a bolus injection at each meal. The basal insulin rate is decreased during the evening and increased slightly prior to the patient awakening in the morning. *(Adapted from Intensive Diabetes Management, 2d ed, R. Farkas-Hirsch (ed). Alexandria, VA, American Diabetes Association, 1998.)*

1.0 U/kg per day of insulin divided into multiple doses. Initial insulin-dosing regimens should be conservative; approximately 40 to 50% of the insulin should be given as basal insulin. A single daily injection of insulin is not appropriate therapy in type 1 DM.

One commonly used regimen consists of twice-daily injections of an intermediate insulin (NPH or lente) mixed with a short-acting insulin before the morning and evening meal (Fig. 17-13*A*). Such regimens usually prescribe two-thirds of the total daily insulin dose in the morning (with about two-thirds given as intermediate-acting insulin and one-third as short-acting) and one-third before the evening meal (with approximately one-half given as intermediate-acting insulin and one-half as short-acting). The drawback to such a regimen is that it enforces a rigid schedule on the patient, in terms of daily activity and the content and timing of meals. Although it is simple and effective at avoiding severe hyperglycemia, it does not generate near-normal glycemic control in most individuals with type 1 DM. Moreover, if the patient's meal pattern or content varies or if physical activity is increased, hyperglycemia or hypoglycemia may result. Moving the intermediate insulin from before the evening meal to bedtime may avoid nocturnal hypoglycemia and provide more insulin as glucose levels rise in the early morning (so-called dawn phenomenon). The insulin dose in such regimens should be adjusted based on SMBG results with the following general assumptions: (1) the fasting glucose is primarily determined by the prior evening intermediate-acting insulin; (2) the pre-lunch glucose is a function of the morning short-acting insulin; (3) the pre-supper glucose is a function of the morning intermediate-acting insulin; and (4) the bedtime glucose is a function of the pre-supper, short-acting insulin.

Multiple-component insulin regimens refer to the combination of basal insulin; preprandial short-acting insulin; and changes in short-acting insulin doses to accommodate the results of frequent SMBG, anticipated food intake, and physical activity. Also referred to as MDI, such regimens offer the patient more flexibility in terms of lifestyle and the best chance for achieving near normoglycemia. One such regimen, shown in Fig. 17-13*B*, consists of a basal insulin with glargine at bedtime and preprandial lispro or insulin aspart. The lispro or insulin aspart dose is based on individualized algorithms that integrate the preprandial glucose and the anticipated carbohydrate intake. An alternative regimen is two equal doses of ultralente (breakfast and evening; 10 to 12 h apart) and preprandial lispro or insulin aspart. Another alternative multiple-component insulin regimen consists of bedtime intermediate insulin, a small dose of intermediate insulin at breakfast (20 to 30% of bedtime dose), and preprandial short-acting insulin. There are numerous variations of these regimens that can be optimized for individual patients. Frequent SMBG (four to eight times per day) is absolutely essential for these types of insulin regimens.

Continuous subcutaneous insulin infusion (CSII) is another multiple-component insulin regimen (Fig. 17-13*C*). Sophisticated insulin infusion devices can accurately deliver small doses of insulin (microliters per hour). For example, multiple basal infusion rates can be programmed to: (1) accommodate nocturnal versus daytime basal insulin requirement, (2) alter infusion rate during periods of exercise, or (3) select different waveforms of insulin infusion. A preprandial insulin ("bolus") is delivered by the insulin infusion device based on instructions from the patient, which follow individualized algorithms that account for preprandial plasma glucose and anticipated carbohydrate intake. These devices require a health professional with considerable experience with insulin infusion devices and very frequent patient interactions with the diabetes management team. Insulin infusion devices present unique challenges, such as infection at the infusion site, unexplained hyperglycemia because the infusion set becomes obstructed, or diabetic ketoacidosis if the pump becomes disconnected. Since most physicians use lispro or insulin aspart in CSII, the extremely short half-life of these insulins quickly lead to insulin deficiency if the delivery system is interrupted. Essential to the safe use of infusion devices is thorough patient education about pump function and frequent SMBG.

TYPE 2 DIABETES MELLITUS

GENERAL ASPECTS

The goals of therapy for type 2 DM are similar to those in type 1. While glycemic control tends to dominate the management of type 1 DM, the care of individuals with type 2 DM must also include attention to the treatment of conditions associated with type 2 DM (obesity, hypertension, dyslipidemia, cardiovascular disease) and detection/management of DM-related complications (**Fig. 17-14**). DM-specific complications may be present in up to 20 to 50% of individuals with newly diagnosed type 2 DM. Reduction in cardiovascular risk is of paramount importance as this is the leading cause of mortality in these individuals.

Diabetes management should begin with MNT (discussed above). An exercise regimen to increase insulin sensitivity and promote weight loss should also be instituted. After MNT and increased physical activity have been instituted, glycemic control should be reassessed; if the patient's glycemic target is not achieved after 3 to 4 weeks of MNT, pharmacologic therapy is indicated. Pharmacologic approaches to the management of type 2 DM include both oral glucose-lowering agents and insulin; most physicians and patients prefer oral glucose-lowering agents as the initial choice. Any therapy that improves glycemic control reduces "glucose toxicity" to the islet cells and improves endogenous insulin secretion. However, type 2 DM is a progressive disorder and ultimately requires multiple therapeutic agents and often insulin.

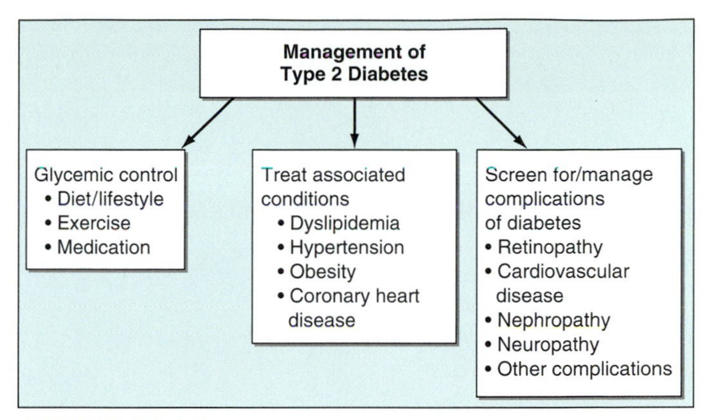

FIGURE 17-14
Essential elements in comprehensive diabetes care of type 2 diabetes.

GLUCOSE-LOWERING AGENTS

Advances in the therapy of type 2 DM have generated considerable enthusiasm for oral glucose-lowering agents that target different pathophysiologic processes in type 2 DM. Based on their mechanisms of action, oral glucose-lowering agents are subdivided into agents that increase insulin secretion, reduce glucose production, or increase insulin sensitivity (**Table 17-12**). Oral glucose-lowering agents (with the exception of α-glucosidase inhibitors) are ineffective in type 1 DM and should not be used for glucose management of severely ill individuals with type 2 DM. Insulin is sometimes the initial glucose-lowering agent.

Insulin Secretagogues Insulin secretagogues stimulate insulin secretion by interacting with the ATP-sensitive potassium channel on the beta cell (Fig. 17-1). These drugs are most effective in individuals with type 2 DM of relatively recent onset (<5 years), who tend to be obese and have residual endogenous insulin production.

TABLE 17-12

ORAL GLUCOSE-LOWERING THERAPIES IN TYPE 2 DIABETES

	MECHANISM OF ACTION	EXAMPLES	ANTICIPATED REDUCTION IN A1C, %	AGENT-SPECIFIC ADVANTAGES	AGENT-SPECIFIC DISADVANTAGES	CONTRA-INDICATIONS
Insulin secretagogues	↑ Insulin		1–2			
Sulfonylureas		See Table 17-13		Lower fasting blood glucose	Hypoglycemia weight gain, hyperinsulinemia	Renal/liver disease
Nonsulfonylureas		See Table 17-13		Short onset of action, lower postprandial glucose	Hypoglycemia	Renal/liver disease
Biguanides	↓ Hepatic glucose production, weight loss, ↑ glucose utilization, ↓ insulin resistance	Metformin	1–2	Weight loss, improved lipid profile, no hypoglycemia	Lactic acidosis, diarrhea, nausea	Serum creatinine >1.5 mg/dL (men), >1.4 mg/dL, (women), radiographic contrast studies, seriousl ill patients, acidosis
α-Glucosidase inhibitors	↓ Glucose absorption	Acarbose, miglitol	0.5–1.0	No risk of hypoglycemia	GI flatulence, ↑ liver function tests	Renal/liver disease
Thiazolidinediones	↓ Insulin resistance, ↑ glucose utilization	Rosiglitazone, pioglitazone	1–2	↓ Insulin and sulfonylurea requirements, ↓ triglycerides	Frequent hepatic monitoring for idiosyncratic hepatocellular injury (see text)	Liver disease congestive heart failure
Medical nutrition therapy and physical activity	↓ Insulin resistance	Low-calorie, low-fat diet, exercise	1–2	Other health benefits	Compliance difficult, long-term success low	

Note: A1C, hemoglobin A1c.

At maximum doses, first-generation sulfonylureas are similar in potency to second-generation agents but have a longer half-life, a greater incidence of hypoglycemia, and more frequent drug interactions (**Table 17-13**). Thus, second-generation sulfonylureas are generally preferred. An advantage to a more rapid onset of action is better coverage of the postprandial glucose rise, but the shorter half-life of such agents requires more than once-a-day dosing. Sulfonylureas reduce both fasting and postprandial glucose and should be initiated at low doses and increased at 1- to 2-week intervals based on SMBG. In general, sulfonylureas increase insulin acutely and thus should be taken shortly before a meal; with chronic therapy, though, the insulin release is more sustained. Repaglinide and nateglinide are not sulfonylureas but also interact with the ATP-sensitive potassium channel. Because of their short half-life, these agents are given with each meal or immediately before to reduce meal-related glucose excursions.

Insulin secretagogues are generally well tolerated. All of these agents, however, have the potential to cause profound and persistent hypoglycemia, especially in elderly individuals. Hypoglycemia is usually related to delayed meals, increased physical activity, alcohol intake, or renal insufficiency. Individuals who ingest an overdose of some agents develop prolonged and serious hypoglycemia and should be monitored closely in the hospital (Chap. 19). Most sulfonylureas are metabolized in the liver to compounds that are cleared by the kidney. Thus, their use in individuals with significant hepatic or renal dysfunction is not advisable. Weight gain, a common side effect of sulfonylurea therapy, results from the increased insulin levels and improvement in glycemic control. Some sulfonylureas have significant drug interactions with alcohol and some

TABLE 17-13

CHARACTERISTICS OF AGENTS THAT INCREASE INSULIN SECRETION

GENERIC NAME	APPROVED DAILY DOSAGE RANGE, MG	DURATION OF ACTION, H	CLEARANCE
Sulfonylurea—first generation			
Chlorpropamide	100–500	>48	Renal
Tolazamide	100–1000	12–24	Hepatic, renal
Tolbutamide	500–3000	6–12	Hepatic
Sulfonylurea—second generation			
Glimepiride	1–8	24	Hepatic, renal
Glipizide	2.5–40	12–18	Hepatic
Glipzide (extended release)	5–10	24	Hepatic
Glyburide	1.25–20	12–24	Hepatic, renal
Glyburide (micronized)	0.75–12	12–24	Hepatic, renal
Nonsulfonylureas			
Repaglinide	0.5–16	2–6	Hepatic
Nateglinide	180–360	2–4	Renal

Source: Adapted from BR Zimmerman (ed): *Medical Management of Type 2 Diabetes*, 4th ed. Alexandria, VA, American Diabetes Association, 1998.

medications including warfarin, aspirin, ketoconazole, α-glucosidase inhibitors, and fluconazole. Despite prior concerns that use of sulfonylureas might increase cardiovascular risk, most recent trials have refuted this claim.

Biguanides Metformin is representative of this class of agents. It reduces hepatic glucose production through an undefined mechanism and improves peripheral glucose utilization slightly (Table 17-12). Metformin reduces fasting plasma glucose and insulin levels, improves the lipid profile, and promotes modest weight loss. The initial starting dose of 500 mg once or twice a day can be increased to 1000 mg bid. An extended-release form and a combination formulation with glyburide and glipizide are available. Because of its relatively slow onset of action and gastrointestinal symptoms with higher doses, the dose should be escalated every 2 to 3 weeks based on SMBG measurements. The major toxicity of metformin, lactic acidosis, can be prevented by careful patient selection. Metformin should not be used in patients with renal insufficiency [serum creatinine >133 μmol/L (1.5 mg/dL) in men or >124 μmol/L (1.4 mg/dL) in women, with adjustments for age], any form of acidosis, congestive heart failure, liver disease, or severe hypoxia. Metformin should be discontinued in patients who are seriously ill, in patients who can take nothing orally, and in those receiving radiographic contrast material. Insulin should be used until metformin can be restarted. Though well tolerated in general, some individuals develop gastrointestinal side effects (diarrhea, anorexia, nausea, and metallic taste) that can be minimized by gradual dose escalation. Because the drug is metabolized in the liver, it should not be used in patients with liver disease or heavy ethanol intake.

α-Glucosidase Inhibitors α-Glucosidase inhibitors (acarbose and miglitol) reduce postprandial hyperglycemia by delaying glucose absorption; they do not affect glucose utilization or insulin secretion (Table 17-12). Postprandial hyperglycemia, secondary to impaired hepatic and peripheral glucose disposal, contributes significantly to the hyperglycemic state in type 2 DM. These drugs, taken just before each meal, reduce glucose absorption by inhibiting the enzyme that cleaves oligosaccharides into simple sugars in the intestinal lumen. Therapy should be initiated at a low dose (25 mg of acarbose or miglitol) with the evening meal and may be increased to a maximal dose over weeks to months (50 to 100 mg for acarbose or 50 mg for miglitol with each meal). The major side effects (diarrhea, flatulence, abdominal distention) are related to increased delivery of oligosaccharides to the large bowel and can be reduced somewhat by gradual upward dose titration. α-Glucosidase inhibitors may increase levels of sulfonylureas and increase the incidence of hypoglycemia. Simultaneous treatment with bile acid resins and antacids should be avoided. These agents should not be used in individuals with inflammatory bowel disease, gastroparesis, or a serum creatinine >177 μmol/L (2.0 mg/dL). This class of agents is not as potent as other oral agents in lowering the hemoglobin A1C but is unique because it reduces the postprandial glucose rise even in individuals with type 1 DM. If hypoglycemia occurs while taking these agents, the patient should consume glucose since the degradation and absorption of complex carbohydrates will be retarded.

Thiazolidinediones Thiazolidinediones reduce insulin resistance. These drugs bind to the PPAR-γ (peroxisome proliferator-activated receptor-γ) nuclear receptor. The PPAR-γ receptor is found at highest levels in adipocytes but is expressed at lower levels in many other tissues. Agonists of this receptor promote adipocyte differentiation and may reduce insulin resistance indirectly because of enhanced fatty acid uptake and storage (Table 17-12). Circulating insulin levels decrease with use of the thiazolidinediones, indicating a reduction in insulin resistance. Although direct comparisons are not available, the two currently available thiazolidinediones appear to have similar efficacy; the therapeutic range for pioglitazone is 15 to 45 mg/d in a single daily dose and for rosiglitazone the total daily dose is 2 to 8 mg/d administered either once daily or twice daily in divided doses. The ability of thiazolidinediones to influence other features of the insulin resistance syndrome is under investigation.

The prototype of this class of drugs, troglitazone, was withdrawn from the U.S. market after reports of hepatotoxicity and an association with an idiosyncratic liver reaction that sometimes led to hepatic failure. Although rosiglitazone and pioglitazone do not appear to induce the liver abnormalities seen with troglitazone, the FDA recommends measurement of liver function tests prior to initiating therapy with a thiazolidinedione and at regular intervals (every 2 months for the first year and then periodically). The thiazolidinediones raise LDL and HDL slightly and lower triglycerides by 10 to 15%, but the clinical significance of these changes is not known. Thiazolidinediones are associated with minor weight gain (1 to 2 kg), a small reduction in the hematocrit, and a mild increase in plasma volume. Cardiac function is not affected, but peripheral edema CHF may occur and is more common in individuals treated with insulin. They are contraindicated in patients with liver disease or congestive heart failure (class III or IV). Thiazolidinediones have been shown to induce ovulation in premenopausal women with PCOS. Women should be warned about the risk of pregnancy, since the safety of thiazolidinediones in pregnancy is not established.

Insulin Therapy In Type 2 DM Insulin should be considered as the initial therapy in type 2 DM, particularly in lean individuals or those with severe weight loss, in individuals with underlying renal or hepatic disease that precludes oral glucose-lowering agents, or in individuals who are hospitalized or acutely ill. Insulin therapy is ultimately required by a substantial number of individuals with type 2 DM because of the progressive nature of the disorder and the relative insulin deficiency that develops in patients with long-standing diabetes.

Because endogenous insulin secretion continues and is capable of providing some coverage of mealtime caloric intake, insulin is usually initiated in a single dose of intermediate- or long-acting insulin (0.3 to 0.4 U/kg per day), given either before breakfast (NPH, lente, or ultralente) or just before bedtime (NPH, lente, ultralente, or glargine). Since fasting hyperglycemia and increased hepatic glucose production are prominent features of type 2 DM, bedtime insulin is more effective in clinical trials than a single dose of morning insulin. Some physicians prefer a relatively low, fixed starting dose of intermediate-acting insulin (~15 to 20 units in the morning and 5 to 10 units at bedtime) to avoid hypoglycemia. The insulin dose may then be adjusted in 10% increments as dictated by SMBG results. Both morning and bedtime intermediate insulin may be used in combination with oral glucose-lowering agents (biguanides, α-glucosidase inhibitors, or thiazolidinediones).

Choice of Initial Glucose-Lowering Agent

The level of hyperglycemia should influence the initial choice of therapy. Assuming maximal benefit of MNT and increased physical activity has been realized, patients with mild to moderate hyperglycemia [fasting plasma glucose <11.1 to 13.9

mmol/L (200 to 250 mg/dL)] often respond well to a single oral glucose-lowering agent. Patients with more severe hyperglycemia [fasting plasma glucose >13.9 mmol/L (250 mg/dL)] may respond partially but are unlikely to achieve normoglycemia with oral monotherapy. A stepwise approach that starts with a single agent and adds a second agent to achieve the glycemic target can be used (see "Combination Therapy," below). Insulin can be used as initial therapy in individuals with severe hyperglycemia [fasting plasma glucose >13.9 to 16.7 mmol/L (250 to 300 mg/dL)]. This approach is based on the rationale that more rapid glycemic control will reduce "glucose toxicity" to the islet cells, improve endogenous insulin secretion, and possibly allow oral glucose-lowering agents to be more effective. If this occurs, the insulin may be discontinued.

Insulin secretagogues, biguanides, α-glucosidase inhibitors, thiazolidinediones, and insulin are approved for monotherapy of type 2 DM. Although each class of oral glucose-lowering agents has unique advantages and disadvantages, certain generalizations apply: (1) insulin secretagogues, biguanides, and thiazolidinediones improve glycemic control to a similar degree (1 to 2% reduction in A1C) and are more effective than α-glucosidase inhibitors; (2) assuming a similar degree of glycemic improvement, no clinical advantage to one class of drugs has been demonstrated, and any therapy that improves glycemic control is likely beneficial; (3) insulin secretagogues and α-glucosidase inhibitors begin to lower the plasma glucose immediately, whereas the glucose-lowering effects of the biguanides and thiazolidinediones are delayed by several weeks to months; (4) not all agents are effective in all individuals with type 2 DM (primary failure); (5) biguanides, α-glucosidase inhibitors, and thiazolidinediones do not directly cause hypoglycemia; and (6) most individuals will eventually require treatment with more than one class of oral glucose-lowering agents or insulin, reflecting the progressive nature of type 2 DM.

Considerable clinical experience exists with sulfonylureas and metformin because they have been available for several decades. It is assumed that the α-glucosidase inhibitors and thiazolidinediones, which are newer classes of oral glucose-lowering drugs, will reduce DM-related complications by improving glycemic control, although long-term data are not yet available. The thiazolidinediones are theoretically attractive because they target a fundamental abnormality in type 2 DM, namely insulin resistance. However, these agents are currently more costly than others and require liver function monitoring.

A reasonable treatment algorithm for initial therapy proposes either a sulfonylurea or metformin as initial therapy because of their efficacy, known side-effect profile, and relatively low cost (Fig. 17-14). Metformin has the advantage that it promotes mild weight loss, lowers insulin levels, improves the lipid profile slightly, and may have a lower secondary failure rate. Metformin is the initial choice of many physicians for the treatment of the obese, type 2 diabetic. However, there is no difference in response rate or degree of glycemic control when metformin and sulfonylureas are compared in randomized, prospective clinical trials. Based on SMBG results and the A1C, the dose of either the sulfonylurea or metformin should be increased until the glycemic target is achieved. Thiazolidinediones are alternative, initial agents, but are much more expensive; α-glucosidase inhibitors are the least potent agents and not as desirable for monotherapy (**Fig. 17-15**).

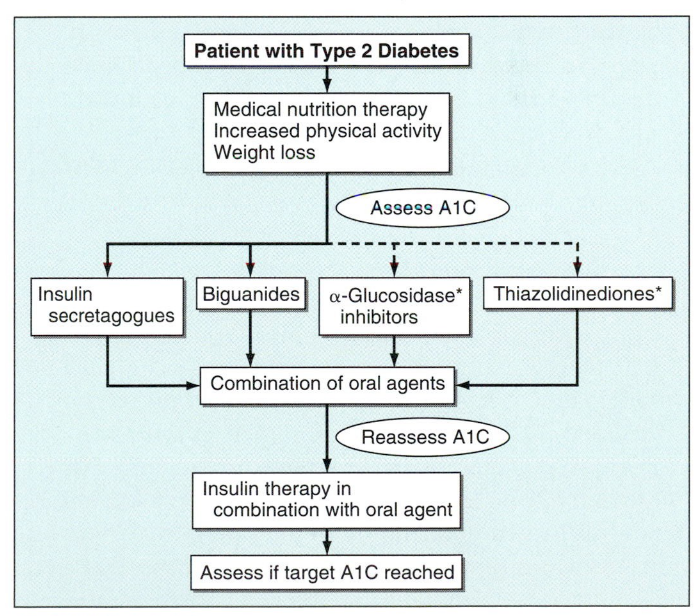

FIGURE 17-15

Glycemic management of type 2 diabetes. See text for discussion. *See text about use as monotherapy. The broken line indicates that biguanides or insulin secretagogues, but not α glucosidase inhibitors or thiazolidinediones, are preferred for initial therapy. A1C, hemoglobin A1c.

Approximately one-third of individuals will reach their target glycemic goal using either a sulfonylurea or metformin as monotherapy. Approximately 25% of individuals will not respond to sulfonylureas or metformin; under these circumstances, the drug usually should be discontinued. Some individuals respond to one agent but not the other. The remaining individuals treated with either sulfonylureas or metformin alone will exhibit some improvement in glycemic control but will not achieve their glycemic target and should be considered for combination therapy.

Combination Therapy with Glucose-Lowering Agents A number of combinations of therapeutic agents are successful in type 2 DM, and the dosing of agents in combination is the same as when the agents are used alone. Because mechanisms of action of the first and second agents are different, the effect on glycemic control is usually additive. Commonly used regimens include: (1) insulin secretagogue with metformin or thiazolidinedione, (2) sulfonylurea with α-glucosidase inhibitor, and (3) insulin with metformin or thiazolidinedione. The combination of metformin and a thiazolidinedione is also effective and complementary. If adequate control is not achieved with two oral agents, bedtime insulin or a third oral agent may be added stepwise. However, long-term experience with any triple combination is lacking, and experience with two-drug combinations is relatively limited.

Insulin becomes required as type 2 DM enters the phase of relative insulin deficiency (as seen in long-standing DM) and is signaled by inadequate glycemic control with one or two oral glucose-lowering agents. Insulin can be used in combination with any of the oral agents in patients who fail to reach the glycemic target. For example, a single dose of intermediate- or long-acting insulin at bedtime is effective in combination with metformin. As endogenous insulin production falls further, multiple injections of intermediate-acting and short-acting insulin regimens are necessary to control postprandial glucose excursions. These combination regimens are identical to the intermediate-, long-acting, and short-acting combination regimens discussed above for type 1 DM. Since the hyperglycemia of type 2 DM tends to be more "stable," these regimens can be increased in 10% increments every 2 to 3 days using SMBG results. The daily insulin dose required can become quite large (1 to 2 units/kg per day) as endogenous insulin production falls and insulin resistance persists. Individuals who require >1 unit/kg per day of intermediate-acting insulin should be considered for combination therapy with metformin or a thiazolidinedione. The addition of metformin or a thiazolidinedione can reduce insulin requirements in some individuals with type 2 DM, while maintaining or even improving glycemic control.

Intensive diabetes management (Table 17-10) is a treatment option in type 2 patients who cannot achieve optimal glycemic control and are capable of implementing such regimens. A recent study from the Veterans Administration found that intensive diabetes management is not associated with a greater degree of side effects (hypoglycemia, weight gain) than standard insulin therapy. The effect of higher insulin levels associated with intensive diabetes management on the prognosis of diseases commonly associated with type 2 DM (cardiovascular disease, hypertension) is still debated. In selected patients with type 2 DM, insulin pumps improve glycemic control and are well tolerated.

EMERGING THERAPIES

Whole pancreas transplantation (conventionally performed concomitantly with a renal transplant) may normalize glucose tolerance and is an important therapeutic option in type 1 DM, though it requires substantial expertise and is associated with the side effects of immunosuppression. Pancreatic islet transplantation has been plagued by limitations in pancreatic islet isolation and graft survival, but recent advances in specific immunomodulation have greatly improved the results. Islet transplantation is an area of active clinical investigation.

New insights into normal mechanisms of glucose homeostasis have led to a number of emerging therapies for diabetes and its complications. For example, glucagon-like peptide 1, a potent insulin secretagogue, may be efficacious in type 2 DM. Inhaled insulin and additional insulin analogues are in advanced stages of clinical trials. Aminoguanidine, an inhibitor of the formation of advanced glycosylation end products, and inhibitors of protein kinase C may reduce the complications of DM. Closed-loop pumps that infuse the appropriate amount of insulin in response to changing glucose levels are potentially feasible now that continuous glucose-monitoring technology has been developed.

COMPLICATIONS OF THERAPY FOR DIABETES MELLITUS

As with any therapy, the benefits of efforts directed towards glycemic control must be weighed against the risks of treatment. Side effects of intensive treatment include an increased frequency of serious hypoglycemia, weight gain, increased economic costs, and greater demands on the patient. In the DCCT, quality of life was very similar in the intensive and standard therapy groups. The most serious complication of therapy for DM is hypoglycemia (Chap. 19). Weight gain occurs with most (insulin, insulin secretagogues, thiazolidinediones) but not all (metformin and α-glucosidase inhibitors) therapies that improve glycemic control. It is due to the anabolic effects of insulin and the reduction in glucosuria without a corresponding decrease in caloric intake. In the DCCT, individuals with the greatest weight gain exhibited increases in LDL cholesterol and triglycerides as well as increases in blood pressure (both systolic and diastolic) similar to those seen in individuals with type 2 DM and insulin resistance. These effects could increase the risk of cardiovascular disease in intensively managed patients. As discussed previously, transient worsening of diabetic retinopathy or neuropathy sometimes accompanies improved glycemic control.

ONGOING ASPECTS OF COMPREHENSIVE DIABETES CARE

The morbidity and mortality of DM-related complications can be greatly reduced by timely and consistent surveillance procedures (**Table 17-14**). These screening procedures are indicated for all individuals with DM, but numerous studies have documented that most individuals with diabetes do not receive comprehensive diabetes care. Screening for dyslipidemia and hypertension should be performed annually. In addition to routine health maintenance, individuals with diabetes should also receive the pneumococcal and tetanus vaccines (at recommended intervals) and the influenza vaccine (annually). As discussed above, aspirin therapy should be considered in many patients with diabetes.

TABLE 17-14

GUIDELINES FOR ONGOING MEDICAL CARE FOR PATIENTS WITH DIABETES

- Self-monitoring of blood glucose (individualized frequency)
- A1C testing (2–4 times/year)
- Patient education in diabetes management (annual)
- Medical nutrition therapy and education (annual)
- Eye examination (annual)
- Foot examination (1–2 times/year by physician; daily by patient)
- Screening for diabetic nephropathy (annual; see Fig. 17–11)
- Blood pressure measurement (quarterly)
- Lipid profile (annual)
- Influenza/pneumococcal immunizations
- Consider antiplatelet therapy (see text)

Note: A1C, hemoglobin A1c.

An annual comprehensive eye examination should be performed by a qualified optometrist or ophthalmologist. If abnormalities are detected, further evaluation and treatment require an ophthalmologist skilled in diabetes-related eye disease. Because many individuals with type 2 DM have had asymptomatic diabetes for several years before diagnosis, the ADA recommends the following ophthalmologic examination schedule: (1) individuals with onset of DM at <29 years should have an initial eye examination within 3 to 5 years of diagnosis, (2) individuals with onset of DM at >30 years should have an initial eye examination at the time of diabetes diagnosis, and (3) women with DM who are contemplating pregnancy should have an eye examination prior to conception and during the first trimester.

An annual foot examination should: (1) assess blood flow, sensation (monofilament testing), and nail care; (2) look for the presence of foot deformities such as hammer or claw toes and Charcot foot; and (3) identify sites of potential ulceration. Calluses and nail deformities should be treated by a podiatrist; the patient should be discouraged from self-care of even minor foot problems. The ADA advises a visual foot inspection for potential problems at each outpatient visit.

An annual microalbuminuria measurement (albumin-to-creatinine ratio in spot urine) is advised in individuals with type 1 or type 2 DM and no protein on a routine urinalysis (Fig. 17-10). If the urinalysis detects proteinuria, the amount of protein should be quantified by standard urine protein measurements. If the urinalysis was negative for protein in the past, microalbuminuria should be the annual screening examination. Routine urine protein measurements do not detect low levels of albumin excretion. Screening should commence 5 years after the onset of type 1 DM and at the time of onset of type 2 DM.

SPECIAL CONSIDERATIONS IN DIABETES MELLITUS

PSYCHOSOCIAL ASPECTS

As with any chronic, debilitating disease, the individual with DM faces a series of challenges that affect all aspects of daily life. The individual with DM must accept that he or she may develop complications related to DM. Even with considerable effort, normoglycemia can be an elusive goal, and solutions to worsening glycemic control may not be easily identifiable. The patient should view him- or herself as an essential member of the diabetes care team and not as someone who is cared for by the diabetes team. Emotional stress may provoke a change in behavior so that individuals no longer adhere to a dietary, exercise, or therapeutic regimen. This can lead to the appearance of either hyper- or hypoglycemia. Depression and eating disorders, including binge eating disorders, bulimia, and anorexia nervosa, appear to occur more frequently in individuals with type 1 or type 2 DM.

MANAGEMENT IN THE HOSPITALIZED PATIENT

Virtually all medical and surgical subspecialties may be involved in the care of hospitalized patients with diabetes. Hyperglycemia, whether in an individual with known diabetes or in one without diabetes, may be a predictor of poor outcome in hospitalized patients. General anesthesia, surgery, and concurrent illness raise the levels of counterregulatory hormones (cortisol, growth hormone, catecholamines, and glucagon), and infection may lead to transient insulin resistance and hyperglycemia. These factors increase insulin requirements by increasing glucose production and impairing glucose utilization and thus may worsen glycemic control. The concurrent illness or surgical procedure may lead to variable insulin absorption and also prevent the patient with DM from eating normally and may promote hypoglycemia. Glycemic control should be assessed (with A1C) and, if feasible, should be optimized prior to surgery. Electrolytes, renal function, and intravascular volume status should be assessed as well. The high prevalence of asymptomatic cardiovascular disease in individuals with DM (especially in type 2 DM) may require preoperative cardiovascular evaluation. Maintenance of a near normal glucose with insulin reduced the risk of postoperative infection after CABG, and in one study, reduced the morbidity and mortality in patients in a surgical intensive care unit.

The goals of diabetes management during hospitalization are avoidance of hypoglycemia, optimization of glycemic control, and transition back to the outpatient diabetes treatment regimen. Optimal glycemic control in the hospitalized patient is <6.1 mmol/L (100 mg/dL, preprandial) and <10 mmol/L (180 mg/dL, postprandial). Attention to each stage in this process requires integrating information regarding the plasma glucose, diabetes treatment regimen, and clinical status of the patient. For example, some surgical procedures utilizing local anesthesia or epidural anesthesia may have minimal effects on glycemic control. If the patient is eating soon after the procedure and there is no disruption of the patient's regular meal plans, then glycemic control is usually maintained. A "consistent-carbohydrate diabetes meal plan" for hospitalized patients provides a similar amount of carbohydrate for a particular meal each day (but not necessarily the same amount for breakfast, lunch, and supper). The hospital diet should be determined by a nutritionist; terms such as "ADA diet" or "low-sugar diet" are no longer used.

The physician caring for an individual with diabetes in the perioperative period, during times of infection or serious physical illness, or simply when fasting for a diagnostic procedure must monitor the plasma glucose vigilantly, adjust the diabetes treatment regimen, and provide glucose infusion as needed. Several different treatment regimens (intravenous or subcutaneous insulin regimens) can be employed successfully. Individuals with type 1 DM require continued insulin administration to maintain the levels of circulating insulin necessary to prevent DKA. Prolongation of a surgical procedure or delay in the recovery room is not uncommon and may result in periods of insulin deficiency. Even relatively brief periods without insulin may lead to mild DKA. Individuals with type 1 DM who are undergoing general anesthesia and surgery, or who are seriously ill, should receive continuous insulin, either through an intravenous insulin infusion or by subcutaneous administration of a reduced dose of long-acting insulin. Short-acting insulin alone is insufficient.

Perioperative Management

Insulin infusions can effectively control plasma glucose in the perioperative period and when the patient is unable to take anything by mouth. The absorption of subcutaneous insulin may be variable in such situations because of changes in blood flow. The physician must consider carefully the clinical setting in which an insulin infusion will be utilized, including whether adequate ancillary personnel are available to monitor the plasma glucose frequently and whether they can adjust the insulin infusion rate, either based on an algorithm or in consultation with the physician. The initial rate for an insulin infusion may range from 0.5 to 5 units/h, depending on the degree of insulin resistance and the clinical situation. Based on hourly capillary glucose measurements, the insulin infusion rate is adjusted to maintain the plasma glucose within the optimal range. The insulin infusion can be temporarily discontinued if hypoglycemia occurs and may be resumed at a lower infusion rate once the plasma glucose exceeds 5.6 mmol/L (100 mg/dL).

Insulin infusion is the preferred method for managing patients with type 1 DM in the perioperative period or when serious concurrent illness is present (0.5 to 1.0 units/h of regular insulin). Insulin-infusion algorithms jointly developed and implemented by nursing and physician staff are advised. If the diagnostic or surgical procedure is brief and performed under local or regional anesthesia, a reduced dose of subcutaneous, long-acting insulin may suffice. This approach facilitates the transition back to the long-acting insulin after the procedure. The dose of long-acting insulin should be reduced by 30 to 40%, and short-acting insulin is either held or, likewise, reduced by 30 to 40%. Glucose may be infused to prevent hypoglycemia.

Individuals with type 2 DM can be managed with either regular insulin infusion 0.5 to 2 units/h or a reduced dose of subcutaneous intermediate- or long-acting insulin supplemented with short-acting insulin. Oral glucose-lowering agents are discontinued upon admission. Oral glucose-lowering agents are not useful in regulating the plasma glucose in clinical situations where the insulin requirements and glucose intake are changing rapidly. Moreover, these oral agents may be dangerous if the patient is fasting (e.g., hypoglycemia with sulfonylureas). Metformin should be withheld when radiographic contrast media will be given or if severe congestive heart failure, acidosis, or declining renal function is present.

Total Parenteral Nutrition

Total parenteral nutrition (TPN) greatly increases insulin requirements. In addition, individuals not previously known to have DM may become hyperglycemic during TPN and require insulin treatment. Intravenous insulin infusion is the preferred treatment for hyperglycemia, and rapid titration to the required insulin dose is done most efficiently using a separate insulin infusion. After the total insulin dose has been determined, insulin may be added directly to the TPN solution or, preferably, given as a separate infusion. Often, individuals receiving either TPN or enteral nutrition receive their caloric loads continuously and not at "meal times"; consequently, subcutaneous insulin regimens must be adjusted.

GLUCOCORTICOIDS

Glucocorticoids increase insulin resistance, decrease glucose utilization, increase hepatic glucose production, and impair insulin secretion. These changes lead to a worsening of glycemic control in individuals with DM and may precipitate diabetes in other individuals ("steroid-induced diabetes"). The effects of glucocorticoids on glucose homeostasis are dose-related, usually reversible, and most pronounced in the postprandial period. If the fasting plasma glucose is near the normal range, oral diabetes agents (e.g., sulfonylureas, metformin) may be sufficient to reduce hyperglycemia. If the fasting plasma glucose >11.1 mmol/L (200 mg/dL), oral agents are usually not efficacious and insulin therapy is required. Short-acting insulin may be required to supplement long-acting insulin in order to control postprandial glucose excursions.

REPRODUCTIVE ISSUES

Reproductive capacity in either men or women with DM appears to be normal. Menstrual cycles may be associated with alterations in glycemic control in women with DM. Pregnancy is associated with marked insulin resistance; the increased insulin requirements often precipitate DM and lead to the diagnosis of GDM. Glucose, which at high levels is a teratogen to the developing fetus, readily crosses the placenta, but insulin does not. Thus, hyperglycemia from the maternal circulation may stimulate insulin secretion in the fetus. The anabolic and growth effects of insulin may result in macrosomia. GDM complicates approximately 4% of pregnancies in the United States. The incidence of GDM is greatly increased in certain ethnic groups, including African Americans and Hispanic Americans, consistent with a similar increased risk of type 2 DM. Current recommendations advise screening for glucose intolerance between weeks 24 and 28 of pregnancy in women with high risk for GDM (≥25 years; obesity; family history of DM; member of an ethnic group such as Hispanic American, Native American, Asian American, African American, or Pacific Islander). Therapy for GDM is similar to that for individuals with pregnancy-associated diabetes and involves MNT and insulin, if hyperglycemia persists. Oral glucose-lowering agents have not been approved for use during pregnancy. With current practices, the morbidity and mortality of the mother with GDM and the fetus are no different from those in the nondiabetic population. Individuals who develop GDM are at marked increased risk for developing type 2 DM in the future and should be screened periodically for DM. After delivery, glucose homeostasis should be reassessed in the mother. Most individuals with GDM revert to normal glucose tolerance, but some will continue to have overt diabetes or impairment of glucose tolerance. In addition, children of women with GDM appear to be at risk for obesity and glucose intolerance and have an increased risk of diabetes beginning in the later stages of adolescence.

Pregnancy in individuals with known DM requires meticulous planning and adherence to strict treatment regimens. Intensive diabetes management and normalization of the A1C are the standard of care for individuals with existing DM who are planning pregnancy. The most crucial period of glycemic control is soon after fertilization. The risk of fetal malformations is increased 4 to 10 times in individuals with uncontrolled DM at the time of conception and normal plasma glucose during the preconception period and throughout the periods of organ development in the fetus should be maintained.

LIPODYSTROPHIC DM

Lipodystrophy, or the loss of subcutaneous fat tissue, may be generalized in certain genetic conditions such as leprechaunism. Generalized lipodystrophy is associated with severe insulin resistance and is often accompanied by acanthosis nigricans and dyslipidemia. Localized lipodystrophy associated with insulin injections has been reduced considerably by the use of human insulin.

Protease Inhibitors and Lipodystrophy

Protease inhibitors used in the treatment of HIV disease have been associated with a centripetal accumulation of fat (visceral and abdominal area), accumulation of fat in the dorsocervical region, loss of extremity fat, decreased insulin sensitivity (elevations of the fasting insulin level and reduced glucose tolerance on intravenous glucose tolerance testing), and dyslipidemia. Although many aspects of the physical appearance of these individuals resemble Cushing's syndrome, increased cortisol levels do not account for this appearance. The possibility remains that this is related to HIV infection by some undefined mechanism, since some features of the syndrome were observed before the introduction of protease inhibitors. Therapy for HIV-related lipodystrophy is not well established.

FURTHER READINGS

American Diabetes Association: Clinical practice recommendations 2002. Diabetes Care 27:51, 2004

Clement S et al: Management of diabetes and hyperglycemia in hospitals. Diabetes Care 27:553, 2004

DeFronzo R et al: Effects of exenatide (Exendin-4) on glycemic control and weight over 30 weeks in metformin-treated patients with type 2 diabetes. Diabetes Care 28:1092, 2005

This study showed that exenatide, a recently approved drug for the treatment of type 2 diabetes, flattened post-meal glucose spikes and reduced hemoglobin A1c in patients already taking metformin.

Flaherty JD et al: Diabetes and coronary revascularization. JAMA 293:1501, 2005

Patients with diabetes mellitus account for ~25% of the coronary revascularization procedures performed each year in the United States and experience worse outcomes compared with nondiabetic patients. The era of drug-eluting stents and glycoprotein IIb/IIIa inhibitors are modifying the management of cardiovascular disease in patients with type 2 diabetes.

Inzucchi SE: Oral antihyperglycemic therapy for type 2 diabetes: Scientific review. JAMA 287:360, 2002

Kahn SE: The importance of beta-cell failure in the development and progression of type 2 diabetes. J Clin Endocrinol Metab 86:4047, 2001

Lien LF et al: In-hospital management of type 2 diabetes mellitus. Med Clin North Am 88:1085, 2004

Improved glycemic control improves morbidity and mortality in hospitalized patients with hyperglycemia. This review summarizes practical regimens for subcutaneous insulin administration, intravenous insulin infusion, and inpatient use of oral agents in hospitalized patients with type 2 diabetes.

Permutt MA et al: Genetic epidemiology of diabetes. J Clin Invest 115:1431, 2005

This review discusses the epidemiology of diabetes and provides approaches for accelerated accumulation of clinically useful genetic information.

Stumvoll M et al: Type 2 diabetes: Principles of pathogenesis and therapy. Lancet 365:1333, 2005

Although insulin resistance is an early feature of diabetes that is related to obesity, pancreas beta-cell function declines gradually over time already before the onset of clinical hyperglycemia. This review summarizes mechanisms that underlie the pathogenesis of type 2 diabetes, including increased non-esterified fatty acids, inflammatory cytokines, adipokines, and mitochondrial dysfunction for insulin resistance, and glucotoxicity, lipotoxicity, and amyloid formation in beta-cells.

van den Berghe G et al: Intensive insulin therapy in the critically ill patients. N Engl J Med 345:1359, 2001

◩ WILLIAMSON DF et al: Primary prevention of type 2 diabetes mellitus by lifestyle intervention: Implications for health policy. Ann Intern Med 140:951, 2004

A review of evidence from randomized, controlled trials demonstrating that maintenance of modest weight loss through diet and physical activity reduces the incidence of type 2 diabetes in high-risk persons by about 40 to 60% over 3 to 4 years.

ZIMMET P et al: Global and societal implications of the diabetes epidemic. Nature 414:782, 2001

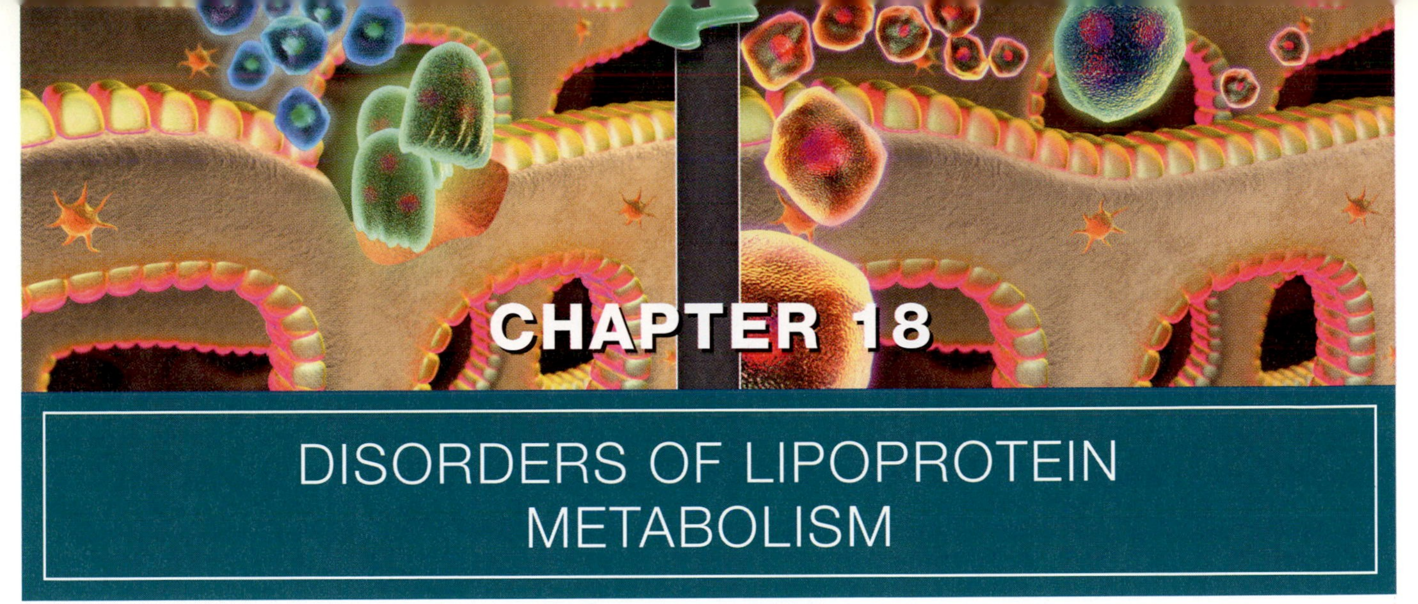

DISORDERS OF LIPOPROTEIN METABOLISM

Daniel J. Rader
Helen H. Hobbs

Lipoproteins are complexes of lipids and proteins that are essential for the transport of cholesterol, triglycerides, and fat-soluble vitamins. Until recently, lipoprotein disorders were the purview of lipidologists, but the demonstration that lipid-lowering therapy significantly reduces the clinical complications of atherosclerotic cardiovascular disease (ASCVD) has brought the diagnosis and treatment of these disorders into the domain of the general internist. The metabolic consequences associated with changes in diet and lifestyle have increased the number of hyperlipidemic individuals who could benefit from lipid-lowering therapy. The development of safe, effective, and well-tolerated pharmacologic agents has greatly expanded the therapeutic armamentarium available to the physician to treat disorders of lipid metabolism. Therefore, the appropriate diagnosis and management of lipid disorders is critically important to the practice of medicine. This chapter reviews normal lipoprotein physiology, the pathophysiology of the known single-gene disorders of lipoprotein metabolism, the environmental factors that influence lipoprotein metabolism, and the practical approaches to their diagnosis and management.

LIPOPROTEIN METABOLISM

LIPOPROTEIN CLASSIFICATION AND COMPOSITION

Lipoproteins are large, mostly spherical complexes that transport lipids (primarily triglycerides, cholesteryl esters, and fat-soluble vitamins) through body fluids (plasma, interstitial fluid, and lymph) to and from tissues. Lipoproteins play an essential role in the absorption of dietary cholesterol, long-chain fatty acids, and fat-soluble vitamins; the transport of triglycerides, cholesterol, and fat-soluble vitamins from the liver to peripheral tissues; and the transport of cholesterol from peripheral tissues to the liver.

Lipoproteins contain a core of hydrophobic lipids (triglycerides and cholesteryl esters) surrounded by hydrophilic lipids (phospholipids, unesterified cholesterol) and proteins that interact with body fluids. The plasma lipoproteins are divided into five major classes based on their relative densities (**Fig. 18-1** and **Table 18-1**): chylomicrons, very low density lipoproteins (VLDL), intermediate-density lipoproteins (IDL), low-density lipoproteins (LDL), and high-density lipoproteins (HDL). Each lipoprotein class comprises a family of

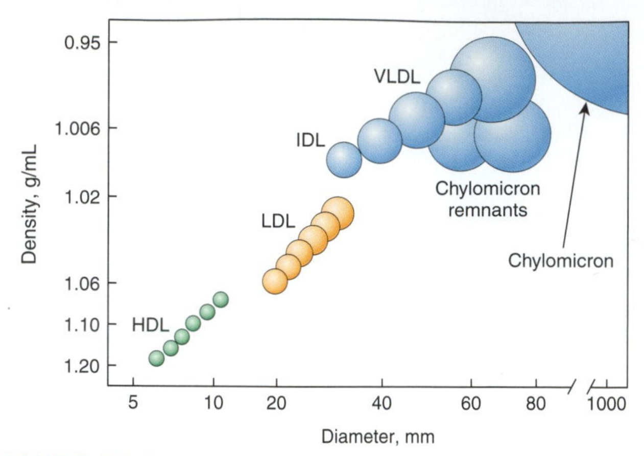

FIGURE 18-1

The density and size-distribution of the major classes of lipoprotein particles. Lipoproteins are classified by density and size, which are inversely related. VLDL, very low density lipoproteins; IDL, intermediate-density lipoproteins; LDL, low-density lipoproteins; HDL, high-density lipoproteins.

particles that vary slightly in density, size, migration during electrophoresis, and protein composition. The density of a lipoprotein is determined by the amount of lipid and protein per particle. HDL is the smallest and most dense lipoprotein, whereas chylomicrons and VLDL are the largest and least dense lipoprotein particles. Most triglyceride is transported in chylomicrons or VLDL, and most cholesterol is carried as cholesteryl esters in LDL and HDL.

The apolipoproteins are required for the assembly and structure of lipoproteins (**Table 18-2**). Apolipoproteins also serve to activate enzymes important in lipoprotein metabolism and to mediate the binding of lipoproteins to cell-surface receptors. ApoA-I, which is synthesized in the liver and intestine, is found on virtually all HDL particles. ApoA-II is the second most abundant HDL apolipoprotein and is found on approximately two-thirds of all HDL particles. ApoB is the major structural protein of chylomicrons, VLDL, IDL, and LDL; one molecule of apoB, either apoB-48 (chylomicrons) or apoB-100 (VLDL, IDL, or LDL), is present on each lipoprotein particle. The human liver makes only apoB-100, and the intestine makes apoB-48, which is derived from the same gene by mRNA editing. ApoE is present in multiple copies on chylomicrons, VLDL, and IDL and plays a critical role in the metabolism and clearance of triglyceride-rich particles. Three apolipoproteins of the C-series (apoC-I, -II, and -III) also participate in the metabolism of triglyceride-rich lipoproteins. The other apolipoproteins are listed in Table 18-2.

TRANSPORT OF DIETARY LIPIDS (EXOGENOUS PATHWAY)

The exogenous pathway of lipoprotein metabolism permits efficient transport of dietary lipids (**Fig. 18-2**). Dietary triglycerides are hydrolyzed by pancreatic lipases within the intestinal lumen and are emulsified with bile acids to form micelles. Dietary cholesterol and retinol are esterified (by the addition of a fatty acid) in the enterocyte to form cholesteryl esters and

TABLE 18-1

MAJOR LIPOPROTEIN CLASSES[a]

LIPOPROTEIN	DENSITY, G/ML[b]	SIZE NM[c]	ELECTROPHORETIC MOBILITY[d]	APOLIPOPROTEINS		OTHER CONSTITUENTS
				MAJOR	OTHER	
Chylomicrons	0.930	75–1200	Origin	ApoB-48	A-I, A-IV, C-I, C-II, C-III	Retinyl esters
Chylomicron remnants	0.930–1.006	30–80	Slow pre-β	ApoB-48	E, A-I, A-IV, C-I, C-II, C-III	Retinyl esters
VLDL	0.930–1.006	30–80	Pre-β	ApoB-100	E, A-I, A-II, A-V, C-I, C-II, C-III	Vitamin E
IDL	1.006–1.019	25–35	Slow pre-β	ApoB-100	E, C-I, C-II, C-III	Vitamin E
LDL	1.019–1.063	18–25	β	ApoB-100		Vitamin E
HDL	1.063–1.210	5–12	α	ApoA-I	A-II, A-IV, E, C-III	LCAT, CETP paroxonase
Lp(a)	1.050–1.120	25	Pre-β	ApoB-100	Apo(a)	

[a]All of the lipoprotein classes contain phospholipids, esterified and unesterified cholesterol, and triglycerides to varying degrees.
[b]The density of the particle is determined by ultracentrifugation.
[c]The size of the particle is measured using gel electrophoresis.
[d]The electrophoretic mobility of the particle on agarose gel electrophoresis reflects the size and surface charge of the particle, with β being the position of LDL and α the position of HDL.

Note: VLDL, very low density lipoprotein; IDL, intermediate-density lipoprotein; LDL, low-density lipoprotein: HDL, high-density lipoprotein; Lp(a), lipoprotein A; LCAT, lecithin-cholesterol acyltransferase; CETP, cholesteryl ester transfer protein.

TABLE 18-2

MAJOR APOLIPOPROTEINS

APOLIPOPROTEIN	PRIMARY SOURCE	LIPOPROTEIN ASSOCIATION	FUNCTION
ApoA-I	Intestine, liver	HDL, chylomicrons	Structural protein for HDL, activates LCAT
ApoA-II	Liver	HDL, chylomicrons	Structural protein for HDL
ApoA-IV	Intestine	HDL, chylomicrons	Unknown
ApoA-V	Liver	VLDL	Unknown
ApoB-48	Intestine	Chylomicrons	Structural protein for chylomicrons
ApoB-100	Liver	VLDL, IDL, LDL, LP(a)	Structural protein for VLDL, LDL, IDL, LP(a); ligand for binding to LDL, receptor
ApoC-I	Liver	Chylomicrons VLDL, HDL	Unknown
ApoC-II	Liver	Chylomicrons VLDL, HDL	Cofactor for LPL
ApoC-III	Liver	Chylomicrons VLDL, HDL	Inhibits lipoprotein binding to receptors
ApoD	Spleen, brain, testes, adrenals	HDL	Unknown
ApoE	Liver	Chylomicron remnants, IDL, HDL	Ligand for binding to LDL receptor
ApoH	Liver	Chylomicrons VLDL, LDL, HDL	B_2 glycoprotein I
ApoJ	Liver	HDL	Unknown
ApoL	Unknown	HDL	Unknown
Apo(a)	Liver	Lp(a)	Unknown

Note: HDL, high-density lipoprotein; LCAT, lecithin-cholesterol acyltransferase; VLDL, very low density lipoprotein; IDL, intermediate-density lipoprotein; LDL, low-density lipoprotein; Lp(a), lipoprotein A; LPL, lipoprotein lipase.

retinyl esters, respectively. Longer-chain fatty acids (>12 carbons) are incorporated into triglycerides and packaged with apoB-48, cholesteryl esters, retinyl esters, phospholipids, and cholesterol to form chylomicrons. Nascent chylomicrons are secreted into the intestinal lymph and delivered directly to the systemic circulation, where they are extensively processed by peripheral tissues before reaching the liver. The particles encounter lipoprotein lipase (LPL), which is anchored to proteoglycans that decorate the capillary endothelial surfaces of adipose tissue, heart, and skeletal muscle (Fig. 18-2). The triglycerides of chylomicrons are hydrolyzed by LPL, and free fatty acids are released; apoC-II, which is transferred to circulating chylomicrons, acts as a cofactor for LPL in this reaction. The released free fatty acids are taken up by adjacent myocytes or adipocytes and either oxidized or reesterified and stored as triglyceride. Some free fatty acids bind albumin and are transported to other tissues, especially the liver. The chylomicron particle progressively shrinks in size as the hydrophobic core is hydrolyzed and the hydrophilic lipids (cholesterol and phospholipids) on the particle surface are transferred to HDL. The resultant smaller, more cholesterol ester–rich particles are referred to as *chylomicron remnants*. The remnant particles are rapidly removed from the circulation by the liver in a process that requires apoE. Consequently, few, if any, chylomicrons are present in the blood after a 12-h fast, except in individuals with disorders of chylomicron metabolism.

TRANSPORT OF HEPATIC LIPIDS (ENDOGENOUS PATHWAY)

The *endogenous pathway of lipoprotein metabolism* refers to the hepatic secretion and metabolism of VLDL to IDL and LDL (Fig. 18-2). VLDL particles resemble chylomicrons in protein composition but contain apoB-100 rather than apoB-48 and have a higher ratio of cholesterol to triglyceride (~1 mg of cholesterol for every 5 mg of triglyceride). The triglycerides of VLDL are derived predominantly from the esterification of long-chain fatty acids. The packaging of hepatic triglycerides with the other major components of the nascent VLDL particle (apoB-100, cholesteryl esters, phospholipids, and vitamin E) requires the action of the enzyme microsomal transfer protein (MTP). After secretion into the plasma, VLDL acquires multiple copies of apoE and apolipoproteins of the C series. The triglycerides of VLDL are hydrolyzed by LPL, especially in muscle and adipose tissue. As VLDL remnants undergo further hydrolysis, they continue to shrink in size and become

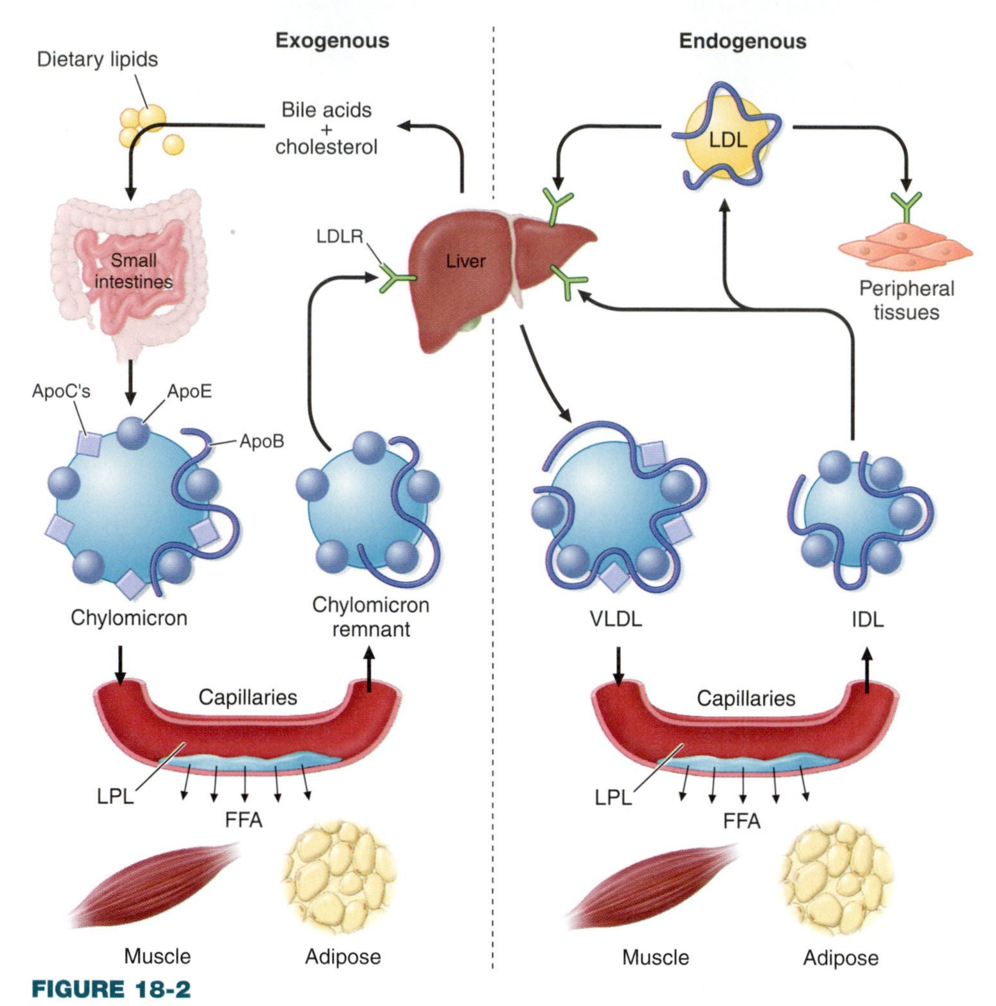

FIGURE 18-2

The exogenous and endogenous lipoprotein metabolic pathways. The exogenous pathway transports dietary lipids to the periphery and the liver. The exogenous pathway transports hepatic lipids to the periphery. LPL, lipoprotein lipase; FFA, free fatty acids; VLDL, very low density lipoproteins; IDL, intermediate-density lipoproteins; LDL, low-density lipoproteins; LDLR, low-density lipoprotein receptor.

IDL, which contain similar amounts of cholesterol and triglyceride. The liver removes ~40 to 60% of VLDL remnants and IDL by LDL receptor–mediated endocytosis via binding to apoE. The remainder of IDL is remodeled by hepatic lipase (HL) to form LDL; during this process, most of the triglyceride in the particle is hydrolyzed and all apolipoproteins except apoB-100 are transferred to other lipoproteins. The cholesterol in LDL accounts for ~70% of the plasma cholesterol in most individuals. Approximately 70% of circulating LDLs are cleared by LDL receptor–mediated endocytosis in the liver. Lipoprotein(a) [Lp(a)] is a lipoprotein similar to LDL in lipid and protein composition, but it contains an additional protein called apolipoprotein(a) [apo(a)]. Apo(a) is synthesized in the liver and is attached to apoB-100 by a disulfide linkage. The mechanism by which Lp(a) is removed from the circulation is not known.

HDL METABOLISM AND REVERSE CHOLESTEROL TRANSPORT

All nucleated cells synthesize cholesterol but only hepatocytes can efficiently metabolize and excrete cholesterol from the body. The predominant route of cholesterol elimination is by excretion into the bile, either directly or after conversion to bile acids. Cholesterol in peripheral cells is transported from the plasma membranes of peripheral cells to the liver by an HDL-mediated process termed *reverse cholesterol transport* (**Fig. 18-3**).

Nascent HDL particles are synthesized by the intestine and the liver. The newly formed discoidal HDL particles contain apoA-I and phospholipids (mainly lecithin) but rapidly acquire unesterified cholesterol and additional phospholipids from peripheral tissues via transport by the membrane protein ATP-binding

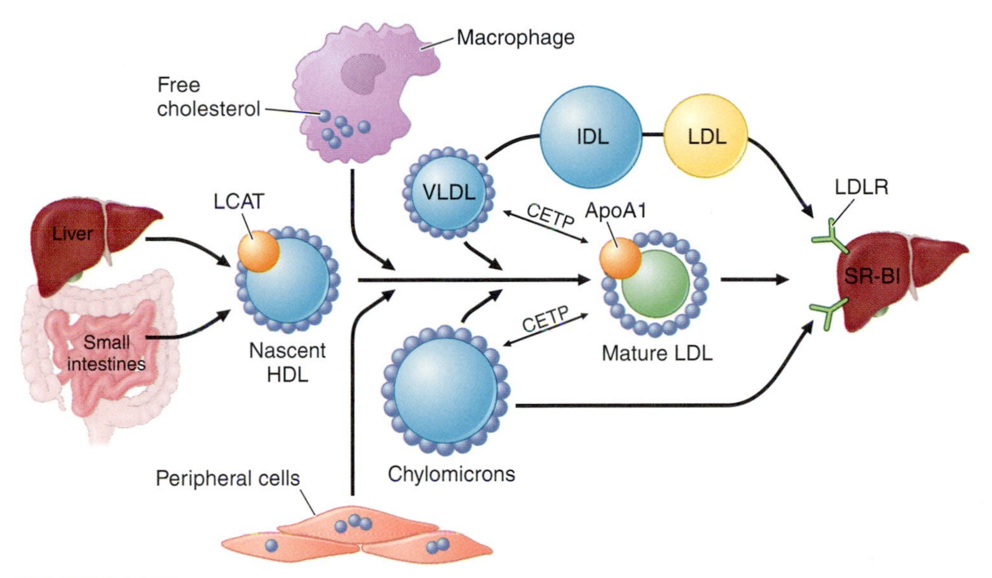

FIGURE 18-3

HDL metabolism and reverse cholesterol transport. This pathway transports excess cholesterol from the periphery back to the liver for excretion in the bile. The liver and the intestine produce nascent HDL. Free cholesterol is acquired from macrophages and other peripheral cells and esterfied by LCAT, forming mature HDL. HDL cholesterol can be selectively taken up by the liver via SR-BI. Alternatively, HDL cholesteryl ester can be transferred by CETP from HDL to VLDL and chylomicrons, which can then be taken up by the liver. LCAT, lecithin-cholesterol acyltransferase; CETP, cholesteryl ester transfer protein; VLDL, very low density lipoproteins; IDL, intermediate-density lipoproteins; LDL, low-density lipoproteins; HDL, high-density lipoproteins; LDLR, low-density lipoprotein receptor; TG, triglycerides; SR-B1, scavenger receptor class B1.

cassette protein A1 (ABCA1). Once incorporated in the HDL particle, cholesterol is esterified by lecithin-cholesterol acyltransferase (LCAT), a plasma enzyme associated with HDL. As HDL acquires more cholesteryl ester it becomes spherical, and additional apolipoproteins and lipids are transferred to the particles from the surfaces of chylomicrons and VLDL during lipolysis.

HDL cholesterol is transported to hepatoctyes by both an indirect and a direct pathway. HDL cholesteryl esters are transferred to apoB-containing lipoproteins in exchange for triglyceride by the cholesteryl ester transfer protein (CETP). The cholesteryl esters are then removed from the circulation by LDL receptor–mediated endocytosis. HDL cholesterol can also be taken up directly by hepatocytes via the scavenger receptor class BI (SR-BI), a cell-surface receptor that mediates the selective transfer of lipids to cells.

HDL particles undergo extensive remodeling within the plasma compartment as they transfer lipids and proteins to lipoproteins and cells. For example, after CETP-mediated lipid exchange, the triglyceride-enriched HDL becomes a substrate for HL, which hydrolyzes the triglycerides and phospholipids to generate smaller HDL particles.

DISORDERS OF LIPOPROTEIN METABOLISM

The identification and characterization of genes responsible for the genetic forms of hyperlipidemia have provided important molecular insight into the critical roles of apolipoproteins, enzymes, and receptors in lipid metabolism.

PRIMARY DISORDERS OF ApoB-CONTAINING LIPOPROTEIN BIOSYNTHESIS CAUSING LOW PLASMA CHOLESTEROL LEVELS (KNOWN ETIOLOGY)

The synthesis and secretion of apoB-containing lipoproteins in the enterocytes of the proximal small bowel and in the hepatocytes of the liver involve a complex series of events that coordinate the coupling of various lipids with apoB-48 and apoB-100, respectively.

Abetalipoproteinemia

Abetalipoproteinemia is a rare autosomal recessive disease caused by mutations in the gene encoding MTP, which transfers lipids to nascent chylomicrons and VLDL in the intestine and liver, respectively. Plasma cholesterol and triglyceride levels are extremely low in this disorder, and no chylomicrons, VLDL, LDL, or apoB are detectable. The parents of patients with abetalipoproteinemia (who are obligate heterozygotes) have normal plasma lipid and apoB levels. Abetalipoproteinemia usually presents in early childhood with diarrhea and failure to thrive and is characterized clinically by fat malabsorption, spinocerebellar degeneration, pigmented retinopathy, and acanthocytosis. The initial neurologic manifestations are loss of deep-tendon reflexes, followed by decreased distal lower extremity vibratory and proprioceptive sense, dysmetria, ataxia, and the development of a spastic gait, often by the third or fourth decade. Patients with abetalipoproteinemia also develop a progressive pigmented retinopathy presenting with decreased night and color vision, followed by reductions in daytime visual acuity and ultimately progressing to near blindness. The presence of spinocerebellar degeneration and pigmented retinopathy in this disease has resulted in misdiagnosis of Friedreich's ataxia. Rarely, patients with abetalipoproteinemia develop a cardiomyopathy with associated life-threatening arrhythmias.

Most clinical manifestations of abetalipoproteinemia result from defects in the absorption and transport of fat-soluble vitamins. Vitamin E and retinyl esters are normally transported from enterocytes to the liver by chylomicrons, and vitamin E is dependent on VLDL for transport out of the liver and into the circulation. Patients with abetalipoproteinemia are markedly deficient in vitamin E and are also mildly to moderately deficient in vitamin A and vitamin K. Treatment of abetalipoproteinemia consists of a low-fat, high-caloric, vitamin-enriched diet accompanied by large supplemental doses of vitamin E. It is imperative for treatment to be initiated as soon as possible to obviate the development of neurologic sequelae.

Familial Hypobetalipoproteinemia

Familial homozygous hypobetalipoproteinemia has a clinical picture similar to abetalipoproteinemia but is autosomal codominant in inheritance pattern. The disease can be differentiated from abetalipoproteinemia since the parents of the probands with this disorder have levels of plasma LDL-C and apoB that are less than half of the normal levels. Mutations in the gene encoding apoB-100 that interfere with protein synthesis are common causes of this disorder. These patients, like those with abetalipoproteinemia, should be referred to specialized centers for confirmation of the diagnosis and appropriate therapy.

PRIMARY DISORDERS OF ApoB-CONTAINING LIPOPROTEIN CATABOLISM CAUSING ELEVATED PLASMA CHOLESTEROL LEVELS (KNOWN ETIOLOGY)

Single-gene defects can result in the accumulation of specific classes of lipoprotein particles. Mutations in genes encoding key proteins in the metabolism and clearance of apoB-containing lipoproteins cause type I (chylomicronemia), type II (elevations in LDL) and type III (elevations in IDL) hyperlipoproteinemias (**Table 18-3**).

Lipoprotein Lipase and ApoC-II Deficiency (Familial Chylomicronemia Syndrome; Type I Hyperlipoproteinemia)

LPL is required for the hydrolysis of triglycerides in chylomicrons and VLDL. ApoC-II is a cofactor for LPL (Fig. 18-2). Genetic deficiency of either LPL or apoC-II results in impaired lipolysis and profound elevations in plasma chylomicrons. These patients also have elevations in plasma VLDL, but chylomicronemia predominates. Normally chylomicrons are delipidated and removed from the circulation within 12 h of the last meal, but in LPL-deficient patients, the triglyceride-rich chylomicrons persist in the circulation for days. The fasting plasma is turbid, and if left at 4^0C for a few hours, the chylomicrons float to the top and form a creamy supernatant. In these disorders, called *familial chylomicronemia syndromes,* fasting triglyceride levels are almost invariably >11.3 μmol/L (1000 mg/dL). Fasting cholesterol levels are also usually elevated, but to a much less severe degree.

LPL deficiency is autosomal recessive and has a population frequency of ~1 in 1 million. ApoC-II deficiency is also recessive in inheritance pattern and is even less common than LPL deficiency. Multiple mutations in the LPL and apoC-II genes cause these diseases. Obligate LPL heterozygotes have normal or mild to moderate elevations in plasma triglyceride levels, whereas individuals heterozygous for mutation in apoC-II are not hypertriglyceridemic.

Both LPL and apoC-II deficiency usually present in childhood with recurrent episodes of severe abdominal pain caused by acute pancreatitis. On fundoscopic examination the retinal blood vessels are opalescent (*lipemia retinalis*). Eruptive xanthomas, which are small yellowish-white papules, often appear in clusters on the back, buttocks, and extensor surfaces of the arms and legs. These typically painless skin lesions may become pruritic as they regress. Hepatosplenomegaly results from the uptake of circulating chylomicrons by reticuloendothelial cells in the liver and spleen. For reasons unknown, some patients with persistent and pronounced chylomicronemia never develop pancreatitis, eruptive xanthomas, or hepatosplenomegaly. Premature

TABLE 18-3

PRIMARY HYPERLIPOPROTEINEMIAS CAUSED BY KNOWN SINGLE-GENE MUTATIONS

GENETIC DISORDER	GENE DEFECT	LIPOPROTEINS ELEVATED	CLINICAL FINDINGS	GENETIC TRANSMISSION	ESTIMATED INCIDENCE
Lipoprotein lipase deficiency	LPL(*LPL*)	Chylomicrons	Eruptive xanthomas, hepatosplenomegaly pancreatitis	AR	1/1,000,000
Familial apolipoprotein C-II deficiency	ApoC-II (*APOC2*)	Chylomicrons	Eruptive xanthomas, hepatosplenomegaly pancreatitis	AR	<1/1,000,000
Familial hepatic lipase deficiency	Hepatic lipase (*LIPC*)	VLDL remnants	Premature atherosclerosis	AR	<1/1,000,000
Familial dysbetalipoproteinemia	ApoE(*APOE*)	Chylomicron and VLDL remnants	Palmar and tuberoeruptive xanthomas, CHD, PVD	AR AD	1/10,000
Familial hypercholesterolemia	LDL receptor (*LDLR*)	LDL	Tendon xanthomas, CHD	AD	1/500
Familial defective apoB-100	ApoB-100 (*APOB*) ($Arg_{1500} \rightarrow Gln$)	LDL	Tendon xanthomas, CHD	AD	1/1000
Autosomal recessive hypercholesterolemia	ARH (*ARH*)	LDL	Tendon xanthomas, CHD	AR	<1/1,000,000
Sitosterolemia	*ABCG5* or *ABCG8*	LDL	Tendon xanthomas, CHD	AR	<1/1,000,000

Note: AR, autosomal recessive; AD, autosomal dominant; VLDL, very low density lipoprotein; CHD, coronary heart disease; PVD, peripheral vascular disease; LDL, low-density lipoprotein.

ASCVD has not been consistently demonstrated to be a feature of familial chylomicronemia syndromes.

The diagnoses of LPL and apoC-II deficiency are established enzymatically by assaying triglyceride lipolytic activity in post-heparin plasma. Blood is sampled after an intravenous heparin injection to release the endothelial-bound lipases. LPL activity is profoundly reduced in both LPL and apoC-II deficiency; in patients with apoC-II deficiency, the addition of normal pre-heparin plasma (a source of apoC-II) normalizes LPL activity, but this correction does not occur in patients with LPL deficiency.

The major therapeutic intervention in familial chylomicronemia syndromes is dietary fat restriction (to as little as 15 g/d) with fat-soluble vitamin supplementation. Consultation with a registered dietician familiar with this disorder is essential. Caloric supplementation with medium-chain triglycerides, which are absorbed directly into the portal circulation, can be useful but may be associated with hepatic fibrosis if used for prolonged periods. If dietary fat restriction alone is not successful in resolving the chylomicronemia, fish oils have been effective in some patients. In patients with apoC-II deficiency, apoC-II can be provided by infusing fresh-frozen plasma to resolve the chylomicronemia. Management of patients with familial chylomicronemia syndrome is particularly challenging during pregnancy when VLDL production is increased. Plasmapheresis may be required if pancreatitis develops and the chylomicronemia is not responsive to diet therapy.

Hepatic Lipase Deficiency

HL is a member of the same gene family as LPL and hydrolyzes triglycerides and phospholipids in remnant lipoproteins and HDL. HL deficiency is a very rare autosomal recessive disorder characterized by elevated plasma cholesterol and triglycerides (mixed hyperlipidemia) due to the accumulation of lipoprotein remnants. HDL-C is normal or elevated. The diagnosis is confirmed by measuring HL activity in post-heparin plasma. Due to the small number of patients with HL deficiency, the association of this genetic defect with ASCVD is not known, but lipid-lowering therapy is recommended.

Familial Dysbetalipoproteinemia (Type III Hyperlipoproteinemia)

Like HL deficiency, familial dysbetalipoproteinemia (FDBL) (also known as *type III hyperlipoproteinemia* or *familial broad β disease*) is characterized by a mixed hyperlipidemia due to the accumulation of remnant lipoprotein particles. ApoE is present in multiple copies on chylomicron and VLDL remnants and mediates their removal via hepatic lipoprotein receptors (Fig. 18-2). FDBL is due to genetic variations in apoE that interfere with its ability to bind lipoprotein receptors. The *APOE* gene is polymorphic in sequence resulting in the expression of three common isoforms: apoE3, apoE2, and apoE4. Although associated with slightly higher LDL-C levels and increased coronary heart disease (CHD) risk, the apoE4 allele is not associated with FDBL. Patients with apoE4 have an increased incidence of late-onset Alzheimer disease. ApoE2 has a lower affinity for the LDL receptor. Therefore, chylomicron and VLDL remnants containing apoE2 are removed from plasma at a slower rate. Individuals who are homozygous for the E2 allele (the E2/E2 genotype) comprise the most common subset of patients with FDBL.

Approximately 1% of the general population are apoE2/E2 homozygotes but only a small minority of these individuals develop FDBL. In most cases an additional, identifiable factor precipitates the development of hyperlipoproteinemia. The most common precipitating factors are a high-caloric, high-fat diet, diabetes mellitus, obesity, hypothyroidism, renal disease, estrogen deficiency, alcohol use, or the presence of another genetic form of hyperlipidemia, most commonly familial combined hyperlipidemia (FCHL) or familial hypercholesterolemia (FH). Rare mutations in apoE cause dominant forms of FDBL; in this case the hyperlipidemia is fully manifest in the heterozygous state.

Patients with FDBL usually present in adulthood with xanthomas and premature coronary and peripheral vascular disease. The disease seldom presents in women before menopause. Two distinctive types of xanthomas are seen in FDBL patients: tuberoeruptive and palmar xanthomas. *Tuberoeruptive xanthomas* begin as clusters of small papules on the elbows, knees, or buttocks and can grow to the size of small grapes. *Palmar xanthoma* (alternatively called *xanthomata striata palmaris*) are orange-yellow discolorations of the creases in the palms. In FDBL, the plasma cholesterol and triglyceride are elevated to a relatively similar degree until the triglyceride levels reach ~5.6 mol/L (~500 mg/dL), and then the triglycerides tends to be greater than cholesterol.

The traditional approach to diagnose this disorder is to use lipoprotein electrophoresis; in FDBL, the remnant lipoproteins accumulate in a broad β band. The preferred method to confirm the diagnosis of FDBL is to measure VLDL-C by ultracentrifugation and determine the ratio of VLDL-C to total plasma triglyceride; a ratio >0.30 is consistent with the diagnosis of FDBL. Protein methods (apoE phenotyping) or DNA-based methods (apoE genotyping) can be performed to confirm homozygosity for apoE2. However, absence of the apoE2/2 genotype does not rule out the diagnosis of FDBL, since other mutations in apoE can cause this condition.

Because FDBL is associated with increased risk of premature ASCVD, it should be treated aggressively. Other metabolic conditions that can worsen the hyperlipidemia (see above) should be actively treated. Patients with FDBL are typically very diet responsive and can respond dramatically to weight reduction and to low-cholesterol, low-fat diets. Alcohol intake should be curtailed. In postmenopausal women with FDBL, the dyslipidemia responds to estrogen-replacement therapy. HMG-CoA reductase inhibitors, fibrates, and niacin are all generally effective in the treatment of FDBL, and combination drug therapy is sometimes required.

Familial Hypercholesterolemia

FH is an autosomal codominant disorder characterized by elevated plasma LDL-C with normal triglycerides, tendon xanthomas, and premature coronary atherosclerosis. FH is caused by >750 mutations in the LDL receptor gene and has a higher incidence in certain populations, such as Afrikaners, Christian Lebanese, and French Canadians, due to the founder effect. The elevated levels of LDL-C in FH are due to delayed catabolism of LDL and its precursor particles from the blood, resulting in increased rates of LDL production. There is a major gene dose effect, in that individuals with two mutated LDL receptor alleles (FH homozygotes) are much more affected than those with one mutant allele (FH heterozygotes).

Homozygous FH occurs in approximately 1 in 1 million persons world-wide. Patients with homozygous FH can be classified into one of two groups based on the amount of LDL receptor activity measured in their skin fibroblasts: those patients with <2% of normal LDL receptor activity (receptor negative) and those patients with 2 to 25% of normal LDL receptor activity (receptor defective). Most patients with homozygous FH present in childhood with cutaneous xanthomas on the hands, wrists, elbows, knees, heels, or buttocks. Arcus cornea is usually present and some patients have xanthelasmas. Total cholesterol levels are usually >12.93 mmol/L (500 mg/dL) and can be >25.86 mmol/L (1000 mg/dL). Accelerated atherosclerosis is a devastating complication of homozygous FH and can result in disability and death in childhood. Atherosclerosis often develops first in the aortic root and can cause aortic valvular or supravalvular stenosis and typically extends into the coronary ostia. Children with homozygous FH often develop symptomatic vascular disease before puberty, when symptoms can be atypical and sudden death is common. Untreated, receptor-negative patients with homozygous FH rarely survive beyond the second decade; patients with receptor-defective LDL receptor defects have a better prognosis but almost invariably develop clinically apparent atherosclerotic vascular disease by age 30, and often much sooner. Carotid and femoral disease develop later in life and are usually not clinically significant.

A careful family history should be taken, and plasma lipid levels should be measured in the parents and other first-degree relatives of patients with homozygous FH. The diagnosis can be confirmed by obtaining a skin biopsy and measuring LDL receptor activity in cultured skin fibroblasts or by quantifying the number of LDL receptors on the surfaces of lymphocytes using cell-sorting technology.

Combination therapy with an HMG-CoA reductase inhibitor and a bile acid sequestrant sometimes results in modest reductions in plasma LDL-C in the FH homozygote. Patients with homozygous FH invariably require additional lipid-lowering therapy. Since the liver is quantitatively the most important tissue for removing circulating LDL via the LDL receptor, liver transplantation is effective in decreasing plasma LDL-C levels in this disorder. Liver transplantation is, however, associated with substantial risks, including the requirement for long-term immunosuppression. The current treatment of choice for homozygous FH is LDL apheresis (a process where the LDL particles are selectively removed from the circulation), which can promote regression of xanthomas and may slow the progression of atherosclerosis. Initiation of LDL apheresis should be delayed until ~5 years of age except when evidence of atherosclerotic vascular disease is present.

Heterozygous FH is caused by the inheritance of one mutant LDL receptor allele and occurs in ~1 in 500 persons worldwide, making it one of the most common single-gene disorders. It is characterized by elevated plasma LDL-C [usually 5.17 to 10.34 μmol/L (200 to 400 mg/dL)] and normal triglyceride levels. Patients with heterozygous FH have hypercholesterolemia from birth, although the disease is often not detected until adulthood, usually due to the detection of hypercholesterolemia on routine screening, the appearance of tendon xanthomas, or the premature development of symptomatic coronary atherosclerotic disease. Since the disease is codominant in inheritance and has a high penetrance (>90%), one parent and ~50% of the patient's siblings are usually hypercholesterolemic. The family history is frequently positive for premature ASCVD on one side of the family, particularly among male relatives. Corneal arcus is common, and tendon xanthomas involving the dorsum of the hands, elbows, knees, and especially the Achilles tendons are present in ~75% of patients. The age of onset of ASCVD is highly variable and depends in part on the molecular defect in the LDL receptor gene and other coexisting cardiac risk factors. FH heterozygotes with elevated plasma Lp(a) appear to be at greater risk for cardiovascular complications. Untreated men with heterozygous FH have an ~50% chance of having a myocardial infarction before age 60. Although the age of onset of atherosclerotic heart disease is later in women with FH, coronary disease is significantly more common in women with FH than in the general female population.

No definitive diagnostic test for heterozygous FH is available. Although FH heterozygotes tend to have reduced levels of LDL receptor function in skin fibroblasts, there is significant overlap with the levels in normal fibroblasts. The clinical diagnosis is usually not problematic, but it is critical that hypothyroidism, nephrotic syndrome, and obstructive liver disease be excluded before initiating therapy.

FH patients should be treated aggressively to lower plasma levels of LDL-C. Initiation of a low-cholesterol, low-fat diet is recommended, but heterozygous FH patients inevitably require lipid-lowering drug therapy. HMG-CoA reductase inhibitors are especially effective in heterozygous FH, inducing upregulation of the normal LDL receptor allele in the liver. Many heterozygous FH patients can achieve desired LDL-C levels with HMG-CoA reductase inhibitor therapy alone, but combination drug therapy with the addition of a bile acid sequestrant or nicotinic acid is frequently required. Heterozygous FH patients who cannot be adequately controlled on combination drug therapy are candidates for LDL apheresis.

Familial Defective ApoB-100

Familial defective apoB-100 (FDB) is a dominantly inherited disorder that clinically resembles heterozygous FH. FDB occurs with a frequency of ~1 in 1000 in western populations. The disease is characterized by elevated plasma LDL-C levels with normal triglycerides, tendon xanthomas, and an increased incidence of premature ASCVD. FDB is caused by mutations in the LDL receptor–binding domain of apoB-100. Almost all patients with FDB have a substitution of glutamine for arginine at position 3500 in apoB-100, although other rarer mutations have been reported to cause this disease. As a consequence of the mutation in apoB-100, LDL binds the LDL receptor with reduced affinity and LDL is removed from the circulation at a reduced rate. Patients with FDB cannot be clinically distinguished from patients with heterozygous FH, although patients with FDB tend to have lower plasma LDL-C than FH heterozygotes. The apoB-100 gene mutation can be detected directly, but currently genetic diagnosis is not encouraged since the recommended management of FDB and heterozygous FH is identical.

Autosomal Recessive Hypercholesterolemia

Autosomal recessive hypercholesterolemia (ARH) is a rare disorder (except in Sardinia) due to mutations in a protein (ARH) involved in LDL receptor–mediated endocytosis in the liver. ARH clinically resembles homozygous FH and is characterized by hypercholesterolemia, tendon xanthomas, and premature coronary artery disease. The hypercholesterolemia tends to be intermediate between the levels seen in FH homozygotes and FH heterozygotes. LDL receptor function in cultured fibroblasts is normal or only modestly reduced in ARH, whereas LDL receptor function in lymphocytes and the liver is negligible. Unlike FH homozygotes, the hyperlipidemia responds partially to treatment with HMG-CoA reductase inhibitors, but these patients usually require LDL apheresis to lower plasma LDL-C to recommended levels.

Wolman Disease and Cholesteryl Ester Storage Disease

Wolman disease is an autosomal recessive disorder caused by complete deficiency of lysosomal acid lipase. After LDL is taken up from the cell surface by LDL receptor–mediated endocytosis, it is delivered from endosomes to lysosomes. In the acidic environment of the endosome, the particle dissociates from the receptor, which recycles to the cell surface. In the lysosome, apoB-100 is degraded and the cholesteryl esters and triglycerides of LDL are hydrolyzed by lysosomal acid lipase. Patients with Wolman disease fail to hydrolyze the neutral lipids, resulting in their accumulation within cells. The disease presents within the first weeks of life with hepatosplenomegaly, steatorrhea, adrenal calcification, and failure to thrive. The disease is usually fatal within the first year of life and can be diagnosed by measuring acid lipase activity in fibroblasts or liver tissue biopsy specimens. Cholesteryl ester storage disease is a less severe form of the same genetic disorder in which there is low, but detectable, acid lipase activity. Patients with this disorder sometimes present in childhood with hepatomegaly and a mixed hyperlipidemia, due to elevations in the levels of plasma LDL and VLDL. Other patients present later in life with hepatic fibrosis, portal hypertension, or with premature atherosclerosis.

Sitosterolemia

Sitosterolemia is a rare autosomal recessive disease caused by mutations in one of two members of the adenosine triphosphate (ATP)-binding cassette transporter family, ABCG5 and ABCG8. These genes are expressed in the intestine and liver, where they form a functional complex to limit intestinal absorption and promote biliary excretion of plant- and animal-derived neutral sterols. In normal individuals, <5% of dietary plant sterols, of which sitosterol is the most plentiful, are absorbed by the proximal small intestine and delivered to the liver. Plant sterols in the liver are preferentially secreted into the bile, and plasma plant sterol levels are normally very low. In sitosterolemia, the intestinal absorption of plant sterols is increased and biliary excretion of the sterols is reduced, resulting in increased plasma levels of sitosterol and other plant sterols. The trafficking of cholesterol is also impaired. Patients with sitosterolemia can have either normal or elevated plasma levels of cholesterol. Irrespective of the plasma cholesterol level, these patients develop cutaneous and tendon xanthomas as well as premature atherosclerosis. Episodes of hemolysis, presumably secondary to the incorporation of plant sterols into the red blood cell membrane, are a distinctive clinical feature of this disease. The hypercholesterolemia in patients with sitosterolemia is unusually responsive to reductions in dietary cholesterol content. Sitosterolemia should be suspected when the plasma cholesterol level falls by >40% on a low-cholesterol diet (without associated weight loss).

Sitosterolemia is confirmed by demonstrating an elevated plasma sitosterol level. The hypercholesterolemia does not respond to HMG-CoA reductase inhibitors, but bile acid sequestrants and cholesterol-absorption inhibitors, such as ezetimibe, are effective in reducing plasma sterol levels in these patients.

PRIMARY DISORDERS OF ApoB-CONTAINING LIPOPROTEIN METABOLISM (UNKNOWN ETIOLOGY)

A large proportion of patients with elevated levels of apoB-containing lipoproteins have disorders in which the molecular defect has not been defined, largely because multiple other genetic and nongenetic factors contribute to the hyperlipidemia.

Familial Hypertriglyceridemia

Familial hypertriglyceridemia (FHTG) is a relatively common (1 in 500) autosomal dominant disorder of unknown etiology characterized by moderately elevated plasma triglycerides accompanied by more modest elevations in cholesterol. VLDL is the major class of lipoproteins elevated in this disorder, which is often referred to as type IV hyperlipoproteinemia (Frederickson classification, **Table 18-4**). The elevated plasma VLDL is due to increased VLDL production, impaired VLDL catabolism, or a combination of the two. Some patients with FHTG have a more severe form of hyperlipidemia in which both VLDL and chylomicrons are elevated (type V hyperlipidemia), as these two classes of lipopro-

TABLE 18-4

FREDERICKSON CLASSIFICATION OF HYPERLIPOPROTEINEMIAS

PHENOTYPE	I	IIa	IIb	III	IV	V
Lipoprotein elevated	Chylomicrons	LDL	LDL and VLDL	Chylomicron and VLDL remnants	VLDL	Chylomicrons and VLDL
Triglycerides	++++	−−	++	++ to +++	++	++++
Cholesterol	+ to ++	+++	++ to +++	++ to +++	−− to +	++ to +++
LDL-cholesterol	↓	↑	↑	↓	↓	↓
HDL-cholesterol	↓↓↓	↓	↓	−	↓↓	↓↓↓
Plasma appearance	Lactescent	Clear	Clear	Turbid	Turbid	Lactescent
Xanthomas	Eruptive	Tendon, tuberous	None	Palmar, tuberoeruptive	None	Eruptive
Pancreatitis	+++	0	0	0	0	+++
Coronary atherosclerosis	0	+++	+++	+++	+/−	+/−
Peripheral atherosclerosis	0	+	+	++	+/−	+/−
Molecular defects	LPL and apoC-II	LDL receptor and apoB-100	Unknown	ApoE	Unknown	Unknown
Genetic nomenclature	FCS	FH, FDB	FCHL	FDBL	FHTG	FHTG

Note: LPL, lipoprotein lipase; apo, apolipoprotein; FCS, familial chylomicronemia syndrome; FH, familial hypercholesterolemia; FDB, familiar defective apoB; FCHL, familial combined hyperlipidemia; FDBL, familial dysbetalipoproteinemia; FHTG, familial hypertriglyceridemia.

teins compete for the same lipolytic pathway. Increased intake of simple carbohydrates, obesity, insulin resistance, alcohol use, or estrogen treatment, all of which increase VLDL synthesis, can precipitate the development of chylomicronemia. FHTG does not appear to be associated with increased risk of ASCVD in many families.

The diagnosis of FHTG is suggested by the triad of elevated plasma triglycerides [2.8 to 11.3 mmol/L (250 to 1000 mg/dL)], normal or only mildly increased cholesterol levels [<6.5 mmol/L (<250 mg/dL)], and reduced plasma HDL-C. Plasma LDL-C is generally not increased and is often reduced due to defective metabolism of the triglyceride-rich particles. The identification of other first-degree relatives with hypertriglyceridemia is useful in making the diagnosis. FDBL and FCHL should also be ruled out as these two conditions are associated with a significantly increased risk of ASCVD. The plasma apoB levels and the ratio of plasma cholesterol to triglyceride tend to be lower in FHTG than in either FDBL or FCHL.

It is important to exclude secondary causes of the hypertriglyceridemia before making the diagnosis of FHTG. Lipid-lowering drug therapy can frequently be avoided with appropriate dietary and life-style changes. Patients with plasma triglyceride levels >4.5 to 6.8 mmol/L (>400 to 600 mg/dL), after a trial of diet and exercise, should be considered for drug therapy to avoid the development of chylomicronemia and pancreatitis. A fibrate is a reasonable first-line drug for FHTG, and niacin can also be considered in this condition.

Familial Combined Hyperlipidemia

The molecular etiology of FCHL is unknown but is likely to involve defects in several different genes. FCHL is the most common primary lipid disorder, occurring in ~1 in 200 persons. Approximately 20% of patients who develop CHD before age 60 have FCHL.

FCHL is characterized by moderate elevation of plasma triglycerides and cholesterol and reduced plasma HDL-C. The disease is autosomal dominant, and affected family members typically have one of three possible phenotypes: (1) elevated plasma LDL-C, (2) elevated plasma triglycerides and VLDL-C, or (3) elevated plasma LDL-C and VLDL-C. A classic feature of FCHL is that the lipoprotein phenotype can switch among these phenotypes. FCHL can manifest in childhood but is sometimes not fully expressed until adulthood. Visceral obesity, glucose intolerance, insulin resistance, hypertension, and hyperuricemia are often present. These patients do not develop xanthomas.

Patients with FCHL almost always have significantly elevated plasma apoB. The levels of apoB are disproportionately high relative to plasma LDL-C due to the presence of small dense LDL particles, which are characteristic of this syndrome and are highly atherogenic. *Hyperapobetalipoproteinemia* has been used as a term to de-scribe the coupling of elevated plasma apoB with normal plasma cholesterol, and is probably a form of FCHL.

A mixed dyslipidemia [plasma triglyceride levels between 2.3 and 9.0 mmol/L (200 and 800 mg/dL), cholesterol levels between 5.2 and 10.3 mmol/L (200 and 400 mg/dL), and HDL-C levels <10.3 mmol/L (<40 mg/dL)] and a family history of hyperlipidemia and/or premature CHD suggests the diagnosis of FCHL. An elevated plasma apoB level or an increased number of small dense LDL particles in the plasma supports this diagnosis. FDBL should be considered and ruled out by beta-quantification in suspected patients with a mixed hyperlipidemia.

Individuals with FCHL should be treated aggressively due to significantly increased risk of premature CHD. Decreased dietary intake of saturated fat and simple carbohydrates, aerobic exercise, and weight loss have beneficial effects on the lipid profile. Patients with diabetes should be aggressively treated to maintain good glucose control. Most patients with FCHL require lipid-lowering drug therapy to reduce lipoprotein levels to the recommended range. HMG-CoA reductase inhibitors are very effective in lowering plasma levels of LDL-C and can also significantly reduce VLDL-C. Nicotinic acid decreases both LDL-C and VLDL-C, while raising plasma HDL-C, and is frequently effective for this condition when used in combination with HMG-CoA reductase inhibitors.

Polygenic Hypercholesterolemia

Polygenic hypercholesterolemia is characterized by hypercholesterolemia with a normal plasma triglyceride in the absence of secondary causes of hypercholesterolemia. Plasma LDL-C levels are not as elevated as they are in FH and FDB. Family studies are useful to differentiate polygenic hypercholesterolemia from the single-gene disorders described above; half of the first-degree relatives of patients with FH and FDB are hypercholesterolemic, whereas <10% of first-degree relatives of patients with polygenic hypercholesterolemia are hypercholesterolemic. Treatment of polygenic hypercholesterolemia is identical to that of other forms of hypercholesterolemia.

GENETIC DISORDERS OF HDL METABOLISM (KNOWN ETIOLOGY)

Mutations in certain genes encoding critical proteins in HDL synthesis and catabolism cause marked variations in plasma HDL-C levels. Unlike the genetic forms of hypercholesterolemia, which are invariably associated with premature coronary atherosclerosis, genetic forms of hypoalphalipoproteinemia (low HDL-C) are not always associated with accelerated atherosclerosis. Whereas high plasma LDL-C is invariably associated with increased atherosclerosis, the risk associated with low plasma levels of HDL-C depends on the underlying mechanism. Analysis of the genetic disorders of HDL metabolism has provided insights into the less well understood etiologic relationship between plasma HDL-C levels and atherosclerosis.

ApoA-I Deficiency and ApoA-I Mutations

Complete genetic deficiency of apoA-I due to mutations in the apoA-I gene results in the virtual absence of HDL from the plasma. The genes encoding apoA-I, apoC-III, apoA-IV, and apoA-V are clustered together on chromosome 11, and some patients with complete absence of apoA-I have deletions that include more than one of these genes. Because apoA-I is required for LCAT function, plasma and tissue levels of free cholesterol are increased, resulting in the development of corneal opacities and planar xanthomas. Clinically apparent coronary atherosclerosis typically appears between the fourth and seventh decade in the apoA-I-deficient patient.

Although missense mutations in the apoA-I gene have been identified in selected patients with low plasma HDL [usually 0.39 to 0.78 mmol/L (15 to 30 mg/dL)], they are very rare causes of low HDL-C levels in the general population. Patients with apoA-I$_{\text{Milano}}$ have very low plasma levels of HDL due to the rapid catabolism of the apolipoprotein, but these patients do not have an increased risk of premature CHD. Other than corneal opacities, most individuals with low plasma HDL-C levels due to missense mutations in apoA-I have no clinical sequelae. A few specific mutations in apoA-I cause systemic amyloidosis, and the mutant apoA-I has been found as a component of the amyloid plaque.

Tangier Disease

Tangier disease is a rare autosomal codominant form of low plasma HDL-C caused by mutations in the gene encoding ABCA1, a cellular transporter that facilitates efflux of unesterified cholesterol and phospholipids from cells to apoA-I (Fig. 18-3). ABCA1 plays a critical role in the generation and stabilization of the mature HDL particle. In its absence, HDL is rapidly cleared from the circulation. Patients with Tangier disease have plasma HDL-C levels <0.13 mmol/L (<5 mg/dL) and extremely low circulating levels of apoA-I. The disease is associated with cholesterol accumulation in the reticuloendothelial system, resulting in hepatosplenomegaly and pathognomonic enlarged, grayish yellow or orange tonsils. An intermittent peripheral neuropathy (mononeuritis multiplex) or a sphingomyelia-like neurologic disorder can also be seen in this disorder. Tangier disease is associated with premature atherosclerotic disease, but the risk is not as high as might be anticipated given the markedly decreased plasma HDL-C and apoA-I. Plasma LDL-C is also low and this may attenuate the atherosclerotic risk. Obligate heterozygotes for ABCA1 mutations have moderately reduced plasma HDL-C levels and are also at increased risk of premature CHD.

LCAT Deficiency

LCAT deficiency is a rare disorder caused by mutations in lecithin-cholesterol acyltransferase (Fig. 18-3). LCAT is synthesized in the liver and secreted into the plasma, where it circulates associated with lipoproteins. Because the enzyme mediates the esterification of cholesterol, the proportion of free cholesterol in circulating lipoproteins is greatly increased (from ~25% to >70% of total plasma cholesterol). Lack of normal cholesterol esterification impairs the formation of mature HDL particles and leads to rapid catabolism of circulating apoA-I. Two genetic forms of LCAT deficiency have been described in humans—complete deficiency (also called *classic LCAT deficiency*) and partial deficiency (also called *fish-eye disease*). Progressive corneal opacification due to the deposition of free cholesterol in the lens, very low plasma HDL-C [usually <0.26 mmol/L (<10 mg/dL)], and variable hypertriglyceridemia are characteristic of both types. In partial LCAT deficiency, there are no other known clinical sequelae. In contrast, complete LCAT deficiency is characterized by a hemolytic anemia and progressive renal insufficiency that eventually leads to end-stage renal disease (ESRD). Despite the extremely low plasma levels of HDL-C and apoA-I, premature ASCVD is not a feature of either complete or partial LCAT deficiency, once again exemplifying the complex relationship between low plasma levels of HDL-C and the development of ASCVD. The diagnosis can be confirmed by assaying LCAT activity in the plasma.

CETP Deficiency

Mutations in the gene encoding cholesteryl ester transfer protein (CETP) cause a high HDL-C condition called *CETP deficiency*. CETP facilitates the transfer of cholesteryl esters among lipoproteins, especially from HDL to apoB-containing lipoproteins in exchange for triglycerides (Fig. 18-3). Homozygous deficiency of CETP, which occurs predominantly in Japan, results in very high plasma HDL-C [>3.88 mmol/L (>150 mg/dL)] due to accumulation of large, cholesterol-rich HDL particles. Heterozygotes for CETP deficiency have only modestly elevated HDL-C. The relationship of CETP deficiency to risk of ASCVD remains a matter of debate.

PRIMARY DISORDERS OF HDL METABOLISM (UNKNOWN ETIOLOGY)

The gene defect in other individuals with either very high or very low plasma HDL-C is not known.

Primary Hypoalphalipoproteinemia

The most common inherited cause of low plasma HDL-C is termed *primary* or *familial hypoalphalipoproteinemia*. Hypoalphalipoproteinemia is defined as a plasma HDL-C level below the 10th percentile in the setting of relatively normal cholesterol and triglyceride levels, no apparent secondary causes of low plasma HDL-C, and no clinical signs of LCAT deficiency or Tangier disease. This syndrome is often referred to as "isolated low HDL." A family history of low HDL-C facilitates the diagnosis of an inherited condition, which usually follows an autosomal dominant pattern. The metabolic etiology of this disease appears to be primarily accelerated catabolism of HDL and its apolipoproteins. Several kindreds with primary hypoalphalipoproteinemia have been described in association with an increased incidence of premature ASCVD.

Familial Hyperalphalipoproteinemia

Familial hyperalphalipoproteinemia has a dominant inheritance pattern. Plasma HDL-C is usually >2.07 mmol/L (80 mg/dL) in affected women and >1.81 mmol/L (70 mg/dL) in affected men. The genetic basis of primary hyperalphalipoproteinemia is not known, and the condition may be associated with decreased risk of CHD and increased longevity in some cases.

SECONDARY DISORDERS OF LIPOPROTEIN METABOLISM

Significant changes in plasma levels of lipoproteins are seen in a variety of diseases. It is critical that secondary causes of hyperlipidemias (**Table 18-5**) are considered prior to initiation of lipid-lowering therapy.

Obesity

Obesity is frequently, though not invariably, accompanied by hyperlipidemia. The increase in adipocyte mass and accompanying decrease in insulin sensitivity associated with obesity have multiple effects on lipid metabolism.

TABLE 18-5

SECONDARY FORMS OF HYPERLIPIDEMIA

LDL		HDL					
ELEVATED	REDUCED	ELEVATED	REDUCED	VLDL ELEVATED	IDL ELEVATED	CHYLOMICRONS ELEVATED	LP(A) ELEVATED
Hypothyroidism Nephrotic syndrome Cholestasis Acute intermittent porphyria Anorexia nervosa Hepatoma Drugs: thiazides, cyclosporine, tegretol	Severe liver disease Malabsorption Malnutrition Gaucher disease Chronic infectious disease Hyperthyroidisim Drugs: niacin toxicity	Alcohol Exercise Exposure to chlorinated hydrocarbons Drugs: estrogen	Smoking DM type 2 Obesity Malnutrition Gaucher disease Drugs: anabolic steroids, beta blockers	Obesity DM type 2 Glycogen storage disease Hepatitis Alcohol Renal failure Sepsis Stress Cushing syndrome Pregnancy Acromegaly Lipodystrophy Drugs: estrogen, beta blockers, furosemide, glucocrticoids, bile acid –binding resins, retinoic acid, HIV protease inhibitors	Multiple myeloma Monoclonal gammopathy Autoimmune disease Hypothyroidism	Autoimmune disease Drug: Isotretinoin	Renal insufficiency Inflammation Menopause Orchidectomy Hypothyroidism Acromegaly Nephrosis Drugs: growth hormone

Note: LDL, low-density lipoprotein; HDL, high-density lipoprotein; VLDL, very low density lipoprotein; IDL, intermediate-density lipoprotein; Lp(a), lipoprotein A; DM, diabetes mellitus.

More free fatty acids are delivered from the expanded adipose tissue to the liver where they are re-esterified in hepatocytes to form triglycerides, which are packaged into VLDL for secretion into the circulation. High dietary intake of simple carbohydrates also drives hepatic production of VLDL, leading to increases in VLDL and/or LDL in some obese individuals. Plasma HDL-C tends to be low in obesity. Weight loss is often associated with a reduction of plasma apoB-containing lipoproteins and an increase of plasma HDL-C.

Diabetes Mellitus

Patients with type 1 diabetes mellitus are generally not hyperlipidemic if they are under good glycemic control. Diabetic ketoacidosis is frequently accompanied by hypertriglyceridemia due to increased hepatic influx of free fatty acids from adipose tissue. The hypertriglyceridemia responds dramatically to administration of insulin in the insulinopenic diabetic.

Patients with type 2 diabetes mellitus are usually dyslipidemic, even if under relatively good glycemic control. The high levels of insulin and insulin resistance associated with type 2 diabetes have multiple effects on fat metabolism: (1) a decrease in LPL activity resulting in reduced catabolism of chylomicrons and VLDL, (2) an increase in the release of free fatty acid from the adipose tissue, (3) an increase in fatty acid synthesis in the liver, and (4) an increase in hepatic VLDL production. Patients with type 2 diabetes mellitus have several lipid abnormalities, including elevated plasma triglycerides (due to increased VLDL and lipoprotein remnants), elevated dense LDL, and decreased HDL-C. In some diabetic patients, especially those with a genetic defect in lipid metabolism, the triglycerides can be extremely elevated. Elevated plasma LDL-C levels are usually not a feature of diabetes mellitus and suggest the presence of an underlying lipoprotein abnormality or may indicate the development of diabetic nephropathy. Patients with lipodystrophy, who have profound insulin resistance, have markedly elevated VLDL and chylomicrons.

Thyroid Disease

Hypothyroidism is associated with elevated plasma LDL-C due primarily to a reduction in hepatic LDL receptor function and delayed clearance of LDL. Conversely, plasma LDL-C is often reduced in the hyperthyroid patient. Hypothyroid patients may have increased circulating IDL, and some are mildly hypertriglyceridemic [<3.34 μmol/L (<300 mg/dL)]. Because hypothyroidism is easily overlooked, all patients presenting with elevated plasma LDL-C or IDL should be screened for hypothyroidism. Thyroid replacement therapy usually ameliorates the hypercholesterolemia.

Renal Disorders

Nephrotic syndrome is associated with hyperlipoproteinemia, which is usually mixed but can manifest as hypercholesterolemia or hypertriglyceridemia alone. The hyperlipidemia of nephrotic syndrome appears to be due to a combination of increased hepatic production and decreased clearance of VLDL, with increased LDL production. Effective treatment of the underlying renal disease normalizes the lipid profile, but most patients with chronic nephrotic syndrome require lipid-lowering drug therapy.

ESRD is often associated with mild hypertriglyceridemia [<3.34 μmol/L (<300 mg/dL)] due to the accumulation of VLDL and remnant lipoproteins in the circulation. Triglyceride lipolysis and remnant clearance are both reduced in patients with renal failure. Because the risk of ASCVD is increased in hyperlipidemic patients with ESRD, they should be treated aggressively with lipid-lowering agents.

Patients with renal transplants are usually hyperlipidemic due to immunosuppression drugs (cyclosporine and glucocorticoids); they present a difficult management problem as HMG-CoA reductase inhibitors must be used cautiously in these patients.

Liver Disorders

Because the liver is the principal site of formation and clearance of lipoproteins, it is not surprising that liver diseases can profoundly affect plasma lipid levels in a variety of ways. Hepatitis due to infection, drugs, or alcohol is often associated with increased VLDL synthesis and mild to moderate hypertriglyceridemia. Severe hepatitis and liver failure are associated with dramatic reductions in plasma cholesterol and triglycerides due to reduced lipoprotein biosynthetic capacity. Cholestasis is associated with hypercholesterolemia, which sometimes can be very severe. The major pathway by which cholesterol is excreted is via secretion into bile, either directly or after conversion to bile acids. Cholestasis blocks this critical excretory pathway. In cholestasis, free cholesterol coupled with phospholipids are secreted into the plasma as constituents of a lamellar particle called *Lp(X)*. These particles can deposit in skin folds, producing lesions resembling those seen in patients with FDBL (xanthomata strata palmaris). Planar and eruptive xanthomas can also be seen in patients with cholestasis.

Alcohol

Regular alcohol consumption has a variable effect on plasma lipid levels. The most common effect of alcohol is to increase plasma triglyceride levels. Alcohol consumption stimulates hepatic secretion of VLDL, possibly by inhibiting the hepatic oxidation of free fatty acids, which then promote hepatic triglyceride synthesis and VLDL secretion. The usual lipoprotein pattern seen with alcohol consumption is type IV (increased VLDL), but persons with an underlying primary lipid disorder may develop severe hypertriglyceridemia (type V) if they drink alcohol. Regular alcohol use is also associated with a mild to moderate increase in plasma levels of HDL-C.

Estrogen

Estrogen administration is associated with increased VLDL and HDL synthesis resulting in elevated plasma triglycerides and HDL-C. This lipoprotein pattern is distinctive since the levels of plasma triglyceride and HDL-C are typically inversely related. Estrogen treatment may convert a person with type IV to type V hyperlipidemia. Plasma triglyceride levels should be monitored when birth control pills or estrogen replacement therapy is initiated. Use of low-dose estrogen preparations or the estrogen patch can minimize the effect of exogenous estrogen on lipids.

Glycogen Storage Diseases

Other rarer causes of secondary hyperlipidemias include glycogen storage diseases such as *von Gierke's disease,* which is caused by mutations in glucose-6-phosphatase. The inability to mobilize hepatic glucose during fasting results in hypoinsulinemia and increased release of free fatty acids from adipose tissue. Hepatic fatty acids synthesis is also increased, resulting in fat accumulation in the liver and increased VLDL secretion. The hyperlipidemia associated with this disease can be very severe but responds well to treatment of the underlying disorder.

Cushing Syndrome

Glucocorticoid excess is associated with increased VLDL synthesis and hypertriglyceridemia. Patients with Cushing syndrome can also have mild elevations in plasma LDL-C.

Drugs

Many drugs have a significant impact on lipid metabolism and can result in significant alterations in the lipoprotein profile (Table 18-5).

SCREENING

Guidelines for the screening and management of lipid disorders have been provided by an expert Adult Treatment Panel (ATP) convened by the National Cholesterol

Education Program (NCEP) of the National Heart Lung and Blood Institute. The NCEP ATPIII guidelines published in 2001 recommend that all adults over age 20 have plasma levels of cholesterol, triglyceride, LDL-C, and HDL-C measured after a 12-h overnight fast. In most clinical laboratories, the total cholesterol and triglycerides in the plasma are measured enzymatically and then the cholesterol in the supernatant is measured after precipitation of apoB-containing lipoproteins to determine the HDL-C. The LDL-C is estimated using the following equation:

$$\text{LDL-C} = \text{total cholesterol} - (\text{triglycerides}/5) - \text{HDL-C}$$

The VLDL-C is estimated by dividing the plasma triglyceride by 5, reflecting the ratio of cholesterol to triglyceride in VLDL particles. This formula is reasonably accurate if test results are obtained on fasting plasma and if the triglyceride level $<\sim 4.0$ μmol/L (350 mg/dL). The accurate determination of LDL-C levels in patients with triglyceride levels greater than this requires application of ultracentrifugation techniques (beta quantification), although direct assays for LDL-C are also available in some laboratories.

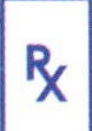

TREATMENT FOR CHD

Multiple epidemiologic studies have demonstrated a strong relationship between serum cholesterol and CHD. Randomized controlled clinical trials have unequivocally documented that lowering plasma cholesterol reduces the risk of clinical events due to atherosclerosis. Although the proportional benefit accrued from reducing plasma LDL-C is similar over the entire range of LDL-C values, the absolute risk reduction depends on the baseline LDL-C, the presence of established CHD, and other cardiovascular risk factors.

Elevated plasma triglyceride levels are also associated with increased risk of CHD, but this relationship weakens considerably when statistical corrections are made for the plasma levels of LDL-C and HDL-C. Plasma levels of HDL-C are strongly and consistently inversely related to the prevalence and incidence of CHD, and yet no clinical trial data are available demonstrating that increasing plasma levels of HDL-C reduces the frequency of cardiovascular events. No pharmacologic agents are available that exclusively either lower plasma triglyceride levels or increase plasma HDL-C levels, contributing to the dearth of clinical trial data addressing the role of treatment of these lipid abnormalities in CHD prevention. Since both hypertriglyceridemia and low plasma levels of HDL-C confer higher ASCVD risk, the NCEP ATPIII recommends more aggressive therapy to lower the plasma LDL-C in patients with these dyslipidemias.

Nonpharmacologic Treatment

DIET

Dietary modification is an important component in the management of hyperlipidemia. In the hypercholesterolemic patient, dietary saturated fat and cholesterol should be restricted. For patients who are hypertriglyceridemic, the intake of simple sugars should also be curtailed. For severe hypertriglyceridemia [>11.3 mmol/L (>1000 mg/dL)], restriction of total fat intake is critical. The most widely used diet to lower the LDL-C level is the "Step 1 diet" developed by the American Heart Association. Most patients have a relatively modest (<10%) decrease in plasma levels of LDL-C on a step I diet in the absence of any associated weight loss. Almost all persons experience a decrease in plasma HDL-C levels with a reduction in the amount of total and saturated fat in their diet.

FOODS AND ADDITIVES

Certain foods and dietary additives are associated with modest reductions in plasma cholesterol levels. Plant stanol and sterol esters are available in a variety of foods such as spreads, salad dressings, and snack bars. They interfere with cholesterol absorption and reduce plasma LDL-C levels by ~10 to 15% when taken three times per day. The addition to the diet of psyllium, soy protein, or Chinese red yeast rice (which contains lovastatin) can have modest cholesterol-lowering effects. Other herbal approaches such as guggulipid require further study to assess their effectiveness.

WEIGHT LOSS AND EXERCISE

The treatment of obesity, if present, can have a favorable impact on plasma lipid levels and should be actively encouraged. Plasma triglyceride and LDL-C levels tend to fall and HDL-C levels tend to increase in obese persons who lose weight. Aerobic exercise has a very modest elevating effect on plasma levels of HDL-C in most individuals but has cardiovascular benefits that extend beyond the effects on plasma lipid levels.

Pharmacologic Treatment

The decision to use drug therapy depends on the cardiovascular risk. An effective way to estimate absolute risk of a cardiovascular event over 10 years is to use a scoring system based on the Framingham Heart Study database. Patients with a 10-year absolute CHD risk of >20% are considered "CHD risk equivalents." Current NCEP ATPIII guidelines call for drug therapy to reduce LDL-C to <2.6 mmol/L (<100 mg/dL) in patients with established CHD, other ASCVD (aortic aneurysm, peripheral vascular disease, or cerebrovascular disease), diabetes mellitus, or CHD risk equivalents. Based on these guidelines, most CHD and CHD risk–equivalent patients require cholesterol-lowering drug therapy. Moderate risk patients with two or more risk factors and a 10-year absolute risk of 10 to 20% should be treated to a goal LDL-C of <3.4 mmol/L (<130 mg/dL). All other individuals have a goal of LDL-C <4.1 mmol/L (<160 mg/dL), but not all persons are candidates for drug therapy to achieve this goal.

Persons with markedly elevated plasma LDL-C levels [>4.9 mmol/L (>190 mg/dL)] should be considered for drug therapy even if their 10-year absolute CHD risk is not particularly elevated. The decision to initiate drug treatment in individuals with plasma LDL-C levels between 3.4 and 4.9 mmol/L (130 and 190 mg/dL) can be difficult. Although it is desirable to avoid drug treatment in patients who are unlikely to develop CHD, a very high proportion of patients who eventually develop CHD have plasma LDL-C levels that are in this range. Other clinical information can assist in the decision-making process. For example, a low plasma HDL-C [<1.0 mmol/L (<40 mg/dL)] supports a decision in favor of more aggressive therapy. The diagnosis of the metabolic syndrome also identifies a higher risk individual who should be targeted for therapeutic life-style changes and might be a candidate for more aggressive drug therapy. Other laboratory tests, such as an elevated plasma Lp(a) or high-sensitivity C-reactive protein, may help to identify additional high-risk individuals. In persons at low risk, the emphasis should primarily be on dietary and life-style modification.

Drug treatment is also indicated in patients with triglycerides >11.3 mmol/L (>1000 mg/dL) who have been screened and treated for secondary causes of chylomicronemia. The goal is to reduce plasma triglycerides to <4.5 mmol/L (400 mg/dL) to prevent the risk of acute pancreatitis. Most major clinical end-point trials with statins have excluded persons with triglyceride levels >3.9 to 5.1 mmol/L (>350 to 450 mg/dL), and therefore there are few data regarding the effectiveness of statins in reducing cardiovascular risk in persons with triglycerides higher than this threshold. Combination therapy is often required for optimal control of mixed dyslipidemia.

HMG-COA REDUCTASE INHIBITORS

3-Hydroxy-3-methylglutaryl coenzyme A (HMG-CoA reductase) is the rate-limiting step in cholesterol biosynthesis, and inhibition of this enzyme decreases cholesterol synthesis. By inhibiting cholesterol biosynthesis, HMG-CoA reductase inhibitors (statins) lead to increased hepatic LDL receptor activity and accelerated clearance of circulating LDL, resulting in a dose-dependent reduction in plasma LDL-C. There is wide interindividual variation in the initial response to a statin, but once a patient is on the medication, the doubling of the dose produces a 6% further reduction of plasma LDL-C. The HMG-CoA reductase inhibitors currently available differ in their LDL-C reducing effects (**Table 18-6**). HMG-CoA reductase inhibitors also reduce plasma triglycerides in a dose-dependent fashion, which is proportional to their LDL-C lowering effects [if the triglycerides are <3.9 mmol/L (<350 mg/dL)]. HMG-CoA reductase inhibitors have a modest HDL-raising effect (5 to 10%), and this effect is not dose-dependent.

HMG-CoA reductase inhibitors are well tolerated and can be taken in tablet form once a day. Potential side effects include dyspepsia, headaches, fatigue, and muscle or joint pains. Severe myopathy and even rhabdomyolysis occurs rarely. The risk of myopathy is increased by the presence of renal insufficiency and by coadministration of drugs that interfere with the metabolism of HMG-CoA reductase inhibitors, such as erythromycin and related antibiotics, antifungal agents, immunosuppressive drugs, and fibric acid derivatives. Severe myopathy can usually be avoided by careful patient selection, avoidance of interacting drugs, and by instructing the patient to contact the physician immediately in the event of unexplained muscle pain. In the event of muscle symptoms, the plasma creatine phosphokinase (CPK) level should be obtained to document the myopathy, but serum CPK levels do not need to

TABLE 18-6

SUMMARY OF THE MAJOR DRUGS USED FOR THE TREATMENT OF HYPERLIPIDEMIA

DRUG	MAJOR INDICATIONS	STARTING DOSE	MAXIMAL DOSE	MECHANISM	COMMON SIDE EFFECTS
HMG-CoA reductase inhibitors (statins)	Elevated LDL			↓ Cholesterol synthesis, ↓ hepatic LDL receptors, ↓ VLDL production	Myalgias, arthralgias, elevated transaminases, dyspepsia
Lovastatin		20 mg daily	80 mg daily		
Pravastatin		40 mg qhs	80 mg qhs		
Simvastatin		20 mg qhs	80 mg qhs		
Fluvastatin		20 mg qhs	80 mg qhs		
Atorvastatin		10 mg qhs	80 mg qhs		
Rosuvastatin		10 mg qhs	40 mg qhs		
Bile acid sequestrants	Elevated LDL			↑ Bile acid excretion ↑ LDL receptors	Bloating, constipation, elevated trigylcerides
Cholestyramine		4 g daily	32 g daily		
Colestipol		5 g daily	40 g daily		
Colesevelam		3750 mg daily	4375 mg daily		
Nicotinic acid	Elevated LDL, low HDL, elevated TG			↓ VLDL hepatic synthesis	Cutaneous flushing; GI upset; elevated glucose, uric acid, and liver function tests
Immediate-release		100 mg tid	2 g tid		
Sustained-release		250 mg bid	1.5 g bid		
Extended-release		500 mg qhs	2 g qhs		
Fibric acid derivatives	Elevated TG, elevated remnants			↑ LPL ↓ VLDL synthesis	Dyspepsia, myalgia, gallstones, elevated transaminases
Gemfibrozil		600 mg bid	600 mg bid		
Fenofibrate		160 mg qd	160 mg qd		
Fish oils	Severely elevated TG	3 g daily	12 g daily	↓ Chylomicron and VLDL production	Dyspepsia, diarrhea, fishy odor to breath
Cholesterol absorption inhibitors					
Ezetimibe	Elevated LDL	10 mg daily	10 mg daily	↓ Intenstinal cholesterol absorption	Elevated transaminases

Note: LDL, low-density lipoprotein; VLDL, very low density lipoprotein; HDL, high-density lipoprotein; TG, triglycerides; LPL, lipoprotein lipase.

be monitored on a routine basis as an elevated CPK in the absence of symptoms does not predict the development of myopathy and does not necessarily suggest the need for discontinuing the drug.

Another side effect of HMG-CoA reductase inhibitor therapy is hepatitis. Liver transaminases (ALT and AST) should be checked before starting therapy, at 8 weeks, and then every 6 months. Substantial (>3 × upper limit of normal) elevation in transaminases is relatively rare, and mild to moderate (1 to 3 × normal) elevation in transaminases in the absence of symptoms need not mandate discontinuing the medication. Severe clinical hepatitis associated with HMG-CoA reductase inhibitors is exceedingly rare, and the trend is toward less frequent monitoring of transaminases in patients taking HMG-CoA reductase inhibitors. The HMG-CoA reductase inhibitor–associated elevation in liver enzymes resolves after discontinuation of the medication.

Overall, HMG-CoA reductase inhibitors appear to be remarkably safe. Over 50,000 patients have been treated with HMG-CoA reductase inhibitors for over 5 to 6 years as a part of large randomized controlled clinical trials and no increase in any major noncardiac diseases have been seen in these individuals. HMG-CoA reductase inhibitors are the drug class of choice for LDL-C reduction and are by far the most widely used class of lipid-lowering drugs.

BILE ACID SEQUESTRANTS (RESINS)

Bile acid sequestrants bind bile acids in the intestine and promote their excretion in the stool. In order to maintain an adequate bile acid pool, the liver diverts cholesterol to bile acid synthesis. The decreased hepatic intracellular cholesterol content upregulates the LDL receptor and enhances LDL clearance from the plasma. Bile acid sequestrants, including cholestyramine, colestipol, and colesevelam (Table 18-6), primarily reduce plasma LDL-C levels but can increase plasma triglycerides. Therefore, patients with hypertriglyceridemia should not be treated with bile acid–binding resins.

Cholestyramine and colestipol are insoluble resins that must be mixed with liquids. Colestipol is also available in large tablets but multiple tablets must be taken to achieve significant lowering of plasma LDL-C levels. The newest bile acid sequestrant, colesevelam, has greater bile acid–binding capacity than traditional resins. The colesevelam tablets are smaller, and fewer tablets per day are required. Most side effects of resins are limited to the gastrointestinal tract and include bloating and constipation. Bile acid sequestrants may bind other drugs (e.g., digoxin, warfarin) and interfere with their absorption. Therefore, all other medications should be taken either 1 h before or 4 h after the bile acid sequestrants.

Bile acid sequestrants are not systemically absorbed and are very safe. They are the cholesterol-lowering drug of choice in children and in women of childbearing age who are lactating, pregnant, or could become pregnant. These drugs can also be useful in young, well-motivated patients with moderate hypercholesterolemia who wish to avoid systemic drug therapy. This class of drugs is also useful in combination with HMG-CoA reductase inhibitors in patients who are unable to reach their LDL-C goal on HMG-CoA reductase inhibitor monotherapy and have relatively normal triglyceride levels.

NICOTINIC ACID (NIACIN)

Nicotinic acid, or niacin, is a B-complex vitamin that reduces plasma triglyceride and LDL-C levels and raises the plasma HDL-C (Table 18-6) in high doses. Niacin is the only currently available lipid-lowering drug that significantly reduces plasma levels of Lp(a). If properly prescribed and monitored, niacin is a safe and effective lipid-lowering agent.

The cheapest form of niacin is immediate-release crystalline niacin. Niacin should be started at a low dose (100 mg three times a day) and taken with meals to delay absorption. The dose of niacin should be increased every 4 to 7 days by 100 mg until a dose of 500 mg tid is obtained. After 1 month on this dose, lipids and pertinent chemistries (glucose, uric acid, liver transaminases) should be measured. The dose can be further increased as needed up to a total dose of 6 g/d. The most frequent side effect is cutaneous flushing, but this improves with continued administration. In many patients, taking an aspirin 30 min prior to the niacin prevents flushing. Over-the-counter sustained-release forms of niacin are generally administered twice a day and are associated with less flushing, but some have been associated with rare cases of severe hepatitis. A clue to the development of niacin-induced hepatitis is a sudden, precipitous drop in the plasma lipid levels. A prescription form of extended-release niacin that is administered once daily at bedtime has not been associated with severe hepatic toxicity. Mild elevations in transaminases occur in up to 15% of patients treated with any form of niacin, but these elevations rarely require discontinuation of the medication. Niacin potentiates the effect of warfarin, and these two drugs should be prescribed together with caution. Acanthosis nigricans and maculopathy are infrequent side effects of niacin. Niacin is contraindicated in patients with peptic ulcer disease and can exacerbate the symptoms of esophageal reflux. Niacin can raise plasma levels of uric acid and precipitate gouty attacks in susceptible patients.

Niacin can raise fasting plasma glucose levels, but concerns regarding the use of niacin in diabetic patients have been allayed by the results of two studies. In one study, short-acting niacin treatment of dyslipidemia was associated with only a slight increase in fasting glucose and no significant change from baseline in the HbA1c. In the other, low-dose niacin was found to reduce triglycerides effectively and raise HDL-C in diabetics without adversely impacting glycemic control.

Successful therapy with niacin requires careful education and motivation of the patient. Its advantages are its low cost and long-term safety. It is the most effective drug currently available for raising HDL-C levels. It is particularly useful in patients with combined hyperlipidemia and low plasma levels of HDL-C and is effective in combination with statins.

FIBRIC ACID DERIVATIVES (FIBRATES)

Fibric acid derivatives, or fibrates, are agonists of PPARα, a nuclear receptor involved in the regulation of carbohydrate and lipid metabolism. Fibrates stimulate LPL activity (enhancing triglyceride hydrolysis), reduce apoC-III synthesis (enhancing lipoprotein remnant clearance), and may reduce VLDL production. Fibrates are the most effective drugs available for reducing triglyceride levels, and they also raise HDL-C levels (Table 18-6). Fibrates have variable effects on LDL-C, and in hypertriglyceridemic patients can sometimes be associated with increases in plasma LDL-C levels.

Fibrates are generally very well tolerated. The most common side effect is dyspepsia. Myopathy and hepatitis occur rarely in the absence of other lipid-lowering agents. Fibrates promote cholesterol secretion into bile and are associated with an increased risk of gallstones. Importantly, fibrates can potentiate the effect of warfarin and certain oral hypoglycemic agents; the anticoagulation status and plasma glucose levels should be closely monitored in patients on these agents.

Fibrates are the drug class of choice in patients with severe hypertriglyceridemia [11.3 mmol/L (>1000 mg/dL)] and are a reasonable consideration in patients with moderate hypertriglyceridemia [4.5 to 11.3 mmol/L (400 to 1000 mg/dL)]. The Veterans Affairs High-Density Lipoprotein Intervention Trial study also suggests that they may have a role in high-risk patients with well-controlled LDL-C levels but elevated plasma triglyceride levels and low plasma levels of HDL-C. The relative indications of fibrates vs. statins and the role of combined therapy will be determined by ongoing and future trials.

OMEGA-3 FATTY ACIDS (FISH OILS)

N-3 polyunsaturated fatty acids (PUFAs) are present in high concentration in fish and in flax seeds. The most widely used n-3 PUFAs for the treatment of hyperlipidemias are the two active molecules in fish oil, eicosapentanoic acid (EPA) and decohexanoic acid (DHA). N-3 PUFAs have been concentrated into tablets and in doses of 3 to 6 g/d decrease fasting and postprandial triglycerides. At least 6 g/d is usually required for a substantial triglyceride-lowering effect, and many patients require 9 to 12 g/d. Fish oil treatment of hypertriglyceridemia can be associated with a significant increase in plasma LDL-C levels. Fish oil supplements can be used in combination with fibrates, niacin, or statins to treat hypertriglyceridemia. In general, fish oils are well tolerated and appear to be safe, at least at doses up to 3 g. The large number of capsules required for a therapeutic effect, the associated dyspepsia, and fishy aftertaste have limited the clinical use of these agents. Although fish oil administration is associated with a prolongation in the bleeding time, no increase in bleeding has been seen in clinical trials.

CHOLESTEROL ABSORPTION INHIBITORS

A new mechanism of cholesterol-lowering is the inhibition of intestinal cholesterol absorption. Ezetimibe (Table 18-6) inhibits the absorption of dietary and biliary cholesterol from the intestinal lumen. It reduces LDL-C cholesterol levels by ~18% as monotherapy or in combination with a statin. Cholesterol absorption inhibitors are particularly useful in combination with a statin in patients unable to reach their LDL-C goal on statin monotherapy.

COMBINATION DRUG THERAPY

Combination drug therapy is frequently used in the following situations: (1) patients unable to reach their LDL-C goal on a single drug, (2) patients with combined hypertriglyceridemia and hypercholesterolemia that cannot be adequately controlled with a single drug, and (3) patients with elevated LDL-C and low HDL-C levels. Inability to achieve LDL-C goal is not uncommon on statin monotherapy. If the patient has a normal plasma triglyceride level, a bile acid sequestrant can be added. A cholesterol absorption inhibitor can also be used in this setting. Combination of niacin with a statin is an attractive option for high-risk patients who do not attain their target LDL-C level on statin monotherapy and who have an HDL-C < 10.3 mmol/L (<40 mg/dL). One product currently available offers the combination of lovastatin and extended-release niacin in a single tablet.

Patients with combined hyperlipidemia frequently have persistent hypertriglyceridemia on statin monotherapy. Addition of niacin or a fibrate can reduce the plasma triglyceride level in these patients. Conversely, hypertriglyceridemic patients treated with a fibrate often fail to reach their LDL-C goal and are therefore candidates for the addition of a statin. Coadministration of statins and fibrates has obvious appeal in patients with combined hyperlipidemia, but no clinical trials have assessed the effectiveness of a statin-fibrate combination compared with either a statin or a fibrate alone in reducing cardiovascular events, and the long-term safety of this combination is not known. Statin-fibrate combinations are known to be associated with an increased incidence of severe myopathy (up to 2.5%) and rhabdomyolysis, and patients treated with these two drugs must be carefully counseled and monitored. This combination of drugs should be used cautiously in patients with underlying renal or hepatic insufficiency; in the elderly, frail, and chronically ill; and in those on multiple medications.

Other Approaches

Occasionally, patients cannot tolerate any of the existing lipid-lowering drugs at doses required for adequate control of their lipid levels. Some patients, mostly those with genetic lipid disorders, remain significantly hypercholesterolemic despite combination drug therapy. These patients are at high risk for development or progression of CHD and clinical CHD events.

LDL APHERESIS

The preferred option for management of patients with refractory or drug-resistant hypercholesterolemia is LDL apheresis. In this process, the patient's plasma is passed over a column that selectively removes the LDL, and the LDL-depleted plasma is returned to the patient. Patients on maximally tolerated combination drug therapy who have CHD and a plasma LDL-C level >5.2 mmol/L (>200 mg/dL) or no CHD and a plasma LDL-C level >7.8 mmol/L (>300 mg/dL), are candidates for every-other-week LDL apheresis.

PARTIAL ILEAL BYPASS

Partial ileal bypass interrupts the enterohepatic circulation of bile acids, resulting in upregulation of the hepatic LDL receptor and reduction in plasma LDL-C levels. Diarrhea is a common side effect, and the incidence of kidney stones, gallstones, and intestinal obstruction is increased after ileal bypass surgery. The clinical utility of partial ileal bypass at this time is limited to severely hypercholesterolemic patients with normal triglycerides who cannot tolerate existing lipid-lowering medications and do not have access to LDL apheresis. Partial ileal bypass has not been proven effective in patients with severe hypercholesterolemia who have not responded adequately to statins.

Management of Low HDL-C

Severely reduced plasma HDL-C [<0.5 mmol/L (<20 mg/dL)] accompanied by triglycerides <4.5 mmol/L (<400 mg/dL) usually indicates the presence of a genetic disorder, such as a mutation in apoA-I, LCAT deficiency, or Tangier disease. HDL-C levels <0.5 mmol/L (<20 mg/dL) are common in the setting of severe hypertriglyceridemia, in which case the primary focus should be on the management of the triglycerides. Secondary causes of more moderate reductions in plasma HDL [0.5 to 10.3 mmol/L (20 to 40 mg/dL)] should be considered (Table 18-5). Smoking should be discontinued, obese persons should be encouraged to lose weight, sedentary persons should be encouraged to exercise, and diabetes should be optimally controlled. When possible, medications associated with reduced plasma levels of HDL-C should be discontinued. The presence of an isolated low plasma HDL-C level in a patient with a borderline plasma LDL-C should prompt consideration of LDL-lowering drug therapy in high-risk individuals. Statins increase plasma levels of HDL-C only modestly (~5 to 10%). Fibrates also have a modest effect on plasma HDL-C levels (increasing levels ~5 to 15%) except in patients with coexisting hypertriglyceridemia, where they can be more effective. Niacin is the most effective therapeutic agent and can increase plasma HDL-C levels by up to ~30%.

The issue of whether pharmacologic intervention should be used to specifically raise HDL-C levels has not been adequately addressed in clinical trials. Pending these studies, it may be reasonable to initiate therapy (with a fibrate or niacin) directed specifically at reducing plasma triglyceride levels and raising the plasma HDL-C level in persons with established CHD and low HDL-C levels whose plasma LDL-C levels are at or below the goal.

FURTHER READINGS

◪ BROUSSEAU ME et al: Effects of an inhibitor of cholesteryl ester transfer protein on HDL cholesterol. N Engl J Med 350:1505, 2004

Inhibition of cholesteryl ester transfer protein (CETP) has been proposed as a strategy to raise HDL cholesterol levels. This study examined the effects of torcetrapib, a potent inhibitor of CETP, on plasma lipoprotein levels in subjects with low HDL cholesterol. Treatment with 120 mg of torcetrapib daily markedly increased HDL cholesterol levels and also decreased LDL cholesterol levels.

◪ CANNON CP et al: Intensive versus moderate lipid lowering with statins after acute coronary syndromes. N Engl J Med 350:1495, 2004

This study compared standard versus intensive lipid-lowering therapy with statins in 4162 patients who had been hospitalized for an acute coronary syndrome. The intensive lipid-lowering statin regimen provided greater protection against death or major cardiovascular events, suggesting that such patients benefit from early and continued lowering of LDL cholesterol to levels substantially below current target levels.

GRUNDY SM et al: Implications of recent clinical trials for the National Cholesterol Education Program Adult Treatment Panel III Guidelines. J Am Coll Cardiol 44:720, 2004

Heart Protection Study Collaborative Group: MRC/BHF Heart Protection Study of cholesterol lowering with simvastatin in 20,536 high-risk individuals: A randomised placebo-controlled trial. Lancet 360:7, 2002

LAROSA JC et al: Past, present, and future standards for management of dyslipidemia. Am J Med 116 Suppl 6A:3S, 2004

LIMA JA et al: Statin-induced cholesterol lowering and plaque regression after 6 months of magnetic resonance imaging-monitored therapy. Circulation 110:2336, 2004

Muldoon MF et al: Cholesterol reduction and non-illness mortality: Meta-analysis of randomised clinical trials. BMJ 322:11, 2001

Executive summary of the third report of the National Cholesterol Education Program (NCEP) expert panel on detection, evaluation, and treatment of high blood cholesterol in adults (Adult Treatment Panel III). JAMA 285:2486, 2001

NISSEN SE et al: Statin therapy, LDL cholesterol, C-reactive protein, and coronary artery disease. N Engl J Med 352:29, 2005.

Recent trials have demonstrated better outcomes with intensive than with moderate statin treatment. This study of patients with coronary artery disease confirmed a reduced rate of progression of atherosclerosis associated with intensive statin treatment, and documented a correlation with greater reductions in the levels of both atherogenic lipoproteins and CRP.

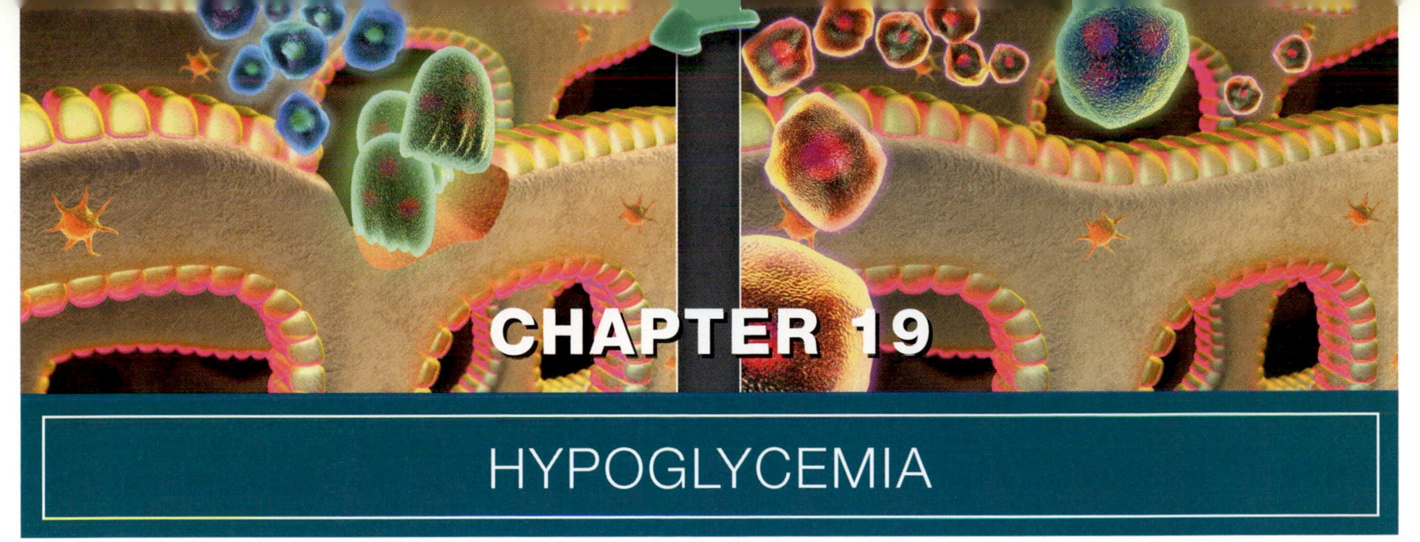

HYPOGLYCEMIA

Philip E. Cryer

Hypoglycemia is most commonly the result of taking drugs used to treat diabetes mellitus or other drugs, including alcohol. However, a number of other disorders, including end-stage organ failure and sepsis, endocrine deficiencies, large mesenchymal tumors, insulinoma, and inherited metabolic disorders are also associated with hypoglycemia (**Table 19-1**). Hypoglycemia is sometimes defined as a plasma glucose level <2.5 to 2.8 mmol/L (<45 to 50 mg/dL). However, glucose thresholds for hypoglycemia-induced symptoms and physiologic responses vary widely, depending on the clinical setting. Therefore, an important framework for making the diagnosis of hypoglycemia is *Whipple's triad*: (1) symptoms consistent with hypoglycemia, (2) a low plasma glucose concentration, and (3) relief of symptoms after the plasma glucose level is raised. Hypoglycemia can cause significant morbidity and can be lethal, if severe and prolonged; it should be considered in any patient with confusion, altered level of consciousness, or seizures.

TABLE 19-1

CAUSES OF HYPOGLYCEMIA
Drugs
Especially insulin, sulfonylureas, ethanol
Sometimes pentamidine, quinine
Rarely salicylates, sulfonamides, and others
Critical illnesses
Hepatic, renal, or cardiac failure
Sepsis
Starvation and inanition
Endocrine deficiencies
Cortisol, growth hormone
Glucagon and epinephrine (type 1 diabetes)
Non-β cell tumors
Fibrosarcoma, mesothelioma, rhabdomyosarcoma, liposarcoma, other sarcomas
Hepatoma, adrenocortical tumors, carcinoid
Leukemia, lymphoma, melanoma, teratoma
Endogenous hyperinsulinism
Insulinoma
Other β cell disorders
Secretagogue (sulfonylurea)
Autoimmune (autoantibodies to insulin, insulin receptor, β cell?)
Ectopic insulin secretion
Disorders of infancy or childhood
Transient intolerance of fasting
Infants of diabetic mothers (hyperinsulinism)
Congenital hyperinsulinism
Inherited enzyme defects
Postprandial
Reactive (after gastric surgery)
Ethanol-induced
Autonomic symptoms without true hypoglycemia
Factitious
Insulin, sulfonylureas

SYSTEMIC GLUCOSE BALANCE AND COUNTERREGULATION

Glucose is an obligate metabolic fuel for the brain under physiologic conditions. By contrast, other organs can use fatty acids, in addition to glucose, to generate energy. The brain cannot synthesize glucose and stores only a few minutes' supply as glycogen and therefore requires a continuous supply of glucose, which is delivered by facilitated diffusion from arterial blood. As the plasma glucose concentration falls below the physiologic range, blood-to-brain glucose transport becomes insufficient for adequate brain energy metabolism and functioning. Fortunately, redundant physiologic mechanisms prevent or rapidly correct hypoglycemia.

Plasma glucose levels are maintained within a narrow range, usually between 3.3 and 8.3 mmol/L (60 and 150 mg/dL), despite wide variation of food intake and activity level. This delicate balance requires dynamic regulation of glucose influx into the circulation as glucose utilization in various tissues can change rapidly. The diet is normally a major source of glucose. However, between meals or during fasting, plasma glucose levels are maintained primarily by the breakdown of glycogen and by gluconeogenesis (**Fig. 19-1**). In most persons, hepatic glycogen stores are sufficient to maintain plasma glucose levels for 8 to 12 h, but this time period can be shorter if glucose demand is increased by exercise or if glycogen stores are depleted by illness or starvation.

As glycogen stores are depleted, glucose is generated by gluconeogenesis, which occurs mainly in the liver but also in the kidneys. Gluconeogenesis requires a coordinated supply of precursors from liver, muscle,

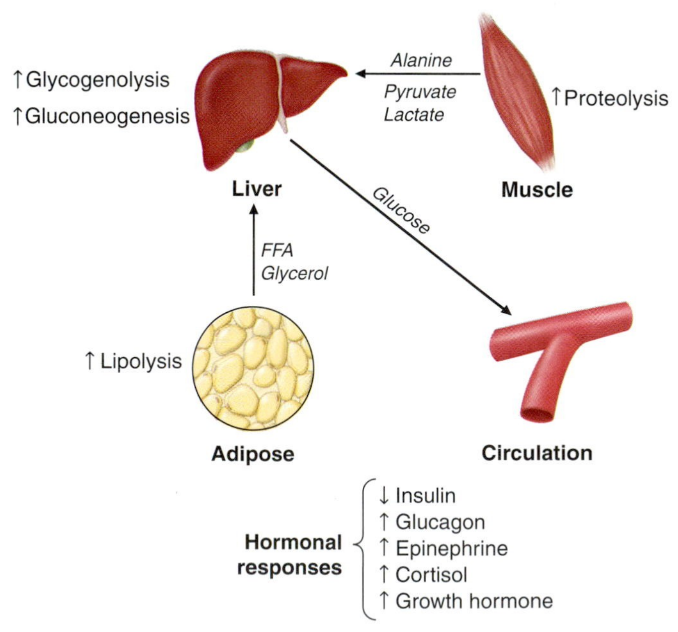

FIGURE 19-1

Overview of glucose metabolism and pathways of counterregulatory responses to fasting and hypoglycemia.

and adipose tissue. Muscle provides lactate, pyruvate, alanine, and other amino acids. Triglycerides in adipose tissue are broken down into glycerol, which is a precursor for gluconeogenesis. Free fatty acids generate acetyl CoA for gluconeogenesis and provide an alternative fuel source to tissues other than the brain.

The balance of glucose production and its uptake and utilization in peripheral tissues are exquisitely regulated by a network of hormones, neural pathways, and metabolic signals (Chap. 17). Among the factors that control glucose production and utilization, insulin plays a dominant and pivotal role. In the fasting state, insulin is suppressed, allowing increased gluconeogenesis in the liver and the kidneys and enhancing glucose generation by the breakdown of liver glycogen. Low insulin levels also reduce glucose uptake and utilization in peripheral tissues and allow lipolysis and proteolysis to occur, which leads to the release of precursors for gluconeogenesis and provides alternative energy sources. In the fed state, insulin release from the pancreatic beta cells reverses this process. Glycogenolysis and gluconeogenesis are inhibited, thereby reducing hepatic and renal glucose output; peripheral glucose uptake and utilization are enhanced; lipolysis and proteolysis are restrained; and energy storage is promoted by the conversion of substrates into glycogen, triglycerides, and proteins. Other hormones, such as glucagon, epinephrine, growth hormone, and cortisol, play less important roles in the control of glucose flux during normal physiologic circumstances. However, these hormones are critically important in the response to hypoglycemia.

As glucose levels approach, and ultimately enter, the hypoglycemic range, a characteristic sequence of *counterregulatory hormone responses* occurs. Glucagon is the first and most important of these responses. It promotes glycogenolysis and gluconeogenesis. Epinephrine can also play an important role in the acute response to hypoglycemia, particularly when glucagon is insufficient. It, too, stimulates glycogenolysis and gluconeogenesis and limits glucose utilization by insulin-sensitive tissues. When hypoglycemia is prolonged, growth hormone and cortisol also reduce glucose utilization and support its production.

The glucose thresholds at which various counterregulatory hormone responses occur are quite similar in healthy subjects (**Table 19-2**). Nevertheless, these thresholds are dynamic and can be influenced by recent metabolic events. A person with poorly controlled diabetes can have symptoms of hypoglycemia at higher-than-normal glucose levels. Recurrent hypoglycemia, which may occur in individuals with diabetes or an insulinoma, shifts thresholds for

TABLE 19-2

PHYSIOLOGIC RESPONSES TO DECREASING PLASMA GLUCOSE CONCENTRATIONS

RESPONSE	GLYCEMIC THRESHOLD, mmol/L (mg/dL)	PHYSIOLOGIC EFFECTS	ROLE IN THE PREVENTION OR CORRECTION OF HYPOGLYCEMIA (GLUCOSE COUNTERREGULATION)
↓ Insulin	4.4–4.7 (80–85)	↑ R_0 (↓ R_d)	Primary glucose regulatory factor/first defense against hypoglyemia
↑ Glucagon	3.6–3.9 (65–70)	↑ R_a	Primary glucose counterregulatory factor
↑ Epinephrine	3.6–3.9 (65–70)	↑ R_a, ↓ R_d	Involved, critical when glucagon is deficient
↑ Cortisol and growth hormone	3.6–3.9 (65–70)	↑ R_a, ↓ R_d	Involved, not critical
Symptoms	2.8–3.1 (50–55)	↑ Exogenous glucose	Prompt behavioral defense (food ingestion)
↓ Cognition	<2.8 (<50)	—	(Compromises behavioral defense)

Note: R_a, rate of glucose appearance, glucose production by the liver and kidneys; R_d, rate of glucose disappearance, glucose utilization by insulin-sensitive tissues such as skeletal muscle. (R_d includes glucose utilization by the central nervous system, but the glucoregulatory hormones have no direct effects on that.)

symptoms and counterregulatory responses to lower glucose levels.

CLINICAL MANIFESTATIONS

Symptoms of hypoglycemia can be divided into two categories, neuroglycopenic and neurogenic (or autonomic) responses. Neuroglycopenic symptoms are a direct result of central nervous system neuronal glucose deprivation. Symptoms include behavioral changes, confusion, fatigue, seizure, loss of consciousness, and, if hypoglycemia is severe and prolonged, death. Hypoglycemia-induced autonomic responses include adrenergic symptoms such as palpitations, tremor, and anxiety as well as cholinergic symptoms such as sweating, hunger, and paresthesia. Adrenergic symptoms are mediated by norepinephrine released from sympathetic postganglionic neurons and the release of epinephrine from the adrenal medullae. Increased sweating is mediated by cholinergic sympathetic nerve fibers. Patients with diabetes mellitus learn to recognize the characteristic symptoms of hypoglycemia, but these are less familiar to individuals with other causes of hypoglycemia. Symptoms may be less pronounced with repeated hypoglycemic episodes (see below).

Common signs of hypoglycemia include pallor and diaphoresis. Heart rate and the systolic blood pressure are typically raised, but these findings may not be prominent. The neuroglycopenic manifestations are valuable, albeit nonspecific, signs. Transient focal neurologic deficits occur occasionally.

CAUSES

Hypoglycemia is traditionally classified as *postprandial* or *fasting*. However, in the clinical setting, hypoglycemia is most commonly a result of diabetes treatment. This topic is therefore addressed before considering the other causes of hypoglycemia.

HYPOGLYCEMIA IN DIABETES

FREQUENCY AND IMPACT

Were it not for hypoglycemia, diabetes would be rather easy to treat by administering enough insulin (or any effective drug) to lower plasma glucose concentrations to, or below, the normal range. But because current insulin-replacement regimens are imperfect, individuals with type 1 diabetes are at ongoing risk for periods of relative hyperinsulinemia with resultant hypoglycemia. Those attempting to achieve near-normal glycemic control may experience several episodes of asymptomatic or symptomatic hypoglycemia each week. Plasma glucose levels may be <2.8 mmol/L (<50 mg/dL) as often as 10% of the time. Such patients suffer an average of one episode of severe, temporarily disabling hypoglycemia, often with seizure or coma, in a given year. Although seemingly complete recovery from the latter is the rule, the possibility of persistent cognitive deficits has been raised, but permanent neurologic defects are rare. About 2 to 4% of deaths associated with type 1 diabetes are estimated to be a result of hypoglycemia. Fear of hypoglycemia can also lead to disabling psychosocial morbidity.

Hypoglycemia is a less frequent problem in type 2 diabetes but still occurs in those treated with insulin or sulfonylureas. Transient, mild hypoglycemia may be seen with the shorter-acting sulfonylureas and repaglinide or nateglinide, which also act by enhancing insulin secretion. Patients who take the long-acting sulfonylureas, chlorpropamide and glyburide, may experience episodes of severe hypoglycemia that last between 24 and 36 h.

CONVENTIONAL RISK FACTORS

Insulin excess is the primary determinant of risk from iatrogenic hypoglycemia. Relative or absolute insulin excess occurs when: (1) insulin (or oral agent) doses are excessive, ill timed, or of the wrong type; (2) the influx of exogenous glucose is reduced (e.g., during an overnight fast or following missed meals or snacks); (3) insulin-independent glucose utilization is increased (e.g., during exercise); (4) insulin sensitivity is increased (e.g., with effective intensive therapy, in the middle of the night, late after exercise, or with increased fitness or weight loss); (5) endogenous glucose production is reduced (e.g., following alcohol ingestion); and (6) insulin clearance is reduced (e.g., in renal failure). However, analyses of the Diabetes Control and Complications Trial (DCCT) indicate that these conventional risk factors explain only a minority of episodes of severe iatrogenic hypoglycemia; other causes are involved in the majority of episodes.

HYPOGLYCEMIA-ASSOCIATED AUTONOMIC FAILURE

It is now clear that inadequate physiologic counterregulatory and behavioral responses greatly compound the problem of hypoglycemia caused by insulin excess. Hypoglycemia-associated autonomic failure has two main components: (1) reduced counterregulatory hormone responses, which result in impaired glucose generation; and (2) hypoglycemia unawareness, which precludes appropriate behavioral responses, such as eating.

Defective Glucose Counterregulation

The counterregulatory hormone response is fundamentally altered in patients with established (e.g., absent C peptide) type 1 diabetes. As insulin deficiency progresses over the first few months or years of the disease, circulating insulin levels are no longer tightly coordinated with glucose levels and are a passive function of administered insulin. Thus, insulin levels do not decline as glucose levels fall; the first defense against hypoglycemia is lost. Over the same time frame, the glucagon response to falling glucose levels diminishes, and the second defense against hypoglycemia is lost. The cause of defective glucagon production by the pancreatic islet alpha cells is unknown, but it is tightly linked to the loss of insulin production by the beta cells. It is a functional abnormality rather than an absolute deficiency of glucagon, as responses to stimuli other than hypoglycemia are intact. The third defense against hypoglycemia is compromised when the epinephrine response to hypoglycemia is reduced. In contrast to the absent glucagon response, epinephrine deficiency is a threshold abnormality; an epinephrine response can still be elicited, but a lower plasma glucose concentration is required. This threshold shift is largely a result of recent antecedent hypoglycemia, although an additional anatomical component may also be present in patients affected by classic diabetic autonomic neuropathy. The development of a reduced epinephrine response is a critical pathophysiologic event. Prospective studies have shown that patients with combined deficiencies of glucagon and epinephrine suffer severe hypoglycemia at rates 25-fold or greater than individuals with absent glucagon but intact epinephrine responses.

Hypoglycemia Unawareness

Hypoglycemia unawareness refers to a loss of the warning symptoms that alert individuals to the presence of hypoglycemia and prompt them to eat and abort the episode. Under these circumstances, the first manifestation of hypoglycemia is neuroglycopenia, when it is often too late for patients to treat themselves. Like defective counterregulation, the presence of hypoglycemia unawareness has been shown in prospective studies to be associated with a high frequency of severe hypoglycemia.

The interplay of factors involved in hypoglycemia-associated autonomic failure in type 1 diabetes, and consequent hypoglycemia unawareness, is summarized in **Fig. 19-2.** Periods of relative or absolute therapeutic insulin excess, in the setting of absent glucagon responses, lead to episodes of iatrogenic hypoglycemia. These episodes, in turn, cause reduced autonomic (including adrenomedullary) responses to falling glucose concentrations. These impaired autonomic responses result in reduced symptoms of impending hypoglycemia (e.g., hypoglycemia unawareness) because epinephrine responses are reduced in the setting of absent glucagon responses. Thus, a vicious cycle of recurrent hypoglycemia is created and perpetuated. The syndrome of hypoglycemia unawareness and the reduced epinephrine component of defective glucose counterregulation are reversible but require >2 weeks of scrupulous avoidance of hypoglycemia. This involves a shift of glycemic thresholds back to higher plasma glucose concentrations.

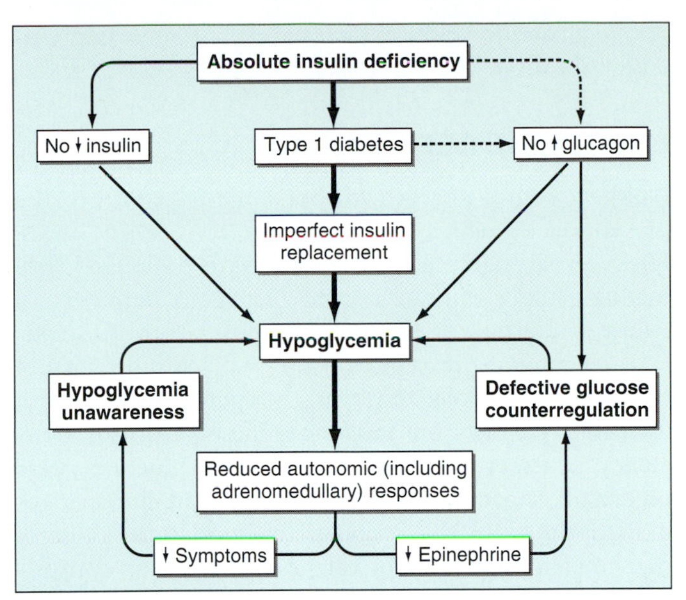

FIGURE 19-2
Hypoglycemia-associated autonomic failure and hypoglycemia unawareness in type 1 diabetes. (*PE Cryer: Diabetes 41:255, 1992.*)

HYPOGLYCEMIA RISK FACTOR REDUCTION

A diagnosis of hypoglycemia unawareness can usually be made from the history. One should note that hypoglycemia unawareness implies that previous episodes of hypoglycemia have occurred, whether these are documented or not. If low glucose levels are not apparent from the patient's self-monitoring log, one should suspect hypoglycemia during the night. The presence of clinical hypoglycemia unawareness makes defective glucose counterregulation likely. It is possible to minimize the risk of hypoglycemia by applying the principles of modern therapy—patient education and empowerment, frequent self-monitoring of blood glucose, flexible insulin (and other drug) regimens, rational glycemic goals, and ongoing professional guidance and support. If hypoglycemia is a recognized problem, first consider each of the conventional risk factors summarized earlier and recommend the appropriate adjustments of medications, diet, and life-style. Nonselective beta blockers may attenuate the recognition of hypoglycemia and they impair glycogenolysis; a relatively selective β_1-antagonist (e.g., metoprolol or atenolol) is preferable when a beta blocker is indicated.

REACTIVE HYPOGLYCEMIA

Postprandial (reactive) hypoglycemia occurs only after meals and is self-limited. Postprandial hypoglycemia occurs in children with certain rare enzymatic defects in carbohydrate metabolism such as hereditary fructose intolerance and galactosemia. Reactive hypoglycemia also occurs in some individuals who have undergone gastric surgery, which allows the rapid passage of food from the stomach to the small intestine. This type of *alimentary hypoglycemia* causes a rapid postprandial rise in plasma glucose levels and the release of gut incretins, which induce an exuberant insulin response and subsequent hypoglycemia. Administration of an α-glucosidase inhibitor, which delays carbohydrate digestion and thus glucose absorption from the intestine, can be considered for treatment of reactive hypoglycemia, although its efficacy remains to be established in controlled trials.

If postprandial symptoms occur as an idiopathic disorder, caution should be exercised before labeling a person with a diagnosis of hypoglycemia. Indeed, a self-diagnosis of hypoglycemia has often been reinforced by the finding of a "low" venous glucose concentration late after glucose ingestion. An oral glucose tolerance test should not be used in this setting. Plasma glucose falls as low as 2.4 mmol/L (43 mg/dL) after a 100-g glucose load in 5% of normal asymptomatic individuals, making it difficult to identify hypoglycemia based on the results of this test. The diagnosis of postprandial hypoglycemia requires documentation of Whipple's triad after a typical mixed meal. The cause of repetitive postprandial symptoms in certain individuals is unknown, but they may be particularly sensitive to the normal autonomic responses that follow ingestion of a meal.

FASTING HYPOGLYCEMIA

There are many causes of fasting hypoglycemia (Table 19-1). In addition to insulin and sulfonylureas used in the treatment of diabetes, ethanol use is a relatively common cause of hypoglycemia. Sepsis and renal failure are often complicated by hypoglycemia. Endocrine deficiencies, non-beta-cell tumors, and endogenous hyperinsulinemia (including that caused by an insulinoma) are rare causes of hypoglycemia. Enzymatic metabolic errors that cause hypoglycemia are also rare but are being recognized more frequently in infants and children.

DRUGS

In contrast to the sulfonylureas and rapid-acting insulin secretagogues (e.g., repaglinide, nateglinide), other oral hypoglycemic agents—biguanides (e.g., metformin), α-glucosidase inhibitors (e.g., acarbose, miglitol), and thiazolidinediones (e.g., rosiglitazone, pioglitazone)—do not act by stimulating insulin secretion. Therefore, with these agents, insulin levels usually decrease appropriately as plasma glucose levels fall. However, these drugs can contribute to hypoglycemia in other ways. Treatment with an α-glucosidase inhibitor alters the management of hypoglycemia; pure glucose should be used rather than ingestion of complex carbohydrates. Thiazolidinediones, as well as metformin, can predispose patients to hypoglycemia if they are receiving combined treatment with insulin or an insulin secretagogue.

Ethanol blocks gluconeogenesis but not glycogenolysis. Thus, alcohol-induced hypoglycemia typically occurs after a several-day ethanol binge during which the person eats little food, thereby causing glycogen depletion. Hypoglycemia in this setting can be profound, with mortality rates as high as 10%. Blood ethanol levels correlate poorly with plasma glucose concentrations at the time of diagnosis, as hypoglycemia occurs late in the sequence and often precludes further alcohol consumption.

Pentamidine, which is used to treat *Pneumocystis* pneumonia and other parasitic infections, is toxic to the pancreatic beta cell. It causes insulin release initially, with hypoglycemia in about 10% of treated patients, and predisposes to the development of diabetes mellitus later. Quinine also stimulates insulin secretion. However, the relative contribution of hyperinsulinemia to the pathogenesis of hypoglycemia in quinine-treated patients who are critically ill with malaria is debated. Salicylates and sulfonamides can cause hypoglycemia, but do so rarely. There are reports of hypoglycemia attributed to nonselective β-adrenergic antagonists (e.g., propranolol) and a variety of other drugs.

CRITICAL ILLNESS

Rapid and extensive hepatic destruction (e.g., severe toxic hepatitis) causes fasting hypoglycemia because the liver is the major site of endogenous glucose production. The mechanism of hypoglycemia reported in patients with cardiac failure is unknown but likely involves hepatic congestion. Although the kidneys are a source of glucose production, it is perhaps too simplistic to attribute hypoglycemia in persons with renal failure to this mechanism alone. The clearance of insulin is reduced substantially in renal failure, and reduced mobilization of gluconeogenic precursors has been reported.

Sepsis is sometimes complicated by hypoglycemia, which is multifactorial in origin. There is impaired endogenous glucose production, perhaps a result of hepatic hypoperfusion, and increased glucose utilization, which is induced by cytokines in macrophage-rich tissues such as the liver, spleen, and ileum and in muscle. Nutrition is also often inadequate in the setting of sepsis. Hypoglycemia can be seen with prolonged starvation, perhaps because of a loss of whole-body fat stores and the subsequent depletion of gluconeogenic precursors (e.g., amino acids), which necessitate increased glucose utilization.

ENDOCRINE DEFICIENCIES

Neither cortisol nor growth hormone is critical to the prevention of acute hypoglycemia, at least in adults. However, hypoglycemia can occur with prolonged fasting in patients with untreated primary adrenocortical failure (Addison's disease) or hypopituitarism. Anorexia and weight loss are typical features of chronic cortisol deficiency and likely result in glycogen depletion with increased reliance on gluconeogenesis. Cortisol deficiency is associated with low levels of gluconeogenic precursors, suggesting that substrate-limited gluconeogenesis, in the setting of glycogen depletion, is the cause of the impaired ability to tolerate fasting in cortisol-deficient individuals. Growth hormone deficiency can cause hypoglycemia in young children. In addition to extended fasting, high rates of glucose utilization (e.g., during exercise, pregnancy) or low rates of glucose production (e.g., following alcohol ingestion) can precipitate hypoglycemia in adults with hypopituitarism. Cortisol and growth hormone secretion should be evaluated in patients with fasting hypoglycemia when the history suggests pituitary or adrenal disease and when other causes of hypoglycemia are not apparent.

Hypoglycemia is not a feature of the epinephrine-deficient state that results from bilateral adrenalectomy when glucocorticoid replacement is adequate, nor does it occur during pharmacologic adrenergic blockage when other glucoregulatory systems are intact. There are case reports of fasting hypoglycemia attributed to isolated glucagon or epinephrine deficiency, although hyperinsulinemia was not excluded convincingly in neonatal cases and other counterregulatory defects may have contributed in the adults. Thus, the regular assessment of glucagon and epinephrine secretion is not warranted.

NON-BETA-CELL TUMORS

Fasting hypoglycemia, often termed *non-islet cell tumor hypoglycemia,* occurs in some patients with large mesenchymal or other tumors (e.g., hepatoma, adrenocortical tumors, carcinoids; Chap. 22). The glucose kinetic patterns resemble those of hyperinsulinism, but insulin secretion is suppressed appropriately during hypoglycemia. In most instances, hypoglycemia is due to overproduction of an incompletely processed form of insulin-like growth factor (IGF) II. Although total IGF-II levels are not consistently elevated, circulating free IGF-II levels are high. Hypoglycemia results from IGF-II actions through the insulin or IGF-I receptors.

ENDOGENOUS HYPERINSULINISM

Hypoglycemia due to excessive endogenous insulin secretion can be caused by: (1) a primary pancreatic islet beta cell disorder, typically a beta cell tumor (insulinoma), sometimes multiple insulinomas, or, especially in infants or young children, a functional beta cell disorder without an anatomical correlate; (2) a beta cell secretagogue, often a sulfonylurea, and, theoretically, a beta cell–stimulating autoantibody; (3) an autoantibody to insulin; or (4) ectopic insulin secretion. None of these disorders is common. Endogenous hyperinsulinism is more likely to occur in an overtly healthy individual without other apparent causes of hypoglycemia such as a relevant drug history, critical illness, endocrine deficiencies, or a non-beta-cell tumor. Accidental, surreptitious, or even malicious administration of a sulfonylurea or insulin should also be considered in such individuals.

The fundamental pathophysiologic feature of endogenous hyperinsulinism is the failure of insulin secretion to fall to very low rates during hypoglycemia. This is assessed by measuring insulin, proinsulin, and C peptide, which is derived from the processing of proinsulin. Critical diagnostic findings are a plasma insulin concentration ≥36 pmol/L (≥6 μU/mL) and a plasma C-peptide concentration ≥0.2 mmol/L (≥0.6 ng/mL) when the plasma glucose concentration is ≤2.5 mmol/L (≤45 mg/dL) in the fasting state with symptoms of hypoglycemia. Insulin and C-peptide levels do not need to be absolutely increased (e.g., relative to euglycemic normal values) but only inappropriately increased in the setting of fasting hypoglycemia. Plasma proinsulin concentrations are also inappropriately elevated, particularly in patients with an insulinoma. Sulfonylureas, because they stimulate insulin secretion, result in a pattern of glucose, insulin, and C-peptide levels that is indistinguishable from that produced by a primary beta cell disorder. The measurement of sulfonylureas in plasma or urine distinguishes these conditions. Antibodies to insulin produce *autoimmune hypoglycemia* following the transition from the postprandial to the postabsorptive state, as insulin slowly dissociates from the antibodies. Total and free plasma insulin concentrations are inappropriately high. The distinguishing feature is the presence of circulating antibodies to insulin, but the need to measure these routinely is debated, since autoimmune hypoglycemia is rare. Autoantibodies to the insulin receptor are another rare cause of hypoglycemia and usually occur in the context of other autoimmune diseases. A few cases of ectopic insulin secretion (from a non-beta-cell tumor) have been reported.

Insulinoma and Other Primary Beta Cell Disorders

Insulinomas are uncommon, but because ~90% are benign, they are a treatable cause of potentially fatal hypoglycemia. The yearly incidence is estimated to be 1 in 250,000. About 60% of cases occur in women. The median age at presentation is 50 years in sporadic cases, but it usually presents in the third decade when associated with multiple endocrine neoplasia type 1 (Chap. 21). Insulinomas arise within the substance of the pancreas in >99% of cases and are usually small (1 to 2 cm). About 5 to 10% of insulinomas are malignant, as evidenced by the presence of metastases.

Insulinomas are almost always recognized because of hypoglycemia rather than mass effects. Unusually low plasma glucose concentrations may be required to produce symptoms and signs of hypoglycemia because recurrent hypoglycemia shifts the glycemic thresholds. Although symptomatic hypoglycemia can occur after an overnight fast, it often follows exercise. Rarely, symptomatic hypoglycemia occurs following meals, but most such patients have evidence of fasting hypoglycemia as well.

Octreotide scans localize approximately half of insulinomas. Arteriography has been used extensively in the past, but false-negative and false-positive results occur, and it is generally preferable to use less invasive computed tomography (CT) or magnetic resonance imaging (MRI) scans, which detect 45 to 75% of tumors. Preoperative ultrasound is valuable for some patients. Intraoperative ultrasonography has high sensitivity and may localize tumors not identified by palpation. Surgical resection of a solitary insulinoma is generally curative. Diazoxide, which inhibits insulin secretion, and the somatostatin analogue, octreotide, can be used to treat hypoglycemia in patients with unresectable insulinomas.

FACTITIOUS HYPOGLYCEMIA

Factitious hypoglycemia, caused by malicious or self-administration of insulin or ingestion of a sulfonylurea, shares many clinical and laboratory features with insulinoma. It is most common among health care workers, patients with diabetes or their relatives, and people with a history of other factitious illnesses. When this diagnosis is suspected, it is useful to seek previous medical records, which may reveal admissions for similar episodes. In individuals taking exogenous insulin, factitious hypoglycemia can be distinguished from insulinoma by the presence of high insulin levels without a concomitant increase in the C-peptide level, which is suppressed by the exogenous insulin. As noted above, sulfonylureas stimulate endogenous insulin and can therefore be detected only by measuring drug levels in plasma or urine. Factitious or surreptitious hypoglycemia should be considered in every patient requiring a fasting test for hypoglycemia. In addition to laboratory tests, observing the patient's behavior may help make this diagnosis.

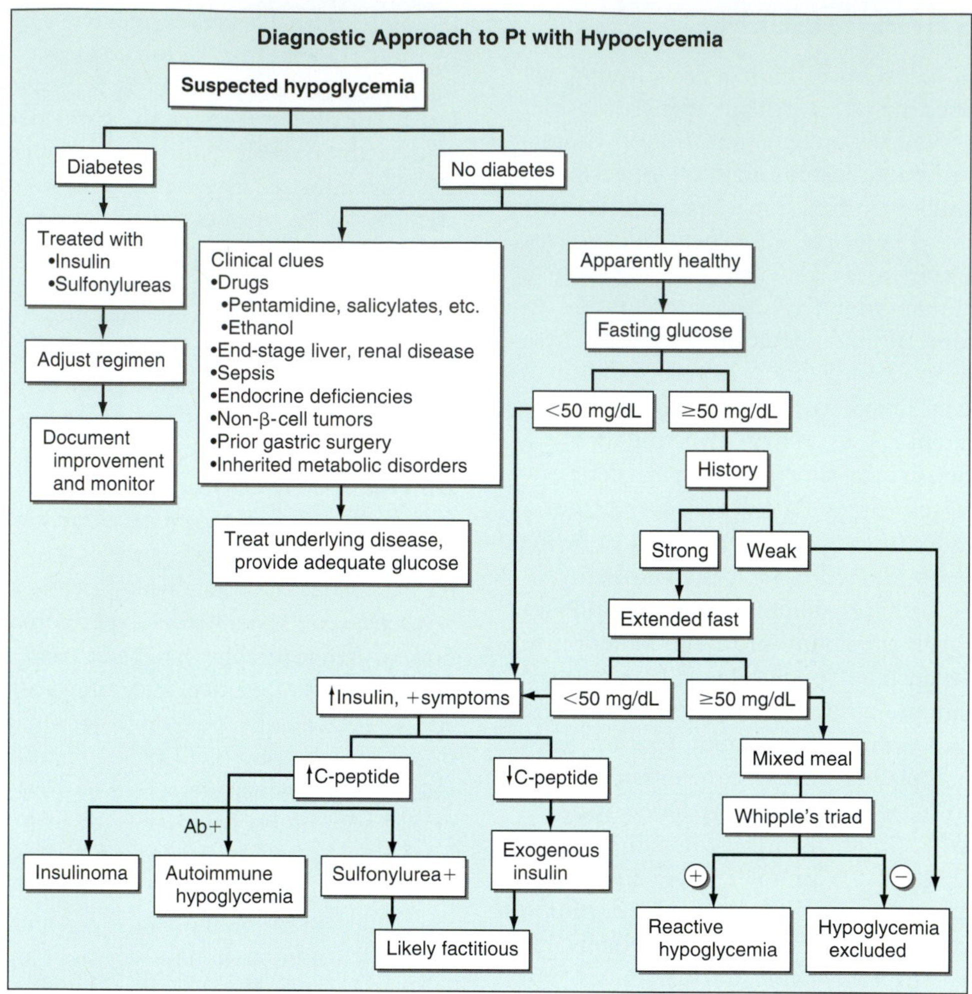

FIGURE 19-3

Diagnostic approach to a patient with suspected hypoglycemia based on a history of symptoms, a low plasma glucose concentration, or both.

APPROACH TO THE PATIENT WITH HYPOGLYCEMIA

In addition to recognition and documentation of hypoglycemia, and often urgent treatment, diagnosis of the hypoglycemic mechanism is critical for choosing a treatment that prevents, or at least minimizes, recurrent hypoglycemia. A diagnostic algorithm is shown in **Fig. 19-3.**

RECOGNITION AND DOCUMENTATION

Urgent treatment is often necessary in patients with suspected hypoglycemia. Blood should be drawn, whenever possible, before the administration of glucose to allow documentation of the plasma glucose level. Convincing documentation of hypoglycemia requires the fulfillment of Whipple's triad. Thus, *the ideal time to test the plasma glucose is during an episode associated with hypoglycemic symptoms.* A normal plasma glucose concentration measured when the patient is free of symptoms does not exclude hypoglycemia at the time of earlier symptoms. When the cause of hypoglycemia is obscure, additional assays should include glucose, insulin, C peptide, sulfonylurea levels, cortisol, and ethanol.

Hypoglycemia is sometimes detected serendipitously. A distinctly low plasma glucose measurement in a person without a history of corresponding symptoms raises the possibility of a laboratory error caused by ongoing metabolism of glucose by the formed elements of the blood after the sample is drawn. This type of artifactually low glucose level is particularly likely when leukocyte, erythrocyte, or platelet counts are abnormally high, but also if separation of the plasma or serum from the formed elements is delayed.

DIAGNOSIS OF THE HYPOGLYCEMIC MECHANISM

In an adult patient with documented hypoglycemia, a plausible hypoglycemic mechanism and further diagnostic evaluation can be guided by the history, physical examination, and available laboratory data (Fig. 19-3). In the absence of documented spontaneous hypoglycemia, overnight fasting, or food deprivation during observation in the outpatient setting, will sometimes elicit hypoglycemia and allow diagnostic evaluation. If there is a high degree of clinical suspicion, an extended fast lasting 48 to 72 h is often required to make the diagnosis. This procedure should be performed in the hospital with careful supervision and should be terminated if the plasma glucose drops to <2.5 mmol/L (<45 mg/dL) and the patient has symptoms. It is essential to draw blood samples for appropriate tests before administering glucose or allowing the patient to eat.

URGENT TREATMENT

Oral treatment with glucose tablets or glucose-containing fluids, candy, or food is appropriate if the patient is able and willing to take these. A reasonable initial dose is 20 g of glucose. If neuroglycopenia precludes oral feedings, parenteral therapy is necessary. Intravenous glucose (25 g) should be given using a 50% solution followed by a constant infusion of 5 or 10% dextrose. If intravenous therapy is not practical, subcutaneous or intramuscular glucagon can be used, particularly in patients with type 1 diabetes mellitus. Because it acts primarily by stimulating glycogenolysis, glucagon is ineffective in glycogen-depleted individuals (e.g., those with alcohol-induced hypoglycemia). It also stimulates insulin secretion and is therefore less useful in type 2 diabetes mellitus. These treatments raise plasma glucose concentrations only transiently, and patients should be encouraged to eat as soon as practical to replete glycogen stores.

PREVENTION OF RECURRENT HYPOGLYCEMIA

Prevention of recurrent hypoglycemia requires an understanding of the hypoglycemic mechanism. Offending drugs can be discontinued or their doses reduced. It should be remembered that hypoglycemia caused by sulfonylureas may recur after a period of several hours or days. Underlying critical illnesses can often be treated. Cortisol and growth hormone can be replaced if deficient. Surgical, radiotherapeutic, or chemotherapeutic reduction of a non-beta-cell tumor can alleviate hypoglycemia, even if the tumor cannot be cured; glucocorticoid or growth hormone administration may also reduce hypoglycemic episodes in such patients. Surgical resection of an insulinoma is often curative; medical therapy with diazoxide or octreotide can be used if resection is not possible and in patients with a nontumor primary beta cell disorder. The treatment of autoimmune hypoglycemia (e.g., with a glucocorticoid) is more problematic, but this disorder is often self-limited. Failing these treatments, frequent feedings and avoidance of fasting may be required. Uncooked cornstarch at bedtime or an overnight infusion of intragastric glucose may be necessary in some patients.

FURTHER READINGS

American Diabetes Association: Defining and reporting hypoglycemia in diabetes: A report from the American Diabetes Association Workgroup on Hypoglycemia. Diabetes Care 28:1245, 2005

Davis S et al: Hypoglycemia as a barrier to glycemic control. J Diabetes Complications 18:60, 2004

This review summarizes the current knowledge on hypoglycemia with a focus on the improvements in insulin therapy that may produce more normal physiologic insulin profiles with an attendant lower risk of hypoglycemia.

Service FJ: Hypoglycemic disorders. Endocrinol Metab Clin North Am 28:467, 1999

Service GJ et al: Hyperinsulinemic hypoglycemia with nesidioblastosis after gastric-bypass surgery. N Engl J Med 353:249, 2005

Bariatric surgery is increasingly used to treat morbidly obese patients. This study describes the development of postprandial hyperinsulinemic hypoglycemia from nesidioblastosis, or hyperplastic beta cells, in six patients who underwent Roux-en-Y bypass surgery. A possible explanation for this association is an increase in gut hormones, specifically glucagon-like peptide-1 (GLP-1), which is increased by rapid intestinal exposure to nutrients, as occurs with the Roux-en-Y procedure.

Section IV

DISORDERS AFFECTING MULTIPLE ENDOCRINE SYSTEMS

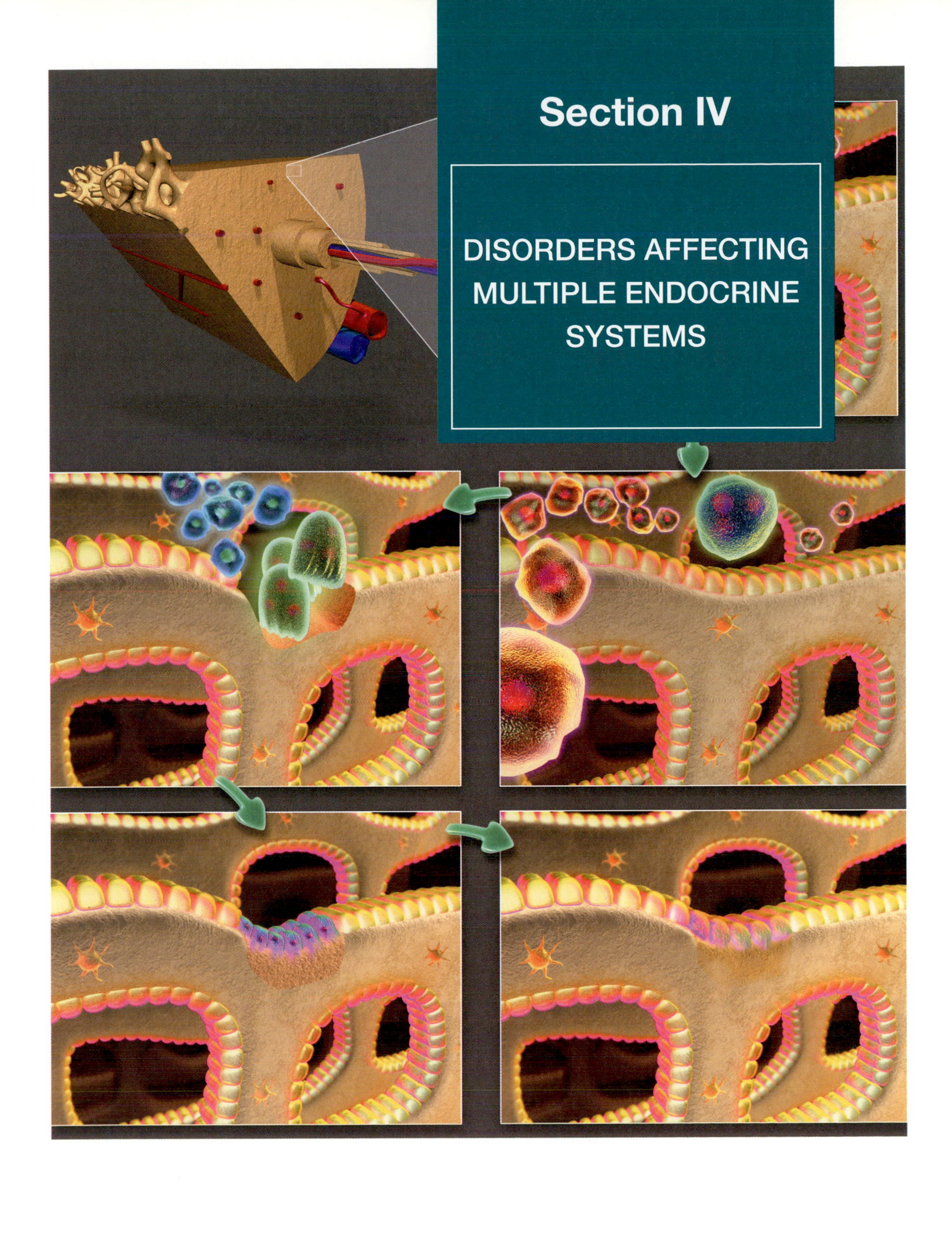

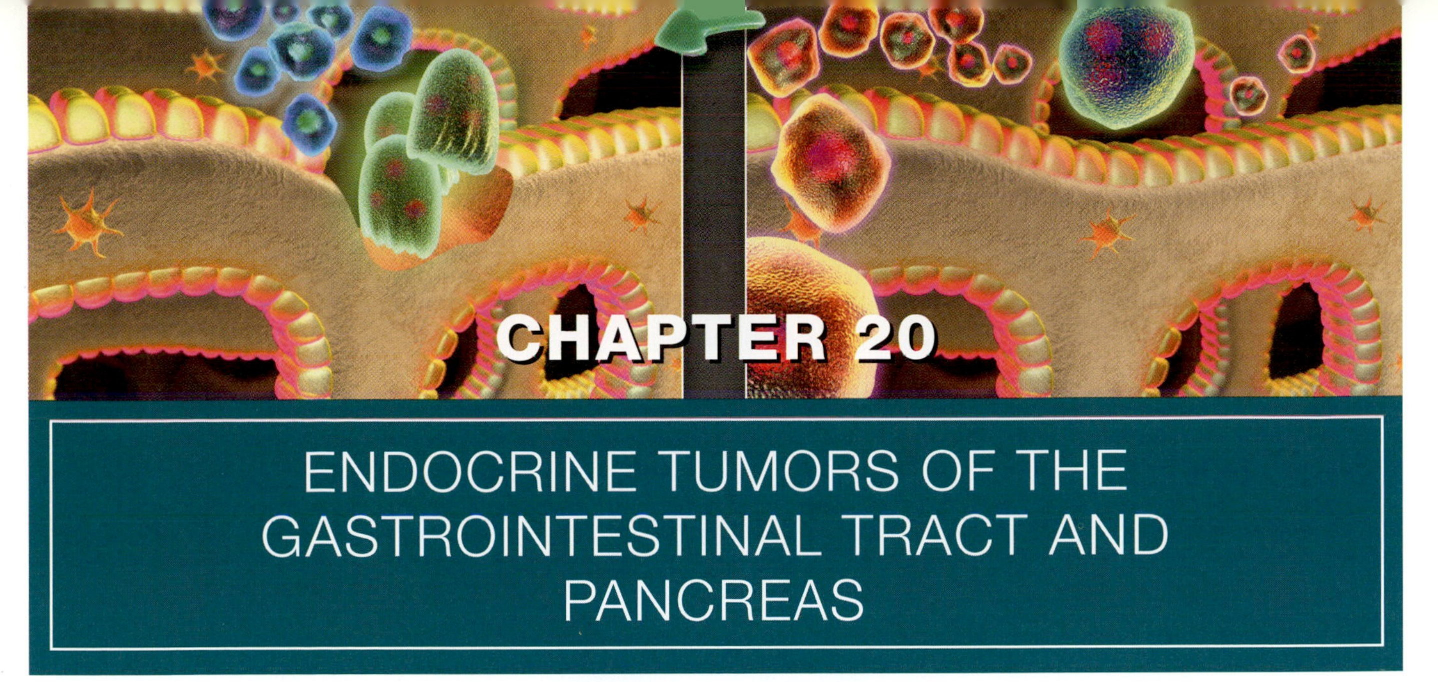

ENDOCRINE TUMORS OF THE GASTROINTESTINAL TRACT AND PANCREAS

Robert T. Jensen

Gastrointestinal neuroendocrine tumors (NETs) are tumors derived from the diffuse neuroendocrine system of the gastrointestinal (GI) tract, which is composed of amine- and acid-producing cells with different hormonal profiles, depending on the site of origin. The tumors they produce can be generally divided into carcinoid tumors and pancreatic endocrine tumors (PETs). These tumors were originally classified as APUDomas (for *a*mine *p*recursor *u*ptake and *d*ecarboxylation), as were pheochromocytomas, melanomas, and medullary thyroid carcinomas because they share certain cytochemical features as well as various pathologic, biologic, and molecular features (**Table 20-1**). APUDomas were thought to have a similar embryonic origin from neural crest cells, but the peptide-secreting cells are not of neuroectodermal origin.

CLASSIFICATION/PATHOLOGY/TUMOR BIOLOGY OF NETS

NETs are composed of monotonous sheets of small round cells with uniform nuclei; mitoses are uncommon. They can be tentatively identified on routine histology; however, these tumors are principally recognized by their histologic staining patterns due to shared cellular proteins. Historically, silver staining was used and tumors were classified as showing an argentaffin reaction if they took up and reduced silver or as being argyrophilic if they did not reduce it. Immunocytochemical localization of chromogranins (A, B, C), neuron-specific enolase, or synaptophysin, which are all neuroendocrine cell markers, are now used (Table 20-1). Chromogranin A is the most widely used.

Ultrastructurally, these tumors possess electron-dense neurosecretory granules and frequently contain small clear vesicles that correspond to synaptic vesicles of neurons. NETs synthesize numerous peptides, growth factors, and bioactive amines that may be ectopically secreted, giving rise to a specific clinical syndrome (**Table 20-2**). The diagnosis of the specific syndrome requires the clinical features of the disease and cannot be made from the immunocytochemistry results only. The presence or absence of a specific clinical syndrome cannot be predicted from the immunocytochemistry (Table 20-1). Furthermore, pathologists cannot distinguish between benign and malignant NETs unless metastases or invasion are present.

Carcinoid tumors are frequently classified according to their anatomical area of origin (i.e., foregut, midgut,

TABLE 20-1

GENERAL CHARACTERISTICS OF GI NEUROENDOCRINE TUMORS [CARCINOIDS, PANCREATIC ENDOCRINE TUMORS (PETs)]

I. Share general neuroendocrine cell markers
   A. Chromogranins (A, B, C) are acidic monomeric soluble proteins found in the large secretory granules; chromogranin A is most widely used
   B. Neuron-specific enolase (NSE) is the γ-γ dimer of the enzyme enolase and is a cytosolic marker of neuroendocrine differentiation
   C. Synaptophysin is an integral membrane glycoprotein of 38,000 molecular weight found in small vesicles of neurons and neuroendocrine tumors
II. Pathologic similarities
   A. All are APUDomas showing *a*mine *p*recursor *u*ptake and *d*ecarboxylation
   B. Ultrastructurally they have dense-core secretory granules (>80nm)
   C. Histologically appear similar with few mitoses and uniform nuclei
   D. Frequently synthesize multiple peptides/amines, which can be detected immunocytochemically but may not be secreted
   E. Presence or absence of clinical syndrome or type cannot be predicted by immunocytochemical studies
   F. Histologic classifications do not predict biologic behavior; only invasion or metastases establishes malignancy
III. Similarities of biologic behavior
   A. Generally slow growing, but a proportion are aggressive
   B. Secrete biologically active peptides/amines, which can cause clinical symptoms
   C. Generally have high densities of somatostatin receptors, which are used for both localization and treatment.
IV. Similarities/differences in molecular abnormalities
   A. Similarities
      1. Uncommon—alterations in common oncogenes (*ras, jun, fos, etc*)
      2. Uncommon—alterations in common tumor-suppressor genes (p53, retinoblastoma).
      3. Alterations at MEN-1 gene locus (11q13) and $p16^{INK4a}$ (9p21) occur in a proportion (10–30%).
   B. Differences
      1. PETs—loss of 3p (8–47%), 3q (8–41%), 11q (21–62%), 6q (18–68%); gains at 17q (10–55%), 7q (16–68%).
      2. Carcinoids—loss of 18q (38–67%) >18p (33–43%) >9p (21%); gains at 17q, 19p (57%).

Note: MEN, multiple endocrine neoplasia; PETs, pancreatic endocrine tumors.

TABLE 20-2

GI NEUROENDOCRINE TUMOR SYNDROMES

NAME	BIOLOGICALLY ACTIVE PEPTIDE(S) SECRETED	INCIDENCE NEW CASES/10^6 POPULATION/YEAR	TUMOR LOCATION	MALIGNANT, %	ASSOCIATED WITH MEN-1, %	MAIN SYMPTOMS/SIGNS
		I. ESTABLISHED SPECIFIC FUNCTIONAL SYNDROME				
Carcinoid tumor Carcinoid syndrome	Serotonin, possibly tachykinins, motilin, prostaglandins	0.5–2	Midgut (75–87%) Foregut (2–33%) Hindgut (1–8%) Unknown (2–15%)	95–100	Rare	Diarrhea (32–84%) Flushing (63– 75%) Pain (10–34%) Asthma (4–18%) Heart disease (11–41%)

(Continued)

TABLE 20-2 ***(Continued)***

GI NEUROENDOCRINE TUMOR SYNDROMES

NAME	BIOLOGICALLY ACTIVE PEPTIDE(S) SECRETED	INCIDENCE NEW CASES/10^6 POPULATION/YEAR	TUMOR LOCATION	MALIGNANT, %	ASSOCIATED WITH MEN-1, %	MAIN SYMPTOMS/SIGNS
Pancreatic endocrine tumor						
Zollinger-Ellison syndrome	Gastrin	0.5–1.5	Duodenum (70%) Pancreas (25%) Other sites (5%)	60–90	20–25	Pain (79–100%) Diarrhea (30–75%) Esophageal symptoms (31–56%)
Insulinoma	Insulin	1–2	Pancreas (>99%)	<10	4–5	Hypoglycemic symptoms (100%)
VIPoma (Verner-Morrison syndrome, pancreatic cholera, WDHA)	Vasoactive intestinal peptide	0.05–0.2	Pancreas (90%, adult) Other (10%, neural, adrenal, periganglionic)	40–70	6	Diarrhea (90–100%) Hypokalemia (80–100%) Dehydration (83%)
Glucagonoma	Glucagon	0.01–0.1	Pancreas (100%)	50–80	1–20	Rash (67–90%) Glucose intolerance (38–87%) Weight loss (66–96%)
Somatostatinoma	Somatostatin	Rare	Pancreas (55%) Duodenum-jejunum (44%)	>70	45	Diabetes mellitus (63–90%) Cholelithiasis (65–90%) Diarrhea (35–90%)
GRFoma	Growth hormone–releasing hormone	Unknown	Pancreas (30%) Lung (54%) Jejunum (7%) Other (13%)	>60	16	Acromegaly (100%)
ACTHoma	ACTH	Rare	Pancreas (4–16%, all ectopic Cushing's)	>95	Rare	Cushing's syndrome (100%)
PET causing carcinoid syndrome	Serotonin, ? tachykinins	Rare (43 cases)	Pancreas (<1% all carcinoids)	60–88	Rare	Same as carcinoid syndrome above
PET causing hypercalcemia	PTHrP, others unknown	Rare	Pancreas (rare cause of hypercalcemia)	84	Rare	Abdominal pain due to hepatic metastases
II. POSSIBLE SPECIFIC FUNCTIONAL SYNDROME						
PET secreting calcitonin	Calcitonin	Rare	Pancreas (rare cause of hypercalci-tonemia)	>80	16	Diarrhea (50%)
PET secreting rennin		Renin	Rare	Pancreas	Unknown	No Hypertension
III. NO FUNCTIONAL SYNDROME						
Ppoma/nonfunctional	None	1–2	Pancreas (100%)	>60	18–44	Weight loss (30–90%) Abdominal mass (10–30%) Pain (30–95%)

Note: MEN, multiple endocrine neoplasia; VIPoma, tumor-secreting vasoactive intestinal peptide; WDHA, watery diarrhea, hypokalemia, and achlorhydria syndrome; ACTH, adrenocorticotrophic hormone; PET, pancreatic endocrine tumor; PTHrP, parathyroid hormone–related peptide; PPoma, tumor secreting pancreatic polypeptide.

hindgut), because tumors with similar areas of origin share functional manifestations, histochemistry, and secretory products (**Table 20-3**). Foregut tumors generally have a low serotonin (5HT) content, are argentaffin-negative but argyrophilic, occasionally secrete adrenocorticotropic hormone (ACTH) or 5-hydroxytryptophan (5HTP) causing an atypical carcinoid syndrome (**Fig. 20-1**), are often multihormonal, and may metastasize to bone. They uncommonly produce a clinical syndrome due to secreted products. Midgut carcinoids are argentaffin-positive, have a high serotonin content, most frequently cause the typical carcinoid syndrome when they metastasize (Table 20-3, Fig. 20-1), release serotonin and tachykinins (substance P, neuropeptide K, substance K), rarely secrete 5HTP or ACTH, and uncommonly metastasize to bone. Hindgut carcinoids (rectum, transverse and descending colon) are argentaffin-negative, often argyrophilic, rarely contain serotonin or cause the carcinoid syndrome (Fig. 20-1, Table 20-3), rarely secrete 5HTP or ACTH, contain numerous peptides, and may metastasize to bone.

PETs can be classified into nine well-established specific functional syndromes, two possible specific functional syndromes (PETs secreting calcitonin or renin), and nonfunctional PETs [pancreatic polypeptide (PP)-secreting tumors; PPomas] (Table 20-2). Each of the functional syndromes is associated with symptoms due to the specific hormone released. In contrast, nonfunctional PETs release no products that cause a specific clinical syndrome. "Nonfunctional" is a misnomer in the strict sense because they frequently secrete a number of peptides (PP, chromogranin A, ghrelin, neurotensin); however, they cause no specific clinical syndrome. The symptoms caused by nonfunctional PETs are entirely due to the tumor per se.

Carcinoid tumors can occur in almost any GI tissue; however, at present most (70%) originate from one of three sites: bronchus, jejuno-ileum, or colon/rectum (Table 20-3). In the past, carcinoid tumors most frequently occurred in the appendix (i.e., 40%); however, the bronchus/lung and small intestine are now the most common sites. Overall, GI carcinoids are the most common site for these tumors, comprising 64%, with the respiratory tract a distant second at 28%.

The term *pancreatic endocrine tumor*, although widely used and therefore retained here, is also a misnomer because these tumors can occur either almost entirely in the pancreas (insulinomas, glucagonomas, nonfunctional PETs, PETs causing hypercalcemia) or at both pancreatic and extrapancreatic sites [gastrinomas, VIPomas (VIP, vasoactive intestinal peptide), somatostatinomas, GRFomas (GRF, growth hormone–releasing factor)]. PETs are also called *islet cell tumors*; however, this

TABLE 20-3

CARCINOID TUMOR LOCATION, FREQUENCY OF METASTASES, AND ASSOCIATION WITH THE CARCINOID SYNDROME

	LOCATION (%OF TOTAL)	INCIDENCE OF METASTASES	INCIDENCE OF CARCINOID SYNDROME
Foregut			
Esophagus	<0.1	—	—
Stomach	4.6	10	9.5
Duodenum	2.0	—	3.4
Pancreas	0.7	71.9	20
Gallbladder	0.3	17.8	5
Bronchus, lung, trachea	27.9	5.7	13
Midgut			
Jejunum	1.8	58.4 (jejunum and ileum)	9
Ileum	14.9		9
Meckel's diverticulum	0.5	—	13
Appendix	4.8	38.8	<1
Colon	8.6	51	5
Liver	0.4	32.2	—
Ovary	1.0	32	50
Testis	<0.1	—	50
Hindgut			
Rectum	13.6	3.9	

Source: Location is from the PAN-SEER data (1973–1999), and incidence of metastases from the SEER data (1992–1999), reported by IM Modlin et al: Cancer 97:934. 2003. Incidence of carcinoid syndrome is from 4349 cases studied from 1950–1971, reported by JD Godwin: Cancer 36:560, 1975.

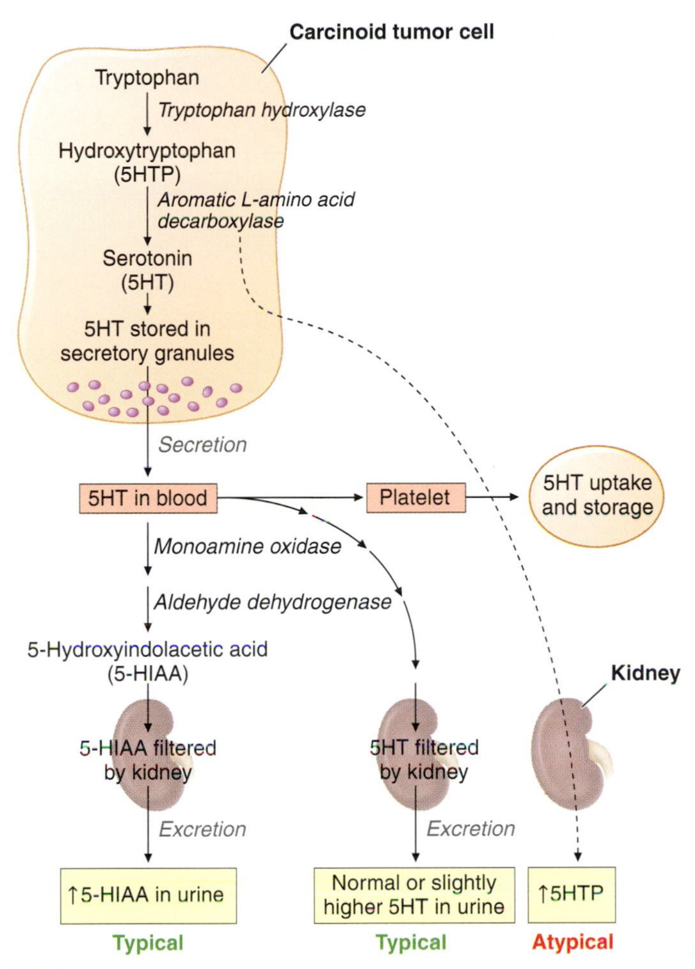

FIGURE 20-1

Synthesis, secretion, and metabolism of serotonin (5HT) in patients with typical and atypical carcinoid syndromes. Abbreviations: 5-HIAA, 5-hydroxyindolacetic acid.

term is discouraged because many do not originate from the islets and they can occur at extrapancreatic sites.

The exact incidence of carcinoid tumors or PETs varies according to whether only symptomatic or all tumors are considered. The incidence of clinically significant carcinoids is 7 to 13 cases per million population per year, whereas any malignant carcinoids at autopsy are reported in 21 to 84 cases per million population per year. Clinically significant PETs have a prevalence of 10 cases per million population, with insulinomas, gastrinomas, and nonfunctional PETs having an incidence of 0.5 to 2 cases per million population per year (Table 20-2). VIPomas are 2- to 8-fold less common, glucagonomas are 17- to 30-fold less common, and somatostatinomas the least common. In autopsy studies 0.5 to 1.5% of all cases have a PET; however, in <1 in 1000 cases was a functional tumor present.

Both carcinoid tumors and PETs commonly show malignant behavior (Tables 20-2, 20-3). Except for insulinomas, in which <10% are malignant, 50 to 100% of PETs are malignant. The fraction of carcinoid tumors showing malignant behavior varies in different locations. For the three most common sites of occurrence the incidence of metastases varies greatly: jejuno-ileum (58%) > lung/bronchus (6%) > rectum (4%). A number of factors influence survival and the aggressiveness of the tumor (**Table 20-4**). The presence of liver metastases is the single most important prognostic factor for both carcinoid tumors and PETs. Particularly important in the development of liver metastases is the size of the primary tumor. For small-intestinal carcinoids, the most frequent cause of the carcinoid syndrome due to metastatic disease in the liver, metastases occur in 15 to 25% if the tumor diameter is <1 cm, 58 to 80% if it is 1 to 2 cm, and >75% if >2 cm. Similar data exist for gastrinomas and other PETs. The presence of lymph node metastases, the depth of invasion, various histologic features (differentiation, mitotic rates, growth indices),

TABLE 20-4

PROGNOSTIC FACTORS IN NEUROENDOCRINE TUMORS

- Both carcinoid tumors and PETs
  - Presence of liver metastases ($p < .001$)
  - Extent of liver metastases ($p < .001$)
  - Presence of lymph node metastases ($p < .001$)
  - Depth of invasion ($p < .001$)
  - Primary tumor site ($p < .001$)
  - Primary tumor size ($p < .005$)
  - Various histologic features
    - Tumor differentiation ($p < .001$)
    - High growth indices (high Ki-67 index, PCNA expression)
    - High mitotic counts ($p < .001$)
    - Vascular or perineural invasion
    - Flow cytometric features (i.e., aneuploidy)
- Carcinoid tumors
  - Presence of carcinoid syndrome
  - Laboratory results [urinary 5-HIAA level ($p < .01$), plasma neuropeptide K ($p < .05$), serum chromogranin A ($p < .01$)]
  - Presence of a secondary malignancy
  - Male gender ($p < .001$)
  - Older age ($p < .01$)
  - Mode of discovery (incidental > symptomatic)
  - Molecular findings [TGF-α expression ($p < .05$), chr 16q LOH or gain chr 4p ($p < .05$)
- PETs
  - *Ha-Ras* oncogene or p53 overexpression
  - Female gender
  - MEN-1 syndrome absent
  - Laboratory findings (increased chromogranin A in some studies; gastrinomas—increased gastrin level)
  - Molecular findings [increased HER2/*neu* expression ($p = .032$), chr 1q, 3p, 3q, or 6q LOH ($p = .0004$), EGF receptor overexpression ($p = .034$), gains in chr 7q, 17q, 17p, 20q]

Note: PET, pancreatic endocrine tumor; Ki-67, proliferation-associated nuclear antigen recognized by Ki-67 monoclonal antibody; PCNA, proliferating cell nuclear antigen; 5-HIAA, 5-hydroxy indolacetic acid; TGF-α, transforming growth factor α; chr, chromosome; LOH, loss of heterozygosity; MEN, multiple endocrine neoplasia; EGF, epidermal growth factor.

and the presence of aneuploidy are all important prognostic factors for the development of metastatic disease (Table 20-4). For patients with carcinoid tumors, additional poor prognosis factors include the development of the carcinoid syndrome, older age, male gender, the presence of a symptomatic tumor, or increases in a number of tumor markers [5-hydroxyindolactic acid (5-HIAA), neuropeptide K, chromogranin A]. With PETs or gastrinomas, the best studied PET, a worse prognosis is associated with female gender, overexpression of the *Ha-Ras* oncogene or p53, the absence of multiple endocrine neoplasia (MEN) type 1, and higher levels of various tumor markers (i.e., chromogranin A, gastrin).

A number of genetic disorders are associated with an increased incidence of NETs (**Table 20-5**). Each is caused by a loss of a putative tumor-suppressor gene. The most important is MEN 1, which is an autosomal dominant disorder due to a defect in a 10-exon gene on 11q13 that encodes for a 610-amino-acid nuclear protein, menin (Chap. 21). In patients with MEN 1, 95 to 100% develop hyperparathyroidism due to parathyroid hyperplasia, 80 to 100% develop PETs, 54 to 80% develop pituitary adenomas, and bronchial carcinoids develop in 8%, thymic carcinoids in 8%, and gastric carcinoids in 13 to 30% of the patients with Zollinger-Ellison syndrome (ZES). In patients with MEN 1, 80 to 100% develop nonfunctional PETs; functional PETs occur in 80%, with 54% developing ZES, 21% insulinomas, 3% glucagonomas, and 1% VIPomas. MEN 1 is present in 20 to 25% of all patients with ZES, in 4% with insulinomas, and in a low percentage (<5%) of the other PETs.

Three phacomatoses associated with NETs are von Hippel–Lindau disease, von Recklinghausen's disease [neurofibromatosis (NF) type 1], and tuberous sclerosis (Bourneville's disease). Von Hippel–Lindau disease is an autosomal dominant disorder due to defects on chromosome 3p25, which encodes for a 213-amino-acid protein that interacts with the elongin family of proteins as a transcriptional regulator. In addition to cerebellar hemangioblastomas, renal cancer, and pheochromocytomas, 10 to 17% of these patients develop a PET. Most are nonfunctional, although insulinomas and VIPomas are reported. Patients with NF-1 have defects in a gene on chromosome 17q11.2 encoding for a 2845-amino-acid protein, neurofibromin, which functions in normal cells as a suppressor of the ras signaling cascade. Up to 12% of these patients develop an upper GI carcinoid tumor, characteristically in the periampullary region (54%). Many are classified as somatostatinomas because they contain somatostatin immunocytochemically; however, they uncommonly secrete somatostatin or produce a clinical somatostatinoma syndrome. NF-1 has rarely been associated with insulinomas and ZES. Tuberous sclerosis is caused by mutations that alter either the 1164-amino-acid protein, hamartin (TSC1), or the 1807-amino-acid protein, tuberin (TSC2). Both hamartin and tuberin interact in a pathway related to cytosolic G protein regulation. A few cases including nonfunctional and functional PETs (insulinomas and gastrinomas) have been reported in these patients.

In contrast to most common nonendocrine tumors such as carcinoma of the breast, colon, lung, or stomach, PETs and carcinoid tumors do not have alterations in common oncogenes (*ras, myc, fos, src, jun*) or common tumor-suppressor genes (p53, retinoblastoma susceptibility gene) (Table 20-1). Alterations that may be important in their pathogenesis include changes in the

TABLE 20-5

GENETIC SYNDROMES ASSOCIATED WITH AN INCREASED INCIDENCE OF NEUROENDOCRINE TUMORS [NETs: CARCINOIDS OR PANCREATIC ENDOCRINE TUMORS (PETs)]

SYNDROME	LOCATION OF GENE MUTATION AND GENE PRODUCT	NETs SEEN/FREQUENCY
Multiple endocrine neoplasia type 1 (MEN-1)	11q13 (encodes 610-aminoacid protein, menin)	80–100% develop PETs: (nonfunctional > gastrinoma > insulinoma) Carcinoids: gastric (13–30%), bronchial/thymic (8%)
von Hippel–Lindau disease	3q25 (encodes 213-amino-acid-protein)	12–17% develop PETs (almost always nonfunctional)
von Recklinghausen's disease [neurofibromatosis1 (NF-1)]	17q11.2 (encodes 2485-amino-acid protein, neurofibromin)	Duodenal somatostatinomas (usually nonfunctional) Rarely insulinoma, gastrinoma
Tuberous sclerosis	9q34 (TSCI) (encodes 1164-amino-acid protein, hamartin) 16p13 (TSC2) (encodes 1807-amino-acid protein, tuberin)	Uncommonly develop PETs [nonfunctional and functional (insulinoma, gastrinoma)]

MEN 1 gene, p16/MTS1 tumor-suppressor gene, and DPC 4/*Smad* 4 gene; amplification of the HER-2/*neu* protooncogene and growth factors and their receptors; and deletions of unknown tumor-suppressor genes as well as gains in other unknown genes. Comparative genomic hybridization and genome-wide allelotyping studies have shown genetic differences between PETs and carcinoids (Table 20-1), some of which have prognostic significance (Table 20-4). Mutations in the *MEN 1* gene are particularly important. Loss of heterozygosity at the MEN 1 locus on chromosome 11q13 occurs in 46% of sporadic PETs (those without MEN 1) and in 26 to 75% of sporadic carcinoid tumors. Mutations in the *MEN 1* gene are reported in 31 to 34% of sporadic gastrinomas. The presence of a number of these molecular alterations correlates with tumor growth, tumor size, and disease extent or invasiveness and may have prognostic significance.

CARCINOID TUMORS AND CARCINOID SYNDROME

GENERAL TUMOR CHARACTERISTICS OF THE MOST COMMON GI CARCINOID TUMORS

Appendiceal Carcinoids

These occur in 1 in every 200 to 300 appendectomies, usually in the appendiceal tip. Most are <1 cm in diameter without metastases; however, up to 35% have metastases (Table 20-3). Among 1570 appendiceal carcinoids, 62% were localized and 27% had regional and 8% had distant metastases. Of tumors 1 to 2 cm in diameter, half metastasized to lymph nodes. The percentage of larger carcinoids has decreased from 43.9% (1950 to 1969) to 2.4% (1992 to 1999).

Small Intestinal Carcinoids

These are frequently multiple; 70 to 80% are present in the ileum and 70% are within 60 cm (24 in.) of the ileocecal valve. Some 40% are <1 cm in diameter, 32% are 1 to 2 cm, and 29% are >2 cm. Between 35 and 70% are associated with metastases (Table 20-3). They characteristically cause a marked fibrotic reaction that can lead to intestinal obstruction. Distant metastases occur to liver in 36 to 60% of patients, to bone in 3%, and to lung in 4%. Even small carcinoid tumors of the small intestine (<1 cm) have metastases in 15 to 25%; the incidence increases to 58 to 100% for tumors 1 to 2 cm in diameter. Carcinoids also occur in the duodenum, with 31% having metastases. No duodenal tumor <1 cm metastasized, whereas 33% of those >2 cm had metastases. Small-intestinal carcinoids are the most common cause (60 to 87%) of the carcinoid syndrome (**Table 20-6**).

Rectal Carcinoids

Rectal carcinoids are found in 1 of every 2500 proctoscopies. Nearly all occur 4 to 13 cm above the dentate line. Most are small, with 66 to 80% being <1 cm in diameter; 5% metastasize. Tumors between 1 and 2 cm

TABLE 20-6

CLINICAL CHARACTERISTICS IN PATIENTS WITH CARCINOID SYNDROME

	AT PRESENTATION	DURING COURSE OF DISEASE
Symptoms/signs		
Diarrhea	32–73%	68–84%
Flushing	23–65%	63–74%
Pain	10%	34%
Asthma/wheezing	4–8%	3–18%
Pellagra	2%	5%
None	12%	22%
Carcinoid heat disease present	11%	14–41%
Demographics		
Male	46–59%	46–61%
Age		
Mean	57 yrs	52–54 yrs
Range	25–79 yrs	9–91 yrs
Tumor location		
Foregut	5–9%	2–33%
Midgut	78–87%	60–87%
Hindgut	1–5%	1–8%
Unknown	2–11%	2–15%

can metastasize in 5 to 30% of patients, and tumors >2 cm, which are uncommon, in >70%.

Bronchial Carcinoids

Bronchial carcinoids are not related to smoking. A number of different classifications have been proposed. In some studies lung NETs are classified into four categories: typical carcinoid [also called bronchial carcinoid tumor, Kulchitsky cell carcinoma (KCC)-I]; atypical carcinoid (also called well-differentiated neuroendocrine carcinoma, KCC-II); intermediate small cell neuroendocrine carcinoma; and small cell neuroendocarcinoma (KCC-III). Another proposed classification includes three categories: benign or low-grade malignant (typical carcinoid); low-grade malignant (atypical carcinoid), and high-grade malignant (poorly differentiated carcinoma of the large cell or small cell type). These different categories of lung NETs have different prognoses varying from excellent for typical carcinoid to poor for small cell neuroendocrine carcinomas.

Gastric Carcinoids

These account for 3 of every 1000 gastric neoplasms. Three different subtypes of gastric carcinoids are observed. Each originates from gastric enterochromaffin-like (ECL) cells in the gastric mucosa. Two subtypes are associated with hypergastrinemic states: (1) chronic atrophic gastritis (type I) (80% of all gastric carcinoids), or (2) ZES, almost always as part of the MEN-1 syndrome (type II) (6% of all cases). These tumors generally pursue a benign course, with 9 to 30% associated with metastases. They are usually multiple and small and infiltrate only to the submucosa. The third subtype of gastric carcinoid (type III) (sporadic) occurs without hypergastrinemia (14% of all carcinoids) and pursues an aggressive course, with 54 to 66% developing metastases. Sporadic carcinoids are usually single, large tumors, 50% have atypical histology, and they can be a cause of the carcinoid syndrome. Gastric carcinoids as a percentage of all carcinoids are increasing in frequency [1.96% (1969 to 1971), 3.6% (1973 to 1991), 5.8% (1991 to 1999)].

CARCINOID TUMORS WITHOUT THE CARCINOID SYNDROME

The age of patients at diagnosis ranges from 10 to 93 years, with a mean age of 63 years for small intestine and 66 years for the rectum. The presentation is diverse and related to the site of origin and extent of malignant spread. In the appendix, carcinoid tumors are usually found incidentally during surgery for suspected appendicitis. Small-intestinal carcinoids in the jejunoileum present with periodic abdominal pain (51%), intestinal obstruction with ileus/invagination (31%), an abdominal tumor (17%), or GI bleeding (11%). Because of the vagueness of the symptoms the diagnosis is usually delayed about 2 years from onset of the symptoms, with a range up to 20 years. Duodenal, gastric, and rectal carcinoids are most frequently found by chance at endoscopy. The most common symptoms of rectal carcinoids are melena/bleeding (39%), constipation (17%), and diarrhea (12%). Bronchial carcinoids are frequently discovered as a lesion on a chest radiograph, and 31% of the patients are asymptomatic. Thymic carcinoids present as anterior mediastinal masses, usually on chest radiograph or computed tomography (CT) scan. Ovarian and testicular carcinoids usually present as masses discovered on physical examination or ultrasound. Metastatic carcinoid tumor in the liver frequently presents as hepatomegaly in a patient who may have minimal symptoms and near-normal liver function tests.

CARCINOID TUMORS WITH SYSTEMIC SYMPTOMS DUE TO SECRETED PRODUCTS

Carcinoid tumors immunocytochemically can contain numerous GI peptides: gastrin, insulin, somatostatin, motilin, neurotensin, tachykinins (substance K, substance P, neuropeptide K), glucagon, gastrin-releasing peptide, VIP, PP, other biologically active peptides (ACTH, calcitonin, growth hormone), prostaglandins, and bioactive amines (serotonin). These substances may or may not be released in sufficient amounts to cause symptoms. In patients with carcinoid tumors, elevated serum levels of PP were found in 43%, motilin in 14%, gastrin in 15%, and VIP in 6%. Foregut carcinoids are more likely to produce various GI peptides than midgut carcinoids. Ectopic ACTH production causing Cushing's syndrome is increasingly seen with foregut carcinoids (respiratory tract primarily) and in some series was the most common cause of the ectopic ACTH syndrome, accounting for 64% of all cases. Acromegaly due to GRF release occurs with foregut carcinoids; the somatostatinoma syndrome with duodenal carcinoids. The most common systemic syndrome with carcinoid tumors is the carcinoid syndrome.

CARCINOID SYNDROME

Clinical Features

The cardinal features at presentation and during the disease course are shown in Table 20-6. Flushing and diarrhea are the two most common symptoms, occurring in up to 73% initially and in up to 89% during the course of the disease. The characteristic flush is of sudden onset; it is a deep red or violaceous erythema of the upper body (especially the neck and face), often associated with a feeling of warmth, and occasionally associated with pruritus, lacrimation, diarrhea, or facial edema. Flushes may be precipitated by stress, alcohol, exercise, or certain foods such as cheese or by certain agents such as catecholamines, pentagastrin, and serotonin reuptake inhibitors. Flushing episodes may be brief, lasting 2 to 5 min, especially initially, or may last hours, especially later in the disease course. Flushing is usually seen with midgut carcinoids but can also occur with foregut carcinoids. With bronchial carcinoids the flushes are frequently prolonged for hours to days, reddish in color, and associated with salivation, lacrimation, diaphoresis, diarrhea, and hypotension. The flush associated with gastric carcinoids is also reddish in color but patchy in distribution over the face and neck. It may be provoked by food and have accompanying pruritus.

Diarrhea is present in 32 to 73% initially and in 68 to 84% at some time in their disease course. Diarrhea usually occurs with flushing (85% of cases). The diarrhea is usually described as watery, with 60% having <1 L per day of diarrhea. Steatorrhea is present in 67%, and in 46% it is >15 g/d (normal <7 g). Abdominal pain may be present with the diarrhea or independently in 10 to 34% of cases.

Cardiac manifestations occur in 11% initially and in 14 to 41% at some time in the disease course. The cardiac disease is due to fibrosis involving the endocardium, primarily on the right side, although left side lesions can occur also. The dense fibrous deposits are most commonly on the ventricular aspect of the tricuspid valve and less commonly on the pulmonary valve cusps. They can result in constriction of the valves and pulmonic stenosis is usually predominant, whereas the tricuspid valve is often fixed open, resulting in regurgitation. Up to 80% of patients with cardiac lesions develop heart failure. Lesions on the left side are much less extensive, occur in 30% at autopsy, and most frequently affect the mitral valve.

Other clinical manifestations include wheezing or asthma-like symptoms (8 to 18%) and pellagra-like skin lesions (2 to 25%). A variety of noncardiac problems due to increased fibrous tissue may be seen including retroperitoneal fibrosis causing urethral obstruction, Peyronie's disease of the penis, intraabdominal fibrosis, and occlusion of the mesenteric arteries or veins.

Pathobiology

In different studies carcinoid syndrome occurred in 8% of 8876 patients with carcinoid tumors, with a rate of 1.4 to 18.4%. It occurs only when sufficient concentrations of products secreted by the tumor reach the systemic circulation. In 91% of cases this occurs after distant metastases to the liver. Rarely primary gut carcinoids with nodal metastases with extensive retroperitoneal invasion, pancreatic carcinoids with retroperitoneal lymph nodes, or carcinoids of the lung or ovary with direct access to the systemic circulation can cause the carcinoid syndrome without hepatic metastases. All carcinoid tumors do not have the same propensity to metastasize and cause the carcinoid syndrome (Table 20-3). Midgut carcinoids account for 60 to 67% of the cases of carcinoid syndrome, foregut tumors for 2 to 33%, hindgut for 1 to 8%, and an unknown primary location for 2 to 15% (Tables 20-2, 20-3).

One of the main secretory products of carcinoid tumors involved in the carcinoid syndrome is serotonin (Fig. 20-1), which is synthesized from tryptophan. Up to 50% of dietary tryptophan can be used in this synthetic pathway by tumor cells, which can result in inadequate supplies for conversion to niacin; thus, some patients (2.5%) develop pellagra-like lesions. Serotonin has numerous biologic effects including stimulating intestinal secretion, inhibition of absorption, increasing intestinal motility, and stimulating fibrogenesis. Serotonin overproduction is found in 56 to 88% of all carcinoid tumors; however, 12 to 26% of patients do not have the carcinoid syndrome. In 90 to 100% of patients with the carcinoid syndrome serotonin is overproduced. Through its effects on gut motility and intestinal secretion, serotonin is thought to be predominantly responsible for the diarrhea. Serotonin receptor antagonists (especially $5HT_3$ antagonists) relieve the diarrhea in most patients. However, prostaglandin E_2 and tachykinins may be important mediators of the diarrhea in some patients. Serotonin does not appear to be involved in the flushing, because flushing is not relieved by serotonin receptor antagonists. In patients with gastric carcinoids the red, patchy pruritic flush is likely due to histamine release, because it can be prevented by H_1 and H_2 receptor antagonists. Numerous studies show tachykinins are stored in carcinoid tumors and released during flushing. However, octreotide can relieve the flushing induced by pentagastrin in these patients without altering the stimulated increase in plasma substance P, suggesting other mediators must be involved in the flushing. Both histamine and serotonin may be responsible for the wheezing as well as the fibrotic reactions involving the heart, Peyronie's disease, and intraabdominal fibrosis. The exact mechanism of the heart disease is unclear. The valvular heart disease caused by the appetite-suppressant drug dexfenfluramine is histologically indistinguishable from that observed in carcinoid disease or after long exposure to $5HT_2$-preferring ergot drugs. Metabolites of fenfluramine have high affinity for $5HT_2$ receptors whose activation is known to cause fibroblast mitogenesis. High levels of $5HT_{2B}$ and $5HT_{2C}$ receptor transcripts are known to occur in heart valves. Studies on sheep aortic valve interstitial cells demonstrate serotonin interacts primarily with $5HT_{2A/2B}$ receptors and stimulates transforming growth factor β and collagen biosynthesis. Thus, serotonin overproduction is important for the valvular changes, possibly by activating $5HT_2$ receptors in the endocardium. Both the magnitude of serotonin overproduction and prior chemotherapy are important predictors of progression of the heart disease. Atrial natriuretic peptide overproduction is also reported in patients with cardiac disease, but its role in the pathogenesis is unknown.

Patients may develop either a typical or atypical carcinoid syndrome (Fig. 20-1). In patients with the typical form, characteristically caused by a midgut carcinoid tumor, the conversion of tryptophan to 5HTP is the rate-limiting step. Once 5HTP is formed it is rapidly converted to 5HT and stored in secretory granules of the tumor or in platelets. A small amount remains in plasma and is converted to 5-HIAA, which appears in large amounts in the urine. These patients have an expanded serotonin pool size, increased blood and platelet serotonin, and increased urinary 5-HIAA. Some carcinoid tumors cause an atypical carcinoid syndrome thought due to a deficiency in the enzyme dopa decarboxylase in which 5HTP cannot be converted to 5HT (serotonin), and 5HTP is secreted into the bloodstream. In these patients plasma serotonin levels are normal but urinary levels may be increased because some 5HTP is converted to 5HT in the kidney. Characteristically, urinary 5HTP and 5HT are increased, but urinary 5-HIAA levels are only slightly elevated. Foregut carcinoids are the most likely to cause an atypical carcinoid syndrome.

One of the most life-threatening complications of the carcinoid syndrome is the development of a carcinoid crisis. This is more frequent in patients who have intense symptoms from foregut tumors or have greatly increased urinary 5-HIAA levels (i.e., >200 mg/d). The crises may occur spontaneously or be provoked by stress, anesthesia, chemotherapy, or a biopsy. Patients develop intense flushing, diarrhea, abdominal pain, and cardiac abnormalities including tachycardia, hypertension, or hypotension. If not adequately treated it can be fatal.

Diagnosis of the Carcinoid Syndrome and Carcinoid Tumors

The diagnosis of carcinoid syndrome relies on measurement of urinary or plasma serotonin or its metabolites in the urine. The measurement of 5-HIAA is most frequently used. False-positive elevations may occur if the patient is eating serotonin-rich foods, such as bananas, pineapple, walnuts, pecans, avocados, or hickory nuts, or taking certain medications (cough syrup containing guaifenesin, acetaminophen, salicylates, or L-dopa). The normal range in daily urinary 5-HIAA excretion is between 2 and 8 mg/d. 5-HIAA has 73% sensitivity and 100% specificity for carcinoid syndrome.

Most physicians use only the urinary 5-HIAA excretion rate; however, plasma and platelet serotonin levels, if available, may give additional information. Platelet serotonin levels are more sensitive than urinary 5-HIAA but are not generally available. Patients with foregut carcinoids may produce an atypical carcinoid syndrome. If this syndrome is suspected and the urinary 5-HIAA is minimally elevated or normal, other urinary metabolites of tryptophan such as 5HTP or 5HT should be measured (Fig. 20-1).

Flushing occurs in a number of other diseases including systemic mastocytosis or chronic myeloid leukemia with increased histamine release; in menopause; as a reaction to alcohol or glutamate; or as side effects of chlorpropamide, calcium channel blockers, and nicotinic acid. None of these conditions cause an increase in urinary 5-HIAA.

The diagnosis of carcinoid tumor can be suggested by the carcinoid syndrome, by recurrent abdominal symptoms in a healthy-appearing individual, or by discovering hepatomegaly or hepatic metastases associated with minimal symptoms. Ileal carcinoids, which make up 25% of all clinically detected carcinoids, should be suspected in patients with bowel obstruction, abdominal pain, flushing, or diarrhea.

Serum chromogranin A levels are elevated in 56 to 100% of patients with carcinoid tumors, and the level correlates with tumor bulk. Serum chromogranin A levels are not specific for carcinoid tumors because they are also elevated in patients with PETs and other NETs. Plasma neuron-specific enolase levels are also used as a marker of carcinoid tumors but are less sensitive than chromogranin A, being increased in only 17 to 47% of patients.

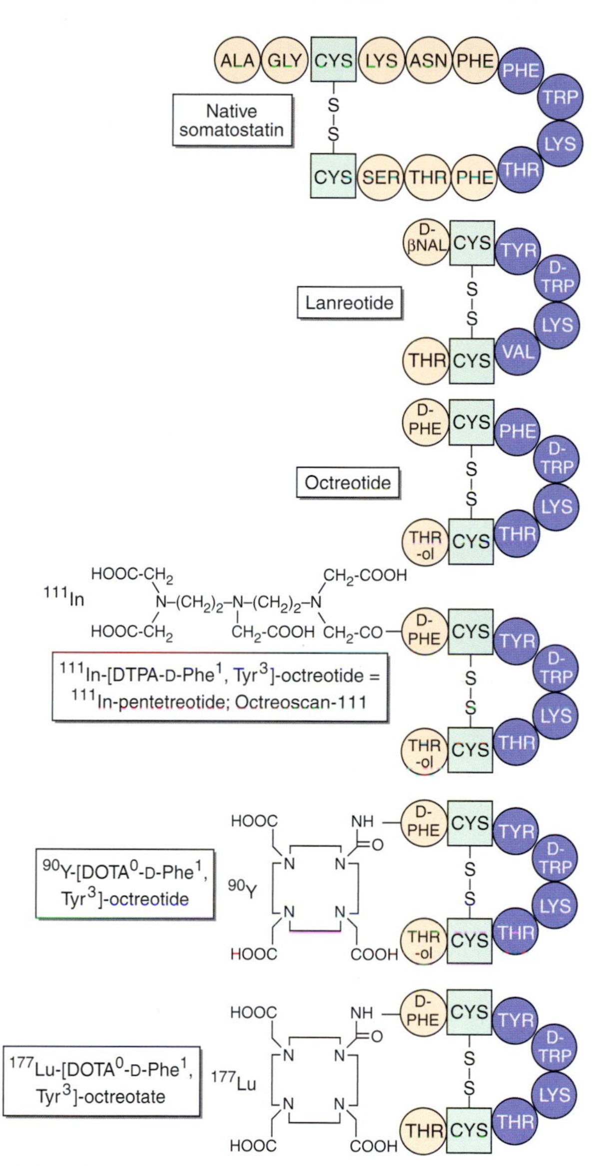

FIGURE 20-2

Structure of somatostatin and synthetic analogues used for diagnostic or therapeutic indications.

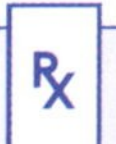

TREATMENT

Carcinoid Syndrome

Treatment includes avoiding conditions that precipitate flushing, dietary supplementation with nicotinamide, treatment of heart failure with diuretics, treatment of wheezing with oral bronchodilators, and controlling the diarrhea with antidiarrheal agents such as loperamide or diphenoxylate. If patients still have symptoms, serotonin receptor antagonists or somatostatin analogues (**Fig. 20-2**) are the drugs of choice.

There are 14 subclasses of serotonin (5HT) receptors; antagonists for most are not available. The $5HT_1$ and $5HT_2$ receptor antagonists methysergide, cyproheptadine, and ketanserin have all been used to control diarrhea but usually do not decrease flushing. The use of methysergide is limited because it can cause or enhance retroperitoneal fibrosis. Ketanserin diminishes diarrhea in 30 to 100% of patients. $5HT_3$ receptor antagonists (ondansetron, tropisetron, alosetron) can control diarrhea and nausea in up to 100% of patients and occasionally ameliorate the flushing. A combination of histamine H_1 and H_2 receptor antagonists (i.e., diphenhydramine and cimetidine or ranitidine) may control flushing in patients with foregut carcinoids.

Synthetic analogues of somatostatin (octreotide, lanreotide) are now the most widely used agents to control the symptoms of patients with carcinoid syndrome (Fig. 20-2). These drugs are effective at relieving symptoms and decreasing urinary 5-HIAA levels in patients with carcinoid syndrome. Octreotide controls symptoms in >80% of patients, including the diarrhea and flushing, and produces a >50% decrease in urinary 5-HIAA excretion in 70% of patients. Patients with mild to moderate symptoms should initially be treated with 100 μg subcutaneously every 8 h. Individual responses vary; doses as high as 3000 μg/d have been given. About 40% of patients escape control after a median 4 months, and the dose may need to be increased. Similar results are reported with lanreotide.

In patients with carcinoid crises, somatostatin analogues are effective at both treating the condition as well as preventing its development during known precipitating events such as surgery, anesthesia, chemotherapy, or stress. Octreotide, 150 to 250 μg subcutaneously every 6 to 8 h, should be used 24 to 48 h before anesthesia and then continued throughout the procedure.

Sustained-release preparations of both octreotide [octreotide-LAR, (long-acting release)] and lanreotide [lanreotide-PR (prolonged release)] have been developed. Octreotide-LAR (30 mg/month) gives a plasma level ≥ 1 ng/mL for 25 days, whereas the non-sustained-release form would need to be injected three to six times a day to achieve this level. Lanreotide-PR is given intramuscularly every 10 to 14 days. Both sustained-release forms are highly effective at controlling the symptoms of the carcinoid syndrome (61 to 85% of patients).

Short-term side effects occur in 40 to 60% of patients receiving subcutaneous somatostatin analogues. Pain at the injection site and side effects related to the GI tract (59% discomfort, 15% nausea, diarrhea) are the most common. They are usually short-lived and do not interrupt treatment. Important long-term side effects include gallstone formation, steatorrhea, and deterioration in glucose tolerance. The overall incidence of gallstones/biliary sludge is 52%, with 7% having symptomatic disease requiring surgical treatment.

Interferon-α controls symptoms of the carcinoid syndrome either alone or combined with hepatic artery embolization. The response rate to interferon-α alone is 42%, and when combined with hepatic artery embolization, diarrhea was controlled for 1 year in 43% and flushing in 86%.

Hepatic artery embolization alone or with chemotherapy (chemoembolization) has been used to control the symptoms of carcinoid syndrome. Embolization alone is reported to control symptoms in up to 76% of patients, and chemoembolization (5-fluorouracil, adriamycin, cisplatin, mitomycin) in 60 to 75% of patients. Hepatic artery embolization can have major side effects including nausea, vomiting, pain, and fever. The mortality rate is 5 to 7%.

Other drugs have been used successfully in small numbers of patients to control the symptoms of carcinoid syndrome. Parachlorophenylanine can inhibit tryptophan hydroxylase and therefore the conversion of tryptophan to 5HTP (Fig. 20-1). However, its severe side effects, including psychiatric disturbances, make it intolerable for long-term use. α-Methyldopa inhibits the conversion of 5HTP to 5HT; however, its effects are only partial.

Carcinoid Tumors (Nonmetastatic)

Surgery is the only potentially curative therapy. Because the probability of metastatic disease increases with increasing primary tumor size, the extent of surgical resection is determined accordingly. With appendiceal carcinoids, simple appendectomy was curative in 103 patients followed for up to 35 years. With rectal carcinoids <1 cm, local resection is curative. With small-intestinal carcinoids <1 cm, consensus has not been reached. Because 15 to 69% of small-intestinal carcinoids this size have metastases in different studies, some recommend a wide resection with en bloc resection of the adjacent lymph-bearing mesentery. If the carcinoid tumor is >2 cm in rectal, appendiceal, or small-intestinal sites, a full cancer operation should be done. This includes a right hemicolectomy for appendiceal carcinoid, an abdominoperineal resection or low anterior resection for rectal carcinoids, and an en bloc resection of adjacent lymph nodes for small-intestinal carcinoids. For carcinoids 1 to 2 cm in the appendix, a simple appendectomy is proposed by some, whereas others favor a formal right hemicolectomy. For rectal carcinoids of 1 to 2 cm, a wide local full-thickness excision is recommended.

With type I or II gastric carcinoids, which are usually <1 cm, endoscopic removal is recommended. For type I or II gastric carcinoids >2 cm or locally invasive, some recommend total gastrectomy; others recommend antrectomy in type 1. For types I and III gastric carcinoids of 1 to 2 cm, some recommend endoscopic treatment, others surgical treatment. With type III gastric carcinoids >2 cm, excision and regional lymph node clearance are recommended. Most tumors <1 cm are treated endoscopically.

Resection of isolated or limited hepatic metastases may be beneficial (see below).

PANCREATIC ENDOCRINE TUMORS

Functional PETs usually present with symptoms due to hormone excess. Only late in the course of the disease does the tumor per se cause prominent symptoms such as abdominal pain. In contrast, all of the symptoms due to nonfunctional PETs are due to the tumor per se. The overall result is that some functional PETs may present with severe symptoms with a small or undetectable primary tumor, whereas nonfunctional tumors almost always present late in their disease course with large tumors that are usually metastatic. The mean delay between onset of continuous symptoms and diagnosis of a functional PET syndrome is 4 to 7 years. Therefore, the diagnoses are frequently missed for extended periods of time.

Treatment of PETs requires two different strategies. Treatment must be directed at the hormone excess state such as the gastric acid hypersecretion in gastrinomas or hypoglycemia in insulinomas. Ectopic hormone secretion usually causes the presenting symptoms and can cause life-threatening complications. Second, with all of the tumors except insulinomas, >50% are malignant (Table 20-2); therefore, treatment must also be directed against the tumor per se. Because these tumors are not frequently surgically curable due to the extent of disease, in many cases surgical resection for cure, which addresses both treatment aspects, is not possible.

GASTRINOMA (ZOLLINGER-ELLISON SYNDROME)

A gastrinoma is a NET that secretes gastrin. The chronic hypergastrinemia results in marked gastric acid hypersecretion (ZES) and growth of the gastric mucosa, with increased numbers of parietal cells and proliferation of gastric ECL cells. The gastric acid hypersecretion characteristically causes peptic ulcer disease (PUD), often refractory and severe, as well as diarrhea. The most common presenting symptoms are abdominal pain (70 to 100%), diarrhea (37 to 73%), and gastroesophageal reflux disease (GERD) (30 to 35%), though 10 to 20% have diarrhea only. Although peptic ulcers may occur in unusual locations, most patients have a typical duodenal ulcer. Important observations that should suggest this diagnosis include PUD with diarrhea; PUD in an unusual location or with multiple lesions; and PUD that is refractory to treatment or persistent, associated with prominent gastric folds, associated with findings suggestive of MEN 1 (endocrinopathy, family history of ulcer or endocrinopathy, nephrolithiasis), or without *Helicobacter pylori* present. *H. pylori* is present in >90% of idiopathic peptic ulcers but is present in <50% of patients with gastrinomas. Chronic unexplained diarrhea should also suggest gastrinoma.

About 20 to 25% of patients have MEN 1, and in most cases the hyperparathyroidism is present before the gastrinoma. These patients are treated differently from those without MEN 1; therefore, MEN 1 should be sought in all patients by family history, by measuring plasma ionized calcium and prolactin levels and plasma hormone levels (parathormone, growth hormone).

Most gastrinomas (50 to 70%) are present in the duodenum, followed by the pancreas (20 to 40%) and other intraabdominal sites (mesentery, lymph nodes, biliary tract, liver, stomach, ovary). Rare cases may originate outside the abdominal cavity. In MEN 1 the gastrinomas are also usually in the duodenum (70 to 90%) or the pancreas (10 to 30%), and they are almost always multiple. Between 60 and 90% of gastrinomas are malignant (Table 20-2), with metastatic spread to lymph nodes and liver. Distant metastases to bone occur in 12 to 30% of patients with liver metastases.

Diagnosis

The diagnosis of gastrinoma requires the demonstration of fasting hypergastrinemia and an increased basal gastric acid output (BAO) (hyperchlorhydria). Nearly all patients with gastrinomas have fasting hypergastrinemia, although in 40 to 60% the level may be elevated by less than a factor of 10. Therefore, when the diagnosis is suspected a fasting gastrin level should be determined first. Potent gastric acid–suppressant drugs such as proton pump inhibitors (omeprazole, pantoprazole, lansoprazole, rabeprazole) can suppress acid secretion sufficiently to cause hypergastrinemia; because of their prolonged duration of action, these drugs need to be discontinued for a week before the gastrin determination. If the gastrin level is elevated, gastric pH should be measured. If gastric pH < 2.0, the hypergastrinemia is not a physiologic response to achlorhydria (atrophic gastritis, pernicious anemia), another common cause of hypergastrinemia. If the fasting gastrin > 1000 μg/L (10 times increased) and the pH < 2.0, which occurs in 40 to 60% of patients with gastrinoma, the diagnosis is established after ruling out the possibility of retained antrum syndrome by history. In patients with hypergastrinemia with fasting gastrin < 1000 μg/L and gastric pH < 2.0, other conditions such as *H. pylori* infections, antral G cell hyperplasia/hyperfunction, gastric outlet obstruction, or, rarely, renal failure can masquerade as a gastrinoma. To establish the diagnosis in this group, a determination of BAO and a secretin provocative test should be done. In patients with gastrinomas, BAO is usually (>80%) elevated (i.e., >15 meq/h) and the secretin provocative test is positive (i.e., >200 μg/L increase in serum gastrin level).

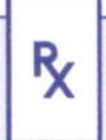

TREATMENT FOR GASTRINOMA

The gastric acid hypersecretion in patients with gastrinomas can be controlled in almost every case by oral gastric antisecretory drugs. Because of their long duration of action and potency, allowing once- or twice-a-day dosing, the proton pump inhibitors (H^+, K^+-ATPase inhibitors) are the drugs of choice. Histamine H_2-receptor antagonists are also effective, although more frequent (every 4 to 8 h) and high doses are usually required. In patients with MEN 1 with hyperparathyroidism, correction of the hyperparathyroidism increases the sensitivity to gastric antisecretory drugs and decreases the BAO.

Although gastric acid secretion can be controlled, more than half the patients who are not cured (>60%) will die from tumor-related causes. Careful imaging studies are essential to localize the extent of the tumor (see below). About one-third of patients present with hepatic metastases; in <15% of those with hepatic metastases, the disease is limited so that surgical resection may be possible. Surgical cure is possible in 30 to 60% of all patients without MEN 1 or liver metastases (40% of all patients). In patients with MEN 1, surgical cure is rare because the tumors are multiple, frequently with lymph node metastases.

INSULINOMAS

An insulinoma is an endocrine tumor of the pancreas derived from beta cells that ectopically secrete insulin, which results in hypoglycemia. The average age of occurrence is in persons 40 to 50 years old. The most common clinical symptoms are due to the effect of the hypoglycemia on the central nervous system (neuroglycemic symptoms) and include confusion, headache, disorientation, visual difficulties, irrational behavior, or even coma. Also, most patients have symptoms due to excess catecholamine release secondary to the hypoglycemia including sweating, tremor, and palpitations. Characteristically these attacks are associated with fasting.

Insulinomas are generally small (>90% are <2 cm), usually not multiple (90%), and only 5 to 15% are malignant. They almost invariably occur only in the pancreas, distributed equally in the pancreatic head, body, and tail. Insulinomas should be suspected in all patients with hypoglycemia, especially those with attacks provoked by fasting or with a family history of MEN 1. Insulin is synthesized as proinsulin which consists of a 21-amino-acid α chain and a 30-amino-acid β chain connected by a 33-amino-acid connecting peptide (C peptide). In insulinomas, in addition to elevated plasma insulin levels, elevated plasma proinsulin levels are found and C-peptide levels can be elevated.

Diagnosis

The diagnosis of insulinoma requires the demonstration of an elevated plasma insulin level at the time of hypoglycemia. Other causes of fasting hypoglycemia include the inadvertent or surreptitious use of insulin or oral hypoglycemic agents, severe liver disease, alcoholism, poor nutrition, or other extrapancreatic tumors. The most reliable test to diagnose insulinoma is a fast up to 72 h with serum glucose, C-peptide, and insulin measurements every 4 to 8 h. If at any point the patient becomes symptomatic or glucose levels are persistently <2.2 mmol/L (<40 mg/dL), the test should be terminated and repeat samples for the above studies obtained before glucose is given. Between 70 and 80% of patients with insulinoma will develop hypoglycemia during the first 24 h and 98% by 48 h. In nonobese normal subjects serum insulin levels should decrease to <43 pmol/L (<6 μU/mL) when blood glucose decreases to ≤2.2 mmol/L (<40 mg/dL) and the ratio of insulin to glucose is <0.3 (in mg/dL). In addition to having an insulin level > 6 μU/mL when blood glucose ≤ 40 mg/dL, some investigators also require an elevated C-peptide and serum proinsulin level and/or insulin:glucose ratio > 0.3 for the diagnosis of insulinoma. Surreptitious use of insulin or hypoglycemic agents may be difficult to distinguish from the symptoms of insulinomas. The combination of proinsulin levels (normal in exogenous insulin/hypoglycemic agent users), C-peptide levels (low in exogenous insulin users), antibodies to insulin (positive in exogenous insulin users), and sulfonylurea levels in serum or plasma will allow the correct diagnosis to be made.

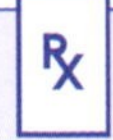

TREATMENT FOR INSULINOMA

Only 5 to 15% of insulinomas are malignant; therefore, after appropriate imaging (see below), surgery should be performed. Some 75 to 95% of patients are cured by surgery. Before surgery, the hypoglycemia can be controlled by frequent small meals and the use of diazoxide (150 to 800 mg/d). Diazoxide is a benzothiadiazide whose hyperglycemic effect is attributed to inhibition of insulin release; 50 to 60% of patients respond to diazoxide. Its side effects are sodium retention and GI symptoms such as nausea. Other agents effective in some patients include verapamil and diphenylhydantoin. Long-acting somatostatin analogues such as octreotide are acutely effective in 40% of patients. However, octreotide needs to be used with care because it inhibits growth hormone secretion and can alter plasma glucagon levels and so worsen the hypoglycemia in some patients.

For the 5 to 15% of patients with malignant insulinomas, the above drugs or somatostatin analogues are used initially. If they are not effective, various antitumor treatments such as hepatic arterial embolization, chemoembolization, or chemotherapy have been used. These will be discussed below.

GLUCAGONOMAS

A glucagonoma is an endocrine tumor of the pancreas that secretes excessive amounts of glucagon, which causes a distinct syndrome characterized by dermatitis, glucose intolerance or diabetes, and weight loss. Glucagonomas occur in persons between 45 and 70 years of age and are clinically heralded by a characteristic dermatitis (migratory necrolytic erythema) (67 to 90%), accompanied by glucose intolerance (40 to 90%), weight loss (66 to 96%), anemia (33 to 85%), diarrhea (15 to 29%), and thromboembolism (11 to 24%). The characteristic rash usually starts as an annular erythema at intertriginous and periorificial sites, especially in the groin or buttock. It subsequently becomes raised, and bullae form and leave erosions when the bullae rupture. The lesions can wax and wane. A characteristic laboratory finding is hypoaminoacidemia, which occurs in 26 to 100% of patients.

Glucagonomas are generally large tumors at diagnosis, with average size of 5 to 10 cm. From 50 to 80% occur in the pancreatic tail, and from 50 to 82% have metastatic spread at presentation, usually to the liver. Glucagonomas are rarely extrapancreatic and usually occur singly.

Diagnosis

The diagnosis is confirmed by demonstrating an increased plasma glucagon level (normal is <150 μg/L). Plasma glucagon levels are >1000 μg/mL in 90%, are between 500 and 1000 μg/mL in 7%, and <500 μg/mL in 3%. A plasma glucagon level > 1000 μg/L is considered diagnostic of glucagonoma. Other diseases causing increased plasma glucagon levels include renal insufficiency, acute pancreatitis, hypercorticism, hepatic insufficiency, prolonged fasting, or familial hyperglucagonomia. These disorders do not increase plasma glucagon to >500 μg/L except cirrhosis.

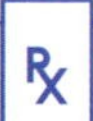

TREATMENT FOR GLUCAGONOMA

In 50 to 80% of patients metastases are present at presentation, so curative surgical resection is not possible. Surgical debulking in patients with advanced disease or other antitumor treatments may be beneficial and will be discussed below. Long-acting somatostatin analogues such as octreotide or lanreotide improve the skin rash in 75% of patients and may improve the weight loss, pain, and diarrhea, but usually do not improve the glucose intolerance.

SOMATOSTATINOMA SYNDROME

The somatostatinoma syndrome is due to a NET that secretes excessive amounts of somatostatin, which causes a distinct syndrome characterized by diabetes mellitus, gallbladder disease, diarrhea, and steatorrhea. Usually no distinction is made between a tumor that contains somatostatin-like immunoreactivity (somatostatinoma) and that does or does not produce a clinical syndrome (somatostatinoma syndrome) by secreting somatostatin (11 to 45% and 55 to 89%, respectively). In one review of 173 cases of somatostatinomas, only 11% were associated with the somatostatinoma syndrome. The mean age of patients is 51 years. Somatostatinomas occur primarily in the pancreas and small intestine, and the frequency of the symptoms differs in each. Each of the usual symptoms is more frequent in pancreatic than intestinal somatostatinomas: diabetes mellitus (95% vs. 21%), gallbladder disease (94% vs. 43%), diarrhea (92% vs. 38%), steatorrhea (83% vs. 12%), hypochlorhydria (86% vs. 12%), and weight loss (90% vs. 69%). Somatostatinomas occur in the pancreas in 56 to 74% of cases, with the primary location being in the pancreatic head. The tumors are usually solitary (90%) and large, with a mean size of 4.5 cm. Liver metastases are frequent (69 to 84% of patients).

Somatostatin is a tetradecapeptide (Fig. 20-2) that is widely distributed in the central nervous system and gastrointestinal tract, where it functions as a neurotransmitter or has paracrine and autocrine actions. It is a potent inhibitor of many processes, including release of almost all hormones, acid secretion, intestinal and pancreatic secretion, and intestinal absorption. Most of the clinical manifestations are directly related to these inhibitory actions.

Diagnosis

In most cases somatostatinomas have been found by accident either at the time of cholecystectomy or during endoscopy. The presence of psammoma bodies in a duodenal tumor should particularly raise suspicion. Duodenal somatostatin-containing tumors are increasingly associated with von Recklinghausen's disease. Most of these do not cause the somatostatinoma syndrome. The diagnosis of the somatostatinoma syndrome requires elevated plasma somatostatin levels.

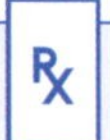

TREATMENT FOR SOMATOSTATINOMA

Pancreatic tumors are frequently metastatic at presentation (70 to 92%), whereas 30 to 69% of small-intestinal somatostatinomas have metastases. Surgery is the treatment of choice for those without widespread hepatic metastases. Symptoms in patients with the somatostatinoma syndrome are also improved by octreotide treatment.

VIPOMAS

VIPomas are endocrine tumors that secrete excessive amounts of VIP, which causes a distinct syndrome characterized by large-volume watery diarrhea, hypokalemia, and dehydration. This syndrome is also called Verner-Morrison syndrome, pancreatic cholera, or WDHA syndrome for *w*atery *d*iarrhea, *h*ypokalemia, and *a*chlorhydria, which some patients develop. The mean age of patients is 49 years; however, it can occur in children, and when it does is usually caused by a ganglioneuroma or ganglioneuroblastoma.

The principal symptoms are large-volume diarrhea (100%) severe enough to cause hypokalemia (80 to 100%), dehydration (83%), hypochlorhydria (54 to 76%), and flushing (20%). The diarrhea is secretory in nature, persists during fasting, and is almost always >1 L/d and >3 L/d in 70%. Most patients do not have accompanying steatorrhea (16%), and the increased stool volume is due to increased excretion of sodium and potassium, which, with the anions, account for the osmolality of the stool. Patients frequently have hyperglycemia (25 to 50%) and hypercalcemia (25 to 50%).

VIP is a 28-amino-acid peptide that is an important neurotransmitter ubiquitously present in the central nervous system and GI tract. Its known actions include stimulation of small-intestinal chloride secretion and effects on smooth-muscle contractility, inhibition of acid secretion, and vasodilatory effects which explain most features of the clinical syndrome.

In adults 80 to 90% of VIPomas are pancreatic in location, with the rest due to VIP-secreting pheochromocytomas, intestinal carcinoids, and rarely ganglioneuromas. These tumors are usually not multiple, 50 to 75% are in the pancreatic tail, and 37 to 68% have hepatic metastases at diagnosis. In children <10 years, the syndrome is usually due to ganglioneuromas or ganglioblastomas, which are less malignant and account for 10% of VIPomas in adults.

Diagnosis

The diagnosis requires the demonstration of an elevated plasma VIP level and the presence of large-volume diarrhea. A stool volume of <700 mL/d excludes the diagnosis of VIPoma. By fasting the patient, a number of causes can be excluded that can cause marked diarrhea. Other diseases that can give a secretory large-volume diarrhea include gastrinomas, chronic laxative abuse, carcinoid syndrome, systemic mastocytosis, rarely medullary thyroid cancer, diabetic diarrhea, and AIDS. Of these conditions, only VIPomas caused a marked increase in plasma VIP.

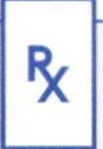

TREATMENT FOR VIPOMAS

The most important initial treatment is to correct the dehydration, hypokalemia, and electrolyte losses with fluid and electrolyte replacement. These patients may require 5 L/d of fluid and >350 meq/d of potassium. Because 37 to 68% of adults with VIPomas have metastatic disease in the liver at presentation, a significant number of patients cannot be cured surgically. In these patients, long-acting somatostatin analogues such as octreotide or lanreotide are the drugs of choice.

Octreotide will control the diarrhea in 87% of patients. In nonresponsive patients, the combination of glucocorticoids and octreotide has proved helpful in a small number of patients. Other drugs reported to be helpful in small numbers of patients include prednisone (60 to 100 mg/d), clonidine, indomethacin, phenothiazines, loperamide, lidamidine, lithium, propranolol, and metochlorpramide.

Treatment of advanced disease with embolization, chemoembolization, and chemotherapy may also be helpful (see below).

NONFUNCTIONAL PANCREATIC ENDOCRINE TUMORS

Nonfunctional PETs are endocrine tumors that originate in the pancreas and either secrete no products or their secreted products do not cause a specific clinical syndrome. The symptoms are due entirely to the tumor per se. Nonfunctional PETs almost always secrete chromogranin A (90 to 100%), chromogranin B (90 to 100%), PP (58%), α-human chorionic gonadotropin (hCG) (40%), and β-hCG (20%), but none cause a specific syndrome. Because the symptoms are due to the tumor per se, patients with nonfunctional PETs usually present late in their disease course with invasive tumors and hepatic metastases (64 to 92%), and the tumors are usually large (72% are >5 cm). These tumors are usually solitary except in patients with MEN 1, where they are multiple, and occur primarily in the pancreatic head. Even though these tumors do not cause a functional syndrome, immunocytochemical studies show that they synthesize numerous peptides and cannot be distinguished from functional tumors by immunocytochemistry.

The most common symptoms are abdominal pain (30 to 80%); jaundice (20 to 35%); and weight loss, fatigue, or bleeding; 10 to 15% are found incidentally. The average time from the beginning of symptoms to diagnosis is 5 years.

Diagnosis

The diagnosis is established by histologic confirmation in a patient with a PET without either clinical symptoms or elevated plasma hormone levels of one of the established syndromes. Even though chromogranin A levels are elevated in almost every patient, this is not specific for this disease as it can be found in functional PETs, carcinoids, and other neuroendocrine disorders. Plasma PP is increased in 22 to 71% of patients and should strongly suggest the diagnosis in a patient with a pancreatic mass because it is usually normal in patients with pancreatic adenocarcinomas. Elevated plasma PP is not diagnostic of this tumor because it is elevated in a number of other conditions such as chronic renal failure, old age, inflammatory conditions, and diabetes.

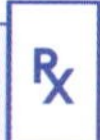

TREATMENT FOR NONFUNCTIONAL PETs

Unfortunately, surgical curative resection can be considered only in the minority of patients because of the high frequency of metastatic disease. Treatment needs to be directed against the tumor per se (see below).

GRFOMAS

GRFomas are endocrine tumors that secrete excessive amounts of GRF, which causes acromegaly. The true frequency of this syndrome is not known. GRF is a 44-amino-acid peptide, and 25 to 44% of PETs have GRF immunoreactivity, although it is uncommonly secreted. GRFomas are lung tumors in 47 to 54% of cases, PETs in 29 to 30%, and small-intestinal carcinoids in 8 to 10%, and up to 12% occur at other sites. Patients have a mean age of 38 years, and the symptoms are usually due to either acromegaly or the tumor per se. The acromegaly caused by GRFomas is indistinguishable from classic acromegaly. The pancreatic tumors are usually large (>6 cm) and liver metastases are present in 39%. They should be suspected in any patient with acromegaly and an abdominal tumor, in a patient with MEN 1 with acromegaly, or in a patient without a pituitary adenoma with acromegaly or associated with hyperprolactinemia, which occurs in 70% of GRFomas. GRFomas are an uncommon cause of acromegaly. The diagnosis is established by performing plasma assays for GRF and growth hormone. The normal level for GRF is <5 μg/L in men and <10 μg/L in women. Most GRFomas have a plasma GRF level ≥300 μg/L. Patients with GRFomas also have increased plasma insulin-like growth factor 1 levels similar to those in classic acromegaly. Surgery is the treatment of choice if diffuse metastases are not present. Long-acting somatostatin analogues such as octreotide or lanreotide are the agents of choice, with 75 to 100% of patients responding.

OTHER RARE PANCREATIC ENDOCRINE TUMOR SYNDROMES

Cushing's (ACTHoma) due to a PET occurs in 4 to 16% of all ectopic Cushing's syndrome cases. It occurs in 5% of cases of sporadic gastrinomas, almost invariably in patients with hepatic metastases, and is an independent, poor prognostic factor. Paraneoplastic hypercalcemia due to PETs releasing parathyroid hormone–related peptide (PTHrP), a parathyroid hormone–like material, or unknown factor is rarely reported. The tumors are usually large, and liver metastases are usually present. Most (88%) appear to be due to release of PTHrP. PETs can occasionally cause the carcinoid syndrome. PETs secreting calcitonin appear to have a specific clinical syndrome. Half the patients have diarrhea, which disappears with resection of the tumor. That this could be a discrete syndrome is supported by finding that 25 to 42% of patients with medullary thyroid cancer with hypercalcitonemia develop diarrhea, likely secondary to a motility disorder. This is classified in Table 20-2 as a possible specific disorder because so few cases have been described. A renin-producing PET has been described in a patient presenting with hypertension (Table 20-2). Ghrelin is a 28-amino-acid peptide with growth hormone–releasing effect and a strong influence on appetite, among other functions. Even though it is detectable immunohistochemically in most PETs, only 1 in 24 patients (4%) with a PET had elevated plasma ghrelin levels and the patient was asymptomatic, suggesting that no specific syndrome is associated with release of ghrelin by a PET.

TUMOR LOCALIZATION

Localization of the primary tumor and determination of the extent of disease are essential to the proper management of all carcinoids and PETs. Without proper localization studies it is not possible (1) to determine whether the patient is a candidate for curative resection or cytoreductive surgery or requires antitumor treatment or (2) to predict the patient's prognosis.

Numerous tumor localization methods are used in both types of NETs including conventional imaging studies [CT scanning, magnetic resonance imaging (MRI), transabdominal ultrasound, selective angiography] and somatostatin receptor scintigraphy (SRS). In PETs, endoscopic ultrasound (EUS) and functional localization by measuring venous hormonal gradients are also useful. Bronchial carcinoids are usually detected by a standard chest radiograph and assessed by CT. Rectal, duodenal, colonic, and gastric carcinoids are usually detected by GI endoscopy.

PETs and carcinoid tumors frequently overexpress high-affinity somatostatin receptors in both their primary and their metastatic tumors. Of the five types of somatostatin receptors (sst_{1-5}), radiolabeled octreotide binds with high affinity to sst_2 and sst_5, lower for sst_3, and has a very low affinity for sst_1 and sst_4. Nearly all carcinoid tumors and PETs express sst_2, and many also have the other four sst subtypes. Interaction with these receptors can be used to localize NETs using [^{111}In-DTPA-D-Phe^1]octreotide (Fig. 20-2) and radionuclide scanning (somatostatin receptor scintigraphy; SRS) as well as for treatment of the hormone excess state with octreotide or lanreotide. Because of its sensitivity and ability to localize tumor throughout the body at one time, SRS is now the initial imaging modality of choice for localizing both primary NETs and metastases. SRS localizes tumor in 73 to 89% of patients with carcinoids and in 56 to 100% of patients with PETs, except for insulinomas. Insulinomas are usually small and have low densities of sst receptors, resulting in SRS being positive in only 12 to 50% of insulinomas. SRS has greater sensitivity than conventional imaging studies in localizing both the primary tumor and metastases. **Figure 20-3** shows an example of the increased sensitivity of SRS in a patient

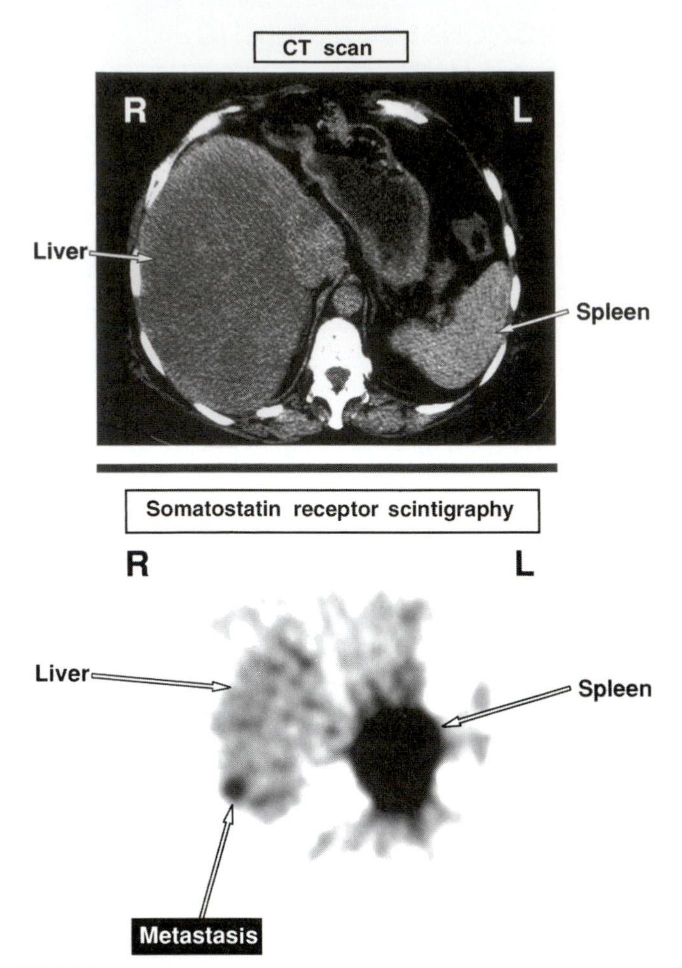

FIGURE 20-3
Ability of computed tomography (*top*) or somatostatin receptor scintigraphy (*bottom*) to localize metastatic gastrinoma in the liver in a patient with Zollinger-Ellison syndrome.

with a gastrinoma. The CT scan (Fig. 20-3, *top*) did not show any disease after resection of the primary tumor; however, hypergastrinemia remained and the SRS demonstrated a metastasis in the liver (Fig. 20-3, *bottom*). Occasional false-positive responses with SRS can occur (12% in one study) because numerous other normal tissues and diseases can have high densities of sst receptors including granulomas (sarcoid, tuberculosis, etc.), thyroid diseases (goiter, thyroiditis), and activated lymphocytes (lymphomas, wound infections). For PETs located in the pancreas, EUS is highly sensitive localizing 77 to 93% of insulinomas, which occur almost exclusively within the pancreas. EUS is less sensitive for extrapancreatic tumors. If liver metastases are identified by SRS, either a CT scan or MRI is then recommended to assess the size and exact location of the metastases because SRS does not give information on tumor size. Functional localization, i.e., by measuring hormone gradients after intraarterial calcium injections in insulinomas (insulin) or gastrin gradients after secretin injections in gastrinoma, is a sensitive method, being positive in 80 to 100% of patients. However, this method gives only regional localization and is reserved for cases where the other imaging modalities are negative.

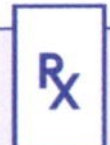

TREATMENT

Advanced Disease (Diffuse Metastatic Disease)

The single most important prognostic factor for survival is the presence of liver metastases (**Fig. 20-4**). For patients with foregut carcinoids without hepatic metastases, the 5-year survival is 95% and with distant metastases is 20% (Fig. 20-4, *bottom*). With gastrinomas the 5-year survival without liver metastases is 98%, with limited metastases in one hepatic lobe it is 78%, and with diffuse metastases it is 16% (Fig. 20-4, *top*). Therefore, treatment for advanced metastatic disease is important. A number of different modalities are effective, including cytoreductive surgery (removal of all visible tumor), treatment with chemotherapy, somatostatin analogues, interferon α, hepatic embolization alone or with chemotherapy (chemoembolization), radiotherapy, and liver transplantation.

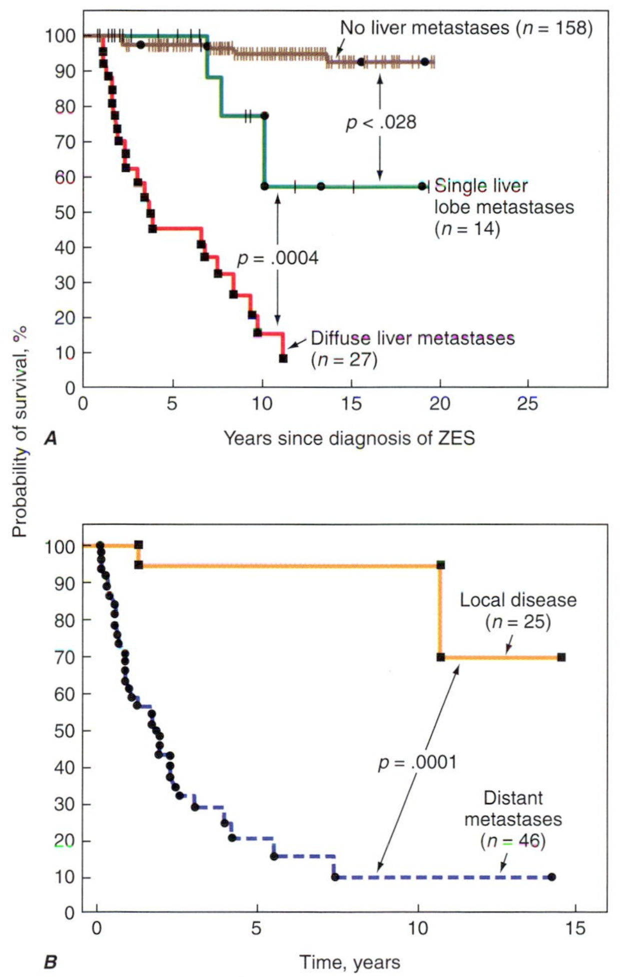

FIGURE 20-4

Effect of the presence and extent of liver metastases on survival in patients with gastrinomas (*top*) or carcinoid tumors (*bottom*). *(Top panel is drawn from data from 199 patients with gastrinomas modified from F Yu et al: J Clin Oncol 17:615, 1999. Bottom panel is drawn from data from 71 patients with foregut carcinoid tumors from EW McDermott et al: Br J Surg 81:1007, 1994.)*

Specific Antitumor Treatments

Cytoreductive surgery, unfortunately, is only possible in 9 to 22% of patients who present with limited hepatic metastases. Although no randomized studies have proven it extends life, results from a number of studies suggest it likely increases survival, and therefore it is recommended if possible.

Chemotherapy for metastatic carcinoid tumors has generally been disappointing, with response rates of 0 to 40% with various two- or three-drug combinations. Chemotherapy for PETs has been more successful with tumor shrinkage reported in 30 to 70% of patients. The current regimen of choice is streptozocin and doxorubicin.

Long-acting somatostatin analogues, such as octreotide and lanreotide, and interferon α rarely decrease tumor size (i.e., 0 to 17%); however, these drugs have tumoristatic effects, stopping additional growth in 26 to 95% of patients with NETs. How long tumor stabilization lasts or whether it prolongs survival has not been established. Somatostatin analogues can induce apoptosis in carcinoid tumors.

Hepatic embolization and chemoembolization (with dacarbazine, cisplatin, doxorubicin, 5-fluorouracil, or streptozocin) may decrease tumor bulk and help control the symptoms of the hormone-excess state. These modalities are generally reserved for cases in which treatment with somatostatin analogues, interferon (carcinoids), or chemotherapy (PETs) fails. Embolization, when combined with treatment with octreotide and interferon α, significantly reduces tumor progression compared to treatment with embolization and octreotide alone in patients with advanced midgut carcinoids.

Radiotherapy with radiolabeled somatostatin analogues (Fig. 20-2) that are internalized by the tumors is an approach being investigated. Three different radionuclides are being used. High doses of [^{111}In-DTPA-D-Phe^{1}]octreotide (emits γ rays, internal conversion, and Auger electrons) and yttrium-90 (emits high energy β-particles) coupled by a DOTA-chelating group (Fig. 20-2) to octreotide or octreotate are being used as well as ^{177}Lu-coupled analogues (emit β- and γ-rays). In one study, treatment with the ^{111}In or ^{177}Lu compounds caused tumor stabilization in 41% and 40%, respectively, and a decrease in tumor size in 30% and 38%, respectively, in patients with advanced metastatic NETs. Hormone-directed radiation therapy may be helpful in patients with advanced, widespread metastatic disease.

The use of liver transplantation has been abandoned for treatment of most metastatic tumors to the liver. However, for metastatic NETs it is still a consideration. In a recent review of 103 cases of malignant NETs (48 PETs, 43 carcinoids) the 2- and 5-year survival rates were 60% and 47%, respectively. However, recurrence-free survival was low (<24%). For younger patients with metastatic NETs limited to the liver, liver transplantation may be justified.

FURTHER READINGS

CORLETO VD et al: Molecular insights into gastrointestinal neuroendocrine tumors: Importance and recent advances. Dig Liver Dis 34:668, 2002

KALTSAS GA et al: The diagnosis and medical management of advanced neuroendocrine tumors. Endocr Rev 25:458, 2004

This article reviews the use of tumor markers and imaging modalities that are useful in the management of neuroendocrine tumors. It also summarizes a multimodal treatment approach that may combine surgery with medical therapy with somatostatin analogues or interferon α, radionuclides and chemotherapy being reserved for poorly differentiated and progressive tumors. The need for individualized therapy is emphasized.

MODLIN IM et al: A 5-decade analysis of 13,715 carcinoid tumors. Cancer 97:934, 2003

OBERG K, ERIKSSON B: Nuclear medicine in the detection, staging and treatment of gastrointestinal carcinoid tumours. Best Pract Res Clin Endocrinol Metab 19:265, 2005

SOGA J: Early-stage carcinoids of the gastrointestinal tract: An analysis of 1914 reported cases. Cancer 103:1587, 2005

WARNER RR: Enteroendocrine tumors other than carcinoid: A review of clinically significant advances. Gastroenterology 128:1668, 2005

This review summarizes advances in the diagnosis and treatment of enteroendocrine tumors [insulinoma (hypoglycemia), gastrinoma (Zollinger-Ellison syndrome; ZES), vasoactive intestinal peptideoma (VIPoma), watery diarrhea, hypokalemia-achlorhydria (WDHA), glucagonoma (glucagonoma syndrome), etc.]. Because their growth rate is often relatively slow relative to patients with more malignant cancers, patients with neuroendocrine tumors often can be palliated and appear to survive longer when managed using sequential multimodality treatment.

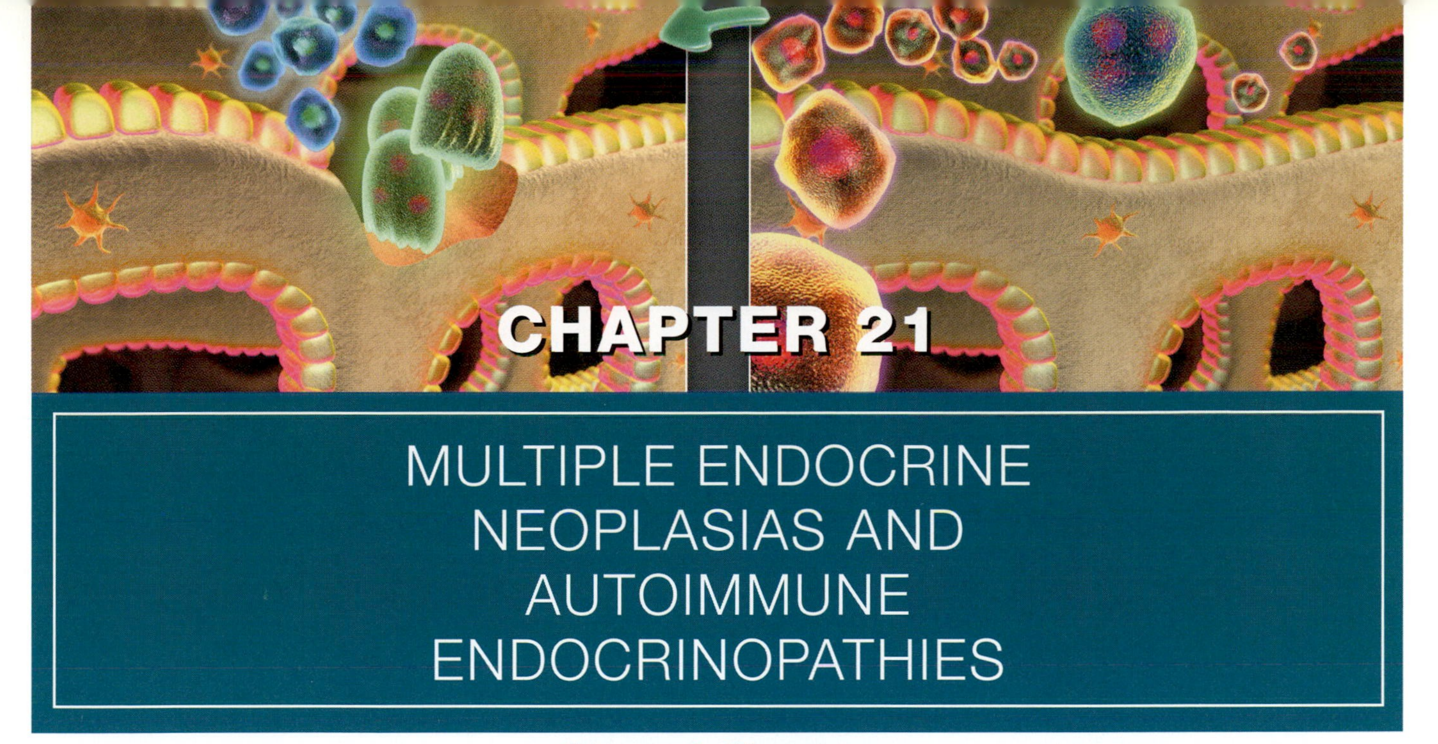

CHAPTER 21

MULTIPLE ENDOCRINE NEOPLASIAS AND AUTOIMMUNE ENDOCRINOPATHIES

Steven I. Sherman
Robert F. Gagel

NEOPLASTIC DISORDERS AFFECTING MULTIPLE ENDOCRINE ORGANS

Several distinct genetic disorders predispose to endocrine gland neoplasia and cause hormone excess syndromes (**Table 21-1**). DNA-based genetic testing is now available for these disorders, but effective management requires an understanding of endocrine neoplasia and the range of clinical features that may be manifest in an individual patient.

MULTIPLE ENDOCRINE NEOPLASIA (MEN) TYPE 1

Clinical Manifestations

MEN 1, or Wermer's syndrome, is an autosomal dominant genetic syndrome characterized by neoplasia of parathyroid, pituitary, pancreatic islet, and other neuroendocrine cell types (Table 21-1). Each child born to an affected parent has a 50% probability of inheriting the gene. The variable penetrance of the several neoplastic components can make the differential diagnosis challenging.

Hyperparathyroidism is the most common manifestation of MEN 1. Hypercalcemia may develop during the teenage years, and most individuals are affected by age 40 (**Fig. 21-1**). The neoplastic changes in hyperparathyroidism exemplify one of the cardinal features of endocrine tumors in MEN 1—multicentricity. The neoplastic changes inevitably affect multiple parathyroid glands, making surgical cure difficult. Screening for hyperparathyroidism involves measurement of either an albumin-adjusted or ionized serum calcium level. The diagnosis is established by demonstrating elevated levels of serum calcium and inappropriately normal or high intact parathyroid hormone. Manifestations of hyperparathyroidism in MEN 1 do not differ substantially from those in sporadic hyperparathyroidism and include calcium-containing kidney stones, bone abnormalities, and gastrointestinal and musculoskeletal complaints (Chap. 24).

Other familial disorders associated with hypercalcemia include familial isolated hyperparathyroidism, a broad categorization that includes at least two types, HRPT1 and HRPT2. The first type, HRPT1, includes familial parathyroid hyperplasia and adenomatosis. The second type, HRPT2, is associated with multiple cystic parathyroid adenomas and ossifying jaw fibromas. Inactivating mutations of the gene that encodes parafibromin were recently identified in nearly all families with HRPT2. Subsequent analysis of this gene in families with HRPT1 indicates that some patients with HRPT1 have mutations of the HRPT2 gene. Inactivating

TABLE 21-1

DISEASE ASSOCIATIONS IN THE MULTIPLE ENDOCRINE NEOPLASIA (MEN) SYNDROMES

MEN 1	MEN 2	MIXED SYNDROMES
Parathyroid hyperplasia or adenoma Islet cell hyperplasia, adenoma, or carcinoma Pituitary hyperplasia or adenoma Other less common manifestations: foregut carcinoid, pheochromocytoma, subcutaneous or visceral lipomas	MEN 2A MTC Pheochromocytoma Parathyroid hyperplasia or adenoma Cutaneous lichen amyloidosis Hirschsprung disease Familial MTC MEN 2B MTC Pheochromocytoma Mucosal and gastro-intestinal neuromas Marfanoid features	von Hippel–Lindau syndrome, pheo-chromocytoma, islet cell tumor, renal cell carcinoma, hemangioblastoma of central nervous system, retinal angiomas Neurofibromatosis with features of MEN 1 or 2 Carney complex Myxomas of heart, skin, and breast Spotty cutaneous pigmentation Testicular, adrenal, and GH-producing pituitary tumors Peripheral nerve schwannomas

Note: MTC, medullary thyroid carcinoma; GH, growth hormone.

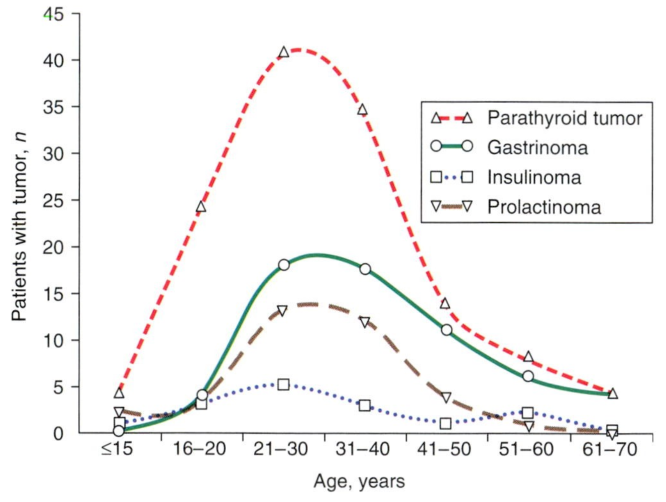

FIGURE 21-1

Age at onset of endocrine tumor expression in multiple endocrine neoplasia type 1 (MEN 1). Data derived from retrospective analysis for each endocrine organ hyperfunction in 130 cases of MEN 1. Age at onset is the age at first symptom or, with tumors not causing symptoms, age at the time of the first abnormal finding on a screening test. The rate of diagnosis of hyperparathyroidism increased sharply between ages 16 and 20 years. *(Reprinted with permission from S Marx et al: Ann Intern Med 129:484, 1998.)*

mutations of HRPT2 are also found commonly in sporadic parathyroid cancers. MEN 2 (to be discussed below) should also be considered in the differential diagnosis. Another cause of familial hypercalcemia is familial hypercalcemic hypocalciuria (FHH), an autosomal dominant form of hypercalcemia caused by inactivating mutations of the calcium sensor, a transmembrane G protein–coupled receptor found in parathyroid tissue and kidney (Chap. 24). Hypercalcemia associated with MEN 1, MEN 2, HRPT1, and HRPT2 is characterized by increased urine calcium excretion (calcium/creatinine clearance ratio > 0.01) whereas in FHH it is associated with low urine calcium excretion (calcium/creatinine clearance ratio < 0.01). Another distinguishing feature is that the serum calcium level is rarely elevated at birth in patients with MEN 1 but is frequently elevated in newborns with FHH.

Differentiation of hyperparathyroidism of MEN 1 from other forms of familial primary hyperparathyroidism is usually based on family history, histologic features of resected parathyroid tissue, and, sometimes, long-term observation to determine whether other manifestations of MEN 1 develop. Parathyroid hyperplasia is the most common cause of hyperparathyroidism in MEN 1, although single and multiple adenomas have been described. Hyperplasia of one or more parathyroid glands is common in younger patients; adenomas are usually found in older patients or those with long-standing disease.

Neoplasia of the pancreatic islets is the second most common manifestation of MEN 1 and tends to occur in parallel with hyperparathyroidism (Fig. 21-1). Increased pancreatic islet cell hormones include pancreatic polypeptide (75 to 85%), gastrin [60%; Zollinger-Ellison syndrome (ZES)], insulin (25 to 35%), vasoactive intestinal peptide (VIP) (3 to 5%; Verner-Morrison, or watery diarrhea, syndrome), glucagon (5 to 10%), and somatostatin (1 to 5%). The tumors rarely produce adrenocorticotropin (ACTH), corticotropin-releasing hormone (CRH), growth hormone–releasing hormone (GHRH), calcitonin gene products, neurotensin, gastric inhibitory peptide, and others. Many of the tumors produce more than one peptide. The pancreatic neoplasms differ from the other components of MEN 1 in that approximately one-hird of the tumors display malignant features, including hepatic metastases (Chap. 20).

Pancreatic islet cell tumors are diagnosed by identification of a characteristic clinical syndrome, hormonal assays with or without provocative stimuli, or radiographic techniques. One approach involves annual screening of individuals at risk with measurement of basal and meal-stimulated levels of pancreatic polypeptide to identify the tumors as early as possible; the rationale of this screening strategy is that surgical removal of islet cell tumors at an early stage will be curative. Other approaches to screening include measurement of serum gastrin and pancreatic polypeptide levels every 2 to 3 years, with the rationale that pancreatic neoplasms will be detected at a later stage but can be managed medically, if possible, or by surgery. High-resolution, early-phase computed tomography (CT) scanning or endoscopic ultrasound provides the best preoperative technique for identification of these tumors; intraoperative ultrasonography is the most sensitive method for detection of small tumors.

ZES is caused by excessive gastrin production and occurs in more than half of MEN 1 patients with pancreatic islet cell tumors or small carcinoid-like tumors in the duodenal wall (Fig. 21-1) (Chap. 20). Approximately one-fourth of all ZES occurs in the context of MEN 1. Clinical features include increased gastric acid production, recurrent peptic ulcers, diarrhea, and esophagitis. The ulcer diathesis is refractory to conservative therapy such as antacids. The diagnosis is made by finding increased gastric acid secretion, elevated basal gastrin levels in serum [generally >115 pmol/L (200 pg/mL)], and an exaggerated response of serum gastrin to either secretin or calcium. Other causes of elevated serum gastrin levels, such as achlorhydria, treatment with H_2 receptor antagonists or omeprazole, retained gastric antrum, small-bowel resection, gastric outlet obstruction, and hypercalcemia, should be excluded.

Insulinoma causes hypoglycemia in about one-third of MEN 1 patients with pancreatic islet cell tumors (Fig. 21-1). The tumors may be benign or malignant (25%). The diagnosis can be established by documenting hypoglycemia during a short fast with simultaneous inappropriate elevation of serum insulin and C-peptide levels. More commonly, it is necessary to subject the patient to a supervised 12- to 72-h fast to provoke hypoglycemia (Chap. 19). Large insulinomas may be identified by CT scanning; small tumors not detected by radiographic techniques may be localized by selective arteriographic injection of calcium into each of the arteries that supply the pancreas and timed sampling of the hepatic vein for insulin to determine the anatomical region containing the tumor. Intraoperative ultrasonography can also be used to localize these tumors, but preoperative calcium injection data are helpful in guiding the appropriate pancreatic surgical procedure if multiple or no abnormalities are detected by intraoperative ultrasonography.

Glucagonoma in occasional MEN 1 patients causes a syndrome of hyperglycemia, skin rash (necrolytic migratory erythema), anorexia, glossitis, anemia, depression, diarrhea, and venous thrombosis. In about half of these patients the plasma glucagon level is high, leading to its designation as the *glucagonoma syndrome,* although elevation of plasma glucagon level in MEN 1 patients is not necessarily associated with these symptoms. Some patients with this syndrome also have elevated plasma ghrelin levels. The glucagonoma syndrome may represent a complex interaction between glucagon and ghrelin overproduction and the nutritional status of the patient.

The *Verner-Morrison syndrome,* or *watery diarrhea syndrome,* consists of watery diarrhea, hypokalemia, hypochlorhydria, and metabolic acidosis. The diarrhea can be voluminous and is almost always found in association with an islet cell tumor, prompting use of the term *pancreatic cholera.* However, the syndrome is not restricted to pancreatic islet tumors and has been observed with carcinoids or other tumors. This syndrome is believed to be due to overproduction of VIP, although plasma VIP levels are not always elevated. Hypercalcemia may be induced by the effects of VIP on bone as well as by hyperparathyroidism. The differential diagnosis includes other causes of chronic diarrhea, infectious or parasitic diseases, inflammatory bowel disease, or sprue or other endocrine causes such as ZES, carcinoid syndrome, or medullary thyroid carcinoma.

Pituitary tumors occur in more than half of patients with MEN 1 and tend to be multicentric, making them difficult to resect (Chap. 2). Prolactinomas are most common (Fig. 21-1) and are diagnosed by finding serum prolactin levels >200 μg/L, with or without a pituitary mass evident by magnetic resonance imaging (MRI). Values <200 μg/L may be due to a prolactin-secreting neoplasm or to compression of the pituitary stalk by a different type of pituitary tumor. Acromegaly due to excessive growth hormone (GH) production is the second most common syndrome caused by pituitary tumors in MEN 1 (Chap. 2) but is rarely caused by production of GHRH by an islet cell tumor (see above). Cushing's disease can be caused by ACTH-producing pituitary tumors or by ectopic production of ACTH or CRH by other components of MEN 1 syndrome including islet cell or carcinoid tumors. Diagnosis of pituitary Cushing's disease is generally best accomplished by a high-dose dexamethasone suppression test or by petrosal venous sinus sampling for ACTH after intravenous injection of CRH (Chap. 2). Differentiation of a primary pituitary tumor from an ectopic CRH-producing tumor may be difficult because the pituitary is the source of ACTH in both disorders; documentation of CRH production by a pancreatic islet or carcinoid tumor may be the only method of proving ectopic CRH production. Adrenal cortical tumors are found in almost one-half of gene carriers but are rarely functional; malignancy in the cortical adenomas is uncommon.

Carcinoid tumors in MEN 1 are of the foregut type and are derived from thymus, lung, stomach, or duodenum; they may metastasize or be locally invasive. These tumors usually produce serotonin, calcitonin, or CRH. The typical carcinoid syndrome with flushing, diarrhea, and bronchospasm is rare (Chap. 20). Mediastinal carcinoid tumors (an upper mediastinal mass) are more common in men; bronchial carcinoid tumors are more common in women. Carcinoid tumors are a late manifestation of MEN 1; screening regularly for mediastinal carcinoid tumors by chest CT scans has been recommended because of the high rate of malignant transformation.

Unusual Manifestations of Men 1 Subcutaneous or visceral lipomas and cutaneous leiomyomas may also be present but rarely undergo malignant transformation. Skin angiofibromas or collagenomas are seen in most patients with MEN 1 when carefully sought.

MEN 1 is transmitted as an autosomal dominant trait, reflecting the fact that the gene that causes MEN 1, located on chromosome 11q13, encodes a tumor-suppressor protein termed *menin* (**Fig. 21-2**). Affected individuals typically harbor a germline mutation in *MEN 1* and acquire a "second hit" in the normal gene as a result of another mutation or, more commonly, loss of the portion of chromosome 11 that contains the MEN 1 locus. Though the function of menin is not well understood, it is a nuclear protein that interacts with at least two transcriptional factors, SMAD 3 and Jun D, suggesting a regulatory role in cell growth.

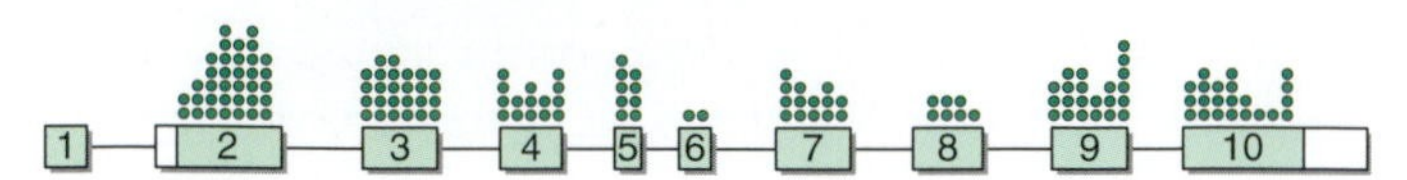

FIGURE 21-2

Schematic depiction of the *MEN 1* gene and the distribution of mutations. The shaded areas show coding sequence. The closed circles show the relative distribution of mutations, mostly inactivating, in each exon. Mutation data are derived from the Human Gene Mutation Database from which more detailed information can be obtained (*www.uwcm.ac.uk/uwcm/mg/hgmd0.html*). (*Data from M Krawczak, DN Cooper: Trends Genet 13:121, 1997.*)

MEN 1 gene mutations are found in >90% of families with the syndrome (Fig. 21-2). Genetic testing can be performed in individuals at risk for the development of MEN 1 and is now commercially available in the United States and Europe. The major value of genetic testing in a kindred with an identifiable mutation is the assignment or exclusion of gene carrier status. In those identified as carrying the mutant gene, routine screening for individual manifestations of MEN 1 should be performed as outlined above. Those with negative genetic test results (in a kindred with an identified mutation) can be excluded from further screening for MEN 1. A significant percentage of sporadic parathyroid, islet cell, and carcinoid tumors also have loss or mutation of *MEN 1*. It is presumed that these mutations are somatic and occur in a single cell, leading to subsequent transformation.

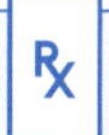

TREATMENT FOR MEN 1

Almost everyone who inherits a mutant *MEN 1* gene develops at least one clinical manifestation of the syndrome. Most develop hyperparathyroidism, 80% develop pancreatic islet cell tumors, and more than half develop pituitary tumors. For most of these tumors, initial surgery is not curative and patients frequently require multiple surgical procedures on two or more endocrine glands during a lifetime. For this reason, it is essential to establish clear goals for management of these patients rather than to recommend surgery casually each time a tumor is discovered. Ranges for acceptable management are discussed below.

Hyperparathyroidism

Individuals with serum calcium levels >3.0 mmol/L (12 mg/dL), evidence of calcium nephrolithiasis or renal dysfunction, neuropathic or muscular symptoms, or bone involvement (including osteopenia) should undergo parathyroid exploration. There is less agreement regarding the necessity for parathyroid exploration in individuals who do not meet these criteria, and observation may be appropriate in the MEN 1 patient with asymptomatic hyperparathyroidism.

When parathyroid surgery is indicated in MEN 1, all parathyroid tissue should be identified and removed at the time of primary operation, and parathyroid tissue should be implanted in the nondominant forearm. Thymectomy should also be performed because of the potential for later development of malignant carcinoid tumors. If reoperation for hyperparathyroidism is necessary at a later date, transplanted parathyroid tissue can be resected from the forearm under local anesthesia with titration of tissue removal to lower the intact parathyroid hormone (PTH) to <50% of basal.

A less desirable approach is to remove 3 to 3.5 parathyroid glands from the neck (leaving ~50 mg of parathyroid tissue), carefully marking the location of residual tissue so that the remaining tissue can be located easily during subsequent surgery. If this approach is utilized, intraoperative PTH measurements should be utilized to monitor adequacy of removal of parathyroid tissue with a goal of reducing postoperative serum intact PTH to ≤50% of basal values.

Pancreatic Islet Tumors

(See Chap. 20 for discussion of pancreatic islet tumors not associated with MEN 1.) Two features of pancreatic islet cell tumors in MEN 1 complicate the management. First, the pancreatic islet cell tumors are multicentric, malignant about a third of the time, and cause death in 10 to 20% of patients. Second, removal of all pancreatic islets to prevent malignancy causes diabetes mellitus, a disease with significant long-term complications that include neuropathy, retinopathy, and nephropathy. These features make it difficult to formulate clear-cut guidelines, but some general concepts appear to be valid. First, islet cell tumors producing insulin, glucagon, VIP, GHRH, or CRH should be resected because medical therapy for the hormonal effects of these tumors is generally ineffective. Second, gastrin-producing islet cell tumors that cause ZES are frequently multicentric. Recent experience suggests that a high percentage of ZES in MEN 1 is caused by duodenal wall tumors and that resection of these tumors improves the cure rate. Treatment with H_2 receptor antagonists (cimetidine or ranitidine) and the H^+, K^+-ATPase inhibitors (omeprazole or lansoprazole) provides an alternative, and some think preferable, therapy to surgery for control of ulcer disease in patients with multicentric tumors or with hepatic metastases. Third, total pancreatectomy at an early age may be justified to prevent malignancy for families who have a high incidence of malignant cell tumors that cause death.

Management of metastatic islet cell carcinoma is unsatisfactory. Hormonal abnormalities can sometimes be controlled. For example, ZES can be treated with H_2 receptor antagonists or H^+, K^+-ATPase inhibitors; the somatostatin analogues, octreotide or lanreotide, are useful in the management of carcinoid and the watery diarrhea syndrome. Bilateral adrenalectomy may be required for ectopic ACTH syndrome if medical therapy is ineffective (Chap. 5). Islet cell carcinomas frequently metastasize to the liver but may grow slowly. Hepatic artery embolization or chemotherapy (5-fluorouracil, streptozocin, chlorozotocin, doxorubicin, or dacarbazine) may reduce tumor mass, control symptoms of hormone excess, and prolong life; however, these treatments are never curative.

Pituitary Tumors

Treatment of prolactinomas with dopamine agonists (bromocriptine, cabergoline, or quinagolide) usually returns the serum prolactin level to normal and prevents further tumor growth (Chap. 2). Surgical resection of a prolactinoma is rarely curative but may relieve mass effects. Transsphenoidal resection is appropriate for neoplasms that secrete ACTH, GH, or the α-subunit of the pituitary glycoprotein hormones. Octreotide reduces tumor mass in one-third of GH-secreting tumors and reduces GH and insulin-like growth factor I levels in >75% of patients. Pegvisomant, a GH receptor antagonist, rapidly lowers insulin-like growth factor 1 levels (IGF-1) and is now approved for treatment of acromegaly. Radiation therapy may be useful for large or recurrent tumors.

Advances in the management of MEN 1, particularly islet cell and pituitary tumors, have improved outcome in these patients substantially. As a result, other neoplastic manifestations that develop later in the course of this disorder, such as carcinoid syndrome, are now seen with increased frequency.

MULTIPLE ENDOCRINE NEOPLASIA TYPE 2

Clinical Manifestations

Medullary thyroid carcinoma (MTC) and pheochromocytoma are associated in two major syndromes: MEN type 2A and MEN type 2B (Table 21-1). MEN 2A is the combination of MTC, hyperparathyroidism, and pheochromocytoma. Three subvariants of MEN 2A are familial medullary thyroid carcinoma (FMTC), MEN 2A with cutaneous lichen amyloidosis, and MEN 2A with Hirschsprung disease. MEN 2B is the combination of MTC, pheochromocytoma, mucosal neuromas, intestinal ganglioneuromatosis, and marfanoid features.

Multiple Endocrine Neoplasia Type 2A MTC is the most common manifestation. This tumor usually develops in childhood, beginning as hyperplasia of the calcitonin-producing cells (C cells) of the thyroid. MTC is typically located at the junction of the upper one-third and lower two-thirds of each lobe of the thyroid, reflecting the high density of C cells in this location; tumors >1 cm in size are frequently associated with local or distant metastases. Measurement of the serum calcitonin level after calcium or pentagastrin injection makes it possible to diagnose this disorder at an early stage in its development (see below).

Pheochromocytoma occurs in ~50% of patients with MEN 2A and causes hypertension with palpitations, nervousness, headaches, and sometimes sweating (Chap. 6). About half the tumors are bilateral. After unilateral adrenalectomy, >50% of patients develop a pheochromocytoma in the contralateral gland within a decade. A second feature of these tumors is a disproportionate increase in the secretion of epinephrine relative to norepinephrine. This characteristic differentiates the MEN 2 pheochromocytomas from sporadic pheochromocytoma and those associated with von Hippel–Lindau (VHL) syndrome, hereditary paraganglioma, or neurofibromatosis. Capsular invasion is common, but metastasis is uncommon. Finally, the pheochromocytomas are almost always found in the adrenal gland, differentiating the pheochromocytomas in MEN 2 from the extraadrenal tumors found in hereditary paraganglioma syndromes.

Hyperparathyroidism occurs in 15 to 20% of patients, with the peak incidence in the third or fourth decade. The manifestations of hyperparathyroidism do not differ from those in other forms of primary hyperparathyroidism (Chap. 24). Diagnosis is established by finding hypercalcemia, hypophosphatemia, hypercalciuria, and an inappropriately high serum level of intact PTH. Multiglandular parathyroid hyperplasia is the most common histologic finding, although with long-standing disease, adenomatous changes may be superimposed on hyperplasia.

The most common subvariant of MEN 2A is familial MTC, an autosomal dominant syndrome in which MTC is the only manifestation (Table 21-1). The clinical diagnosis of FMTC is established by the identification of MTC in multiple generations without a pheochromocytoma. Since the penetrance of pheochromocytoma is 50% in MEN 2A, it is possible that MEN 2A could masquerade as FMTC in small kindreds. It is important to consider this possibility carefully before classifying a kindred as having FMTC; failure to do so could lead to death or serious morbidity from pheochromocytoma in an affected kindred member.

Multiple Endocrine Neoplasia Type 2B The association of MTC, pheochromocytoma, mucosal neuromas, and a marfanoid habitus is designated MEN 2B. MTC in MEN 2B develops earlier and is more aggressive than in MEN 2A. Metastatic disease has been described prior to 1 year of age, and death commonly occurs in the second or third decade of life. However, the prognosis is not invariably bad even in patients with metastatic disease, as evidenced by a number of multigenerational families with this disease.

Pheochromocytoma occurs in more than half of MEN 2B patients and does not differ from that in MEN 2A. Hypercalcemia is rare in MEN 2B, and there are no well-documented examples of hyperparathyroidism.

The mucosal neuromas and marfanoid body habitus are the most distinctive features and are recognizable in childhood. Neuromas are present on the tip of the tongue, under the eyelids, and throughout the gastrointestinal tract and are true neuromas, distinct from neurofibromas. The most common presentation in children relates to gastrointestinal symptomatology, including intermittent colic, pseudoobstruction, and diarrhea.

Mutations of the *RET* protooncogene have been identified in most patients with MEN 2 (**Fig. 21-3**). *RET* encodes a tyrosine kinase receptor that, in combination with a co-receptor, GDNF family-receptor alpha (GFRα), is normally activated by glial cell–derived neurotropic factor or other members of this transforming growth factor–like family of peptides including artemin, persephin, and neurturin. In the C cell there is evidence that persephin normally activates the RET/GFRα-4 receptor complex and is partially responsible for migration of the C cells into the thyroid gland, whereas in the gastrointestinal tract, glial cell–derived neurotrophic factor activates a RET/GFRα-1 complex. *RET* mutations induce constitutive activity of the receptor, explaining the autosomal dominant transmission of the disorder.

Naturally occurring mutations localize to two regions of the RET tyrosine kinase receptor. The first is a cysteine-rich extracellular domain; point mutations in

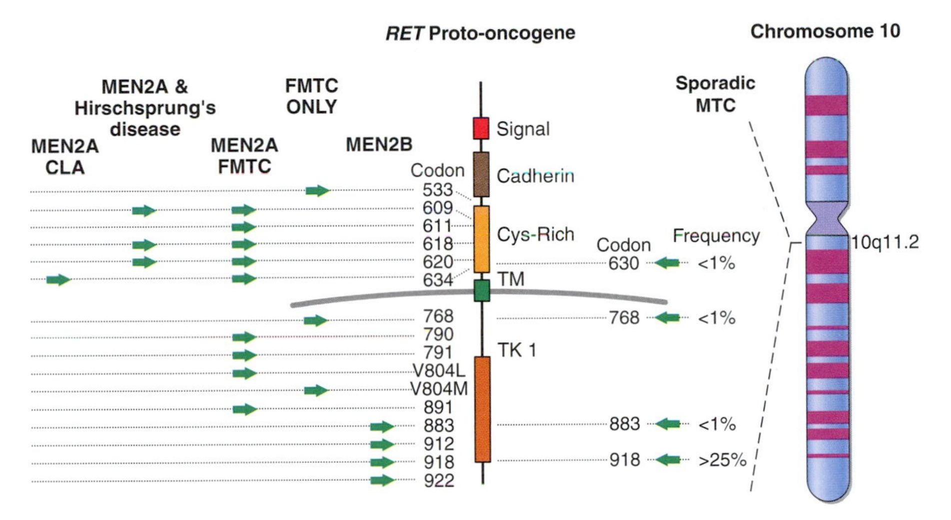

FIGURE 21-3

Schematic diagram of the *RET* protooncogene showing mutations found in MEN type 2 and sporadic medullary thyroid carcinoma (MTC). The *RET* protooncogene is located on the proximal arm of chromosome 10q (10q11.2). Activating mutations of two functional domains of the RET tyrosine kinase receptor have been identified. The first affects a cysteine-rich (Cys-Rich) region in the extracellular portion of the receptor. Each germline mutation changes a cysteine at codons 609, 611, 618, 620, or 634 to another amino acid. The second region is the intracellular tyrosine kinase (TK) domain. Codon 634 mutations account for ~80% of all germline mutations. Mutations of codons 630, 768, 883, and 918 have been identified as somatic (nongermline) mutations that occur in a single parafollicular or C cell within the thyroid gland in sporadic MTC. A codon 918 mutation is the most common somatic mutation. Abbreviations: MEN 2, multiple endocrine neoplasia type 2; CLA cutaneous lichen amyloidosis; FMTC, familial medullary thyroid carcinoma; Signal, the signal peptide; Cadherin, a cadherin-like region in the extracellular domain; TM, transmembrane domain; TK, tyrosine kinase domain.

the coding sequence for one of six cysteines (codons 609, 611, 618, 620, 630, or 634) cause amino acid substitutions that induce receptor dimerization and activation in the absence of its ligand. Codon 634 mutations occur in 80% of MEN 2A kindreds and are most commonly associated with classic MEN 2A features (Figs. 21-3 and 21-2); an arginine substitution at this codon accounts for half of all MEN 2A mutations. All reported families with MEN 2A and cutaneous lichen amyloidosis have a codon 634 mutation. Mutations of codons 609, 611, 618, or 620 occur in 10 to 15% of MEN 2A kindreds and are more commonly associated with FMTC (Fig. 21-3). Mutations in codons 609, 618, and 620 have also been identified in a variant of MEN 2A that includes Hirschsprung disease (Fig. 21-3).

The second region of the RET tyrosine kinase that is mutated in MEN 2 is in the substrate recognition pocket at codon 918 (Fig. 21-3). This activating mutation is present in ~95% of patients with MEN 2B and accounts for 5% of all *RET* protooncogene mutations in MEN 2. Mutations of codons 883 and 922 have also been identified in a few patients with MEN 2B.

Uncommon mutations (initially <5% of the total) include those of codons 533 (exon 8), 768, 790, 791, 804, 891, and 912. Mutations associated with only FMTC include codons 533, 768, V804M, and 912. A cautionary note is that rare mutations that were once associated with FMTC only (791, V804L, and 891) have been found in families with MEN 2A as there are occasional reports of pheochromocytoma. At present it is reasonable to conclude that only kindreds with codon 533, 768, V804M, or 912 mutations are consistently associated with FMTC; in kindreds with all other *RET* mutations, pheochromocytoma is a possibility. Germline mutations occur in at least 6% of patients with apparently sporadic MTC, leading to the recommendation that all patients with MTC should be screened for these mutations. These findings mirror results in other malignancies where germline mutations of cancer-causing genes contribute to a greater percentage of apparently sporadic cancer than previously considered. The recognition of new mutations of *RET* almost 10 years following the initial discovery of *RET* mutations suggests that more will be identified in the future.

Somatic mutations (found only in the tumor and not transmitted in the germline) of the *RET* protooncogene have been identified in sporadic MTC; 25 to 35% of sporadic tumors have codon 918 mutations, and somatic mutations in codons 630, 768, and 804 have also been identified (Fig. 21-3).

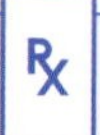

TREATMENT FOR MEN 2

Screening for Multiple Endocrine Neoplasia Type 2

Death from MTC can be prevented by early thyroidectomy. The identification of *RET* protooncogene mutations and the application of DNA-based molecular diagnostic techniques to identify these mutations has simplified the screening process. During the initial evaluation of a kindred, a *RET* protooncogene analysis should be performed on an individual with proven MEN 2A. Establishment of the specific germline mutation facilitates the subsequent analysis of other family members. Each family member at risk should be tested twice for the presence of the specific mutation; the second analysis should be performed on a new DNA sample and, ideally, in a second laboratory to exclude sample mix-up or technical error (see *www.genetests.org* for an up-to-date list of laboratory testing sites). Both false-positive and false-negative analyses have been described; a false-negative test result is of the greatest concern because calcitonin testing is now rarely performed as a diagnostic backup study; if there is a genetic test error, a child may present in the second or third decade with metastatic MTC. Individuals in a kindred with a known mutation who have two normal analyses can be excluded from further screening.

There is general consensus that children with codon 883, 918, and 922 mutations, those associated with MEN 2B, should have a total thyroidectomy and central lymph node dissection (level VI) performed during the first months of life or soon after identification of the syndrome. If local metastasis is discovered, a more extensive lymph node dissection (levels II to V) is generally indicated. In children with codon 611, 618, 620, 630, 634, and 891 mutations, thyroidectomy should be performed before age 6 because of reports of local metastatic disease in children this age. Finally, there are kindreds with codon 609, 768, 790, 791, 804, and 912 mutations where the phenotype of MTC appears to be less aggressive. In kindreds with these mutations, two management approaches have been suggested: (1) perform a total thyroidectomy, with or without central node dissection, at some arbitrary age (perhaps 6 to 10 years of age); or (2) continue annual or biannual calcitonin provocative testing with performance of total thyroidectomy, with or without central neck dissection, when the test becomes abnormal. The pentagastrin test involves measurement of serum calcitonin basally and at 2, 5, 10, and 15 min after a bolus injection of 5 μg pentagastrin per kilogram body weight. Before injection, patients should be warned of epigastric tightness, nausea, warmth, and tingling of extremities and reassured that the symptoms will last ~2 min. The recent unavailability of pentagastrin in the United States has led to use of a short calcium infusion, performed by obtaining a baseline serum calcitonin and then infusing 150 mg calcium salt intravenously over 10 min with measurement of serum calcium and calcitonin at 5, 10, 15, and 30 min after initiation of the infusion.

The *RET* protooncogene analysis should be performed in patients with suspected MEN 2B to detect codon 883, 918, and 922 mutations, especially in newborn children where the diagnosis is suspected but the clinical phenotype is not fully developed. Other family members at risk for MEN 2B should also be tested because the mucosal neuromas can be subtle and not always identified. Most MEN 2B mutations represent de novo germline mutations derived from the paternal allele. In the rare families with proven germline transmission of MTC but no identifiable *RET* protooncogene mutation, annual pentagastrin or calcium-pentagastrin testing should be performed on members at risk.

Annual screening for pheochromocytoma in subjects with germline *RET* mutations should be performed by measuring basal plasma or 24-h urine catecholamines and metanephrines. The goal is to identify a pheochromocytoma before it causes significant symptoms or is likely to cause sudden death, an event most commonly associated with large tumors. Radiographic studies, such as MRI or CT scans, are generally reserved for individuals with abnormal screening tests or with symptoms suggestive of pheochromocytoma (Chap. 6). Women should be tested during pregnancy because undetected pheochromocytoma can cause maternal death during childbirth.

Measurement of serum calcium and parathyroid hormone levels every 2 to 3 years provides an adequate screen for hyperparathyroidism, except in those families in which hyperparathyroidism is a prominent component.

Medullary Thyroid Carcinoma

Hereditary MTC is a multicentric disorder. Total thyroidectomy with a central lymph node dissection should be performed in children who carry the mutant gene. Incomplete thyroidectomy leaves the possibility of later transformation of residual C cells. The goal of early therapy is to cure, and a strategy that does not accomplish this goal is short-sighted. Long-term follow-up studies indicate an excellent outcome with ~90% of children free of disease 15 to 20 years after surgery. In contrast, 15 to 25% of patients whose diagnosis is based on a palpable thyroid nodule die from the disease within 15 to 20 years.

In adults with MTC >1 cm in size, metastases to regional lymph nodes are common (>75%). Total thyroidectomy with central lymph node dissection and selective dissection of other regional chains provide the best chance for cure. In patients with extensive local metastatic disease in the neck, external radiation may prevent local recurrence or reduce tumor mass but is not curative. Chemotherapy with combinations of adriamycin, vincristine, cyclophosphamide, and dacarbazine may provide palliation. The recent success of gleevec for treatment of chronic myelogenous leukemia and gastrointestinal stromal tumors has prompted efforts to develop inhibitors that target the RET tyrosine kinase. Preliminary in vitro studies have identified several promising agents, and human trials are forthcoming.

Pheochromocytoma

The long-term goal for management of pheochromocytoma is to prevent death and cardiovascular complications. Improvements in radiographic imaging of the adrenals make direct examination of the apparently normal contralateral gland during surgery less important, and the rapid evolution of laparoscopic surgery has simplified management of early pheochromocytoma. The major question is whether to remove both adrenal glands or to remove only the affected adrenal at the time of primary surgery. Issues to be considered in this decision include the possibility of malignancy (<15 reported cases), the high probability of developing pheochromocytoma in the apparently unaffected gland over an 8- to 10-year period, and the risks of adrenal insufficiency caused by removal of both glands (at least two deaths related to adrenal insufficiency in MEN 2 patients). Most clinicians recommend removing only the affected gland. If both adrenals are removed, glucocorticoid and mineralocorticoid replacement are mandatory. An alternative approach is to perform a cortical-sparing adrenalectomy, removing the pheochromocytoma and adrenal medulla, leaving the adrenal cortex behind. This approach is usually successful and eliminates the necessity for steroid hormone replacement in most patients, although the pheochromocytoma recurs in a small percentage.

Hyperparathyroidism

Hyperparathyroidism has been managed by one of two approaches. Removal of 3.5 glands with maintenance of the remaining half gland in the neck is the usual procedure. In families in whom hyperparathyroidism is a prominent manifestation (almost always associated with a codon 634 *RET* mutation) and recurrence is common, total parathyroidectomy with transplantation of parathyroid tissue into the nondominant forearm is preferred. This approach is discussed above in the context of hyperparathyroidism associated with MEN 1.

OTHER GENETIC ENDOCRINE TUMOR SYNDROMES

A number of mixed syndromes exist in which the neoplastic associations differ from those in MEN 1 or 2 (Table 21-1).

The cause of VHL syndrome, the association of central nervous system tumors, renal cell carcinoma, pheochromocytoma, and islet cell neoplasms, is a mutation in the *VHL* tumor-suppressor gene. Germline-inactivating mutations of the *VHL* gene cause tumor formation when there is additional loss or somatic mutation of the normal *VHL* allele in brain, kidney, pancreatic islet, or adrenal medullary cells. Missense mutations have been identified in >40% of VHL families with pheochromocytoma, suggesting that families with this type of mutation should be surveyed routinely for pheochromocytoma. A point that may be useful in differentiating VHL from MEN 1 (overlapping features include islet cell tumor and rare pheochromocytoma) or MEN 2 (overlapping feature is pheochromocytoma) is that hyperparathyroidism rarely occurs in VHL.

The molecular defect in type 1 neurofibromatosis inactivates neurofibromin, a cell membrane–associated protein that normally activates a GTPase. Inactivation of this protein impairs GTPase and causes continuous activation of p21 Ras and its downstream tyrosine kinase pathway. Endocrine tumors also form in less common neoplastic genetic syndromes. These include Cowden's disease, Carney complex, familial acromegaly, and familial carcinoid syndrome. Carney complex comprises myxomas of the heart, skin, and breast; peripheral nerve schwannomas; spotty skin pigmentation; and testicular, adrenal, and GH-secreting pituitary tumors. Linkage analysis has identified two loci: chromosome 2p in half of families and 17q in the others. The 17q gene has been identified as the regulatory subunit (type IA) of protein kinase A (PRKA1A).

IMMUNOLOGIC SYNDROMES AFFECTING MULTIPLE ENDOCRINE ORGANS

When immune dysfunction affects two or more endocrine glands and other nonendocrine immune disorders are present, the polyglandular autoimmune (PGA) syndromes should be considered. The PGA syndromes are classified as two main types: the type I syndrome starts in childhood and is characterized by mucocutaneous candidiasis, hypoparathyroidism, and adrenal insufficiency; the type II, or Schmidt, syndrome is more likely to present in adults and most commonly comprises adrenal insufficiency, thyroiditis, and type 1 diabetes mellitus (**Table 21-2**).

POLYGLANDULAR AUTOIMMUNE SYNDROME TYPE I

PGA type I is usually recognized in the first decade of life and requires two of three components for diagnosis: mucocutaneous candidiasis, hypoparathyroidism, and adrenal insufficiency. Mineralocorticoids and glucocorticoids may be lost simultaneously or sequentially. This disorder is also called *autoimmune polyendocrinopathy-candidiasis-ectodermal dystrophy* (APECED). Other endocrine defects can include gonadal failure, hypothyroidism, anterior hypophysitis, and, less commonly, destruction of the beta cells of the pancreatic islets and development of insulin-dependent (type 1) diabetes mellitus. Additional features include hypoplasia of the dental enamel, ungual dystrophy, tympanic membrane sclerosis, vitiligo, keratopathy, and gastric parietal cell dysfunction resulting in pernicious anemia. Some patients develop autoimmune hepatitis, malabsorption (variably attributed to intestinal lymphangiectasia, IgA deficiency, bacterial overgrowth,

TABLE 21-2

FEATURES OF POLYGLANDULAR AUTOIMMUNE (PGA) SYNDROMES

PGA I	PGA II
Epidemiology	
Autosomal recessive Mutations in APECED gene Childhood onset Equal male:female ratio	Polygenic inheritance HLA-DR3 and HLA-DR4 associated Adult onset Female predominance
Disease Associations	
Mucocutaneous candidiasis Hypoparathyroidism Adrenal insufficiency Hypogonadism Alopecia Hypothyroidism Dental enamel hypoplasia Malabsorption Chronic active hepatitis Vitiligo Pernicious anemia	Adrenal insufficiency Hypothyroidism Graves' disease Type 1 diabetes Hypogonadism Hypophysitis Myasthenia gravis Vitiligo Alopecia Pernicious anemia Celiac disease

Note: APECED, autoimmune polyendocrinopathy-candidiasis-ectodermal dystrophy.

or hypoparathyroidism), asplenism, achalasia, and cholelithiasis (Table 21-2). At the outset, only one organ may be involved, but the number increases with time so that patients eventually manifest two to five components of the syndrome.

Most patients initially present with oral candidiasis in childhood; it is poorly responsive to treatment and relapses frequently. Chronic hypoparathyroidism usually occurs before adrenal insufficiency develops. More than 60% of postpubertal women develop premature hypogonadism. The endocrine components, including adrenal insufficiency and hypoparathyroidism, may not develop until the fourth decade, making continued surveillance necessary.

Type I PGA syndrome is usually inherited as an autosomal recessive trait. The responsible gene, designated as either *APECED* or *AIRE,* encodes a transcription factor that is expressed in thymus and lymph nodes; a variety of different mutations have been reported.

POLYGLANDULAR AUTOIMMUNE SYNDROME TYPE II

PGA type II is characterized by two or more of the endocrinopathies listed in Table 21-2. Most often these include primary adrenal insufficiency, Graves' disease or autoimmune hypothyroidism, type 1 diabetes mellitus, and primary hypogonadism. Because adrenal insufficiency is relatively rare, it is frequently used to define the presence of the syndrome. Among patients with adrenal insufficiency, type 1 diabetes mellitus coexists in 52% and autoimmune thyroid disease occurs in 69%. However, many patients with antimicrosomal and antithyroglobulin antibodies never develop abnormalities of thyroid function. Thus, increased antibody titers alone are poor predictors of future disease. Other associated conditions include hypophysitis, celiac disease, atrophic gastritis, and pernicious anemia. Vitiligo, caused by antibodies against the melanocyte, and alopecia are less common than in the type I syndrome. Mucocutaneous candidiasis does not occur. A few patients develop a late-onset, usually transient hypoparathyroidism caused by antibodies that compete with parathyroid hormone for binding to the PTH receptor. Up to 25% of patients with myasthenia gravis, and an even higher percentage who have myasthenia and a thymoma, have PGA type II.

The type II syndrome is familial in nature, often transmitted as an autosomal dominant trait with incomplete penetrance. Like many of the individual autoimmune endocrinopathies, certain HLA-DR3 and HLA-DR4 alleles increase disease susceptibility; several different genes probably contribute to the expression of this syndrome.

A variety of autoantibodies are seen in PGA type II, including antibodies directed against: (1) thyroid antigens such as thyroid peroxidase, thyroglobulin, or the thyroid-stimulating hormone (TSH) receptor; (2) adrenal side chain cleavage enzyme, steroid 21-hydroxylase, or ACTH receptor; and (3) pancreatic islet glutamic acid decarboxylase or the insulin receptor, among others.

DIAGNOSIS

The clinical manifestations of adrenal insufficiency often develop slowly, may be difficult to detect, and can be fatal if not diagnosed and treated appropriately. Thus, prospective screening should be performed routinely in all patients and family members at risk for PGA types I and II. The most effective screening test for adrenal disease is a cosyntropin stimulation test (Chap. 5). A fasting blood glucose level can be obtained to screen for hyperglycemia. Additional screening tests should include measurements of TSH, luteinizing hormone, follicle-stimulating hormone, and, in men, testosterone levels. In families with suspected type I PGA syndrome, calcium and phosphorus levels should be measured. These screening studies should be performed every 1 to 2 years up to about age 50 in families with PGA type II syndrome and until about age 40 in patients with type I syndrome. Screening measurements of autoantibodies against potentially affected endocrine organs are of uncertain prognostic value. The differential diagnosis of PGA syndrome should include the DiGeorge syndrome (hypoparathyroidism due to glandular agenesis and mucocutaneous candidiasis), Kearns-Sayre syndrome (hypoparathyroidism, primary hypogonadism, type 1 diabetes mellitus, and panhypopituitarism), Wolfram's syndrome (congenital diabetes insipidus and diabetes mellitus), IPEX syndrome (*i*mmunodysregulation, *p*olyendocrinopathy, and *e*nteropathy, *X*-linked), and congenital rubella (type 1 diabetes mellitus and hypothyroidism).

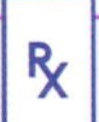

TREATMENT

With the exception of Graves' disease, the management of each of the endocrine components of the disease involves hormone replacement and is covered in detail in the chapters on adrenal, thyroid, gonadal, and parathyroid disease (Chaps. 4, 5, 8, 10, and 24). One aspect of therapy deserves special emphasis. Namely, primary hypothyroidism can mask adrenal insufficiency by prolonging the half-life of cortisol; consequently, administration of thyroid hormone to a patient with unsuspected adrenal insufficiency can precipitate adrenal crisis. Thus, all patients with hypothyroidism in the context of PGA syndrome should be screened for adrenal disease and, if it is present, be treated with glucocorticoids prior to or concurrently with thyroid hormone therapy.

OTHER AUTOIMMUNE ENDOCRINE SYNDROMES

Insulin Receptor Antibodies

Rare insulin-resistance syndromes occur in patients who develop antibodies that block the interaction of insulin with its receptor. Conversely, other classes of anti-insulin receptor antibodies can activate the receptor and can cause hypoglycemia; this disorder should be considered in the differential diagnosis of fasting hypoglycemia (Chap. 19).

Patients with insulin receptor antibodies and acanthosis nigricans are often middle-aged women who acquire insulin resistance in association with other autoimmune disorders such as systemic lupus erythematosus or Sjögren's syndrome. Vitiligo, alopecia, Raynaud's phenomenon, and arthritis may also be seen. Other autoimmune endocrine disorders, including thyrotoxicosis, hypothyroidism, and hypogonadism, occur rarely. Acanthosis nigricans, a velvety, hyperpigmented, thickened skin lesion, is prominent on the dorsum of the neck and other skin fold areas in the axillae or groin and often heralds the diagnosis in these patients. However, acanthosis nigricans also occurs in patients with obesity or polycystic ovarian syndrome, in which insulin resistance appears to be due to a postreceptor defect; thus acanthosis nigricans itself is not diagnostic of the immunologic form of insulin resistance.

Ataxia telangiectasia is an autosomal recessive disorder caused by mutations in *ATM,* a gene involved in cellular responses to ionizing radiation and oxidative damage. This disorder is characterized by ataxia, telangiectasia, immune abnormalities, and an increased incidence of malignancies. Insulin-resistant diabetes mellitus occurs and is associated with anti-insulin antibodies.

Autoimmune Insulin Syndrome with Hypoglycemia

This disorder typically occurs in patients with other autoimmune disorders and is caused by polyclonal insulin-binding autoantibodies that bind to endogenously synthesized insulin. If the insulin dissociates from the antibodies several hours or more after a meal, hypoglycemia can result. Most cases of the syndrome have been described in Japan, and there may be a genetic component. In plasma cell dyscrasias such as multiple myeloma, the plasma cells may produce monoclonal antibodies against insulin and cause hypoglycemia by a similar mechanism.

Antithyroxine Antibodies and Hypothyroidism

Circulating autoantibodies against thyroid hormones in patients with both immune thyroid disease and plasma cell dyscrasias such as Waldenström's macroglobulinemia can bind thyroid hormones, decrease their biologic activity, and result in primary hypothyroidism. In other patients the antibodies simply interfere with thyroid hormone immunoassays and cause false elevations or decreases in measured hormone levels.

Crow-Fukase Syndrome

The features of this syndrome are highlighted by an acronym that emphasizes its important features: *p*olyneuropathy, *o*rganomegaly, *e*ndocrinopathy, *M*-proteins, and *s*kin changes (POEMS). The most important feature is a severe, progressive sensorimotor polyneuropathy associated with a plasma cell dyscrasia. Localized collections of plasma cells (plasmacytomas) can cause sclerotic bone lesions and produce monoclonal IgG or IgA proteins. Endocrine manifestations include amenorrhea in women and impotence and gynecomastia in men, hypogonadism, hyperprolactinemia, type 2 diabetes mellitus, primary hypothyroidism, adrenal insufficiency, and hyperparathyroidism. Skin changes include hyperpigmentation, thickening of the dermis, hirsutism, and hyperhidrosis. Hepatomegaly and lymphadenopathy occur in about two-thirds of patients, and splenomegaly is seen in about one-third. Other manifestations include increased cerebrospinal fluid pressure with papilledema, peripheral edema, ascites, pleural effusions, glomerulonephritis, and fever. Median survival may be >10 years, though shorter in patients with extravascular volume overload or clubbing.

The systemic nature of the disorder may cause confusion with other connective tissue diseases. The endocrine manifestations suggest an autoimmune basis of the disorder, but circulating antibodies against endocrine cells have not been demonstrated. Increased serum and tissue levels of interleukin 6, interleukin 1β, vascular endothelial growth factor, matrix metalloproteins, and tumor necrosis factor α are present, but the pathophysiologic basis for the POEMS syndrome is uncertain. Therapy directed against the plasma cell dyscrasia such as local radiation of bony lesions, chemotherapy, thalidomide, plasmapheresis, bone marrow or stem cell transplantation, and treatment with all-*trans* retinoic acid may result in endocrine improvement.

FURTHER READINGS

BETTERLE C et al: Autoimmune adrenal insufficiency and autoimmune polyendocrine syndromes: Autoantibodies, autoantigens, and their applicability in diagnosis and disease prediction. Endocr Rev 23:327, 2002

COTE GJ, GAGEL RF: Lessons learned from the management of a rare genetic cancer. N Engl J Med 349:1566, 2003

This editorial highlights consensus recommendations for using genetic testing in the management of MEN 2. In addition to specific recommendations, the authors describe how rapidly these guidelines have evolved since the discovery of the RET protooncogene .

KOUVARAKI MA et al: RET proto-oncogene: A review and update of genotype-phenotype correlations in hereditary medullary thyroid cancer and associated endocrine tumors. Thyroid 15:531, 2005

MACHENS A et al: Early malignant progression of hereditary medullary thyroid carcinoma. N Engl J Med 349: 1517, 2003

MARX SJ: Molecular genetics of multiple endocrine neoplasia types 1 and 2. Nat Rev Cancer 5:367, 2005

PERHEENTUPA J: APS-1/APECED: The clinical disease and therapy. Endocrinol Metab Clin North Am 31:295, 2002

SKINNER MA et al: Prophylactic thyroidectomy in multiple endocrine neoplasia type 2A. N Engl J Med 353:1105, 2005

This prospective study of 50 patients with genetic risk of MEN 2A provides evidence that early prophylactic thyroidectomy, performed on the basis of results of genetic testing, may prevent or reduce the likelihood of developing recurrent MTC in individuals who inherit a germline RET mutation associated with MEN 2A.

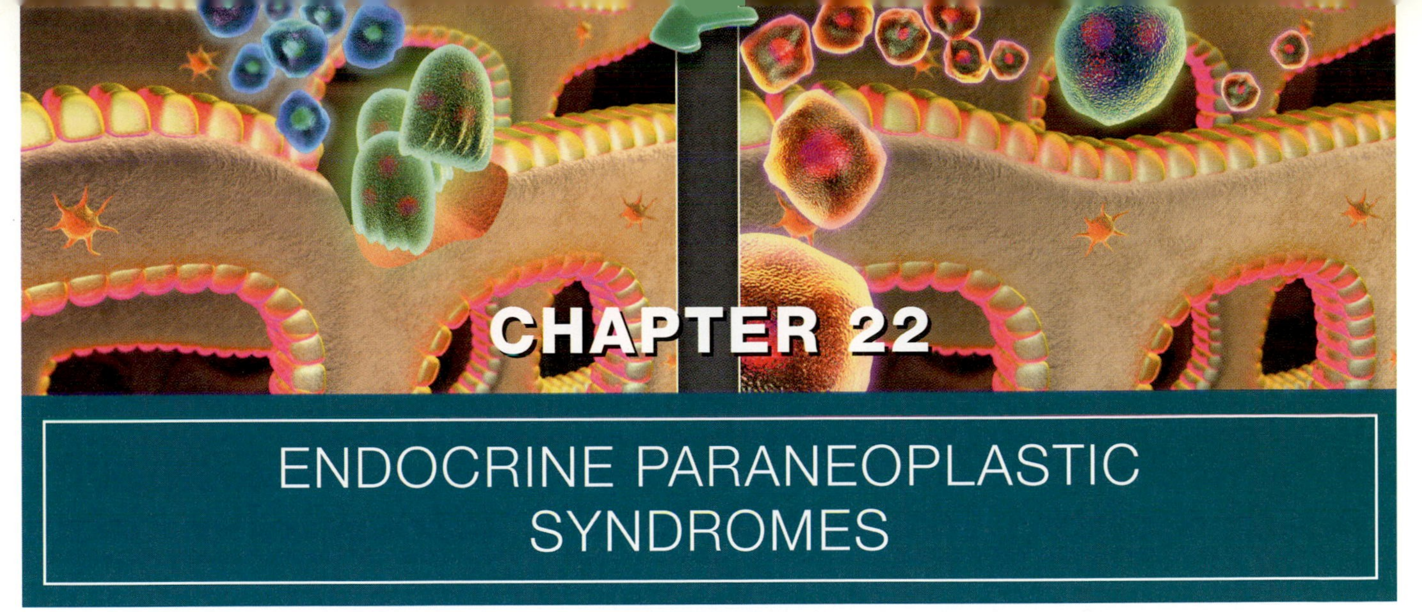

ENDOCRINE PARANEOPLASTIC SYNDROMES

J. Larry Jameson

In addition to local tissue invasion and metastasis, neoplastic cells can produce a variety of peptides that exert biologic actions at local and distant sites and can elicit responses that cause a variety of hormonal, hematologic, dermatologic, and neurologic symptoms. *Paraneoplastic syndromes* refer to the disorders that accompany benign or malignant tumors but are not directly related to mass effects or invasion by the primary tumor or its metastases. Tumors of neuroendocrine origin, such as small cell lung carcinoma (SCLC) and carcinoids, produce a wide array of peptide hormones and are common causes of paraneoplastic syndromes. However, almost every type of malignancy has the potential to produce hormones or cytokines or to induce immunologic responses. Careful studies of the prevalence of paraneoplastic syndromes indicate that they are more common than is generally appreciated. The signs, symptoms, and metabolic alterations associated with paraneoplastic disorders may be overlooked in the context of a malignancy and its treatment. Consequently, atypical clinical manifestations in a patient with cancer should prompt consideration of a paraneoplastic syndrome. In this chapter, we review the most common endocrinologic, hematologic, and dermatologic syndromes associated with underlying neoplasia.

ENDOCRINE PARANEOPLASTIC SYNDROMES

ETIOLOGY

Hormones can be produced from eutopic or ectopic sources. *Eutopic* refers to the expression of a hormone from its normal tissue of origin, whereas *ectopic* refers to hormone production from an atypical tissue source. For example, adrenocorticotropic hormone (ACTH) is expressed eutopically by the corticotrope cells of the anterior pituitary but it can be expressed ectopically in SCLC. As assay methodologies have become more sensitive, it is now apparent that many hormones are produced at low levels from a wide array of tissues, in addition to the classic endocrine source. Thus, ectopic expression is often a quantitative change rather than an absolute change in tissue expression. Nevertheless, the term *ectopic expression* is firmly entrenched and conveys the abnormal physiology associated with neoplastic hormone production. In addition to high levels of hormones, ectopic expression is typically characterized by abnormal regulation of hormone production (e.g., defective feedback control) and peptide processing (resulting in large, unprocessed precursors).

A diverse array of molecular mechanisms has been suggested to cause ectopic hormone production, but this process remains incompletely understood. In rare instances, genetic rearrangements explain aberrant hormone expression. For example, translocation of the *parathyroid hormone (PTH)* gene resulted in high levels of PTH expression in an ovarian carcinoma, presumably because the genetic rearrangement brings the

PTH gene under the control of ovary-specific regulatory elements. A related phenomenon is well documented in many forms of leukemia and lymphoma, in which somatic genetic rearrangements confer a growth advantage and frequently alter cellular differentiation and function. Although genetic rearrangements may cause selected cases of ectopic hormone production, this mechanism is probably unusual, as many tumors are associated with excessive production of a wide variety of peptides. It is likely that cellular dedifferentiation underlies most cases of ectopic hormone production. In support of this idea, many cancers are poorly differentiated histologically, and certain tumor products, such as human chorionic gonadotropin (hCG), parathyroid hormone–related protein (PTHrP), and α fetoprotein, are characteristic of gene expression at earlier developmental stages. On the other hand, the propensity of certain cancers to produce particular hormones (e.g., squamous cell carcinomas produce PTHrP) suggests that dedifferentiation is partial or that selective pathways are derepressed. These expression profiles are likely to be driven by alterations in transcriptional repression, changes in DNA methylation, or other factors that govern cell differentiation. In SCLC, the pathway of differentiation has been relatively well defined. The neuroendocrine phenotype is dictated in part by the basic-helix-loop-helix (bHLH) transcription factor human achaete-scute homologue-1 (hASH1), which is expressed at abnormally high levels in SCLC associated with ectopic ACTH. The activity of hASH-1 is inhibited by hairy enhancer of split-1 (HES-1) and by Notch proteins, which are also capable of inducing growth arrest. Thus, abnormal expression of these developmental transcription factors appears to provide a link between cell proliferation and differentiation.

Ectopic hormone production would only be an epiphenomenon associated with cancer if it did not sometimes result in clinical manifestations. Excessive and unregulated production of hormones such as ACTH, PTHrP, or vasopressin can lead to substantial morbidity and can complicate the cancer treatment plan. Moreover, the paraneoplastic endocrinopathies are sometimes the presenting feature of underlying malignancy and may prompt the search for an unrecognized tumor.

A large number of paraneoplastic endocrine syndromes have been described, linking overproduction of particular hormones with specific types of tumors. However, certain recurring syndromes emerge from this large group (**Table 22-1**). The most common paraneoplastic endocrine syndromes include hypercalcemia from overproduction of PTHrP and other factors, hyponatremia from excess vasopressin, and Cushing's syndrome from ectopic ACTH.

SELECTED PARANEOPLASTIC ENDOCRINE SYNDROMES

HYPERCALCEMIA CAUSED BY ECTOPIC PRODUCTION OF PTHRP

(See also Chap. 24)

Etiology

Humoral hypercalcemia of malignancy (HHM) occurs in up to 5% of patients with cancer. HHM is most common in cancers of the lung, breast, head and neck, genitourinary tract, esophagus, and skin, and in multiple myeloma and lymphomas. There are several humoral causes of HHM but it is most often associated with overproduction of PTHrP. In addition to acting as a circulating humoral factor, many bone metastases (e.g., breast, multiple myeloma) produce PTHrP, leading to local osteolysis and hypercalcemia.

PTHrP is structurally related to PTH and it binds to the PTH receptor, explaining the similar biochemical features of HHM and hyperparathyroidism. PTHrP plays a key role in skeletal development and regulates cellular proliferation and differentiation in other tissues including skin, bone marrow, breast, and hair follicles. The mechanism of PTHrP induction in malignancy is incompletely understood but it is notable that tumor-bearing tissues commonly associated with HHM normally produce PTHrP during development or cellular renewal. Mutations in certain oncogenes, such as *Ras,* can activate PTHrP expression. In adult T cell lymphoma, the transactivating Tax protein produced by human T cell lymphotropic virus I (HTLV-I) stimulates PTHrP promoter activity. Metastatic lesions to bone are more likely to produce PTHrP than are metastases in other tissues, suggesting that bone produces factors that enhance PTHrP production, or that PTHrP-producing metastases have a selective growth advantage in bone. Thus, PTHrP production can be stimulated by mutations in oncogenes, by altered expression of viral or cellular transcription factors, and by local growth factors.

Another relatively common cause of HHM is excess production of 1,25-dihydroxyvitamin D. Like granulomatous disorders associated with hypercalcemia, lymphomas can produce an enzyme that converts 25-hydroxyvitamin D to the more active 1,25-dihydroxyvitamin D, leading to enhanced gastrointestinal calcium absorption. Other causes of HHM include tumor-mediated production of osteolytic cytokines and inflammatory mediators.

Clinical Manifestations

The typical presentation of HHM is a patient with a known malignancy who is found to be hypercalcemic on routine laboratory tests. Less often, hypercalcemia is the initial presenting feature of malignancy. Particularly

TABLE 22-1

PARANEOPLASTIC SYNDROMES CAUSED BY ECTOPIC HORMONE PRODUCTION

PARANEOPLASTIC SYNDROME	ECTOPIC HORMONE	TYPICAL TUMOR TYPES[a]
	Common	
Hypercalcemia of malignancy	Parathyroid hormone-related protein (PTHrP)	Squamous cell (head and neck, lung, skin), breast, genitourinary, gastrointestinal
	1,25 dihydroxyvitamin D	Lymphomas
	Parathyroid hormone (PTH) (rare)	Lung, ovary
	Prostaglandin E2 (PGE2) (rare)	Renal, lung
Syndrome of inappropriate antidiuretic hormone secretion (SIADH)	Vasopressin	Lung (squamous, small cell), gastrointestinal, genitourinary, ovary
Cushing's syndrome	Adrenocorticotropic hormone (ACTH)	Lung (small cell, bronchial carcinoid, adenocarcinoma, squamous), thymus, pancreatic islet, medullary thyroid carcinoma
	Corticotropin-releasing hormone (CRH) (rare)	Pancreatic islet, carcinoid, lung, prostate
	Ectopic expression of gastric inhibitory peptide (GIP), luteinizing hormone (LH)/ human chorionic gonadotropin (hCG), other G protein–coupled receptors (rare)	Macronodular adrenal hyperplasia
	Less Common	
Non-islet cell hypoglycemia	Insulin-like growth factor (IGF-II)	Mesenchymal tumors, sarcomas, adrenal, hepatic, gastrointestinal, kidney, prostate
	Insulin (rare)	Cervix (small cell carcinoma)
Male feminization	hCG[b]	Testis (embryonal, seminomas), germinomas, choriocarcinoma, lung, hepatic, pancreatic islet
Diarrhea or intestinal hypermotility	Calcitonin[c]	Lung, colon, breast, medullary thyroid carcinoma
	Vasoactive intestinal peptide (VIP)	Pancreas, pheochromocytoma, esophagus
	Rare	
Oncogenic osteomalacia	Phosphatonin [fibroblast growth factor 23 (FGF23)]	Hemangiopericytomas, osteoblastomas, fibromas, sarcomas, giant cell tumors, prostate, lung
Acromegaly	Growth hormone–releasing hormone (GHRH)	Pancreatic islet, bronchial and other carcinoids
	Growth hormone (GH)	Lung, pancreatic islet
Hyperthyroidism	Thyroid-stimulating hormone (TSH)	Hydatidiform mole, embryonal tumors, struma ovarii
Hypertension	Renin	Juxtaglomerular tumors, kidney, lung, pancreas, ovary

[a]Only the most common tumor types are listed. For most ectopic hormone syndromes, an extensive list of tumors has been reported to produce one or more hormones.
[b]hCG is produced eutopically by trophoblastic tumors. Certain tumors produce disproportionate amounts of the hCG α or hCG β subunits. High levels of hCG rarely cause hyperthyroidism because of weak binding to the TSH receptor.
[c]Calcitonin is produced eutopically by medullary thyroid carcinoma and is used as a tumor marker.

when calcium levels are markedly increased (>14 mg/dL), patients may experience fatigue, mental status changes, dehydration, or symptoms of nephrolithiasis.

Diagnosis

Features that favor HHM as opposed to primary hyperparathyroidism include known malignancy, recent onset of hypercalcemia, and very high serum calcium levels. Like hyperparathyroidism, hypercalcemia caused by PTHrP is accompanied by hypercalciuria and hypophosphatemia. Measurement of PTH is useful to exclude primary hyperparathyroidism; the PTH level should be suppressed in HHM. An elevated PTHrP level confirms the diagnosis, and it is increased in about 80% of hypercalcemic patients with cancer. 1,25-Dihydroxyvitamin D levels may be increased in patients with lymphoma.

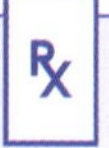

TREATMENT FOR HHM

The management of HHM begins with saline rehydration to dilute serum calcium and promote calciuresis. Forced diuresis with furosemide or other loop diuretics can enhance calcium excretion but provides relatively little value except in life-threatening hypercalcemia. When used, loop diuretics should be administered only after complete rehydration and with careful monitoring of fluid balance. Bisphosphonates such as pamidronate (30 to 90 mg IV) or zoledronate (4 to 8 mg IV) can reduce serum calcium within 1 to 2 days and suppress calcium release for several weeks. Oral bisphosphonates can also be used for chronic treatment. Previously used agents, such as calcitonin and mithramycin, have little utility now that bisphosphonates are available. Calcitonin (2 to 8 U/kg SC every 6 to 12 h) should be considered when rapid correction of severe hypercalcemia is needed. Hypercalcemia associated with lymphomas, multiple myeloma, or leukemia may respond to glucocorticoid treatment (e.g., prednisone 40 to 100 mg PO in four divided doses).

ECTOPIC VASOPRESSIN: TUMOR-ASSOCIATED SIADH

Etiology

Vasopressin is an antidiuretic hormone normally produced by the posterior pituitary gland. Ectopic vasopressin production by tumors is a common cause of the syndrome of inappropriate antidiuretic hormone (SIADH), occurring in at least half of patients with SCLC. Compensatory mechanisms, such as decreased thirst, suppression of aldosterone, and production of atrial natriuretic peptide (ANP), may mitigate the development of hyponatremia in patients who produce excessive vasopressin. Tumors with neuroendocrine features, such as SCLC and carcinoids, are the most common sources of ectopic vasopressin production, but it also occurs in other forms of lung cancer and with central nervous system (CNS) lesions; head and neck cancer; and genitourinary, gastrointestinal, and ovarian cancers. The mechanism of activation of the vasopressin gene in these tumors is unknown but often involves concomitant expression of the adjacent oxytocin gene, suggesting derepression of this locus.

Clinical Manifestations

Most patients with ectopic vasopressin secretion are asymptomatic and are identified because of the presence of hyponatremia on routine chemistry testing. Symptoms may include weakness, lethargy, nausea, confusion, depressed mental status, and seizures. The severity of symptoms reflects the rapidity of onset as well as the extent of hyponatremia. In most cases, hyponatremia develops slowly but may be exacerbated by the administration of intravenous fluids or the institution of new medications. Thirst is typically suppressed.

Diagnosis

The diagnostic features of ectopic vasopressin production are the same as those of other causes of SIADH. Hyponatremia and reduced serum osmolality occur in the setting of an inappropriately normal or increased urine osmolality. Unless there is concomitant volume depletion, urine sodium excretion is normal or increased. Other causes of hyponatremia should be excluded, including renal, adrenal, or thyroid insufficiency. Physiologic sources of vasopressin stimulation (CNS lesions, pulmonary disease, nausea) and adaptive circulatory mechanisms (hypotension, heart failure, hepatic cirrhosis), as well as medications, including many chemotherapeutic agents, should also be considered as possible causes of hyponatremia. Measurement of vasopressin is not usually necessary to make the diagnosis.

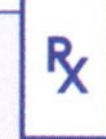

TREATMENT FOR ECTOPIC VASOPRESSIN

Most patients with ectopic vasopressin production develop hyponatremia over several weeks or months and it is reasonable to correct the disorder gradually unless mental status is altered or there is risk of seizures. Treatment of the underlying malignancy may reduce ectopic vasopressin production but this response is slow, if it occurs at all. Fluid restriction to less than urine output, plus insensible losses, is often sufficient to partially correct hyponatremia. However, strict monitoring of the amount and types of liquids consumed or administered intravenously is required for fluid restriction to be effective. Salt tablets or saline are not helpful unless there is concomitant volume depletion. Demeclocycline (150 to 300 mg orally three to four times daily) can be used to inhibit vasopressin action on the renal distal tubule but its onset of action is relatively slow (1 to 2 weeks). Other vasopressin antagonists are under investigation. Severe hyponatremia (Na < 115 meq/L) or mental status changes may require treatment with hypertonic (3%) or normal saline infusion together with furosemide, to enhance free water clearance. The rate of sodium correction should be slow (0.5 to 1 meq/L per h) to prevent rapid fluid shifts and the possible development of central pontine myelinolysis.

CUSHING'S SYNDROME CAUSED BY ECTOPIC ACTH PRODUCTION

(See also Chap. 5)

Etiology

Ectopic production of ACTH accounts for 10 to 20% of Cushing's syndrome. The syndrome is particularly common in neuroendocrine tumors. SCLC (>50%) is by far the most common cause of ectopic ACTH, followed by thymic carcinoid (15%), islet cell tumors (10%), bronchial carcinoid (10%), other carcinoids (5%), and pheochromocytomas (2%). As noted above, the mechanism of ectopic ACTH production in neuroendocrine tumors appears to be linked to the expression of transcription factors that dictate pathways of cell differentiation. Ectopic ACTH production is caused by increased expression of the proopiomelanocortin (POMC) gene, which encodes ACTH, along with melanocyte-stimulating hormone (MSH), β lipotropin, and several other peptides. In many tumors, there is abundant but aberrant expression of the POMC gene from an internal promoter, proximal to the third exon, which encodes ACTH. However, because this product lacks the signal sequence necessary for protein processing, it is not secreted. Increased production of ACTH arises instead from less abundant, but unregulated, POMC expression from the same promoter site used in the pituitary. However, because the tumors lack many of the enzymes needed to process the POMC polypeptide, it is typically released as multiple large, biologically inactive fragments along with relatively small amounts of fully processed, active ACTH.

Rarely, corticotropin-releasing hormone (CRH) is produced by pancreatic islet tumors, SCLC, medullary thyroid cancer, carcinoids, or prostate cancer. When levels are high enough, CRH can cause pituitary corticotrope hyperplasia and Cushing's syndrome. Tumors that produce CRH sometimes also produce ACTH, raising the possibility of a paracrine mechanism for ACTH production.

A distinct mechanism for ACTH-independent Cushing's syndrome involves ectopic expression of various G protein–coupled receptors in the adrenal nodules. Ectopic expression of the gastric inhibitory peptide (GIP) receptor is the best-characterized example of this mechanism. In this case, meals induce GIP secretion, which inappropriately stimulates adrenal growth and glucocorticoid production.

Clinical Manifestations

The clinical features of hypercortisolemia are detected in only a small fraction of patients with documented ectopic ACTH production. However, the ectopic ACTH syndrome is associated with several clinical features that distinguish it from other causes of Cushing's syndrome (e.g., pituitary adenomas, adrenal adenomas, iatrogenic glucocorticoid excess). The metabolic manifestations of ectopic ACTH syndrome are dominated by fluid retention and hypertension, hypokalemia, metabolic alkalosis, glucose intolerance, and, often, steroid psychosis. Patients with ectopic ACTH syndrome generally exhibit less marked weight gain and centripetal fat redistribution, probably because the exposure to excess steroids is relatively short and because cachexia reduces the propensity for weight gain and fat deposition. The very high levels of ACTH often cause increased pigmentation, and melanotrope-stimulating hormone (MSH) activity derived from the POMC precursor peptide is also increased. The extraordinarily high glucocorticoid levels in patients with ectopic sources of ACTH can lead to marked skin fragility and easy bruising. In addition, the high cortisol levels often overwhelm the renal 11β-hydroxysteroid dehydrogenase type II enzyme, which normally inactivates cortisol and prevents it from binding to renal mineralocorticoid receptors. Consequently, in addition to the excess mineralocorticoids produced by ACTH stimulation of the adrenal gland, high levels of cortisol exert activity through the mineralocorticoid receptor, leading to severe hypokalemia.

Diagnosis

The diagnosis of ectopic ACTH syndrome is usually not difficult in the setting of a known malignancy. Urine free cortisol levels fluctuate but are typically greater than

2 to 4 times normal and the plasma ACTH level is usually >100 pg/mL. A suppressed ACTH level excludes this diagnosis and indicates an ACTH-independent cause of Cushing's syndrome (e.g., adrenal or exogenous glucocorticoid). In contrast to pituitary sources of ACTH, most ectopic sources of ACTH do not respond to glucocorticoid suppression. Therefore, high-dose dexamethasone (8 mg PO) suppresses 8:00 A.M. serum cortisol (50% decrease from baseline) in about 80% of pituitary ACTH-producing adenomas but fails to suppress ectopic ACTH in about 90% of cases. Bronchial and other carcinoids are well-documented exceptions to these general guidelines, as these ectopic sources of ACTH may exhibit feedback regulation indistinguishable from pituitary adenomas, including suppression by high-dose dexamethasone, and ACTH responsiveness to adrenal blockade with metyrapone. If necessary, petrosal sinus catheterization can be used to evaluate a patient with ACTH-dependent Cushing's syndrome when the source of ACTH is unclear. After CRH stimulation, a 3:1 petrosal sinus:peripheral ACTH ratio strongly suggests a pituitary ACTH source. Imaging studies are also useful in the evaluation of suspected carcinoid lesions, allowing biopsy and characterization of hormone production using special stains.

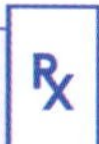

TREATMENT FOR ECTOPIC ACTH

The morbidity associated with the ectopic ACTH syndrome can be substantial. Patients may experience depression or personality changes because of extreme cortisol excess. Metabolic derangements including diabetes mellitus and hypokalemia can worsen fatigue. Poor wound healing and predisposition to infections can complicate the surgical management of tumors, and opportunistic infections, caused by organisms such as *Pneumocystis carinii* and mycoses, are often the cause of death in patients with ectopic ACTH production. Depending on prognosis and treatment plans for the underlying malignancy, measures to reduce cortisol levels are often indicated. Treatment of the underlying malignancy may reduce ACTH levels but is rarely sufficient to reduce cortisol levels to normal. Adrenalectomy is not practical for most of these patients but should be considered if the underlying tumor is not resectable and the prognosis is otherwise favorable (e.g., carcinoid). Medical therapy with ketoconazole (200 to 400 mg PO twice daily), metyrapone (250 to 500 mg PO every 6 h), mitotane (3 to 6 g PO in four divided doses, tapered to maintain low cortisol production), or other agents that block steroid synthesis or action is often the most practical strategy for managing the hypercortisolism associated with ectopic ACTH production (Chap. 2). Glucocorticoid replacement should be provided to avoid adrenal insufficiency. Unfortunately, many patients will eventually escape from medical blockade.

TUMOR-INDUCED HYPOGLYCEMIA CAUSED BY EXCESS PRODUCTION OF IGF-II (See also Chap. 19)

Mesenchymal tumors, hemangiopericytomas, hepatocellular tumors, adrenal carcinomas, and a variety of other large tumors have been reported to produce excessive amounts of insulin-like growth factor type II (IGF-II) precursor, which binds weakly to insulin receptors and strongly to IGF-I receptors, leading to insulin-like actions. The IGF-II gene resides on a locus on chromosome 11p15 that is normally imprinted (that is, expression is exclusively from a single parental allele). There is mounting evidence for biallelic expression of the IGF-II gene in a subset of tumors, suggesting loss of methylation and loss of imprinting as a mechanism for gene induction. In addition to increased IGF-II production, IGF-II bioavailability is increased due to complex alterations in circulating binding proteins. Increased IGF-II suppresses growth hormone (GH) and insulin, resulting in reduced IGF binding protein-3 (IGFBP-3), IGF-I, and acid-labile subunit (ALS). The reduction in ALS and IGFBP-3, which normally sequester IGF-II, causes it to be displaced to a small circulating complex that has greater access to insulin target tissues. For this reason, circulating IGF-II levels may not be markedly increased, despite causing hypoglycemia. In addition to IGF-II–mediated hypoglycemia, tumors may occupy enough of the liver to impair gluconeogenesis.

In most cases, the tumor causing hypoglycemia is clinically apparent and hypoglycemia develops in association with fasting. The diagnosis is made by documenting low serum glucose and suppressed insulin levels in association with symptoms of hypoglycemia. Serum IGF-II levels may not be increased (IGF-II assays may not detect IGF-II precursors). Increased IGF-II mRNA expression is found in most tumors. Any medications associated with hypoglycemia should be eliminated. Treatment of the underlying malignancy, if possible, may reduce the predisposition to hypoglycemia. Frequent meals and intravenous glucose, especially during sleep or fasting, are often necessary to prevent hypoglycemia. Glucagon, GH, and glucocorticoids have also been used to enhance glucose production.

HUMAN CHORIONIC GONADOTROPIN

hCG is composed of α and β subunits and can be produced as intact hormone, which is biologically active, or as uncombined biologically inert subunits. Ectopic production of intact hCG occurs most often in association with testicular embryonal tumors, germ cell tumors, extragonadal germinomas, lung cancer, hepatoma, and pancreatic islet tumors. Eutopic production of hCG occurs with trophoblastic malignancies. Low levels of hCG or its uncombined α or β subunits have been reported in a wide range of tumors. hCG α subunit production is particularly common in lung cancer and pancreatic islet cancer. In men, high hCG levels stimulate steroidogenesis and aromatase activity in testicular Leydig cells, resulting in increased estrogen production and the development of gynecomastia. Precocious puberty in boys or gynecomastia in men should prompt measurement of hCG and consideration of a testicular tumor or another source of ectopic hCG production. Most women are asymptomatic. hCG is easily measured using sensitive immunoradiometric assays. Treatment should be directed at the underlying malignancy.

ONCOGENIC OSTEOMALACIA

Hypophosphatemic oncogenic osteomalacia is characterized by markedly reduced serum phosphorus and renal phosphate wasting, leading to muscle weakness and osteomalacia. Serum calcium and PTH levels are normal and 1,25 dihydroxyvitamin D is low. Oncogenic osteomalacia is usually caused by benign mesenchymal tumors, such as hemangiopericytomas, fibromas, or giant cell tumors, often of the skeletal extremities or head. It has also been described in sarcomas and in patients with prostate and lung cancer. Resection of the tumor reverses the disorder, confirming its humoral basis. The circulating phosphaturic factor is called *phosphatonin*—a factor that inhibits renal tubular reabsorption of phosphate and renal conversion of 25-hydroxyvitamin D to 1,25-dihydroxyvitamin D. Phosphatonin has been identified as fibroblast growth factor 23 (FGF23). The disorder exhibits biochemical features similar to those seen with inactivating mutations in the *PHEX* gene, the cause of hereditary X-linked hypophosphatemia. The *PHEX* gene encodes a protease that activates FGF23. Treatment involves removal of the tumor, if possible, and supplementation with phosphate and vitamin D. Octreotide treatment reduces phosphate wasting in some patients with tumors that express somatostatin receptor subtype 2. Octreotide scans may also be useful to detect these tumors.

FURTHER READINGS

DELELLIS RA, XIA L: Paraneoplastic endocrine syndromes: A review. Endocr Pathol 14: 303, 2003

An update on the pathogenesis and clinical features of paraneoplastic syndromes.

DIRNHOFER S et al: Selective expression of trophoblastic hormones by lung carcinoma: Neurendocrine tumors exclusively produce human chorionic gonadotropin alpha-subunit (hCGalpha). Hum Pathol 31:966, 2000

A clinical case study of tumor-induced osteomalacia (TIO). This article reviews the distinctive clinical characteristics of this syndrome and the advances in diagnosis and pathophysiology of TIO.

Jan de Beur SM: Tumor-induced osteomalacia. JAMA 294:1260, 2005

JONES PA, BAYLIN SB: The fundamental role of epigenetic events in cancer. Nat Rev Genet 3:415, 2002

NEWELL-PRICE J et al: The CpG island promoter of the human proopiomelanocortin gene is methylated in nonexpressing normal tissue and tumors and represses expression. Mol Endocrinol 15:338, 2001

SEUFERT J et al: Octreotide therapy for tumor-induced osteomalacia. N Engl J Med 345:1883, 2001

STEWART AF: Clinical practice. Hypercalcemia associated with cancer. N Engl J Med 352:373, 2005

Hypercalcemia of malignancy is predominantly caused by production of parathyroid hormone–related peptide (PTHrP). PTHrP is structurally related to PTH and binds to the PTH receptor, thereby explaining their similar effects with respect to calcium metabolism. This review summarizes the pathophysiology and management of hypercalcemia associated with malignancy.

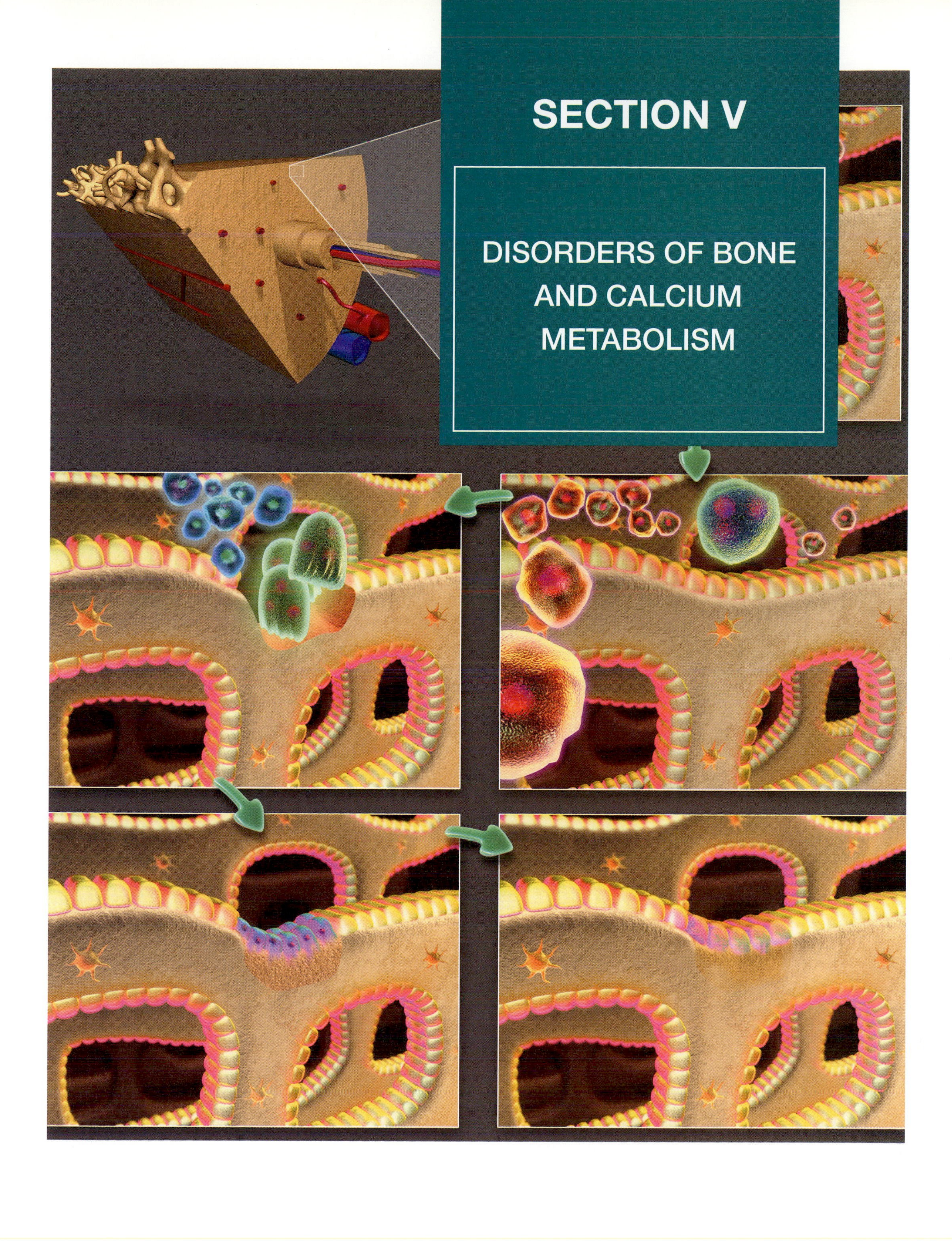

SECTION V

DISORDERS OF BONE AND CALCIUM METABOLISM

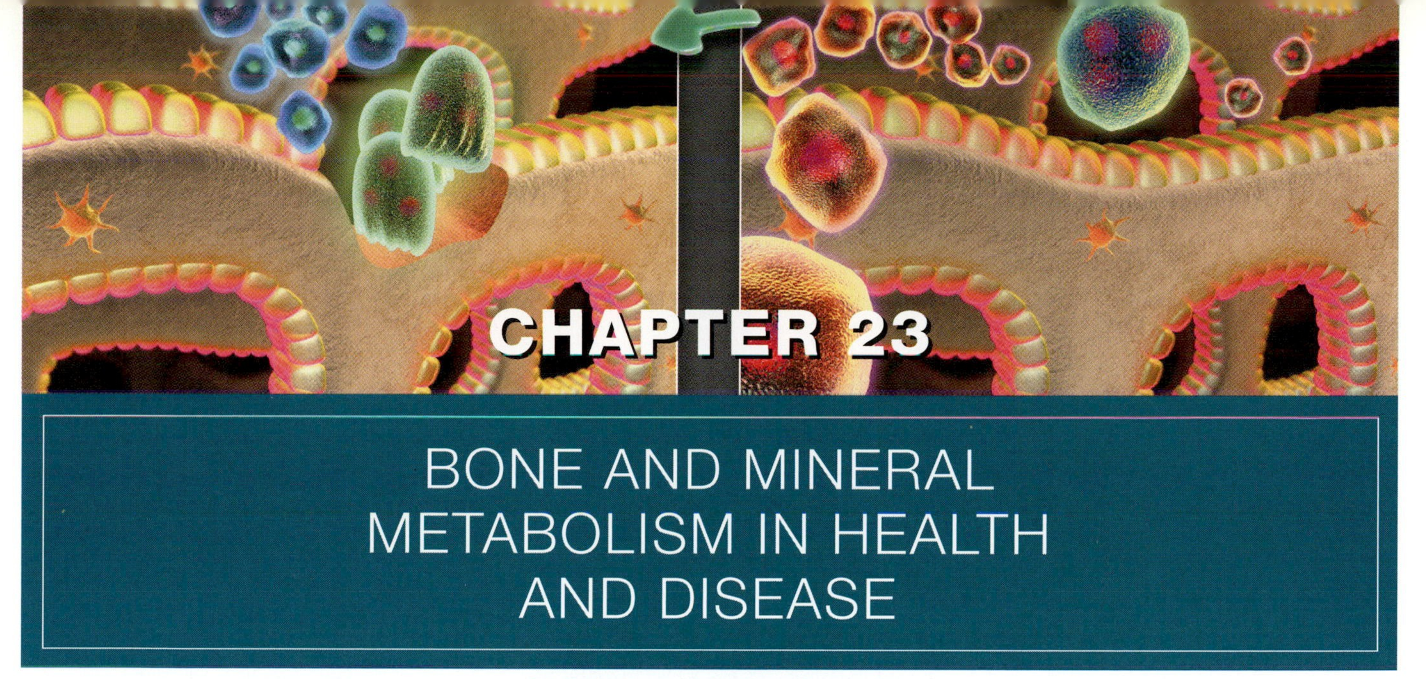

BONE AND MINERAL METABOLISM IN HEALTH AND DISEASE

F. Richard Bringhurst
Marie B. Demay
Stephen M. Krane
Henry M. Kronenberg

BONE STRUCTURE AND METABOLISM

Bone is a dynamic tissue that is remodeled constantly throughout life. The arrangement of compact and cancellous bone provides a strength and density suitable for mobility and protection. In addition, bone provides a reservoir for calcium, magnesium, phosphorus, sodium, and other ions necessary for homeostatic functions. The skeleton is highly vascular and receives about 10% of the cardiac output. Remodeling of bone is accomplished by two distinct cell types: osteoblasts produce bone matrix and osteoclasts resorb the matrix.

The extracellular components of bone consist of a solid mineral phase in close association with an organic matrix, of which 90 to 95% is type I collagen. The noncollagenous portion of the organic matrix is heterogeneous and contains serum proteins, such as albumin, as well as many locally produced proteins, whose functions are incompletely understood. These proteins include cell attachment/signaling proteins, such as thrombospondin, osteopontin, and fibronectin; calcium-binding proteins such as matrix gla protein and osteocalcin; and proteoglycans such as biglycan and decorin. Some of these proteins organize collagen fibrils; others initiate mineralization and binding of the mineral phase to the matrix.

The mineral phase is made up of calcium and phosphate and is best characterized as a poorly crystalline hydroxyapatite. The mineral phase of bone is deposited initially in intimate relation to the collagen fibrils and is found in specific locations in the "holes" between the collagen fibrils. This architectural arrangement of mineral and matrix results in a two-phase material well suited to withstand mechanical stresses. The organization of collagen influences the amount and type of mineral phase formed in bone. Although the primary structures of type I collagen in skin and bone tissues are similar, there are differences in posttranslational modifications and distribution of intermolecular cross-links. The holes in the packing structure of the collagen are larger in mineralized collagen of bone and dentin than in unmineralized collagens such as tendon. Single amino-acid substitutions in the helical portion of either the α1 (*COL1A1*) or α2 (*COL1A2*) chains of type I collagen disrupt the organization of bone in osteogenesis imperfecta. The severe skeletal fragility associated with these disorders highlights the importance of the fibrillar matrix in the structure of bone.

Osteoblasts synthesize and secrete the organic matrix. They are derived from cells of mesenchymal origin (**Fig. 23-1*A***). Active osteoblasts are found on the surface of

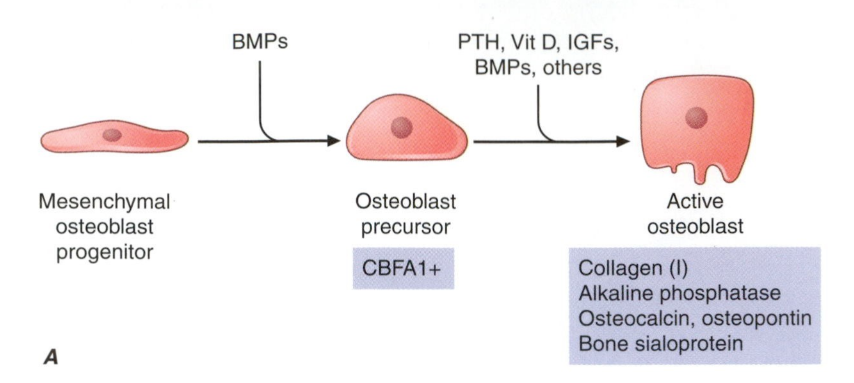

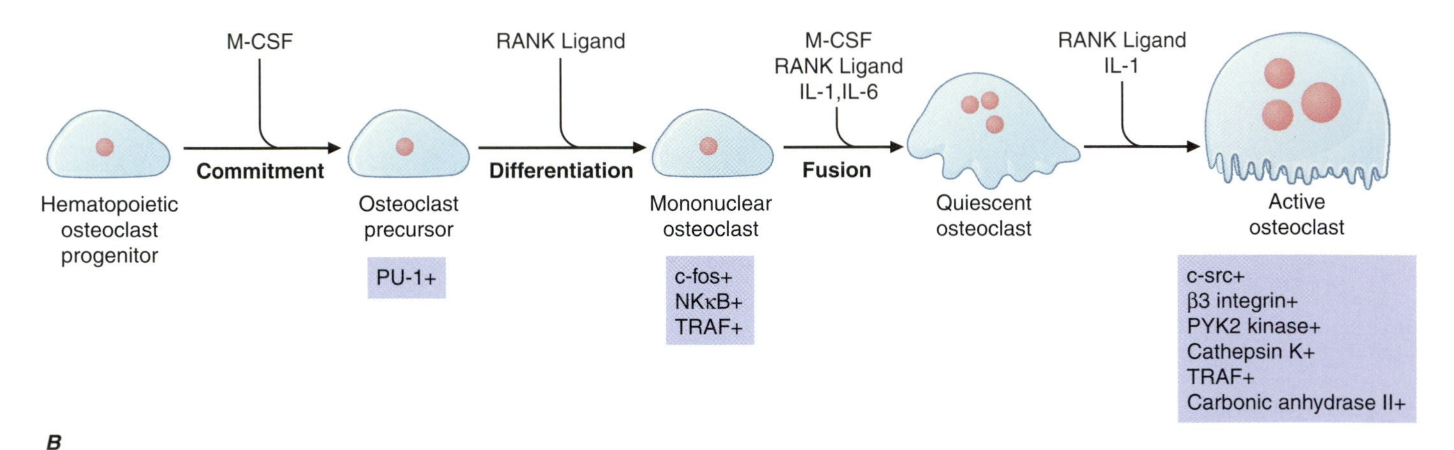

FIGURE 23-1

Pathways regulating development of (*A*) osteoblasts and (*B*) osteoclasts. Hormones, cytokines, and growth factors that control cell proliferation and differentiation are shown above the arrows. Transcription factors and other markers specific for various stages of development are depicted below the arrows. BMPs, bone morphogenic proteins; PTH, parathyroid hormone; Vit D, vitamin D; IGFs, insulin-like growth factors; CBFA1, core binding factor A1; M-CSF, macrophage colony-stimulating factor; PU-1, a monocyte- and B lymphocyte–specific ets family transcription factor; NF*k*B, nuclear factor *k*B; TRAF, tumor necrosis factor receptor –associated factors; RANK ligand, receptor activator of NF*k*B ligand; IL-1, interleukin-1; IL-6, interleukin-6. *(Modified from T Suda et al: Endocr Rev 20: 345, 1999, with permission.)*

newly forming bone. As an osteoblast secretes matrix, which is then mineralized, the cell becomes an *osteocyte,* still connected with its blood supply through a series of canaliculi. Osteocytes represent the vast majority of the cells in bone. They are thought to be the mechanosensors in bone that communicate signals to surface osteoblasts and their progenitors through the canalicular network. Mineralization of the matrix, both in trabecular bone and in osteones of compact cortical bone (*haversian systems*), begins soon after the matrix is secreted (primary mineralization) but is not completed for several weeks or even longer (secondary mineralization). While this mineralization takes advantage of the high concentrations of calcium and phosphate already near saturation in serum, mineralization is a carefully regulated process dependent on the activity of osteoblast-derived alkaline phosphatase, which probably works by hydrolyzing inhibitors of mineralization.

Genetic studies in humans and mice have identified several key genes that control osteoblast development. Core-binding factor A1 (*CBFA1,* also called *RUNX2*), is a transcription factor expressed specifically in chondrocyte (cartilage cells) and osteoblast progenitors, as well as in mature osteoblasts. *CBFA1* regulates the expression of several important osteoblast proteins including osterix (another transcription factor needed for osteoblast maturation), osteopontin, bone sialoprotein, type I collagen, osteocalcin, and receptor-activator of NFκB (RANK) ligand. *CBFA1* expression is regulated, in part, by bone morphogenic proteins (BMPs). *CBFA1*-deficient mice are devoid of osteoblasts, whereas mice with a deletion of only one allele (*CBFA1* +/−) exhibit a delay in formation of the clavicles and some cranial bones. The latter abnormalities are similar to those in the human disorder *cleidocranial dysplasia,* which is also caused by heterozygous inactivating mutations in *CBFA1*.

The paracrine signaling molecule, Indian hedgehog (Ihh), also plays a critical role in osteoblast development, as evidenced by Ihh-deficient mice that lack osteoblasts in bone formed on a cartilage mold (endochondral ossification). Signals originating from members of the wnt (wingless-type mouse mammary tumor virus integration site) family of paracrine factors are also important. Humans and mice missing a wnt-family co-receptor, LRP5 (lipoprotein receptor–related protein 5), have osteoporosis. Remarkably, humans with an overactive form of LPR5 have increased bone mass. Numerous other growth-regulatory factors affect osteoblast function, including the three closely related transforming growth factor βs, fibroblast growth factors (FGFs) 2 and 18, platelet-derived growth factor, and insulin-like growth factors (IGFs) I and II. Hormones, such as parathyroid hormone (PTH) and 1,25-dihydroxyvitamin D [1,25(OH)$_2$D] activate receptors expressed by osteoblasts to assure mineral homeostasis and to influence a variety of bone cell functions.

Resorption of bone is carried out mainly by *osteoclasts,* multinucleated cells that are formed by fusion of cells derived from the common precursor of macrophages and osteoclasts. Multiple factors regulating osteoclast development have been identified (Fig. 23-1*B*). Factors produced by osteoblasts or marrow stromal cells allow osteoblasts to control osteoclast development and activity. Macrophage colony-stimulating factor (M-CSF) plays a critical role during several steps in the pathway and ultimately leads to fusion of osteoclast progenitor cells to form multinucleated, active osteoclasts. RANK ligand, a member of the tumor necrosis factor (TNF) family, is expressed on the surface of osteoblast progenitors and stromal fibroblasts. In a process involving cell-cell interactions, RANK ligand binds to the RANK receptor on osteoclast progenitors, stimulating osteoclast differentiation and activation. Alternatively, a soluble decoy receptor, referred to as *osteoprotegerin,* can bind RANK ligand and inhibit osteoclast differentiation. Several growth factors and cytokines (including interleukins 1, 6, and 11; TNF; and interferon γ) modulate osteoclast differentiation and function. Most hormones that influence osteoclast function do not directly target this cell but instead influence M-CSF and RANK ligand signaling by osteoblasts. Both PTH and 1,25(OH)$_2$D increase osteoclast number and activity, whereas estrogen decreases osteoclast number and activity by this indirect mechanism. Calcitonin, in contrast, binds to its receptor on the basal surface of osteoclasts and directly inhibits osteoclast function.

Osteoclast-mediated resorption of bone takes place in scalloped spaces (*Howship's lacunae*) where the osteoclasts are attached through a specific $\alpha_v\beta_3$ integrin to components of the bone matrix such as osteopontin. The osteoclast forms a tight seal to the underlying matrix and secretes protons, chloride, and proteinases into a confined space likened to an extracellular lysosome. The active osteoclast surface forms a ruffled border that contains a specialized proton-pump ATPase, which secretes acid and solubilizes the mineral phase. Carbonic anhydrase (type II isoenzyme) within the osteoclast generates the needed protons. The bone matrix is resorbed in the acid environment adjacent to the ruffled border by proteases that act at low pH, such as cathepsin K.

In the embryo and in the growing child, bone develops by remodeling and replacing previously calcified cartilage (endochondral bone formation) or is formed without a cartilage matrix (intramembranous bone formation). Chondrocytes proliferate, secrete and mineralize a matrix, enlarge (hypertrophy), and then die, thereby enlarging bone and providing the matrix and factors that stimulate endochondral bone formation. This program is regulated by both local factors, such as IGF-I and -II, parathyroid hormone–related peptide (PTHrP), and FGFs, and by systemic hormones such as growth hormone, glucocorticoids, and estrogen.

New bone, whether formed in infants or in adults during repair, has a relatively high ratio of cells to matrix and is characterized by coarse fiber bundles of collagen that are interlaced and randomly dispersed (woven bone). In adults, the more mature bone is organized with fiber bundles regularly arranged in parallel or concentric sheets (lamellar bone). In long bones, deposition of lamellar bone in a concentric arrangement around blood vessels forms the haversian systems. Growth in length of bones is dependent on proliferation of cartilage cells and on the endochondral sequence at the growth plate. Growth in width and thickness is accomplished by formation of bone at the periosteal surface and by resorption at the endosteal surface, with the rate of formation exceeding that of resorption. In adults, after the growth plates close, growth in length and endochondral bone formation cease, except for some activity in the cartilage cells beneath the articular surface. Even in adults, however, remodeling of bone (within haversian systems as well as trabecular bone) continues throughout life. In adults, ~4% of the surface of trabecular bone (such as iliac crest) is involved in active resorption, whereas 10 to 15% of trabecular surfaces is covered with osteoid. Radioisotope studies indicate that as much as 18% of the total skeletal calcium is deposited and removed each year. Thus, bone is an active metabolizing tissue that requires an intact blood supply. The cycle of bone resorption and formation is a highly orchestrated process carried out by the basic multicellular unit, composed of a group of osteoclasts and osteoblasts (**Fig. 23-2**).

The response of bone to fractures, infection, and interruption of blood supply and to expanding lesions is relatively limited. Dead bone must be resorbed, and

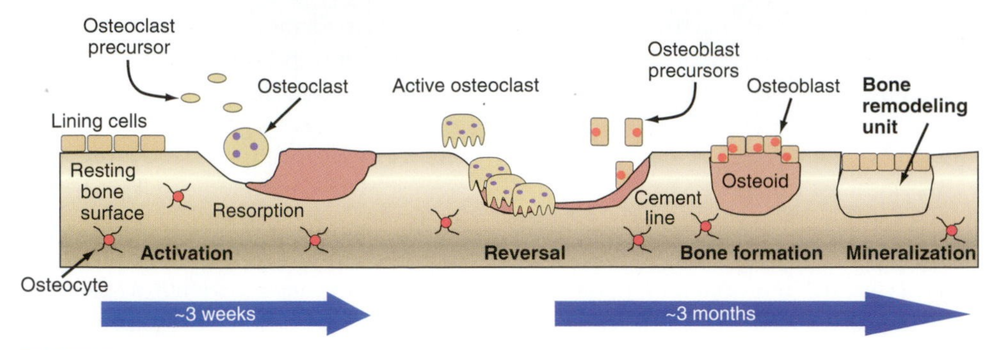

FIGURE 23-2

Schematic representation of bone remodeling. The cycle of bone remodeling is carried out by the basic multicellular unit (BMU), comprising a group of osteoclasts and osteoblasts. In cortical bone, the BMUs tunnel through the tissue, whereas in cancellous bone, they move across the trabecular surface. The process of bone remodeling is initiated by contraction of the lining cells and the recruitment of osteoclast precursors. These precursors fuse to form multinucleated, active osteoclasts that mediate bone resorption. Osteoclasts adhere to bone and subsequently remove it by acidification and proteolytic digestion. As the BMU advances, osteoclasts leave the resorption site and osteoblasts move in to cover the excavated area and begin the process of new bone formation by secreting osteoid, which is eventually mineralized into new bone. After osteoid mineralization, osteoblasts flatten and form a layer of lining cells over new bone.

new bone must be formed, a process carried out in association with growth of new blood vessels into the involved area. In injuries that disrupt the organization of the tissue, such as a fracture in which apposition of fragments is poor or when motion exists at the fracture site, the progenitor stromal cells differentiate into cells with functional capacities different from those of osteoblasts, and varying amounts of fibrous tissue and cartilage are formed. When there is good apposition with fixation and little motion at the fracture site, repair occurs predominantly by formation of new bone without other scar tissue.

Remodeling of bone occurs along lines of force generated by mechanical stress. The signals from these mechanical stresses are sensed by osteocytes, which transmit signals to osteoclasts or osteoblasts, or their precursors. A bowing deformity increases new bone formation at the concave surface and resorption at the convex surface, seemingly designed to produce the strongest mechanical structure. Expanding lesions in bone, such as tumors, induce resorption at the surface in contact with the tumor, by producing ligands, such as PTHrP, that stimulate osteoclast differentiation and function. Even in a disorder as architecturally disruptive as Paget's disease, remodeling is dictated by mechanical forces. Thus, bone plasticity reflects the interaction of cells with each other and with the environment.

The products of osteoblast and osteoclast activity can assist in the diagnosis and management of bone diseases. Osteoblast activity can be assessed by measuring serum bone-specific alkaline phosphatase. Similarly, osteocalcin, a protein secreted from osteoblasts, is made virtually only by osteoblasts. Osteoclast activity can be assessed by measurement of products of collagen degradation. Collagen molecules are covalently linked to each other in the extracellular matrix through the formation of hydroxypyridinium crosslinks. These crosslinked peptides can be measured both in urine and in blood.

CALCIUM METABOLISM

Over 99% of the 1 to 2 kg of calcium present normally in the adult human body resides in the skeleton, where it provides mechanical stability and serves as a reservoir sometimes needed to maintain extracellular fluid (ECF) calcium concentration (**Fig. 23-3**). Skeletal calcium accretion first becomes significant during the third trimester of fetal life, accelerates throughout childhood and adolescence, reaches a peak in early adulthood, and gradually declines thereafter at rates that rarely exceed 1 to 2% per year. These slow changes in total skeletal calcium content contrast with relatively high daily rates of closely matched fluxes of calcium into and out of bone (~250 to 500 mg each), a process mediated by coupled osteoblastic and osteoclastic activity. Another 0.5 to 1% of skeletal calcium is freely exchangeable (e.g., in chemical equilibrium) with that in the ECF.

The concentration of ionized calcium in the ECF must be maintained within a narrow range because of the critical role it plays in a wide array of cellular

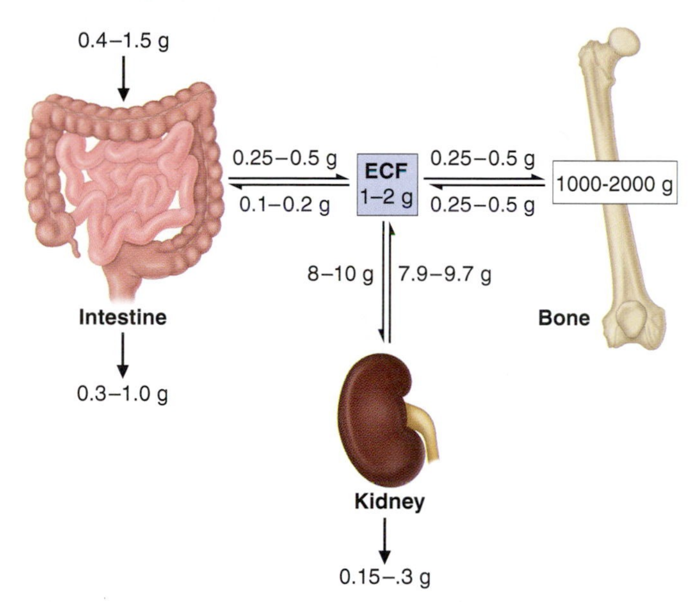

FIGURE 23-3

Calcium homeostasis. Schematic illustration of calcium content of extracellular fluid (ECF) and bone as well as of diet and feces; magnitude of calcium flux per day as calculated by various methods is shown at sites of transport in intestine, kidney, and bone. Ranges of values shown are approximate and chosen to illustrate certain points discussed in text. In conditions of calcium balance, rates of calcium release from and uptake into bone are equal.

functions, especially those involved in neuromuscular activity, secretion, and signal transduction. Intracellular cytosolic free calcium levels are ~100 nmol/L and are 10,000-fold lower than ionized calcium concentration in the blood and ECF (1.1 to 1.3 mmol/L). This steep chemical gradient promotes rapid calcium influx through various membrane calcium channels that can be activated by hormones, metabolites, or neurotransmitters, swiftly changing cellular function. In blood, total calcium concentration is normally 2.2 to 2.6 mM (8.5 to 10.5 mg/dL), of which ~50% is ionized. The remainder is bound ionically to negatively charged proteins (predominantly albumin and immunoglobulins) or loosely complexed with phosphate, citrate, sulfate, or other anions. Alterations in serum protein concentrations directly affect the total blood calcium concentration, even if the ionized calcium concentration remains normal. An algorithm to correct for protein changes adjusts the total serum calcium (in mg/dL) upward by 0.8 times the deficit in serum albumin (g/dL) or by 0.5 times the deficit in serum immunoglobulin (in g/dL). Such corrections provide only rough approximations of actual free calcium concentrations, however, and may be misleading. Acidosis also alters ionized calcium by reducing its association with proteins. The best practice is to measure blood ionized calcium directly by a method that employs calcium-selective electrodes.

Control of the ionized calcium concentration in the ECF ordinarily is accomplished by adjusting the rates of calcium movement across intestinal and renal epithelia. These adjustments are mediated mainly via changes in blood levels of the hormones PTH and $1,25(OH)_2D$. Blood-ionized calcium directly suppresses PTH secretion by activating parathyroid calcium-sensing receptors (CaSRs). Also, ionized calcium indirectly affects PTH secretion via effects on $1,25(OH)_2D$ production. This active vitamin D metabolite inhibits PTH production by an incompletely understood mechanism of negative feedback (Chap. 24).

Normal dietary calcium intake in the United States varies widely, ranging from 10 to 37 mmol/d (400 to 1500 mg/d). Many individuals, in an effort to prevent osteoporosis, routinely supplement this further with oral calcium salts to a total intake of 37 to 50 mmol/d (1500 to 2000 mg/d). Intestinal absorption of ingested calcium involves both active (transcellular) and passive (paracellular) mechanisms. Passive calcium absorption is nonsaturable and approximates 5% of daily calcium intake, whereas the active mechanism, controlled principally by $1,25(OH)_2D$, normally ranges from 20 to 70%. Active calcium transport occurs mainly in the proximal small bowel (duodenum and proximal jejunum), although some active calcium absorption occurs in most segments of the small intestine. Optimal rates of calcium absorption require gastric acid. This is especially true for weakly dissociable calcium supplements such as calcium carbonate. In fact, large boluses of calcium carbonate are poorly absorbed because of their neutralizing effect upon gastric acid. In achlorhydric subjects or for those taking drugs that inhibit gastric acid secretion, supplements should be taken with meals to optimize their absorption. Use of calcium citrate may be preferable in these circumstances. Calcium absorption may also be blunted in disease states such as pancreatic or biliary insufficiency, where ingested calcium remains bound to unabsorbed fatty acids or other food constituents. At high levels of calcium intake, synthesis of $1,25(OH)_2D$ is reduced, which decreases the rate of active intestinal calcium absorption. The opposite occurs with dietary calcium restriction. Some calcium, ~2.5 to 5.0 mmol/d (100 to 200 mg/d), is excreted as an obligate component of intestinal secretions and is not regulated by calciotropic hormones.

The feedback-controlled hormonal regulation of intestinal absorptive efficiency results in a relatively constant daily net calcium absorption of ~5 to 7.5 mmol/d (200 to 400 mg/d), despite large changes in daily dietary calcium intake. This daily load of absorbed calcium is excreted by the kidneys in a manner that is also tightly regulated by the concentration of ionized calcium in the blood. Approximately 8 to 10 g/d of calcium are filtered by the glomeruli, of which only 2 to 3% appears in the urine. Most filtered calcium (65%) is reabsorbed in the proximal tubules via a passive, paracellular route that is coupled to concomitant NaCl reabsorption and not specifically regulated. The cortical thick ascending limb of Henle's loop (cTAL) reabsorbs roughly another 20% of filtered calcium, also via a paracellular mechanism. Calcium reabsorption in the cTAL requires a tight-junctional protein called *paracellin-1* and is inhibited by increased blood concentrations of calcium or magnesium, acting via the CaSR, which is highly expressed on basolateral membranes in this nephron segment. Operation of the renal CaSR provides a mechanism, independent of those engaged directly by PTH or $1,25(OH)_2D$, whereby serum ionized calcium can control renal calcium reabsorption. Finally, ~10% of filtered calcium is reabsorbed in the distal convoluted tubules (DCT) by a transcellular mechanism. Calcium enters the luminal surface of the cell through specific apical calcium channels, whose number is regulated. It then moves across the cell in association with a specific calcium-binding protein (calbindin-D28k) that buffers cytosolic calcium concentrations from the large mass of transported calcium. Ca^{2+}-ATPases and Na/Ca^{2+} exchangers actively extrude calcium across the basolateral surface and thereby maintain the transcellular calcium gradient. All of these steps are increased, directly or indirectly, by PTH. The DCT is also the site of action of thiazide diuretics, which lower urinary calcium excretion by blocking a NaCl transporter expressed on the apical surface of these cells. Conversely, dietary sodium loads, or increased distal sodium delivery caused by loop diuretics or saline infusion, reduce DCT calcium reabsorption by an action opposite to that of thiazides.

The homeostatic mechanisms that normally maintain a constant serum ionized calcium concentration may fail at extremes of calcium intake or when the hormonal systems or organs involved are compromised. Thus, even with maximal activity of the vitamin D–dependent intestinal active transport system, sustained calcium intakes <5 mmol/d (<200 mg/d) cannot provide enough net calcium absorption to replace obligate losses via the intestine, kidney, sweat, or other secretions. In this case, increased blood levels of PTH and $1,25(OH)_2D$ activate osteoclastic bone resorption to obtain needed calcium from bone, which leads to progressive bone loss and negative calcium balance. Increased PTH and $1,25(OH)_2D$ also enhance renal calcium reabsorption, and $1,25(OH)_2D$ enhances calcium absorption in the gut. At very high calcium intakes (>100 mmol/d; >4 g/d), passive intestinal absorption continues to deliver calcium into the ECF, despite maximally downregulated intestinal active transport and renal tubular calcium reabsorption. This can cause severe hypercalciuria, nephrocalcinosis, progressive renal failure, and hypercalcemia (e.g., "milk alkali syndrome"). Deficiency or excess of PTH or vitamin D, intestinal disease, and renal failure represent other commonly encountered challenges to normal calcium homeostasis (Chap. 24).

PHOSPHORUS METABOLISM

Although 85% of the ~600 g of body phosphorus is present in bone mineral, phosphorus is also a major intracellular constituent, both as the free anion(s) and as a component of numerous organophosphate compounds including structural proteins, enzymes, transcription factors, carbohydrate and lipid intermediates, high-energy stores (ATP, creatine phosphate), and nucleic acids. Unlike calcium, phosphorus exists intracellularly at concentrations close to those present in ECF (e.g., 1 to 2 mmol/L). In cells and in the ECF, phosphorus exists in several forms, predominantly as $H_2PO_4^-$ or $NaHPO_4^-$, with perhaps 10% as HPO_4^{2-}. This mixture of anions will be referred to here as "phosphate." In serum, about 12% of phosphorus is bound to proteins. Concentrations of phosphates in blood and ECF are generally expressed in terms of elemental phosphorus, the normal range in adults being 0.75 to 1.45 mmol/L (2.5 to 4.5 mg/dL). Because the volume of the intracellular fluid compartment is twice that of the ECF, measurements of ECF phosphate may not accurately reflect phosphate availability within cells that follows even modest shifts of phosphate from one compartment to the other.

Phosphate is widely available in foods and is efficiently absorbed (65%) by the small intestine, even in the absence of vitamin D. On the other hand, phosphate absorptive efficiency may be further enhanced (to 85 to 90%) via active transport mechanisms that are stimulated by $1,25(OH)_2D$. These involve activation of Na^+/PO_4^{2-} co-transporters that move phosphate into intestinal cells against an unfavorable electrochemical gradient. Daily net intestinal phosphate absorption varies widely according to the composition of the diet but is generally in the range of 500 to 1000 mg/d. Phosphate absorption can be inhibited by large doses of calcium salts or by sevelamer hydrochloride (Renagel), strategies commonly used to control levels of serum phosphate in renal failure. Aluminum hydroxide antacids also reduce phosphate absorption but are less commonly used because of the potential for aluminum toxicity. Low serum phosphate directly stimulates renal proximal tubular synthesis of $1,25(OH)_2D$.

Serum phosphate levels vary by as much as 50% on a normal day. This reflects the effect of food intake but also an underlying circadian rhythm that produces a nadir between 7 and 10 A.M. Carbohydrate administration, especially as intravenous dextrose solutions in fasting subjects, can decrease serum phosphate by >0.7 mmol/L (2 mg/dL) due to rapid uptake into, and utilization by, cells. A similar response is observed in the treatment of diabetic ketoacidosis and during metabolic or respiratory alkalosis. Because of this wide variation in serum phosphate, it is best to perform measurements in the basal, fasting state.

Control of serum phosphate is determined mainly by the rate of renal tubular reabsorption of the filtered load, which approximates 4 to 6 g/d. Because intestinal phosphate absorption is highly efficient, urinary excretion is not constant but varies directly with dietary intake. The fractional excretion of phosphate (ratio of phosphate to creatinine clearance) is generally in the range of 10 to 15%. The proximal tubule is the principal site at which renal phosphate reabsorption is regulated. This is accomplished by changes in the apical expression and activity of a specific Na^+/PO_4^{2-} co-transporter (NaPi-2) in the proximal tubule. Apical expression of NaPi-2 is rapidly reduced by PTH, the major known hormonal regulator of renal phosphate excretion. FGF23 can dramatically impair phosphate reabsorption. Activating *FGF23* mutations cause the rare disorder autosomal dominant hypophosphatemic rickets. In contrast to PTH, this molecule also leads to reduced synthesis of $1,25(OH)_2D$, which may worsen the resulting hypophosphatemia by lowering intestinal phosphate absorption. Renal reabsorption of phosphate is responsive to changes in dietary intake, such that experimental dietary phosphate restriction leads to a dramatic lowering of urinary phosphate within hours, preceding any decline in serum phosphate (e.g., filtered load). This physiologic renal adaptation to changes in dietary phosphate availability occurs independently of PTH. Findings in *FGF23*-knockout mice suggest that FGF23 normally acts to lower blood phosphate and $1,25(OH)_2D$ levels.

Renal phosphate reabsorption is impaired by hypocalcemia, hypomagnesemia, and severe hypophosphatemia. Phosphate clearance is enhanced by ECF volume expansion and impaired by dehydration. Phosphate retention is an important pathophysiologic feature of renal insufficiency.

HYPOPHOSPHATEMIA

Causes

Hypophosphatemia can occur by one or more of three primary mechanisms: (1) inadequate intestinal phosphate absorption, (2) excessive renal phosphate excretion, or (3) rapid redistribution of phosphate from the ECF into bone or soft tissue (**Table 23-1**). Because phosphate is so abundant in foods, inadequate intestinal absorption is almost never observed now that aluminum hydroxide antacids, which bind phosphate in the gut, are no longer commonly used. Fasting or starvation, however, may result in depletion of body phosphate and predispose to subsequent hypophosphatemia during refeeding, especially if this is accomplished with intravenous glucose alone.

Chronic hypophosphatemia usually signifies a persistent renal tubular phosphate-wasting disorder. Excessive activation of PTH/PTHrP receptors in the proximal tubule, because of primary or secondary hyperparathyroidism or because of the PTHrP-mediated hypercalcemia syndrome in malignancy (Chap. 24), is among the more common causes of renal hypophosphatemia, especially because of the high prevalence of vitamin D deficiency in older Americans. Familial hypocalciuric hypercalcemia and Jansen's chondrodystrophy are rare examples of genetic disorders in this category (Chap. 24). Several genetic diseases cause PTH/PTHrP-independent tubular phosphate wasting, with associated rickets and osteomalacia. The most common of these is X-linked hypophosphatemic rickets (XLHR), which results from inactivating mutations in an endopeptidase termed *PHEX* (*p*hosphate-regulating gene with *h*omologies to *e*ndopeptidases on the *X* chromosome) that is most abundantly expressed on the surface of mature osteoblasts. It is believed that PHEX normally inactivates a phosphaturic hormone (phosphatonin) that impairs both renal tubular phosphate reabsorption and $1,25(OH)_2D$ synthesis in the proximal renal tubules. Disorders likely to share a related pathophysiology with XLHR are autosomal dominant hypophosphatemic rickets (ADHR) and tumor-induced osteomalacia (TIO). All of these manifest severe hypophosphatemia; renal phosphate wasting, sometimes accompanied by aminoaciduria; low blood levels of $1,25(OH)_2D$; low or low-normal serum levels of calcium; and evidence of impaired cartilage or bone mineralization. ADHR results from activating mutations in the gene encoding FGF23, which is phosphaturic when administered to mice. TIO is an acquired disorder in which tumors, usually of mesenchymal origin and generally histologically benign, secrete a phosphatonin-like molecule (Chap. 22). The hypophosphatemic syndrome resolves completely within hours to days following successful resection of the responsible tumor. Such tumors express large amounts of FGF23 mRNA, raising the possibility that FGF23 may be a phosphatonin. It is not yet clear if FGF23 is a physiologic substrate for PHEX, however. Dent's disease is an X-linked recessive disorder caused by inactivating mutations in CLCN5, a chloride transporter expressed in endosomes of the proximal tubule; features include hypercalciuria, hypophosphatemia, and recurrent kidney stones. Renal phosphate wasting is common among

TABLE 23-1

CAUSES OF HYPOPHOSPHATEMIA

1. Reduced renal tubular phosphate reabsorption
- A. PTH/PTHrP-dependent
  - 1. Primary hyperparathyroidism
  - 2. Secondary hyperparathyroidism
    - a. Vitamin D deficiency/resistance
    - b. Calcium starvation/malabsorption
    - c. Bartter syndrome
    - d. Autosomal recessive renal hypercalciuria with hypomagnesemia
  - 3. PTHrP-dependent hypercalcemia of malignancy
  - 4. Familial hypocalciuric hypercalcemia
- B. PTH/PTHrP independent
  - 1. Genetic hypophosphatemia
    - a. X-linked hypophosphatemic rickets
    - b. Dent disease
    - c. Autosomal dominant hypophosphatemic rickets
    - d. Fanconi syndrome(s)
    - e. Cystinosis
    - f. Wilson disease
    - g. McCune-Albright syndrome (fibrous dysplasia)
    - h. Idiopathic hypercalciuria (absorptive subtype)
    - i. Hereditary hypophosphatemia with hypercalciuria (Bedouins)
  - 2. Tumor-induced osteomalacia
  - 3. Other systemic disorders
    - a. Poorly controlled diabetes mellitus
    - b. Alcoholism
    - c. Hyperaldosteronism
    - d. Hypomagnesemia
    - e. Amyloidosis
    - f. Hemolytic uremic syndrome
    - g. Renal transplantation or partial liver resection
    - h. Rewarming or induced hyperthermia
  - 4. Drugs of toxins
    - a. Ethanol
    - b. Acetazolamide, other diuretics
    - c. High-dose estrogens or glucocorticoids
    - d. Heavy metals (lead, cadmium)
    - e. Toluene, *N*-methyl formamide
    - f. Cisplatin, ifosfamide, foscarnet, rapamycin
    - g. Calcitonin, pamidronate

II. Impaired intestinal phosphate absorption
- A. Aluminum-containing antacids
- B. Servalamer

III. Shifts of extracellular phosphate into cells
- A. Intravenous glucose
- B. Insulin therapy of prolonged hyperglycemia or diabetic ketoacidosis
- C. Catecholamines (epinephrine, dopamine, albuterol)
- D. Acute respiratory alkalosis
- E. Grain-negative sepsis, toxic shock syndrome
- F. Recovery from starvation or acidosis
- G. Rapid cellular proliferation
  - 1. Leukemic blast crisis
  - 2. Intensive erythropoetin, other CSF therapy

IV. Accelerated net bone formation
- A. Following parathyroidectomy
- B. Treatment of vitamin D deficiency, Paget disease
- C. Osteoblastic metastases

Note: CSF, cerebrospinal fluid.

poorly controlled diabetics and alcoholics, who therefore are at risk for iatrogenic hypophosphatemia when treated with insulin or intravenous glucose, respectively. Diuretics and certain other drugs and toxins can cause defective renal tubular phosphate reabsorption (Table 23-1).

In hospitalized patients, hypophosphatemia is often attributable to massive redistribution of phosphate from the ECF into cells. Insulin therapy of diabetic ketoacidosis is a paradigm for this phenomenon, in which the severity of the hypophosphatemia is related to the extent of antecedent depletion of phosphate and other electrolytes (Chap. 17). The hypophosphatemia is usually greatest at a point many hours after initiation of insulin therapy and is difficult to predict from baseline measurements of serum phosphate at the time of presentation, when prerenal azotemia can obscure significant phosphate depletion. Other factors that may contribute to such acute redistributive hypophosphatemia include antecedent starvation or malnutrition, administration of intravenous glucose without other nutrients, elevated blood catecholamines (endogenous or exogenous), respiratory alkalosis, and recovery from metabolic acidosis.

Hypophosphatemia can also occur transiently (over weeks to months) during the phase of accelerated net bone formation following parathyroidectomy for severe primary hyperparathyroidism or during treatment of vitamin D deficiency or lytic Paget's disease. This is usually most prominent in patients who preoperatively have evidence of high bone turnover (e.g., high serum levels of alkaline phosphatase). Osteoblastic metastases can also lead to this syndrome.

Clinical and Laboratory Findings

The clinical manifestations of severe hypophosphatemia reflect a generalized defect in cellular energy metabolism because of ATP depletion, a shift from oxidative phosphorylation toward glycolysis, and associated tissue or organ dysfunction. Acute, severe hypophosphatemia occurs mainly or exclusively in hospitalized patients with underlying serious medical or surgical illness and preexisting phosphate depletion due to excessive urinary losses, severe malabsorption, or malnutrition. Chronic hypophosphatemia tends to be less severe, with a clinical presentation dominated by musculoskeletal complaints such as bone pain, pseudofractures, and proximal muscle weakness or, in children, rickets and short stature.

Neuromuscular manifestations of severe hypophosphatemia are variable but may include muscle weakness, lethargy, confusion, disorientation, hallucinations, dysarthria, dysphagia, oculomotor palsies, anisocoria, nystagmus, ataxia, cerebellar tremor, ballismus, hyporeflexia, impaired sphincter control, distal sensory deficits, paresthesia, hyperesthesia, generalized or Guillain Barré–like ascending paralysis, seizures, coma, and death. Serious sequelae such as paralysis, confusion, and seizures are likely only at phosphate concentrations <0.25 mmol/L (<0.8 mg/dL). Rhabdomyolysis may develop during rapidly progressive hypophosphatemia. The diagnosis of hypophosphatemia-induced rhabdomyolysis may be overlooked, as up to 30% of patients with acute hypophosphatemia (<0.7 m*M*) have creatine phosphokinase elevations that peak 1 to 2 days after the nadir in serum phosphate, when the release of phosphate from injured myocytes may have led to a near-normalization of circulating levels of phosphate.

Respiratory failure and cardiac dysfunction, reversible with phosphate treatment, may occur at serum phosphate levels of 0.5 to 0.8 mmol/L (1.5 to 2.5 mg/dL). Renal tubular defects, including tubular acidosis, glycosuria, and impaired reabsorption of sodium and calcium, may occur. Hematologic abnormalities correlate with reductions in intracellular ATP and 2,3-diphosphoglycerate and may include erythrocyte microspherocytosis and hemolysis; impaired oxyhemoglobin dissociation; defective leukocyte chemotaxis, phagocytosis, and bacterial killing; and platelet dysfunction with spontaneous gastrointestinal hemorrhage.

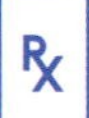

TREATMENT FOR SEVERE HYPOPHOSPHATEMIA

Severe hypophosphatemia [<0.75 mmol/L (<2 mg/dL)], particularly in the setting of underlying phosphate depletion, constitutes a dangerous electrolyte abnormality that should be corrected promptly. Unfortunately, the cumulative deficit in body phosphate cannot be easily predicted from knowledge of the circulating level of phosphate, and therapy must be approached empirically. The threshold for intravenous phosphate therapy and the dose administered should reflect consideration of renal function, the likely severity and duration of the underlying phosphate depletion, and the presence and severity of symptoms consistent with those of hypophosphatemia. In adults, phosphate may be safely administered intravenously as neutral mixtures of sodium and potassium phosphate salts at initial doses of 0.2 to 0.8 mmol/kg of elemental phosphorus over 6 h (e.g., 10 to 50 mmol over 6 h), with doses >20 mmol/6 h reserved for those who have serum levels <0.5 mmol/L (1.5 mg/dL) and normal renal function. A suggested approach is

TABLE 23-2

INTRAVENOUS THERAPY OF HYPOPHOSPHATEMIA

Consider

- Likely severity of underlying phosphate depletion
- Concurrent parenteral glucose administration
- Presence of neuromuscular, cardiopulmonary, or hematologic complications of hypophosphatemia
- Renal function [reduce dose by 50% if serum creatinine > 220 μmol/L (>2.5 mg/dL)]
- Serum calcium level (correct hypocalcemia first; reduce dose by 50% in hypercalcemia)

Guidelines[a]

SERUM PHOSPHORUS, MM (MG/DL)	RATE OF INFUSION MMOL/H	DURATION, H	TOTAL ADMINISTERED, MMOL
<0.8(<2.5)	2.0	6	12
<0.5(<1.5)	4.0	6	24
<0.3(<1.0)	8.0	6	48

[a]Rates shown are calculated for a 70-kg person; levels of serum calcium and phosphorus must be measured every 6 to 12 h during therapy; infusions can be repeated to achieve stable serum phosphorus levels > 0.8 mmol/L (>2.5 mg/dL); most formulations available in the United States provide 3 mmol/mL of sodium or potassium phosphate.

presented in **Table 23-2.** Serum levels of phosphate and calcium must be monitored closely (every 6 to 12 h) throughout treatment. It is necessary to avoid a serum calcium-phosphorus product >50 to reduce the risk of heterotopic calcification. Hypocalcemia, if present, should be corrected before administering intravenous phosphate. Less severe hypophosphatemia, in the range of 0.5 to 0.8 mmol/L (1.5 to 2.5 mg/dL), can usually be treated with oral phosphate in divided doses of 750 to 2000 mg/d, as elemental phosphorus; higher doses can cause bloating and diarrhea.

Management of chronic hypophosphatemia requires knowing the cause(s) of the disorder. Hypophosphatemia related to the secondary hyperparathyroidism of vitamin D deficiency usually responds to treatment with vitamin D and calcium alone. XLHR, ADHR, TIO, and related renal tubular disorders are usually managed with divided oral doses of phosphate, often with calcium and $1,25(OH)_2D$ supplements to bypass the block in renal $1,25(OH)_2D$ synthesis and prevent secondary hyperparathyroidism caused by suppression of ECF calcium levels. Thiazide diuretics may be used to prevent nephrocalcinosis in patients who are managed this way. Complete normalization of hypophosphatemia is generally not possible in these conditions. Optimal therapy of TIO is extirpation of the responsible tumor, which may be localized by radiographic skeletal survey or bone scan (many are located in bone) or by radionuclide scanning using sestamibi or labeled octreotide. Successful treatment of TIO-induced hypophosphatemia with octreotide has been reported in a small number of patients.

HYPERPHOSPHATEMIA

Causes

When the filtered load of phosphate and glomerular filtration rate (GFR) are normal, control of serum phosphate levels is achieved by adjusting the rate at which phosphate is reabsorbed by the proximal tubular NaPi-2 co-transporter. The principal hormonal regulator of NaPi-2 activity is PTH. Hyperphosphatemia, defined in adults as a fasting serum phosphate concentration >1.8 mmol/L (5.5 mg/dL), usually results from impaired glomerular filtration, hypoparathyroidism, excessive delivery of phosphate into the ECF (from bone, gut, or parenteral phosphate therapy), or some combination of these factors (**Table 23-3**). The upper limit of normal serum phosphate concentrations is higher in children and neonates [2.4 mmol/L (7 mg/dL)]. It is useful to distinguish hyperphosphatemia caused by impaired renal phosphate excretion from that which results from excessive delivery of phosphate into the ECF (Table 23-3).

TABLE 23-3

CAUSES OF HYPERPHOSPHATEMIA

- **I. Impaired renal phosphate excretion**
  - A. Renal insufficiency
  - B. Hypoparathyroidism
    - 1. Developmental
    - 2. Autoimmune
    - 3. After neck surgery or radiation
    - 4. Activating mutations of the calcium-sensing receptor
  - C. Parathyroid suppression
    - 1. Parathyroid-independent hypercalcemia
      - a. Vitamin D or vitamin A intoxication
      - b. Sarcoidosis, other granulomatous diseases
      - c. Immobilization, osteolytic metastases
      - d. Milk-alkali syndrome
    - 2. Severe hypermagnesemia or hypomagnesemia
  - D. Pseudohypoparathyroidism
  - E. Acromegaly
  - F. Tumoral calcinosis
  - G. Heparin therapy
- **II. Massive extracellular fluid phosphate loads**
  - A. Rapid administration of exogenous phosphate (intravenous, oral, rectal)
  - B. Extensive cellular injury or necrosis
    - 1. Crush injuries
    - 2. Rhabdomyolysis
    - 3. Hyperthermia
    - 4. Fulminant hepatitis
    - 5. Cytotoxic therapy
    - 6. Severe hemolytic anemia
  - C. Transcellular phosphate shifts
    - 1. Metabolic acidosis
    - 2. Respiratory acidosis

In chronic renal insufficiency, reduced GFR leads to phosphate retention. Hyperphosphatemia, in turn, further impairs renal synthesis of $1{,}25(OH)_2D$ and stimulates PTH secretion and hypertrophy, both directly and indirectly (by lowering blood ionized calcium levels). Thus, hyperphosphatemia is a major cause of the secondary hyperparathyroidism of renal failure and must be addressed early in the course of the disease.

Hypoparathyroidism leads to hyperphosphatemia via increased expression of NaPi-2 co-transporters in the proximal tubule. Hypoparathyroidism, or parathyroid suppression, has multiple potential causes including autoimmune disease; developmental, surgical, or radiation-induced absence of functional parathyroid tissue; vitamin D intoxication or other causes of PTH-independent hypercalcemia; cellular PTH resistance (pseudohypoparathyroidism or hypomagnesemia); infiltrative disorders such as Wilson disease and hemochromatosis; and impaired PTH secretion caused by hypermagnesemia, severe hypomagnesemia, or activating mutations in the CaSR. Hypocalcemia may also contribute directly to impaired phosphate clearance, as calcium infusion can induce hyperphosphaturia in hypoparathyroid patients. Increased tubular phosphate reabsorption also occurs in acromegaly, during heparin administration, and in tumoral calcinosis. Tumoral calcinosis is a rare genetic disorder in which elevated serum $1{,}25(OH)_2D$, parathyroid suppression, increased intestinal calcium absorption, and focal hyperostosis with large, lobulated periarticular heterotopic ossifications (especially at shoulders or hips) are accompanied by hyperphosphatemia. In some forms of tumoral calcinosis serum phosphorus levels are normal.

When large amounts of phosphate are rapidly delivered into the ECF, hyperphosphatemia can occur despite normal renal function. Examples include overzealous intravenous phosphate therapy, oral or rectal administration of large amounts of phosphate-containing laxatives or enemas (especially in children), extensive soft tissue injury or necrosis (crush injuries, rhabdomyolysis, hyperthermia, fulminant hepatitis, cytotoxic chemotherapy), extensive hemolytic anemia, or transcellular phosphate shifts induced by severe metabolic or respiratory acidosis.

Clinical Findings

The clinical consequences of acute, severe hyperphosphatemia are due mainly to the formation of widespread calcium phosphate precipitates and resulting hypocalcemia. Thus, tetany, seizures, accelerated nephrocalcinosis (with renal failure, hyperkalemia, hyperuricemia, and metabolic acidosis), and pulmonary or cardiac calcifications (including development of acute heart block) may occur. The severity of these complications relates to the elevation of serum phosphate levels, which can reach concentrations as high as 7 mmol/L (20 mg/dL) in instances of massive soft tissue injury or tumor lysis syndrome.

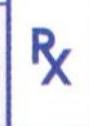

TREATMENT FOR SEVERE HYPERPHOSPHATEMIA

Therapeutic options for management of severe hyperphosphatemia are limited. Volume expansion may enhance renal phosphate clearance. Aluminum hydroxide antacids or sevalamer may be helpful in chelating and limiting absorption of offending phosphate salts present in the intestine. Hemodialysis is the most effective therapeutic strategy and should be considered early in the course of severe hyperphosphatemia, especially in the setting of renal failure and symptomatic hypocalcemia.

MAGNESIUM METABOLISM

Magnesium is the major intracellular divalent cation. Normal concentrations of extracellular magnesium and calcium are crucial for normal neuromuscular activity. Intracellular magnesium forms a key complex with ATP and is an important cofactor for a wide range of enzymes, transporters, and nucleic acids required for normal cellular function, replication, and energy metabolism. The concentration of magnesium in serum is closely regulated within the range of 0.7 to 1.0 mmol/L (1.5 to 2.0 meq/L; 1.7 to 2.4 mg/dL), of which 30% is protein-bound and another 15% is loosely complexed to phosphate and other anions. Half of the 25 g (1000 mmol) of total body magnesium is located in bone, only half of which is insoluble in the mineral phase. Almost all extraskeletal magnesium is present within cells, where the total concentration is 5 m*M*, 95% of which is bound to proteins and other macromolecules. Because only 1% of body magnesium resides in the ECF, measurements of serum magnesium levels may not accurately reflect the level of total body magnesium stores.

Dietary magnesium content normally ranges from 6 to 15 mmol/d (140 to 360 mg/d), of which 30 to 40% is absorbed, mainly in the jejunum and ileum. Intestinal magnesium absorptive efficiency is stimulated by $1,25(OH)_2D$ and can reach 70% during magnesium deprivation. Urinary magnesium excretion normally matches net intestinal absorption and is ~4 mmol/d (100 mg/d). Regulation of serum magnesium concentrations is achieved mainly by control of renal magnesium reabsorption. Only 20% of filtered magnesium is reabsorbed in the proximal tubule, whereas 60% is reclaimed in the cTAL and another 5 to 10% in the DCT. Magnesium reabsorption in the cTAL occurs via a paracellular route that requires both a lumen-negative potential, created by NaCl reabsorption, and the tight-junction protein, paracellin-1. Magnesium reabsorption in the cTAL is increased by PTH but inhibited by hypercalcemia or hypermagnesemia, both of which activate the CaSR in this nephron segment.

HYPOMAGNESIA

Causes

Hypomagnesemia usually signifies substantial depletion of body magnesium stores (0.5 to 1 mmol/kg). Hypomagnesemia can result from intestinal malabsorption; protracted vomiting, diarrhea, or intestinal drainage; defective renal tubular magnesium reabsorption; or rapid shifts of magnesium from the ECF into cells, bone, or third spaces (**Table 23-4**). Dietary magnesium deficiency

TABLE 23-4

CAUSES OF HYPOMAGNESEMIA

- **I. Impaired intestinal absorption**
  - A. Primary infantile hypomagnesemia
  - B. Malabsorption syndromes
  - C. Vitamin D deficiency
- **II. Increased intestinal losses**
  - A. Protracted vomiting/diarrhea
  - B. Intestinal drainage, fistulae
- **III. Impaired renal tubular reabsorption**
  - A. Genetic magnesium-wasting syndromes
    1. Gitelman syndrome
    2. Bartter syndrome
    3. Paracellin-1 mutations
    4. Na-K-ATPase g-subunit mutations (FXYD2)
    5. Autosomal dominant, with low bone mass
  - B. Acquired renal disease
    1. Tubulointerstitial disease
    2. Postobstruction, ATN (diuretic phase)
    3. Renal transplantation
  - C. Drugs and toxins
    1. Ethanol
    2. Diuretics (loop, thiazide, osmotic)
    3. Cisplatin
    4. Pentamidine, foscarnet
    5. Cyclosporine
    6. Aminoglycosides, amphotericin B
  - D. Other
- **IV. Extracellular fluid volume expansion**
  - A. Hyperaldosteronism
  - B. SIADH
  - C. Diabetes mellitus
  - D. Hypercalcemia
  - E. Phosphate depletion
  - F. Metabolic acidosis
  - G. Hyperthyroidism
- **V. Rapid shifts from extracellular fluid**
  - A. Intracellular redistribution
    1. Recovery from diabetic ketoacidosis
    2. Refeeding syndrome
    3. Correction of respiratory acidosis
    4. Catecholamines
  - B. Accelerated bone formation
    1. Post parathyroidectomy
    2. Treatment of vitamin D deficiency
    3. Osteoblastic metastases
  - C. Other
    1. Pancreatitis, burns, excessive sweating
    2. Pregnancy (3rd trimester) and lactation

Note: ATN, acute tubular necrosis; SIADH, syndrome of inappropriate anti-diuretic hormone.

is unlikely except possibly in the setting of alcoholism. A rare genetic disorder causing selective intestinal magnesium malabsorption has been described (primary infantile hypomagnesemia). Malabsorptive states, often compounded by vitamin D deficiency, can critically limit magnesium absorption and produce hypomagnesemia, despite the compensatory effects of secondary hyperparathyroidism and of hypocalcemia and hypomagnesemia to enhance cTAL magnesium reabsorption. Diarrhea or surgical drainage fluid may contain ≥5 mmol/L of magnesium.

Several genetic magnesium-wasting syndromes are described, including inactivating mutations of genes encoding the DCT NaCl co-transporter (Gitelman syndrome), proteins required for cTAL Na-K-Cl_2 transport (Bartter syndrome), paracellin-1 (autosomal recessive renal hypomagnesemia with hypercalciuria), and a DCT Na-K-ATPase γ-subunit (autosomal dominant renal hypomagnesemia with hypocalciuria). ECF expansion, hypercalcemia, and severe phosphate depletion may impair magnesium reabsorption, as can various forms of renal injury, including those caused by drugs such as cisplatin, cyclosporine, aminoglycosides, and pentamidine (Table 23-4). A rising blood concentration of ethanol directly impairs tubular magnesium reabsorption, and persistent glycosuria with osmotic diuresis leads to magnesium wasting and likely contributes to the high frequency of hypomagnesemia in poorly controlled diabetics. Magnesium depletion is aggravated by metabolic acidosis, which causes intracellular losses as well.

Hypomagnesemia due to rapid shifts of magnesium from ECF into the intracellular compartment can occur during recovery from diabetic ketoacidosis, from starvation, or from respiratory acidosis. Less acute shifts may be seen during rapid bone formation after parathyroidectomy, with treatment of vitamin D deficiency, or with osteoblastic metastases. Large amounts of magnesium may be lost with acute pancreatitis, extensive burns, protracted and severe sweating, and during pregnancy and lactation.

Clinical and Laboratory Findings

Hypomagnesemia may cause generalized alterations in neuromuscular function, including tetany, tremor, seizures, muscle weakness, ataxia, nystagmus, vertigo, apathy, depression, irritability, delirium, and psychosis. Patients are usually asymptomatic when serum magnesium concentrations are >0.5 mmol/L (1 meq/L; 1.2 mg/dL), although the severity of symptoms may not correlate with serum magnesium levels. Cardiac arrhythmias may occur, including sinus tachycardia, other supraventricular tachycardias, and ventricular arrhythmias. Electrocardiographic abnormalities may include prolonged PR or QT intervals, T-wave flattening or inversion, and ST straightening. Sensitivity to digitalis toxicity may be enhanced.

Other electrolyte abnormalities often seen with hypomagnesemia, including hypocalcemia (with hypocalciuria) and hypokalemia, may not be easily corrected unless magnesium is administered as well. The hypocalcemia may be a result of concurrent vitamin D deficiency, although hypomagnesemia can cause impaired synthesis of $1,25(OH)_2D$, cellular resistance to PTH and, at very low serum magnesium [<0.4 mmol/L (<0.8 meq/L; <1 mg/dL)], a defect in PTH secretion; these abnormalities are reversible with therapy.

℞ TREATMENT FOR HYPOMAGNESEMIA

Mild, asymptomatic hypomagnesemia may be treated with oral magnesium salts [$MgCl_2$, MgO, $Mg(OH)_2$] in divided doses totaling 20 to 30 mmol/d (40 to 60 meq/d). Diarrhea may occur with larger doses. More severe hypomagnesemia should be treated parenterally, preferably with intravenous $MgCl_2$, which can be administered safely as a continuous infusion of 50 mmol/d (100 meq Mg^{2+}/d) if renal function is normal. If GFR is reduced, the infusion rate should be lowered by 50 to 75%. Use of intramuscular $MgSO_4$ is discouraged; the injections are painful and provide relatively little magnesium (2 mL of 50% $MgSO_4$ supplies only 4 mmol). $MgSO_4$ may be given intravenously instead of $MgCl_2$, although the sulfate anions may bind calcium in serum and urine and aggravate hypocalcemia. Serum magnesium should be monitored at intervals of 12 to 24 h during therapy, which may continue for several days because of impaired renal conservation of magnesium (only 50 to 70% of the daily intravenous magnesium dose is retained) and delayed repletion of intracellular deficits, which may be as high as 1 to 1.5 mmol/kg (2 to 3 meq/kg).

It is important to consider the need for calcium, potassium, and phosphate supplementation in patients with hypomagnesemia. Vitamin D deficiency frequently coexists and should be treated with oral or parenteral vitamin D or 25(OH)D [but not $1,25(OH)_2D$, which may impair tubular magnesium reabsorption, possibly via PTH suppression]. In severely hypomagnesemic patients with concomitant hypocalcemia and hypophosphatemia, administration of intravenous magnesium alone may worsen hypophosphatemia, provoking neuromuscular symptoms or rhabdomyolysis, due to rapid stimulation of PTH secretion. This is avoided by administering both calcium and magnesium.

HYPERMAGNESEMIA

Causes

Hypermagnesemia is rarely seen in the absence of renal insufficiency, as normal kidneys can excrete large amounts (250 mmol/d) of magnesium. Mild hypermagnesemia due to excessive reabsorption in the cTAL occurs with calcium-sensing receptor mutations in familial hypocalciuric hypercalcemia and has been described in some patients with adrenal insufficiency, hypothyroidism, or hypothermia. Massive exogenous magnesium exposures, usually via the gastrointestinal tract, can overwhelm renal excretory capacity and cause life-threatening hypermagnesemia (**Table 23-5**). A notable example of this is prolonged retention of even normal amounts of magnesium-containing cathartics in patients with intestinal ileus, obstruction, or perforation. Extensive soft tissue injury or necrosis can also deliver large amounts of magnesium into the ECF in patients who have suffered trauma, shock, sepsis, cardiac arrest, or severe burns.

Clinical and Laboratory Findings

The most prominent clinical manifestations of hypermagnesemia are vasodilation and neuromuscular blockade, which may appear at serum magnesium concentrations >2 mmol/L (>4 meq/L; >4.8 mg/dL). Hypotension, refractory to vasopressors or volume expansion, may be an early sign. Nausea, lethargy, and weakness may progress to respiratory failure, paralysis, and coma, with hypoactive tendon reflexes, at serum magnesium levels >4 mmol/L. Other findings may include gastrointestinal hypomotility or ileus; facial flushing; pupillary dilation; paradoxical bradycardia; prolongation of PR, QRS, and QT intervals, heart block; and, at serum magnesium levels approaching 10 mmol/L, asystole.

Hypermagnesemia, acting via the CaSR, causes hypocalcemia and hypercalciuria due to both parathyroid suppression and impaired cTAL calcium reabsorption.

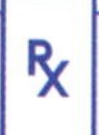

TREATMENT FOR HYPERMAGNESEMIA

Successful treatment of hypermagnesemia generally involves identifying and interrupting the source of magnesium and employing measures to increase magnesium clearance from the ECF. Use of magnesium-free cathartics or enemas may be helpful in clearing ingested magnesium from the gastrointestinal tract. Vigorous intravenous hydration should be attempted, if appropriate. Hemodialysis is effective and may be required in patients with significant renal insufficiency. Calcium, administered intravenously in doses of 100 to 200 mg over 1 to 2 h, has been reported to provide temporary improvement in signs and symptoms of hypermagnesemia.

TABLE 23-5

CAUSES OF HYPERMAGNESEMIA

Impaired Mg excretion	Rapid Mg mobilization from soft tissues
Renal failure	Trauma
Familial hypocalciuric hypercalcemia	Extensive burns
Excessive Mg intake	Shock, sepsis,
Cathartics	Post cardiac arrest
Intestinal obstruction/perforation following magnesium ingestion	Other disorders
Parenteral magnesium administration	Adrenal insufficiency
Magnesium rich urologic irrigants	Hypothyroidism
	Hypothermia

VITAMIN D

SYNTHESIS AND METABOLISM

1,25-Dihydroxyvitamin D [1,25(OH)$_2$D] is the major steroid hormone involved in mineral ion homeostasis regulation. Vitamin D and its metabolites are hormones and hormone precursors rather than vitamins, since in the proper biologic setting, they can be synthesized endogenously (**Fig. 23-4**). In response to ultraviolet radiation of the skin, a photochemical cleavage results in the formation of vitamin D from 7-dehydrocholesterol. Cutaneous production of vitamin D is decreased by melanin and high solar protection factor sunblocks, which effectively impair skin penetration of ultraviolet light. The increased use of sunblocks in North America and Western Europe and a reduction in the magnitude of solar exposure of the general population over the past several decades has led to an increased reliance on dietary sources of vitamin D. In the United States and Canada, these sources largely consist of fortified cereals and dairy products, in addition to fish oils and egg yolks. Vitamin D from plant sources is in the form of vitamin D_2, whereas that from animal sources is vitamin D_3. These two forms have equivalent biologic activity and are activated equally well by the vitamin D hydroxylases in humans. Vitamin D enters the circulation, whether absorbed from the intestine or synthesized cutaneously, bound to vitamin D–binding protein, an α-globulin synthesized in the liver. Vitamin D is subsequently 25-hydroxylated in the liver by cytochrome P450–like enzymes in the mitochondria and microsomes. The activity of this hydroxylase is not tightly regulated, and the resultant metabolite, 25-hydroxyvitamin D [25(OH)D], is the major circulating and storage form of vitamin D. Approximately 88% of 25(OH)D circulates bound to the vitamin D–binding protein, 0.03% is free, and the rest circulates bound to albumin. The half-life of 25(OH)D is ~2 to 3 weeks; however, it is dramatically shortened when vitamin D–binding protein levels are reduced, as can occur with increased urinary losses in the nephrotic syndrome.

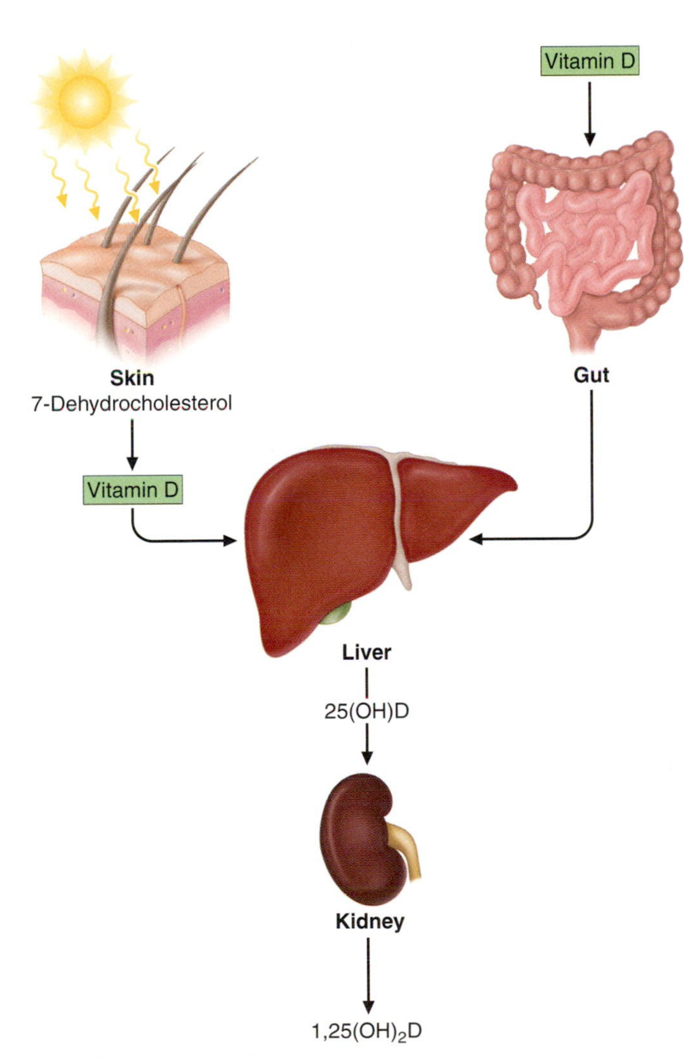

FIGURE 23-4
Vitamin D synthesis and activation. Vitamin D is synthesized in the skin in response to ultraviolet radiation and is also absorbed from the diet. It is then transported to the liver, where it undergoes 25-hydroxylation. This metabolite is the major circulating form of vitamin D. The final step in hormone activation, 1α-hydroxylation, occurs in the kidney.

The final hydroxylation required for mature hormone formation occurs in the kidney (**Fig. 23-5**). The 25(OH)D-1α-hydroxylase is a tightly regulated cytochrome P450–like mixed function oxidase expressed in proximal convoluted tubule cells. PTH stimulates this microsomal enzyme, whereas calcium and the product of the enzyme's action, 1,25(OH)$_2$D, repress it. The 25(OH)D-1α-hydroxylase is also present in epidermal keratinocytes, but keratinocyte production of 1,25(OH)$_2$D is not thought to contribute to circulating levels of this hormone. The 1α-hydroxylase is present in the trophoblastic layer of the placenta and is produced in the granulomas of sarcoidosis, tuberculosis, and berylliosis as well as in lymphomas. In these latter pathologic states, the activity of the enzyme is induced by interferon γ and TNF but is not regulated by calcium or 1,25(OH)$_2$D; therefore, hypercalcemia may occur because of elevated levels of 1,25(OH)$_2$D. Treatment of sarcoidosis-associated hypercalcemia with glucocorticoids, ketoconazole, or chloroquine has been shown to lower serum 1,25(OH)$_2$D levels.

The major pathway for inactivation of vitamin D metabolites is an additional hydroxylation step by vitamin D–24-hydroxylase, an enzyme that is expressed in most tissues. 1,25(OH)$_2$D, the major inducer of vitamin D–24-hydroxylase, thus promotes its own inactivation, thereby limiting its biologic effects. Polar metabolites of

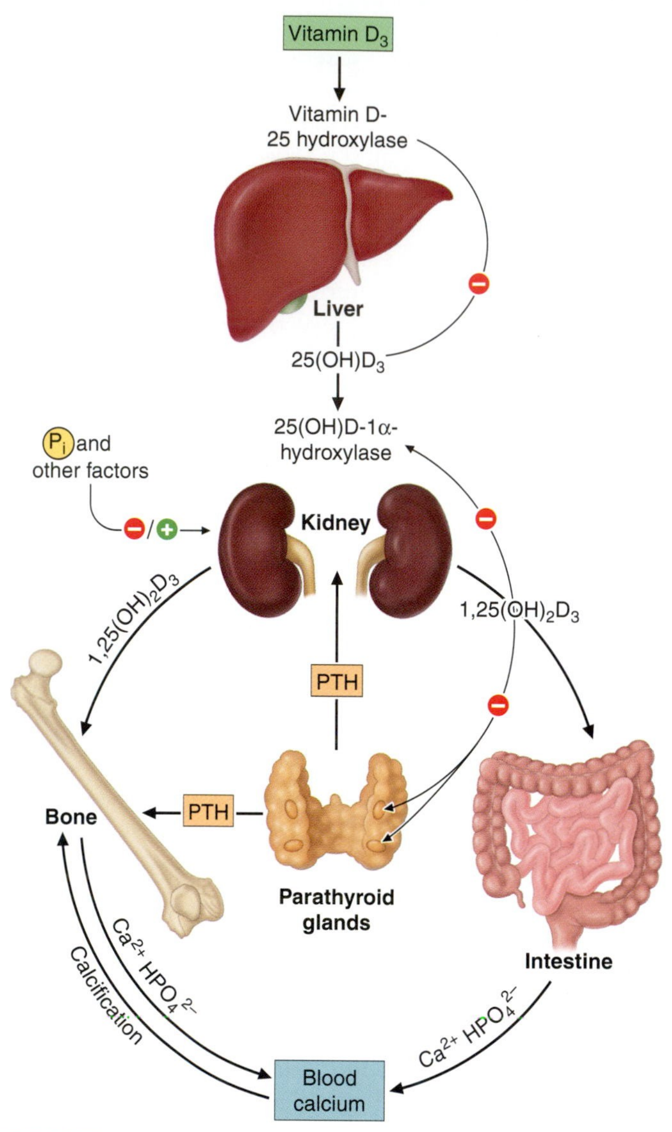

FIGURE 23-5

Schematic representation of the hormonal control loop for vitamin D metabolism and function. A reduction in the serum calcium below ~2.2 mmol/L (8.8 mg/dL) prompts a proportional increase in the secretion of parathyroid hormone (PTH) and so mobilizes additional calcium from the bone. PTH promotes the synthesis of $1,25(OH)_2D$ in the kidney, which, in turn, stimulates the mobilization of calcium from bone and intestine and regulates the synthesis of PTH by negative feedback.

$1,25(OH)_2D$ are secreted into the bile and reabsorbed via the enterohepatic circulation. Impairment of this circulation, seen with diseases of the terminal ileum, leads to accelerated losses of vitamin D metabolites.

ACTIONS OF $1,25(OH)_2D$

$1,25(OH)_2D$ mediates its biologic effects by binding to a member of the nuclear receptor superfamily, the vitamin D receptor (VDR). This receptor belongs to the subfamily that includes the thyroid hormone receptors, the retinoid receptors, and the peroxisome proliferator–activated receptors (Chap. 1). In contrast to the other members of this subfamily, however, only one VDR isoform has been isolated. The VDR binds to target DNA sequences as a heterodimer with the retinoid X receptor, recruiting a series of coactivators that result in the induction of target gene expression. When the VDR causes repression of target gene expression, it either interferes with the action of activating transcription factors or recruits novel proteins to the VDR complex that cause transcriptional repression.

The affinity of the VDR for $1,25(OH)_2D$ is approximately three orders of magnitude higher than for the other vitamin D metabolites. Under normal physiologic circumstances, these other metabolites do not stimulate receptor-dependent actions. However, in states of vitamin D toxicity, the markedly elevated levels of 25(OH)D may lead to hypercalcemia by interacting directly with the VDR and by displacing $1,25(OH)_2D$ from serum vitamin D–binding protein, resulting in increased bioavailability of the active hormone.

The VDR is expressed in a wide range of cells and tissues. The molecular actions of $1,25(OH)_2D$ have been most extensively studied in tissues involved in the regulation of mineral ion homeostasis. This hormone is a major inducer of calbindin 9K, a calcium-binding protein expressed in the intestine, which is thought to play an important role in the active transport of calcium across the enterocyte. The two major calcium transporters expressed by intestinal epithelia, ECaC and ICaC, are also vitamin D responsive. By inducing the expression of these and other genes in the small intestine, $1,25(OH)_2D$ increases the efficiency of intestinal calcium absorption.

The VDR regulates the expression of several genes in osteoblasts. Target genes include the bone matrix proteins, osteocalcin and osteopontin, which are upregulated by $1,25(OH)_2D$, in addition to type I collagen, which is transcriptionally repressed by $1,25(OH)_2D$. $1,25(OH)_2D$, as well as PTH, induces the expression of RANK ligand, which promotes osteoclast differentiation and increases osteoclast activity.

In the parathyroid gland, the VDR exerts antiproliferative effects on parathyroid cells and suppresses the transcription of the PTH gene. These effects of $1,25(OH)_2D$ on the parathyroid gland provide part of the rationale for current therapies directed at preventing and treating hyperparathyroidism associated with renal insufficiency.

The VDR is also expressed in tissues and organs that do not play a role in mineral ion homeostasis. Notable in this respect is the observation that $1,25(OH)_2D$ has an antiproliferative effect on several cell types, including keratinocytes, breast cancer cells, and prostate cancer cells. Alopecia is seen in humans and mice with mutant VDRs, but alopecia is not a feature of vitamin D deficiency, suggesting hormone-independent effects of the receptor.

VITAMIN D DEFICIENCY

The mounting concern about the relationship between solar exposure and the development of skin cancer has led to increased reliance on dietary sources of vitamin D. Although the prevalence of vitamin D deficiency varies, the third National Health and Nutrition Examination Survey (NHANES III) revealed that vitamin D deficiency is common throughout the United States. The clinical syndrome of vitamin D deficiency can result from deficient production of vitamin D in the skin, lack of dietary intake, accelerated losses of vitamin D, impaired vitamin D activation, or resistance to the biologic effects of 1,25$(OH)_2$D (**Table 23-6**). The elderly and nursing home residents are particularly at risk for vitamin D deficiency, since both the efficiency of vitamin D synthesis in the skin and the absorption of vitamin D from the intestine decline with age.

Intestinal malabsorption of dietary fats can also lead to vitamin D deficiency. This is further exacerbated in the presence of terminal ileal disease, which results in impaired enterohepatic circulation of vitamin D metabolites. In addition to intestinal diseases, accelerated inactivation of vitamin D metabolites can be seen with drugs such as barbiturates, phenytoin, and rifampin, which induce hepatic cytochrome P450 mixed function oxidases. Impaired 25-hydroxylation, associated with severe liver disease or isoniazid, is an infrequent cause of vitamin D deficiency. Impaired 1α-hydroxylation is prevalent in the population with profound renal dysfunction, and therapeutic interventions should be considered in patients whose creatinine clearance is <0.5 mL/s (30 mL/min).

Mutations in the renal 1α-hydroxylase are the basis for the genetic disorder, pseudo-vitamin D–deficiency rickets. This autosomal recessive disorder presents with the syndrome of vitamin D deficiency in the first year of life. Affected children manifest growth retardation, rickets, and hypocalcemic seizures. Serum 1,25$(OH)_2$D levels are low, despite normal 25(OH)D levels and elevated PTH levels. Treatment with vitamin D metabolites that do not require 1α-hydroxylation corrects this disorder and must be continued throughout life. A second autosomal recessive disorder, hereditary vitamin D–resistant rickets, is caused by VDR mutations. Affected children present in a similar fashion during the first year of life, but alopecia often accompanies the disorder, demonstrating a functional role of the VDR in postnatal hair regeneration. Serum levels of 1,25$(OH)_2$D are dramatically elevated in these individuals, both because of increased production due to stimulation of 1α-hydroxylase activity as a consequence of secondary hyperparathyroidism and because of impaired inactivation, since induction of the 24-hydroxylase by 1,25$(OH)_2$D requires an intact VDR. Since the receptor mutation results in hormone resistance, daily calcium and phosphorus infusions may be required to bypass the defect in intestinal mineral ion absorption.

Regardless of the cause, the clinical manifestations of vitamin D deficiency are largely a consequence of impaired intestinal calcium absorption. Mild to moderate vitamin D deficiency is asymptomatic, whereas long-standing vitamin D deficiency results in hypocalcemia accompanied by secondary hyperparathyroidism, impaired mineralization of the skeleton (osteopenia on x-ray or decreased bone mineral density), and proximal myopathy. In the absence of an intercurrent illness, the hypocalcemia associated with long-standing vitamin D deficiency rarely presents with acute symptoms of hypocalcemia, such as numbness, tingling, or seizures. The concurrent development of hypomagnesemia, however, which impairs parathyroid gland function, or the

TABLE 23-6

CAUSES OF IMPAIRED VITAMIN D ACTION

Vitamin D deficiency	Impaired 1α-hydroxylation
Impaired cutaneous production	Hypoparathyroidism
Dietary absence	Renal failure
Malabsorption	Ketoconazole
Accelerated loss of vitamin D	1α-hydroxylase mutation
Increased metabolism (barbiturates, phenytoin, rifampin)	Oncogenic osteomalacia
Impaired enterohepatic circulation	X-linked hypophosphatemic rickets
Impaired 25-hydroxylation	Target organ resistance
Liver disease	Vitamin D receptor mutation
Isoniazid	Phenytoin

administration of potent bisphosphonates, which impairs bone resorption, can lead to acute symptomatic hypocalcemia in vitamin D–deficient individuals.

RICKETS AND OSTEOMALACIA

In children, prior to epiphyseal fusion, vitamin D deficiency results in growth retardation associated with an expansion of the growth plate known as *rickets.* Three layers of chondrocytes are present in the normal growth plate: the reserve zone, the proliferating zone, and the hypertrophic zone. Rickets, associated with impaired vitamin D action, is characterized by expansion of the hypertrophic chondrocyte layer. The expansion of the growth plate is thought to be a result of impaired apoptosis of the late hypertrophic chondrocytes, an event that precedes replacement of these cells by osteoblasts during endochondral bone formation. Investigations in mice lacking the VDR have demonstrated that maintenance of normal mineral ion homeostasis prevents the development of rickets. The observation that phosphate promotes chondrocyte apoptosis, combined with the presence of rickets in syndromes associated with renal phosphate wasting, suggests that hypophosphatemia, which in vitamin D deficiency is a consequence of secondary hyperparathyroidism, is a key etiologic factor in the development of the rachitic growth plate.

The hypocalcemia and hypophosphatemia that accompany vitamin D deficiency result in impaired mineralization of bone matrix, a condition known as *osteomalacia.* Osteomalacia is also a feature of long-standing hypophosphatemia, which may be a consequence of renal phosphate wasting or chronic use of etidronate or phosphate-binding antacids. This hypomineralized matrix is biomechanically inferior to normal bone and, as a result, patients with vitamin D deficiency are prone to bowing of weight-bearing extremities because of abnormal remodeling and to skeletal fractures. Vitamin D and calcium supplementation have been shown to decrease the incidence of hip fracture among ambulatory nursing home residents in France, suggesting that undermineralization of bone contributes significantly to morbidity in the elderly. Proximal myopathy is a striking feature of severe vitamin D deficiency, both in children and in adults. Rapid resolution of the myopathy is observed after vitamin D repletion.

Though vitamin D deficiency is the most common cause of rickets and osteomalacia, many disorders lead to inadequate mineralization of the growth plate and bone. Calcium deficiency without vitamin D deficiency, the disorders of vitamin D metabolism previously discussed, and hypophosphatemia can all lead to inefficient mineralization. Even in the presence of normal calcium and phosphate levels, chronic acidosis and drugs such as bisphosphonates can lead to osteomalacia. The inorganic calcium/phosphate mineral phase of bone cannot form at low pH, and bisphosphonates bind to and prevent mineral crystal growth. Since alkaline phosphatase is necessary for normal mineral deposition, probably because the enzyme can hydrolyze inhibitors of mineralization such as inorganic pyrophosphate, genetic inactivation of the alkaline phosphatase gene (hereditary hypophosphatasia) can also lead to rickets and osteomalacia in the setting of normal calcium and phosphate levels.

DIAGNOSIS OF VITAMIN D DEFICIENCY, RICKETS, AND OSTEOMALACIA

The most specific screening test for vitamin D deficiency in otherwise healthy individuals is a serum 25(OH)D level. While the normal ranges vary, levels of 25(OH)D < 37 nmol/L (<15 ng/mL) are associated with increasing PTH levels and lower bone density, suggesting the need to revise normative values. Vitamin D deficiency leads to impaired intestinal absorption of calcium, resulting in decreased serum total and ionized calcium levels. Hypocalcemia results in secondary hyperparathyroidism, a homeostatic response that initially maintains serum calcium levels at the expense of the skeleton. Alkaline phosphatase levels are often increased because of the PTH-induced increase in bone turnover. In addition to increasing bone resorption, PTH decreases urinary calcium excretion, while promoting phosphaturia. This results in hypophosphatemia, which exacerbates the mineralization defect in the skeleton. With prolonged vitamin D deficiency resulting in osteomalacia, calcium stores in the skeleton become relatively inaccessible, since osteoclasts cannot resorb unmineralized osteoid, and frank hypocalcemia ensues. Since PTH is a major stimulus for the renal 1α-hydroxylase, there is increased synthesis of the active hormone, $1,25(OH)_2D$. Paradoxically, levels of this hormone may be normal in vitamin D deficiency. Measurements of $1,25(OH)_2D$, therefore, do not provide an accurate index of vitamin D stores and should not be used to diagnose vitamin D deficiency in patients with normal renal function.

Radiologic features of vitamin D deficiency in children include a widened, expanded growth plate, characteristic of rickets. These findings are apparent not only in the long bones, but also at the costochondral junctions, where the expansion of the growth plate leads to swellings known as "rachitic rosaries." Impairment of intramembranous bone mineralization leads to delayed fusion of the calvarial sutures and a decrease in the radio-opacity of cortical bone in the long bones. If vitamin D deficiency occurs after epiphyseal fusion, the

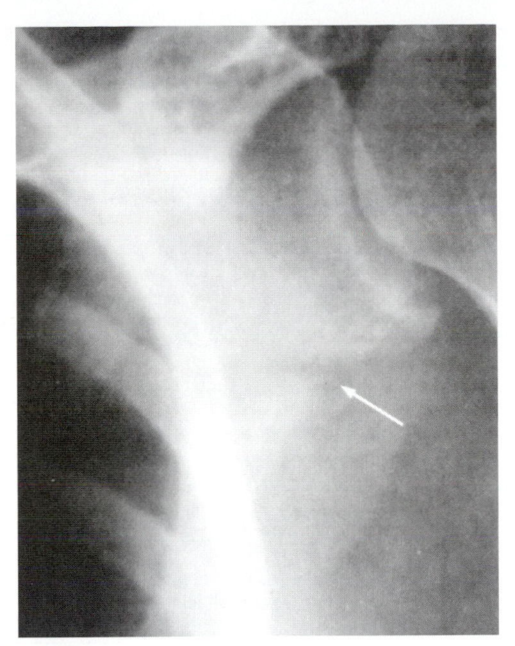

FIGURE 23-6
Radiograph of the scapula of a 58-year-old woman with phosphaturia as a cause of osteomalacia. The presence of a pseudofracture or Looser's zone is indicated by an arrow.

main radiologic finding is a decrease in cortical thickness and relative radiolucency of the skeleton. A specific radiologic feature of osteomalacia, whether associated with phosphate wasting or vitamin D deficiency, is pseudofractures or Looser's zones (**Fig. 23-6**). These are radiolucent lines that occur where large arteries are in contact with the underlying skeletal elements; it is believed that the arterial pulsations lead to the radiolucencies. As a result, these pseudofractures are usually a few millimeters wide, several centimeters long, and are seen particularly in the scapula, the pelvis, and the femoral neck.

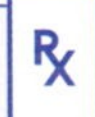

TREATMENT FOR VITAMIN D DEFICIENCY

Daily intake of a multivitamin preparation that contains 400 IU of vitamin D is often insufficient to prevent vitamin D deficiency. Based on the observation that 800 IU of vitamin D, with calcium supplementation, decreases the risk of hip fractures in elderly women, 800 IU is considered to be a more appropriate daily dosage for prevention of vitamin D deficiency. The safety margin for vitamin D is large, and vitamin D toxicity is usually observed only in patients taking doses >40,000 IU daily. Treatment of vitamin D deficiency should be directed at the underlying disorder, if possible, and tailored to the severity of the condition. Vitamin D should always be repleted in conjunction with calcium supplementation since most, if not all, of the consequences of vitamin D deficiency are a result of impaired mineral ion homeostasis.

In patients whose 1α-hydroxylation is impaired, vitamin D analogues not requiring this activation step are preferred. These include dihydrotachysterol (DHT, 0.2 to 1.0 mg daily), $1,25(OH)_2D_3$ [calcitriol (Rocaltrol), 0.25 to 0.5 μg daily], and 1α-hydroxyvitamin D_2 [doxercalciferol (Hectorol), 2.5 to 5 μg daily]. If the pathway required for activation of vitamin D is intact, severe vitamin D deficiency can be treated with pharmacologic repletion initially (50,000 IU weekly for 3 to 12 weeks), followed by maintenance therapy (800 IU daily). Pharmacologic doses may be required for maintenance therapy in patients who are taking drugs such as barbiturates or phenytoin that accelerate the metabolism of, or cause resistance to, 1,25-dihydroxyvitamin D. If intestinal malabsorption is a contributing factor, up to tenfold higher doses of vitamin D may be needed, or repletion can be performed with intramuscular vitamin D (250,000 IU biannually). Calcium supplementation should include 1.5 to 2.0 g of elemental calcium daily. Normocalcemia is usually observed within 1 week of institution of therapy, although increases in PTH and alkaline phosphatase levels may persist for 3 to 6 months.

The most efficacious methods to monitor treatment and resolution of vitamin D deficiency are serum and urinary calcium measurements. For patients who are vitamin D replete and are taking adequate calcium supplementation, the 24-h urinary calcium excretion should be in the range of 100 to 250 mg/24 h. Lower levels suggest problems with adhering to the treatment regimen or with absorption of calcium or vitamin D supplements. The 25(OH)D level can be remeasured to address the latter, although the half-life of this metabolite is long (3 weeks) and levels may continue to increase for many months on a stable regimen. Urinary calcium excretion >250 mg/24 h predisposes to nephrolithiasis and should prompt a reduction in vitamin D dosage and/or calcium supplementation.

FURTHER READINGS

BOYDEN LM et al: High bone density due to a mutation in LDL-receptor-related protein 5. N Engl J Med 346:1513, 2002

DELUCA HF: Overview of general physiologic features and functions of vitamin D. Am J Clin Nutr 80:1689S, 2004

An overview of the physiologic, endocrinologic, and molecular biologic characteristics of vitamin D, including selective analogues of 1α,25-dihydroxyvitamin D_3.

HEANEY RP: Vitamin D, nutritional deficiency, and the medical paradigm. J Clin Endocrinol Metab 88:5107, 2003

KANTOROVICH V et al: Genetic heterogeneity in familial magnesium wasting. J Clin Endocrinol Metab 87:612, 2002

KOBAYASHI T et al: Minireview: Transcriptional regulation in development of bone. Endocrinology 146:1012, 2005

Three lineages of bone cells, chondrocytes, osteoblasts, and osteoclasts, develop and differentiate according to their distinct developmental programs. This review summarizes selected transcription factors that have been demonstrated to critically affect bone cell development.

QUARLES LD, DREZNER MK: Pathophysiology of X-linked hypophosphatemia, tumor-induced osteomalacia, and autosomal dominant hypophosphatemia: A perPHEXing problem. J Clin Endocrinol Metab 86: 494, 2001

SEUFERT J et al: Octreotide therapy for tumor-induced osteomalacia. N Engl J Med 345:1883, 2001

SHIMADA T et al: Cloning and characterization of FGF23 as a causative factor of tumor-induced osteomalacia. Proc Natl Acad Sci USA 98:6500, 2001

WHARTON B et al: Rickets. Lancet 362:1389, 2003

Rickets, once thought vanquished, is reappearing. Rickets can be secondary to disorders of the gut, pancreas, liver, kidney, or metabolism; however, it is mostly due to nutrient deficiency. This review focuses on molecular mechanism of vitamin D deficiency and strategies to ensure adequate replacement.

YAMAGUCHI T et al: G protein–coupled extracellular Ca^{2+} (Ca^{2+})-sensing receptor (CaR) in cell signaling and control of diverse cellular functions. Adv Pharmacol 47:209, 2000

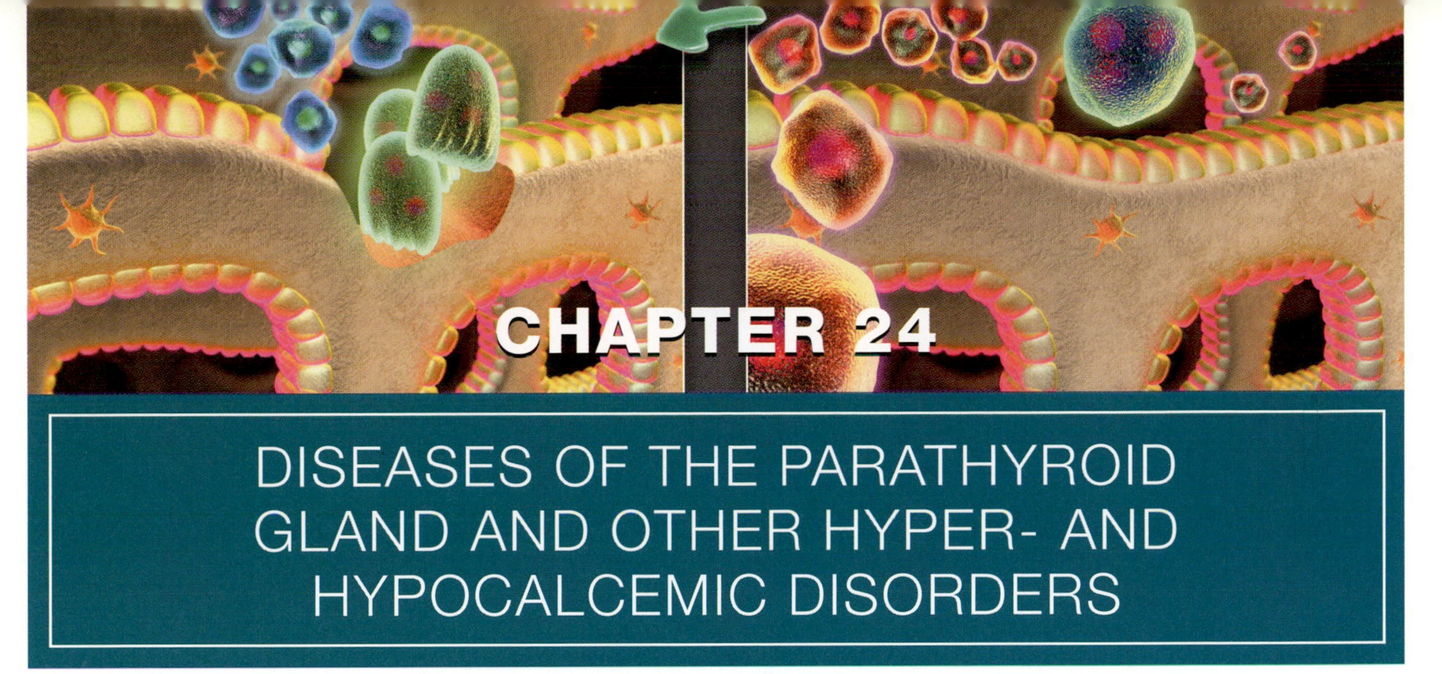

CHAPTER 24

DISEASES OF THE PARATHYROID GLAND AND OTHER HYPER- AND HYPOCALCEMIC DISORDERS

John T. Potts, Jr

The four parathyroid glands are located posterior to the thyroid gland. They produce parathyroid hormone (PTH), which is the primary regulator of calcium physiology. PTH acts directly on bone, where it induces calcium resorption, and on the kidney, where it stimulates calcium reabsorption and synthesis of 1,25-dihydroxyvitamin D [$1,25(OH)_2D$], a hormone that stimulates gastrointestinal calcium absorption. Serum PTH levels are tightly regulated by a negative feedback loop. Calcium, acting through the calcium-sensing receptor, and vitamin D, acting through its nuclear receptor, inhibit PTH release and synthesis. Understanding the hormone pathways that regulate calcium levels and bone metabolism is essential for effective diagnosis and management of a wide array of hyper- and hypocalcemic disorders.

Hyperparathyroidism, characterized by excess production of PTH, is a common cause of hypercalcemia and is usually the result of autonomously functioning adenomas or hyperplasia. Surgery for this disorder is highly effective and has been shown to reverse some of the deleterious effects of long-standing PTH excess on bone density. Hypercalcemia of malignancy is also common and is usually due to the overproduction of parathyroid hormone–related peptide (PTHrP) by cancer cells. The similarities in the biochemical characteristics of hyperparathyroidism and hypercalcemia of malignancy, first noted by Albright in 1941, are now known to reflect the actions of PTH and PTHrP through the same G protein–coupled PTH/PTHrP receptor.

The genetic basis of multiple endocrine neoplasia (MEN) types 1 and 2, familial hypocalciuric hypercalcemia (FHH), the different forms of pseudohypoparathyroidism (PHP), Jansen's syndrome, disorders of vitamin D synthesis and action, and the molecular events associated with parathyroid gland neoplasia have provided new insights into calcium metabolism. The advent of new drugs, including bisphosphonates and selective estrogen receptor modulators (SERMs), offers new avenues for the treatment and prevention of metabolic bone disease. PTH analogues are promising therapeutic agents for the treatment of postmenopausal or senile osteoporosis, and calcimimetic agents, which act through the calcium-sensing receptor, may provide new approaches for PTH suppression.

PARATHYROID HORMONE

PHYSIOLOGY

The primary function of PTH is to maintain the extracellular fluid (ECF) calcium concentration within a narrow normal range. The hormone acts directly on bone and kidney and indirectly on intestine through its effects on synthesis of 1,25$(OH)_2$D to increase serum calcium concentrations; in turn, PTH production is closely regulated by the concentration of serum ionized calcium. This feedback system is the critical homeostatic mechanism for maintenance of ECF calcium. Any tendency toward hypocalcemia, as might be induced by calcium-deficient diets, is counteracted by an increased secretion of PTH. This in turn (1) increases the rate of dissolution of bone mineral, thereby increasing the flow of calcium from bone into blood; (2) reduces the renal clearance of calcium, returning more of the calcium filtered at the glomerulus into ECF; and (3) increases the efficiency of calcium absorption in the intestine by stimulating the production of 1,25$(OH)_2$D. Immediate control of blood calcium is due to PTH effects on bone and, to a lesser extent, on renal calcium clearance. Maintenance of steady-state calcium balance, on the other hand, probably results from the effects of 1,25$(OH)_2$D on calcium absorption (Chap. 23). The renal actions of the hormone are exerted at multiple sites and include inhibition of phosphate transport (proximal tubule), increased reabsorption of calcium (distal tubule), and stimulation of the renal 25(OH)D-1α-hydroxylase. As much as 12 mmol (500 mg) calcium is transferred between the ECF and bone each day (a large amount in relation to the total ECF calcium pool), and PTH has a major effect on this transfer. The homeostatic role of the hormone can preserve calcium concentration in blood at the cost of bone destruction.

PTH has multiple actions on bone, some direct and some indirect. PTH-mediated changes in bone calcium release can be seen within minutes. The chronic effects of PTH are to increase the number of bone cells, both osteoblasts and osteoclasts, and to increase the remodeling of bone; these effects are apparent within hours after the hormone is given and persist for hours after PTH is withdrawn. Continuous exposure to elevated PTH (as in hyperparathyroidism or long-term infusions in animals) leads to increased osteoclast-mediated bone resorption. However, the intermittent administration of PTH, elevating hormone levels for 1 to 2 h each day, leads to a net stimulation of bone formation rather than bone breakdown. Striking increases, especially in trabecular bone in the spine and hip, have been reported with the use of PTH in combination with estrogen. PTH as monotherapy caused a highly significant reduction in fracture incidence in a worldwide placebo-controlled trial.

Osteoblasts (or stromal cell precursors), which have PTH receptors, are crucial to this bone-forming effect of PTH; osteoclasts, which mediate bone breakdown, lack PTH receptors. PTH-mediated stimulation of osteoclasts is believed to be indirect, acting in part through cytokines released from osteoblasts to activate osteoclasts; in experimental studies of bone resorption in vitro, osteoblasts must be present for PTH to activate osteoclasts to resorb bone (Chap. 23).

STRUCTURE

PTH is an 84-amino-acid single-chain peptide. The amino acid portion, PTH(1–34), is highly conserved and is critical for the biologic actions of the molecule. Modified synthetic fragments of the amino-terminal sequence as small as PTH(1–11) are sufficient to activate the major receptor (see below). The carboxyl-terminal region of PTH binds to a separate receptor (cPTH-R), but it has not yet been cloned. Fragments shortened at the amino terminus bind to cPTH-R and inhibit the actions of the full-length PTH(1–84) or the PTH(1–34) active fragments.

BIOSYNTHESIS, SECRETION, AND METABOLISM

Synthesis

Parathyroid cells have multiple methods of adapting to increased needs for PTH production. Most rapid (within minutes) is secretion of preformed hormone in response to hypocalcemia. Second, within hours, PTH mRNA expression is induced by sustained hypocalcemia. Finally, protracted challenge leads within days to cellular replication to increase gland mass.

PTH is initially synthesized as a larger molecule (preproparathyroid hormone, consisting of 115 amino acids), which is then reduced in size by a second cleavage (proparathyroid hormone, 90 amino acids) before secretion as the 84-amino-acid peptide. In one kindred with hypoparathyroidism, a mutation in the preprotein region of the gene interferes with hormone transport and secretion.

Transcriptional suppression of the PTH gene by calcium is nearly maximal at physiologic calcium concentrations. Hypocalcemia increases transcriptional activity within hours. 1,25$(OH)_2D_3$ strongly suppresses PTH gene transcription. In patients with renal failure, intravenous administration of supraphysiologic levels of 1,25$(OH)_2D_3$ or analogues of the active metabolite can dramatically suppress PTH overproduction, which is sometimes difficult to control due to severe secondary hyperparathyroidism. Regulation of proteolytic destruction of preformed hormone (posttranslational regulation of hormone production) is an important mechanism for mediating rapid (minutes) changes in hormone availability. High calcium increases and low calcium inhibits the proteolytic destruction of hormone stores.

Regulation of PTH Secretion

PTH secretion increases steeply to a maximum value of five times the basal rate of secretion as calcium concentration falls from normal to the range of 1.9 to 2.0 mmol/L (7.5 to 8.0 mg/dL) (measured as total calcium). The ionized fraction of blood calcium is the important determinant of hormone secretion. Severe intracellular magnesium deficiency impairs PTH secretion (see below).

ECF calcium controls PTH secretion by interaction with a calcium sensor, a G protein–coupled receptor (GPCR) for which Ca^{2+} ions act as the ligand (see below). This receptor is a member of a distinctive subfamily of the GPCR superfamily that is characterized by a large extracellular domain suitable for "clamping" the small-molecule ligand. Stimulation of the receptor by high calcium levels suppresses PTH secretion. The receptor is present in parathyroid glands and the calcitonin-secreting cells (C cells) of the thyroid, as well as in other sites such as brain and kidney. Genetic evidence has revealed a key biologic role for the calcium-sensing receptor in parathyroid gland responsiveness to calcium and in renal calcium clearance. Point mutations associated with loss of function cause the syndrome FHH resembling hyperparathyroidism but with hypocalciuria. On the other hand, gain-of-function mutations cause a form of hypocalcemia resembling hypoparathyroidism (see below).

Metabolism

The secreted form of PTH is indistinguishable by immunologic criteria and by molecular size from the 84-amino-acid peptide (PTH 1–84) extracted from glands. However, much of the immunoreactive material found in the circulation is smaller than the extracted or secreted hormone. The principal circulating fragments of immunoreactive hormone lack a portion of the critical amino-terminal sequence required for biologic activity and, hence, are biologically inactive fragments (so-called middle- and carboxyl-terminal fragments). Much of the proteolysis of hormone occurs in the liver and kidney. Peripheral metabolism of PTH does not appear to be regulated by physiologic states (high versus low calcium, etc.); hence peripheral metabolism of hormone, although responsible for rapid clearance of secreted hormone, appears to be a high-capacity, metabolically invariant catabolic process.

The rate of clearance of the secreted 84-amino-acid peptide from blood is more rapid than the rate of clearance of the biologically inactive fragment(s) corresponding to the middle- and carboxyl-terminal regions of PTH. Consequently, the interpretation of PTH immunoassays is influenced by the nature of the peptide fragments detected by the antibodies.

Although the problems inherent in PTH measurements have been largely circumvented by use of double-antibody assays that detect only the intact molecule, new evidence has revealed the existence of a hitherto unappreciated larger PTH fragment that may affect the interpretation of most currently available double-antibody assays. A large amino-terminally truncated form of PTH, possibly PTH(7–84), is present in normal and uremic individuals in addition to PTH(1–84). The concentration of the putative (7–84) fragment relative to that of intact PTH(1–84) is higher with induced hypercalcemia than in eucalcemic or hypocalcemic conditions and is higher in patients with renal failure. Growing evidence suggests that the PTH(7–84)-like amino-terminally truncated fragments can act as an inhibitor of PTH action and may be of clinical significance, particularly in renal failure. Efforts to prevent secondary hyperparathyroidism by a variety of measures (vitamin D analogues, higher calcium intake, and phosphate-lowering strategies) may have led to oversuppression of biologically active intact PTH since the amino-terminally truncated PTH reacts in many first-generation double-antibody PTH assays. The role, if any, of excessive PTH suppression due to inaccurate measurement of PTH in adynamic bone disease in renal failure (see below) is unknown. Newer assays with extreme amino-terminal epitopes that detect only full-length PTH(1–84) are being studied intensively.

PARATHYROID HORMONE–RELATED PROTEIN

The paracrine factor termed *PTHrP* is responsible for most instances of hypercalcemia of malignancy (Chap. 22), a syndrome that resembles hyperparathyroidism. Many different cell types produce PTHrP, including brain, pancreas, heart, lung, mammary tissue, placenta, endothelial cells, and smooth muscle. In fetal animals, PTHrP directs transplacental calcium transfer, and high concentrations of PTHrP are produced in mammary tissue and secreted into milk. Human and bovine milk contain very high concentrations of the hormone, the biologic significance of which is unknown. PTHrP may also play a role in uterine contraction and other biologic functions.

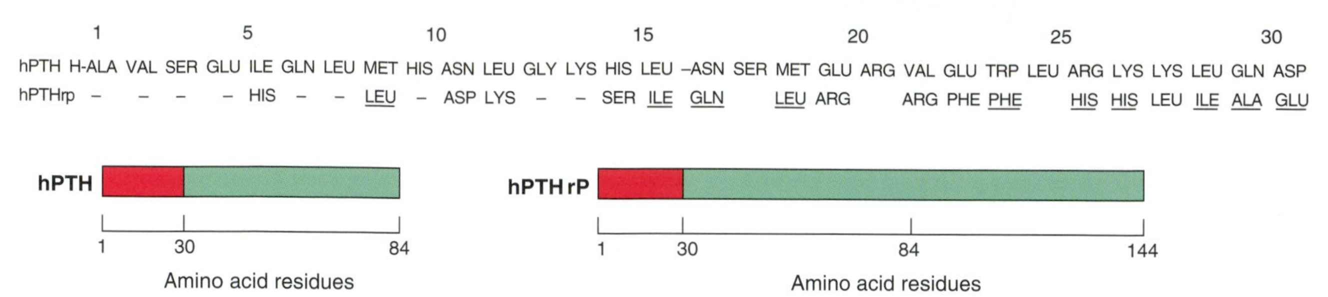

FIGURE 24-1

Schematic diagram to illustrate similarities and differences in structure of human parathyroid hormone (PTH) and human PTH-related peptide (PTHrP). Close structural (and functional) homology exists between the first 30 amino acids of hPTH and hPTHrP. The PTHrP sequence may be ≥144 amino acid residues in length. PTH is only 84 residues long; after residue 30, there is little structural homology between the two. Dashed lines in the PTHrP sequence indicate identity; underlined residues, although different from those of PTH, still represent conservative changes (charge or polarity preserved). Eleven amino acids are identical, and a total of 21 of 30 are homologues.

PTH and PTHrP, although distinctive products of different genes, exhibit considerable functional and structural homology (**Fig. 24-1**) and may have evolved from a shared ancestral gene. The structure of the gene for human PTHrP, however, is more complex than that of PTH, containing multiple exons and multiple sites for alternate splicing patterns during formation of the mature mRNA. Protein products of 141, 139, and 173 amino acids are produced, and other molecular forms may result from tissue-specific degradation at accessible internal cleavage sites. The biologic roles of these various molecular species and the nature of the circulating forms of PTHrP are unclear. It is uncertain whether PTHrP circulates at any significant level in adults; as a paracrine factor, PTHrP may be produced, act, and be destroyed locally within tissues. In adults PTHrP appears to have little influence on calcium homeostasis, except in disease states, when large tumors, especially of the squamous cell type, lead to massive overproduction of the hormone.

PTH AND PTHrP HORMONE ACTION

Both PTH and PTHrP bind to and activate the PTH/PTHrP receptor. The 500-amino-acid PTH/PTHrP receptor (also known as the PTH-1 receptor, PTH1R) belongs to a subfamily of GPCRs that includes those for glucagon, secretin, and vasoactive intestinal peptide. The extracellular regions are involved in hormone binding, and the intracellular domains, after hormone activation, bind G protein subunits to transduce hormone signaling into cellular responses through stimulation of second messengers. A second receptor that binds PTH, termed the *PTH-2 receptor* (PTH2R), is expressed in brain, pancreas, and several other tissues. PTH1R responds equivalently to PTH and PTHrP, whereas PTH2R responds only to PTH. The endogenous ligand of this receptor is now believed to be a peptide distinct from PTH, a 39-amino-acid hypothalamic peptide (*tubular infundibular peptide*, TIP-39). PTH1R and PTH2R can be traced backward in evolutionary time to fish. Zebrafish PTH1R and PTH2R exhibit the same selective responses to PTH and PTHrP as do human PTH1R and PTH2R. The evolutionary conservation of structure and function suggests unique biologic roles for these receptors.

Studies using cloned PTH1R confirm that it can be coupled to more than one G protein and second-messenger kinase pathway, apparently explaining the multiplicity of pathways stimulated by PTH. Stimulation of protein kinases (A and C) and calcium transport channels is associated with a variety of hormone-specific tissue responses. These responses include inhibition of phosphate and bicarbonate transport, stimulation of calcium transport, and activation of renal 1α-hydroxylase in the kidney. The responses in bone include effects on collagen synthesis; increased alkaline phosphatase, ornithine decarboxylase, citrate decarboxylase, and glucose-6-phosphate dehydrogenase activities; DNA, protein, and phospholipid synthesis; and calcium and phosphate transport. Ultimately, these biochemical events lead to an integrated hormonal response in bone turnover and calcium homeostasis. PTH also activates Na^+/Ca^{2+} exchanges in renal distal tubular sites and stimulates translocation of preformed calcium transport channels, moving them from the interior to the apical surface to mediate increased tubular uptake of calcium. PTH-dependent stimulation of phosphate excretion (blocking reabsorption—the opposite effect from actions on calcium in the kidney) involves the sodium-dependent phosphate cotransporter, NPT-2, lowering its apical membrane content (and therefore function). Similar shifts may be involved in other renal tubular transport effects of PTH.

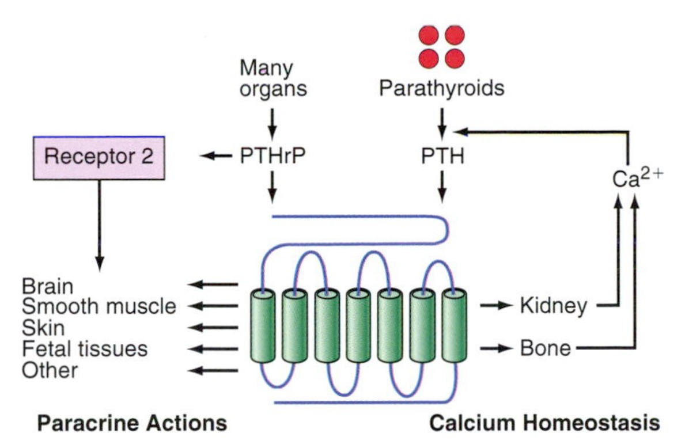

FIGURE 24-2

Dual role for the actions of the PTH/PTHrP receptor (PTH1R). Parathyroid hormone (PTH; endocrine-calcium homeostasis) and PTH-related peptide (PTHrP; paracrine–multiple tissue actions including growth plate cartilage in developing bone) use the single receptor for their disparate functions mediated by the amino-terminal 30 residues of either peptide. Other regions of both ligands interact with other receptors (not shown).

PTHrP exerts important developmental influences on fetal bone development and in adult physiology. A homozygous knockout of the PTHrP gene (or the gene for the PTH receptor) in mice causes a lethal deformity in which animals are born with severe skeletal deformities resembling chondrodysplasia (**Fig. 24-2**).

CALCITONIN (See also Chap. 21)

Calcitonin is a hypocalcemic peptide hormone that in several mammalian species acts as an antagonist to PTH. Calcitonin seems to be of limited physiologic significance in humans, however, at least in calcium homeostasis. It is of medical significance because of its role as a tumor marker in sporadic and hereditary cases of medullary carcinoma and its medical use as an adjunctive treatment in severe hypercalcemia and in Paget's disease of bone.

The hypocalcemic activity of calcitonin is accounted for primarily by inhibition of osteoclast-mediated bone resorption and secondarily by stimulation of renal calcium clearance. These effects are mediated by receptors on osteoclasts and renal tubular cells. Calcitonin exerts additional effects through receptors present in brain, gastrointestinal tract, and the immune system. The hormone, for example, exerts analgesic effects directly on cells in the hypothalamus and related structures, possibly by interacting with receptors for related peptide hormones, such as calcitonin gene–related peptide (CGRP) or amylin. The latter ligands have specific high-affinity receptors and can also bind to and trigger calcitonin receptors. The calcitonin receptors are homologous in structure to PTH1R.

The thyroid is the major source of the hormone, and the cells involved in calcitonin synthesis arise from neural crest tissue. During embryogenesis, these cells migrate into the ultimobranchial body, derived from the last branchial pouch. In submammalian vertebrates, the ultimobranchial body constitutes a discrete organ, anatomically separate from the thyroid gland; in mammals, the ultimobranchial gland fuses with and is incorporated into the thyroid gland.

The naturally occurring calcitonins consist of a peptide chain of 32 amino acids. There is considerable sequence variability among species. Calcitonin from salmon, which is used therapeutically, is 10 to 100 times more potent than mammalian forms in lowering serum calcium.

There are two calcitonin genes, α and β; the transcriptional control of these genes is complex. Two different mRNA molecules are transcribed from the α gene; one is translated into the precursor for calcitonin, and the other message is translated into an alternative product, CGRP. CGRP is synthesized wherever the calcitonin mRNA is expressed, e.g., in medullary carcinoma of the thyroid. The β, or CGRP-2, gene is transcribed into the mRNA for CGRP in the central nervous system (CNS); this gene does not produce calcitonin, however. CGRP has cardiovascular actions and may serve as a neurotransmitter or play a developmental role in the CNS.

The circulating level of calcitonin in humans is lower than that in many other species. In humans, even extreme variations in calcitonin production do not change calcium and phosphate metabolism; no definite effects are attributable to calcitonin deficiency (totally thyroidectomized patients receiving only replacement thyroxine) or excess (patients with medullary carcinoma of the thyroid, a calcitonin-secreting tumor) (Chap. 21). Calcitonin has been a useful pharmacologic agent to suppress bone resorption in Paget's disease (Chap. 26) and osteoporosis (Chap. 25) and in the treatment of hypercalcemia of malignancy (see below). However, the physiologic role, if any, of calcitonin in humans is uncertain.

HYPERCALCEMIA

Hypercalcemia can be a manifestation of a serious illness such as malignancy or can be detected coincidentally by laboratory testing in a patient with no obvious illness. The number of patients recognized with asymptomatic hypercalcemia, usually hyperparathyroidism, increased in the late twentieth century but is now declining somewhat, perhaps due to decreased use of routine blood calcium measurements or for other unknown reasons.

Whenever hypercalcemia is confirmed, a definitive diagnosis must be established. Although hyperparathyroidism, a frequent cause of asymptomatic hypercalcemia, is a chronic disorder in which manifestations, if any, may be expressed only after months or years, hypercalcemia can also be the earliest manifestation of malignancy, the second most common cause of hypercalcemia in the adult. The causes of hypercalcemia are numerous (**Table 24-1**), but hyperparathyroidism and cancer account for 90% of cases.

Before undertaking a diagnostic workup, it is essential to be sure that true hypercalcemia, not a false-positive laboratory test, is present. A false-positive diagnosis of hypercalcemia is usually the result of inadvertent hemoconcentration during blood collection or elevation in serum proteins such as albumin. Hypercalcemia is a chronic problem, and it is cost-effective to obtain several serum calcium measurements; these tests need not be in the fasting state.

Clinical features are helpful in differential diagnosis. Hypercalcemia in an adult who is asymptomatic is usually due to primary hyperparathyroidism. In malignancy-associated hypercalcemia the disease is usually not occult; rather, symptoms of malignancy bring the patient to the physician, and hypercalcemia is discovered during the evaluation. In such patients the interval between detection of hypercalcemia and death is often <6 months. Accordingly, if an asymptomatic individual has had hypercalcemia or some manifestation of hypercalcemia, such as kidney stones, for >1 or 2 years, it is unlikely that malignancy is the cause. Nevertheless, differentiating primary hyperparathyroidism from *occult* malignancy can occasionally be difficult, and careful evaluation is required, particularly when the duration of the hypercalcemia is unknown. Hypercalcemia not due to hyperparathyroidism or malignancy can result from excessive vitamin D action, high bone turnover from any of several causes, or from renal failure (Table 24-1). Dietary history and a history of ingestion of vitamins or drugs are often helpful in diagnosing some of the less frequent causes. PTH immunoassays based on double-antibody methods serve as the principal laboratory test in differential diagnosis.

Hypercalcemia from any cause can result in fatigue, depression, mental confusion, anorexia, nausea, vomiting, constipation, reversible renal tubular defects, increased urination, a short QT interval in the electrocardiogram, and, in some patients, cardiac arrhythmias. There is a variable relation from one patient to the next between the severity of hypercalcemia and the symptoms. Generally, symptoms are more common at calcium levels >2.9 to 3 mmol/L (11.5 to 12.0 mg/dL), but some patients, even at this level, are asymptomatic. When the calcium level is >3.2 mmol/L (13 mg/dL), calcification in kidneys, skin, vessels, lungs, heart, and stomach occurs and renal insufficiency may develop, particularly if blood phosphate levels are normal or elevated due to impaired renal function. Severe hypercalcemia, usually defined as ≥3.7 to 4.5 mmol/L (15 to 18 mg/dL), can be a medical emergency; coma and cardiac arrest can occur.

TABLE 24-1

CLASSIFICATION OF CAUSES OF HYPERCALCEMIA

I. Parathyroid-related
   A. Primary hyperparathyroidism
      1. Solitary adenomas
      2. Multiple endocrine neoplasia
   B. Lithium therapy
   C. Familial hypocalciuric hypercalcemia
II. Malignancy-related
   A. Solid tumor with metastases (breast)
   B. Solid tumor with humoral mediation of hypercalcemia (lung, kidney)
   C. Hematologic malignancies (multiple myeloma, lymphoma, leukemia)
III. Vitamin D—related
   A. Vitamin D intoxication
   B. ↑ 1,25 $(OH)_2D$; sarcoidosis and other granulomatous diseases
   C. Idiopathic hypercalcemia of infancy
IV. Associated with high bone turnover
   A. Hyperthyroidism
   B. Immobilization
   C. Thiazides
   D. Vitamin A intoxication
V. Associated with renal failure
   A. Severe secondary hyperparathyroidism
   B. Aluminum intoxication
   C. Milk-alkali syndrome

Acute management of the hypercalcemia is usually successful. The type of treatment is based on the severity of the hypercalcemia and the nature of associated symptoms, as outlined below.

PRIMARY HYPERPARATHYROIDISM

Natural History and Incidence

Primary hyperparathyroidism is a generalized disorder of calcium, phosphate, and bone metabolism due to an increased secretion of PTH. The elevation of circulating hormone usually leads to hypercalcemia and hypophosphatemia. There is great variation in the manifestations. Patients may present with multiple signs and symptoms, including recurrent nephrolithiasis, peptic ulcers, mental changes, and, less frequently, extensive bone resorption. However, with greater awareness of the disease and wider use of multiphasic screening tests, including measurements of blood calcium, the diagnosis is frequently made in patients who have no symptoms and minimal, if any, signs of the disease other than hypercalcemia and elevated levels of PTH. The manifestations may be subtle, and the disease may have a benign course for many years or a lifetime. This milder form of the disease is usually termed *asymptomatic hyperparathyroidism*. Rarely, hyperparathyroidism develops or worsens abruptly and causes severe complications, such as marked dehydration and coma, so-called hypercalcemic parathyroid crisis.

The annual incidence of the disease is calculated to be as high as 0.2% in patients >60, with an estimated prevalence, including undiscovered asymptomatic patients, of ≥1%; some reports suggest the incidence may be declining, perhaps reflecting earlier overestimates. The disease has a peak incidence between the third and fifth decades but occurs in young children and in the elderly.

Etiology

Solitary Adenomas The cause of hyperparathyroidism is one or more hyperfunctioning glands. A single abnormal gland is the cause in ~80% of patients; the abnormality in the gland is usually a benign neoplasm or adenoma and rarely a parathyroid carcinoma. Some surgeons and pathologists report that the enlargement of multiple glands is common; double adenomas are reported. In ~15% of patients, all glands are hyperfunctioning; *chief cell parathyroid hyperplasia* is usually hereditary and frequently associated with other endocrine abnormalities.

Multiple Endocrine Neoplasia Hereditary hyperparathyroidism can occur without other endocrine abnormalities but is usually part of a *multiple endocrine neoplasia* syndrome (Chap. 21). MEN 1 (Wermer's syndrome) consists of hyperparathyroidism and tumors of the pituitary and pancreas, often associated with gastric hypersecretion and peptic ulcer disease (Zollinger-Ellison syndrome). MEN 2A is characterized by pheochromocytoma and medullary carcinoma of the thyroid, as well as hyperparathyroidism; MEN 2B has additional associated features such as multiple neuromas but usually lacks hyperparathyroidism. Each of these MEN syndromes is transmitted in an apparent autosomal dominant manner, although, as noted below, the genetic basis does not always involve a dominant allele.

Pathology

Adenomas are most often located in the inferior parathyroid glands, but in 6 to 10% of patients, parathyroid adenomas may be located in the thymus, the thyroid, the pericardium, or behind the esophagus. Adenomas are usually 0.5 to 5 g in size but may be as large as 10 to 20 g (normal glands weigh 25 mg on average). Chief cells are predominant in both hyperplasia and adenoma. With chief cell hyperplasia, the enlargement may be so asymmetric that some involved glands appear grossly normal. If generalized hyperplasia is present, however, histologic examination reveals a uniform pattern of chief cells and disappearance of fat even in the absence of an increase in gland weight. Thus, microscopic examination of biopsy specimens of several glands is essential to interpret findings at surgery.

Parathyroid carcinoma is usually not aggressive. Long-term survival without recurrence is common if at initial surgery the entire gland is removed without rupture of the capsule. Recurrent parathyroid carcinoma is usually slow-growing with local spread in the neck, and surgical correction of recurrent disease may be feasible. Occasionally, however, parathyroid carcinoma is more aggressive, with distant metastases (lung, liver, and bone) found at the time of initial operation. It may be difficult to appreciate initially that a primary tumor is carcinoma; increased numbers of mitotic figures and increased fibrosis of the gland stroma may precede invasion. The diagnosis of carcinoma is often made in retrospect. Hyperparathyroidism from a parathyroid carcinoma may be indistinguishable from other forms of primary hyperparathyroidism; a potential clue to the diagnosis, however, is provided by the degree of calcium elevation. Calcium values of 3.5 to 3.7 mmol/L (14 to 15 mg/dL) are frequent with carcinoma and may alert the surgeon to remove the abnormal gland with care to avoid capsular rupture.

Defects Associated with Hyperparathyroidism

As in many other types of neoplasia, two fundamental types of genetic defects have been identified in parathyroid gland tumors: (1) overactivity of protooncogenes, and (2) loss of function of tumor-suppressor genes. The former, by definition, can lead to uncontrolled cellular growth and function by activation (gain-of-function mutation) of a single allele of the responsible gene, whereas the latter requires loss of function of both allelic copies.

Mutations in the *MENIN* gene locus on chromosome 11q13 are responsible for causing MEN 1; the normal allele of this gene fits the definition of a tumor-suppressor gene. A mutation of one allele is inherited; loss of the other allele via somatic cell mutation leads to monoclonal expansion and tumor development. In ~20% of sporadic parathyroid adenomas, the *MENIN* locus on chromosome 11 is deleted, implying that the same defect responsible for MEN 1 can also cause the sporadic disease (**Fig. 24-3*A***). Consistent with the Knudson hypothesis for two-step neoplasia in certain inherited cancer syndromes, the earlier onset of hyperparathyroidism in the hereditary syndromes reflects the need for only one mutational event to trigger the monoclonal outgrowth. In sporadic adenomas, typically occurring later in life, two different somatic events must occur before the *MENIN* gene is silenced.

Other presumptive antioncogenes involved in hyperparathyroidism include a gene mapped to chromosome 1p seen in 40% of sporadic parathyroid adenomas and a gene mapped to chromosome Xp11 in patients with secondary hyperparathyroidism and renal failure, who progressed to "tertiary" hyperparathyroidism, now known to reflect monoclonal outgrowths within previously hyperplastic glands.

The *Rb* gene, a tumor-suppressor gene located on chromosome 13q14, was initially associated with retinoblastomas but has since been implicated in many other forms of neoplasia including parathyroid carcinoma. Allelic deletion (with a presumed point mutation in the second allele) has been identified in all parathyroid carcinomas examined; there is also an abnormal staining pattern of the protein product of the gene. Allelic deletion is also seen in 10% of parathyroid adenomas, although the abnormal staining pattern of the Rb protein

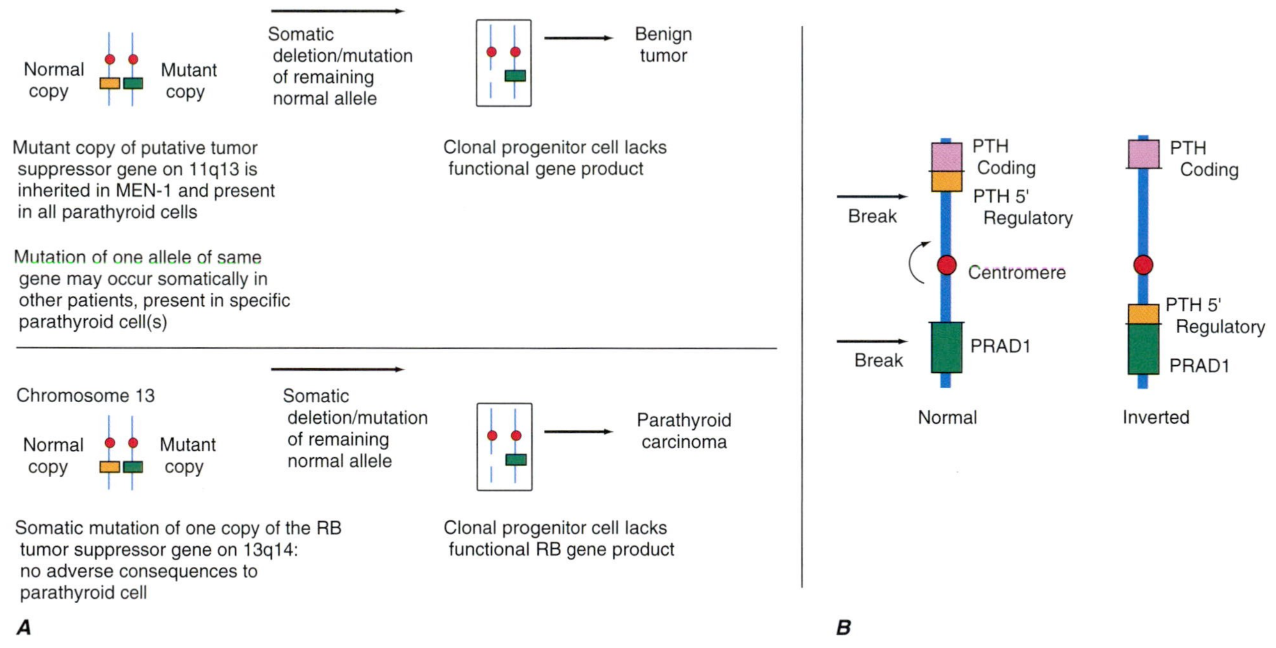

FIGURE 24-3

A. Schematic diagram indicating concept of autosomal recessive rather than autosomal dominant inheritance of tumor susceptibility. The patient with the hereditary abnormality (multiple endocrine neoplasia, or MEN) is envisioned as having one defective gene inherited from the affected parent on chromosome 11, but one copy of the normal gene is present from the other parent. In the monoclonal tumor (benign tumor), a somatic event, here partial chromosomal deletion, removes the remaining normal gene from a cell. In nonhereditary tumors, two successive somatic mutations must occur, a process that takes a longer time. By either pathway, the cell, deprived of growth-regulating influence from this gene, has unregulated growth and becomes a tumor. A different genetic locus also involving loss of a tumor-suppressor gene on chromosome 13 is involved in the pathogenesis of parathyroid carcinoma. ***B.*** Schematic illustration of the mechanism and consequences of gene rearrangement and overexpression of the PRAD 1 protooncogene (pericentromeric inversion of chromosome 11) in parathryoid adenomas. The excessive expression of PRAD 1 (a cell cycle control protein, cyclin D1) by the highly active PTH gene promoter in the parathyroid cell contributes to excess cellular proliferation. [*From J Habener et al, in L DeGroot, JL Jameson (eds): Endocrinology, 4th ed. Philadelphia, Saunders, 2001, with permission.*]

is not seen. Other gene loci on chromosome 13 may be involved in addition to the *Rb* locus.

There are two rare syndromes associated with hyperparathyroidism that involve one or more genes located on chromosome 1q. The hereditary *hyperparathyroidism jaw tumor* (HPT-JT) syndrome shows an autosomal dominant inheritance pattern; the jaw tumors are benign, but the parathyroid pathology may involve carcinoma as well as adenoma. Parathyroid carcinoma may also appear in the other syndrome, *familial isolated primary hyperparathyroidism* (FIPH). Both syndromes have been mapped through linkage studies to the chromosome 1q21-q31 region. Certain findings have led to speculation that this chromosome region might contain a protooncogene rather than a tumor-suppressor gene.

In some parathyroid adenomas, activation of a protooncogene has been identified (Fig. 24-3B). A reciprocal translocation involving chromosome 11 has been identified that juxtaposes the PTH gene promoter upstream of a gene product termed *PRAD-1*, a cyclin D protein that plays a key role in normal cell division. This translocation is found in as many as 15% of parathyroid adenomas, usually in larger tumors. Targeted overexpression of cyclin D_1 in the parathyroid glands of transgenic mice causes the development of hyperparathyroidism, consistent with the role of this cell cycle control protein in parathyroid neoplasia.

A mutated protooncogene, *RET*, is involved in each of the clinical variants of MEN 2 (Chap. 21). *RET* encodes a tyrosine kinase–type receptor; specific mutations lead to constitutive activity of the receptor, thereby explaining the autosomal dominant mode of transmission and the relatively early onset of neoplasia.

Signs and Symptoms

Half or more of patients with hyperparathyroidism are asymptomatic. In series in which patients are followed without operation, as many as 80% are classified as without symptoms. Manifestations of hyperparathyroidism involve primarily the kidneys and the skeletal system. Kidney involvement, due either to deposition of calcium in the renal parenchyma or to recurrent nephrolithiasis, was present in 60 to 70% of patients prior to 1970. With earlier detection, renal complications occur in <20% of patients in many large series. Renal stones are usually composed of either calcium oxalate or calcium phosphate. In occasional patients, repeated episodes of nephrolithiasis or the formation of large calculi may lead to urinary tract obstruction, infection, and loss of renal function. Nephrocalcinosis may also cause decreased renal function and phosphate retention.

The distinctive bone manifestation of hyperparathyroidism is *osteitis fibrosa cystica*, which occurred in 10 to 25% of patients in series reported 50 years ago. Histologically, the pathognomonic features are an increase in the giant multinucleated osteoclasts in scalloped areas on the surface of the bone (Howship's lacunae) and a replacement of the normal cellular and marrow elements by fibrous tissue. X-ray changes include resorption of the phalangeal tufts and replacement of the usually sharp cortical outline of the bone in the digits by an irregular outline (subperiosteal resorption). In recent years, osteitis fibrosa cystica is very rare in primary hyperparathyroidism, probably due to the earlier detection of the disease.

With the use of multiple markers of bone turnover, such as formation indices (bone-specific alkaline phosphatase, osteocalcin, and type I procollagen peptides) and bone resorption indices (including hydroxypyridinium collagen cross-links and telopeptides of type I collagen), increased skeletal turnover is detected in essentially all patients with established hyperparathyroidism.

Computed tomography (CT) scan and dual-energy x-ray absorptiometry (DEXA) of the spine provide reproducible quantitative estimates (within a few percent) of spinal bone density (Chap. 25). Similarly, bone density in the extremities can be quantified by densitometry of the hip or of the distal radius at a site chosen to be primarily cortical. Cortical bone density is reduced while cancellous bone density, especially in the spine, is relatively preserved. Serial studies in patients who choose to be followed without surgery have indicated that in the majority there is little further change over a number of years, consistent with laboratory data indicating relatively unchanged blood calcium and PTH levels. After an initial loss of bone mass in patients with mild asymptomatic hyperparathyroidism, a new equilibrium may be reached, with bone density and biochemical manifestations of the disease remaining relatively unchanged.

In symptomatic patients, dysfunctions of the CNS, peripheral nerve and muscle, gastrointestinal tract, and joints also occur. It has been reported that severe neuropsychiatric manifestations may be reversed by parathyroidectomy; it remains unclear, in the absence of controlled studies, whether this improvement has a defined cause-and-effect relationship. Generally, the fact that hyperparathyroidism is common in elderly patients, in whom there are often other problems, suggests the possibility that such coexisting problems as hypertension, renal deterioration, and depression may not be parathyroid-related and suggests caution in recommending parathyroid surgery as a cure for these manifestations.

When present, neuromuscular manifestations may include proximal muscle weakness, easy fatigability, and atrophy of muscles and may be so striking as to suggest a primary neuromuscular disorder. The distinguishing feature is the complete regression of neuromuscular disease after surgical correction of the hyperparathyroidism.

Gastrointestinal manifestations are sometimes subtle and include vague abdominal complaints and disorders of the stomach and pancreas. Again, cause and effect are unclear. In MEN 1 patients with hyperparathyroidism, duodenal ulcer may be the result of associated pancreatic tumors that secrete excessive quantities of gastrin (Zollinger-Ellison syndrome). Pancreatitis has been reported in association with hyperparathyroidism, but the incidence and the mechanism are not established.

DIAGNOSIS

The diagnosis is typically made by detecting an elevated immunoreactive PTH level in a patient with asymptomatic hypercalcemia (see "Differential Diagnosis: Special Tests," below). Serum phosphate is usually low but may be normal, especially if renal failure has developed.

Many tests based on renal responses to excess PTH (renal calcium and phosphate clearance; blood phosphate, chloride, magnesium; urinary or nephrogenous cyclic AMP) were used in earlier decades. These tests have low specificity for hyperparathyroidism and are therefore not cost-effective; they have been replaced by PTH immunoassays.

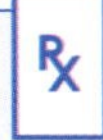

TREATMENT FOR HYPERPARATHYROIDISM

Medical Surveillance versus Surgical Treatment

The critical management question is whether the disease should be treated surgically. If severe hypercalcemia [3.7 to 4.5 mmol/L (15 to 18 mg/dL)] is present, surgery is mandatory as soon as the diagnosis can be confirmed by a PTH immunoassay. However, in most patients with hyperparathyroidism, hypercalcemia is mild and does not require urgent surgical or medical treatment.

The National Institutes of Health (NIH) held a Consensus Conference on Management of Asymptomatic Hyperparathyroidism in 1990. *Asymptomatic hyperparathyroidism* was defined as documented (presumptive) hyperparathyroidism without signs or symptoms attributable to the disease. The consensus was that patients <50 should undergo surgery, given the long surveillance that would be required. Other considerations that favored surgery included concern that consistent follow-up would be unlikely or that coexistent illness would complicate management. Patients >50 were deemed appropriate for medical monitoring if certain criteria were met, the patients wished to avoid surgery, or the guidelines for recommending surgery were not present (**Table 24-2**). Careful evaluation of patients over the subsequent dozen years has both provided reassurance that in some patients medical monitoring rather than surgery is still prudent yet has promoted new questions about the natural history of the disease with or without surgery.

Data developed since the Consensus Conference indicated that a subgroup of patients had selective vertebral osteopenia out of proportion to bone loss at other sites and responded to surgery with striking restoration of bone mass (average >20%). In addition, as much as a 5% increase in bone mineral density in the spine and hip have been reported with alendronate use in asymptomatic hyperparathyroid patients. In light of this new information, the NIH convened a Workshop on Asymptomatic Hyperparathyroidism in 2002, and an independent (non-NIH) panel offered a revised set

TABLE 24-2

GUIDELINES FOR PARATHYROID SURGERY IN ASYMPTOMATIC PRIMARY HYPERPARATHYROIDISM[a]

MEASUREMENT	GUIDELINES, 1990	GUIDELINES, 2002
Serum calcium (above upper limit of normal)	0.3–0.4 mmol/L (1–6 mg/dL)	0.3 mmol/L (1.0 mg/dL)
24-h urinary calcium	>400 mg	>400 mg
Creatinine clearance	Reduced by 30%	Reduced by 30%
Bone mineral density	Z-score <−2.0 (forearm)	T-score <−2.5 at any site
Age	<50	<50

[a]Surgery is also indicated in patients for whom medical surveillance is neither desired nor possible.
Source: From JP Bilezikian et al: J Clin Endocrinol Metab 87:5353, 2002.

of recommendations. The changes reflect both practical considerations (such as the difficulty in creatinine clearance measurements and therefore substituting calculations based on serum creatinine) and concerns regarding potential deleterious skeletal effects in untreated patients (**Tables** 24-2 and **24-3**). Accordingly, indication for surgical intervention was lowered (i.e., stricter serum calcium and bone density criteria). Asymptomatic patients should be monitored regularly. Surgical correction of hyperparathyroidism can always be undertaken when indicated, since the success rate is high (>90%), mortality is low, and morbidity is minimal. The goals of monitoring are early detection of worsening hypercalcemia, deteriorating bone or renal status, or other complications of hyperparathyroidism. No specific recommendations about medical therapy were made, but the promise of the newer agents was stressed, with the prediction that they would be used in clinical practice to increase bone mass in patients not electing surgery as further experience is gained. Neither panel recommended estrogen use in patients for whom surgery was not elected because there was insufficient cumulative experience with such therapy to balance theoretical risks (breast and endometrial cancer) versus benefits. Raloxifene (Evista), the first of the SERMS, has been shown to have many of the bone-protective effects of estrogen in osteoporotic individuals yet at the same time lowers the incidence of breast cancer; preliminary use of this agent in a small series of hyperparathyroid patients led to increased bone density. Experience with calcimimetics, drugs that selectively stimulate the calcium sensor and suppress PTH secretion, indicates that these agents decrease calcium levels to normal and lower PTH levels by at least 50% for >1 year of continuous use.

Surgical Treatment

Parathyroid exploration is challenging and should be undertaken by an experienced surgeon. Certain features help in predicting the pathology (e.g., multiple abnormal glands in familial cases). However, some critical decisions regarding management can be made only during the operation.

As discussed above, there are many unresolved issues to consider in surgery for this disease. One surgical strategy is based on the view that typically only one gland (the adenoma) is abnormal. If an enlarged gland is found, a normal gland should be sought. In this view, if a biopsy of a normal-sized second gland confirms its histologic (and presumed functional) normality, no further exploration, biopsy, or excision is needed. At the other extreme is the minority viewpoint that all four glands be sought and that most of the total parathyroid tissue mass should be removed. The concern with the former approach is that the recurrence rate of hyperparathyroidism may be high if a second abnormal gland is missed; the latter approach could involve unnecessary surgery and an unacceptable rate of hypoparathyroidism. The majority viewpoint favors conservative surgery, i.e., removal of what is usually only one enlarged gland but only after four-gland exploration to eliminate the possibility that more than one gland is abnormal. When normal glands are found in association with one enlarged gland, excision of the single adenoma usually leads to cure or at least years free of symptoms.

TABLE 24-3

MANAGEMENT GUIDELINES FOR PATIENTS WITH ASYMPTOMATIC PRIMARY HYPERPARATHYROIDISM WHO DO NOT UNDERGO PARATHYROID SURGERY

MEASUREMENT	OLDER GUIDELINES	NEW GUIDELINES
Serum calcium	Biannually	Biannually
24-h urinary calcium	Annually	Not recommended[a]
Creatinine clearance	Annually	Not recommended[a]
Serum creatinine	Annually	Annually[b]
Bone density	Annually	Annually (lumber spine, hip, forearm)
Abdominal x-ray (+/− ultrasound)	Annually	Not recommended[a]

[a]Except at the time of initial evaluation.

[b]If the serum creatinine concentration suggests a change in the creatinine clearance when the Cockcroft-Gault equation is applied, further, more direct assessments of the creatinine clearance are recommended.

Source: From JP Bilezikian et al: J Clin Endocrinol Metab 87:5353, 2002.

Long-term follow-up studies are limited to establish true rates of recurrence.

Recently, there has been growing experience with new surgical strategies that feature a minimally invasive approach guided by improved preoperative localization and intraoperative monitoring by PTH assays. Preoperative ^{99m}Tc sestamibi scans with positron emission computed tomography (SPECT) are used to predict the location of an abnormal gland and intraoperative sampling of PTH before and at 5-min intervals after removal of a suspected adenoma to confirm a rapid fall (>50%) to normal levels of PTH. In several centers, a combination of preoperative sestamibi imaging, cervical block anesthesia, minimal surgical incision, and intraoperative PTH measurements has allowed successful outpatient surgical management with a clear-cut cost benefit compared to general anesthesia and more extensive neck surgery. The use of these minimally invasive approaches requires clinical judgment to select patients unlikely to have multiple gland disease (e.g., MEN or secondary hyperparathyroidism). The growing acceptance of the technique and its relative ease for the patient has lowered the threshold for surgery.

When parathyroid carcinoma is encountered, the tissue should be widely excised; care must be taken to avoid rupture of the capsule to prevent local seeding of tumor cells.

Multiple gland hyperplasia, as predicted in familial cases, poses more difficult questions of surgical management. Once a diagnosis of hyperplasia is established, all the glands must be identified. Two schemes have been proposed for surgical management. One is to totally remove three glands with partial excision of the fourth gland; care is taken to leave a good blood supply for the remaining gland. Other surgeons advocate total parathyroidectomy with immediate transplantation of a portion of a removed, minced parathyroid gland into the muscles of the forearm, with the view that surgical excision is easier from the ectopic site in the arm if there is recurrent hyperfunction.

In a minority of cases, if no abnormal parathyroid glands are found in the neck, the issue of further exploration must be decided. There are documented cases of five or six parathyroid glands and of unusual locations for adenomas, such as in the mediastinum.

When a second parathyroid exploration is indicated, the minimally invasive techniques such as ultrasound, CT scan, and isotope scanning may be combined with venous sampling and/or selective digital arteriography in one of the centers specializing in these techniques. Intraoperative monitoring of PTH levels by rapid PTH immunoassays may be useful in guiding the surgery, especially in patients who are reexplored after an initial unsuccessful operation. At one center, long-term cures have been achieved with selective embolization or injection of large amounts of contrast material into the end-arterial circulation feeding the parathyroid tumor.

A decline in serum calcium occurs within 24 h after successful surgery; usually blood calcium falls to low-normal values for 3 to 5 days until the remaining parathyroid tissue resumes hormone secretion. Severe postoperative hypocalcemia is likely only if osteitis fibrosa cystica is present or if injury to all the normal parathyroid glands occurs during surgery. In general, patients with uncomplicated disease such as a single adenoma (the clear majority) who do not have symptomatic bone disease or a large deficit in bone mineral and who have good renal and gastrointestinal function have few problems with postoperative hypocalcemia. The extent of postoperative hypocalcemia varies with the surgical approach. If all glands are biopsied, hypocalcemia may be transiently symptomatic and more prolonged. Hypocalcemia is more likely to be symptomatic after second parathyroid explorations, particularly when normal parathyroid tissue was removed at the initial operation and when the manipulation and/or biopsy of the remaining normal glands is more extensive in the search for the missing adenoma.

Patients with hyperparathyroidism have efficient intestinal calcium absorption due to the increased levels of $1,25(OH)_2D$ stimulated by PTH excess. Once hypocalcemia signifies successful surgery, patients can be put on a high-calcium intake or be given oral calcium supplements. Despite mild hypocalcemia, most patients do not require parenteral therapy. If the serum calcium falls to <2 mmol/L (8 mg/dL), *and if the phosphate level rises simultaneously*, the possibility that surgery has caused hypoparathyroidism must be considered. With unexpected hypocalcemia, coexistent hypomagnesemia should be considered, as it interferes with PTH secretion and causes functional hypoparathyroidism (see below). Signs of hypocalcemia include symptoms such as muscle twitching, a general sense of anxiety, and positive Chvostek and Trousseau signs coupled with serum calcium consistently <2 mmol/L (8 mg/dL). Parenteral calcium replacement at a low level should be instituted when hypocalcemia is symptomatic. The rate and duration of intravenous therapy are determined by the severity of the symptoms and the response of the serum calcium to treatment. An infusion of 0.5 to 2 (mg/kg)/h or 30 to 100 mL/h of a 1-mg/mL solution usually suffices to relieve symptoms. Usually, parenteral therapy is required for only a few days. If symptoms worsen or if parenteral calcium is needed for >2 to 3 days, therapy with a vitamin D analogue and/or oral calcium (2 to 4 g/d) should be started (see below). It is cost-effective to use calcitriol (doses of 0.5 to 1.0 μg/d) because of the rapidity of onset of effect and prompt cessation of action when stopped, in comparison to other forms of vitamin D (see below). A rise in blood calcium after several months of vitamin D replacement may indicate restoration of parathyroid function to normal. It is also appropriate to monitor serum PTH serially to estimate gland function in such patients.

Magnesium deficiency may also complicate the postoperative course. Magnesium deficiency impairs the secretion of PTH, and so hypomagnesemia should be corrected whenever detected. Magnesium chloride is effective by mouth, but this compound is not widely available. Repletion is usually parenteral. Because the depressant effect of magnesium on central and peripheral nerve functions does not occur at levels <2 mmol/L (normal range 0.8 to 1.2 mmol/L), parenteral replacement can be given rapidly. A cumulative dose as great as 0.5 to 1 mmol/kg of body weight can be administered if severe hypomagnesemia is present; often, however, total doses of 20 to 40 mmol are sufficient. The magnesium is given either as an intravenous infusion over 8 to 12 h or in divided doses intramuscularly (magnesium sulfate, USP).

OTHER PARATHYROID-RELATED CAUSES OF HYPERCALCEMIA

Lithium Therapy

Lithium, used in the management of bipolar depression and other psychiatric disorders, causes hypercalcemia in ~10% of treated patients. The hypercalcemia is dependent on continued lithium treatment, remitting and recurring when lithium is stopped and restarted. The parathyroid adenomas reported in some hypercalcemic patients with lithium therapy may reflect the presence of an independently occurring parathyroid tumor; a permanent effect of lithium on parathyroid gland growth need not be implicated as most patients have complete reversal of hypercalcemia when lithium is stopped. However, long-standing stimulation of parathyroid cell replication by lithium may predispose to development of adenomas (as is documented in secondary hyperparathyroidism and renal failure).

At the levels achieved in blood in treated patients, lithium can be shown in vitro to shift the PTH secretion curve to the right in response to calcium; i.e., higher calcium levels are required to lower PTH secretion, probably acting at the calcium sensor (see below); this effect can cause elevated PTH levels and consequent hypercalcemia in otherwise normal individuals. Fortunately, there are alternative medications for the underlying psychiatric illness. Parathyroid surgery should not be recommended unless hypercalcemia and elevated PTH levels persist after lithium is discontinued.

GENETIC DISORDERS CAUSING HYPERPARATHYROID-LIKE SYNDROMES

Familial Hypocalciuric Hypercalcemia

FHH (also called *familial benign hypercalcemia*) is inherited as an autosomal dominant trait. Affected individuals are discovered because of asymptomatic hypercalcemia. This disorder and Jansen's disease (discussed below) are variants of hyperparathyroidism. FHH involves excessive secretion of PTH, whereas Jansen's disease is caused by excessive biologic activity of the PTH receptor in target tissues. Neither disorder, however, involves a primary growth disorder of the parathyroids.

The pathophysiology of FHH is now understood. The primary defect is abnormal sensing of the blood calcium by the parathyroid gland and renal tubule, causing inappropriate secretion of PTH and excessive renal reabsorption of calcium. The calcium sensor is a member of the third family of GPCRs (type C, or III). The receptor responds to the ECF calcium concentration, suppressing PTH secretion through second messenger signaling, thereby providing negative-feedback regulation of PTH secretion. Many different mutations in the calcium-sensing receptor have been identified in patients with FHH (**Fig. 24-4**). These mutations lower the capacity of the sensor to bind calcium, and the mutant receptors function as though blood calcium levels were low; excessive secretion of PTH occurs from an otherwise normal gland. Approximately two-thirds of patients with FHH have mutations within the protein-coding region of the gene. The remaining one-third of kindreds may have mutations in the gene promoter or may involve still unknown mechanisms in other regions of the genome identified through mapping studies (e.g., chromosome 19).

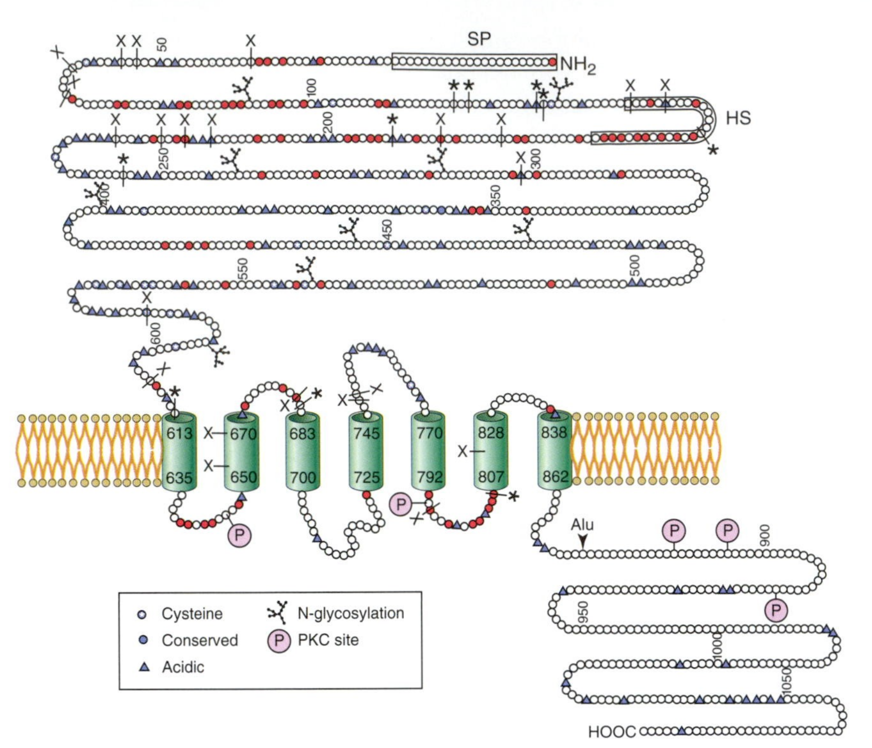

FIGURE 24-4
Mutations in the calcium sensor receptor. The extracellular domain binds calcium, leading to conformational changes that stimulate Gq-coupled activation of the phospholipase C and suppression of PTH. The identified sequence alterations (X) cause loss of function and lead to inadequate suppression of parathyroid hormone release and, therefore, mild hypercalcemia (FHH); *, a gain-of-function mutation that causes hypocalcemia; ●, conserved residues; ▲, acidic residues. (*From EM Brown et al: J Nutr 125:1965S, 1995, with permission.*)

Even before elucidation of the pathophysiology of FHH, abundant clinical evidence served to separate the disorder from primary hyperparathyroidism. Patients with primary hyperparathyroidism have <99% renal calcium reabsorption, whereas most patients with FHH have >99% reabsorption. The hypercalcemia in FHH is often detectable in affected members of the kindreds in the first decade of life, whereas hypercalcemia rarely occurs in patients with primary hyperparathyroidism or the MEN syndromes who are <10. PTH may be elevated in FHH, but the values are usually normal or lower for the same degree of calcium elevation than in patients with primary hyperparathyroidism. Parathyroid surgery in a few patients with FHH led to permanent hypoparathyroidism, but hypocalciuria persisted nevertheless, establishing that hypocalciuria, therefore, is not PTH-dependent (now known to be due to the abnormal calcium sensor in the kidney).

Few clinical signs or symptoms are present in patients with FHH, and other endocrine abnormalities are not present. Most patients are detected as a result of family screening after hypercalcemia is detected in a proband. In those patients inadvertently operated upon, the parathyroids appeared normal or moderately hyperplastic. Parathyroid surgery is not appropriate, nor, in view of the lack of symptoms, does medical treatment seem needed to lower the calcium. Calcimimetic agents that bind to the calcium sensor and elevate the set point are under investigation.

One striking exception to the rule against parathyroid surgery in this syndrome is the occurrence, usually in consanguineous marriages (due to the rarity of the gene mutation), of a homozygous or compound heterozygote state, resulting in complete loss of the calcium sensor function. In this condition, neonatal severe hypercalcemia, total parathyroidectomy is mandatory.

Jansen's Disease

Mutations in the PTH1R have been identified as responsible for this rare autosomal dominant syndrome (Fig. 24-4). Because the mutations lead to constitutive receptor function, one abnormal copy of the mutant receptor is sufficient to cause the disease, thereby accounting for its dominant mode of transmission. The disorder leads to short-limbed dwarfism due to abnormal regulation of the bone growth plate. In adult life, there are numerous abnormalities in bone, including multiple cystic resorptive areas resembling those seen in severe hyperparathyroidism. Hypercalcemia and hypophosphatemia with undetectable or low PTH levels are typically seen. The pathogenesis of the disease has been confirmed by transgenic experiments in which targeted expression of the mutant receptor to the growth plate emulated several features of the disorder.

MALIGNANCY-RELATED HYPERCALCEMIA

Clinical Syndromes and Mechanisms of Hypercalcemia

Hypercalcemia due to malignancy is common (occurring with 10 to 15% of certain types of tumor, such as lung carcinoma), often severe and difficult to manage, and occasionally difficult to distinguish from primary hyperparathyroidism. Although malignancy is often clinically obvious or readily detectable by medical history, hypercalcemia can occasionally be due to an occult tumor. Previously, hypercalcemia associated with malignancy was thought to be due to local invasion and destruction of bone by tumor cells; many cases are now known to result from the elaboration by the malignant cells of humoral mediators of hypercalcemia. PTHrP is the responsible humoral agent in most solid tumors that cause hypercalcemia.

The histologic character of the tumor is more important than the extent of skeletal metastases in predicting hypercalcemia. Small-cell carcinoma (oat cell) and adenocarcinoma of the lung, although the most common lung tumors associated with skeletal metastases, rarely cause hypercalcemia. By contrast, as many as 10% of patients with squamous cell carcinoma of the lung develop hypercalcemia. Histologic studies of bone in patients with squamous cell or epidermoid carcinoma of the lung, in sites invaded by tumor as well as areas remote from tumor invasion, reveal increased bone remodeling, including osteoclastic and osteoblastic activity.

Two main mechanisms of hypercalcemia are operative in cancer hypercalcemia. Many solid tumors associated with hypercalcemia, particularly squamous cell and renal tumors, produce and secrete PTHrP that causes increased bone resorption and mediate the hypercalcemia through systemic actions on the skeleton. Alternatively, direct bone marrow invasion occurs with hematologic malignancies such as leukemia, lymphoma, and multiple myeloma. Lymphokines and cytokines produced by cells involved in the marrow response to the tumors promote resorption of bone through local destruction. Several hormones, hormone analogues, cytokines, and growth factors have been implicated as the result of clinical assays, in vitro tests, or chemical isolation. The etiologic factor produced by activated normal lymphocytes and by myeloma and lymphoma cells, termed *osteoclast activation factor*, now appears to represent the biologic action of several different cytokines, probably interleukin 1 and lymphotoxin or tumor necrosis factor. In some lymphomas, typically B cell lymphomas, there is a third mechanism, caused by an increased blood level of $1,25(OH)_2D$, which is probably produced by lymphocytes.

In the more common mechanism, usually termed *humoral hypercalcemia of malignancy*, solid tumors (cancers of the lung and kidney, in particular), in which bone metastases are absent, minimal, or not detectable clinically, secrete PTHrP measurable by immunoassay. Secretion by the tumors of the PTH-like factor, PTHrP, activates the PTH1R, resulting in a pathophysiology closely resembling hyperparathyroidism. The clinical picture resembles primary hyperparathyroidism (hypophosphatemia accompanies hypercalcemia), and elimination or regression of the primary tumor leads to disappearance of the hypercalcemia.

As in hyperparathyroidism, patients with the humoral hypercalcemia of malignancy have elevated urinary nephrogenous cyclic AMP excretion, hypophosphatemia, and increased urinary phosphate clearance. However, in humoral hypercalcemia of malignancy, immunoreactive PTH is undetectable or suppressed, making the differential diagnosis easier. Other features of the disorder differ from those of true hyperparathyroidism. Patients may have high, rather than low, renal calcium clearance (relative to serum calcium when compared to true hyperparathyroidism, unlike the expected elevation) and low to normal levels of $1,25(OH)_2D$. The reason that the humoral syndrome differs from hyperparathyroidism in these parameters is unclear since the biologic actions of PTH and PTHrP are presumably exerted through the same receptor. Other cytokines elaborated by the malignancy may be responsible for these variations from hyperparathyroidism. In some patients with the humoral hypercalcemia of malignancy, osteoclastic resorption is unaccompanied by an osteoblastic or bone-forming response, implying inhibition of the normal coupling of bone formation and resorption. Thus the interaction of more than one substance may determine whether hypercalcemia develops in a particular patient.

Several different assays (single- or double-antibody, different epitopes) have been developed to detect PTHrP. Most data indicate that circulating PTHrP levels are undetectable (or low) in normal individuals, elevated in most cancer patients with the humoral syndrome, and high in human milk. The etiologic mechanisms in cancer hypercalcemia may be multiple in the same patient. For example, in breast carcinoma (metastatic to bone) and in a distinctive type of T cell lymphoma/leukemia initiated by human T cell lymphotropic virus I, hypercalcemia is caused by direct local lysis of bone as well as by a humoral mechanism involving excess production of PTHrP.

Diagnostic Issues

Levels of PTH measured by the double-antibody technique are undetectable or extremely low in tumor hypercalcemia, as would be expected with the mediation of the hypercalcemia by a factor other than PTH (the hypercalcemia suppresses the normal parathyroid glands). In a patient with minimal symptoms referred for hypercalcemia, low or undetectable PTH levels would focus attention on a possible occult malignancy.

Ordinarily, the diagnosis of cancer hypercalcemia is not difficult because tumor symptoms are prominent when hypercalcemia is detected. Indeed, hypercalcemia may be noted incidentally during the workup of a patient with known or suspected malignancy. Clinical suspicion that malignancy is the cause of the hypercalcemia is heightened when there are other paraneoplastic signs or symptoms, such as weight loss, fatigue, muscle weakness, or unexplained skin rash, or when symptoms specific for a particular tumor are present. Squamous cell tumors are most frequently associated with hypercalcemia, particularly tumors of the lung, kidney, head and neck, and urogenital tract. Radiologic examinations can focus on these areas when clinical evidence is unclear. Bone scans with technetium-labeled bisphosphonate are useful for detection of osteolytic metastases; the sensitivity is high, but specificity is low; results must be confirmed by conventional x-rays to be certain that areas of increased uptake are due to osteolytic metastases per se. Bone marrow biopsies are helpful in patients with anemia or abnormal peripheral blood smears.

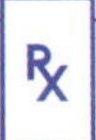

TREATMENT FOR HYPERCALCEMIA

Treatment for the hypercalcemia of malignancy is first directed to control of tumor; reduction of tumor mass usually corrects hypercalcemia. If a patient has severe hypercalcemia yet has a good chance for effective tumor therapy, treatment of the hypercalcemia should be vigorous while awaiting the results of definitive therapy. If hypercalcemia occurs in the late stages of a tumor that is resistant to anti-tumor therapy, the treatment for the hypercalcemia should be judicious as high calcium levels can have a mild sedating effect. Standard therapies for hypercalcemia (discussed below) are applicable to patients with malignancy.

VITAMIN D–RELATED HYPERCALCEMIA

Hypercalcemia caused by vitamin D can be due to excessive ingestion or abnormal metabolism of the vitamin. Abnormal metabolism of the vitamin is usually acquired in association with a widespread granulomatous disorder. Vitamin D metabolism is carefully regulated, particularly the activity of renal 1α-hydroxylase, the enzyme responsible for the production of 1,25$(OH)_2$D (Chap. 23). The regulation of 1α-hydroxylase and the normal feedback suppression by 1,25$(OH)_2$D seem to work less well in infants than in adults and to operate poorly, if at all, in sites other than the renal tubule; these phenomena explain the occurrence of hypercalcemia secondary to excessive 1,25$(OH)_2D_3$ production in infants with Williams' syndrome (see below) and in adults with sarcoidosis or lymphoma.

Vitamin D Intoxication

Chronic ingestion of 50 to 100 times the normal physiologic requirement of vitamin D (amounts >50,000 to 100,000 U/d) is usually required to produce significant hypercalcemia in normal individuals. An upper limit of dietary intake of 2000 U/d (50 μg/d) in adults is now recommended because of concerns about potential toxic effects of cumulative supraphysiologic doses. Vitamin D excess increases intestinal calcium absorption and, if severe, also increases bone resorption.

Hypercalcemia in vitamin D intoxication is due to an excessive biologic action of the vitamin, perhaps the consequence of increased levels of 25(OH)D rather than merely increased levels of the active metabolite 1,25$(OH)_2$D (the latter may not be elevated in vitamin D intoxication). 25(OH)D has definite, if low, biologic activity in intestine and bone. The production of 25(OH)D is less tightly regulated than is the production of 1,25$(OH)_2$D. Hence concentrations of 25(OH)D are elevated several-fold in patients with excess vitamin D intake.

The diagnosis is substantiated by documenting elevated levels of 25(OH)D $>$ 100 ng/mL. Hypercalcemia is usually controlled by restriction of dietary calcium intake and appropriate attention to hydration. These measures, plus discontinuation of vitamin D, usually lead to resolution of hypercalcemia. However, vitamin D stores in fat may be substantial, and vitamin D intoxication may persist for weeks after vitamin D ingestion is terminated. Such patients are responsive to glucocorticoids, which in doses of 100 mg/d of hydrocortisone or its equivalent, usually return serum calcium levels to normal over several days; severe intoxication may require intensive therapy.

Sarcoidosis and Other Granulomatous Diseases

In patients with sarcoidosis and other granulomatous diseases, such as tuberculosis and fungal infections, excess 1,25$(OH)_2$D is synthesized in macrophages or other cells in the granulomas. Indeed, increased 1,25$(OH)_2$D levels have been reported in anephric patients with sarcoidosis and hypercalcemia. Macrophages obtained from granulomatous tissue convert 25(OH)D to 1,25$(OH)_2$D at an increased rate. There is a positive correlation in patients with sarcoidosis between 25(OH)D levels (reflecting vitamin D intake) and the circulating concentrations of 1,25$(OH)_2$D, whereas normally there is no increase in 1,25$(OH)_2$D with increasing 25(OH)D levels due to multiple feedback controls on renal 1α-hydroxylase (Chap. 23). The usual regulation of active metabolite production by calcium or PTH does not operate in these patients; hypercalcemia does not lead to a reduction in the blood levels of

$1,25(OH)_2D$ in patients with sarcoidosis. Clearance of $1,25(OH)_2D$ from blood may be decreased in sarcoidosis as well. PTH levels are usually low and $1,25(OH)_2D$ levels are elevated, but primary hyperparathyroidism and sarcoidosis may coexist in some patients.

Management of the hypercalcemia can often be accomplished by avoiding excessive sunlight exposure and limiting vitamin D and calcium intake. Presumably, however, the abnormal sensitivity to vitamin D and abnormal regulation of $1,25(OH)_2D$ synthesis will persist as long as the disease is active. Alternatively, glucocorticoids in the equivalent of $\leq$100 mg/d of hydrocortisone control hypercalcemia. Glucocorticoids appear to act by blocking excessive production of $1,25(OH)_2D$ as well as the response to it in target organs.

Idiopathic Hypercalcemia of Infancy

This rare disorder, usually referred to as *Williams' syndrome*, is an autosomal dominant disorder characterized by multiple congenital development defects, including supravalvular aortic stenosis, mental retardation, and an elfin facies, in association with hypercalcemia due to abnormal sensitivity to vitamin D. The syndrome was first recognized in England after the fortification of milk with vitamin D. Levels of $1,25(OH)_2D$ are elevated, ranging from 46 to 120 nmol/L (150 to 500 pg/mL). The mechanism of the abnormal sensitivity to vitamin D and of the increased circulating levels of $1,25(OH)_2D$ is still unclear. Studies suggest that mutations involving the elastin locus and perhaps other genes on chromosome 7 may play a role in the pathogenesis.

HYPERCALCEMIA ASSOCIATED WITH HIGH BONE TURNOVER

Hyperthyroidism

As many as 20% of hyperthyroid patients have high-normal or mildly elevated serum calcium concentrations; hypercalciuria is even more common. The hypercalcemia is due to increased bone turnover, with bone resorption exceeding bone formation. Severe calcium elevations are not typical, and the presence of such suggests a concomitant disease such as hyperparathyroidism. Usually, the diagnosis is obvious, but signs of hyperthyroidism may occasionally be occult, particularly in the elderly (Chap. 4). Hypercalcemia is managed by treatment of the hyperthyroidism.

Immobilization

Immobilization is a rare cause of hypercalcemia in adults in the absence of an associated disease but may cause hypercalcemia in children and adolescents, particularly after spinal cord injury and paraplegia or quadriplegia. With resumption of ambulation, the hypercalcemia in children usually returns to normal.

The mechanism appears to involve a disproportion between bone formation and bone resorption. Hypercalciuria and increased mobilization of skeletal calcium can develop in normal volunteers subjected to extensive bed rest, although hypercalcemia is unusual. Immobilization of an adult with a disease associated with high bone turnover, however, such as Paget's disease, may cause hypercalcemia.

Thiazides

Administration of benzothiadiazines (thiazides) can cause hypercalcemia in patients with high rates of bone turnover, such as patients with hypoparathyroidism treated with high doses of vitamin D. Traditionally, thiazides are associated with aggravation of hypercalcemia in primary hyperparathyroidism, but this effect can be seen in other high-bone-turnover states as well. The mechanism of thiazide action is complex. Chronic thiazide administration leads to reduction in urinary calcium; the hypocalciuric effect appears to reflect the enhancement of proximal tubular resorption of sodium and calcium in response to sodium depletion. Some of this renal effect is due to augmentation of PTH action and is more pronounced in individuals with intact PTH secretion. However, thiazides cause hypocalciuria in hypoparathyroid patients on high-dose vitamin D and oral calcium replacement if sodium intake is restricted. This finding is the rationale for the use of thiazides as an adjunct to therapy in hypoparathyroid patients, as discussed below. Thiazide administration to normal individuals causes a transient increase in blood calcium (usually within the high-normal range) that reverts to preexisting levels after a week or more of continued administration. If hormonal function and calcium and bone metabolism are normal, homeostatic controls are reset to counteract the calcium-elevating effect of the thiazides. In the presence of hyperparathyroidism or increased bone turnover from another cause, homeostatic mechanisms are ineffective. The abnormal effects of the thiazide on calcium metabolism disappear within days of cessation of the drug.

Vitamin A Intoxication

Vitamin A intoxication is a rare cause of hypercalcemia and is most commonly a side effect of dietary faddism. Calcium levels can be elevated into the 3 to 3.5 mmol/L (12 to 14 mg/dL) range after the ingestion of 50,000 to 100,000 units of vitamin A daily (10 to 20 times the minimum daily requirement). Typical features of severe hypercalcemia include fatigue, anorexia, and, in some, severe muscle and bone pain. Excess vitamin A intake is presumed to increase bone resorption.

The diagnosis can be established by history and by measurement of vitamin A levels in serum. Occasionally, skeletal x-rays reveal periosteal calcifications, particularly in the hands. Withdrawal of the vitamin is usually associated with prompt disappearance of the hypercalcemia and reversal of the skeletal changes. As in vitamin D intoxication, administration of 100 mg/d hydrocortisone or its equivalent leads to a rapid return of the serum calcium to normal.

HYPERCALCEMIA ASSOCIATED WITH RENAL FAILURE

Severe Secondary Hyperparathyroidism

Secondary hyperparathyroidism occurs when partial resistance to the metabolic actions of PTH leads to excessive production of the hormone. Parathyroid gland hyperplasia occurs because resistance to the normal level of PTH leads to hypocalcemia, which, in turn, is a stimulus to parathyroid gland enlargement.

Secondary hyperparathyroidism occurs not only in patients with renal failure but also in those with osteomalacia due to multiple causes (Chap. 23), including deficiency of vitamin D action, and PHP (deficient response to PTH at the level of the receptor). Hypocalcemia seems to be the common denominator in initiating secondary hyperparathyroidism. Primary and secondary hyperparathyroidism can be distinguished conceptually by the autonomous growth of the parathyroid glands in primary hyperparathyroidism (presumably irreversible) and the adaptive response of the parathyroids in secondary hyperparathyroidism (typically reversible). In fact, reversal over weeks from an abnormal pattern of secretion, presumably accompanied by involution of parathyroid gland mass to normal, occurs in patients who have been treated effectively to reverse the resistance to PTH (such as with calcium and vitamin D in osteomalacia).

Patients with secondary hyperparathyroidism may develop bone pain, ectopic calcification, and pruritus. The bone disease seen in patients with secondary hyperparathyroidism and renal failure is termed *renal osteodystrophy*. Osteomalacia (predominantly due to vitamin D and calcium deficiency) and/or osteitis fibrosa cystica (excessive PTH action on bone) may occur.

Two other skeletal disorders are associated with long-term dialysis in patients with renal failure. Aluminum deposition (see below) is associated with an osteomalacia-like picture. The other entity is a low-bone-turnover state termed "aplastic" or "adynamic" bone disease; PTH levels are lower than in typical secondary hyperparathyroidism. It is believed that the condition is caused, at least in part, by excessive PTH suppression, which may be even greater than previously appreciated in light of evidence that some of the immunoreactive PTH detected by most commercially available PTH assays is not the full-length biologically active molecule (as discussed above).

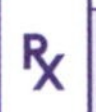

TREATMENT FOR SECONDARY HYPERPARATHYROIDISM

Medical therapy to reverse secondary hyperparathyroidism includes reduction of excessive blood phosphate by restriction of dietary phosphate, the use of nonabsorbable antacids, and careful, selective addition of calcitriol (0.25 to 2.0 μg/d); calcium carbonate is preferred over aluminum-containing antacids to prevent aluminum toxicity. Intravenous calcitriol, administered as several pulses each week, helps control secondary hyperparathyroidism. Aggressive but carefully administered medical therapy can often, but not always, reverse hyperparathyroidism and its symptoms and manifestations.

Occasional patients develop severe manifestations of secondary hyperparathyroidism, including hypercalcemia, pruritus, extraskeletal calcifications, and painful bones, despite aggressive medical efforts to suppress the hyperparathyroidism. PTH hypersecretion no longer responsive to medical therapy, a state of severe hyperparathyroidism in patients with renal failure that requires surgery, has been referred to as *tertiary hyperparathyroidism*. Parathyroid surgery is necessary to control this condition. Based on genetic evidence from examination of tumor samples in these patients, the emergence of autonomous parathyroid function is due to a monoclonal outgrowth of one or more previously hyperplastic parathyroid glands. The adaptive response has become an independent contributor to disease; this finding seems to emphasize the importance of optimal medical management to reduce the proliferative response of the parathyroid cells that enables the irreversible genetic change.

Aluminum Intoxication

Aluminum intoxication (and often hypercalcemia as a complication of medical treatment) may occur in patients on chronic dialysis; manifestations include acute dementia and unresponsive and severe osteomalacia. Bone pain, multiple nonhealing fractures, particularly of the ribs and pelvis, and a proximal myopathy may occur. Hypercalcemia develops when these patients are treated with vitamin D or calcitriol because of impaired skeletal responsiveness. Aluminum is present at the site of osteoid mineralization, osteoblastic activity is minimal, and calcium incorporation into the skeleton is impaired. Prevention is accomplished by avoidance of aluminum excess in the dialysis regimen; treatment of established disease involves mobilizing aluminum through the use of the chelating agent deferoxamine.

Milk-Alkali Syndrome

The milk-alkali syndrome is due to excessive ingestion of calcium and absorbable antacids such as milk or calcium carbonate. It is much less frequent since nonabsorbable antacids and other treatments became available for peptic ulcer disease. However, the increased use of calcium carbonate in the management of osteoporosis has led to reappearance of the syndrome. Several clinical presentations—acute, subacute, and chronic—have been described, all of which feature hypercalcemia, alkalosis, and renal failure. The chronic form of the disease, termed *Burnett's syndrome*, is associated with irreversible renal damage. The acute syndromes reverse if the excess calcium and absorbable alkali are stopped.

Individual susceptibility is important in the pathogenesis, as many patients are treated with calcium carbonate alkali regimens without developing the syndrome. One variable is the fractional calcium absorption as a function of calcium intake. Some individuals absorb a high fraction of calcium, even with intakes as high as 2 g or more of elemental calcium per day, instead of reducing calcium absorption with high intake, as occurs in most normal individuals. Resultant mild hypercalcemia after meals in such patients is postulated to contribute to the generation of alkalosis. Development of hypercalcemia causes increased sodium excretion and some depletion of total-body water. These phenomena and perhaps some suppression of endogenous PTH secretion due to mild hypercalcemia lead to increased bicarbonate resorption and to alkalosis in the face of continued calcium carbonate ingestion. Alkalosis per se selectively enhances calcium resorption in the distal nephron, thus aggravating the hypercalcemia. The cycle of mild hypercalcemia → bicarbonate retention → alkalosis → renal calcium retention → severe hypercalcemia perpetuates and aggravates hypercalcemia and alkalosis as long as calcium and absorbable alkali are ingested.

DIFFERENTIAL DIAGNOSIS: SPECIAL TESTS

Differential diagnosis of hypercalcemia is best achieved by using clinical criteria, but the immunoassay for PTH is especially useful in distinguishing among major causes (**Fig. 24-5**). The clinical features that deserve emphasis are the presence or absence of symptoms or signs of disease and evidence of chronicity. If one discounts fatigue or depression, >90% of patients with primary hyperparathyroidism

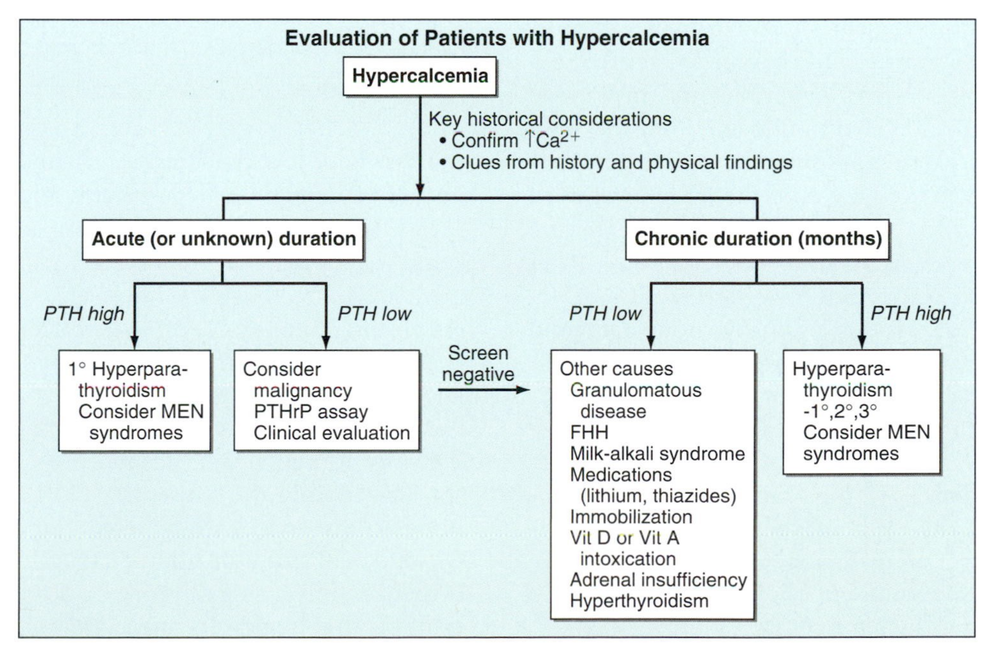

FIGURE 24-5

Algorithm for the evaluation of patients with hypercalcemia. See text for details. FHH, familial hypocalciuric hypercalcemia; MEN, multiple endocrine neoplasia; PTH, parathyroid hormone; PTHrP, parathyroid hormone–related peptide.

have *asymptomatic hypercalcemia;* symptoms of malignancy are usually present in cancer-associated hypercalcemia. Disorders other than hyperparathyroidism and malignancy cause <10% of cases of hypercalcemia, and some of the nonparathyroid causes are associated with clear-cut manifestations such as renal failure.

Hyperparathyroidism is the likely diagnosis in patients with *chronic hypercalcemia*. If hypercalcemia has been manifest for >1 year, malignancy can usually be excluded as the cause. A striking feature of malignancy-associated hypercalcemia is the rapidity of the course, whereby signs and symptoms of the underlying malignancy are evident within months of the detection of hypercalcemia. Although clinical considerations are helpful in arriving at the correct diagnosis of the cause of hypercalcemia, appropriate laboratory testing is essential for definitive diagnosis. The immunoassay for PTH should separate hyperparathyroidism from all other causes of hypercalcemia. Patients with hyperparathyroidism have elevated PTH levels despite hypercalcemia, whereas patients with malignancy and the other causes of hypercalcemia (except for disorders mediated by PTH such as lithium-induced hypercalcemia) have levels of hormone below normal or undetectable. Assays based on the double-antibody method for PTH exhibit very high sensitivity (especially if serum calcium is simultaneously evaluated) and specificity for the diagnosis of primary hyperparathyroidism (**Fig. 24-6**).

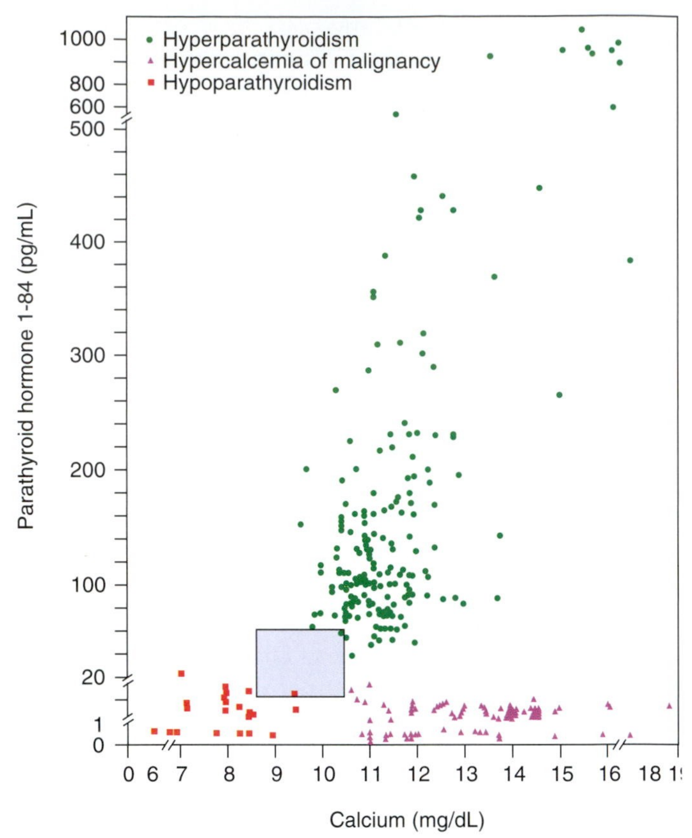

FIGURE 24-6

Levels of immunoreactive parathyroid hormone (PTH) detected in patients with primary hyperparathyroidism, hypercalcemia of malignancy, and hypoparathyroidism. Boxed area represents the upper and normal limits of blood calcium and/or immunoreactive PTH. [*From SR Nussbaum, JT Potts, Jr, in L DeGroot, JL Jameson (eds): Endocrinology, 4th ed. Philadelphia, Saunders, 2001, with permission.*]

In summary, PTH values are elevated in >90% of parathyroid-related causes of hypercalcemia, undetectable or low in malignancy-related hypercalcemia, and undetectable or normal in vitamin D–related and high-bone-turnover causes of hypercalcemia. In view of the specificity of the PTH immunoassay and the high frequency of hyperparathyroidism in hypercalcemic patients, it is cost-effective to measure the PTH level in all hypercalcemic patients unless malignancy or a specific nonparathyroid disease is obvious. False-positive PTH assay results are rare. There are very rare reports of ectopic production of excess PTH by nonparathyroid tumors. Immunoassays for PTHrP are helpful in diagnosing certain types of malignancy-associated hypercalcemia. Although FHH is parathyroid-related, the disease should be managed distinctively from hyperparathyroidism. Clinical features and the low urinary calcium excretion can help make the distinction. Because the incidence of malignancy and hyperparathyroidism both increase with age, they can coexist as two independent causes of hypercalcemia.

$1,25(OH)_2D$ levels are elevated in many (but not all) patients with primary hyperparathyroidism. In other disorders associated with hypercalcemia, concentrations of $1,25(OH)_2D$ are low or, at the most, normal. However, this test is of low specificity and is not cost-effective, as not all patients with hyperparathyroidism have elevated $1,25(OH)_2D$ levels, and not all nonparathyroid hypercalcemic patients have suppressed $1,25(OH)_2D$. Measurement of $1,25(OH)_2D$ is, however, critically valuable in establishing the cause of hypercalcemia in sarcoidosis and certain B cell lymphomas.

A useful general approach is outlined in Fig. 24-5. If the patient is *asymptomatic* and there is evidence of *chronicity* to the hypercalcemia, hyperparathyroidism is almost certainly the cause. If PTH levels (usually measured at least twice) are elevated, the clinical impression is confirmed and little additional evaluation is necessary. If there is only a short history or no data as to the duration of the hypercalcemia, *occult malignancy* must be considered; if the PTH levels are not elevated, then a thorough workup must be undertaken for malignancy, including chest x-ray, CT of chest and abdomen, and bone scan. Immunoassays for PTHrP may be especially useful in such situations. Attention should also be paid to clues for underlying hematologic disorders such as anemia, increased plasma globulin, and abnormal serum immunoelectrophoresis; bone scans can be negative in some patients with metastases, such as in multiple myeloma. Finally, if a patient with chronic hypercalcemia is asymptomatic and malignancy therefore seems unlikely on clinical grounds, but PTH values are not elevated, it is useful to search for other chronic causes of hypercalcemia, such as occult sarcoidosis. A careful history of dietary supplements and drug use may suggest intoxication with vitamin D or vitamin A or the use of thiazides.

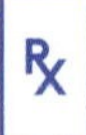

TREATMENT FOR HYPERCALCEMIA

Hypercalcemic States

The approach to medical treatment of hypercalcemia varies with its severity (**Table 24-4**). Mild hypercalcemia, <3.0 mmol/L (12 mg/dL), can be managed by hydration. More severe hypercalcemia [levels of 3.2 to 3.7 mmol/L (13 to 15 mg/dL)] must be managed aggressively; above that level, hypercalcemia can be life-threatening and requires emergency measures. By using a combination of

TABLE 24-4

THERAPIES FOR SEVERE HYPERCALCEMIA

TREATMENT	ONSET OF ACTION	DURATION OF ACTION	ADVANTAGES	DISADVANTAGES
		MOST USEFUL THERAPIES		
Hydration with saline	Hours	During infusion	Rehydration invariably needed	Volume overload, cardiac decompensation, intensive monitoring, electrolyte disturbance, inconvenience
Forced diuresis; saline plus loop diuretic	Hours	During treatment	Rapid action	
Bisphosphonates 1st generation: etidronate	1–2 days	5–7 days in doses used	First available bisphosphonate; intermediate onset of action	Less effective than other bisphosphonates
2d generation: pamidronate	1–2 days	10–14 days to weeks	High potency; intermediate onset of action	Fever in 20% hypophosphatemia, hypocalcemia, hypomagnesemia
3d generation: zolendronate	1–2 days	> 3 weeks	High potency; rapid infusion; prolonged duration of action	Minor; fever, rarely hypocalcemia or hypophosphatemia
Calcitonin	Hours	1–2 days	Rapid onset of action; useful as adjunct in severe hypercalcemia	Rapid tachyphylaxis
		SPECIAL USE THERAPIES		
Phosphate Oral	24 h	During use	Chronic management (with hypophosphatemia); low toxicity if P < 4 mg/dL	Limited use except as adjuvant or chronic therapy
Intravenous	Hours	During use and 24–48 h afterward	Rapid action, highly potent but *rarely used* except with severe hypercalcemia and cardiac and renal decompensation present	Ectopic calcification; renal damage, fatal hypocalcemia
Glucocorticoids	Days	Days, weeks	Oral therapy, antitumor agent	Active only in certain malignancies; glucocorticoid side effects
Dialysis	Hours	During use and 24–48 h afterward	Useful in renal failure; onset of effect in hours; can immediately reverse life-threatening hypercalcemia	Complex procedure, reserved for extreme or special circumstances

approaches in severe hypercalcemia, the serum calcium concentration can be decreased by 0.7 to 2.2 mmol/L (3 to 9 mg/dL) within 24 to 48 h in most patients, enough to relieve acute symptoms, prevent death from hypercalcemic crisis, and permit diagnostic evaluation. Therapy can then be directed at the underlying disorder—the second priority.

Hypercalcemia develops because of excessive skeletal calcium release, increased intestinal calcium absorption, or inadequate renal calcium excretion. Understanding the particular pathogenesis helps guide therapy. For example, hypercalcemia in patients with malignancy is primarily due to excessive skeletal calcium release and is, therefore, minimally improved by restriction of dietary calcium. On the other hand, patients with vitamin D hypersensitivity or vitamin D intoxication have excessive intestinal calcium absorption, and restriction of dietary calcium is beneficial. Decreased renal function or ECF depletion decreases urinary calcium excretion. In such situations, rehydration may rapidly reduce or reverse the hypercalcemia, even though increased bone resorption persists. As outlined below, the more severe the hypercalcemia, the greater the number of combined therapies that should be used. Rapid acting (hours) approaches—rehydration, forced diuresis, and calcitonin—can be used with the most effective antiresorptive agents, such as bisphosphonates (since severe hypercalcemia usually involves excessive bone resorption).

HYDRATION, INCREASED SALT INTAKE, MILD AND FORCED DIURESIS

The first principle of treatment is to restore normal hydration. Many hypercalcemic patients are dehydrated because of vomiting, inanition, and/or hypercalcemia-induced defects in urinary concentrating ability. The resultant drop in glomerular filtration rate is accompanied by an additional decrease in renal tubular sodium and calcium clearance. Restoring a normal ECF volume corrects these abnormalities and increases urine calcium excretion by 2.5 to 7.5 mmol/d (100 to 300 mg/d). Increasing urinary sodium excretion to 400 to 500 mmol/d increases urinary calcium excretion even further than simple rehydration. After rehydration has been achieved, saline can be administered or furosemide or ethacrynic acid can be given twice daily to depress the tubular reabsorptive mechanism for calcium (care must be taken to prevent dehydration). The combined use of these therapies can increase urinary calcium excretion to ≥12.5 mmol/d (500 mg/d) in most hypercalcemic patients. Since this is a substantial percentage of the exchangeable calcium pool, the serum calcium concentration usually falls 0.25 to 0.75 mmol/L (1 to 3 mg/dL) within 24 h. Precautions should be taken to prevent potassium and magnesium depletion; calcium-containing renal calculi are a potential complication.

Under life-threatening circumstances, the preceding approach can be pursued more aggressively, giving as much as 6 L isotonic saline (900 mmol sodium) daily plus furosemide or equivalent in doses up to 100 mg every 1 to 2 h or ethacrynic acid in doses to 40 mg every 1 to 2 h. Urinary calcium excretion may exceed 25 mmol/d (1000 mg/d), and the serum calcium may decrease by ≥1 mmol/L (4 mg/dL) within 24 h. Depletion of potassium and magnesium is inevitable unless replacements are given; pulmonary edema can be precipitated. The potential complications can be reduced by careful monitoring of central venous pressure and plasma or urine electrolytes; catheterization of the bladder may be necessary. This treatment approach should be supplemented with agents to block bone resorption. Though these agents do not become effective for several days, forced diuresis is difficult to sustain even in patients with good cardiopulmonary and renal function.

BISPHOSPHONATES

The bisphosphonates are analogues of pyrophosphate, with high affinity for bone, especially in areas of increased bone turnover, where they are powerful inhibitors of bone resorption. These bone-seeking compounds are stable in vivo because phosphatase enzymes cannot hydrolyze the central carbon-phosphorus-carbon bond. The bisphosphonates are concentrated in areas of high bone turnover and are taken up by and inhibit osteoclast action; the mechanism of action is complex. Bisphosphonates alter osteoclast proton pump function or impair the release of acid hydrolases into the extracellular lysosomes contiguous with mineralized bone. They may also inhibit the differentiation of monocyte-macrophage precursors into osteoclasts and possibly have effects on osteoblasts as well. The bisphosphonate molecules that contain amino groups in the side chain structure (see below) interfere with prenylation of proteins and can lead to cellular apoptosis. The highly active non-amino group–containing bisphosphonates are also metabolized to cytotoxic products.

The initial bisphosphonate widely used in clinical practice, etidronate, was effective but had several disadvantages, including the capacity to inhibit bone formation as well as blocking resorption. Subsequently, a number of second-generation compounds have become the mainstays of antiresorptive therapy for treatment of hypercalcemia and osteoporosis. The newer bisphosphonates have a highly favorable ratio of blocking resorption versus inhibiting bone formation; they inhibit osteoclast-mediated skeletal resorption yet do not cause mineralization defects at ordinary doses. Though the bisphosphonates have similar structures, the routes of administration, efficacy, toxicity, and side effects vary. The potency of the compounds for inhibition of bone resorption varies a thousandfold, increasing in the order of etidronate, tiludronate, pamidronate, alendronate, and risedronate. Oral alendronate and risedronate are approved for the therapy of osteoporosis in the United States, but in Europe only for the chronic treatment of hypercalcemia. Only the intravenous use of pamidronate is approved for the treatment of hypercalcemia in the United States; between 30 and 90 mg pami-dronate, given as a single intravenous dose over a few hours, returns serum calcium to normal within 24 to 48 h with an effect that lasts for weeks in 80 to 100% of patients.

Even more potent third-generation bisphosphonates have been recently introduced into clinical practice. Zolendronate, said to be severalfold more potent than second-generation compounds, is reported in preliminary trials to be superior in treatment of hypercalcemia, normalizing calcium faster and for longer periods of time after infusion. Doses of 1 to 4 mg can be given over a few minutes intravenously.

CALCITONIN

Calcitonin acts within a few hours of its administration, through receptors on osteoclasts, to block bone resorption and, in addition, to increase urinary calcium excretion by inhibition of renal tubular calcium reabsorption. Results with calcitonin, particularly after 24 h of use, are variable, with minimal lowering of calcium. Tachyphylaxis, a known phenomenon with this drug, may explain the results. However, in life-threatening hypercalcemia, calcitonin can be used effectively within the first 24 h in combination with rehydration and saline diuresis while waiting for more sustained effects from a simultaneously administered bisphosphonate such as pamidronate. Usual doses of calcitonin are 2 to 8 U/kg of body weight intravenously, subcutaneously, or intramuscularly every 6 to 12 h.

OTHER THERAPIES

Plicamycin (formerly mithramycin), which inhibits bone resorption, has been a useful therapeutic agent but is now seldom used because of its toxicity and the effectiveness of bisphosphonates. Plicamycin must be given intravenously, either as a bolus or by slow infusion; the usual dose is 25 μg/kg body weight. *Gallium nitrate* exerts a hypocalcemic action by inhibiting bone resorption and altering the structure of bone crystals. It is not often used now because of superior alternatives.

Glucocorticoids have utility, especially in hypercalcemia complicating certain malignancies. They increase urinary calcium excretion and decrease intestinal calcium absorption when given in pharmacologic doses, but they also cause negative skeletal calcium balance. In normal individuals and in patients with primary hyperparathyroidism, glucocorticoids neither increase nor decrease the serum calcium concentration. In patients with hypercalcemia due to certain osteolytic malignancies, however, glucocorticoids may be effective as a result of antitumor effects. The malignancies in which hypercalcemia responds to glucocorticoids include multiple myeloma, leukemia, Hodgkin's disease, other lymphomas, and carcinoma of the breast, at least early in the course of the disease. Glucocorticoids are also effective in treating hypercalcemia due to vitamin D intoxication and sarcoidosis. In all the preceding situations, the hypocalcemic effect develops over several days, and the usual glucocorticoid dosage is 40 to 100 mg prednisone (or its equivalent) daily in four divided doses. The side effects of chronic glucocorticoid therapy may be acceptable in some circumstances.

Dialysis is often the treatment of choice for severe hypercalcemia complicated by renal failure, which is difficult to manage medically. Peritoneal dialysis with calcium-free dialysis fluid can remove 5 to 12.5 mmol (200 to 500 mg) of calcium in 24 to 48 h and lower the serum calcium concentration by 0.7 to 3 mmol/L (3 to 12 mg/dL). Large quantities of phosphate are lost during dialysis, and serum inorganic phosphate concentrations usually fall, thus aggravating hypercalcemia. Therefore, the serum inorganic phosphate concentration should be measured after dialysis, and phosphate supplements should be added to the diet or to dialysis fluids if necessary.

Phosphate therapy, oral or intravenous, has a limited role in certain circumstances. Correcting hypophosphatemia lowers the serum calcium concentration by several mechanisms, including bone/calcium exchange. The usual oral treatment is 1 to 1.5 g phosphorus per day for several days, given in divided doses. It is generally believed, but not established, that toxicity does not occur if therapy is limited to restoring serum inorganic phosphate concentrations to normal.

Raising the serum inorganic phosphate concentration above normal decreases serum calcium levels, sometimes strikingly. Intravenous phosphate is one of the most dramatically effective treatments available for severe hypercalcemia but is toxic and even dangerous (fatal hypocalcemia). For these reasons, it is used rarely and only in severely hypercalcemic patients with cardiac or renal failure. A phosphate phosphorus dose of ≥1500 mg intravenously over 6 to 8 h leads to a prompt decrease in serum calcium of as much as 1.2 to 2.5 mmol/L (5 to 10 mg/dL) in patients with initially normal serum inorganic phosphate concentrations. This therapy should be employed only in extreme emergencies. Inorganic phosphate is commercially available for oral use in liquid, powder, and capsule form and as a liquid for intravenous use. If used, it is important to calculate doses in terms of phosphate phosphorus.

Summary

The various therapies for hypercalcemia are listed in Table 24-4. The choice depends on the underlying disease, the severity of the hypercalcemia, the serum inorganic phosphate level, and the renal, hepatic, and bone marrow function. Mild hypercalcemia [≤3 mmol/L (12 mg/dL)] can usually be managed by hydration. Severe hypercalcemia [≥3.7 mmol/L (15 mg/dL)] requires rapid correction. Calcitonin should be given for its rapid, albeit short-lived, blockade of bone resorption, and intravenous pamidronate or zolendronate should be administered, although its onset of action is delayed for 1 to 2 days. In addition, for the first 24 to 48 h, aggressive sodium-calcium diuresis with intravenous saline and large doses of furosemide or ethacrynic acid following initial hydration should be initiated, but only if appropriate monitoring is available and cardiac and renal function are adequate. Otherwise, dialysis may be necessary. Intermediate degrees of hypercalcemia between 3.0 and 3.7 mmol/L (12 and 15 mg/dL) should be approached with vigorous hydration and then the most appropriate selection for the patient of the combinations used with severe hypercalcemia.

HYPOCALCEMIA

PATHOPHYSIOLOGY OF HYPOCALCEMIA: CLASSIFICATION BASED ON MECHANISM

Chronic hypocalcemia is less common than hypercalcemia; causes include chronic renal failure, hereditary and acquired hypoparathyroidism, vitamin D deficiency, PHP, and hypomagnesemia.

Acute rather than chronic hypocalcemia is seen in critically ill patients or as a consequence of certain medications and often does not require specific treatment. Transient hypocalcemia is seen with severe sepsis, burns, acute renal failure, and extensive transfusions with citrated blood. Although as many as half of patients in an intensive care setting are reported to have calcium concentrations <2.1 mmol/L (8.5 mg/dL), most do not have a reduction in ionized calcium. Patients with severe sepsis may have a decrease in ionized calcium (true hypocalcemia), but in other severely ill individuals, hypoalbuminemia is the primary cause of the reduced total calcium concentration. Alkalosis increases calcium binding to proteins, and in this setting direct measurements of ionized calcium should be made.

Medications such as protamine, heparin, and glucagon may cause transient hypocalcemia. These forms of hypocalcemia are usually not associated with tetany and resolve with improvement in the overall medical condition. The hypocalcemia after repeated transfusions of citrated blood usually resolves quickly.

Patients with *acute pancreatitis* have hypocalcemia that persists during the acute inflammation and varies in degree with the severity of the pancreatitis. The cause of hypocalcemia remains unclear. PTH values are reported to be low, normal, or elevated, and both resistance to PTH and impaired PTH secretion have been postulated. Occasionally, a chronic low total calcium and low ionized calcium concentration are detected in an elderly patient without obvious cause and with a paucity of symptoms; the pathogenesis is unclear.

Chronic hypocalcemia, however, is usually symptomatic and requires treatment. Neuromuscular and neurologic manifestations of chronic hypocalcemia include muscle spasms, carpopedal spasm, facial grimacing, and, in extreme cases, laryngeal spasm and convulsions. Respiratory arrest may occur. Increased intracranial pressure occurs in some patients with long-standing hypocalcemia, often in association with papilledema. Mental changes include irritability, depression, and psychosis. The QT interval on the electrocardiogram is prolonged, in contrast to its shortening with hypercalcemia. Arrhythmias occur, and digitalis effectiveness may be reduced. Intestinal cramps and chronic malabsorption may occur. Chvostek's or Trousseau's sign can be used to confirm latent tetany.

TABLE 24-5

FUNCTIONAL CLASSIFICATION OF HYPOCALCEMIA (EXCLUDING NEONATAL CONDITIONS)

PTH ABSENT	
Hereditary hypoparathyroidism	Hypomagnesemia
Acquired hypoparathyroidism	
PTH INEFFECTIVE	
Chronic renal failure	Active vitamin D ineffective
Active vitamin D lacking	Intestinal malabsorption
↓ Dietary intake or sunlight	Vitamin D–dependent rickets type II
Defective metabolism:	Pseudohypoparathyroidism
Anticonvulsant therapy	
Vitamin D–dependent rickets type I	
PTH OVERWHELMED	
Severe, acute hyperphosphatemia	Osteitis fibrosa after parathyroidectomy
Tumor lysis	
Acute renal failure	
Rhabdomyolysis	

Note: PTH, parathyroid hormone.

The classification of hypocalcemia shown in **Table 24-5** is based on an organizationally useful premise that PTH is responsible for minute-to-minute regulation of plasma calcium concentration and, therefore, that the occurrence of hypocalcemia must mean a failure of the homeostatic action of PTH. Failure of the PTH response can occur if there is hereditary or acquired parathyroid gland failure, if PTH is ineffective in target organs, or if the action of the hormone is overwhelmed by the loss of calcium from the ECF at a rate faster than it can be replaced.

PTH ABSENT

Whether hereditary or acquired, hypoparathyroidism has a number of common components. Symptoms of untreated hypocalcemia are shared by both types of hypoparathyroidism, although the onset of hereditary hypoparathyroidism is more gradual and is often associated with other developmental defects. Basal ganglia calcification and extrapyramidal syndromes are more common and earlier in onset in hereditary hypoparathyroidism. In earlier decades, acquired hypoparathyroidism secondary to surgery in the neck was more common than hereditary hypoparathyroidism, but the frequency of surgically induced parathyroid failure has diminished as a result of improved surgical techniques that spare the parathyroid glands and increased use of nonsurgical therapy for hyperthyroidism. PHP, an example of ineffective PTH action rather than a failure of parathyroid gland production, may share several features with hypoparathyroidism, including extraosseous calcification and extrapyramidal manifestations such as choreoathetotic movements and dystonia.

Papilledema and raised intracranial pressure may occur in both hereditary and acquired hypoparathyroidism, as do chronic changes in fingernails and hair and lenticular cataracts, the latter usually reversible with treatment of hypocalcemia. Certain skin manifestations, including alopecia and candidiasis, are characteristic of hereditary hypoparathyroidism associated with autoimmune polyglandular failure (Chap. 21).

Hypocalcemia associated with hypomagnesemia is associated with both deficient PTH release and impaired responsiveness to the hormone. Patients with hypocalcemia secondary to hypomagnesemia have absent or low levels of circulating PTH, indicative of diminished hormone release despite maximum physiologic stimulus by hypocalcemia. Plasma PTH levels return to normal with correction of the hypomagnesemia. Thus hypoparathyroidism with low levels of PTH in blood can be due to hereditary gland failure, acquired gland failure, or acute but reversible gland dysfunction (hypomagnesemia).

Genetic Abnormalities and Hereditary Hypoparathyroidism

Hereditary hypoparathyroidism can occur as an isolated entity without other endocrine or dermatologic manifestations (idiopathic hypoparathyroidism). More typically, it occurs in association with other abnormalities such as defective development of the thymus or failure of other endocrine organs such as the adrenal, thyroid, or ovary (Chap. 21). Idiopathic and hereditary hypoparathyroidism are often manifest within the first decade but may appear later.

A rare form of hypoparathyroidism associated with defective development of both the thymus and the parathyroid glands is termed the *DiGeorge syndrome*, or the *velocardiofacial syndrome*. Congenital cardiovascular, facial, and other developmental defects are present, and most patients die in early childhood with severe infections, hypocalcemia and seizures, or cardiovascular complications. Some survive into adulthood, and milder, incomplete forms occur. Most cases are sporadic, but an autosomal dominant form involving microdeletions of chromosome 22q11.2 has been described. Smaller deletions in this region are seen in incomplete forms of the DiGeorge syndrome, appearing in childhood or adolescence, that are manifest primarily by parathyroid gland failure.

Hypoparathyroidism can occur in association with a complex hereditary autoimmune syndrome involving failure of the adrenals, the ovaries, the immune system, and the parathyroids in association with recurrent mucocutaneous candidiasis, alopecia, vitiligo, and pernicious anemia (Chap. 21). The responsible gene on chromosome 21q22.3 has been identified. The protein product, which resembles a transcription factor, has been termed the *autoimmune regulator*, or AIRE. A stop codon mutation occurs in many Finnish families with the disorder, commonly referred to as *polyglandular autoimmune type 1 deficiency*.

Gain-of-function mutations in the calcium-sensing receptor cause *autosomal dominant hypocalcemia*. These mutations induce constitutive receptor functions that lead to features that are the inverse of FHH. The activated receptor suppresses PTH secretion, leading to hypocalcemia; receptor activation in the kidney results in excessive renal calcium excretion. Recognition of the syndrome is important because efforts to treat the hypocalcemia of these patients with vitamin D analogues and increased oral calcium exacerbate the already excessive urinary calcium secretion (several grams or more per 24 h), leading to irreversible renal damage from stones and ectopic calcification.

Hypoparathyroidism is seen in two disorders associated with mitochondrial dysfunction and myopathy, one termed the *Kearns-Sayre syndrome* (KSS), with ophthalmoplegia and pigmentary retinopathy, and the other termed the *MELAS syndrome*, *m*itochondrial *e*ncephalopathy, *l*actic *a*cidosis, and *s*troke-like episodes. Mutations or deletions in mitochondrial genes have been identified.

The two other rare forms of hypoparathyroidism with other multisystem developmental abnormalities follow either an autosomal dominant pattern, with deafness and/or renal dysplasia, or an autosomal recessive pattern, with growth retardation and dysmorphic features.

Hereditary hypoparathyroidism occurs also as an isolated entity without any other defects. The pattern of inheritance varies and includes autosomal dominant, autosomal recessive, and X-linked inheritance patterns. In one family in which the disorder is transmitted as an autosomal dominant trait, a structural abnormality in the PTH gene has been identified. A defect in the signal sequence needed for processing of the hormone impairs PTH secretion. In another kindred with autosomal recessive inheritance, the mutant allele in the first intron of the PTH gene causes a splicing defect in mRNA production. An X-linked recessive form of hypoparathyroidism has been described in males and the defect has been localized to chromosome Xq26-q27.

Acquired Hypoparathyroidism

Acquired chronic hypoparathyroidism is usually the result of inadvertent surgical removal of all the parathyroid glands; in some instances, not all the tissue is removed, but the remainder undergoes vascular supply compromise secondary to fibrotic changes in the neck after surgery. In the past, the most frequent cause of acquired hypoparathyroidism was surgery for hyperthyroidism. Hypoparathyroidism now usually occurs after surgery for hyperparathyroidism when the surgeon, facing the dilemma of removing too little tissue and thus not curing the hyperparathyroidism, removes too much. Parathyroid function may not be totally absent in all patients with postoperative hypoparathyroidism.

Even rarer causes of acquired chronic hypoparathyroidism include radiation-induced damage subsequent to radioiodine therapy of hyperthyroidism and glandular damage in patients with hemochromatosis or hemosiderosis after repeated blood transfusions. Infection may involve one or more of the parathyroids but usually does not cause hypoparathyroidism because all four glands are rarely involved.

Transient hypoparathyroidism is frequent following surgery for hyperparathyroidism. After a variable period of hypoparathyroidism, normal parathyroid function may return due to hyperplasia or recovery of remaining tissue. Occasionally, recovery occurs months after surgery.

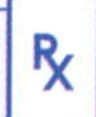

TREATMENT FOR HYPOPARATHYROIDISM

Treatment of acquired and hereditary hypoparathyroidism involves replacement with vitamin D or 1,25$(OH)_2D_3$ (calcitriol) combined with a high oral calcium intake. In most patients, blood calcium and phosphate levels are satisfactorily regulated, but some patients show resistance and a brittleness, with a tendency to alternate between hypocalcemia and hypercalcemia. For many patients, vitamin D in doses of 40,000 to 120,000 U/d (1 to 3 mg/d) combined with ≥1 g elemental calcium is satisfactory. The wide dosage range reflects the variation encountered from patient to patient; precise regulation of each patient is required. Compared to typical daily requirements in euparathyroid patients of 200 U/d, the high dose of vitamin D reflects the reduced conversion of vitamin D to 1,25(OH)$_2$D. Many physicians now use 0.5 to 1.0 μg of calcitriol in management of such patients, especially if they are difficult to control. Because of its storage in fat, when vitamin D is withdrawn, weeks are required for the disappearance of the biologic effects, compared with a few days for calcitriol, which has a rapid turnover.

Oral calcium and vitamin D restore the overall calcium-phosphate balance but do not reverse the lowered urinary calcium reabsorption typical of hypoparathyroidism. Therefore, care must be taken to avoid excessive urinary calcium excretion after vitamin D and calcium replacement therapy; otherwise, kidney stones can develop. Thiazide diuretics lower urine calcium by as much as 100 mg/d in hypoparathyroid patients on vitamin D, provided they are maintained on a low-sodium diet. Use of thiazides seems to be of benefit in mitigating hypercalciuria and easing the daily management of these patients.

Hypomagnesemia

Severe hypomagnesemia (<0.4 mmol/L; <0.8 meq/L) is associated with hypocalcemia (Chap. 23). Restoration of the total-body magnesium deficit leads to rapid reversal of hypocalcemia. There are at least two causes of the hypocalcemia—impaired PTH secretion and reduced responsiveness to PTH. For discussion of causes and treatment of hypomagnesemia, see Chap. 23.

The effects of magnesium on PTH secretion are similar to those of calcium; hypermagnesemia suppresses and hypomagnesemia stimulates PTH secretion. The effects of magnesium on PTH secretion are normally of little significance, however, because the calcium effects dominate. Greater change in magnesium than in calcium is needed to influence hormone secretion. Nonetheless, hypomagnesemia might be expected to increase hormone secretion. It is therefore surprising to find that severe hypomagnesemia is associated with blunted secretion of PTH. The explanation for the paradox is that severe, chronic hypomagnesemia leads to intracellular magnesium deficiency, which interferes with secretion and peripheral responses to PTH. The mechanism of the cellular abnormalities caused by hypomagnesemia is unknown, although effects on adenylate cyclase (for which magnesium is a cofactor) have been proposed.

PTH levels are undetectable or inappropriately low in severe hypomagnesemia despite the stimulus of severe hypocalcemia, and acute repletion of magnesium leads to a rapid increase in PTH level. Serum phosphate levels are often not elevated, in contrast to the situation with acquired or idiopathic hypoparathyroidism, probably because phosphate deficiency is a frequent accompaniment of hypomagnesemia.

Diminished peripheral responsiveness to PTH also occurs in some patients, as documented by subnormal response in urinary phosphorus and urinary cyclic AMP excretion after administration of exogenous PTH to patients who are hypocalcemic and hypomagnesemic. Both blunted PTH secretion and lack of renal response to administered PTH can occur in the same patient. When acute magnesium repletion is undertaken, the restoration of PTH levels to normal or supranormal may precede restoration of normal serum calcium by several days.

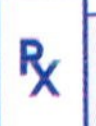

TREATMENT FOR HYPOMAGNESEMIA

Repletion of magnesium cures the condition. Repletion should be parenteral. Attention must be given to restoring the intracellular deficit, which may be considerable. After intravenous magnesium administration, serum magnesium may return transiently to the normal range, but unless replacement therapy is adequate serum magnesium will again fall. If the cause of the hypomagnesemia is renal magnesium wasting, magnesium may have to be given chronically to prevent recurrence (Chap. 23).

PTH INEFFECTIVE

PTH is ineffective when the hormone receptor–guanyl nucleotide–binding protein complex is defective (PHP, discussed below), when PTH action to promote calcium absorption from the diet is impaired because of vitamin D deficiency or because vitamin D is ineffective (receptor or synthesis defects), or in chronic renal failure in which the calcium-elevating action of PTH is impaired.

Typically, hypophosphatemia is more severe than hypocalcemia in vitamin D deficiency states because of the increased secretion of PTH, which, although only partly effective in elevating blood calcium, is capable of promoting phosphaturia.

PHP, on the other hand, has a pathophysiology different from the other disorders of ineffective PTH action. PHP resembles hypoparathyroidism (in which PTH synthesis is deficient) and is manifested by hypocalcemia and hyperphosphatemia. The cause of the disorder is defective hormone activation of guanyl nucleotide–binding proteins, resulting in failure of PTH to increase intracellular cyclic AMP (see below).

Chronic Renal Failure

Improved medical management of chronic renal failure (CRF) now allows many patients to survive for years and hence time enough to develop features of renal osteodystrophy, which must be controlled to avoid its morbidity. Phosphate retention and impaired production of $1,25(OH)_2D$ are the principal factors that cause calcium deficiency, secondary hyperparathyroidism, and bone disease. Low levels of $1,25(OH)_2D$ due to hyperphosphatemia and destruction of renal tissue are critical in the development of hypocalcemia. The uremic state also causes impairment of intestinal absorption by mechanisms other than defects in vitamin D metabolism. Nonetheless, treatment with supraphysiologic amounts of vitamin D or calcitriol corrects the impaired calcium absorption.

Hyperphosphatemia in renal failure lowers blood calcium levels by several mechanisms, including extraosseous deposition of calcium and phosphate, impairment of the bone-resorbing action of PTH, and reduction in $1,25(OH)_2D$ production by remaining renal tissue.

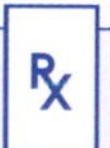

TREATMENT FOR CRF

Therapy of chronic renal failure involves appropriate management of patients prior to dialysis and adjustment of regimens once dialysis is initiated. Attention should be paid to restriction of phosphate in the diet; avoidance of aluminum-containing phosphate-binding antacids to prevent the problem of aluminum intoxication; provision of an adequate calcium intake by mouth, usually 1 to 2 g/d; and supplementation with 0.25 to 1.0 μg/d calcitriol. Each patient must be monitored closely. The aim of therapy is to restore normal calcium balance to prevent osteomalacia and secondary hyperparathyroidism and, in light of evidence of genetic changes and monoclonal outgrowths of parathyroid glands in renal failure patients, to prevent secondary from becoming autonomous hyperparathyroidism. Reduction of hyperphosphatemia and restoration of normal intestinal calcium absorption by calcitriol can improve blood calcium levels and reduce the manifestations of secondary hyperparathyroidism. Since adynamic bone disease can occur in association with low PTH levels, it is important to avoid excessive suppression of the parathyroid glands while recognizing the beneficial effects of controlling the secondary hyperparathyroidism. These patients should probably be closely monitored with PTH assays that detect only the full-length PTH(1–84) to ensure that biologically active PTH and not inactive, inhibitory PTH fragments are measured.

Vitamin D Deficiency due to Inadequate Diet and/or Sunlight

Vitamin D deficiency due to inadequate intake of dairy products enriched with vitamin D, lack of vitamin supplementation, and reduced sunlight exposure in the elderly, particularly during winter in northern latitudes, is more common in the United States than previously recognized. Biopsies of bone in elderly patients with hip fracture (documenting osteomalacia) and abnormal levels of vitamin D metabolites, PTH, calcium, and phosphate indicate that vitamin D deficiency may occur in as many as 25% of elderly patients, particularly in northern latitudes in the United States. Concentrations of 25(OH)D are low or low-normal in these patients. Quantitative histomorphometry of bone biopsy specimens reveals widened osteoid seams consistent with osteomalacia (Chap. 23). PTH hypersecretion compensates for the tendency for the blood calcium to fall but also induces renal phosphate wasting and results in osteomalacia.

Treatment involves adequate replacement with vitamin D and calcium until the deficiencies are corrected. Severe hypocalcemia rarely occurs in moderately severe vitamin D deficiency of the elderly, but vitamin D deficiency must be considered in the differential diagnosis of mild hypocalcemia.

Defective Vitamin D Metabolism

Anticonvulsant Therapy Anticonvulsant therapy with any of several agents induces acquired vitamin D deficiency by increasing the conversion of vitamin D to inactive compounds. The more marginal the vitamin D intake in the diet, the more likely that anticonvulsant therapy will lead to abnormal mineral and bone metabolism For discussion of treatment, see Chap. 23.

Vitamin D–Dependent Rickets Type I Rickets can be due to *resistance to the action* of vitamin D as well as to vitamin D deficiency. Vitamin D–dependent rickets type I, previously termed *pseudo-vitamin D–resistant rickets*, differs from true vitamin D–resistant rickets (vitamin D–dependent rickets type II, see below) in that it is less severe and the biochemical and radiographic abnormalities can be reversed with appropriate doses of the vitamin or the active metabolite, $1{,}25(OH)_2D_3$. Physiologic amounts of calcitriol cure the disease (Chap. 23). This finding fits with the pathophysiology of the disorder, which is autosomal recessive, and is now known to be caused by mutations in the gene encoding 25(OH)D-1α-hydroxylase. Both alleles are inactivated in all patients, and compound heterozygotes, harboring distinct mutations, are common.

Clinical features include hypocalcemia, often with tetany or convulsions, hypophosphatemia, secondary hyperparathyroidism, and osteomalacia, often associated with skeletal deformities and increased alkaline phosphatase. Treatment involves physiologic replacement doses of $1{,}25(OH)_2D_3$ (Chap. 23).

Vitamin D Ineffective

Intestinal Malabsorption Mild hypo-calcemia, secondary hyperparathyroidism, severe hypophosphatemia, and a variety of nutritional deficiencies occur with gastrointestinal diseases. Hepatocellular dysfunction can lead to reduction in 25(OH)D levels, as in portal or biliary cirrhosis of the liver, and malabsorption of vitamin D and its metabolites, including $1{,}25(OH)_2D$, may occur in a variety of bowel diseases, hereditary or acquired. Hypocalcemia itself can lead to steatorrhea, due to deficient production of pancreatic enzymes and bile salts. Depending on the disorder, vitamin D or its metabolites can be given parenterally, guaranteeing adequate blood levels of active metabolites.

Vitamin D-Dependent Rickets Type II Vitamin D–dependent rickets type II results from end-organ resistance to the active metabolite $1{,}25(OH)_2D_3$. The clinical features resemble those of the type I disorder and include hypocalcemia, hypophosphatemia, secondary hyperparathyroidism, and rickets but also partial or total alopecia. Plasma levels of $1{,}25(OH)_2D$ are at least three times normal, in keeping with the refractoriness of the end organs. All of the genetically characterized phenotypes have mutations in the gene for the vitamin D receptor. Treatment is difficult, given the receptor defect (Chap. 23).

Pseudohypoparathyroidism

PHP is a hereditary disorder characterized by symptoms and signs of hypoparathyroidism, typically in association with distinctive skeletal and developmental defects. The hypoparathyroidism is due to a deficient end-organ response to PTH. Hyperplasia of the parathyroids, a response to hormone resistance, causes elevation of PTH levels. Studies, both clinical and basic, have clarified some aspects of this syndrome, including the variable clinical spectrum, the pathophysiology, the genetic defects, and the inheritance.

A working classification of the various forms of PHP is given in **Table 24-6.** The classification scheme is based on the signs of ineffective PTH action (low calcium and high phosphate), urinary cyclic AMP response to exogenous PTH, the presence or absence of *Albright's hereditary osteodystrophy* (AHO), and assays of the concentration of the $G_s\alpha$ subunit of the adenylate cyclase enzyme. Using these criteria, there are four types: PHP type I, subdivided into a and b categories; PHP-II; and pseudopseudohypoparathyroidism (PPHP).

PHP-IA and PHP-IB Individuals with PHP-I, the most common of the disorders, show a deficient urinary cyclic AMP response to administration of exogenous PTH. Patients with PHP-I are divided into type a, who have reduced amounts of $G_s\alpha$ in in vitro assays with erythrocytes, and type b, with normal amounts of $G_s\alpha$ in erythrocytes. There is a third type (PHP-Ic, reported in a few patients) that differs from PHP-Ia only in having normal erythroycte levels of $G_s\alpha$ despite having AHO, hypocalcemia, and decreased urinary cyclic

TABLE 24-6

CLASSIFICATION OF PSEUDOHYPOPARATHYROIDISM (PHP) AND PSEUDOPSEUDOHYPOPARATHYROIDISM (PPHP)

TYPE	HYPOCALCEMIA, HYPERPHOSPHATEMIA	RESPONSE OF URINARY cAMP TO PTH	SERUM PTH	$G_S\alpha$ SUBUNIT DEFICIENCY	AHO	RESISTANCE TO HORMONES IN ADDITION TO PTH
PHP-Ia	Yes	↓	↑	Yes	Yes	Yes
PHP-Ib	Yes	↓	↑	No	No	No
PHP-II	Yes	Normal	↑	No	No	No
PPHP	No	Normal	Normal	Yes	Yes	±

Note: ↓, decreased; ↑, increased; AHO, Albright's hereditary osteodystrophy; PTH, parathyroid hormone.

AMP responses to PTH (presumably with a post-$G_s\alpha$ defect in adenyl cyclase stimulation).

Most patients show characteristic features of AHO, consisting of short stature, round face, skeletal anomalies (brachydactyly), and heterotopic calcification. Patients have low calcium and high phosphate levels, as with true hypoparathyroidism. PTH levels, however, are elevated, reflecting resistance to hormone action.

Amorphous deposits of calcium and phosphate are found in the basal ganglia in about half of patients. The defects in metacarpal and metatarsal bones are sometimes accompanied by short phalanges as well, possibly reflecting premature closing of the epiphyses. The typical findings are short fourth and fifth metacarpals and metatarsals. The defects are usually bilateral. Exostoses and radius curvus are frequent. Impairments in olfaction and taste and unusual dermatoglyphic abnormalities have been reported.

PPHP Multiple defects have now been identified in the *GNAS-1* gene in PHP-Ia and PPHP patients. This gene, which is located on chromosome 20q13, encodes the stimulatory G protein subunit $G_s\alpha$, among other products (see below). Mutations include abnormalities in splice junctions associated with deficient mRNA production and point mutations that result in a protein with defective function as well as a 50% reduction in $G_s\alpha$ levels in erythrocytes.

Detailed analyses of disease transmission in affected kindreds have clarified many features of PHP-Ia, PPHP, and PHP-Ib (**Fig. 24-7**). The former two entities, traced through multiple kindreds, have an inheritance pattern consistent with gene imprinting—only females, not males, can transmit the full disease with hypocalcemia—and PHP and PPHP do not coexist in the same generation. The phenomenon of gene imprinting involves selective inactivation of either the maternal or the paternal allele. In the case of the $G_s\alpha$ gene, it is paternally imprinted (silenced) so that the disease PHP-Ia is never inherited from the father carrying the defective allele but only from the mother. On the other hand, the defective allele is not imprinted or silenced in all tissues. It seems possible, therefore, that the AHO phenotype recognized in PPHP as well as PHP-Ia reflects haplotype insufficiency during embryonic development. In the renal cortex, however, it is postulated that only the maternal allele is normally active, such that lack of activity from a defective paternal allele is not of consequence. This explains the occurrence in PHP-Ia of hypocalcemia, hyperphosphatemia, and other stigmata such as variable resistance to other hormones (if similar tissue-specific imprinting occurs in other organs). Strong evidence favoring this overall hypothesis comes from gene knockout studies in the mouse (ablating exon 2 of the gene).

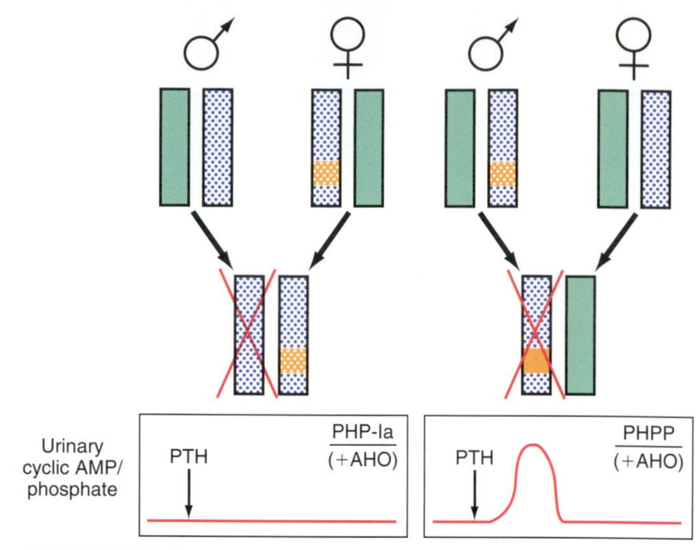

FIGURE 24-7

Paternal imprinting of renal parathyroid hormone (PTH) resistance (*GNAS-1* gene for $G_s\alpha$ subunit) in pseudohypoparathyroidism (PHP). An impaired excretion of urinary cyclic AMP and phosphate is observed in patients with PHP. In the renal cortex, there is selective silencing of the paternal $G_s\alpha$ gene mRNA. The disease becomes manifest only in patients who inherit the defective gene from an obligate female carrier (***left***). If the genetic defect is inherited from an obligate male gene carrier, there is no biochemical abnormality; administration of PTH causes an appropriate increase in the urinary cyclic AMP and phosphate concentration [pseudo-PHP (PPHP); ***right***]. Both patterns of inheritance lead to Albright's hereditary osteodystrophy (AHO), perhaps because of haplotype insufficiency—i.e., both copies of $G_s\alpha$ must be active in the fetus for normal bone development.

Mice inheriting the mutant allele from the female had undetectable $G_s\alpha$ protein in renal cortex and were hypocalcemic and resistant to renal actions of PTH. Offspring inheriting the mutant allele from the male showed no evidence of PTH resistance or hypercalcemia.

The complex mechanisms that control the *GNAS-1* gene also contribute to challenges involved in unraveling the pathogenesis of these disorders. Alternative splicing patterns produce three different transcripts that encode distinct proteins. In addition to $G_s\alpha$, this gene encodes a second protein product with a unique NH_2-terminus (the XL exon); $XL_\alpha s$ includes exons 2–13. It is unknown whether this protein can function as a stimulatory G protein, but the mRNA encoding it is expressed in numerous endocrine tissues and is transcribed from only the paternal allele. A third transcript is transcribed from only the maternal allele and encodes the protein product, NESP55, which contains no homology with $XL_\alpha s$ or $G_s\alpha$.

PHP-Ib, lacking the AHO phenotype, shares with PHP-Ia the resistance to PTH action and a blunted urinary cyclic AMP response to administered PTH, a standard test for hormone resistance (Table 24-6). PHP-Ib patients, however, show normal levels of $G_s\alpha$ in erythrocytes. Bone responsiveness may be excessive rather than blunted in PHP-Ib compared to PHP-Ia patients, based on case reports that have emphasized an osteitis fibrosa–like pattern in some PHP patients who lack the AHO phenotype. The inheritance patterns in PHP-Ib kindreds are clearly consistent with paternal imprinting and lack male transmission of symptomatic disease; gene cloning studies have narrowed the responsible region to chromosome 20, close to—if not within—the *GNAS-1* gene locus. Elucidation of the responsible genetic and pathogenetic mechanisms in this disorder may further illuminate the function of the complex *GNAS-1* gene and the role of its products in hormonal signaling.

PHP-II refers to patients with hypocalcemia and hyperphosphatemia who have a normal urinary cyclic AMP response to PTH. These patients are assumed to have a defect in the response to PTH at a locus distal to cyclic AMP production, although at least some patients may instead have occult vitamin D deficiency.

The diagnosis of these hormone-resistant states can usually be made without difficulty when there is a positive family history for developmental defects and/or the presence of developmental anomalies, including brachydactyly, in association with the signs and symptoms of hypoparathyroidism. In all categories—PHP-Ia, -Ib, and -II—serum PTH levels are elevated, particularly when patients are hypocalcemic. However, patients with PHP-Ib or PHP-II do not have phenotypic abnormalities, only hypocalcemia with high PTH levels, confirming hormone resistance. In PHP-Ib, the response of urinary cyclic AMP to the administration of exogenous PTH is blunted. Levels of $G_s\alpha$ subunits in erythrocyte membranes are, however, normal in those with PHP-Ib. The diagnosis of PHP-II is more complex, in that cyclic AMP responses in urine are, by definition, normal. Since vitamin D deficiency itself can dissociate phosphaturic and urinary cyclic AMP responses to exogenous PTH, vitamin D deficiency must be excluded before the diagnosis of PHP-II can be entertained.

TREATMENT FOR PHP

Treatment for PHP is similar to that of hypoparathyroidism, except that the doses of vitamin D and calcium are usually lower than those required in true hypoparathyroidism, presumably because the defect in PHP is only partial because of imprinting in specific tissues (renal cortex vs. renal medulla). Variability in response makes it necessary to establish the optimal regimen for each patient, based on maintaining the appropriate blood calcium level and urinary calcium excretion.

PTH Overwhelmed

Occasionally, loss of calcium from the ECF is so severe that PTH cannot compensate. Such situations include acute pancreatitis and severe, acute hyperphosphatemia, often in association with renal failure, conditions in which there is rapid efflux of calcium from the ECF. Severe hypocalcemia can occur quickly; PTH rises in response to hypocalcemia but does not return blood calcium to normal.

Severe, Acute Hyperphosphatemia

Severe hyperphosphatemia is associated with extensive tissue damage or cell destruction (Chap. 23). The combination of increased release of phosphate from muscle and impaired ability to excrete phosphorus because of renal failure causes moderate to severe hyperphosphatemia, the latter causing calcium loss from the blood and mild to moderate hypocalcemia. Hypocalcemia is usually reversed with tissue repair and restoration of renal function as phosphorus and creatinine values return to normal. There may even be a mild hypercalcemic period in the oliguric phase of renal function recovery. This sequence, severe hypocalcemia followed by mild hypercalcemia, reflects widespread deposition of calcium in muscle and subsequent redistribution of some of the calcium to the ECF after phosphate levels return to normal.

Other causes of hyperphosphatemia include hypothermia, massive hepatic failure, and hematologic malignancies, either because of high cell turnover of malignancy or because of cell destruction by chemotherapy.

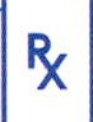

TREATMENT FOR ACUTE HYPERPHOSPHATEMIA

Treatment is directed toward lowering of blood phosphate by the administration of phosphate-binding antacids or dialysis, often needed for the management of renal failure. Although calcium replacement may be necessary if hypocalcemia is severe and symptomatic, calcium administration during the hyperphosphatemic period tends to increase extraosseous calcium deposition and aggravate tissue damage. The levels of $1,25(OH)_2D$ may be low during the hyperphosphatemic phase and return to normal during the oliguric phase of recovery.

Osteitis Fibrosis after Parathyroidectomy

Severe hypocalcemia after parathyroid surgery is rare now that osteitis fibrosa cystica is an infrequent manifestation of hyperparathyroidism. When osteitis fibrosa cystica is severe, however, bone mineral deficits can be large. After parathyroidectomy, hypocalcemia can persist for days if calcium replacement is inadequate. Treatment may require parenteral administration of calcium; addition of calcitriol and oral calcium supplementation is sometimes needed for weeks to a month or two until bone defects are filled (which, of course, is of therapeutic benefit in the skeleton), making it possible to discontinue parenteral calcium and/or reduce the amount.

DIFFERENTIAL DIAGNOSIS OF HYPOCALCEMIA

Care must be taken to ensure that true hypocalcemia is present; in addition, acute transient hypocalcemia can be a manifestation of a variety of severe, acute illnesses, as discussed above. *Chronic hypocalcemia*, however, can usually be ascribed to a few disorders associated with absent or ineffective PTH. Important clinical criteria include the duration of the illness, signs or symptoms of associated disorders, and the presence of features that suggest a hereditary abnormality. A nutritional history can be helpful in recognizing a low intake of vitamin D and calcium in the elderly, and a history of excessive alcohol intake may suggest magnesium deficiency.

Hypoparathyroidism and PHP are typically lifelong illnesses, usually (but not always) appearing by adolescence; hence a recent onset of hypocalcemia in an adult is more likely due to nutritional deficiencies, renal failure, or intestinal disorders that result in deficient or ineffective vitamin D. Neck surgery, even long past, however, can be associated with a delayed onset of postoperative hypoparathyroidism. A history of seizure disorder raises the issue of anticonvulsive medication. Developmental defects may point to the diagnosis of PHP. Rickets and a variety of neuromuscular syndromes and deformities may indicate ineffective vitamin D action, either due to defects in vitamin D metabolism or to vitamin D deficiency.

A pattern of *low calcium with high phosphorus* in the absence of renal failure or massive tissue destruction almost invariably means hypoparathyroidism or PHP. A *low calcium and low phosphorus* points to absent or ineffective vitamin D, thereby impairing the action of PTH on calcium metabolism (but not phosphate clearance). The relative ineffectiveness of PTH in calcium homeostasis in vitamin D deficiency, anticonvulsant therapy, gastrointestinal disorders, or hereditary defects in vitamin D metabolism leads to secondary hyperparathyroidism as a compensation. The excess PTH on renal tubule phosphate transport accounts for renal phosphate wasting and hypophosphatemia.

Exceptions to these patterns may occur. Most forms of hypomagnesemia are due to long-standing nutritional deficiency as seen in chronic alcoholics. Despite the fact that the hypocalcemia is principally due to an acute absence of PTH, phosphate levels are usually low, rather than elevated as in hypoparathyroidism. Chronic renal failure is often associated with hypocalcemia and hyperphosphatemia, despite secondary hyperparathyroidism.

Diagnosis is usually established by application of the PTH immunoassay, tests for vitamin D metabolites, and measurements of the urinary cyclic AMP response to exogenous PTH. In hereditary and acquired hypoparathyroidism and in severe hypomagnesemia, PTH is either undetectable or in the normal range. This finding in a hypocalcemic patient is supportive of hypoparathyroidism, as distinct from ineffective PTH action, in which even mild hypocalcemia is associated with elevated PTH levels. Hence a failure to detect elevated PTH levels establishes the diagnosis of hypoparathyroidism; elevated levels suggest the presence of secondary hyperparathyroidism, as found in many of the situations in which the hormone is ineffective due to associated abnormalities in vitamin D action. Assays for 25(OH)D and $1,25(OH)_2D$ can be helpful. Low or low-normal 25(OH)D indicates vitamin D deficiency due to lack of sunlight, inadequate vitamin D intake, or intestinal malabsorption. A low level of $1,25(OH)_2D$ in the presence of elevated concentrations of PTH suggests ineffective PTH action in disorders such as chronic renal failure, severe vitamin D deficiency, vitamin D–dependent rickets type I, and PHP. Recognition that mild hypocalcemia, rickets, and hypophosphatemia are due to anticonvulsant therapy is made by history.

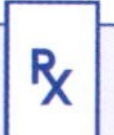

TREATMENT FOR DEFECTS IN VITAMIN D METABOLISM

HYPOCALCEMIC STATES

The management of hypoparathyroidism, PHP, chronic renal failure, and hereditary defects in vitamin D metabolism involves the use of vitamin D or vitamin D metabolites and calcium supplementation. Vitamin D itself is the least expensive form of vitamin D replacement and is frequently used in the management of uncomplicated hypoparathyroidism and some disorders associated with ineffective vitamin D action. When vitamin D is used prophylactically, as in the elderly or in those with chronic anticonvulsant therapy, there is a wider margin of safety than with the more potent metabolites. However, most of the conditions in which vitamin D is administered chronically for hypocalcemia require amounts 50 to 100 times the daily replacement dose because the formation of $1,25(OH)_2D$ is deficient. In such situations, vitamin D is no safer than the active metabolite because intoxication can occur with high-dose therapy (because of storage in fat). Calcitriol is more rapid in onset of action and also has a short biologic half-life.

Vitamin D [200 U (5 μg/d)] or calcifediol and lower doses of calcitriol (0.25 to 1.0 μg/d) are required to prevent rickets in normal individuals. In contrast, 40,000 to 12,000 U (1 to 3 mg) of vitamin D_2 or D_3 is typically required in hypoparathyroidism; doses of calcifediol are also high (several hundred micrograms per day). The dose of calcitriol is unchanged in hypoparathyroidism, since the defect is in hydroxylation by the 25(OH)D-1α-hydroxylase.

Patients with hypoparathyroidism should be given 2 to 3 g elemental calcium by mouth each day. The two agents, vitamin D or calcitriol and oral calcium, can be varied independently. If hypocalcemia alternates with episodes of hypercalcemia in more brittle patients with hypoparathyroidism, administration of calcitriol and use of thiazides, as discussed above, may make management easier.

FURTHER READINGS

BILEZIKIAN JP, POTTS JT Jr: Asymptomatic primary hyperparathyroidism: New issues and new questions—bridging the past with the future. J Bone Min Res 17(Suppl 2):N57, 2002

——— et al: Clinical practice. Asymptomatic primary hyperparathyroidism. N Engl J Med 350:1746, 2004

The 2002 NIH Workshop on asymptomatic PHPT has led to revised guidelines to help determine which patients should have parathyroid surgery. In this NIH workshop, a number of items were highlighted for further investigation such as pharmacological approaches to controlling hypercalcemia, elevated PTH levels, and maintaining bone density.

MAJOR P et al: Zoledronic acid is superior to pamidronate in the treatment of hypercalcemia of malignancy: A pooled analysis of two randomized, controlled clinical trials. J Clin Oncol 19:558, 2001

REID R et al: Intravenous zoledronic acid in postmenopausal women with low bone mineral density. N Engl J Med 346:653, 2002

STEWART AF: Clinical practice. Hypercalcemia associated with cancer. N Engl J Med 352:373, 2005

Hypercalcemia of malignancy is predominantly caused by production of parathyroid hormone–related peptide (PTHrP). PTHrP is structurally related to PTH and binds to the PTH receptor, thereby explaining their similar effects with respect to calcium metabolism. This review summarizes the pathophysiology and management of hypercalcemia associated with malignancy.

THAKKER RV: Genetics of endocrine and metabolic disorders: Parathyroid. Rev Endocr Metab Disord 5:37, 2004

THOMPSON SD ET AL: The management of parathyroid carcinoma. Curr Opin Otolaryngol Head Neck Surg 12:93, 2004

WEINSTEIN LS ET AL: Minireview: *GNAS:* Normal and abnormal functions. Endocrinology 145:5459, 2004

GNAS is a complex imprinted gene that uses multiple promoters to generate several gene products, including the G protein alpha-subunit ($G_s\alpha$) that couples $G_s\alpha$ seven-transmembrane receptors to the cyclic AMP-generating enzyme adenylyl cyclase. Somatic activating $G_s\alpha$ mutations are present in various endocrine tumors and fibrous dysplasia of bone and in patients with Mc-Cune- Albright syndrome. Heterozygous inactivating $G_s\alpha$ mutations lead to Albright hereditary osteodystrophy (AHO). Maternally inherited mutations lead to AHO plus PTH, TSH, and gonadotropin resistance (pseudohypoparathyroidism type 1A), whereas paternally inherited mutations lead to AHO alone.

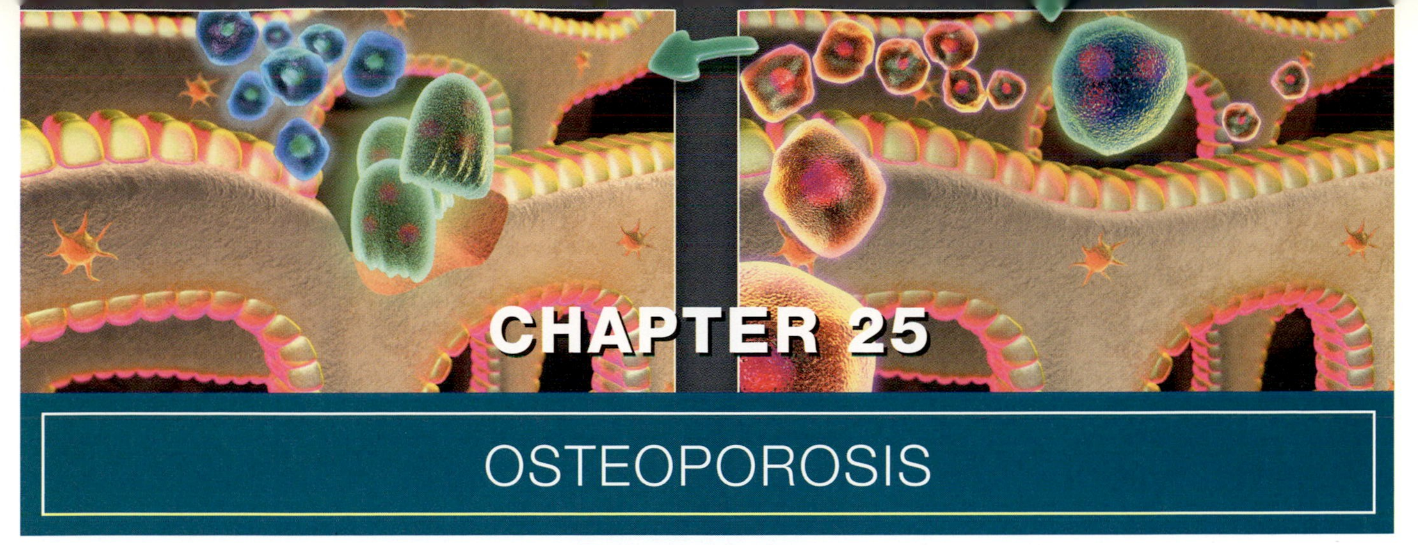

OSTEOPOROSIS

Robert Lindsay
Felicia Cosman

Osteoporosis, a condition characterized by decreased bone strength, is prevalent among postmenopausal women but also occurs in men and women with underlying conditions or major risk factors associated with bone demineralization. Its chief clinical manifestations are vertebral and hip fractures, although fractures can occur at any skeletal site. Osteoporosis affects >10 million individuals in the United States, but only a small proportion are diagnosed and treated.

DEFINITION

Osteoporosis is defined as a reduction of bone mass (or density) or the presence of a fragility fracture. Loss of bone tissue causes deterioration in the architecture of the skeleton, the combination leading to a markedly increased risk of fracture. Based on the recommendation of a WHO committee, osteoporosis is defined operationally as a bone density that falls 2.5 standard deviations (SD) below the mean for young healthy adults of the same race and gender—also referred to as a *T-score* of −2.5. Those who fall at the lower end of the young normal range (a T-score of >1 SD below the mean) are defined as having low bone density and are considered to be at increased risk of osteoporosis.

EPIDEMIOLOGY

In the United States, as many as 8 million women and 2 million men have osteoporosis (T-score < −2.5), and an additional 18 million individuals have bone mass levels that put them at increased risk of developing osteoporosis (e.g., bone mass T-score < −1.0). Osteoporosis occurs more frequently with increasing age as bone tissue is progressively lost. In women, the loss of ovarian function at menopause (typically about age 50) precipitates rapid bone loss such that most women meet the diagnostic criteria for osteoporosis by age 70 to 80.

The epidemiology of fractures follows similar trends as bone density loss. Fractures of the distal radius increase in frequency before age 50 and plateau by age 60, with only a modest age-related increase thereafter. In contrast, incidence rates for hip fractures double every 5 years after age 70 (**Fig. 25-1**). This distinct epidemiology may be related to the way people fall as they age, with fewer falls on an outstretched hand and more directly on the hip. At least 1.5 million fractures occur each year in the United States as a consequence of osteoporosis. As the population continues to age, the total number of fractures will continue to escalate.

About 300,000 hip fractures occur each year in the United States, most of which require hospital admission and surgical intervention. The probability that a 50-year-old white individual will have a hip fracture during his or her lifetime is 14% for women and 5% for men;

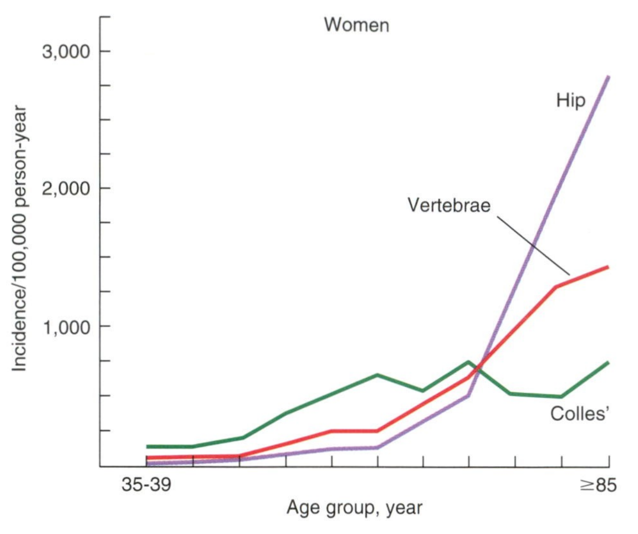

FIGURE 25-1
Epidemiology of vertebral, hip, and Colles' fractures with age. [*Adapted from LJ Melton III, in BL Riggs, LJ Melton II (eds): Osteoporosis: Etiology, Diagnosis and Management, 2d ed. Rochester, MN, Mayo Foundation, 1995.*]

the risk for African Americans is lower (about half these rates). Hip fractures are associated with a high incidence of deep-vein thrombosis and pulmonary embolism (20 to 50%) and a mortality rate between 5 and 20% during the year after surgery.

There are about 700,000 vertebral crush fractures per year in the United States. Only a fraction of these are recognized clinically, since many are relatively asymptomatic and are identified incidentally during radiography for other purposes (**Fig. 25-2**). Vertebral fractures rarely

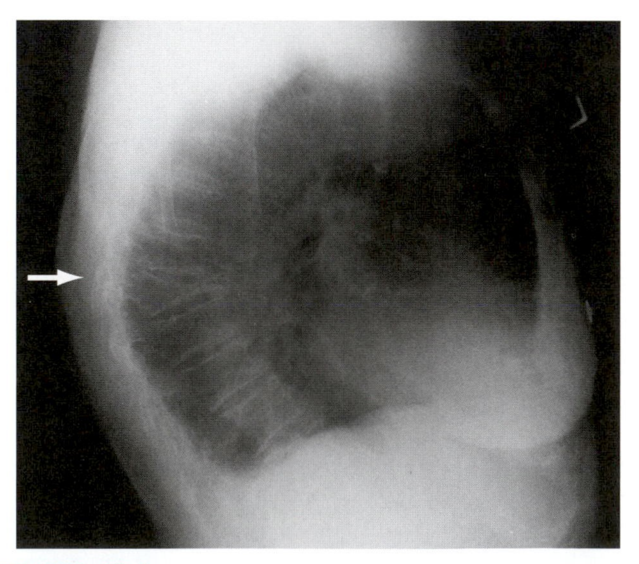

FIGURE 25-2
Lateral spine x-ray showing severe osteopenia and a severe wedge-type deformity (severe anterior compression).

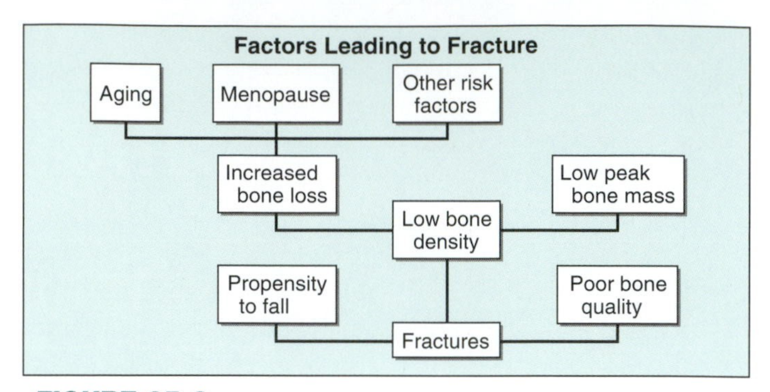

FIGURE 25-3
Factors leading to osteoporotic fractures.

require hospitalization but are associated with long-term morbidity and a slight increase in mortality. Multiple fractures lead to height loss (often of several inches), kyphosis, and secondary pain and discomfort related to altered biomechanics of the back. Thoracic fractures can be associated with restrictive lung disease, whereas lumbar fractures are associated with abdominal symptoms including distention, early satiety, and constipation.

Approximately 250,000 wrist fractures occur in the United States each year. Fractures of other bones (estimated to be about 300,000 per year) also occur with osteoporosis, which is not surprising given that bone loss is a systemic phenomenon. Fractures of the pelvis and proximal humerus are clearly associated with osteoporosis. Although some fractures are the result of major trauma, the threshold for fracture is reduced for an osteoporotic bone (**Fig. 25-3**). A list of common risk factors for osteoporotic fractures is summarized in **Table 25-1.** Prior fractures, a family history of osteoporotic fractures, and low body weight are each independent predictors of fracture. Chronic diseases that increase the

TABLE 25-1

RISK FACTORS FOR OSTEOPOROSIS FRACTURE	
Nonmodifiable	Estrogen deficiency
Personal history of fracture as an adult	Early menopause (<45 years) or bilateral ovariectomy
History of fracture in first-degree relative	Prolonged premenstrual amenorrhea (>1 year)
Female sex	Low calcium intake
Advanced age	Alcoholism
Caucasian race	Impaired eyesight despite adequate correction
Dementia	Recurrent falls
Potentially modifiable	Inadequate physical activity
Current cigarette smoking	Poor health/frailty
Low body weight [<58 kg (127 lb)]	

risk of falling or frailty, including dementia, Parkinson's disease, and multiple sclerosis, also increase fracture risk.

In the United States and Europe, osteoporosis-related fractures are more common among women than men, presumably due to a lower peak bone mass as well as postmenopausal bone loss in women. However, this gender difference in bone density and age-related increase in hip fractures is not as apparent in some other cultures, possibly due to genetics, physical activity level, or diet.

PATHOPHYSIOLOGY

BONE REMODELING

Osteoporosis results from bone loss due to normal age-related changes in bone remodeling as well as extrinsic and intrinsic factors that exaggerate this process. These changes may be superimposed on a low peak bone mass. Consequently, understanding the bone remodeling process is fundamental to understanding the pathophysiology of osteoporosis (Chap. 23). The skeleton increases in size by linear growth and by apposition of new bone tissue on the outer surfaces of the cortex (**Fig. 25-4**). This latter process is called *modeling*, a process that also allows the long bones to adapt in shape to the stresses placed on them. Increased sex hormone production at puberty is required for skeletal maturation, which reaches maximum mass and density in early adulthood. Nutrition and lifestyle also play an important role in growth, although genetic factors are the major determinants of peak skeletal mass and density. Numerous genes control skeletal growth, peak bone mass, and body size, but it is likely that separate genes control skeletal structure and density. Heritability estimates of 50 to 80% for bone density and size have been derived based on twin studies. Though peak bone mass is often lower among individuals with a family history of osteoporosis, association studies of candidate genes [vitamin D receptor; type I collagen, the estrogen receptor (ER), interleukin (IL) 6; and insulin-like growth factor (IGF) I] and bone mass, bone turnover, and fracture prevalence have been inconsistent. Linkage studies suggest that a genetic locus on chromosome 11 is associated with high bone mass. Recently, a family with extremely high bone mass was identified with a point mutation in LRP 5, a low-density lipoprotein receptor–related protein.

Bone remodeling has two primary functions: (1) to repair microdamage within the skeleton to maintain skeletal strength, and (2) to supply calcium from the skeleton to maintain serum calcium. Remodeling may be activated by microdamage to bone as a result of excessive or accumulated stress. Acute demands for calcium involve osteoclast-mediated resorption as well as calcium transport by osteocytes.

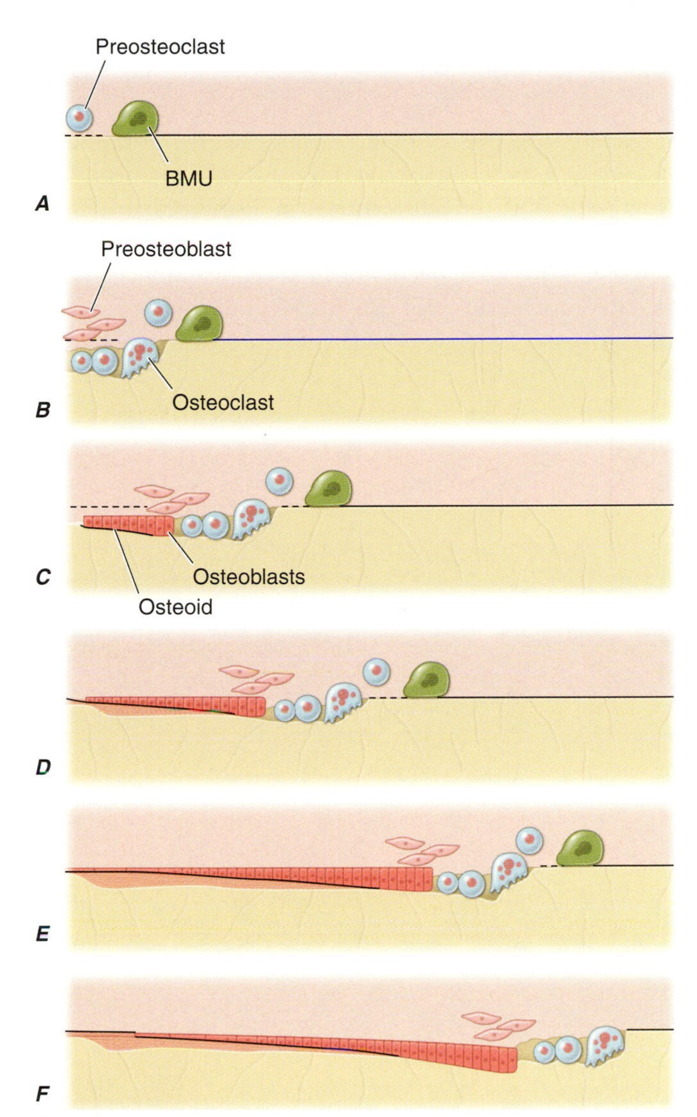

FIGURE 25-4

Mechanism of bone remodeling. The basic molecular unit (BMU) moves along the trabecular surface at a rate of about 10 μm/d. The figure depicts remodeling over ~120 days. ***A.*** BMU-lining cells contract to expose collagen and attract preosteoclasts. ***B.*** Osteoclasts fuse into multinucleated cells that resorb a cavity. Mononuclear cells continue resorption and preosteoblasts are stimulated to proliferate. ***C.*** Osteoblasts align at bottom of cavity and start forming osteoid (black). ***D.*** Osteoblasts continue formation and mineralization. Previous osteoid starts to mineralize (horizontal lines). ***E.*** Osteoblasts begin to flatten. ***F.*** Osteoblasts turn into lining cells; bone remodeling at initial surface (left of drawing) is now complete, but BMU is still advancing (to the right). *[Adapted from: SM Ott, in JP Bilezikian et al (eds): Principles of Bone Biology, vol. 18. San Diego, Academic Press, 1996, pp 231–241.]*

Bone remodeling is also regulated by several circulating hormones, including estrogens, androgens, vitamin D, and parathyroid hormone (PTH), as well as locally produced growth factors such as IGF-I and -II, transforming growth factor (TGF) β, parathyroid hormone–related peptide (PTHrP), ILs, prostaglandins, and tumor necrosis factor (TNF). The cytokine responsible for communication between the osteoblast and osteoclast has been identified as RANK or osteoprotegerin ligand (Chap. 23). The osteoclast receptor for this protein is referred to as RANK. A humoral decoy for RANK ligand is referred to as osteoprotegerin (**Fig. 25-5**). Modulation of osteoclast recruitment and activity appears to be related to the interplay among these three factors.

Additional influences include nutrition (particularly calcium intake) and physical activity level. The end result of this remodeling process is that the resorbed bone is replaced by an equal amount of new bone tissue. Thus, the mass of the skeleton remains constant after peak bone mass is achieved in adulthood. After age 30 to 45, however, the resorption and formation processes become imbalanced, and resorption exceeds formation. This imbalance may begin at different ages and varies at different skeletal sites; it becomes exaggerated in women after menopause. Excessive bone loss can be due to an

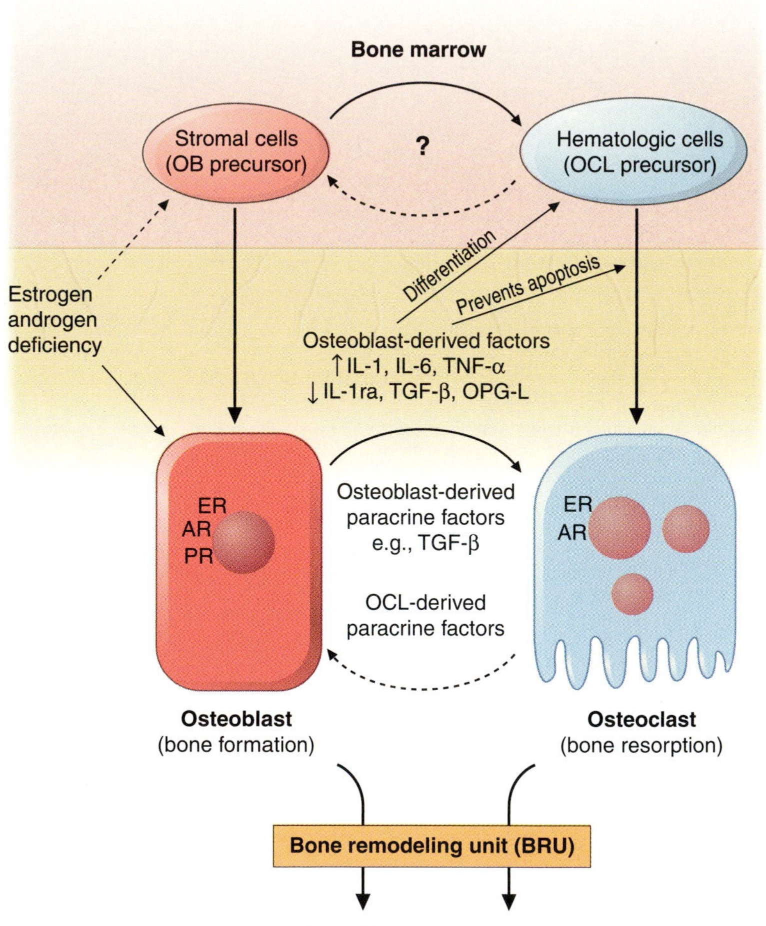

FIGURE 25-5

Steroid actions and interactions with growth factors/cytokines in bone cells at bone resorption and formation sites. Estrogen inhibits osteoclasts (OCL), cells that mediate bone resorption; estrogen stimulates osteoblasts (OB), cells that mediate bone formation. OBs produce many growth factors and cytokines that mediate estrogen action, some of which regulate the OCL indirectly. Estrogen deficiency stimulates OB production of IL-1, IL-6, and TNF-α (and inhibits apoptosis and extends the life span of OCLs). Estrogen deficiency decreases IL-1ra leading to enhanced OCL sensitivity to IL-1. Estrogen deficiency also decreases production of TGF-β and OPG-L, factors that mediate osteoclast apoptosis. Solid lines indicate well-documented pathways. Dashed lines indicate less well-defined pathways. ER, estrogen receptor; AR, androgen receptor; OPG, osteoprotegerin; OPG-L, osteoprotegerin-ligand; IL, interleukin; IL-1ra, interleukin 1 receptor antagonist; TGF-β, transforming growth factor β; TNF-α, tumor necrosis factor α. (*Adapted from TC Spelsberg et al: Mol Endocrinol 13:819, 1999.*)

increase in osteoclastic activity and/or a decrease in osteoblastic activity. In addition, an increase in remodeling activation frequency can magnify the small imbalance seen at each remodeling unit.

In trabecular bone, if the osteoclasts penetrate trabeculae, they leave no template for new bone formation to occur and, consequently, may cause rapid bone loss. In cortical bone, increased activation of remodeling creates more porous bone. The effect of this increased porosity on cortical bone strength may be modest if the overall diameter of the bone is not changed. However, decreased apposition of new bone on the periosteal surface coupled with increased endocortical resorption of bone decreases the biomechanical strength of long bones. Even a slight exaggeration in normal bone loss increases the risk of osteoporotic fracture.

CALCIUM NUTRITION

Peak bone mass may be impaired by inadequate calcium intake during growth among other nutritional factors (calories, protein, and other minerals), thereby leading to increased risk of osteoporosis later in life. During the adult phase of life, insufficient calcium intake induces secondary hyperparathyroidism and an increase in the rate of remodeling to maintain normal serum calcium levels. PTH stimulates the hydroxylation of vitamin D in the kidney, leading to increased levels of 1,25-dihydroxyvitamin D [1,25$(OH)_2$D] and enhanced gastrointestinal calcium absorption. PTH also reduces renal calcium loss. Although these are appropriate short-term homeostatic responses for adjusting calcium economy, the long-term effects are detrimental to the skeleton because of the ongoing imbalance at remodeling sites.

Total daily calcium intakes of <400 mg are likely to be detrimental to the skeleton, but there are fewer data about intakes in the 600- to 800-mg range, which is the average intake among adults in the United States. The recommended daily required intake of 1000 to 1200 mg for adults accommodates population heterogeneity in controlling calcium balance (Chap. 60 in HPIM, 16e).

VITAMIN D (See also chap. 23)

Severe vitamin D deficiency causes rickets in children or osteomalacia in adults. There is accumulating evidence that vitamin D deficiency may be more prevalent than previously thought, particularly among individuals at increased risk, such as the elderly; those living in northern latitudes; and in individuals with poor nutrition, malabsorption, or chronic liver or renal disease. Modest vitamin D deficiency [25-hydroxyvitamin D levels ≤50 nmol/L (20 ng/mL)] leads to compensatory secondary hyperparathyroidism and is an important risk factor for osteoporosis and fractures. Some studies have shown that >50% of inpatients on a general medical service exhibit biochemical features of vitamin D deficiency, including increased levels of PTH and alkaline phosphatase and lower levels of ionized calcium. In women living in northern latitudes, it has been shown that vitamin D levels decline during the winter months. This is associated with a striking seasonal bone loss, reflecting increased bone turnover. Even among healthy ambulatory individuals, mild vitamin D deficiency is increasing in prevalence. Treatment with vitamin D can return vitamin D levels to normal [>50 μmol/L (20 ng/mL)] and prevent the associated increase in bone remodeling, bone loss, and fractures. Reduced fracture rates have also been documented among individuals in northern latitudes who have greater vitamin D intake and have higher 25-hydroxyvitamin D [25(OH)D] levels (see below).

ESTROGEN STATUS

Estrogen deficiency probably causes bone loss by two distinct but interrelated mechanisms: (1) activation of new bone remodeling sites, and (2) exaggeration of the imbalance between bone formation and resorption. The change in activation frequency causes a transient bone loss until a new steady state between resorption and formation is achieved. The remodeling imbalance, however, results in a permanent decrement in mass that can be corrected only by a remodeling event during which bone formation exceeds resorption. In addition, the very presence of more remodeling sites in the skeleton increases the probability that trabeculae will be penetrated, thereby eliminating the template upon which new bone can be formed and accelerating the loss of bony tissue.

The most frequent estrogen-deficient state is the cessation of ovarian function at the time of menopause, which occurs on average at the age of 51. Thus, with current life expectancy, an average woman will spend about 30 years without ovarian supply of estrogen. The mechanism by which estrogen deficiency causes bone loss is summarized in Fig. 25-5. Marrow cells (macrophages, monocytes, osteoclast precursors, mast cells) as well as bone cells (osteoblasts, osteocytes, osteoclasts) express ERs α and β. The net effect of estrogen deficiency is increased osteoclast recruitment and perhaps activity. Estrogen may also play an important role in determining the life span of bone cells by controlling the rate of apoptosis. Thus, in situations of estrogen deprivation, the life span of osteoblasts may be decreased whereas the longevity of osteoclasts is increased.

Since remodeling is initiated at the surface of bone, it follows that trabecular bone—which has a considerably larger surface area (80% of the total) than cortical bone—will be preferentially affected by estrogen deficiency. Fractures occur earliest at sites where trabecular bone contributes most to bone strength; consequently, vertebral fractures are the most common early consequence of estrogen deficiency.

PHYSICAL ACTIVITY

Inactivity, such as prolonged bed rest or paralysis, results in significant bone loss. Concordantly, athletes have higher bone mass than the general population. These changes in skeletal mass are most marked when the stimulus begins during growth and before the age of puberty. Adults are less capable than children of increasing bone mass following restoration of physical activity. Epidemiologic data support the beneficial effects on the skeleton of chronic high levels of physical activity. Fracture risk is lower in rural communities and in countries where physical activity is maintained into old age. However, when exercise is initiated during adult life, the effects of moderate exercise are modest, with a bone mass increase of 1 to 2% in short-term studies of <2 years duration. It is argued that more active individuals are less likely to fall and are more capable of protecting themselves upon falling, thereby reducing fracture risk.

CHRONIC DISEASE

Various genetic and acquired diseases are associated with an increase in the risk of osteoporosis (**Table 25-2**). Mechanisms that contribute to bone loss are unique for each disease and typically result from multiple factors including nutrition, reduced physical activity levels, and factors that affect bone-remodeling rates.

MEDICATIONS

A large number of medications used in clinical practice have potentially detrimental effects on the skeleton (**Table 25-3**). *Glucocorticoids* are the most common cause of medication-induced osteoporosis. It is often not possible to determine the extent to which osteoporosis is related to the glucocorticoid or to other factors, as treatment is superimposed on

TABLE 25-2

DISEASES ASSOCIATED WITH AN INCREASED RISK OF GENERALIZED OSTEOPOROSIS IN ADULTS

Hypogonadal states	**Hematologic disorders/malignancy**
Turner syndrome	Multiple myeloma
Klinefelter syndrome	Lymphoma and leukemia
Anorexia nervosa	Malignancy-associated parathyroid hormone (PTHrP) production
Hypothalamic amenorrhea	Mastocytosis
Hyperprolactinemia	Hemophilia
Other primary or secondary hypogonadal states	Thalassemia
Endocrine disorders	**Selected inherited disorders**
Cushing's syndrome	Osteogenesis imperfecta
Hyperparathyroidism	Marfan syndrome
Thyrotoxicosis	Hemochromatosis
Type 1 diabetes mellitus	Hypophosphatasia
Acromegaly	Glycogen storage diseases
Adrenal insufficiency	Homocystinuria
Nutritional and gastrointestinal disorders	Ehlers-Danlos syndrome
Malnutrition	Porphyria
Parenteral nutrition	Menkes' syndrome
Malabsorption syndromes	Epidermolysis bullosa
Gastrectomy	**Other disorders**
Severe liver disease, especially biliary cirrhosis	Immobilization
Pernicious anemia	Chronic obstructive pulmonary disease
Rheumatologic disorders	Pregnancy and lactation
Rheumatoid arthritis	Scoliosis
Ankylosing spondylitis	Multiple sclerosis
	Sarcoidosis
	Amyloidosis

TABLE 25-3

DRUGS ASSOCIATED WITH AN INCREASED RISK OF GENERALIZED OSTEOPOROSIS IN ADULTS	
Glucocorticoids	Excessive thyroxine
Cyclosporine	Aluminum
Cytotoxic drugs	Gonadotropin-releasing hormone agonists
Anticonvulsants	Heparin
Excessive alcohol	Lithium

the effects of the primary disease, which may in itself be associated with bone loss (e.g., rheumatoid arthritis). Excessive doses of thyroid hormone can accelerate bone remodeling and result in bone loss.

Other medications have less detrimental effects upon the skeleton than pharmacologic doses of glucocorticoids. *Anticonvulsants* are thought to increase the risk of osteoporosis, although many affected individuals have concomitant vitamin D insufficiency, as some anticonvulsants induce the cytochrome P450 system and vitamin D metabolism. Patients undergoing transplantation are at high risk for rapid bone loss and fracture not only from glucocorticoids but also from treatment with other *immunosuppressants*, such as cyclosporine and tacrolimus (FK506). In addition, these patients often have underlying metabolic abnormalities, such as hepatic or renal failure, that predispose to bone loss.

CIGARETTE CONSUMPTION

The use of cigarettes over a long period has detrimental effects on bone mass. These effects may be mediated directly, by toxic effects on osteoblasts, or indirectly by modifying estrogen metabolism. On average, cigarette smokers reach menopause 1 to 2 years earlier than the general population. Cigarette smoking also produces secondary effects that can modulate skeletal status, including intercurrent respiratory and other illnesses, frailty, decreased exercise, poor nutrition, and the need for additional medications (e.g., glucocorticoids for lung disease).

MEASUREMENT OF BONE MASS

Several noninvasive techniques are now available for estimating skeletal mass or density. These include dual-energy x-ray absorptiometry (DXA), single-energy x-ray absorptiometry (SXA), quantitative computed tomography (CT), and ultrasound.

DXA is a highly accurate x-ray technique that has become the standard for measuring bone density in most centers. Although it can be used for measurements of any skeletal site, clinical determinations are usually made of the lumbar spine and hip. Portable DXA machines have been developed that measure the heel (calcaneus), forearm (radius and ulna), or finger (phalanges). DXA can also be used to measure body composition. In the DXA technique, two x-ray energies are used to estimate the area of mineralized tissue, and the mineral content is divided by the area, which partially corrects for body size. However, this correction is only partial since DXA is a two-dimensional scanning technique and cannot estimate the depths or posteroanterior length of the bone. Thus, small people tend to have lower-than-average bone mineral density (BMD). Bone spurs, which are frequent in osteoarthritis, tend to falsely increase bone density of the spine. Because DXA instrumentation is provided by several different manufacturers, the output varies in absolute terms. Consequently, it has become standard practice to relate the results to "normal" values using T-scores, which compare individual results to those in a young population that is matched for race and gender. Z-scores compare individual results to those of an age-matched population that is also matched for race and gender. Thus, a 60-year-old woman with a Z-score of -1 (1 SD below mean for age) has a T-score of -2.5 (2.5 SD below mean for a young control group) (**Fig. 25-6**).

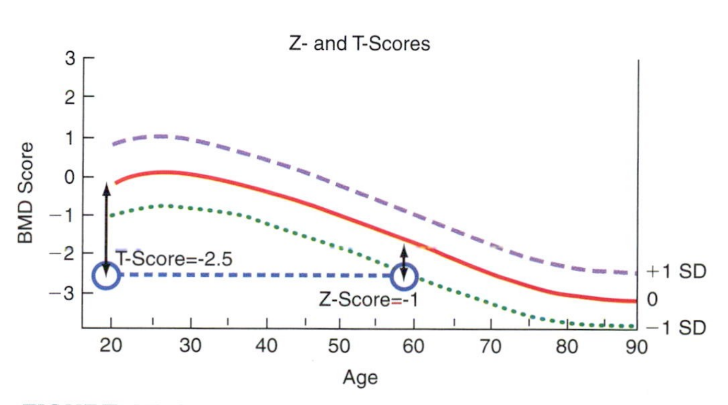

FIGURE 25-6
Relationship between Z-scores and T-scores in a 60-year-old woman. BMD, bone mineral density; SD, standard deviation.

CT is used primarily to measure the spine, and peripheral CT is used to measure bone in the forearm or tibia. Research into the use of CT for measurement of the hip is ongoing. The results obtained from CT are different from all others currently available since this technique specifically analyzes trabecular bone in vertebrae, eliminating posterior cortical elements of the spine, and can provide a true density (mass of bone per unit volume) measurement. However, CT remains expensive, involves greater radiation exposure, and is less reproducible.

Ultrasound is used to measure bone mass by calculating the attenuation of the signal as it passes through bone or the speed with which it traverses the bone. It is unclear whether ultrasound assesses bone quality, but this may be an advantage of the technique. Because of its relatively low cost and mobility, ultrasound is amenable for use as a screening procedure.

All of these techniques for measuring BMD have been approved by the U.S. Food and Drug Administration (FDA) based on their capacity to predict fracture risk. The hip is the preferred site of measurement in most individuals, since it predicts the risk of hip fracture, the most important consequence of osteoporosis, better than any other bone density measurement site. When hip measurements are performed by DXA, the spine can be measured at the same time. In younger individuals, such as perimenopausal or early postmenopausal women, spine measurements may be the most sensitive indicator of bone loss.

WHEN TO MEASURE BONE MASS

Clinical guidelines developed by the National Osteoporosis Foundation recommend bone mass measurements in postmenopausal women, assuming they have risk factors for osteoporosis in addition to age, gender, and estrogen deficiency. The guidelines further recommend that bone mass measurement be considered in *all* women by age 65, a position ratified by the U.S. Preventive Health Services Task Force. Criteria approved for Medicare reimbursement of BMD are summarized in **Table 25-4.**

WHEN TO TREAT BASED ON BONE MASS RESULTS

Several guidelines suggest that patients be considered for treatment when BMD is >2.5 SD below the mean value for young adults (T-score ≤ −2.5). Treatment should also be considered in postmenopausal women with risk factors if BMD of the hip is <−2.0. Because the fracture risk increases continuously as T-scores decline, there is no critical threshold and treatment decisions must be individualized. Clearly clinical status must be evaluated carefully, considering age, prior fracture history, weight, and family history of osteoporosis. Moreover, high bone turnover, particularly in older individuals, should be considered an independent risk factor for fracture and should prompt treatment at a higher BMD level.

TABLE 25-4

FDA-APPROVED INDICATIONS FOR BMD TESTS[a]
Estrogen-deficient women at clinical risk of osteoporosis
Vertebral abnormalities on x-ray suggestive of osteoporosis (osteopenia, vertebral fracture)
Glucocorticoid treatment equivalent to ≥7.5 mg of prednisone, or duration of therapy >3 months
Primary hyperparathyroidism
Monitoring response to an FDA-approved medication for osteoporosis
Repeat BMD evaluations at >23-month intervals, or more frequently, if medically justified

[a]Criteria adapted from the 1998 Bone Mass Measurement Act.

Note: FDA, U.S. Food and Drug Administration; BMD, bone mineral density.

APPROACH TO THE PATIENT WITH OSTEOPOROSIS

The perimenopausal transition is a good opportunity to initiate discussion about risk factors for osteoporosis and to consider indications for a BMD test. A careful history and physical examination should be performed to identify risk factors for osteoporosis. A low Z-score increases the suspicion of a secondary disease. Height loss >2.5 to 3.8 cm (>1 to 1.5 in.) is an indication for radiography to rule out asymptomatic vertebral fractures, as is the presence of significant kyphosis or back pain, particularly if it began after menopause. For patients who present with fractures, it is important to ensure that the fractures are not caused by an underlying malignancy. Usually this is clear on routine radiography, but on occasion, CT, magnetic resonance imaging, or radionuclide scans may be necessary.

Routine Laboratory Evaluation

There is no established algorithm for the evaluation of women presenting with osteoporosis. A general evaluation that includes complete blood count, serum calcium, and perhaps urine calcium is helpful for identifying selected secondary causes of low bone mass, particularly for women with fractures or very low Z-scores. An elevated serum calcium level suggests hyperparathyroidism or malignancy, whereas a reduced serum calcium level may reflect malnutrition and osteomalacia. In the presence of hypercalcemia, a serum PTH level differentiates between hyperparathyroidism (PTH↑) and malignancy (PTH↓), and a high PTHrP level can help document the presence of humoral hypercalcemia of malignancy (Chap. 24). A low urine calcium (<50 mg/24 h) suggests osteomalacia, malnutrition, or malabsorption; a high urine calcium (>300 mg/24 h) is indicative of hypercalciuria and must be investigated further. Hypercalciuria occurs primarily in three situations: (1) a renal calcium leak, which is more frequent in males with osteoporosis; (2) absorptive hypercalciuria, which can be idiopathic or associated with increased $1,25(OH)_2D$ in granulomatous disease; or (3) hematologic malignancies or conditions associated with excessive bone turnover such as Paget's disease, hyperparathyroidism, and hyperthyroidism.

Possible hyperthyroidism can be evaluated by measuring thyroid-stimulating hormone (TSH). When there is clinical suspicion of Cushing's syndrome, urinary free cortisol levels or a fasting serum cortisol should be measured after overnight dexamethasone. When bowel disease, malabsorption, or malnutrition is suspected, serum albumin, cholesterol, and a complete blood count should be checked. Asymptomatic malabsorption might be heralded by anemia (macrocytic-vitamin B_{12} or folate deficiency; or microcytic-iron deficiency) or low serum cholesterol or urinary calcium levels. If these or other features suggest malabsorption, further evaluation is required. Asymptomatic celiac disease with selective malabsorption is being found with increasing prevalence; the diagnosis can be made by testing for antigliadin, antiendomysial, or transglutaminase antibodies but may require endoscopic biopsy. A trial of a gluten-free diet can be confirmatory (Chap. 275, HPIM, 16e). When osteoporosis is found associated with symptoms of rash, multiple allergies, diarrhea, or flushing, mastocytosis should be excluded using 24-h urine histamine collection or serum tryptase.

Myeloma can masquerade as generalized osteoporosis, although it more commonly presents with bone pain and characteristic "punched-out" lesions on radiography. Serum and urine electrophoresis and evaluation for light chains in urine are required to exclude this diagnosis. A bone marrow biopsy may be required to rule out myeloma (in patients with equivocal electrophoretic results) and can also be used to exclude mastocytosis, leukemia, and other marrow infiltrative disorders, such as Gaucher disease.

Bone Biopsy

Tetracycline labeling of the skeleton allows determination of the rate of remodeling as well as evaluation for other metabolic bone diseases. The current use of BMD tests, in combination with hormonal evaluation and biochemical markers of bone remodeling, has largely replaced bone biopsy.

Biochemical Markers

Several biochemical tests are now available that provide an index of the overall rate of bone remodeling (**Table 25-5**). Biochemical markers are usually characterized as those related primarily to *bone formation* or *bone resorption*. These tests measure the overall state of bone remodeling at a single point in time. Clinical use of these tests has been hampered by biologic variability (in part related to circadian rhythm) as well as to analytical variability.

For the most part, remodeling markers do not predict rates of bone loss well enough to use this information clinically. However, markers of bone resorption may help in the prediction of fracture risk, particularly in older individuals. In women ≥65 years, when bone density results are greater than the usual treatment thresholds noted above, a high level of bone resorption should prompt consideration of treatment. The primary use of biochemical markers is for monitoring the response to treatment. With the introduction of antiresorp-

TABLE 25-5

BIOCHEMICAL MARKERS OF BONE METABOLISM IN CLINICAL USE

Bone formation
Serum bone-specific alkaline phosphatase
Serum osteocalcin
Serum propeptide of type I procollagen
Bone resorption
Urine and serum cross-linked N-telopeptide
Urine and serum cross-linked C-telopeptide
Urine total free deoxypyridinoline
Urine hydroxyproline
Serum tartrate-resistant acid phosphatase
Serum bone sialoprotein
Urine hydroxylysine glycosides

tive therapeutic agents, bone remodeling declines rapidly, with the fall in resorption occurring earlier than the fall in formation. Inhibition of bone resorption is maximal within 3 to 6 months. Thus, measurement of bone resorption prior to initiating therapy and 4 to 6 months after starting therapy provides an earlier estimate of patient response than does bone densitometry. A decline in resorptive markers can be ascertained after treatment with bisphosphonates or estrogen; this effect is less marked after treatment with either raloxifene or intranasal calcitonin. A biochemical marker response to therapy is particularly useful for asymptomatic patients and might help to ensure long-term compliance. Bone turnover markers are also useful in monitoring the effects of PTH, or teriparatide, which rapidly increases bone formation and later bone resorption.

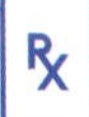

TREATMENT FOR OSTEOPOROSIS

Management of Osteoporotic Fractures

Treatment of the patient with osteoporosis frequently involves management of acute fractures as well as treatment of the underlying disease. Hip fractures almost always require surgical repair if the patient is to become ambulatory again. Depending on the location and severity of the fracture, condition of the neighboring joint, and general status of the patient, procedures may include open reduction and internal fixation with pins and plates, hemiarthroplasties, and total arthroplasties. These surgical procedures are followed by intense rehabilitation in an attempt to return patients to their prefracture functional level. Long bone fractures often require either external or internal fixation. Other fractures (e.g., vertebral, rib, and pelvic fractures) are usually managed with only supportive care, requiring no specific orthopedic treatment.

Only ~25 to 30% of vertebral compression fractures present with sudden-onset back pain. For acutely symptomatic fractures, treatment with analgesics is required, including nonsteroidal anti-inflammatory agents and/or acetaminophen, sometimes with the addition of a narcotic agent (codeine or oxycodone). A few small, randomized clinical trials suggest that calcitonin may reduce pain related to acute vertebral compression fracture. A recently developed technique involves percutaneous injection of artificial cement (polymethylmethacrylate) into the vertebral body (vertebroplasty or kyphoplasty); this has been reported to offer significant immediate pain relief in the majority of patients. Long-term effects are unknown, and conclusions are based on observational studies in patients with severe persistent back pain from acute or subacute vertebral fractures. There have been no randomized controlled trials of either vertebroplasty or kyphoplasty to date. Short periods of bed rest may be helpful for pain management, but, in general, early mobilization is recommended as it helps prevent further bone loss associated with immobilization. Occasionally, use of a soft elastic-style brace may facilitate earlier mobilization. Muscle spasms often occur with acute compression fractures and can be treated with muscle relaxants and heat treatments.

Severe pain usually resolves within 6 to 10 weeks. Chronic pain is probably not bony in origin; instead, it is related to abnormal strain on muscles, ligaments, and tendons and to secondary facet-joint arthritis associated with alterations in thoracic and/or abdominal shape. Chronic pain is difficult to treat effectively and may require analgesics, sometimes including narcotic analgesics. Frequent intermittent rest in a supine or semireclining position is often required to allow the soft tissues, which are under tension, to relax. Back-strengthening exercises (paraspinal) may be beneficial. Heat treatments help relax muscles and reduce the muscular component of discomfort. Various physical modalities, such as ultrasound and transcutaneous nerve stimulation, may be beneficial in some patients. Pain also occurs in the neck region, not as a result of compression fractures (which almost never occur in the cervical spine as a result of osteoporosis) but because of chronic strain associated from trying to elevate the head in a person with a severe thoracic kyphosis.

Multiple vertebral fractures are often associated with psychological symptoms, not always commonly appreciated. The changes in body configuration and back pain can lead to marked loss of self-image and a secondary depression. Altered balance, precipitated by the kyphosis and the anterior movement of the body's center of gravity, leads to a fear of falling, a consequent tendency to remain indoors, and the onset of social isolation. These symptoms can sometimes be alleviated by family support and/or psychotherapy. Medication may be necessary when depressive features are present.

Management of the Underlying Disease

RISK FACTOR REDUCTION

Patients should be thoroughly educated to reduce the likelihood of risk factors associated with bone loss and falling. Medications should be reviewed to ensure that any glucocorticoid medication is truly indicated and is being given in doses as low as possible. For those on thyroid hormone replacement, TSH testing should be performed to determine that an excessive dose is not being used, as thyrotoxicosis can be associated with increased bone loss. In patients who smoke, efforts should be made to facilitate smoking cessation. Reducing risk factors for falling also includes alcohol abuse treatment and a review of the medical regimen for any drugs that might be associated with orthostatic hypotension and/or sedation, including hypnotics and anxiolytics. If nocturia occurs, the frequency should be reduced, if possible (e.g., by decreasing or modifying diuretic use), as arising in the middle of sleep is a common precipitant of a fall. Patients should be instructed about environmental safety with regard to eliminating exposed wires, curtain strings, slippery rugs, and mobile tables. Avoiding stocking feet on wood floors, checking carpet condition (particularly on stairs), and providing good light in paths to bathrooms and outside the home are important preventive measures. Treatment for impaired vision is recommended, particularly a problem with depth perception, which is specifically associated with increased falling risk. Elderly patients with neurologic impairment (e.g., stroke, Parkinson's disease, Alzheimer's disease) are particularly at risk of falling and require specialized supervision and care.

NUTRITIONAL RECOMMENDATIONS

Calcium A large body of data indicates that optimal calcium intake reduces bone loss and suppresses bone turnover. Recommended intakes from a recent report from the Institute of Medicine are shown in **Table 25-6.** The National Health and Nutritional Evaluation Studies (NHANES) have consistently documented that average calcium intakes fall considerably short of these recommendations. The preferred source of calcium is from dairy products and other foods, but many patients require calcium supplementation. Food sources of calcium are dairy products (milk, yogurt, and cheese) and fortified foods such as certain cereals, waffles, snacks, juices, and crackers. Some of these fortified foods contain as much calcium per serving as milk.

If a calcium supplement is required, it should be taken in doses ≤600 mg at a time, as the calcium absorption fraction decreases at higher doses. Calcium supplements should be calculated based on the elemental calcium content of the supplement, not the weight of the calcium salt (**Table 25-7**). Calcium supplements containing carbonate are best taken with food since they require acid for solubility. Calcium citrate supplements can be taken at any time.

Several controlled clinical trials of calcium plus vitamin D have confirmed reductions in clinical fractures, including fractures of the hip (~20 to 30% risk reduction). All recent studies of pharmacologic

TABLE 25-6

ADEQUATE CALCIUM INTAKE

LIFE STAGE GROUP	ESTIMATED ADEQUATE DAILY CALCIUM INTAKE, MG/D
Young children (1–3 years)	500
Older children (4–8 years)	800
Adolescents and young adults (9–18 years)	1300
Men and women (19–50 years)	1000
Men and women (51 and older)	1200

Note: Pregnancy and lactation needs are the same as for nonpregnant women (e.g., 1300 mg/d for adolescents/young adult and 1000 mg/d for ≥19 years).

Source: Adapted from the Standing Committee on the Scientific Evaluation of Dietary Reference Intakes. Food and Nutrition Board. Institute of Medicine. Washington, DC, 1997. National Academy Press.

TABLE 25-7

ELEMENTAL CALCIUM CONTENT OF VARIOUS ORAL CALCIUM PREPARATIONS

CALCIUM PREPARATION	ELEMENTAL CALCIUM CONTENT
Calcium citrate	60 mg/300 mg
Calcium lactate	80 mg/600 mg
Calcium gluconate	40 mg/500 mg
Calcium carbonate	400 mg/g
Calcium carbonate +5 μg vitamin D_2 (OsCal 250)	250 mg/tablet
Calcium carbonate (Tums 500)	500 mg/tablet

Source: Adapted from SM Krane and MF Holick, Chap. 355 in *HPIM, 14e,* 1998.

agents have been conducted in the context of calcium replacement (± vitamin D). Thus, it is standard practice to ensure an adequate calcium and vitamin D intake in patients with osteoporosis, whether they are receiving additional pharmacologic therapy or not.

Although side effects from supplemental calcium are minimal, individuals with a history of kidney stones should have a 24-h urine calcium determination before starting increased calcium to avoid hypercalciuria.

Vitamin D Vitamin D is synthesized in skin under the influence of heat and ultraviolet light (Chap. 23). However, large segments of the population do not obtain sufficient vitamin D to maintain what is now considered an adequate supply [serum 25(OH)D consistently >50 μmol/L (20 ng/mL)]. Since vitamin D supplementation at doses that would achieve these serum levels is safe and inexpensive, the Institute of Medicine recommends daily intakes of 200 IU for adults <50 years of age, 400 IU for those from 50 to 70 years, and 600 IU for those >70 years. Multivitamin tablets usually contain 400 IU, and many calcium supplements also contain vitamin D. Some data suggest that higher doses may be required in the elderly and chronically ill.

Other Nutrients Other nutrients such as salt and caffeine may have modest effects on calcium excretion or absorption. Adequate vitamin K status is required for optimal carboxylation of osteocalcin. States in which vitamin K nutrition or metabolism is impaired, such as with long-term warfarin therapy, have been associated with reduced bone mass.

Magnesium is abundant in foods, and magnesium deficiency is quite rare in the absence of a serious chronic disease. Magnesium supplementation may be warranted in patients with inflammatory bowel disease, celiac disease, chemotherapy, severe diarrhea, malnutrition, or alcoholism. Dietary phytoestrogens, which are derived primarily from soy products and legumes (e.g., chickpeas, and lentils), exert some estrogenic activity but are insufficiently potent to justify their use in place of a pharmacologic agent in the treatment of osteoporosis.

Patients with hip fracture are often frail and relatively malnourished. Some data suggest an improved outcome in such patients when they are provided calorie and protein supplementation. Excessive protein intake can increase renal calcium excretion but this can be corrected by an adequate calcium intake.

EXERCISE

Exercise in young individuals increases the likelihood that they will attain the maximal genetically determined peak bone mass. Meta-analyses of studies performed in postmenopausal women indicate that weight-bearing exercise prevents bone loss but does not appear to result in substantial gain of bone mass. This beneficial effect wanes if exercise is discontinued. Exercise also has beneficial effects on neuromuscular function, and it improves coordination, balance, and strength, thereby reducing the risk of falling. A walking program is a practical way to start. Other activities such as dancing, racquet sports, cross-country skiing, and use of gym equipment also are recommended, depending on the patient's personal preference. Even women who cannot walk benefit from swimming or water exercises, not so much for the effects on bone, which are quite minimal, but because of effects on muscle. Exercise habits should be consistent, optimally at least three times a week.

Pharmacologic Therapies

Until fairly recently, estrogen treatment, either by itself or in concert with a progestin, was the primary therapeutic agent for prevention or treatment of osteoporosis. Over the past 10 years, a number of new drugs have appeared, and more are expected in the near future. Some are agents that specifically treat osteoporosis (bisphosphonates, calcitonin, PTH); others, such as selective estrogen receptor modulators (SERMs), have broader effects. The availability of these drugs allows therapy to be tailored to the needs of an individual patient.

ESTROGENS

A large body of clinical trial data indicates that various types of estrogens (conjugated equine estrogens, estradiol, estrone, esterified estrogens, ethinyl estradiol, and mestranol) reduce bone turnover, prevent bone loss, and induce small increases in bone mass of the spine, hip, and total body. The effects of estrogen are seen in women with natural or surgical menopause and in late postmenopausal women with or without established osteoporosis. Estrogens are efficacious when administered orally or transdermally. For both oral and transdermal routes of administration, combined estrogen/progestin preparations are now available in many countries, obviating the problem of taking two tablets or using a patch and oral progestin. One large study, referred to as PEPI (Postmenopausal Estrogen/Progestin Intervention Trial), indicated that C-21 progestins alone do not augment the effect of standard estrogen doses on bone mass (**Fig. 25-7**).

Dose of Estrogen For oral estrogens, the standard recommended doses are 0.3 mg/d for esterified estrogens, 0.625 mg/d for conjugated equine estrogens, and 5 μg/d for ethinyl estradiol. For transdermal estrogen, the commonly used dose supplies 50 μg estradiol per day, but a lower dose may be appropriate for some individuals. Dose response data for conjugated equine estrogens indicate that lower doses are effective.

Fracture Data Epidemiologic databases indicate that women who take estrogen replacement have a 50% reduction, on average, of osteoporotic fractures, including hip fractures. The beneficial effect of estrogen is greatest among those who start replacement early and continue the treatment; the benefit declines after discontinuation such that there is no residual protective effect against fracture by 10 years after discontinuation. The first

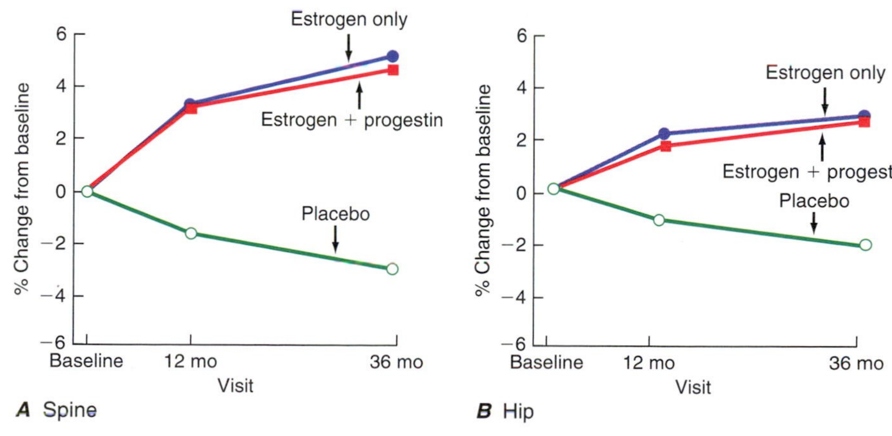

FIGURE 25-7

Results of hormone therapy regimens on bone mineral density (BMD) of the spine (*A*) and hip (*B*). Unadjusted mean percent change in BMD in the hip by treatment assignment and visit: adherent PEPI participants only. Results from the Postmenopausal Estrogen/Progestin Interventions (PEPI) trial. Estrogen, conjugated equine estrogen 0.625 mg/d; progestin, medroxyprogesterone acetate 10 mg/d. (*Adapted from TL Bush et al: JAMA 276:1389, 1996.*)

clinical trial evaluating fractures as secondary outcomes, the Heart and Estrogen-Progestin Replacement Study (HERS) trial, showed no effect of hormone therapy against hip or other clinical fractures in women with established coronary artery disease. These data made the results of the Women's Health Initiative (WHI) exceedingly important (Chap. 11). The estrogen-progestin arm of the WHI in >16,000 postmenopausal healthy women indicated that hormone therapy reduces the risk of hip fracture by 34% and all clinical fractures by 24%.

A few clinical trials have evaluated spine fracture occurrence as an outcome with estrogen therapy. One that used high doses of estrogen (2.5 mg/d conjugated equine estrogen) indicated marked vertebral fracture reduction in estrogen-treated women. Several other small studies, using lower estrogen doses, have consistently shown that estrogen treatment reduces the incidence of vertebral compression fracture.

The WHI has now provided a vast amount of data on the multisystemic effects of hormone therapy. Although earlier observational studies suggested that estrogen replacement might reduce heart disease, the WHI showed that combined estrogen-progestin treatment increased risk of fatal and nonfatal myocardial infarction by about 29%, confirming data from the HERS study. Other important relative risks included a 40% increase in stroke, a 100% increase in venous thromboembolic disease, and a 26% increase in risk of breast cancer. Subsequent analyses have confirmed the increased risk of stroke and shown a twofold increase in dementia. Benefits other than the fracture reductions noted above included a 37% reduction in risk of colon cancer. These relative risks have to be interpreted in light of absolute risk (**Fig. 25-8**). For example, out of 10,000 women treated with estrogen-progestin for 1 year, there will be 8 excess heart attacks, 8 excess breast cancers, 18 excess venous thromboembolic events, 5 fewer hip fractures, 44 fewer clinical fractures, and 6 fewer colorectal cancers. These numbers must be multiplied by years of hormone treatment. There was no effect of hormone treatment on risk of uterine cancer or total mortality.

It is important to note that the WHI findings apply specifically to hormone treatment in the form of conjugated equine estrogen plus medroxyprogesterone acetate. Furthermore, the relative benefits and risks of unopposed estrogen in women who had hysterectomy are still being evaluated in the estrogen-only arm of the WHI.

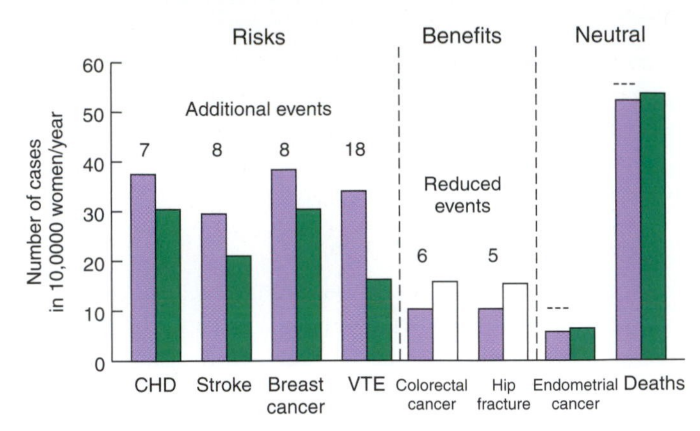

FIGURE 25-8

Effects of hormone therapy on event rates. CHD, coronary heart disease; VTE, venous thromboembolic events. (*Adapted from: Women's Health Initiative. WHI HRT Update. Available at http://www.nhlbi.nih.gov/health/women/upd2002.htm.*)

Mode of Action of Estrogens Two subtypes of ERs, α and β, have been identified in bone and other tissues. Cells of monocyte lineage express both ERα and -β, as do osteoblasts. Estrogen-mediated effects vary depending on the receptor type. Using ER knockout mouse models, elimination of ERα produces a modest reduction in bone mass, whereas mutation of ERβ has less effect on bone. A male patient with a homozygous mutation of ERα had markedly decreased bone density as well as abnormalities in epiphyseal closure, confirming the important role of ERα in bone biology. The mechanism of estrogen action in bone is an area of active investigation (Fig. 25-5). Although data are conflicting, estrogens may inhibit osteoclasts directly. However, the majority of estrogen (and androgen) effects on bone resorption are mediated indirectly through paracrine factors produced by osteoblasts. These actions include: (1) increasing IGF-I and TGF-β, and (2) suppressing IL-1 (α and β), IL-6, TNF-α, and osteocalcin synthesis. The indirect estrogen actions primarily decrease bone resorption.

PROGESTINS

In women with a uterus, daily progestin or cyclical progestins at least 12 days per month are prescribed in combination with estrogens to reduce the risk of uterine cancer. Medroxyprogesterone acetate and norethindrone acetate blunt the high-density lipoprotein response to estrogen, but micronized progesterone does not. Neither medroxyprogesterone acetate nor micronized progesterone appears to have an independent effect on bone; at lower doses, norethindrone acetate might have an additive benefit. On breast tissue, progestins may increase the risk of breast cancer.

SERMS

Two SERMs are currently being used in postmenopausal women: raloxifene, which is approved for prevention and treatment of osteoporosis, and tamoxifen, which is approved for the prevention and treatment of breast cancer.

Tamoxifen reduces bone turnover and bone loss in postmenopausal women compared with placebo groups. These findings support the concept that tamoxifen acts as an estrogenic agent in bone. There are limited data on the effect of tamoxifen on fracture risk, but the Breast Cancer Prevention study indicated a possible reduction in clinical vertebral, hip, and Colles' fractures. The major benefit of tamoxifen is on breast cancer occurrence. The breast cancer prevention trial indicated that tamoxifen administration over 4 to 5 years reduced the incidence of new invasive and noninvasive breast cancer by ~45% in women at increased risk of breast cancer. The incidence of ER-positive breast cancers was reduced by 65%.

Raloxifene (60 mg/d) has effects on bone turnover and bone mass that are very similar to those of tamoxifen, indicating that this agent is also estrogenic on the skeleton. The effect of raloxifene on bone density (+1.4 to 2.8% versus placebo in the spine, hip, and total body) is somewhat less than that seen with standard doses of estrogens. Raloxifene reduces the occurrence of vertebral fracture by 30 to 50%, depending on the subpopulation; however, there are no data confirming that raloxifene can reduce the risk of nonvertebral fractures.

Raloxifene, like tamoxifen and estrogen, has effects in other organ systems. The most beneficial effect appears to be a reduction in invasive breast cancer (mainly decreased ER-positive) occurrence of about 65% in women who take raloxifene compared with placebo. In contrast to tamoxifen, raloxifene is not associated with an increase in the risk of uterine cancer or benign uterine disease. Raloxifene increases the occurrence of hot flashes but reduces serum total and low-density lipoprotein cholesterol, lipoprotein(a), and fibrinogen. In women at high risk of heart disease, preliminary data suggest that raloxifene may reduce the occurrence of heart disease and stroke outcomes by about 40%. A large ongoing pivotal study, called Raloxifene Use for the Heart (RUTH), will further evaluate vascular disease and breast cancer outcomes.

Mode of Action of Serms All SERMs bind to the ER, but each agent produces a unique receptor conformation. As a result, specific coactivator or co-repressor proteins are bound to the receptor (Chap. 1), resulting in differential effects on gene transcription that vary depending on other transcription factors present in the cell. Another aspect of selectivity is the affinity of each SERM for the different ERα and -β subtypes, which are expressed differentially in various tissues. These tissue-selective effects of SERMs offer the possibility of tailoring estrogen therapy to best meet the needs and risk factor profile of an individual patient.

BISPHOSPHONATES

Both alendronate and risedronate are approved for the prevention and treatment of postmenopausal osteoporosis and treatment of steroid-induced osteoporosis. Risedronate is also approved for the prevention of steroid-induced osteoporosis. Alendronate is approved for treatment of osteoporosis in men.

Alendronate has been shown to decrease bone turnover and increase bone mass in the spine by up to 8% versus placebo and by 6% versus placebo in the hip. Multiple trials have evaluated its effect on fracture occurrence. The Fracture Intervention Trial provided evidence in >2000 women with prevalent vertebral fractures that daily alendronate treatment (5 mg/d for 2 years and 10 mg/d for 9 months afterwards) reduces vertebral fracture risk by about 50%, multiple vertebral fractures by up to 90%, and hip fractures by up to 50% (**Fig. 25-9**). Several subsequent trials have confirmed these findings. For example, in a study of >1900 women with low bone mass treated with alendronate (10 mg/d) versus placebo, the incidence of all nonvertebral fractures was reduced by ~47% after only 1 year.

Trials comparing once-weekly alendronate, 70 mg, with daily 10-mg dosing have shown equivalence with regard to bone mass and bone turnover

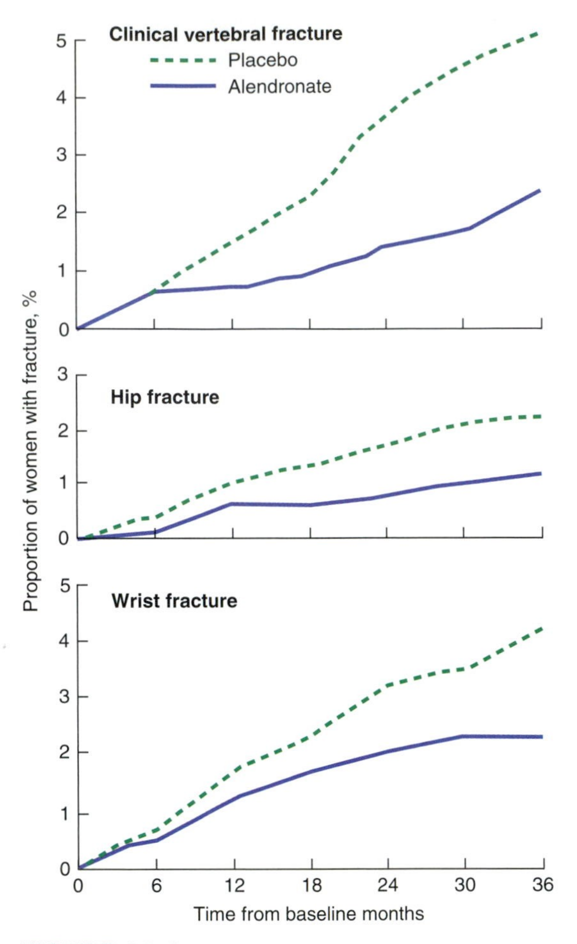

FIGURE 25-9

Cumulative proportions of women with osteoporosis who suffered clinical vertebral, hip, or wrist fracture during 3 years of treatment with alendronate or placebo (FIT 1). (*From DM Black et al: Lancet 348:1535, 1996.*)

responses. Consequently, once-weekly therapy is generally preferred because of low incidence of gastrointestinal side effects and ease of administration. Alendronate should be given with a full glass of water before breakfast, as bisphosphonates are poorly absorbed. Because of the potential for esophageal irritation, alendronate is contraindicated in patients who have stricture or inadequate emptying of the esophagus. It is recommended that patients remain upright for at least 30 min after taking the medication to avoid esophageal irritation. Cases of esophagitis, esophageal ulcer, and esophageal stricture have been described, but the incidence appears to be low. In clinical trials, overall gastrointestinal symptomatology was no different with alendronate compared with placebo.

Risedronate also reduces bone turnover and increases bone mass. Controlled clinical trials have demonstrated a 40 to 50% reduction in vertebral fracture risk over 3 years, accompanied by a 40% reduction in clinical nonspine fractures. The only clinical trial specifically designed to evaluate hip fracture outcome (HIP) indicated that risedronate reduced hip fracture risk in women in their seventies with confirmed osteoporosis by 40%. In contrast, risedronate was not effective at reducing hip fracture occurrence in older women without proven osteoporosis. Studies have shown that 35 mg of risedronate administered once weekly is therapeutically equivalent to 5 mg/d. Patients should take risedronate with a full glass of plain water [0.18 to 0.25 L (6 to 8 oz)], to facilitate delivery to the stomach, and should not lie down for 30 min after taking the drug. The incidence of gastrointestinal side effects in trials with risedronate was similar to that of placebo.

Etidronate was the first bisphosphonate to be approved, initially for use in Paget disease and hypercalcemia. This agent has also been used in osteoporosis trials of smaller magnitude than those performed for alendronate and risedronate but is not approved by the FDA for treatment of osteoporosis. Etidronate probably has some efficacy against vertebral fracture when given as an intermittent cyclical regimen (2 weeks on, 2 1/2 months off). There has not been any study of its effectiveness against nonvertebral fractures.

Zoledronate and ibandronate are potent bisphosphonates with unique administration regimens (once yearly intravenously, once monthly orally) and are currently in clinical development.

Mode of Action of Bisphosphonates Bisphosphonates are structurally related to pyrophosphates, compounds that are incorporated into bone matrix. Bisphosphonates specifically impair osteoclast function and reduce osteoclast number, in part by the induction of apoptosis. Recent evidence suggests that the nitrogen-containing bisphosphonates also inhibit protein prenylation, one of the end products in the mevalonic acid pathway. This effect disrupts intracellular protein trafficking and may ultimately lead to apoptosis. Some bisphosphonates have very long retention in the skeleton and may exert long-term effects.

CALCITONIN

Calcitonin is a polypeptide hormone produced by the thyroid gland (Chap. 24). Its physiologic role is unclear as no skeletal disease has been described in association with calcitonin deficiency or calcitonin excess. Calcitonin preparations are approved by the FDA for Paget disease, hypercalcemia, and osteoporosis in women >5 years past menopause.

Injectable calcitonin produces small increments in bone mass of the lumbar spine. However, difficulty of administration and frequent reactions, including nausea and facial flushing, make general use limited. In 1995, a nasal spray containing calcitonin (200 IU/d) was approved for treatment of osteoporosis in postmenopausal women. One study suggests that nasal calcitonin produces small increments in bone mass and a small reduction in new vertebral fractures in calcitonin-treated patients versus those on calcium alone. There has been no proven effectiveness against nonvertebral fractures.

Calcitonin is not indicated for prevention of osteoporosis and is not sufficiently potent to prevent bone loss in early postmenopausal women. As mentioned above, calcitonin might have an analgesic effect on bone pain, both in the subcutaneous and possibly the nasal form.

Mode of Action of Calcitonin Calcitonin suppresses osteoclast activity by direct action on the osteoclast calcitonin receptor. Osteoclasts exposed to calcitonin cannot maintain their active ruffled border, which normally maintains close contact with underlying bone.

PARATHYROID HORMONE

Endogenous PTH is an 84-amino-acid peptide that is largely responsible for calcium homeostasis (Chap. 24). Although chronic elevation of PTH, as occurs in hyperparathyroidism, is associated with bone loss (particularly cortical bone), PTH can also exert anabolic effects on bone. Consistent with this, some observational studies have indicated that mild elevations in PTH are associated with maintenance of trabecular bone mass. On the basis of these findings, preclinical and early clinical studies have been performed using an exogenous PTH analogue (1-34 PTH). The first randomized controlled trial in postmenopausal women showed that PTH, when superimposed on ongoing estrogen therapy, produced substantial increments in bone mass (13% over a 3-year period compared with estrogen alone) and reduced the risk of vertebral compression deformity. In one study (median 19 months' duration), 20 μg PTH (1-34) reduced vertebral fractures by 65% and nonvertebral fractures by 45% (**Fig. 25-10**). PTH (1-34) has now been approved by the FDA for treatment of patients with osteoporosis (both women and men) at high risk of fracture. Treatment is administered as a single daily injection given for a maximum of 2 years. Antiresorptive agents after PTH withdrawal

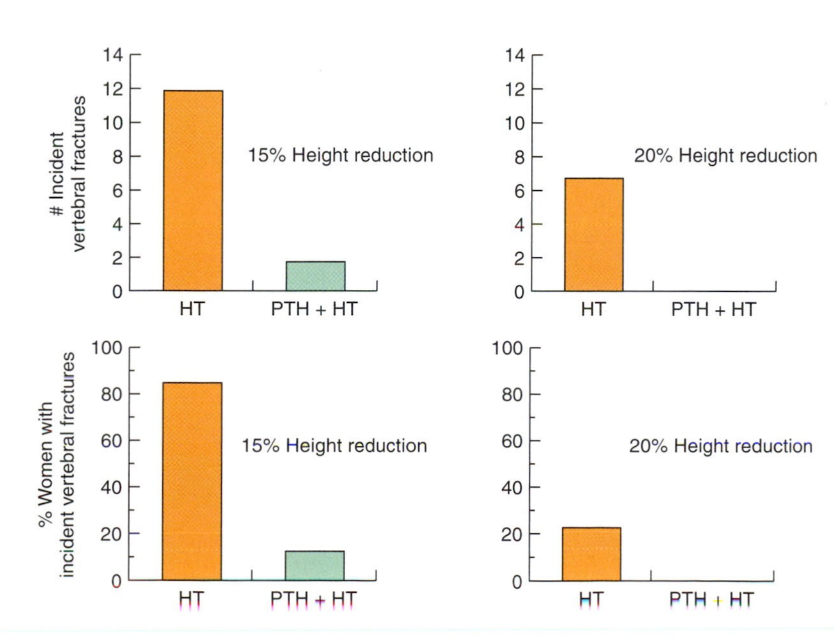

FIGURE 25-10
Number of incident vertebral deformities (15% and 20% reductions) in women with osteoporosis on hormone therapy (HT), compared to HT + PTH over 3 years. HT, hormone therapy; PTH, parathyroid hormone. (*From F Cosman et al: J Bone Miner Res 16:925, 2001, with permission.*)

appear to maintain PTH-induced benefits on bone mass and fracture.

Side effects are generally mild and can include muscle pains, weakness, dizziness, headache, and nausea. Rodents given prolonged treatment with PTH in relatively high doses developed osteogenic sarcomas. It is not believed that this finding has any relevance to humans.

PTH use may be limited by its mode of administration; alternative modes of delivery are being investigated. The optimal frequency of administration also remains to be established, and it is possible that PTH might also be effective when used intermittently. Cost also may be a limiting factor.

Mode of Action of Parathyroid Hormone Exogenously administered PTH appears to have direct actions on osteoblast activity, with biochemical and histomorphometric evidence of de novo bone formation early in response to PTH, prior to activation of bone resorption. Subsequently, PTH activates bone remodeling but still appears to favor bone formation over bone resorption. PTH stimulates IGF-I and collagen production and appears to increase osteoblast number by stimulating replication, enhancing osteoblast recruitment, and inhibiting apoptosis. Unlike all other treatments, PTH produces a true increase in bone tissue and an apparent restoration of bone microarchitecture (**Fig. 25-11**).

FLUORIDE

Fluoride has been available for many years and is a potent stimulator of osteoprogenitor cells when studied in vitro. It has been used in multiple osteoporosis studies with conflicting results, in part related to use of varying doses and preparations. Despite increments in bone mass of up to 10%, there are no consistent effects of fluoride on vertebral or nonvertebral fracture, which might actually increase when high doses of fluoride are used. Fluoride remains an experimental agent, despite its long history and multiple studies.

OTHER POTENTIAL ANABOLIC AGENTS

Several small studies of growth hormone (GH), alone or in combination with other agents, have not shown consistent or substantial positive effects on skeletal mass. Many of these studies are relatively short-term, and the effects of GH, growth hormone–releasing hormone, and the IGFs are still under investigation. Anabolic steroids, mostly derivatives of testosterone, act primarily as antiresorptive agents to reduce bone turnover but may also stimulate osteoblastic activity. Effects on bone mass remain unclear but appear weak, in general, and use is limited by masculinizing side effects. Several recent observational studies suggest that the statin drugs, currently used to treat hypercholesterolemia, may be associated with increased bone mass and reduced fractures, but conclusions from clinical trials are mixed.

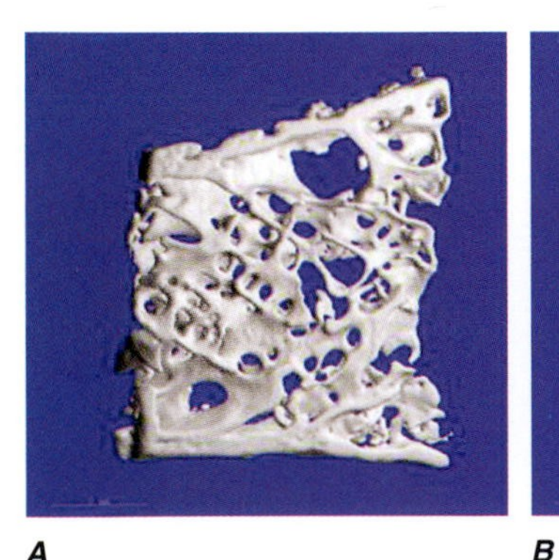

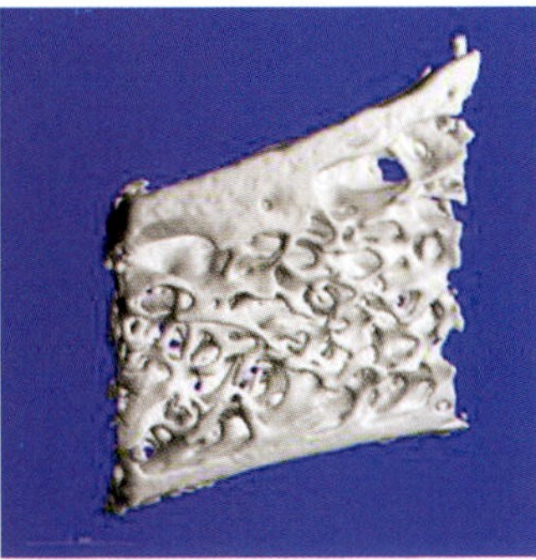

A *B*

FIGURE 25-11

Effect of parathyroid hormone (PTH) treatment on bone microarchitecture. Paired biopsy specimens from a 64-year-old woman before (*A*) and after (*B*) treatment with PTH. (*From DW Dempster et al: J Bone Miner Res 16:1846, 2001.*)

Nonpharmacologic Approaches

Protective pads worn around the outer thigh, which cover the trochanteric region of the hip, can prevent hip fractures in elderly residents in nursing homes. The use of hip protectors is limited largely by compliance and comfort, but new devices are being developed that may circumvent these problems and provide adjunctive treatments.

Kyphoplasty and *vertebroplasty* also are useful nonpharmacologic approaches for the treatment of painful vertebral fractures. However, no long-term data are available.

Treatment Monitoring

There are currently no well-accepted guidelines for monitoring treatment of osteoporosis. Because most osteoporosis treatments produce small or moderate bone mass increments on average, it is reasonable to consider BMD as a monitoring tool. Changes must exceed ~4% in the spine and 6% in the hip to be considered significant in any individual. The hip is the preferred site due to larger surface area and greater reproducibility. Medication-induced increments may require several years to produce changes of this magnitude (if they do at all). Consequently, it can be argued that BMD should not be repeated at intervals <2 years. Only significant BMD reductions should prompt a change in medical regimen, as it is expected that many individuals will not show responses greater than the detection limits of the current measurement techniques.

Biochemical markers of bone turnover may prove useful for treatment monitoring, but there is currently little hard evidence to support this concept; it remains unclear which endpoint is most useful. If bone turnover markers are used, a determination should be made before starting therapy and repeated ≥4 months after therapy is initiated. In general, a change in bone turnover markers must be 30 to 40% lower than the baseline to be significant because of the biologic and technical variability in these tests. A positive change in biochemical markers and/or bone density can be useful to help patients adhere to treatment regimens.

GLUCOCORTICOID-INDUCED OSTEOPOROSIS

Osteoporotic fractures are a well-characterized consequence of the hypercortisolism associated with Cushing's syndrome. However, the therapeutic use of glucocorticoids is by far the most common form of glucocorticoid-induced osteoporosis. Glucocorticoids are widely used in the treatment of a variety of disorders, including chronic lung disorders, rheumatoid arthritis and other connective tissue diseases, inflammatory bowel disease, and posttransplantation. Osteoporosis and related fractures are serious side effects of chronic glucocorticoid therapy. Because the effects of glucocorticoids on the skeleton are often superimposed on the consequences of aging and menopause, it is not surprising that women and the elderly are most frequently affected. The skeletal response to steroids is remarkably heterogeneous, however, and even young, growing individuals treated with glucocorticoids can present with fractures.

The risk of fractures depends on the dose and duration of glucocorticoid therapy, although recent data suggest that there may be no completely safe dose. Bone loss is more rapid during the early months of treatment, and trabecular bone is more severely affected than cortical bone. As a result, fractures have been shown to increase within 3 months of steroid treatment. There is an increase in fracture risk in both the axial and appendicular skeleton, including risk of hip fracture. Bone loss can occur with any route of steroid administration including high-dose inhaled glucocorticoids and intra-articular injections. Alternate-day delivery does not appear to ameliorate the skeletal effects of glucocorticoids.

PATHOPHYSIOLOGY

Glucocorticoids increase bone loss by multiple mechanisms including (1) inhibition of osteoblast function and an increase in osteoblast apoptosis, resulting in impaired synthesis of new bone; (2) stimulation of bone resorption, probably as a secondary effect; (3) impairment of the absorption of calcium across the intestine, probably by a vitamin D–independent effect; (4) increase of urinary calcium loss and induction of some degree of secondary hyperparathyroidism; (5) reduction of adrenal androgens and suppression of ovarian and testicular secretion of estrogens and androgens; and (6) induction of glucocorticoid myopathy, which may exacerbate effects on skeletal and calcium homeostasis as well as increase the risk of falls.

EVALUATION OF THE PATIENT

Because of the prevalence of glucocorticoid-induced bone loss, it is important to evaluate the status of the skeleton in all patients starting or already receiving long-term glucocorticoid therapy. Modifiable risk factors should be identified, including those for falls. Examination should include height and muscle strength testing. Laboratory evaluation should include an assessment of 24-h urinary calcium. All patients on long-term (>3 months) glucocorticoids have measurement of bone mass at both the spine and hip using DXA. If only one skeletal site can be measured, it is best to assess the spine in individuals <60 years and the hip for those >60 years.

PREVENTION

Bone loss caused by glucocorticoids can be prevented, and the risk of fractures significantly reduced. Strategies must include using the lowest dose of glucocorticoid for disease management. Topical and inhaled routes of administration are preferred, where appropriate. Risk factor reduction is important, including smoking cessation, limitation of alcohol consumption, and participation in weight-bearing exercise, when appropriate. All patients should receive an adequate calcium and vitamin D intake from the diet or from supplements.

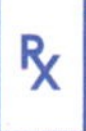

TREATMENT FOR GLUCOCORTICOID-INDUCED OSTEOPOROSIS

Only bisphosphonates have been demonstrated in large clinical trials to reduce the risk of fractures in patients being treated with glucocorticoids. Risedronate prevents bone loss and reduces vertebral fracture risk by about 70%. Similar beneficial effects are observed in studies of alendronate and etidronate. Controlled trials of hormone therapy have shown bone-sparing effects, and calcitonin also has some protective effect in the spine. Thiazides reduce urine calcium loss, but their role in prevention of fractures is unclear. PTH has also been studied in a small group of women with glucocorticoid-induced osteoporosis. Bone mass increased substantially, but no fracture data are available.

FURTHER READINGS

Black D et al: One year of alendronate after one year of parathyroid hormone (1–84) for osteoporosis. N Engl J Med 353:555, 2005

Women with postmenopausal osteoporosis received combinations of PTH (1–84) and alendronate. At 24 months, the largest increase in vertebral and hip BMD from baseline occurred in women who received PTH (1–84) for 12 months followed by alendronate monotherapy for 12 months.

Cosman F et al: Daily and cyclic parathyroid hormone in women receiving alendronate. N Engl J Med 353:566, 2005

A study of daily and cyclical PTH (1–34) as adjuvant therapy in 126 osteoporotic women who were already taking alendronate. Bone mineral density increased in both the daily and cyclical PTH groups.

Guyatt G et al: Meta-analyses of therapies for postmenopausal osteoporosis. Endocr Rev 23:495, 2002

Neer RM et al: Effect of parathyroid hormone (1–34) on fractures and bone mineral density in postmenopausal women with osteoporosis. N Engl J Med 344:1434, 2001

Raisz LG: Clinical practice. Screening for osteoporosis. N Engl J Med 353:164, 2005

A practical summary of bone mineral density testing and laboratory tests used to identify patients with osteoporosis.

Rosen CJ: Clinical practice. Postmenopausal osteoporosis. N Engl J Med 353:595, 2005

A review of the nonpharmacologic and pharmacologic management of osteoporosis, emphasizing the need to individualize therapy for patients with different risk factors.

Rossouw JE et al: Risks and benefits of estrogen plus progestin in healthy postmenopausal women: Principal results from the Women's Health Initiative randomized controlled trial. Writing Group for the Women's Health Initiative Investigators. JAMA 288:321, 2002

Wasnich RD et al: Antifracture efficacy of antiresorptive agents are related to changes in bone density. J Clin Endocrinol Metab 85:231, 2000

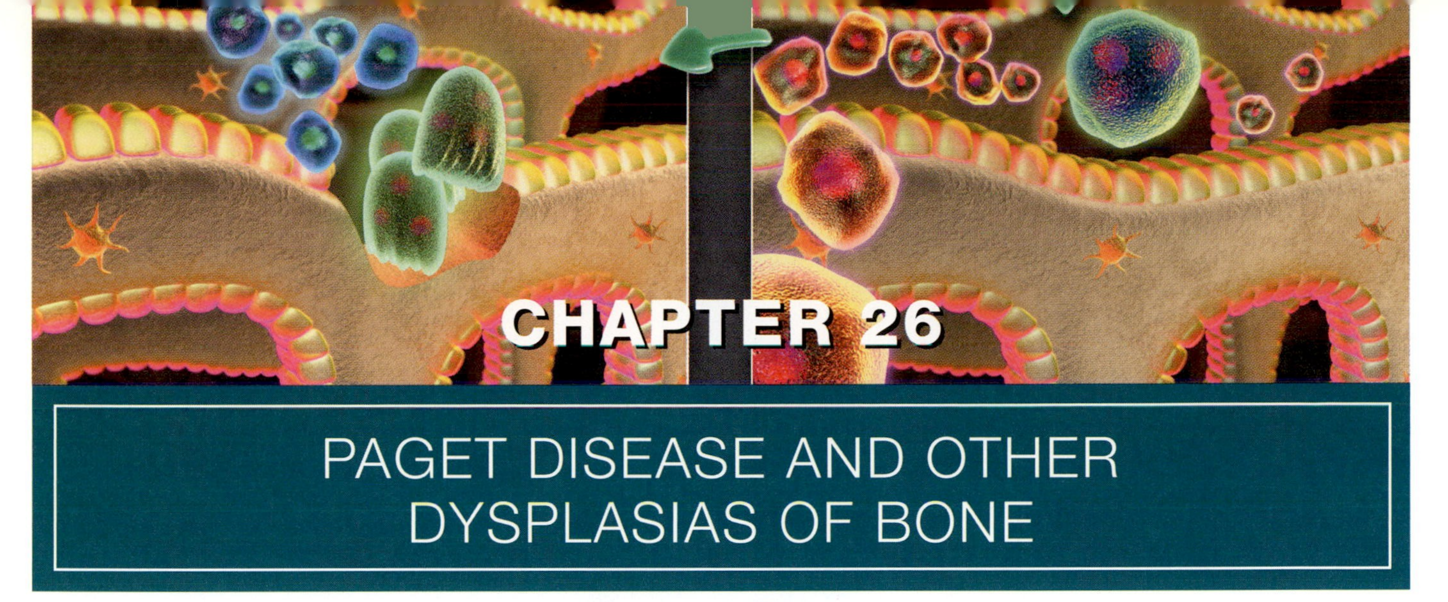

PAGET DISEASE AND OTHER DYSPLASIAS OF BONE

Murray J. Favus
Tamara J. Vokes

PAGET DISEASE OF BONE

Paget disease is a localized bone disorder that often affects widespread areas of the skeleton through increased bone remodeling. The pathologic process is initiated by overactive osteoclastic bone resorption followed by a compensatory increase in osteoblastic new bone formation. New pagetic bone is structurally disorganized and more susceptible to deformities and fractures. Although most patients are asymptomatic, a variety of symptoms and complications may result directly from bony involvement or secondarily from the expansion of bone and subsequent compression of surrounding neural tissue.

EPIDEMIOLOGY

There is a marked geographic variation in the frequency of Paget disease, with high prevalence in Western Europe (Great Britain, France, and Germany but not Switzerland or Scandinavia) and among those who have immigrated to Australia, New Zealand, South Africa, and North and South America. The disease is rare in native populations of the Americas, Africa, Asia, and the Middle East. The prevalence is greater in males and increases with age. Autopsy series reveal Paget disease in about 3% of those over age 40. Prevalence of positive skeletal radiographs in patients over age 55 is 2.5% for men and 1.6% for women. Elevated alkaline phosphatase (ALP) levels in asymptomatic patients has an age-adjusted incidence of 12.7 and 7 per 100,000 person-years in men and women, respectively. The frequency of diagnosis by either radiographic or biochemical criteria has decreased during the past 20 years.

ETIOLOGY

The etiology of Paget disease of bone remains unknown, but evidence supports both genetic and viral etiologies. A positive family history is found in 5 to 25% of patients and, when present, raises the prevalence of the disease seven- to tenfold among first-degree relatives. Familial patterns of disease in several large kindred are consistent with an autosomal dominant pattern of inheritance with variable penetrance. A susceptibility locus for Paget disease has been mapped to chromosome 18q21-22, a region that contains the gene responsible for a rare Paget disease–like skeletal disorder known as familial expansile osteolysis. The gene encodes the receptor activator of nuclear factor-κB (RANK), a member of the tumor necrosis factor superfamily critical for osteoclast differentiation (**Fig. 26-1**). In other families, susceptibility loci have been mapped to loci on chromosomes 18q23, 6p21.3, 5q31, and 5q35. A homozygous deletion of the *TNFRSF11B* gene, which encodes osteoprotegerin (Fig. 26-1), causes juvenile Paget disease, a disorder characterized by uncontrolled osteoclastic differentiation and resorption. Thus, it is likely that Paget disease is genetically heterogeneous with divergent pathogenetic mechanisms in sporadic and familial forms.

Several lines of evidence suggest a viral etiology of Paget disease, including (1) the presence of cytoplasmic and nuclear inclusions resembling paramyxoviruses (measles and respiratory syncytial virus) in pagetic osteoclasts, and (2) viral mRNA in precursor and mature osteoclasts. The viral etiology is further supported by conversion of osteoclast precursors to pagetic-like osteoclasts by vectors containing the measles virus nucleocapsid or matrix genes. However, the viral etiology has been questioned by the inability to culture a live virus from pagetic bone and by failure to clone the full-length viral genes from material obtained from patients with Paget disease.

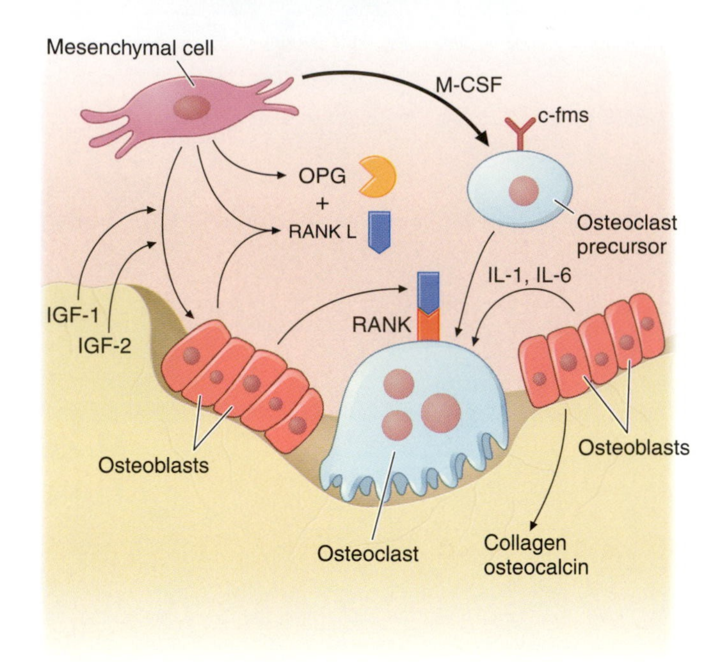

FIGURE 26-1
Diagram illustrating factors that promote differentiation and function of osteoclasts and osteoblasts and the role of the RANK pathway. Stromal bone marrow (mesenchymal) cells and differentiated osteoblasts produce multiple growth factors and cytokines, including macrophage colony-stimulating factor (M-CSF), to modulate osteoclastogenesis. RANKL (receptor activator of NFκB ligand) is produced by osteoblast progenitors and mature osteoblasts and can bind to a soluble decoy receptor known as OPG (osteoprotegerin) to inhibit RANKL action. Alternatively, a cell-cell interaction between osteoblast and osteoclast progenitors allows RANKL to bind to its membrane-bound receptor, RANK, thereby stimulating osteoclast differentiation and function. RANK binds intracellular proteins called TRAFS (tumor necrosis factor receptor-associated factors) that mediate receptor signaling through transcription factors such as NFκB. M-CSF binds to its receptor, c-fms, which is the cellular homologue of the *fms* oncogene. See text for the potential role of these pathways in disorders of osteoclast function such as Paget disease and osteopetrosis.

PATHOPHYSIOLOGY

The principal abnormality in Paget disease is the increased number and activity of osteoclasts. Pagetic osteoclasts are large, increased 10- to 100-fold in number, and have a greater number of nuclei (as many as 100 compared with 3 to 5 nuclei in the normal osteoclast). The overactive osteoclasts create a sevenfold increase in resorptive surfaces and an erosion rate of 9 μg/d (normal is 1 μg/d). Several causes for the increased number and activity of pagetic osteoclasts have been identified: (1) osteoclastic precursors are hypersensitive to $1,25(OH)_2D_3$; (2) osteoclasts are hyperresponsive to RANK ligand (RANKL), the osteoclast stimulatory factor that mediates the effects of most osteotropic factors on osteoclast formation; (3) marrow stromal cells from pagetic lesions have increased RANKL expression; (4) osteoclast precursor recruitment is increased by interleukin (IL) 6, which is increased in the blood of patients with active Paget disease and is overexpressed in pagetic osteoclasts; (5) expression of the proto-oncogene *c-fos,* which increases osteoclastic activity, is increased; and (6) the antiapoptotic oncogene *Bcl-2* in pagetic bone is overexpressed. Numerous osteoblasts are recruited to active resorption sites and produce large amounts of new bone matrix. As a result, bone turnover is high and bone mass is normal or increased, not reduced.

The characteristic feature of Paget disease is increased bone resorption accompanied by accelerated bone formation. An initial osteolytic phase involves prominent bone resorption and marked hypervascularization. Radiographically, this manifests as an advancing lytic wedge, or "blade of grass" lesion. The second phase is a period of very active bone formation and resorption that replaces normal lamellar bone with haphazard (woven) bone. The mosaic pattern of woven bone is structurally inferior and can bow and fracture more readily. At the same time, fibrous connective tissue may replace normal bone marrow. In the final sclerotic phase, bone resorption declines progressively and leads to a hard, dense, less vascular pagetic or mosaic bone, which represents the so-called burned-out phase of Paget disease. All three phases may be present at the same time at different skeletal sites.

CLINICAL MANIFESTATIONS

Asymptomatic patients are often diagnosed by discovery of an elevated ALP level on routine blood chemistry testing or from an abnormality on a skeletal radiograph obtained for another indication. The skeletal sites most commonly involved are the pelvis, vertebral bodies, skull, femur, and tibia. Numerous active sites of skeletal involvement are more common in familial cases with an early presentation.

Pain is the most common presenting symptom. It results from increased bony vascularity, expanding lytic lesions, fractures, bowing, or other deformities of the extremities. Bowing of the femur or tibia causes gait abnormalities and abnormal mechanical stresses with secondary osteoarthritis of the hip or knee joints. Long bone bowing also causes extremity pain by stretching the muscles attached to the bone softened by the pagetic process. Back pain results from enlarged pagetic vertebrae, vertebral compression fractures, spinal stenosis, degenerative changes of the joints, and altered body mechanics with kyphosis and forward tilt of the upper back. Rarely, spinal cord compression may result from bone enlargement or from the vascular steal syndrome. Skull involvement may cause headaches, symmetric or asymmetric enlargement of the parietal or frontal bones (frontal bossing), and increased head size. Cranial expansion may narrow cranial foramina and cause neurologic complications including hearing loss from cochlear nerve damage from temporal bone involvement, cranial nerve palsies, and softening of the base of the skull (*platybasia*) and the risk of brainstem compression. Pagetic involvement of the facial bones may cause facial deformity, loss of teeth and other dental conditions, and, rarely, airway compression.

Fractures are serious complications of Paget disease and usually occur in long bones at areas of active or advancing lytic lesions. Common fracture sites are the femoral shaft and subtrochanteric regions. Neoplasms arising from pagetic bone are rare. The incidence of sarcoma appears to be decreasing, possibly because of earlier, more effective treatment with potent antiresorptive agents. The majority of tumors are osteosarcomas, which usually present with new pain in a long-standing pagetic lesion. Osteoclast-rich benign giant cell tumors may arise in areas adjacent to pagetic bone and respond to glucocorticoid therapy.

Cardiovascular complications may occur in patients with involvement of large (15 to 35%) portions of the skeleton and a high degree of disease activity (ALP four times above normal). The extensive arteriovenous shunting and marked increases in blood flow through the vascular pagetic bone lead to a high-output state and cardiac enlargement. However, high-output heart failure is relatively rare and usually develops in patients with concomitant cardiac pathology. In addition, calcific aortic stenosis and diffuse vascular calcifications have been associated with Paget disease.

DIAGNOSIS

The diagnosis may be suggested on clinical examination by the presence of enlarged skull with frontal bossing, bowing of an extremity, or short stature with simian posturing. An extremity with an area of warmth and tenderness to palpation may suggest an underlying pagetic lesion. Other findings include bony deformity of the pelvis, skull, spine, and extremities; arthritic involvement of the joints adjacent to lesions; and leg length discrepancy resulting from deformities of the long bones.

Paget disease is usually diagnosed from radiologic and biochemical abnormalities. Radiographic findings typical of Paget disease include enlargement or expansion of an entire bone or area of a long bone, cortical thickening, coarsening of trabecular markings, and typical lytic and sclerotic changes. Skull radiographs (**Fig. 26-2**) reveal regions of "cotton wool," or osteoporosis circumscripta; thickening of diploic areas; and enlargement and sclerosis of a portion or all of one or more skull bones. Vertebral cortical thickening of the superior and inferior end plates creates a "picture frame" vertebra. Diffuse radiodense enlargement of a vertebra is referred to as "ivory vertebra." Pelvic radiographs may demonstrate disruption or fusion of the sacroiliac joints; porotic and radiodense lesions of the ilium with whorls of coarse trabeculation; thickened and sclerotic iliopectineal line (Brim sign); and softening with protrusio acetabuli, with axial migration of the hips and functional flexion contracture. Radiographs of long bones reveal bowing deformity and typical pagetic changes of cortical thickening and expansion and areas of lucency and sclerosis (**Fig. 26-3**). Radionuclide ^{99m}Tc bone scans are less specific but are more sensitive than standard radiographs for identifying sites of active skeletal lesions. Suspected areas of malignant transformation are best distinguished from pagetic bone by computed tomography (CT) or magnetic resonance imaging (MRI). Definitive diagnosis of malignancy requires bone biopsy.

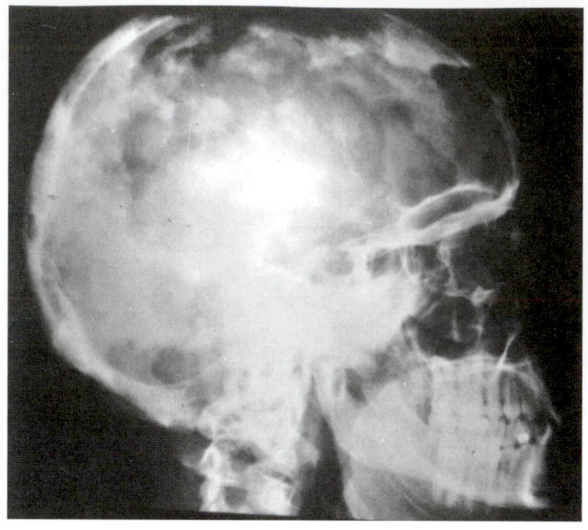

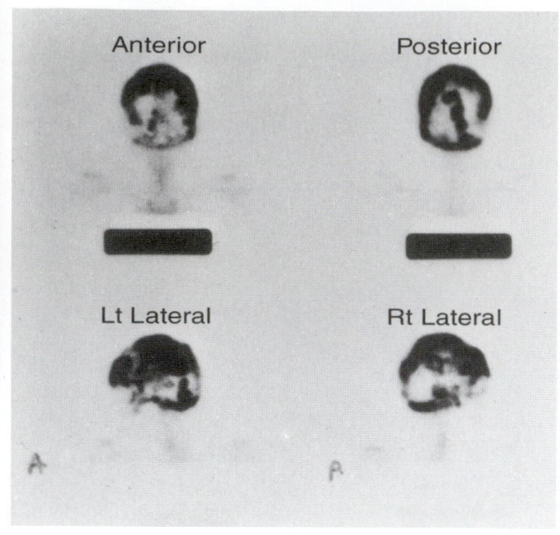

FIGURE 26-2
A 48-year-old woman with Paget disease of the skull. ***Left***. Lateral radiograph showing areas of both bone resorption and sclerosis. ***Right***. ^{99m}Tc HDP bone scan with anterior, posterior, and lateral views of the skull showing diffuse isotope uptake by the frontal, parietal, occipital, and petrous bones.

Biochemical evaluation is useful in the diagnosis and management of Paget disease. The marked increase in bone turnover can be monitored using biochemical markers of bone formation and resorption. The parallel rise in serum ALP and urinary hydroxyproline levels, markers of bone formation and resorption, respectively, confirm the coupling of bone formation and resorption in Paget disease. The degree of bone marker elevation reflects the extent and severity of the disease. Patients with the highest elevation of ALP (10 times the upper limit of normal) typically have involvement of the skull and at least one other skeletal site. Lower values suggest less extensive involvement or a quiescent phase of the disease. For most patients, serum total ALP remains the test of choice both for diagnosis and for assessing response to therapy. Occasionally, a symptomatic patient with evidence of progression at a single site may have a normal total ALP level but increased bone-specific ALP. Serum osteocalcin, a marker of bone formation, is not always elevated in patients with active Paget disease and is not recommended for use in diagnosis or management.

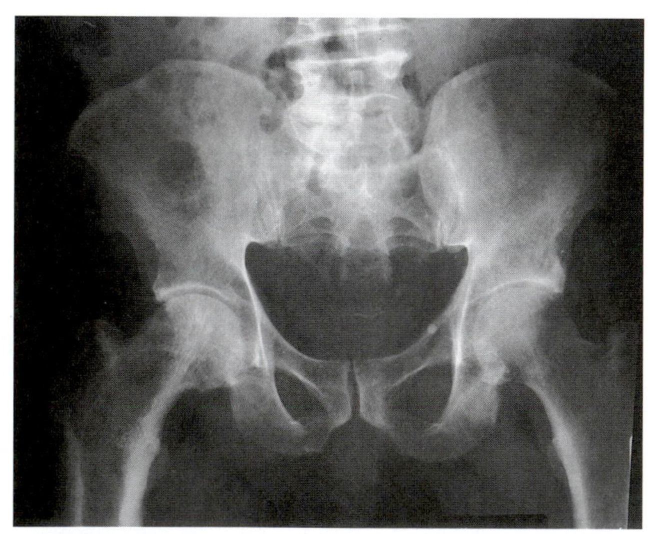

FIGURE 26-3
Radiograph of a 73-year-old man with Paget disease of the right proximal femur. Note the coarsening of the trabecular pattern with marked cortical thickening and narrowing of the joint space consistent with osteoarthritis secondary to pagetic deformity of the right femur.

Urinary and serum deoxypyridinoline, N-telopeptide, and C-telopeptide levels are products of type I collagen degradation and are more specific for bone resorption than hydroxyproline. These newer bone resorption markers have distinct advantages over measurement of 24-h or second-morning void hydroxyproline/creatinine ratio, which requires control of dietary gelatin intake and precise urine collection and analysis. The new resorption markers decrease more rapidly in response to therapy than does ALP.

Serum calcium and phosphate levels are normal in Paget disease. Immobilization of a patient with active Paget disease may rarely cause hypercalcemia and hypercalciuria and increase the risk for nephrolithiasis. However, the discovery of hypercalcemia, even in the presence of immobilization, should prompt a search for another cause of hypercalcemia. In contrast, hypocalcemia or mild secondary hyperparathyroidism may develop in Paget patients with very active bone formation and insufficient dietary calcium intake. Hypocalcemia can occur during bisphosphonate therapy when bone resorption is rapidly suppressed and active bone formation continues. Hypocalcemia may be prevented by adequate calcium and vitamin D intake.

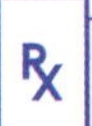

TREATMENT FOR PAGET DISEASE

The development of effective and potent pharmacologic agents (**Table 26-1**) has changed the treatment philosophy from treating only symptomatic patients to treating asymptomatic patients who are at risk for complications. Pharmacologic therapy is indicated in the following circumstances: to control symptoms caused by metabolically active Paget disease such as bone pain, fracture, headache, pain from pagetic radiculopathy or arthropathy, or neurologic complications; to decrease local blood flow and minimize operative blood loss in patients undergoing surgery at an active pagetic site; to reduce hypercalciuria that may occur during immobilization; and to decrease the risk of complications when disease activity is high (elevated ALP) and when the site of involvement involves weight-bearing bones, areas adjacent to major joints, vertebral bodies, and skull. Whether early therapy prevents late complications remains to be determined. However, the restoration of normal bone architecture following suppression of pagetic activity suggests that treatment may prevent further deformities and complications.

Agents approved for treatment of Paget disease suppress the very high rates of bone resorption and secondarily decrease the high rates of bone formation (Table 26-1). As a result of decreasing bone turnover, pagetic structural patterns, including areas of poorly mineralized woven bone, are replaced by more normal cancellous or lamellar bone. The improvement in skeletal structure can be demonstrated on standard radiographs and ^{99m}Tc bone scans, which show decreased isotope accumulation in pagetic sites. Reduced bone turnover can be documented by a decline in urine or serum resorption markers (pyridinoline, deoxypyridinoline, N-telopeptide, C-telopeptide) and serum markers of bone formation (ALP, osteocalcin).

The potencies of various bisphosphonates are expressed relative to that of etidronate, the first clinically useful agent in this class. Etidronate use is now limited as the doses required to suppress bone resorption may impair mineralization. Thus, etidronate is administered in 6-month treatment cycles followed by a 6-month drug-free period. Failure to adhere to the cyclic regimen can pro-

TABLE 26-1

PHARMACOLOGIC AGENTS APPROVED FOR TREATMENT OF PAGET DISEASE

NAME (BRAND)	POTENCY[a]	DOSE	MODE OF ADMINISTRATION[b]
Etidronate (Didronel)	1	400 mg/d for 6 mos	Fasting with 6 oz tap water 2 h before or after a meal
Tiludronate (Skelid)	10	400 mg/d for 3 mos	Fasting with 6 oz tap water and wait 45 min before food, liquids are taken
Pamidronte (Aredia)	100	30 mg IV daily for 3 days or 60 to 90 mg IV at various intervals as determined by disease	
Alendronate (Fosamax)	700	40 mg/d for 6 mos	Fasting with 6 oz tap water and wait 45 min before food, liquids are taken
Risedronate (Actonel)	1000	30 mg/d for 2 mos	Fasting with 6 oz tap water and wait 45 min before food, liquids are taken
Calcitonin (Miacalcin)	NA	100 U sc daily	Dose may be reduced to 50 U qod for 6–18 mos

[a]Potency is relative to etidronate. For each tablet, etidronate strength is 400 mg; tiludronate is 200 mg; alendronate is 40 mg; and risedronate is 30 mg. Miacalcin nasal spray is not approved for use in Paget disease.
[b]6 oz is 175 mL.

duce osteomalacia manifested by bone pain and fractures. Etidronate should not be used in patients with advanced lytic lesions in weight-bearing bones. The major advantage of etidronate is that it is relatively well tolerated and only occasionally causes transient diarrhea or bone pain.

The second-generation oral bisphosphonates tiludronate, alendronate, and risedronate are more potent than etidronate in controlling bone turnover and thus induce a longer remission at a lower dose. The lower doses reduce the risks of impaired mineralization and osteomalacia. Oral bisphosphonates are poorly absorbed and have a potential to produce esophageal ulceration, reflux, and, rarely, perforation. They should be taken first thing in the morning on an empty stomach, followed by maintenance of upright posture with no food or drink for 30 to 60 min. Other medications, liquids, and food should be delayed for at least 30 to 60 min after taking bisphosphonates to optimize absorption. Tiludronate daily for 3 months normalizes ALP in 24 to 35% of moderately affected patients. In patients with moderate to severe disease, alendronate for 6 months normalizes ALP in >67% of patients, with an overall fall in ALP of 79% compared to 44% with etidronate. In patients with moderately active disease, risedronate daily for 2 to 3 months reduces serum ALP by 80% and normalizes indices of bone turnover in 73% of patients compared to 15% of those receiving etidronate.

Pamidronate is the only bisphosphonate currently approved for intravenous use in Paget disease. The recommended dose is 30 mg dissolved in 500 mL of normal saline or dextrose intravenously over 4 h on 3 consecutive days. The dose can be adjusted to each patient's requirements. A single 60-mg dose of pamidronate intravenously may normalize bone turnover in patients with mild disease. In contrast, patients with moderate to severe disease (elevation of ALP of three to four times normal) may require two to four doses of pamidronate, 60 to 90 mg intravenously, every 1 to 2 weeks. Patients with very severe disease may require a total dose of pamidronate of 300 to 500 mg given weekly over several weeks. Although suppression of urinary bone markers occurs after a few days to weeks, normalization of serum ALP levels often requires at least 3 months. Consequently, the effects of pamidronate are best evaluated 3 months after the initial dose. Pamidronate is generally well tolerated; however, a small number of patients experience a flulike syndrome that may begin 24 h after the first infusion. In patients with high bone turnover, vitamin D (400 to 800 IU daily) and calcium (500 mg three times daily) should be provided to prevent hypocalcemia and secondary hyperparathyroidism. Indications for intravenous therapy include mild disease and normalization of bone turnover after a single infusion, previous prevention of disease progression, refractoriness to oral therapy, need for rapid response such as for those with neurologic symptoms or with severe bone pain due to a lytic lesion, risk of an impending fracture, and as pretreatment prior to elective surgery in an area of active disease. Remission following pamidronate therapy may persist for as long as 1 year. Other bisphosphonate agents are in development.

The subcutaneous injectable form of salmon calcitonin is approved for the treatment of Paget disease. Intranasal calcitonin spray is approved for osteoporosis at a dose of 200 U/d; however, the efficacy of this dose in Paget disease has not been thoroughly studied. The usual starting dose of injectable calcitonin (100 U/d) reduces ALP by 50% and may relieve skeletal symptoms. The dose may be reduced to 50 U/d three times weekly after an initial favorable response to 100 U daily; however, the lower dose may require long-term use to sustain efficacy. The common side effects of calcitonin therapy are nausea and facial flushing. Secondary resistance after prolonged use may be due to either the formation of anticalcitonin antibodies or downregulation of osteoclastic cell-surface calcitonin receptors. The lower potency and injectable mode of delivery make this agent a less attractive treatment option that should be reserved for patients who either do not tolerate or do not respond to bisphosphonates.

SCLEROSING BONE DISORDERS

OSTEOPETROSIS

Osteopetrosis refers to a group of disorders caused by severe impairment of osteoclast-mediated bone resorption. Other terms that are often used include marble bone disease, which captures the solid x-ray appearance of the involved skeleton, and Albers-Schonberg disease, which refers to the milder, adult form of osteopetrosis also known as autosomal dominant osteopetrosis type II.

The major types of osteopetrosis include malignant (severe, infantile, autosomal recessive) osteopetrosis and benign (adult, autosomal dominant) osteopetrosis types I and II. A rare autosomal recessive intermediate form has a more benign prognosis. Autosomal recessive carbonic anhydrase (CA) II deficiency produces osteopetrosis of intermediate severity associated with renal tubular acidosis and cerebral calcification.

Etiology and Genetics

Naturally occurring and gene knockout animal models with phenotypes similar to those of the human disorders have been used to explore the genetic basis of osteopetrosis. The primary defect in osteopetrosis is the loss of osteoclastic bone resorption and preservation of normal osteoblastic bone formation. Osteoprotegerin (OPG) is a soluble decoy receptor that binds osteoblast-derived RANK ligand, which mediates osteoclast differentiation and activation (Fig. 26-1). Transgenic mice that overexpress OPG develop osteopetrosis, presumably by blocking RANK ligand. Mice deficient in RANK lack osteoclasts and develop severe osteopetrosis.

Recessive mutations of CA II prevent osteoclasts from generating an acid environment in the clear zone between its ruffled border and the adjacent mineral surface. Absence of CA II, therefore, impairs osteoclastic bone resorption. Other forms of human disease have less clear genetic defects. About one-half of the patients with malignant infantile osteopetrosis have a mutation in the *TCIRG1* gene encoding the osteoclast-specific subunit of the vacuolar proton pump, which mediates the acidification of the interface between bone mineral and the osteoclast ruffled border. Mutations in the *CICN7* chloride channel gene cause autosomal dominant osteopetrosis type II.

Clinical Presentation

The incidence of autosomal recessive severe (malignant) osteopetrosis ranges from 1 in 200,000 to 1 in 500,000 live births. As bone and cartilage fail to undergo modeling, paralysis of one or more cranial nerves may occur due to narrowing of the cranial foramina. Failure of skeletal modeling also results in inadequate marrow space, leading to extramedullary hematopoiesis with hypersplenism and pancytopenia. Hypocalcemia due to lack of osteoclastic bone resorption may occur in infants and young children. The untreated infantile disease is fatal, often before age 5.

Adult (benign) osteopetrosis is an autosomal dominant disease that is usually diagnosed by the discovery of typical skeletal changes in young adults who undergo radiologic evaluation of a fracture. The prevalence is 1 in 100,000 to 1 in 500,000 adults. The course is not always benign, as fractures may be accompanied by loss of vision, deafness, psychomotor delay, mandibular osteomyelitis, and other complications usually associated with the juvenile form. In some kindred, nonpenetrance skips generations, while in other families severely affected children are born into families with benign disease. The milder form of the disease does not usually require treatment.

Radiography

Typically, there are generalized symmetric increases in bone mass with thickening of both cortical and trabecular bone. Diaphyses and metaphyses are broadened, and alternating sclerotic and lucent bands may be seen in the iliac crests, at the ends of long bones, and in vertebral bodies. The cranium is usually thickened, particularly at the base of the skull, and the paranasal and mastoid sinuses are underpneumatized.

Laboratory Findings

The only significant laboratory findings are elevated serum levels of osteoclast-derived tartrate-resistant acid phosphatase (TRAP) and the brain isoenzyme of creatine kinase. Serum calcium may be low in severe disease, and parathyroid hormone and 1,25-dihydroxyvitamin D levels may be elevated in response to hypocalcemia.

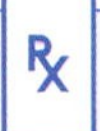

TREATMENT FOR OSTEOPETROSIS

Allogeneic HLA-identical bone marrow transplantation has been successful in some children. Following transplantation, the marrow contains progenitor cells and normally functioning osteoclasts. A cure is most likely when children are transplanted before age 4. Marrow transplantation from nonidentical HLA-matched donors has a much higher failure rate. Limited studies in small numbers of patients have suggested variable benefits following treatment with interferon γ-1b, 1,25-dihydroxyvitamin D (which stimulates osteoclasts directly), methylprednisolone, and a low-calcium/high-phosphate diet.

Surgical intervention is indicated to decompress optic or auditory nerve compression. Orthopedic management is required for the surgical treatment of fractures and their complications including malunion and postfracture deformity.

PYKNODYSOSTOSIS

This is an autosomal recessive form of osteosclerosis that is believed to have affected the French impressionist painter Henri de Toulouse-Lautrec. The molecular basis involves mutations in the gene that encodes cathepsin K, a lysosomal metalloproteinase highly expressed in osteoclasts and important for bone matrix degradation. Osteoclasts are present but do not function normally. Pyknodysostosis is a form of short-limb dwarfism that presents with frequent fractures but usually normal life span. Clinical features include short stature; kyphoscoliosis and deformities of the chest; high arched palate; proptosis; blue sclerae; dysmorphic features including small face and chin, frontooccipital prominence, pointed beaked nose, large cranium, and obtuse mandibular angle; and small square hands with hypoplastic nails. Radiographs demonstrate a generalized increase in bone density, but in contrast to osteopetrosis, the long bones are normally shaped. Separated cranial sutures, including the persistent patency of the anterior fontanel, are characteristic of the disorder. There may also be hypoplasia of the sinuses, mandible, distal clavicles, and terminal phalanges. Persistence of deciduous teeth and sclerosis of the calvarium and base of the skull also are common. Histologic evaluation shows normal cortical bone architecture with decreased osteoblastic and osteoclastic activities. Serum chemistries are normal, and unlike osteopetrosis, there is no anemia. There is no known treatment for this condition, and no reports of attempted bone marrow transplant.

PROGRESSIVE DIAPHYSEAL DYSPLASIA

Also known as Camurati-Engelmann disease, progressive diaphyseal dysplasia is an autosomal dominant disorder that is characterized radiographically by diaphyseal hyperostosis and a symmetric thickening and increased diameter of the endosteal and periosteal surfaces of the diaphyses of the long bones, particularly the femur and tibia, and, less often, the fibula, radius, and ulna. The genetic defect responsible for the disease has been localized to the area of chromosome 19q13.2 encoding tumor growth factor (TGF) β1. The mutation promotes activation of TGF-β1. The clinical severity is variable. The most common presenting symptoms are pain and tenderness of the involved areas, fatigue, muscle wasting, and gait disturbance. The weakness may be mistaken for muscular dystrophy. Characteristic body habitus includes thin limbs with little muscle mass yet prominent and palpable bones and, when the skull is involved, large head with prominent forehead and proptosis. Patients may also display signs of cranial nerve palsies, hydrocephalus, central hypogonadism, and Raynaud's phenomenon. Radiographically, patchy progressive endosteal and periosteal new bone formation is observed along the diaphyses of the long bones. Bone scintigraphy shows increased radiotracer uptake in involved areas.

Treatment with low-dose glucocorticoids relieves bone pain and may reverse the abnormal bone formation. Intermittent bisphosphonate therapy has produced clinical improvement in a limited number of patients.

HYPEROSTOSIS CORTICALIS GENERALISATA

This is also known as Van Buchem disease; it is an autosomal recessive disorder characterized by endosteal hyperostosis in which osteosclerosis involves the skull, mandible, clavicles, and ribs. The major manifestations are due to narrowed cranial foramina with neural compressions that may result in optic atrophy, facial paralysis, and deafness. Adults may have an enlarged mandible. Serum ALP levels may be elevated, which reflects the uncoupled bone remodeling with high osteoblastic formation rates and low osteoclastic resorption. As a result, there is increased accumulation of normal bone. Endosteal hyperostosis with syndactyly, known as *sclerosteosis,* is a more severe form. The genetic defects for both sclerosteosis and van Buchem disease have been assigned to the same region of the chromosome 17q12-q21. It is possible that both conditions may have deactivating mutations in the *BEER* (bone-expressed equilibrium regulator) gene.

MELORHEOSTOSIS

Melorheostosis (Greek, "flowing hyperostosis") may occur sporadically or follow a pattern consistent with an autosomal recessive disorder. The major manifestation is progressive linear hyperostosis in one or more bones of one limb, usually a lower extremity. The name comes from the radiographic appearance of the involved bone, which resembles melted wax that has dripped down a candle. Symptoms appear during childhood as pain or stiffness in the area of sclerotic bone. There may be associated ectopic soft tissue masses, composed of cartilage or osseous tissue, and skin changes overlying the involved bone, consisting of scleroderma-like areas and hypertrichosis. The disease does not progress in adults, but pain and stiffness may persist. Laboratory tests are unremarkable. No specific etiology is known. There is no specific treatment. Surgical interventions to correct contractures are often unsuccessful.

OSTEOPOIKILOSIS

The literal translation of osteopoikilosis is "spotted bones"; it is a benign autosomal dominant condition in which numerous small, variably shaped (usually round or oval) foci of bony sclerosis are seen in the epiphyses and adjacent metaphyses. The lesions may involve any bone except the skull, ribs, and vertebrae. They may be misidentified as metastatic lesions. The main differentiating points are that bony lesions of osteopoikilosis are stable over time and do not accumulate radionucleotide on bone scanning. In some kindred, osteopoikilosis is associated with connective tissue nevi known as *dermatofibrosis lenticularis disseminata,* also known as *Buschke-Ollendorf syndrome.* Histologic inspection reveals thickened but otherwise normal trabeculae and islands of normal cortical bone. No treatment is indicated.

DISORDERS ASSOCIATED WITH DEFECTIVE MINERALIZATION

HYPOPHOSPHATASIA

This is a rare inherited disorder that presents as rickets in infants and children or osteomalacia in adults with paradoxically low serum levels of ALP. The frequency of the severe neonatal and infantile forms is about 1 in 100,000 live births in Canada, where the disease is most common because of its high prevalence among Mennonites and Hutterites. It is rare in African Americans. The severity of the disease is remarkably variable, ranging from intrauterine death associated with profound skeletal hypomineralization at one extreme, to premature tooth loss as the only manifestation in some adults. Severe cases are inherited in an autosomal recessive manner, but the genetic patterns are less clear for the milder forms. The disease is caused by a deficiency of tissue-nonspecific (bone/liver/kidney) ALP (*TNSALP*), which, although ubiquitous, results only in bone abnormalities. Protein levels and functions of the other ALP isozymes (germ cell, intestinal, placental) are normal. Defective ALP permits accumulation of its major naturally occurring substrates including phosphoethanolamine (PEA), inorganic pyrophosphate (PPi), and pyridoxal 5′-phosphate (PLP). The accumulation of PPi interferes with mineralization through its action as a potent inhibitor of hydroxyapatite crystal growth.

Perinatal hypophosphatasia becomes manifest during pregnancy and is often complicated by polyhydroamnios and intrauterine death. The infantile form becomes clinically apparent before age 6 months with failure to thrive, rachitic deformities, functional craniosynostosis despite widely open fontanels (which are actually hypomineralized areas of the calvarium), raised intracranial pressure, and flail chest and predisposition to pneumonia. Hypercalcemia and hypercalciuria are common. This form has a mortality rate of about 50%. Prognosis seems to improve for the children who survive infancy. Childhood hypophosphatasia has variable clinical presentation. Premature loss of deciduous teeth (before age 5 years) is the hallmark of the disease. Rickets causes delayed walking with waddling gait, short stature, and dolichocephalic skull with frontal bossing. The disease often improves during puberty but may recur in adult life. Adult hypophosphatasia presents during middle age with painful, poorly healing metatarsal stress fractures or thigh pain due to femoral pseudofractures.

Laboratory investigation reveals low ALP levels and normal or elevated levels of serum calcium and phosphorus despite clinical and radiologic evidence of rickets or osteomalacia. Serum parathyroid hormone, 25-hydroxyvitamin D, and 1,25-dihydroxyvitamin D levels are normal. The elevation of PLP is specific for the disease and may even be present in asymptomatic parents of severely affected children. As vitamin B_6 increases PLP levels, vitamin B_6 supplements should be discontinued 1 week before testing.

There is no established medical therapy. In contrast to other forms of rickets and osteomalacia, calcium and vitamin D supplementation should be avoided as they may aggravate hypercalcemia and hypercalciuria. A low-calcium diet, glucocorticoids, and calcitonin have been used in a small number of patients with variable responses. Because fracture healing is poor, placement of intramedullary rods is best for acute fracture repair and for prophylactic prevention of fractures.

AXIAL OSTEOMALACIA

This is a rare disorder characterized by defective skeletal mineralization despite normal serum calcium and phosphate levels. Clinically, the disorder presents in middle-aged or elderly men with chronic axial skeletal discomfort. Cervical spine pain may also be present. Radiographic findings are mainly osteosclerosis due to coarsened trabecular patterns typical of osteomalacias. Spine, pelvis, and ribs are most commonly affected. Histologic changes show defective mineralization and flat, inactive osteoblasts. The primary defect appears to be an acquired defect in osteoblast function. The course is benign and there is no established treatment. Calcium and vitamin D therapies are not effective.

FIBROGENESIS IMPERFECTA OSSIUM

The is a rare condition of unknown etiology. It presents in both sexes, in middle age or later, with progressive, intractable skeletal pain and fractures, worsening immobilization, and a debilitating course. Radiographic evaluation reveals generalized osteomalacia, osteopenia, and occasional pseudofractures. Histologic features include a tangled pattern of collagen fibrils with abundant osteoblasts and osteoclasts. There is no effective treatment. Spontaneous remission has been reported in a small number of patients. Calcium and vitamin D have not been beneficial.

FIBROUS DYSPLASIA AND McCUNE ALBRIGHT SYNDROME

Fibrous dysplasia is a sporadic disorder characterized by the presence of one (monoostotic) or more (polyostotic) expanding fibrous skeletal lesions composed of bone-forming mesenchyme. The association of the polyostotic form with café-au-lait spots and hyperfunction of an endocrine system such as pseudo-precocious puberty of ovarian origin is known as *McCune-Albright syndrome* (MAS). A spectrum of the phenotypes is caused by activating mutations in the *GNAS1* gene, which encodes the α subunit of the stimulatory G protein ($G_s\alpha$). As the postzygotic mutations occur at different stages of early development, the extent and type of tissue affected are variable and explain the mosaic pattern of skin and bone changes. GTP binding activates the $G_s\alpha$ regulatory protein and mutations in regions of $G_s\alpha$ that selectively inhibit GTPase activity, which results in constitutive stimulation of the cyclic AMP–protein kinase A signal transduction pathway. Such mutations of the $G_s\alpha$ protein–coupled receptor may cause autonomous function in bone (parathyroid hormone receptor); skin (melanocyte-stimulating hormone receptor); and various endocrine glands including ovary (follicle-stimulating hormone receptor), thyroid (thyroid-stimulating hormone receptor), adrenal (adrenocorticotropic hormone receptor), and pituitary (growth hormone–releasing hormone receptor). The skeletal lesions are composed largely of mesenchymal cells that do not differentiate into osteoblasts, resulting in the formation of imperfect bone. In some areas of bone, fibroblast-like cells develop features of osteoblasts in that they produce extracellular matrix that organizes into woven bone. Calcification may occur in some areas. In other areas, cells have features of chondrocytes and produce cartilage-like extracellular matrix.

CLINICAL PRESENTATION

Fibrous dysplasia occurs with equal frequency in both sexes, whereas MAS with precocious puberty is more common (10:1) in girls. The monoostotic form is the most common and is usually diagnosed in patients between 20 and 30 years of age without associated skin lesions. The polyostotic form typically manifests in children <10 years of age and may progress with age. Early-onset disease is generally more severe. Lesions may become quiescent in puberty and progress during pregnancy or with estrogen therapy. In polyostotic fibrous dysplasia, the lesions most commonly involve the maxilla and other craniofacial bones, ribs, and metaphyseal or diaphyseal portions of the proximal femur or tibia. Expanding bone lesions may cause pain, deformity, fractures, and nerve entrapment. Sarcomatous degeneration involving the facial bones or femur is infrequent (<1%). The risk of malignant transformation is increased by radiation, which has proved to be ineffective treatment. In rare patients with widespread lesions, renal phosphate wasting and hypophosphatemia may cause rickets or osteomalacia. Hypophosphatemia may be due to production of a phosphaturic factor by the abnormal fibrous tissue.

MAS patients may have café-au-lait spots, which are flat, hyperpigmented skin lesions that have rough borders ("coast of Maine") in contrast to the café-au-lait lesions of neurofibromatosis that have smooth borders ("coast of California"). The most common endocrinopathy is isosexual pseudo-precocious puberty in girls. Other less common endocrine disorders include thyrotoxicosis, Cushing's syndrome, acromegaly, hyperparathyroidism, hyperprolactinemia, and pseudo-precocious puberty in boys.

RADIOGRAPHIC FINDINGS

In long bones, the fibrous dysplastic lesions are typically well-defined, radiolucent areas with thin cortices and a ground-glass appearance. Lesions may be lobulated with trabeculated areas of radiolucency (**Fig. 26-4**). Involve-

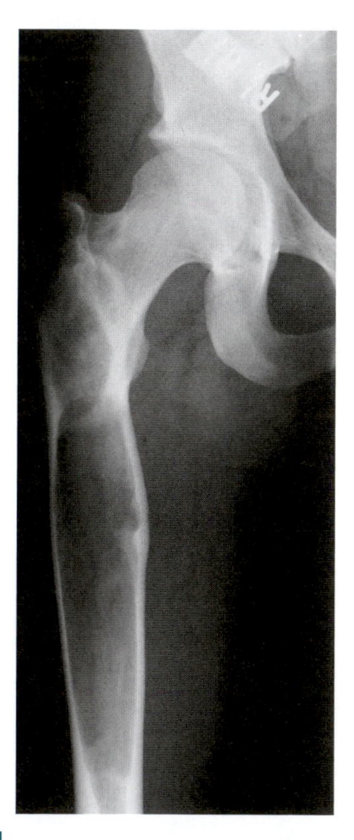

FIGURE 26-4
Radiograph of a 16-year-old male with fibrous dysplasia of the right proximal femur. Note the multiple cystic lesions, including the large lucent lesion in the proximal mid-shaft with scalloping of the interior surface. The femoral neck contains two lucent cystic lesions.

ment of facial bones usually presents as radiodense lesions, which may create a leonine appearance (leontiasis ossea). Expansile cranial lesions may narrow foramina and cause optic lesions, reduce hearing, and create other manifestations of cranial nerve compression.

LABORATORY RESULTS

Serum ALP is occasionally elevated but calcium, parathyroid hormone, 25-hydroxyvitamin D, and 1,25-dihydroxyvitamin D levels are normal. Patients with extensive polyostotic lesions may have hypophosphatemia, hyperphosphaturia, and osteomalacia. Biochemical markers of bone turnover may be elevated.

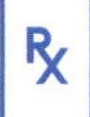

TREATMENT FOR FIBROUS DYSPLASIA AND MCCUNE ALBRIGHT SYNDROME

Spontaneous healing of the lesions does not occur, and there is no established effective treatment. Improvement in bone pain and partial or complete resolution of radiographic lesions have been reported after intravenous bisphosphonate therapy. Surgical stabilization is used to prevent pathologic fracture or destruction of a major joint space, and to relieve nerve root or cranial nerve compression or sinus obstruction.

OTHER DYSPLASIAS OF BONE AND CARTILAGE

PACHYDERMOPERIOSTOSIS

Pachydermoperiostosis, or hypertrophic osteoarthropathy (primary or idiopathic), is an autosomal dominant disorder characterized by periosteal new bone formation that involves the distal extremities. The lesions present as clubbing of the digits and hyperhydrosis and thickening of the skin, primarily of the face and forehead. The changes usually appear during adolescence, progress over the next decade, and then become quiescent. During the active phase, progressive enlargement of the hands and feet produces a pawlike appearance, which may be mistaken for acromegaly. Arthralgias, pseudogout, and limited mobility may also occur. The disorder must be differentiated from secondary hypertrophic osteopathy that develops during the course of serious pulmonary disorders. The two conditions can be differentiated by standard radiography of the digits in which secondary pachydermoperiostosis has exuberant periosteal new bone formation and a smooth and undulating surface. In contrast, primary hypertrophic osteopathy has an irregular periosteal surface.

There are no diagnostic blood or urine tests. Synovial fluid does not have an inflammatory profile. There is no specific therapy, although a limited experience with colchicine suggests some benefit in controlling the arthralgias.

OSTEOCHONDRODYSPLASIAS

These include several hundred heritable disorders of connective tissue. These primary abnormalities of cartilage manifest as disturbances in cartilage and bone growth. Selected growth plate chondrodysplasias are described here.

Achondrodysplasia

This is a relatively common form of short-limb dwarfism that occurs in 1 in 15,000 to 1 in 40,000 live births. The disease is caused by a mutation of the fibroblast growth factor receptor 3 (*FGFR3*) gene that results in a gain-of-function state. Most cases are sporadic mutations. However, when the disorder appears in families, the inheritance pattern is consistent with an autosomal dominant disorder. The primary defect is abnormal chondrocyte proliferation at the growth plate that causes development of short but proportionately thick long bones. Other regions of the long bones may be relatively unaffected. The disorder is manifest by the presence of short limbs (particularly the proximal portions), normal trunk, large head, saddle nose, and an exaggerated lumbar lordosis. Severe spinal deformity may lead to cord compression. The homozygous disorder is more serious than the sporadic form and may cause neonatal death. Pseudoachondroplasia clinically resembles achondroplasia but has no skull abnormalities.

Enchondromatosis

This is also called dyschondroplasia, or Ollier disease; it is also a disorder of the growth plate in which the primary cartilage is not resorbed. Cartilage ossification proceeds normally but it is not resorbed normally, leading to cartilage accumulation. The changes are most marked at the ends of long bones where the highest growth rates occur. Chondrosarcoma develops infrequently. The association of enchondromatosis and cavernous hemangiomas of the skin and soft tissues is known as *Maffucci syndrome.* Both Ollier disease and Maffucci syndrome are associated with various malignancies, including granulosa cell tumor of the ovary and cerebral glioma.

Multiple Exostoses

This is also called diaphyseal aclasis, or osteochondromatosis; it is a genetic disorder that follows an autosomal dominant pattern of inheritance. In this condition, areas of growth plates become displaced, presumably by growing through a defect in the perichondrium. The lesion begins with vascular invasion of the growth plate cartilage, resulting in a characteristic radiographic finding of a mass that is in direct communication with the marrow cavity of the parent bone. The underlying cortex is resorbed. The disease is caused by inactivating mutations of the *EXT1* and *EXT2* genes, whose products normally regulate processing of chondrocyte cytoskeletal proteins. The products of the *EXT* gene likely function as tumor suppressors, with the loss-of-function mutation resulting in abnormal proliferation of growth plate cartilage. Solitary or multiple lesions are located in the metaphyses of long bones. Although usually asymptomatic, the lesions may interfere with joint or tendon function or compress peripheral nerves. The lesions stop growing when growth ceases but may recur during pregnancy. There is a small risk for malignant transformation into chondrosarcoma.

EXTRASKELETAL (ECTOPIC) CALCIFICATION AND OSSIFICATION

Deposition of calcium phosphate crystals (*calcification*) or formation of true bone (*ossification*) in nonosseous soft tissue may occur by one of three mechanisms: (1) metastatic calcification due to a supranormal calcium × phosphate concentration product in extracellular fluid; (2) dystrophic calcification due to mineral deposition into metabolically impaired or dead tissue despite normal serum levels of calcium and phosphate; and (3) ectopic ossification, or true bone formation. Disorders that may cause extraskeletal calcification or ossification are listed in **Table 26-2.**

METASTATIC CALCIFICATION

Soft tissue calcification may complicate diseases associated with significant hypercalcemia, hyperphosphatemia, or both. In addition, vitamin D and phosphate treatments or calcium administration in the presence of mild hyperphosphatemia, such as during hemodialysis, may induce ectopic calcification. Calcium phosphate precipitation may complicate any disorder when the serum calcium × phosphate concentration product is >75. The initial calcium phosphate deposition is in the form of small, poorly organized crystals, which subsequently organize into hydroxyapatite crystals. Calcifications that occur in hypercalcemic states with normal or low phosphate have a predilection for kidney, lungs, and gastric mucosa. Hyperphosphatemia with normal or low serum calcium may promote soft tissue calcification with predilection for the kidney and arteries. The disturbances of calcium and phosphate in renal failure and hemodialysis are common causes of soft tissue (metastatic) calcification.

TABLE 26-2

DISEASES AND CONDITIONS ASSOCIATED WITH ECTOPIC CALCIFICATION AND OSSIFICATION

Metastatic calcification	**Dystrophic calcification**
Hypercalcemic states	Inflammatory disorders
Primary hyperparathyroidism	Scleroderma
Sarcoidosis	Dermatomyositis
Vitamin D intoxication	Systemic lupus erythematosus
Milk-alkali syndrome	Trauma-induced
Renal failure	**Ectopic ossification**
Hyperphosphatemia	Myositis ossificans
Tumoral calcinosis	Post surgery
Secondary hyperparathyroidism	Burns
Pseudohypoparathyroidism	Neurologic injury
Renal failure	Other trauma
Hemodialysis	Fibrodysplasia ossificans progressiva
Cell lysis following chemotherapy	
Therapy with vitamin D and phosphate	

TUMORAL CALCINOSIS

This is a rare genetic disorder characterized by masses of metastatic calcifications in soft tissues around major joints, most often shoulders, hips, and ankles. Tumoral calcinosis differs from other disorders in that the periarticular masses contain hydroxyapatite crystals or amorphous calcium phosphate complexes, while in fibrodysplasia ossificans progressiva (below), true bone is formed in soft tissues. About one-third of tumoral calcinosis cases are familial, with both autosomal recessive and autosomal dominant modes of inheritance reported. The disease is also associated with a variably expressed abnormality of dentition marked by short bulbous roots, pulp calcification, and radicular dentin deposited in swirls. The primary defect responsible for the metastatic calcification appears to be hyperphosphatemia resulting from the increased capacity of the renal tubule to reabsorb filtered phosphate. Spontaneous soft tissue calcification is related to the elevated serum phosphate, which along with normal serum calcium exceeds the concentration product of 75.

All of the North American patients reported have been African-American. The disease usually presents in childhood and continues lifelong. The calcific masses are typically painless and grow at variable rates, sometimes becoming large and bulky. The masses are often located near major joints but remain extracapsular. Joint range of motion is not usually restricted unless the tumors are very large. Complications include compression of neural structures and ulceration of the overlying skin with drainage of chalky fluid and risk of secondary infection. Small deposits not detected by standard radiographs may be detected by ^{99m}Tc bone scanning. The most common laboratory findings are hyperphosphatemia and elevated serum 1,25-dihydroxyvitamin D levels. Serum calcium, parathyroid hormone, and ALP levels are usually normal. Renal function also is usually normal. Urine calcium and phosphate excretions are low, and calcium and phosphate balances are positive.

An acquired form of the disease may occur with other causes of hyperphosphatemia, such as secondary hyperparathyroidism associated with hemodialysis, hypoparathyroidism, pseudohypoparathyroidism, and massive cell lysis following chemotherapy for leukemia. Tissue trauma from joint movement may contribute to the periarticular calcifications. Metastatic calcifications are also seen in conditions associated with hypercalcemia, such as in sarcoidosis, vitamin D intoxication, milk-alkali syndrome, and primary hyperparathyroidism. In these conditions, however, mineral deposits are more likely to occur in proton-transporting organs such as kidney, lungs, and gastric mucosa in which an alkaline milieu is generated by the proton pumps.

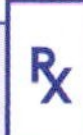

TREATMENT FOR METASTATIC CALCIFICATION

Therapeutic successes have been achieved with surgical removal of subcutaneous calcified masses, which tend not to recur if all calcification is removed from the site. Reduction of serum phosphate by chronic phosphorus restriction may be accomplished using low dietary phosphorus intake alone or in combination with oral phosphate binders. The addition of the phosphaturic agent acetazolamide may be useful. Limited experience using the phosphaturic action of calcitonin deserves further testing.

DYSTROPHIC CALCIFICATION

Posttraumatic calcification may occur with normal serum calcium and phosphate levels and normal ion solubility product. The deposited mineral is either in the form of amorphous calcium phosphate or hydroxyapatite crystals. Soft tissue calcification complicating connective tissue disorders such as scleroderma, dermatomyositis, and systemic lupus erythematosus may involve localized areas of the skin or deeper subcutaneous tissue and is referred to as *calcinosis circumscripta*. Mineral deposition at sites of deeper tissue injury including periarticular sites is called *calcinosis universalis*.

ECTOPIC OSSIFICATION

True extraskeletal bone formation that begins in areas of fasciitis following surgery, trauma, burns, or neurologic injury is referred to as *myositis ossificans*. The bone formed is organized as lamellar or trabecular, with normal osteoblasts and osteoclasts conducting active remodeling. Well-developed Haversian systems and marrow elements may be present. A second cause of ectopic bone formation occurs in an inherited disorder, *fibrodysplasia ossificans progressiva*.

FIBRODYSPLASIA OSSIFICANS PROGRESSIVA

This is also called *myositis ossificans progressiva*; it is a rare autosomal dominant disorder characterized by congenital deformities of the hands and feet and episodic soft tissue swellings that ossify. Ectopic bone formation occurs in fascia, tendons, ligaments, and connective tissue within voluntary muscles. Tender, rubbery induration, sometimes precipitated by trauma, develops in the soft tissue and gradually calcifies. Eventually, heterotopic bone forms at these sites of soft tissue trauma. Morbidity results from heterotopic bone interfering with normal movement and function of muscle and other soft tissues. Mortality is usually related to restrictive lung disease caused by an inability of the chest to expand. Laboratory tests are unremarkable.

There is no effective medical therapy. Bisphosphonates, glucocorticoids, and a low-calcium diet have largely been ineffective in halting progression of the ossification. Surgical removal of ectopic bone is not recommended, as the trauma of surgery may precipitate formation of new areas of heterotopic bone. Dental complications including frozen jaw may occur following injection of local anesthetics. Thus, CT imaging of the mandible should be undertaken to detect early sites of soft tissue ossification before they are appreciated by standard radiography.

ACKNOWLEDGMENT

The authors wish to acknowledge the contributions of Dr. Stephen M. Krane to this chapter in previous editions of Harrison's.

FURTHER READINGS

Campos-Xavier B et al: Phenotypic variability at the TGF-beta 1 locus in Camurati-Engelmann disease. Hum Genet 109:653, 2001

Hocking LJ et al: Domain-specific mutations in sequestosome 1 (SQSTM1) cause familial and sporadic Paget disease. Hum Mol Genet 11:2735, 2002

Isaia GC et al: Bone turnover in children and adolescents with McCune-Albright syndrome treated with pamidronate for bone fibrous dysplasia. Calcif Tissue Int 71:121, 2002

Reddy SV: Etiology of Paget's disease and osteoclast abnormalities. J Cell Biochem 93:688, 2004

Genetic linkage analysis indicates that 40% of patients with Paget disease have an affected first-degree relative, consistent with an autosomal dominant trait with genetic heterogeneity. Recurrent mutations in the ubiquitin-associated (UBA) domain of sequestosome 1 (SQSTM1/p62) have been identified in patients with Paget disease, but the etiology of Paget disease remains uncertain in the majority of patients. This review summarizes the known genetic and pathologic features of the disease.

Roodman GD et al: Paget disease of bone. J Clin Invest 115:200, 2005

This review of the pathophysiology of Paget disease summarizes evidence for both a genetic and a viral etiology.

Takata S et al: Evolution of understanding of genetics of Paget's disease of bone and related diseases. J Bone Miner Metab 22:519, 2004

Whyte MP et al: Osteoprotegerin deficiency and juvenile Paget disease. N Engl J Med 347:175, 2002

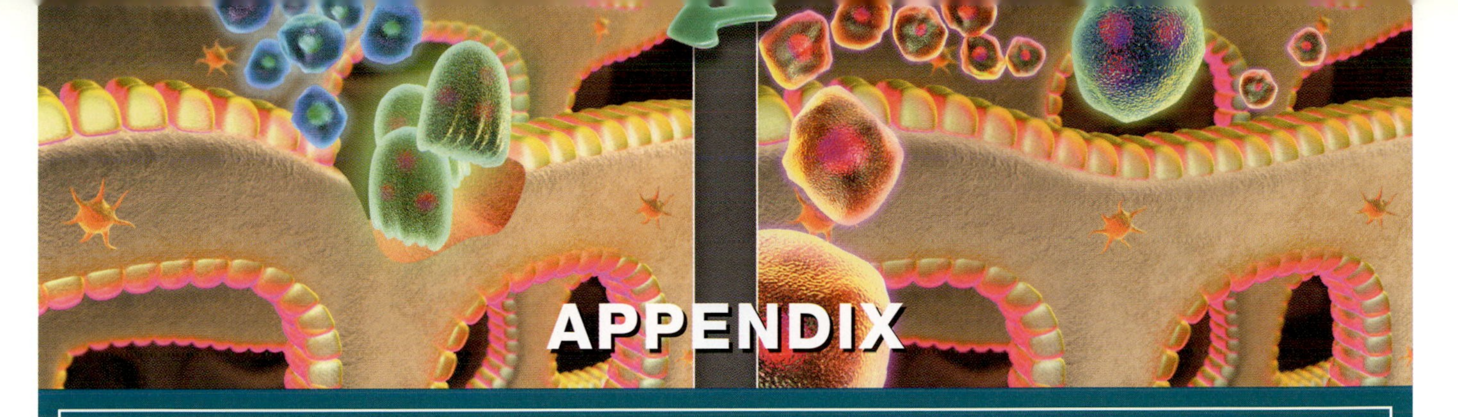

LABORATORY VALUES OF CLINICAL IMPORTANCE

In preparing the Appendix, the authors have taken into account the fact that the system of international units (SI, système international d'unités) is used in most countries and in some medical journals. However, clinical laboratories may continue to report values in conventional units. Therefore, both systems are provided in the Appendix.

Conversion from one system to another can be made as follows:

$$\text{mmol/L} = \frac{\text{mg/dL} \times 10}{\text{atomic weight (or molecular weight)}}$$

$$\text{mg/dL} = \frac{\text{mmol/L} \times \text{atomic weight (or molecular weight)}}{10}$$

For a more complete list of laboratory values, consult the Appendices of *Harrison's, 16e.*[a]

REFERENCE VALUES FOR LABORATORY TESTS

TABLE A-1

HEMATOLOGY AND COAGULATION

ANALYTE	SI UNITS	CONVENTIONAL UNITS
Antithrombin III		
Antigenic	220–390 mg/L	22–39 mg/dL
Functional	0.8–1.30 U/L	80–130%
Bleeding time (adult)	2–9.5 min	2–9.5 min
Carboxyhemoglobin		
Nonsmoker	0–0.023	0–2.3%
Smoker	0.021–0.042	2.1–4.2%
D-Dimer	<0.5 mg/L	<0.5 μg/mL
Differential blood count		
Neutrophils	0.40–0.70	40–70%
Bands	0.0–0.10	0–10%
Lymphocytes	0.22–0.44	22–44%
Monocytes	0.04–0.11	4–11%

(continued)

[a]A variety of factors can influence reference values. Values supplied in this Appendix reflect typical reference ranges in adults. Pediatric reference ranges may vary significantly from adult values. Whenever possible, reference values provided by the laboratory performing the testing should be utilized in the interpretation of laboratory data.

TABLE A-1 *(Continued)*

HEMATOLOGY AND COAGULATION

ANALYTE	SI UNITS	CONVENTIONAL UNITS
Eosinophils	0.0–0.8	0–8%
Basophils	0.0–0.03	0–3%
Erythrocyte count		
Adult males	4.50–5.90 × 10^{12}/L	4.50–5.90 × 10^6/mm^3
Adult females	4.00–5.20 × 10^{12}/L	4.00–5.20 × 10^6/mm^3
Erythrocyte sedimentation rate		
Females	1–25 mm/h	1–25 mm/h
Males	0–17 mm/h	0–17 mm/h
Ferritin		
Male	30–300 μg/L	30–300 ng/mL
Female	10–200 μg/L	10–200 ng/mL
Fibrin(ogen) degradation products	<2.5 mg/L	<2.5 μg/mL
Fibrinogen	1.50–4.00 g/L	150–400 mg/dL
Folate (folic acid): Normal	7.0–39.7 nmol/L	3.1–17.5 ng/mL
Haptoglobin	0.16–1.99 g/L	16–199 mg/dL
Hematocrit		
Adult males	0.41–0.53	41.0–53.0
Adult females	0.36–0.46	36.0–46.0
Hemoglobin		
Plasma	0.01–0.05 g/L	1–5 mg/dL
Whole blood:		
Adult males	8.4–10.9 mmol/L	13.5–17.5 g/dL
Adult females	7.4–9.9 mmol/L	12.0–16.0 g/dL
Hemoglobin electrophoresis		
Hemoglobin A	0.95–0.98	95–98%
Hemoglobin A_2	0.015–0.035	1.5–3.5%
Hemoglobin F	0–0.02	0–2.0%
Homocysteine	0–12 μmol/L	0–12 μmol/L
Iron	5.4–28.7 μmol/L	30–160 μg/dL
Iron binding capacity	40.8–76.7 μmol/L	228–428 μg/dL
Mean corpuscular hemoglobin (MCH)	26.0–34.0 pg/cell	26.0–34.0 pg/cell
Mean corpuscular hemoglobin concentration (MCHC)	310–370 g/L	31.0–37.0 g/dL
Mean corpuscular volume (MCV)		
Male (adult)	78–100 fl	78–100 μm^3
Female (adult)	78–102 fl	78–102 μm^3
Methemoglobin		Up to 1% of total hemoglobin
Partial thromboplastin time, activated	22.1–35.1 s	22.1–35.1 s
Plasminogen		
Antigen	84–140 mg/L	8.4–14.0 mg/dL
Functional	0.80–1.30	80–130%
Plasminogen activator inhibitor 1	4–43 μg/L	4–43 ng/mL
Platelet count	150–350×10^9/L	150–350 × 10^3/mm^3
Protein C	0.70–1.40	70–140%
Protein S	0.70–1.40	70–140%
Prothrombin time	11.1–13.1 s	11.1–13.1 s
Reticulocyte count	0.005–0.025 red cells	0.5–2.5 % red cells
Thrombin time	16–24 s	16–24 s
Total eosinophils	70–140 × 10^6/L	70–440/mm^3
Vitamin B_{12}	185 pmol/L	>250 pg/mL

TABLE A-2

CLINICAL CHEMISTRY

CONSTITUENT	SI UNITS	CONVENTIONAL UNITS
Albumin	35–55 g/L	3.5–5.5 g/dL
Aldolase	0–100 nkat/L	0–6 U/L
α_1 Antitrypsin	0.8–2.1 g/L	85–213 mg/dL
Alpha fetoprotein (adult)	<15 μg/L	<15 ng/mL
Aminotransferases		
Aspartate (AST, SGOT)	0–0.58 μkat/L	0–35 U/L
Alanine (ALT, SGPT)	0–0.58 μkat/L	0–35 U/L
Ammonia, as NH_3	6–47 μmol/L	10–80 μg/dL
Amylase	0.8–3.2 μkat/L	60–180 U/L
Angiotensin-converting enzyme (ACE)	<670 nkat/L	<40 U/L
Anion gap	7–16 mmol/L	7–16 mmol/L
Arterial blood gases		
$[HCO_3^-]$	21–28 mmol/L	21–30 meq/L
P_{CO_2}	4.7–5.9 kPa	35–45 mmHg
pH	7.38–7.44	
P_{O_2}	11–13 kPa	80–100 mmHg
β-2-Microglobulin	1.2–2.8 mg/L ≤200 μg/L	1.2–2.8 mg/L ≤200 μg/L
Bilirubin		
Total	5.1–1.7 μmol/L	0.3–1.0 mg/dL
Direct	1.7–5.1 μmol/L	0.1–03 mg/dL
Indirect	3.4–12 μmol/L	0.2–0.7 mg/dL
Brain type natriuetic peptide (BNP)	Age and gender specific: <167 ng/L	Age and gender specific: <167 pg/mL
Calcium, ionized	1.1–1.4 mmol/L	4.5–5.6 mg/dL
Calcium	2.2–2.6 mmol/L	9–10.5 mg/dL
CA-15-3	0–30 kU/L	0–30 U/mL
CA 19-9	0–37 kU/L	0–37 U/mL
CA 27-29	0–32 kU/L	0–32 U/mL
CA 125	0–35 kU/L	0–35 U/mL
Calcitonin		
Male	3–26 ng/L	3–26 pg/mL
Female	2–17 ng/L	2–7 pg/mL
Carbon dioxide tension (P_{CO_2})	4.7–5.9 kPa	35–45 mmHg
Carbon monoxide content	Symptoms with 20% saturation of hemoglobin	
Carcinoembryonic antigen (CEA)	0.0–3.4 ug/L	0.0–3.4 ng/mL
Chloride	98–106 mmol/L	98–106 meq/L
C-peptide		
Creatine kinase (CK) (total)		
Females	0.67–2.50 μkat/L	40–150 U/L
Males	1.00–6.67 μkat/L	60–400 U/L
Creatine kinase-MB	0–7 μg/L	0–7 ng/mL
Creatinine	<133 μmol/L	<1.5 mg/dL
Erythropoietin	5–36 U/L	
Ferritin		
Female	10–200 μg/L	10–200 ng/mL
Male	15–400 μg/L	15–400 ng/mL

(*continued*)

TABLE A-2 (*Continued*)

CLINICAL CHEMISTRY		
CONSTITUENT	SI UNITS	CONVENTIONAL UNITS
Gamma glutamyltransferase	1–94 U/L	1–94 U/L
Glucose (fasting)		
Normal	4.2–6.4 mmol/L	75–115 mg/dL
Diabetes mellitus	>7.0 mmol/L	>125 mg/dL
Glucose, 2 h postprandial	<6.7 mmol/L	<120 mg/dL
Hemoglobin A_{1c}	0.038–0.064 Hb fraction	3.8–6.4%
Homocysteine	4–12 μmol/L	4–12 μmol/L
Iron	9–27 μmol/L	50–150 μg/dL
Iron-binding capacity	45–66 μmol/L	250–370 μg/dL
Iron-binding capacity saturation	0.2–0.45	20–45%
Lactate dehydrogenase	1.7–3.2 μkat/L	100–190 U/L
Lactate	0.6–1.7 mmol/L	5–15 mg/dL
Lipase	0–2.66 μkat/L	0–160 U/L
Lipoprotein (a)	0–300 mg/L	0–30 mg/dL
Magnesium	0.8–1.2 mmol/L	1.8–3 mg/dL
Microalbumin urine		
24-h urine	<0.2 g/L or <0.031 g/24 h	<20 mg/L or <31 mg/24 h
Spot AM urine	<0.03 g albumin/g creatinine	<0.03 mg albumin/mg creatinine
Myoglobin		
Male	19–92 μg/L	
Female	12–76 μg/L	
Osmolality	285–295 mmol/kg serum water	285–295 mosmol/kg serum water
Osteocalcin	3.1–14 μg/L	3.1–14 ng/mL
Oxygen percent saturation (sea level)	0.97 mol/mol 0.60–0.85 mol/mol	97% 60–85 %
Oxygen tension (P_{O_2})	11–13 kPa	80–100 mmHg
pH	7.38–7.44	
Parathyroid hormone-related peptide	<1.3 pmol/L	<1.3 pmol/L
Phosphatase, acid	0.90 nkat/L	0–5.5 U/L
Phosphatase, alkaline	0.5–2.0 nkat/L	30–120 U/L
Phosphorus, inorganic	1.0–1.4 mmol/L	3–4.5 mg/dL
Potassium	3.5–5.0 mmol/L	3.5–5.0 meq/L
Prostate-specific antigen (PSA)		
Female	<0.5μg/L	<0.5 ng/mL
Male		
<40 years	0.0–2.0 μg/L	0.0.–2.0 ng/mL
>40 years	0.0–4.0 μg/L	0.0–4.0 ng/mL
PSA, free, in males 45–75 years, with PSA values between 4 and 20 μg/L	>0.25 associated with benign prostatic hyperplasia (BPH)	>25% associated with BPH
Protein, total	55–80 g/L	5.5–8.0 g/dL
Protein fractions:		
Albumin	35–55 g/L	3.5–5.5 g/dL (50–60%)
Globulin	20–35 g/L	2.0–3.5 g/dL (40–50%)
$Alpha_1$	2–4 g/L	0.2–0.4 g/dL (4.2–7.2%)
$Alpha_2$	5–9 g/L	0.5–0.9 g/dL (6.8–12%)
Beta	6–11 g/L	0.6–1.1 g/dL (9.3–15%)
Gamma	7–17 g/L	0.7–1.7 g/dL (13–23%)

(*continued*)

TABLE A-2 (*Continued*)

CLINICAL CHEMISTRY

CONSTITUENTS	SI UNITS	CONVENTIONAL UNITS
Sodium	136–145 mmol/L	136–145 meq/L
Transferrin	2.3–3.9 g/L	230–390 mg/dL
Triglycerides	<1.8 mmol/L	<160 mg/dL
Troponin I	0–0.4 μg/L	0–0.4 ng/mL
Troponin T	0–0.1 μg/L	0–0.1 ng/mL
Urea nitrogen	3.6–7.1 mmol/L	10–20 mg/dL
Uric acid		
Males	150–480 μmol/L	2.5–8.0 mg/dL
Females	90–360 μmol/L	1.5–6.0 mg/dL

TABLE A-3

METABOLIC AND ENDOCRINE TESTS

ANALYTE	SI UNITS	CONVENTIONAL UNITS
Adrenocorticotropin (ACTH)	1.3–16.7 pmol/L	6.0–76.0 pg/mL
Aldosterone (adult)		
Supine, normal sodium diet	55–250 pmol/L	2–9 ng/dL
Upright, normal sodium diet		2- to 5-fold increase over supine value
Supine, low-sodium diet		2- to 5-fold increase over normal sodium diet level
Cortisol		
Fasting, 8 AM–Noon	138–690 nmol/L	5–25 μg/dL
Noon–8 PM	138–414 nmol/L	5–15 μg/dL
8 PM–8 AM	0–276 nmol/L	0–10 μg/dL
Cortisol, free (urine)	55–193 nmol/24 h	20–70 μg/24 h
Epinephrine (urine)	0–109 nmol/d	0–20 μg/d
Estradiol		
Female		
Menstruating		
Follicular phase	184–532 pmol/L	20–145 pg/mL
Midcycle peak	411–1626 pmol/L	112–443 pg/mL
Luteal phase	184–885 pmol/L	20–241 pg/mL
Postmenopausal	<217 pmol/L	<59 pg/mL
Male	<184 pmol/L	<20 pg/mL
Follicle-stimulating hormone (FSH)		
Female		
Menstruating		
Follicular phase	3.0–20.0 IU/L	3.0–20.0 U/L
Ovulatory phase	9.0–26.0 IU/L	9.0–26.0 U/L
Luteal phase	1.0–12.0 IU/L	1.0–12.0 U/L
Postmenopausal	18.0–153.0 IU/L	18.0–153.0 U/L
Male	1.0–12.0 IU/L	1.0–12.0 U/L
Gastrin	<100 ng/L	<100 pg/mL
Growth hormone (resting)	0.5–17.0 μg/L	0.5–17.0 ng/mL
Human chorionic gonadotropin (HCG) (nonpregnant)	<5 IU/L	<5 mIU/mL

(*continued*)

TABLE A-3 *(Continued)*

METABOLIC AND ENDOCRINE TESTS

ANALYTE	SI UNITS	CONVENTIONAL UNITS
17-Hydroxyprogesterone (adult)		
Male	0.15 nmol/L	5–250 ng/dL
Female		
Follicular phase	0.6–3.0 nmol/L	20–100 ng/dL
Midcycle peak	3–7.5 nmol/L	100–250 ng/dL
Luteal phase	3–15 nmol/L	100–500 ng/dL
Postmenopausal	≤2.1 nmol/L	≤70 ng/dL
5-Hydroindoleacetic Acid [5-HIAA] (urine)	10.5–36.6 μmol/d	2–7 mg/d
17 Ketosteroids (urine)	10–42 μmol/d	3–12 mg/d
Luteinizing hormone (LH)		
Female		
Menstruating		
Follicular phase	2.0–15.0 U/L	2.0–15.0 U/L
Ovulatory phase	22.0–105.0 U/L	22.0–105.0 U/L
Luteal phase	0.6–19.0 U/L	0.6–19.0 U/L
Postmenopausal	16.0–64.0 U/L	16.0–64.0 U/L
Male	2.0–12.0 U/L	2.0–12.0 U/L
Metanephrine (urine)	0.03–0.69 mmol/mol creatinine	0.05–1.20 μg/mg creatinine
Norepinephrine (urine)	89–473 nmol/d	15–80 μg/d
Parathyroid hormone (PTH)	10–60 ng/L	10–60 pg/mL
Progesterone		
Female		
Follicular	<3.18 nmol/L	<1.0 ng/mL
Midluteal	9.54–63.6 nmol/L	3–20 ng/mL
Male	<3.18 nmol/L	<1.0 ng/mL
Prolactin		
Female	0–20 μg/L	1.9–25.9 ng/mL
Male	0–15 μg/L	1.6–23.0 ng/mL
Renin (adult, normal sodium diet)		
Supine	0.08–0.83 ng/(L-s)	0.3–3.0 ng/(mL/h)
Upright	0.28–2.5 ng(L-s)	1–9.0 ng/(mL/h)
Somatomedin-C (IGF-1) (adult)		
16–24 years	182–780 μg/L	182–780 ng/mL
25–39 years	114–492 μg/L	114–492 ng/mL
40–54 years	90–360 μg/L	90–360 ng/mL
>54 years	71–290 μg/L	71–290 ng/mL
Testosterone, total, morning sample		
Female	0.21–2.98 nmol/L	6–86 ng/dL
Male	9.36–37.10 nmol/L	270–1070 ng/dL
Thyroglobulin	0–60 μg/L	0–60 ng/mL
Thyroid hormone binding index (THBI or T_3RU)	0.83–1.17 mol ratio	0.83–1.17
(Free) thyroxine index	4.2–13	4.2–13
Thyroid stimulating hormone	0.5–4.7 mU/L	0.5–4.7 μU/mL
Thyroxine, total (T4)	58–140 nmol/L	4.5–10.9 μg/dL
Triiodothyronine, total (T3)	0.92–2.78 nmol/L	60–181 ng/dL
Thyroxine, free (fT4)	10.3–35 pmol/L	0.8–2.7 ng/dL
Triiodothyronine, free (fT3)	0.22–6.78 pmol/L	1.4–4.4 pg/mL
Vanillylmandelic Acid (VMA) (urine)	7.6–37.9 μmol/d	0.15–1.2 mg/d

Note: P, plasma; S, serum; U, urine; WB, whole blood.

TABLE A-4

VITAMINS AND SELECTED TRACE MINERALS

SPECIMEN	SI UNITS	CONVENTIONAL UNITS
Aluminum	<0.2 μmol/L	<5.41 μg/L
	5–30 μg/L	0.19–1.11 μmol/L
Arsenic	0.03–0.31 μmol/L	2–23 μg/L
	0.07–0.67 μmol/d	5–50 μg/d
Folic acid	7–36 nmol/L cells	3–16 ng/mL cells
Lead (adult)	<0.5–1 μmol/L	<10–20 μg/dL
Mercury	3.0–294 nmol/L	0.6–59 μg/L
Vitamin A	0.7–3.5 μmol/L	20–100 μg/dL
Vitamin B_1 (thiamine)	0–75 nmol/L	0–2 μg/dL
Vitamin B_2 (riboflavin)	106–638 nmol/L	4–24 μg/dL
Vitamin B_6	20–121 nmol/L	5–30 ng/mL
Vitamin B_{12}	148–590 pmol/L	200–800 pg/mL
Vitamin C (ascorbic acid)	23–57 μmol/L	0.4–1.0 mg/dL
Vitamin D_3, 1,25-dihydroxy	60–108 pmol/L	25–45 pg/mL
Summer	37.4–200 nmol/L	15–80 ng/mL
Winter	34.9–105 nmol/L	14–42 ng/mL
Vitamin E	12–42 μmol/L	5–18 μg/mL
Vitamin K	0.29–2.64 nmol/L	0.13–1.19 ng/mL
Zinc	11.5–18.5 μmol/L	75–120 μg/dL

TABLE A-5

CLASSIFICATION OF LDL, TOTAL, AND HDL CHOLESTEROL

LDL cholesterol	
<100	Optimal
100–129	Near or above normal
130–159	Borderline high
160–189	High
≥190	Very high
Total cholesterol	
<200	Desirable
200–239	Borderline high
≥240	High
HDL cholesterol	
<40	Low
≥60	High

Note: HDL, high-density lipoprotien; LDL, low-density lipoprotein.
Source: Executive summary of the third report of the national cholesterol education program (NCEP) expert panel on detection, evaluation, and treatment of high blood cholesterol in adults (adult treatment panel III): JAMA 285:2486, 2001.

REVIEW AND SELF-ASSESSMENT

QUESTIONS

DIRECTIONS: Each question below contains five or six suggested responses. Choose the **one best** response to each question.

1. A 31-year-old female complains of a 2-month history of a 15-lb unintentional weight loss, anxiety, and "feeling jittery." The neck examination is unremarkable. Physical examination shows tachycardia and hyperreflexia. Thyroid-stimulating hormone (TSH) is below 0.01. Total T_4 is elevated. Whole-body radionuclide iodine scan shows only low uptake in the region of the thyroid. Serum thyroglobulin levels are within the normal range. What is the most likely diagnosis?

   A. Graves' disease
   B. Struma ovarii
   C. Subacute thyroiditis
   D. Lymphocytic thyroiditis
   E. Thyrotoxicosis factitia

2. The World Health Organization (WHO) recently defined osteoporosis operationally as

   A. a patient with a bone density less than the mean of age-, race-, and gender-matched controls
   B. a patient with a bone density less than 1.0 standard deviation (SD) below the mean of race- and gender-matched controls
   C. a patient with a bone density less than 1.0 SD below the mean of age-, race-, and gender-matched controls
   D. a patient with a bone density less than 2.5 SD below the mean of race- and gender-matched controls
   E. a patient with a bone density less than 2.5 SD below the mean of age-, race-, and gender-matched controls

3. A 40-year-old female complains of low-grade fevers and anterior neck pain for 6 days. She denies tremor, weight loss, or visual changes. Examination shows a tender and slightly enlarged thyroid gland. There is no bruit. The rest of the examination is unremarkable. TSH is low. T_4 and T_3 are both elevated. A radionuclide scan shows low uptake. Anti-TPO antibodies are negative. What would be the most appropriate therapy at this point?

   A. Radioiodine ablation
   B. Methimazole

3. *(Continued)*

   C. Change to salicylates or NSAIDs
   D. Levothyroxine
   E. Surgery

4. Which of the following statements regarding hypothyroidism is true?

   A. Hashimoto's thyroiditis is the most common cause of hypothyroidism worldwide.
   B. The annual risk of developing overt clinical hypothyroidism from subclinical hypothyroidism in patients with positive thyroid peroxidase (TPO) antibodies is 20%.
   C. Histologically, Hashimoto's thyroiditis is characterized by marked infiltration of the thyroid with activated T cells and B cells.
   D. A low TSH level excludes the diagnosis of hypothyroidism.
   E. Thyroid peroxidase antibodies are present in less than 50% of patients with autoimmune hypothyroidism.

5. A 40-year-old female with Graves' disease was recently started on methimazole. One month later she comes to the clinic for a routine follow-up. She notes some lowgrade fevers, arthralgias, and general malaise. Laboratories are notable for a mild transaminitis and a glucose of 150 mg/dL. All the following are known side effects of methimazole *except*

   A. agranulocytosis
   B. rash
   C. arthralgia
   D. hepatitis
   E. insulin resistance

6. A 23-year-old female nursing student is brought to the emergency room by her parents after being found unconscious at home. She is noted to have a fingerstick glucose of 29 mg/dL. After administration of intravenous D50, she rapidly regains consciousness. Her parents state that this is the fourth time in a month that this has occurred. She is not taking any medications. The medical history is unremarkable except for a history of depression and a mother with diabetes mellitus. Examination is unremarkable. During an observed period in the hospital,

6. *(Continued)*
the patient is noted to have a symptomatic glucose level of 31 mg/dL. Plasma insulin levels are elevated, and C-peptide levels are low. Which of the following is the most likely cause of her hypoglycemia?

A. Glipizide overdose
B. Surreptitious insulin use
C. Insulinoma
D. Glucagonoma
E. Diabetic ketoacidosis

7. A 52-year-old female is admitted to the hospital for weight loss, diarrhea, and dehydration. She reports 1 to 2 months of watery diarrhea that is unrelated to food intake. Concurrent with the diarrhea she often has cramping abdominal pain and flushing of the neck and face. The onset of these symptoms is often sudden and is preceded by stress, alcohol intake, or eating cheese. Initially the flushing lasted approximately 5 min, but it now lasts up to an hour. The flushing episodes are usually followed by diarrhea. The symptoms have not improved despite the elimination of all dairy products from her diet. The physical examination is notable for a blood pressure of 90/70 mmHg and a heart rate of 95/min. The patient's blood pressure falls and her heart rate increases when she sits. The patient also has hepatomegaly, with a liver span of 15 cm. An ultrasound demonstrates lesions in the liver consistent with metastases. Which of the following tests is most likely to yield the diagnosis?

A. Flow cytometry of a bone marrow aspirate
B. Serum α fetoprotein
C. Serum cortisol
D. Serum glucose
E. Urinary 5-HIAA

8. This patient probably will demonstrate a neoplasm originating in the

A. adrenal gland
B. bone marrow
C. bronchus
D. ileum
E. pancreas

9. A 25-year-old female notes increasing facial hair and acne for the last 4 months. She has noticed some deepening of her voice but denies changes in her libido or genitalia. She weighs 94 kg and is 5 feet 5 inches tall. Blood pressure is 126/70 mmHg. Examination is notable for moderate obesity. There is no evidence of abdominal striae or bruising. All the following would be important initial steps in the clinical assessment of this patient *except*

9. *(Continued)*
A. medication history
B. family history
C. serum testosterone level
D. serum dehydroepiandrosterone sulfate (DHEAS) level
E. abdominal ultrasound

10. Which of the following is consistent with a diagnosis of subacute thyroiditis?

A. A 38-year-old female with a 2-week history of a painful thyroid, elevated T_4, elevated T_3, low TSH, and an elevated radioactive iodine uptake scan
B. A 42-year-old male with a history of a painful thyroid 4 months ago, fatigue, malaise, low free T_4, low T_3, and elevated TSH.
C. A 31-year-old female with a painless enlarged thyroid, low TSH, elevated T_4, elevated free T_4, and an elevated radioiodine uptake scan
D. A 50-year-old male with a painful thyroid, slightly elevated T_4, normal TSH, and an ultrasound showing a mass
E. A 46-year-old female with 3 weeks of fatigue, low T_4, low T_3, and low TSH

11. Which of the following is the most common site for a fracture associated with osteoporosis?

A. Femur
B. Hip
C. Radius
D. Vertebra
E. Wrist

12. All the following are risk factors for the development of osteoporotic fractures *except*

A. African-American race
B. current cigarette smoking
C. female sex
D. low body weight
E. physical inactivity

13. All the following drugs are associated with an increased risk of osteoporosis in adults *except*

A. cyclosporine
B. dilantin
C. heparin
D. prednisone
E. ranitidine

14. A 44-year-old male is involved in a motor vehicle collision. He sustains multiple injuries to the face, chest, and pelvis. He is unresponsive in the field and

14. *(Continued)*
is intubated for airway protection. An intravenous line is placed. The patient is admitted to the intensive care unit (ICU) with multiple orthopedic injuries. He is stabilized medically and on hospital day 2 undergoes successful open reduction and internal fixation of the right femur and right humerus. After his return to the ICU, you review his laboratory values. TSH is 0.3 mU/L, and the total T_4 level is normal. T_3 is 0.6 μg/dL. What is the most appropriate next management step?

A. Initiation of levothyroxine
B. A radioiodine uptake scan
C. A thyroid ultrasound
D. Observation
E. Initiation of prednisone

15. All the following are pharmacologic therapies for androgen excess *except*

A. glucocorticoids
B. oral contraceptives
C. spironolactone
D. cyproterone acetate
E. fludracortisone

16. All the following biochemical markers are a measure of bone resorption *except*

A. serum alkaline phosphatase
B. serum cross-linked N-telopeptide
C. serum cross-linked C-telopeptide
D. urine hydroxyproline
E. urine total free deoxypyridonoline

17. All but which of the following statements about osteoporosis and bone fractures are true?

A. Osteoporosis is defined as a bone density that is 1.5 standard deviations (SD) below the mean for young healthy adults of the same race and gender.
B. Up to 2 million men in the United States have osteoporosis.
C. The risk of hip fracture is higher in whites than in African Americans.
D. The incidence of deep venous thrombosis in patients with hip fractures is more than 20%.
E. More than 10% of white women over age 50 years will have a hip fracture.

18. All the following are associated with bone loss *except*

A. vitamin D deficiency
B. menopause

18. *(Continued)*
C. glucocorticoids
D. tobacco use
E. running

19. A 51-year-old Asian female comes to your clinic for routine health screening. She is otherwise healthy and takes no medications. The family history is notable only for a mother with osteoporosis. A review of systems is notable for hot flashes and mood changes over the last year. The patient's last menstrual period was 3 months ago. The examination is unremarkable. You make arrangements for age-appropriate cancer screening, measure her cholesterol, and order a bone densitometry scan (DEXA). The DEXA shows multiple sites with *t*-scores more than -2.5 SD below the mean. All the following are reasonable treatment recommendations *except*

A. calcium supplementation
B. vitamin D supplementation
C. weekly alendronate
D. tamoxifen
E. exercise

20. A 35-year-old male is referred to your clinic for evaluation of hypercalcemia noted during a health insurance medical screening. He has noted some fatigue, malaise, and a 4-lb weight loss over the last 2 months. He also has noted constipation and "heartburn." He is occasionally nauseated after large meals and has water brash and a sour taste in his mouth. The patient denies vomiting, dysphagia, or odynophagia. He also notes decreased libido and a depressed mood. Vital signs are unremarkable. Physical examination is notable for a clear oropharynx, no evidence of a thyroid mass, and no lymphadenopathy. Jugular venous pressure is normal. Heart sounds are regular with no murmurs or gallops. The chest is clear. The abdomen is soft with some mild epigastric tenderness. There is no rebound or organomegaly. Stool is guaiac-positive. Neurologic examination is nonfocal. Laboratory values are notable for a normal complete blood count. Calcium is 11.2 mg/dL, phosphate is 2.1 mg/dL, and magnesium is 1.8 meq/dL. Albumin is 3.7 g/dL, and total protein is 7.0 g/dL. TSH is 3 μIU/mL, prolactin is 250 μg/L, testosterone is 320 ng/dL, and serum insulin-like growth factor 1 (IGF-1) is normal. Serum intact parathyroid hormone level is 135 pg/dL. In light of the patient's abdominal discomfort and heme-positive stool, you perform an abdominal computed tomography (CT) scan that shows a lesion measuring 2 cm by 2 cm in the head of the pancreas. What is the diagnosis?

20. *(Continued)*
    A. Multiple endocrine neoplasia (MEN) type 1
    B. MEN type 2a
    C. MEN type 2b
    D. Polyglandular autoimmune syndrome
    E. Von Hippel–Lindau (VHL) syndrome

21. Postmenopausal estrogen therapy has been shown to increase a female's risk of all the following clinical outcomes *except*

    A. breast cancer
    B. hip fracture
    C. myocardial infarction
    D. stroke
    E. venous thromboembolism

22. Using available data on morbidity and mortality, the most widely used definition threshold for obesity is

    A. weight more than 2 standard deviations above the mean for age, sex, and race
    B. a waist-to-hip ratio above 1.0 in men and 0.9 in women
    C. a body mass index (BMI) higher than 30
    D. weight more than 100 kg for women and 120 kg for men
    E. electrical impedance more than 2 standard deviations above the mean for age, sex, and race

23. Obesity is associated with an increased incidence of all the following *except*

    A. diabetes mellitus
    B. cancer
    C. hypertension
    D. biliary disease
    E. chronic obstructive lung disease

24. All but which of the following statements regarding diabetes mellitus (DM) are true?

    A. Scandinavia has the highest incidence of type 1 DM.
    B. Up to 60% of women with gestational diabetes mellitus (GDM) go on to develop overt diabetes mellitus.
    C. Hispanic Americans are the ethnic group that has the highest prevalence of DM in the United States.
    D. The prevalence of DM is rising worldwide.
    E. The concordance of type 2 DM in identical twins is higher than the concordance of type 1 DM in identical twins.

25. All the following are direct actions of parathyroid hormone (PTH) *except*

    A. increased calcium resorption from bone
    B. increased calcium resorption from the kidney

25. *(Continued)*
    C. increased calcium resorption from the gastrointestinal tract
    D. increased synthesis of 1,25 dihydroxyvitamin D
    E. decreased phosphate resorption from the kidney

26. A 50-year-old male presents to the clinic for a routine health examination. A comprehensive metabolic panel shows a serum calcium level of 11.2 mg/dL. Serum phosphate is 3.0 mg/dL. Serum creatinine is normal. He denies bone pain, lethargy, weakness, or weight loss. What is the most common cause of hypercalcemia in outpatients?

    A. Malignancy
    B. Medications
    C. Milk-alkali syndrome
    D. Primary hyperparathyroidism
    E. Granulomatous disease

27. All the following are effects of hypercalcemia *except*

    A. diarrhea
    B. confusion
    C. polyuria
    D. a shortened QT interval
    E. nephrolithiasis

28. Which of the following statements is true about familial hypocalciuric hypercalcemia (FHH)?

    A. It is inherited in an autosomal recessive pattern.
    B. The cause is a defect in the parathyroid hormone receptor.
    C. Clinical symptoms first manifest in the third and fourth decades of life.
    D. Treatment is rarely necessary.
    E. Renal calcium reabsorption is more than 99%.

29. All the following are causes of hypocalcemia *except*

    A. hypomagnesemia
    B. sepsis
    C. burn injury
    D. tumor lysis syndrome
    E. immobilization

30. All but which of the following statements about pheochromocytoma are true?

    A. The majority are malignant.
    B. Up to 25% of cases are associated with an inherited form of the disease.
    C. It occurs more frequently in patients under age 50.

30. *(Continued)*
    D. Diagnosis is made by 24-h urine collection of catecholamines.
    E. α-Adrenergic blockade is mandatory before surgical excision.

31. All the following are features of abetalipoproteinemia *except*

    A. autosomal recessive inheritance
    B. spinocerebellar degeneration
    C. retinopathy
    D. childhood presentation
    E. elevated cholesterol levels

32. All the following are features of lipoprotein lipase deficiency *except*

    A. low levels of plasma chylomicrons
    B. acute pancreatitis
    C. hepatosplenomegaly
    D. xanthomas
    E. autosomal recessive inheritance

33. All the following are side effects of HMG-CoA reductase inhibitors (statins) *except*

    A. hepatitis
    B. myopathy
    C. dyspepsia
    D. headache
    E. pulmonary fibrosis

34. A 55-year-old male is admitted to the intensive care unit with 1 week of fever and cough. He was well until 1 week before admission, when he noted progressive shortness of breath, cough, and productive sputum. On the day of admission the patient was noted by his wife to be lethargic and unresponsive. 911 was called, and the patient was intubated in the field and then brought to the emergency department. His medications include insulin. The past medical history is notable for alcohol abuse, diabetes mellitus, and chronic renal insufficiency. Temperature is 38.9°C (102°F). He is hypotensive with a blood pressure of 76/40 mmHg. Oxygen saturation is 86% on room air. On examination, the patient is sedated and intubated. Jugular venous pressure is normal. There are decreased breath sounds at the right lung base with egophony. Heart sounds are normal. The abdomen is soft. There is no peripheral edema. Chest radiography shows a right lower lobe infiltrate with a moderate pleural effusion. An electrocardiogram is normal. Sputum Gram stain shows gram-positive diplococci. White blood cell count is $23 \times 10^3/\mu L$, with 70% polymorphonuclear cells and 6% bands. Blood urea nitrogen is 80 mg/dL, and creatinine is 6.1 mg/dL. Plasma glucose is 425 mg/dL. He is started on broad-spectrum antibiotics, intravenous fluids, omeprazole, and an insulin drip. A nasogastric tube is inserted, and tube feedings are started. On hospital day 2 plasma phosphate is 1.0 mg/dL. All of following are causes of hypophosphatemia *except*

    A. sepsis
    B. renal failure
    C. insulin
    D. alcoholism
    E. malnutrition

35. A 21-year-old competitive runner is evaluated for irregular menstruation. She had menses at age 14 and normally has a 28-day cycle with 5 days of menses. Over the last 4 months she has noted irregularity in her cycles. Menses may last between 2 and 7 days, and she has not had a period for the last month. There is no change in cramping or abdominal symptoms. Pelvic examination is normal. Urine and blood tests for pregnancy are negative. What is the most appropriate management step?

    A. Progesterone challenge
    B. Hysterosalpingography
    C. CT scan of the abdomen with contrast
    D. Serum prolactin
    E. Chromosome analysis

36. A 48-year-old female is undergoing evaluation for flushing and diarrhea. Physical examination is normal except for nodular hepatomegaly. A CT scan of the abdomen demonstrates multiple nodules in both lobes of the liver consistent with metastases in the liver and a 2-cm mass in the ileum. The 24-h urinary 5-HIAA excretion is markedly elevated. All the following treatments are appropriate *except*

    A. diphenhydramine
    B. interferon-α
    C. octreotide
    D. odansetron
    E. phenoxybenzamine

37. While undergoing a physical examination during medical student clinical skills, this patient develops severe flushing, wheezing, nausea, and light-headedness. Vital signs are notable for a blood pressure of 70/30 mmHg and a heart rate of 135/min. Which of the following is the most appropriate therapy?

37. *(Continued)*
   A. Albuterol
   B. Atropine
   C. Epinephrine
   D. Hydrocortisone
   E. Octreotide

38. A 31-year-old female is evaluated for amenorrhea for the last 6 months. Her height is 170 cm, and her weight is 50 kg. Pelvic examination is unremarkable. A pregnancy test is negative. Serum LH and follicle-stimulating hormone (FSH) are elevated. Estradiol is low. What is the most likely diagnosis?

   A. Polycystic ovarian disease
   B. Panhypopituitarism
   C. Asherman's syndrome
   D. Ovarian failure
   E. Turner syndrome

39. A 21-year-old female with a history of type 1 diabetes mellitus is brought to the emergency room with nausea, vomiting, lethargy, and dehydration. Her mother notes that she stopped taking insulin 1 day before presentation. She is lethargic, has dry mucous membranes, and is obtunded. Blood pressure is 80/40 mmHg, and heart rate is 112 beats/min. Heart sounds are normal. Lungs are clear. The abdomen is soft, and there is no organomegaly. She is responsive and oriented ×3 but diffusely weak. Serum sodium is 126 meq/L, potassium is 4.3 meq/L, magnesium is 1.2 meq/L, blood urea nitrogen is 76 mg/dL, creatinine is 2.2 mg/dL, bicarbonate is 10 meq/L, and chloride is 88 meq/L. Serum glucose is 720 mg/dL. All the following are appropriate management steps *except*

   A. arterial blood gas
   B. intravenous insulin
   C. intravenous potassium
   D. 3% sodium solution
   E. intravenous fluids

40. The Diabetes Control and Complications Trial (DCCT) provided definitive proof that reduction in chronic hyperglycemia

   A. improves microvascular complications in type 1 diabetes mellitus
   B. improves macrovascular complications in type 1 diabetes mellitus
   C. improves microvascular complications in type 2 diabetes mellitus
   D. improves macrovascular complications in type 2 diabetes mellitus
   E. improves both microvascular and macrovascular complications in type 2 diabetes mellitus

41. All the following therapies have been shown to reduce the risk of hip fractures in postmenopausal women with osteoporosis *except*

   A. alendronate
   B. estrogen
   C. parathyroid hormone
   D. raloxifene
   E. risedronate
   F. vitamin D plus calcium

42. A 64-year-old male with COPD has been treated frequently with prednisone for exacerbations. Bone densitometry reveals a *z*-score of −3.0. Which of the following is the most appropriate treatment to reduce the risk of fractures?

   A. Calcitonin
   B. Estrogen
   C. Hydrochlorothiazide
   D. Risedronate
   E. Vitamin D

43. A 33-year-old male with end-stage renal disease who is on hemodialysis complains of decreased libido, inability to maintain erections, increasing fatigue, and mild weakness. He has been on a stable hemodialysis regimen for 8 years, and all his electrolytes are normal. Further evaluation reveals a reduced serum testosterone level. Measurement of which of the following will distinguish primary from secondary hypogonadism?

   A. Aldosterone
   B. Cortisol
   C. Estradiol
   D. Luteinizing hormone
   E. Thyroid-stimulating hormone

44. All the following drugs may interfere with testicular function *except*

   A. cyclophosphamide
   B. ketoconazole
   C. metoprolol
   D. prednisone
   E. spironolactone

45. A 55-year-old female comes to her primary care physician's office for evaluation of episodes of flushing. The symptoms started about 1 year ago when she noted occasional night sweats as well as daily facial flushing lasting 3 to 5 min and vaginal dryness. Her menses have become irregular, with the last menstrual period having occurred 6 months ago.

45. *(Continued)*
Past medical history is notable for rheumatoid arthritis and frequent urinary tract infections since young adulthood. Current medications are etanercept and occasional ibuprofen. She quit smoking cigarettes 20 years ago and has no other habits. The following laboratory data are obtained:
TSH 1.23 mIU/mg normal 0.5 to 4.5
FSH 35 mIU/mL upper limit of normal 10
She is interested in discussing the benefits of estrogen-progesterone replacement therapy. Her physician can tell her that there is scientific evidence that this therapy will decrease all the following *except*

A. progression of bone loss
B. incidence of urinary tract infections
C. incidence of myocardial infarction
D. vaginal dryness
E. vasomotor symptoms

46. A 35-year-old male with no significant past medical history complains of 6 weeks of abdominal pain, watery diarrhea, and heartburn. These symptoms were not relieved by a 2-week course of omeprazole. He has no anorexia but has lost 10 lb. He is on no medications currently, does not smoke cigarettes, and does not use alcohol. Further investigation by endoscopy reveals prominent gastric folds and three duodenal ulcers. Fasting serum gastrin is elevated. Which of the following results is most likely to provide a diagnosis in this case?

A. An elevated serum chromogranin A
B. An increase in serum gastrin 15 min after intravenous infusion of secretin
C. A positive antigliadin antibody test
D. A positive gastric biopsy urease test
E. A positive periodic acid–Schiff (PAS) stain on duodenal biopsy

47. A 47-year-old nurse complains of episodic confusion, headaches, disorientation, sweating, and tremors that occur approximately three times a week, usually at work. These episodes began about 4 months ago. She notes they occur more frequently during stressful times at work when she has to skip lunch. The episodes resolve after a few minutes, often after the patient drinks some juice. There is no past medical history except a history of irritable bowel syndrome. During a recent episode at work in the hospital, her serum glucose was found to be 40 mg/dL. Which of the following serum tests should be done during a hypoglycemic episode to determine the etiology of her symptoms?

47. *(Continued)*
A. Cortisol
B. C peptide
C. Glucagon
D. Hemoglobin A_{1C}
E. Serotonin

48. A 49-year-old male is brought to the hospital by his family because of confusion and dehydration. The family reports that for the last 3 weeks he has had persistent copious watery diarrhea that has not abated with the use of over-the-counter medications. The diarrhea has been unrelated to food intake and has persisted during fasting. The stool does not appear fatty and is not malodorous. The patient works as an attorney, is a vegetarian, and has not traveled recently. No one in the household has had similar symptoms. Before the onset of diarrhea, he had mild anorexia and a 5-lb weight loss. Since the diarrhea began, he has lost at least 10 pounds. The physical examination is notable for blood pressure of 100/70, heart rate of 110/min, and temperature of 36.8°C (98.2°F). Other than poor skin turgor, confusion, and diffuse muscle weakness, the physical examination is unremarkable. Laboratory studies are notable for a normal complete blood count and the following chemistry results:

Na^+	146 meq/L
K^+	3.0 meq/L
Cl^-	96 meq/L
HCO_3^-	36 meq/L
BUN	32 mg/dL
Creatinine	1.2 mg/dL

A 24-h stool collection yields 3 L of tea-colored stool. Stool sodium is 50 meq/L, potassium is 25 meq/L, and stool osmolality is 170 mosmol/L. Which of the following diagnostic tests is most likely to yield the correct diagnosis?

A. Serum cortisol
B. Serum TSH
C. Serum VIP
D. Urinary 5-HIAA
E. Urinary metanephrine

49. A 63-year-old male seeks medical attention for a 6-month history of lack of libido and generalized malaise. He has a history of mild obstructive sleep apnea and is trying to lose weight. After a complete evaluation, the patient is found to have a reduced serum testosterone of 150 ng/dL. Testosterone replacement therapy probably will have all the following effects *except*

A. improved libido
B. improved sleep apnea symptoms

49. *(Continued)*
   C. increased bone density
   D. increased energy
   E. increased lean muscle mass

50. A patient is seen in the clinic for routine follow-up for hypertension. A basic metabolic panel is ordered along with a lipid profile while the patient is fasting. The lipid profile is normal. Electrolytes, blood urea nitrogen (BUN), and creatinine are normal. Glucose is 111 mg/dL. On recheck, fasting glucose is 113 mg/dL. The patient can be told which of the following?

   A. A hemoglobin A_{1C} will need to be checked to ensure that he does not have diabetes mellitus.
   B. He has diabetes mellitus.
   C. He has impaired fasting glucose.
   D. His laboratory work is normal.
   E. He will need an oral glucose tolerance test to evaluate for impaired glucose tolerance.

51. Which of the following statements about the possible diagnosis of impaired fasting glucose is correct?

   A. Impaired fasting glucose can be diagnosed when the fasting glucose ranges from 115 mg/dL to 125 mg/dL.
   B. Patients with impaired fasting glucose are at increased risk for cardiovascular disease.
   C. Patients with impaired fasting glucose have a minimally increased risk for developing diabetes mellitus over the next decade.
   D. Patients with impaired fasting glucose should be tested for anti–islet cell antibodies to diagnose autoimmune diabetes mellitus early and prevent severe complications.
   E. Patients with impaired fasting glucose should have regular checks of their hemoglobin A_{1C}.

52. During an employment physical examination, an 18-year-old male is found to have a 1.5-cm nodule in the apex of the left lobe of the thyroid. A fine-needle aspiration reveals malignant C cells that stain positive for calcitonin. All but which of the following statements regarding this patient's condition are true?

   A. He is likely to have distant metastases.
   B. He is at risk of developing hyperparathyroidism.
   C. He is at risk of developing a pancreatic cell tumor.
   D. He is at risk of developing a pheochromocytoma.
   E. It is likely that other members of his family have the same malignancy.

53. A 23-year-old female is admitted to the hospital with 1 day of diffuse abdominal pain. She has no past medical history and takes no medications. Physical examination shows tachycardia, mild hypotension, a fruity odor to her breath, and a mildly diffusely tender abdomen. Blood chemistries show a sodium of 136 meq/L, a potassium of 5.6 meq/L, a chloride of 101 meq/L, and an undetectable bicarbonate. The glucose is 551 mg/dL. Blood ketones are positive at a 1:8 dilution. Three hours after the initiation of intravenous insulin and normal saline, the laboratories are as follows: sodium 140 meq/L, potassium 4.1 meq/L, chloride 106 meq/L, bicarbonate 14 meq/L, and glucose 190 mg/dL. The most appropriate next step in management is to

   A. discontinue intravenous fluids
   B. discontinue insulin infusion and administer subcutaneous insulin
   C. discontinue insulin infusion and begin 5% dextrose normal saline infusion
   D. discontinue normal saline and begin 5% dextrose normal saline infusion
   E. measure a follow-up serum ketone level before making decisions about insulin or fluid management

54. A patient is seen in the clinic for follow-up of type 2 diabetes mellitus. Her hemoglobin A_{1C} has been poorly controlled at 9.4% recently. The patient can be counseled to expect all the following improvements with improved glycemic control *except*

   A. decreased microalbuminuria
   B. decreased risk of nephropathy
   C. decreased risk of neuropathy
   D. decreased risk of peripheral vascular disease
   E. decreased risk of retinopathy

55. The patient's blood pressure is 163/94 mmHg. With improved blood pressure control, the patient can expect all the following *except*

   A. Decreased risk of death
   B. Decreased risk of neuropathy
   C. Decreased risk of retinopathy
   D. Decreased risk of stroke
   E. All of the above

56. Which of the following statements regarding dyslipidemia and diabetes mellitus is correct?

   A. In diabetic individuals, LDL cholesterol is structurally similar to LDL cholesterol in normal individuals.
   B. In diabetic individuals without coronary artery disease, the goal LDL level is below 120 mg/dL.
   C. LDL particles in type 2 diabetic patients are less susceptible to oxidation than they are in individuals without diabetes.

56. *(Continued)*
   D. Male patients with diabetes mellitus have a goal HDL of over 55 mg/dL.
   E. The most common forms of dyslipidemia in diabetic patients are elevated triglycerides and reduced HDL levels.

57. A 59-year-old female is seen in the clinic regarding her diagnosis of type 2 diabetes mellitus. She has attempted diet control and exercise for the last 6 months; however, her hemoglobin A_{1C}, is 8.6%, and it is now recommended that she begin medication for diabetes. The patient takes lisinopril and aspirin and has no allergies. Her other medical problems are mild congestive heart failure and hypertension. Blood work is notable for a creatinine of 1.5 mg/dL. Which of the following medications is it appropriate to start at this time?

   A. Metformin
   B. Glipizide
   C. Insulin
   D. Pioglitazone
   E. Metformin and glipizide

58. Which of the following studies is most sensitive for detecting diabetic nephropathy?

   A. Serum creatinine level
   B. Creatinine clearance
   C. Urine albumin
   D. Glucose tolerance test
   E. Ultrasonography

59. A 61-year-old female noticed severe sharp pain in her back after lifting a suitcase. A compression fracture of the T11 vertebral body is identified on x-ray examination. Routine laboratory evaluation discloses a serum calcium concentration of 2 mmol/L (8.0 mg/dL), a serum phosphorus concentration of 0.77 mmol/L (2.4 mg/dL), and increased serum alkaline phosphatase activity. The serum parathyroid hormone level subsequently is found to be elevated as well. The most likely diagnosis is

   A. Paget's disease of bone
   B. ectopic parathyroid hormone secretion
   C. primary hyperparathyroidism
   D. postmenopausal osteoporosis
   E. vitamin D deficiency

60. Which of the following conditions is most likely to be associated with a normal serum 25(OH) vitamin D level?

60. *(Continued)*
   A. Dietary deficiency of vitamin D
   B. Chronic severe cholestatic liver disease
   C. Chronic renal failure
   D. Anticonvulsant therapy with phenobarbital or phenytoin
   E. High-dose glucocorticoid therapy

61. Four weeks postpartum, a 32-year-old female develops palpitations, heat intolerance, and nervousness. She is diagnosed with hyperthyroidism. Her thyroid is not enlarged or tender. The 24-h uptake of radioactive iodine is 1%. The most appropriate treatment for this patient is

   A. radioactive iodine ablation of the thyroid gland
   B. methimazole
   C. prednisone 60 mg a day followed by a rapid taper
   D. a beta blocker
   E. iodine drops (SSKI)

62. Which of the following statements concerning patients with polyglandular autoimmune syndrome type II (Schmidt's syndrome) is true?

   A. The onset of this disease typically occurs during childhood.
   B. It has an autosomal recessive mode of inheritance.
   C. After Addison's disease, the second most common endocrine abnormality is hypothyroidism.
   D. Mucocutaneous candidiasis is a typical hallmark of this syndrome.
   E. Hypoparathyroidism is a common feature.

63. Which of the following statements regarding erectile dysfunction is correct?

   A. Patients with testosterone deficiency are able to achieve erections with visual stimuli.
   B. Patients with psychogenic erectile dysfunction have excess parasympathetic stimulation that decreases penile smooth muscle tone.
   C. Both beta blockers and α-adrenergic blockers are commonly implicated in erectile dysfunction.
   D. Individuals with diabetes mellitus have normal levels of nitric oxide synthase in both endothelial and neural tissues.
   E. Increased prolactin levels cause erectile dysfunction by directly reducing testicular androgen synthesis.

64. Which of the following statements concerning the use of sildenafil for the treatment of erectile dysfunction is correct?

   A. Sildenafil inhibits phosphodiesterase isoenzyme type V levels, thus increasing the concentration of cyclic AMP.
   B. Sildenafil may cause a transient alteration in color vision.

64. *(Continued)*
 C. Sildenafil may increase a patient's libido.
 D. Sildenafil is hepatically cleared, and therefore no dose reduction is required for patients with impaired renal function.
 E. Sildenafil is ineffective in the treatment of patients with diabetes mellitus who also have erectile dysfunction.

65. A 30-year-old male, the father of three children, has had progressive breast enlargement during the last 6 months. He does not use any drugs. Laboratory evaluation reveals that both LH and testosterone are low.

65. *(Continued)*
Further evaluation of this patient should include which of the following?

 A. Blood sampling for serum glutamic-oxaloacetic transaminase (SGOT) and serum alkaline phosphatase and bilirubin levels
 B. Measurement of estradiol and human chorionic gonadotropin (hCG) levels
 C. A 24-h urine collection for the measurement of 17-ketosteroids
 D. Karyotype analysis to exclude Klinefelter syndrome
 E. Breast biopsy

ANSWERS

1. The answer is E.
Discussion: *(Chap. 4)* Thyrotoxicosis factitia is caused by excess amounts of exogenous thyroid hormone. Radionuclide scans show low uptake because TSH is suppressed. Unlike the situation in subacute thyroiditis, serum thyroglobulin levels are low or normal because there is no inflammatory release of thyroid gland proteins. Struma ovarii and ectopic thyroid tissue are identified by evidence of radioiodine uptake on whole-body scans. Graves' disease is characterized by diffuse thyroid enlargement and increased uptake on iodine scanning.

2. The answer is D.
Discussion: *(Chap. 25)* Osteoporosis is defined as a reduction of bone mass or density or the presence of a fragility fracture. Operationally, the WHO defines osteoporosis as a bone density more than 2.5 SD less than the mean for young healthy adults of the same race and sex. Dual-energy x-ray absorptiometry (DXA) is the most widely used study to determine bone density. Bone density is expressed as a *t*-score, that is, the SD below the mean of young adults of the same race and gender. A *t*-score higher than 2.5 characterizes osteoporosis, and a *t*-score less than 1 identifies patients at risk of osteoporosis. The *z*-score compares individuals with those in an age-, race-, and gender-matched population. The figure shows the relationship between *z*-scores and *t*-scores.

3. The answer is C.
Discussion: *(Chap. 4)* This patient's history is most consistent with the thyrotoxic phase of subacute thyroiditis. The peak incidence occurs between ages 30 and 50. The etiology is usually viral. There is a significant female predominance. The low uptake on a radionuclide scan in the setting of a recent onset of a painful thyroid clearly points to subacute thyroiditis. Elevation in T_4 and T_3 points to the thyrotoxic phase rather than the hypothyroid phase. The patient would be expected to improve over the course of months, and so permanent ablation with radioiodine or surgery is inappropriate. Antithyroid medications such as methimazole and propylthiouracil (PTU) have no role because the pathophysiology of thyroiditis relates to destruction of the gland and hormonal release, not hyperactivity, as in the case of Graves' disease and multinodular goiter. Levothyroxine may play a role in the hypothyroid phase, but not while the patient is acutely thyrotoxic. Anti-inflammatory medications such as salicylates nonsteroidal anti-inflammatory drugs (NSAIDs) or possibly steroids are most appropriate. Beta blockers would be appropriate if the patient were having more symptoms of thyrotoxicosis.

4. The answer is C.
Discussion: *(Chap. 4)* Iodine deficiency is the most common worldwide cause of hypothyroidism. Autoimmune, or Hashimoto's, thyroiditis is a common cause in developed countries with dietary iodine supplementation. Histologically, it is characterized by lymphocytic infiltration of the thyroid with activated T cells and B cells. Thyroid cell destruction is thought to be mediated by cytotoxic CD8+ T lymphocytes. Primary hypothyroidism is characterized by an elevation in TSH as the feedback inhibition of the anterior pituitary is diminished. However, patients with hypothyroidism may have low TSH in the setting of secondary hypothyroidism. In this case, a clinical and radiologic evaluation of the pituitary is required. Subclinical hypothyroidism is characterized by abnormalities in the serum levels of TSH but minimal symptoms and often minimal change in the free T_4 level. The rate of development of overt, symptomatic hypothyroidism is about 4% per year, especially in the case of positive TPO antibodies, which are present in 90 to 95% of patients with autoimmune hypothyroidism.

5. The answer is E.
Discussion: *(Chap. 4)* The thionamides propylthiouracil (PTU), carbimazole, and methimazole are the main antithyroid medications used for the treatment of hyperthyroidism. They all inhibit the function of thyroid peroxidase, reducing oxidation and organification of iodide. PTU also inhibits the deiodination of T_4 to T_3. PTU

has a half-life much shorter than that of methimazole. Rash, urticaria, fever, and arthralgias are common side effects, occurring in up to 5% of these patients. They may resolve spontaneously. Major side effects are rare but include hepatitis, agranulocytosis, and a systemic lupus erythematosus (SLE)-like syndrome. If major side effects are noted, it is essential that antithyroid medications be stopped.

6. The answer is B.
Discussion: *(Chap. 19)* Factitious hypoglycemia from self-administration of insulin or ingestion of a sulfonylurea shares clinical and laboratory features with insulinoma. The absence of an elevated C peptide distinguishes exogenous insulin use from insulinoma. An undetectable sulfonylurea level works against a diagnosis of sulfonylurea toxicity. Factitious hypoglycemia is more common in health care workers, patients with diabetes and their relatives, and patients with psychiatric histories.

7. and 8. The answers are E and D.
Discussion: *(Chap. 20)* The cardinal features of the carcinoid syndrome include diarrhea, flushing, and abdominal pain (see table). Other features, such as wheezing, pellagra, and heart failure, are less common. These patients are typically in their fifties, but the range of presentation spans adulthood to old age. Carcinoid tumors may secrete a variety of substances, including gastrointestinal (GI) peptides [gastrin, insulin, vasoactive intestinal peptide (VIP), glucagons], other peptides (ACTH, calcitonin), and bioactive amines (serotonin). Cardiac involvement is present in up to 40% of cases during the course of disease. Endocardial fibrosis, predominantly on the right side, is most common. This can result in pulmonic stenosis, tricuspid regurgitation, and right-sided heart failure. The carcinoid syndrome occurs when a sufficient concentration of secreted substance reaches the systemic circulation. This most commonly occurs (over 90% of cases) once there are metastases to the liver. Serotonin is a major product of carcinoid tumors that causes the typical carcinoid syndrome. In these patients increased amounts of the serotonin metabolite 5-HIAA is excreted in the urine and is the most frequently used diagnostic test. False positives may occur if the patient is eating serotonin-rich foods such as bananas, pineapple, and walnuts or is taking a medication such as guaifenesin, salicylates, acetaminophen, or L-dopa. Chronic myelogenous leukemia or systemic mastocytosis should be included in the differential diagnosis of typical carcinoid syndrome. The most common origin of liver metastases in the carcinoid syndrome is the ileum. Overall, carcinoid most commonly originates in the bronchi or lung, and this site may cause the carcinoid syndrome; however, bronchial/lung carcinoid does not usually cause metastatic disease (see table).

CLINICAL CHARACTERISTICS IN PATIENTS WITH CARCINOID SYNDROME

	AT PRESENTATION	DURING COURSE OF DISEASE
Symptoms/signs		
Diarrhea	32–73%	68–84%
Flushing	23–65%	63–74%
Pain	10%	34%
Asthma/wheezing	4–8%	3–18%
Pellagra	2%	5%
None	12%	22%
Carcinoid heart disease present	11%	14–41%
Demographics		
Male	46–59%	46–61%
Age		
Mean	57 yr	52–54 yr
Range	25–79 yr	9–91 yr
Tumor location		
Foregut	5–9%	2–33%
Midgut	78–87%	60–87%
Hindgut	1–5%	1–8%
Unknown	2–11%	2–15%

9. The answer is E.
Discussion: *(Chap. 12)* Hirsutism is defined as excessive male-pattern hair growth. It may represent a variation on the norm or be a prelude to a more serious underlying condition. Virilization refers to the state in which androgen levels are elevated enough to cause signs and symptoms of changes in voice, enlargement of genitalia, and increased libido. Virilization is a concerning sign for an ovarian or adrenal cause of excess androgen production. This patient's change in voice and body habitus heightens one's concern about a virilizing process. A thorough medication history is indicated because drugs such as phenytoin, minoxidil, and cyclosporine have been associated with androgen-dependent hair growth. Family history is critical in that some families have a higher incidence of hirsutism than others do. Congenital conditions such as congenital adrenal hyperplasia can show distinct patterns of inheritance. Androgens are secreted by both the ovaries and the adrenal glands. An elevation in plasma total testosterone above 12 nmol/L usually indicates a virilizing tumor. A basal DHEAS level above 18.5 μmol/L suggests an adrenal source. Therefore, checking both levels is a useful initial hormonal screen in evaluating virilization. Although polycystic ovarian syndrome is by far the most common cause of ovarian androgen excess, initial screening with ultrasound is not recommended. Polycystic ovaries may be found in females without any evidence of excess androgen secretion. Likewise, females may have an ovarian source of androgen secretion with only slightly enlarged ovaries on ultrasound. Therefore, ultrasound is an insensitive and nonspecific test.

CARCINOID TUMOR LOCATION, FREQUENCY OF METASTASES, AND ASSOCIATION WITH THE CARCINOID SYNDROME

	LOCATION (% OF TOTAL)	INCIDENCE OF METASTASES	INCIDENCE OF CARCINOID SYNDROME
Foregut			
Esophagus	<0.1	—	—
Stomach	4.6	10	9.5
Duodenum	2.0	—	3.4
Pancreas	0.7	71.9	20
Gallbladder	0.3	17.8	5
Bronchus, lung, trachea	27.9	5.7	13
Midgut			
Jejunum	1.8	} 58.4	9
Ileum	14.9		9
Meckel's diverticulum	0.5	—	13
Appendix	4.8	38.8	<1
Colon	8.6	51	5
Liver	0.4	32.2	—
Ovary	1.0	32	50
Testis	<0.1	—	50
Hindgut			
Rectum	13.6	3.9	—

Source: Location is from the PAN-SEER data (1973–1999), and incidence of metastases from the SEER data (1992–1999), reported by IM Modlin et al: A 5-decade analysis of 13,715 carcinoid tumors. Cancer 97:934, 2003. Incidence of carcinoid syndrome is from 4349 cases studied from 1950–1971, reported by JD Godwin: Carcinoid tumors. An analysis of 2837 cases. Cancer 36:560, 1975.

10. The answer is B.

Discussion: *(Chap. 4)* Subacute thyroiditis, also known as de Quervain's thyroiditis, granulomatous thyroiditis, and viral thyroiditis, is characterized clinically by fever, constitutional symptoms, and a painful enlarged thyroid. The etiology is thought to be a viral infection. The peak incidence is between 30 and 50 years of age, and women are affected more frequently than are men. The symptoms depend on the phase of the illness. During the initial phase of follicular destruction, there is a release of thyroglobulin and thyroid hormones. As a result, there is increased circulating T_4 and T_3, with concomitant suppression of TSH. Symptoms of thyrotoxicosis predominate at this point. Radioiodine uptake is low or undetectable. After several weeks, thyroid hormone is depleted and a phase of hypothyroidism ensues, with low unbound T_4 levels and moderate elevations of TSH. Radioiodine uptake returns to normal. Finally, after 4 to 6 months, thyroid hormone and TSH levels return to normal as the disease subsides. Patient A is consistent with the thyrotoxic phase of subacute thyroiditis except for the increased radioiodine uptake scan. Patient C is more consistent with Graves' disease with suppression of TSH, an elevated uptake scan, and elevated thyroid hormones as a result of stimulating immunoglobulin. Patient D is consistent with a neoplasm. Patient E is consistent with central hypothyroidism.

11. The answer is D.

Discussion: *(Chap. 25)* The epidemiology of fractures follows trends similar to those for loss of bone density. Fractures of the radius increase until age 50 and then plateau by age 60. There are approximately 250,000 wrist fractures each year in the United States. However, there are approximately 300,000 hip fractures annually, with incidence rates doubling every 5 years after age 70. The shift from arm and wrist fractures to hip fractures may be related to the way elderly people fall, with less frequent landing on the hands and more frequent direct hip trauma with increasing age. There are approximately 700,000 vertebral fractures each year in the United States. Most are clinically silent and rarely require hospitalization. They may lead to height loss, kyphosis, and pain secondary to altered biomechanics.

12. and 13. The answers are A and E.

Discussion: *(Chap. 25)* Nonmodifiable risk factors for the development of osteoporosis include a personal history of fracture or a history of fracture in a first-degree relative, female sex, advanced age, and white race. African Americans have approximately one-half the risk of osteoporotic fractures as whites. Diseases that increase the risk of falls or frailty, such as dementia and Parkinson's disease, also increase fracture risk. Cigarette smoking, low body weight, low calcium intake, alcoholism, and lack of physical activity are all associated with increased bone loss and fractures. Multiple drugs are associated with an increased risk of osteoporosis. In addition to those listed, other anticonvulsants, cytotoxic drugs, excessive thyroxine, aluminum, gonadotropin-releasing hormone agonists, and lithium are associated with decreased bone mass and osteoporosis. Histamine antagonists are not associated with osteoporosis.

14. The answer is D.

Discussion: *(Chap. 4)* Sick-euthyroid syndrome, or nonthyroidal illness, can occur in the setting of any acute, severe illness. Abnormalities in the levels of circulating TSH and thyroid hormone are thought to result from the release of cytokines in response to severe stress. Multiple abnormalities may occur. The most common hormone pattern is a decrease in total and unbound T_3 levels as peripheral conversion of T_4 to T_3 is impaired. Teleologically, the fall in T_3, the most active thyroid hormone, is thought to limit catabolism in starved or ill patients. TSH levels may vary, from 0.1 to >20 mU/L, depending on when they are measured during the course of illness. Very sick patients may have a decrease in T_4 levels. This patient has abnormal thyroid function tests as a result of his injuries from the motor vehicle accident. There is no indication for obtaining further imaging in this case. Steroids have no role. The most appropriate management consists of simple observation. Over the course of weeks to months, as the patient recovers, thyroid function will return to normal.

15. The answer is E.

Discussion: *(Chaps. 5 and 7)* Virilization secondary to androgen excess typically has an ovarian or adrenal source in response to the respective tropic hormones, luteinizing hormone (LH) and adrenocorticotropic hormone (ACTH). Optimal pharmacologic treatment depends on the source of excess androgens. In the case of congenital adrenal hyperplasia, an enzymatic defect impedes the ability of the adrenal glands to secrete glucocorticoids efficiently. This results in decreased negative feedback inhibition of ACTH and subsequent adrenal hyperplasia. Therefore, replacement with a glucocorticoid such as prednisone or dexamethasone is the mainstay of treatment for congenital adrenal hyperplasia (CAH). Oral contraceptives suppress the secretion of LH and are the mainstay of treatment for polycystic ovarian syndrome. In patients with a contraindication to oral contraceptive therapy, such as thromboembolic disease or breast cancer, direct antiandrogen therapy may be indicated. Cyproterone acetate directly inhibits the binding of testosterone and dihydrotestosterone to the androgen receptor. Spironolactone has weak antiandrogen properties but is effective at elevated doses. Fludracortisone is a direct mineralocorticoid and has no role in the treatment of androgen excess.

16. The answer is A.

Discussion: *(Chap. 25)* A number of biochemical tests are used to assess the rate of bone remodeling. Bone remodeling is related to the rate of formation and resorption. Remodeling markers do not predict bone loss well enough to be applied clinically. However, measures of bone resorption may help in the prediction of risk of fracture in older patients. In women over 65 years old, even in the presence of normal bone density, a high index of bone resorption should prompt consideration for treatment. Measures of bone resportion fall quickly after the initiation of antiresorptive therapy (bisphosphonates, estrogen, raloxifene, calcitonin) and provide an earlier measure of response than does bone densitometry. Serum alkaline phosphatase is a measure of bone formation, not resorption, as are serum osteocalcin and serum propeptide of type I procollagen.

BIOCHEMICAL MARKERS OF BONE METABOLISM IN CLINICAL USE

Bone formation
- Serum bone-specific alkaline phosphatase
- Serum osteocalcin
- Serum propeptide of type I procollagen

Bone resorption
- Urine and serum cross-linked N-telopeptide
- Urine and serum cross-linked C-telopeptide
- Urine total free deoxypyridinoline
- Urine hydroxyproline
- Serum tartrate-resistant acid phosphatase
- Serum bone sialoprotein
- Urine hydroxylysine glycosides

17. The answer is A.

Discussion: *(Chap. 25)* Osteoporosis is defined as a reduction of bone mass or the presence of a fragility fracture. A more specific definition is a bone density that is 2.5 SD below the mean for young healthy adults of the same race and gender. This is referred to as the *t*-score. Individuals with t-scores below 1 SD are at increased risk of osteoporosis. As many as 8 million to 10 million women and 2 million men in the United States have osteoporosis. Another 15 million to 20 million people are at risk (*t*-score more than 1 SD below the mean). Increasing age, white race, and female sex are the main predictors. Hip fracture is a common occurrence in the elderly. Up to 300,000 hip fractures occur yearly in the United States.

The probability that a 50-year-old white female will have a hip fracture during her lifetime is up to 14%. Infection and thromboembolism are major causes of morbidity and mortality in patients with hip fractures, with between 20 and 50% of these patients having a deep venous thrombosis or pulmonary embolism.

18. The answer is E.
Discussion: *(Chap. 25)* Osteoporosis results from bone loss caused by normal age-related changes in bone remodeling as well as extrinsic and intrinsic factors. Bone remodeling is regulated by several circulating hormones, including estrogens, androgens, vitamin D, and parathyroid hormone. Bone loss decreases calcium intake. The recommended daily intake is 1000 to 1200 mg for adults. Daily calcium intakes below 400 mg are associated with decreases in bone density. Vitamin D causes increased bone absorption in the intestine. Deficiency of vitamin D causes rickets in children and osteomalacia in adults. There is evidence that vitamin D deficiency may be more prevalent than previously was thought. Estrogen regulates the activation of bone remodeling sites and affects the balance between osteoblast and osteoclast activity. Deficiency secondary to ovarian failure promotes rapid bone loss and is responsible for the increased incidence of osteoporosis in women relative to men. Replacement is associated with bone remodeling, but recent studies have indicated a negative effect on cardiovascular health. Many medications result in bone loss. Glucocorticoids, anticonvulsants, and immunosuppressants are thought to contribute significantly to early bone loss. Physical activity is associated with higher bone mass than is inactivity. Fracture risk is lower in rural communities and in countries where physical activity is maintained into old age. Tobacco use is associated with bone loss.

19. The answer is D.
Discussion: *(Chap. 25)* A large body of evidence shows that optimal calcium intake reduces bone loss and suppresses bone turnover. The preferred source of calcium is dairy products and other foods, but many patients require supplementation. Supplementation should be in doses of less than 600 mg at a time because absorption decreases at higher doses. The addition of vitamin D is beneficial, as has been shown in multiple trials. Exercise in younger individuals promotes the achievement of maximal bone mass. Although in older individuals exercise does not promote a large increase in bone mass, there probably is an improvement in neuromuscular function that aids in the prevention of falls and subsequent fractures. Although estrogen is effective in promoting bone mass and formation, multiple trials have suggested an adverse effect on cardiovascular morbidity and mortality, and there is considerable debate about the indications for estrogen replacement therapy. Selective estrogen receptor modulators (SERMs) have been shown to be useful in the prevention and treatment of osteoporosis. Raloxifene has beneficial effects on bone density and help prevent bone loss. Raloxifene reduces the risk of vertebral fractures in certain populations and may not have the adverse cardiovascular effects of estrogen. It increases the occurrence of hot flashes and may not be optimal in women with significant menopausal symptoms. Tamoxifen also has beneficial effects on bone density. However, its use is restricted to patients with breast cancer. It has stimulating effects on the uterus and increases the risk of endometrial cancer. It has no role in the routine treatment of osteoporosis. Bisphosphonates are emerging as the first-line therapy for osteoporosis. They act to stabilize osteoclast activity and reduce bone resorption. Weekly alendronate has been shown to be equivalent to daily alendronate. Bisphosphonates must be given with a full glass of water and on an empty stomach to improve absorption. Some patients may experience esophageal irritation from reflux esophagitis. Other formulations of bisphosphonates are also effective (risidronate, zolendronate, etc.).

20. The answer is A.
Discussion: *(Chap. 21)* This patient's clinical scenario is most consistent with MEN 1, or the "3 Ps": parathyroid, pituitary, and pancreas. MEN 1 is an autosomal dominant genetic syndrome characterized by neoplasia of the parathyroid, pituitary, and pancreatic islet cells. Hyperparathyroidism is the most common manifestation of MEN 1. The neoplastic changes affect multiple parathyroid glands, making surgical care difficult. Pancreatic islet cell neoplasia is the second most common manifestation of MEN 1. Increased pancreatic islet cell hormones include pancreatic polypeptide, gastrin, insulin, vasoactive intestinal peptide, glucagons, and somatostatin. Pancreatic tumors may be multicentric, and up to 30% are malignant, with the liver being the first site of metastases. The symptoms depend on the type of hormone secreted. Elevations of gastrin result in the Zollinger-Ellison syndrome (ZES). Gastrin levels are elevated, resulting in an ulcer diathesis. Conservative therapy is often unsuccessful. Insulinoma results in documented hypoglycemia with elevated insulin and C-peptide levels. Glucagonoma results in hyperglycemia, skin rash, anorexia, glossitis, and diarrhea. Elevations in vasoactive intestinal peptide result in profuse watery diarrhea. Pituitary tumors occur in up to half of patients with MEN 1. Prolactinomas are the most common. The multicentricity of the tumors makes resection difficult. Growth hormone-secreting tumors are the next most common, with ACTH- and corticotropin-releasing hormone (CRH)-secreting tumors being more rare. Carcinoid tumors may also occur in the thymus, lung, stomach, and duodenum.

21. The answer is B.
Discussion: *(Chap. 25)* The Women's Health Initiative (WHI) demonstrated that estrogen-progestin therapy can reduce the risk of hip fractures by 34%. Other clinical trials have shown a decrease in all osteoporotic fractures, including vertebral compression fractures. The beneficial effect of estrogen appears to be maximal in those who start therapy early and continue taking the medication. The benefit declines after discontinuation, and there is no net benefit by 10 years after discontinuation. These effects are present for oral and transdermal formulations. However, the WHI also demonstrated that estrogens are associated with a 30% increase in myocardial infarction, a 40% increase in stroke, a 100% increase in venous thromboembolism, and a 25% increase in breast cancer. In the WHI study there was no overall effect of estrogen-progestin therapy on mortality, probably because of the balance between the detrimental cardiovascular effects and the beneficial effects (in addition to fractures, there was a beneficial effect on the development of colon cancer).

22. The answer is C.
Discussion: *(Chap. 16)* Obesity is a state of excess adipose tissue mass. Although body weight is often viewed as equivalent to adipose tissue mass, this is not always the case. Therefore, more objective measurements linked to morbidity and mortality have been formulated to provide a more accurate and practical guideline for physicians and patients. Body mass index is the most commonly used index to gauge obesity. It is equal to weight/height^2. Other methods, such as skin-fold measurements, underwater weighing, and electrical impedance, are used to varying degrees; however, because of its usefulness, ease of calculation, and correlation with outcome, BMI is the most widely used method to measure obesity. A BMI above 25 is associated with a substantially increased risk of all-cause, metabolic, cancer, and cardiovascular mortality. A BMI more than 30 is the formal definition of obesity. At this threshold, the risk of a poor outcome dramatically rises. A BMI between 25 and 30 is termed *overweight* by some authorities, although there is a movement to change the definition of obesity to a BMI over 25.

23. The answer is E.
Discussion: *(Chap. 16)* Obesity leads to a major increase in morbidity and mortality. Individuals who are more than 150% of their ideal body weight have as much as a 12-fold increase in mortality. Insulin resistance leading to diabetes mellitus is one of the most prominent features of obesity. The vast majority of patients with type 2 diabetes are obese. Weight loss to a moderate degree may be associated with improvements in insulin sensitivity. Obesity is an independent risk factor for cardiovascular disease. Obesity is associated with hypertension. The impact of obesity on cardiovascular mortality may be seen in persons with BMIs above 25. Obesity is associated with an increased incidence of cholesterol stones. Periodic fasting may increase the supersaturation of bile by decreasing the phospholipid component. Multiple studies have indicated increased mortality from cancer in obese individuals. Some of this increase may result from the increased conversion of androstenedione to estrone in adipose tissue. Obesity decreases chest wall compliance. Restrictive lung defects may occur in these individuals. Sleep apnea and obesity hypoventilation syndrome may occur. Although obesity may be associated with obstructive sleep apnea, it is not typically associated with other forms of chronic obstructive lung disease (COPD).

24. The answer is C.
Discussion: *(Chap. 17)* Diabetes mellitus is classified on the basis of the pathogenic process that leads to hyperglycemia. Type 1 DM results from destruction of the pancreas and impaired insulin secretion, typically through autoimmune processes. This usually occurs early in life and may be associated with certain autoantibodies. Type 2 DM is a heterogeneous group of disorders characterized by variable degrees of insulin resistance, impaired insulin secretion, and increased glucose production. Other etiologies for DM include specific genetic defects in insulin secretion or action, metabolic abnormalities, mitochondrial diseases, and other rare conditions that affect glucose tolerance. DM is increasing worldwide. Most of this increase is due to a rise in the prevalence of type 2 DM. There is significant geographic diversity in the prevalence of cases, with regions such as Scandinavia having the highest incidence of type 1 DM and the Pacific islands having the highest incidence of type 2 DM. There is clearly an interplay between genetic and environmental factors. The concordance of type 2 DM in identical twins ranges from 70 to 90%. The concordance of type 1 DM in identical twins is 30 to 70%. The reasons are unclear. In the United States, certain ethnic groups have a high prevalence of DM. African Americans and Hispanic Americans have high rates, but Native Americans have the highest, with a prevalence of nearly 15%. Similarly, although only a small percentage of females develop gestational diabetes during pregnancy, those females are at a much higher risk of developing overt DM.

25. The answer is C.
Discussion: *(Chap. 24)* The four parathyroid glands are located posterior to the thyroid gland. Parathyroid hormone is the primary regulator of calcium. PTH acts directly on bone and the kidney and indirectly, through the action of vitamin D, on the GI tract. PTH induces calcium absorption from the kidney and bone. It stimulates hydroxylation of 25-hydroxyvitamin D, resulting in the more active form. Vitamin D stimulates calcium resorption from the GI tract. Calcium and vitamin D are part of a feedback loop that inhibits PTH release and synthesis. PTH prevents resorption of phosphate from the kidney.

26. The answer is D.
Discussion: *(Chap. 24)* Primary hyperparathyroidism and malignancy account for over 90% of cases of hypercalcemia. In asymptomatic patients, primary hyperparathyroidism is the most common cause. In patients admitted to the hospital with symptomatic hypercalcemia, malignancy is the most common cause. Calcium is regulated in bone, the gastrointestinal tract, and the kidney. Other causes of increased bone turnover include Paget's disease, immobilization, hyperthyroidism, hypervitaminosis A, and adrenal insufficiency. Causes of increased GI absorption include vitamin D intoxication and milk-alkali syndrome. Hypercalcemia from thiazide diuretics and familial hypocalciuric hypercalcemia result from disordered regulation of calcium in the kidney.

27. The answer is A.
Discussion: *(Chap. 24)* Hypercalcemia manifests in a variety of ways. "Stones, bones, groans, and psychiatric overtones" often is used on rounds as a way to remember the clinical symptoms and signs. Neurologic changes may range from depression to confusion and frank coma. These patients often are constipated and may have nausea, vomiting, and abdominal pain. Increased calcium may affect the genitourinary tract with nephrolithiasis, renal tubular acidosis, and polyuria. A shortened QT interval may result in cardiac arrhythmias.

28. The answer is D.
Discussion: *(Chap. 24)* FHH is inherited as an autosomal dominant trait. It results from a defect in serum calcium sensing by the parathyroid gland and renal tubule, causing inappropriate secretion of PTH and excessive renal reabsorption of calcium. The calcium-sensing receptor is sensitive to extracellular calcium concentration, suppressing PTH secretion and therefore resulting in negative-feedback regulation. Many different mutations in the calcium-sensing receptor have been described in patients with FHH. These mutations lower the ability of the sensor to bind calcium, resulting in excessive secretion of PTH and subsequent hypercalcemia. Urinary excretion of calcium is very low, with reabsorption more than 99%. The hypercalcemia is often detected in the first decade of life. This contrasts with primary hyperparathyroidism, which rarely occurs before age 10. Few clinical signs or symptoms are present in patients with FHH. These patients have excellent outcomes, and surgery or medical therapy is rarely necessary. Jansen's disease refers to mutations in the PTH receptor.

29. The answer is E.
Discussion: *(Chap. 24)* Causes of hypocalcemia may be classified on the basis of the action of parathyroid hormone (PTH). PTH is the primary regulator of calcium; therefore, for hypocalcemia to occur, the action of PTH must be ineffective. PTH may be absent in hereditary forms of hypoparathyroidism, acquired hypoparathyroidism, and hypomagnesemia. Magnesium affects the secretion of PTH, and correction of hypomagnesemia results in the return of plasma PTH levels to normal. Hereditary hypoparathyroidism may occur as an isolated entity or result from congenital malformations such as di-George syndrome. The action of PTH may be ineffective in cases of chronic renal failure, lack of dietary vitamin D, and receptor defects that cause pseudohypoparathyroidism. In cases of massive cell injury such as rhabdomyolysis and tumor lysis syndrome, the action of PTH may be overwhelmed.

30. The answer is A.
Discussion: *(Chap. 6)* Pheochromocytomas are derived from the adrenal medulla or the chromaffin cells in or about sympathetic ganglia. They produce, store, and secrete catecholamines. Therefore, the symptoms and signs result from the excessive release of catecholamines. The symptoms include hypertension, headache, anxiety, tachycardia, and an increased metabolic rate. Symptoms may be episodic. In adults, the majority of pheochromocytomas (more than 80%) are unilateral, solitary, and benign. There is an inexplicable predominance of right-sided lesions. Occurrence is more common in women and younger adults. Rarely, extraadrenal pheochromocytomas occur, usually in the abdomen in association with celiac, superior mesenteric, and inferior mesenteric ganglia. Pheochromocytomas produce both norepinephrine and epinephirine. Diagnosis is made by measuring urinary catecholamine metabolites such as vanillylmandelic acid, metanephrines, and other unconjugated catecholamines. Up to one-fourth of cases are associated with familial syndromes such as multiple endocrine neoplasia, von Hippel–Lindau syndrome, and neurofibromatosis. Features that suggest familial disease include bilaterality, multicentricity, and age of onset over 30 years. The treatment is primarily surgical. Surgery or mechanical manipulation can result in a hypertensive crisis. α-Adrenergic blockade is essential before successful surgical treatment. Phenoxybenzamine is the most useful long-lasting, noncompetitive α-receptor blocker. Phenoxybenzamine should be administered up to 2 weeks before surgery. Beta blockers should be administered only after alpha blockade has been achieved because unopposed alpha stimulation and subsequent hypertensive emergency may occur. Malignant pheochromocytoma frequently recurs in the retroperitoneum and commonly metastasizes to the lung and bone. It is typically resistant to radiotherapy. Combination chemotherapy may be beneficial.

31. The answer is E.
Discussion: *(Chap. 18)* Abetalipoproteinemia results from a mutation in the gene that encodes microsomal transfer protein (MTP). MTP is essential for the packaging of hepatic triglycerides with other major components of very low density lipoproteins (VLDLs). This autosomal

recessive disease results in extremely low cholesterol and triglyceride levels and an absence of chylomicrons, VLDL, and low-density lipoproteins (LDLs). The clinical manifestations stem from defects in the absorption and transport of fat-soluble vitamins. Lack of vitamin E results in spinocerebellar degeneration, which is clinically manifested by decreased vibratory and proprioceptive sense, dysmetria, ataxia, and the development of a spastic gait. Other clinical features include diarrhea, fat malabsorption, failure to thrive, pigmented retinopathy, and acanthocytosis. Symptoms and signs develop in childhood. Treatment consists of low-fat, high-calorie diets that are enriched with large supplemental doses of fat-soluble vitamins.

32. The answer is A.
Discussion: *(Chap. 18)* Lipoprotein lipase (LPL) and its cofactor apo CII are required for the hydrolysis of triglycerides in chylomicrons and very low density lipoproteins (VLDLs). A genetic deficiency of either protein impairs lypolysis and results in an elevation in plasma chylomicrons. VLDL is also elevated. The triglyceride-rich proteins persist for days in the circulation, causing fasting levels higher than 1000 mg/dL. The inheritance pattern is autosomal recessive. Heterozygotes have normal or mildly elevated plasma triglyceride levels. Clinically, these patients may have repeated episodes of pancreatitis secondary to hypertriglyceridemia. Eruptive xanthomas may appear on the back, the buttocks, and the extensor surfaces of the arms and legs. Hepatosplenomegaly may result from the uptake of circulating chylomicrons by the reticuloendothelial cells. The diagnosis is made by assaying triglyceride lipolytic activity in plasma. Dietary fat restriction is the treatment of choice.

33. The answer is E.
Discussion: *(Chap. 18)* Statins have emerged over the last decade as one of the most clinically important classes of medications. Numerous studies have indicated important benefits in both primary and secondary prevention of cardiovascular disease. Statins act by inhibiting HMG-CoA reductase, the rate-limiting step in cholesterol biosynthesis. Statins are generally well tolerated, with an excellent safety profile over the years. However, attention must be paid to the side effects. Dyspepsia, headache, fatigue, and myalgias may occur and are generally well tolerated. Myopathy and rhabdomyolysis are rare but serious side effects. The risk of myopathy is increased in the presence of renal insufficiency and with concomitant use of certain medications, including some antibiotics, antifungal agents, some immunosuppressive drugs, and fibric acid derivatives. Hepatitis is another side effect. Liver transaminases should be checked before therapy is started and 4 to 8 weeks afterward. Elevations more than three times the normal range may mandate stopping therapy.

34. The answer is B.
Discussion: *(Chap. 23)* Hypophosphatemia results from one of three mechanisms: inadequate intestinal phosphate absorption, excessive renal phosphate excretion, and rapid redistribution of phosphate from the extracellular space into bone or soft tissue. Inadequate intestinal absorption is rare. Malnutrition from fasting or starvation may result in depletion of phosphate, causing hypophosphatemia during refeeding. In hospitalized patients, redistribution is the main cause. Insulin drives phosphate into cells. Sepsis may cause destruction of cells and metabolic acidosis, resulting in a net shift of phosphate from the extracellular space into cells. Renal failure is associated with hyperphosphatemia, not hypophosphatemia.

35. The answer is A.
Discussion: *(Chap. 10)* This patient has dysfunctional uterine bleeding. The most likely cause in a woman with a prior history of normal menses is anovulatory cycles. This is not due to a structural abnormality in the uterus or cervix but instead to an interruption in the normal sequence of the follicular and luteal phases of the menstrual cycle. Primary dysfunctional uterine bleeding may result from one of three disorders: estrogen withdrawal bleeding, estrogen breakthrough bleeding, and progesterone breakthrough bleeding. Estrogen withdrawal bleeding occurs when estrogen is given to a castrate or postmenopausal female and then withdrawn. Estrogen breakthrough bleeding occurs when there is continuous estrogen stimulation of the endometrium without interruption by cyclic progesterone secretion and withdrawal. This is the most common presentation and usually results from anovulatory cycles. This patient's running may be the etiology. Polycystic ovarian syndrome is another common cause in young females. Other causes include estrogen-secreting tumors and chronic estrogen replacement therapy. Progesterone withdrawal bleeding may occur in patients taking chronic low-dose oral contraceptives. In this case, administration of progesterone or oral contraceptives may serve to regulate the cycle and stimulate proper ovulation and menses. Withdrawal of progesterone will cause menstrual bleeding and confirm that anovulation with estrogen present is the cause. Evaluation for a structural defect, pituitary tumor, or genetic abnormality is not warranted in the initial workup.

36. and 37. The answers are E and E.
Discussion: *(Chap. 20)* In patients with a nonmetastatic carcinoid, surgery is the only potentially curative therapy. The extent of surgical resection depends on the size of the primary tumor because the risk of metastasis is related to the size of the tumor. Symptomatic treatment is aimed at decreasing the amount and effect of circulating substances. Drugs that inhibit the serotonin 5-HT_1 and 5-HT_2 receptors (methysergide, cyproheptadine, ketanserin) may control diarrhea but not flushing. 5-HT_3 receptor antagonists (odansetron, tropisetron, alosetron) control

nausea and diarrhea in up to 100% of these patients and may alleviate flushing. A combination of histamine H_1 and H_2 receptor antagonists may control flushing, particularly in patients with foregut carcinoid tumors. Somatostatin analogues (octreotide, lanreotide) are the most effective and widely used agents to control the symptoms of carcinoid syndrome, decreasing urinary 5-HIAA excretion and symptoms in 70 to 80% of patients. Interferon α, alone or combined with hepatic artery embolization, controls flushing and diarrhea in 40 to 85% of these patients. Phenoxybenzamine is an α_1-adrenergic receptor blocker that is used in the treatment of pheochromocytoma.

Carcinoid crisis is a life-threatening complication of carcinoid syndrome. It is most common in patients with intense symptoms from foregut tumors or markedly high levels of urinary 5-HIAA. The crisis may be provoked by surgery, stress, anesthesia, chemotherapy, or physical trauma to the tumor (biopsy or, in this case, physical compression of liver lesions). These patients develop severe typical symptoms plus systemic symptoms such as hypotension and hypertension with tachycardia. Synthetic analogues of somatostatin (octreotide, lanreotide) are the treatment of choice for carcinoid crisis. They are also effective in preventing crises when administered before a known inciting event. Octreotide 150 to 250 μg subcutaneously every 6 to 8 h should be started 24 to 48 h before a procedure that is likely to precipitate a carcinoid crisis.

38. The answer is D.
Discussion: *(Chap. 10)* Premature ovarian failure is used to describe women who cease menstruating before age 40. The ovaries in those women contain few or no follicles as a result of accelerated atresia. This may also result from autoimmune processes either alone or as part of a polyglandular failure. Low output of estrogens from the ovary results in increased FSH and LH levels from the pituitary. The elevated FSH and LH are not consistent with a pituitary process. Asherman's syndrome results from destruction and fibrosis of the endometrium and does not cause a hormone imbalance. A genetic cause such as Turner syndrome typically has a characteristic body habitus and presents early in life, typically with primary amenorrhea. Patients with polycystic ovarian syndrome typically have menstrual abnormalities from childhood, have elevated estrogen levels, and have an increased ratio of LH to FSH because of positive feedback on LH secretion and negative feedback on FSH secretion.

39. The answer is D.
Discussion: *(Chap. 17)* Diabetic ketoacidosis is an acute complication of diabetes mellitus. It results from a relative or absolute deficiency of insulin combined with a counterregulatory hormone excess. In particular, a decrease in the ratio of insulin to glucagon promotes gluconeogenesis, glycogenolysis, and the formation of ketone bodies in the liver. Ketosis results from an increase in the release of free fatty acids from adipocytes, with a resultant shift toward ketone body synthesis in the liver. This is mediated by the relationship between insulin and the enzyme carnitine palmitoyltransferase I. At physiologic pH, ketone bodies exist as ketoacids, which are neutralized by bicarbonate. As bicarbonate stores are depleted, acidosis develops. Clinically, these patients have nausea, vomiting, and abdominal pain. They are dehydrated and may be hypotensive. Lethargy and severe central nervous system depression may occur. The treatment centers on replacement of the body's insulin, which will result in cessation of the formation of ketoacids and improvement of the acidotic state. Assessment of the level of acidosis may be done with an arterial blood gas. These patients have an anion gap acidosis and often a concomitant metabolic alkalosis resulting from volume depletion. Volume resuscitation with intravenous fluids is critical. Many electrolyte abnormalities may occur. Patients are total body sodium-, potassium-, and magnesium-depleted. As a result of the acidosis, intracellular potassium may shift out of cells and cause a normal or even elevated potassium level. However, with improvement in the acidosis, the serum potassium rapidly falls. Therefore, potassium repletion is critical despite the presence of a "normal" level. Because of the osmolar effects of glucose, fluid is drawn into the intravascular space. This results in a drop in the measured serum sodium. There is a drop of 1.6 meq/L in serum sodium for each rise of 100 mg/dL in serum glucose. In this case, the serum sodium will improve with hydration alone. The use of 3% saline is not indicated because the patient has no neurologic deficits, and the expectation is for rapid resolution with intravenous fluids alone.

40. The answer is A.
Discussion: *(Chap. 17)* The DCCT found definitive proof that reduction in chronic hyperglycemia can prevent many of the early complications of type 1 DM. This multicenter randomized trial enrolled over 1400 patients with type 1 DM to either intensive or conventional diabetes management and prospectively evaluated the development of retinopathy, nephropathy, and neuropathy. The intensive group received multiple administrations of insulin daily along with education and psychological counseling. The intensive group achieved a mean hemoglobin A_{1C} of 7.3% versus 9.1% in the conventional group. Improvement in glycemic control resulted in a 47% reduction in retinopathy, a 54% reduction in nephropathy, and a 60% reduction in neuropathy. There was a nonsignificant trend toward improvement in macrovascular complications. The results of the DCCT showed that individuals in the intensive group would attain up to 7 more years of intact vision and up to 5 more years free from lower limb amputation. Later, the United Kingdom Prospective Diabetes Study (UKPDS) studied over 5000 individuals with type 2 DM. Individuals receiving intensive glycemic control had a reduction in microvascular events but no significant change in macrovascular complications. These

two trials were pivotal in showing a benefit of glycemic control in reducing microvascular complications in patients with type 1 and type 2 DM, respectively. Another result from the UKPDS was that strict blood pressure control resulted in an improvement in macrovascular complications.

41. The answer is D.
Discussion: *(Chap. 25)* The selective estrogen receptor modulators (SERMs) tamoxifen and raloxifene act in a fashion similar to that of estrogen in decreasing bone turnover and bone loss in postmenopausal women. These agents have been shown to decrease the risk of invasive breast cancer. Raloxifene, which is approved for the prevention of osteoporosis, reduces the risk of vertebral fractures by 30 to 50%. There are no data confirming a similar effect on nonvertebral fractures. Optimal calcium intake reduces bone loss and suppresses bone turnover. Vitamin D plus calcium supplements have been shown to reduce the risk of hip fractures by 20 to 30%. The bisphosphonates alendronate and risedronate are structurally related to pyrophosphate and are incorporated into bone matrix. They reduce the number of osteoclasts and impair the function of those already present. Both have been shown to reduce the risk of vertebral and hip fractures by 40 to 50%. One trial found that risedronate reduced hip fractures in osteoporotic women in their seventies but not in older women without osteoporosis. Risedronate may be administered weekly. The newer bisphosphonates zoledronate and ibandronate may be dosed yearly or monthly. A daily injection of exogenous parathyroid hormone analogue superimposed on estrogen therapy produced increases in bone mass and decreased vertebral and nonvertebral fractures by 45 to 65%.

42. The answer is D.
Discussion: *(Chap. 25)* Glucocorticoid-induced osteoporosis and subsequent fractures are among the most devastating complications of long-term steroid therapy. Glucocorticoids increase bone loss through inhibition of osteoblast function, inhibition of osteoblast apoptosis, stimulation of bone resorption, impairment of intestinal absorption of calcium, increases in urinary excretion of calcium, suppression of normal estrogen and androgen secretion, and induction of steroid myopathy that decreases physical activity. It is important that patients receiving glucocorticoids have adequate calcium and vitamin D intake. Patients receiving long-term (more than 6 months) glucocorticoids should have measurements of bone density. Only bisphosphonates have reduced the risk of fractures in patients receiving glucocorticoids. Calcitonin has some beneficial effect on spine density. Thiazide diuretics reduce urinary calcium excretion but do not have a proven role in reducing fractures. Estrogen is not advised for use in men simply to reduce bone loss.

43. The answer is D.
Discussion: *(Chap. 8)* Measurement of luteinizing hormone (LH) or follicle stimulating hormone (FSH) will distinguish primary from secondary hypogonadism in men with reduced serum testosterone levels. Elevations in LH and FSH suggest primary gonadal dysfunction, whereas normal or reduced LH and FSH suggest a central hypothalamic pituitary defect. Patients with chronic illness such as HIV, end-stage renal disease, COPD, and cancer and patients receiving chronic glucocorticoids have a high frequency of hypogonadism that is associated with muscle wasting. There are some reports of reversal of hypogonadism in patients with end-stage renal disease on hemodialysis after a renal transplant.

44. The answer is C.
Discussion: *(Chap. 8)* Many drugs may interfere with testicular function through a variety of mechanisms. Cyclophosphamide damages the seminiferous tubules in a dose- and time-dependent fashion and causes azospermia within a few weeks of initiation. This effect is reversible in approximately half these patients. Ketoconazole inhibits testosterone synthesis. Spironolactone causes a blockade of androgen action. Glucocorticoids lead to hypogonadism predominantly through inhibition of hypothalamic-pituitary function. Sexual dysfunction has been described as a side effect of therapy with beta blockers. However, there is no evidence of an effect on testicular function. Most reports of sexual dysfunction were in patients receiving older beta blockers such as propranolol and timolol.

45. The answer is C.
Discussion: *(Chap. 11)* Menopause is characterized by several symptoms, including hot flashes, vaginal dryness, depression, and cessation of menstrual cycles for 12 months. Laboratory evaluation is imperfect; however, in general, a high FSH level coupled with a low estradiol level predicts ovarian failure and menopause. LH also rises in menopause, but it can be elevated during the preovulatory gonadotropin surge during a normal menstrual cycle. Symptoms of menopause can be debilitating for some women. Furthermore, hormone replacement therapy (HRT), which reduces symptoms, including hot flashes and vaginal dryness, has been said to offer many benefits to postmenopausal women other than symptom relief. Data from randomized clinical trials support the statement that HRT reduces symptoms of menopause, including vasomotor symptoms and genitourinary symptoms. The Women's Health Initiative study demonstrated significantly fewer hip and total fractures among patients randomly assigned to continuous combination therapy versus placebo. Similar randomized controlled trials have shown decreased urinary tract infections in HRT-treated women versus those receiving placebo. Decreased cardiovascular mortality was touted as a benefit of HRT for many years. However, recent data derived from the HERS trial, in

which women were randomized to estrogen-progestin therapy or placebo and followed prospectively for 4 years, showed a 50% increase in the risk of coronary events in the first year in the treatment arm of the cohort. Other trials in both primary and secondary prevention of cardiovascular disease suggest that HRT may cause an increased risk of cardiovascular events and certainly is not better than placebo. Thus, HRT can no longer be recommended to decrease the incidence or progression of cardiovascular disease.

46. The answer is B.

Discussion: *(Chap. 20)* The Zollinger-Ellison syndrome (ZES) is caused by a neuroendocrine tumor that secretes gastric Chronic hypergastrinemia causes acid hypersecretion, growth of gastric mucosa, an increased number of parietal cells, and proliferation of gastric enterochromaffin-like (ECL) cells. The acid hypersecretion usually causes severe peptic ulcer disease that is often refractory to treatment. At endoscopy, the ulcers are usually duodenal but may be multiple and in unusual locations. Prominent gastric folds are also a typical feature of gastrinoma. Diarrhea is common in patients with gastrinoma, and the combination of duodenal ulcer and diarrhea should raise the suspicion of this diagnosis. Approximately 20 to 25% of patients with gastrinoma have the multiple endocrine neoplasia syndrome type 1 (MEN 1). *Helicobacter pylori* is present in less than 50% of patients with peptic ulcer disease caused by gastrinoma in contrast to its presence in more than 90% of patients with typical peptic ulcer disease. The diagnosis of ZES requires demonstration of fasting hypergastrinemia and increased basal acid output. The differential diagnosis includes *H. pylori* infection, antral G cell hyperplasia, gastric outlet obstruction, and renal failure. The secretin provocative test can confirm the diagnosis of gastrinoma. Normally, an intravenous infusion of secretin causes a decrease in serum gastrin concentration; however, gastrinoma cells respond paradoxically with an increase in serum gastrin. Serum chromogranin A may be elevated in any GI neuroendocrine tumor and is not specific for gastrinoma. Antigliadin antibodies are present in gluten-sensitive enteropathy. The urease test on gastric biopsies is used to detect the presence of *H. pylori*. A positive PAS stain on duodenal biopsy is diagnostic of Whipple disease.

47. The answer is B.

Discussion: *(Chap. 20)* The differential diagnosis of a patient with symptomatic hypoglycemia during fasting includes insulinoma and surreptitious insulin (or oral hypoglycemic agents) use. Insulinomas occur typically in patients 40 to 50 years old and present with neuropsychiatric symptoms consistent with hypoglycemia. Coma may occur in severe cases. Symptoms caused by the appropriate catecholamine response are also usually present. The catecholamine response is responsible for the ability of the symptoms to resolve without therapy. Insulinomas arise in the pancreas and are usually small, solitary, and not malignant (85 to 95%). They may be associated with MEN 1. Insulin is synthesized as proinsulin with α and β chains connected by C peptide. In insulinomas, during episodes of hypoglycemia (usually provoked by a monitored fast), serum insulin and C-peptide levels are elevated. Exogenous insulin does not include the C-peptide fraction. Surreptitious insulin use is characterized by hypoglycemia, elevated serum insulin, and low C peptide. It most commonly occurs as a component of psychiatric illness in health care workers who have access to insulin or oral hypoglycemic agents.

48. The answer is C.

Discussion: *(Chap. 20)* This patient presents with the classic findings of a VIPoma, including large-volume watery diarrhea, hypokalemia, dehydration, and hypochlorhydria (WDHA, or Verner-Morrison, syndrome). Abdominal pain is unusual. The presence of a secretory diarrhea is confirmed by a stool osmolal gap [2(stool Na + stool K) − (stool osmolality)]< 35 and persistence during fasting. In osmotic or laxative-induced diarrhea, the stool osmolal gap is over 100. In adults, over 80% of VIPomas are solitary pancreatic masses that usually are larger than 3 cm at diagnosis. Metastases to the liver are common and preclude curative surgical resection. The differential diagnosis includes gastrinoma, laxative abuse, carcinoid syndrome, and systemic mastocytosis. Diagnosis requires the demonstration of large-volume secretory diarrhea (over 700 mL/d) and elevated serum VIP. CT scan of the abdomen will often demonstrate the pancreatic mass and liver metastases.

CONTRAINDICATIONS FOR ANDROGEN REPLACEMENT

- The presence or history of prostate cancer
- Baseline PSA ≥ 4 ng/mL or a palpable abnormality of the prostate without urologic evaluation to rule out prostate cancer
- Severe symptoms of lower urinary tract obstruction as indicated by IPSS or AUA symptom score of ≥22
- Baseline hematocrit >52%
- Severe sleep apnea
- Class IV congestive heart failure

Note: PSA, prostate-specific antigen; IPSS, International Prostate Symptom Score; AUA, American Urological Association.

49. The answer is B.

Discussion: *(Chap. 8)* Testosterone replacement therapy is indicated in men with testosterone levels below 250 ng/dL. This treatment can improve libido, increase bone density, increase energy and well-being, and increase lean muscle mass. These effects have been found only in men with documented androgen deficiency. The aim of therapy is to restore testosterone levels to the midnormal range. Oral agents do not provide adequate sustained levels for chronic replacement. Transdermal patches, gel formulations, and injectable formulations provide sustained adequate levels. Testosterone replacement is contraindicated in patients with prostate carcinoma because the androgens may promote tumor growth. Other adverse effects and potential contraindications (see table) include worsening of prostatic hypertrophy, increased hematocrit (3 to 5%), and worsening of sleep apnea symptoms.

50. and 51. The answers are C and B.

Discussion: *(Chap. 17)* Screening for diabetes mellitus with fasting plasma glucose measurement is indicated in all adults over 45 years old every 3 years and earlier in individuals with additional risk factors. Once the results are obtained, they can interpreted in light of the revised diagnostic criteria issued by the National Diabetes Data Group and the World Health Organization. Currently, normal fasting plasma glucose is less than 110 mg/dL. Impaired fasting glucose is defined by values greater than 110 mg/dL but less than 126 mg/dL. Diabetes mellitus is diagnosed when fasting plasma glucose is 126 mg/dL or higher. In addition, any individual with symptoms of hyperglycemia and a random glucose >200 mg/dL can be diagnosed as having diabetes mellitus. Hemoglobin A_{1C}, though a useful marker of glycemic control in individuals who have a diagnosis of diabetes, is not used in screening or diagnosing diabetes mellitus. This patient meets the criteria for impaired fasting glucose. The diagnosis of impaired fasting glucose is important to make, as it is associated with an increased risk of cardiovascular disease. Furthermore, 40% of individuals with impaired fasting glucose levels will develop frank diabetes in the next decade; thus, close observation is indicated. It is important to note that screening for diabetes mellitus is aimed at identifying persons with type 2 disease. Patients with type 1 diabetes mellitus have a relatively short time delay between pancreatic pathology and the development of symptoms and thus have early presentations. Screening is not indicated for this population. However, many patients with type 2 diabetes mellitus have a long period of asymptomatic hyperglycemia. It is preferable to identify these patients earlier to prevent microvascular complications in the future.

52. The answer is C.

Discussion: *(Chap. 21)* A thyroid nodule containing malignant C cells that stain positive for calcitonin is diagnostic of medullary thyroid carcinoma (MTC). These tumors typically arise in the upper regions of the thyroid where most C cells are located and metastasize early to regional lymph nodes in the neck. Most (80%) MTCs occur sporadically, typically in patients 40 to 50 years old. Occurrence in a young patient makes MEN 2A or MEN 2B likely. MEN 2A is an autosomal dominant syndrome characterized by MTC, hyperparathyroidism, and pheochromocytoma (see table). Pheochromocytoma occurs in approximately 50% of patients with MEN 2A, and half of those pheochromocytomas are bilateral. Hyperparathyroidism occurs in 15 to 20% of these patients and clinically is indistinguishable from primary hyperparathyroidism. Familial MTC is a subvariant of MEN 2A without pheochromocytoma. MEN 2B is also autosomal dominant and is characterized by MTC, pheochromocytoma, mucosal neuromas, intestinal ganglioneuromatosis, and marfanoid features. MEN 2B develops at a younger age and is more aggressive than MEN 2A. Death from MTC can be prevented with early thyroidectomy, and so early diagnosis and screening of family members is indicated. MEN 2 is associated with mutations in the *RET* protooncogene. Screening for pheochromocytoma in asymptomatic patients with known MEN 2 is also indicated because of the risk of morbidity during surgery. Children with identified *RET* mutations characteristic for MEN 2B should be considered for early thyroidectomy. In patients with extensive metastatic disease, radiation or chemotherapy may provide palliative, not curative, relief.

53. The answer is D.

Discussion: *(Chap. 17)* The patient is admitted with diabetic ketoacidosis as manifest by an anion gap acidosis that features positive serum ketones and hyperglycemia. Insulin is administered to allow cells to take up glucose and, perhaps more important, interrupt the process of fatty acid breakdown in the liver that results in ketogenesis. In addition, hyperglycemia results in an osmotic diuresis, and patients with this disorder are generally profoundly dehydrated and require intravenous hydration. Concomitant electrolyte disorders are common. Appropriately, this patient is given both intravenous insulin and normal saline. Decisions regarding further management of diabetic ketoacidosis are guided by blood chemistries. The insulin infusion, which disrupts ketogenesis, must not be discontinued until the anion gap has been closed. In this case, the anion gap persists at the time of the second blood chemistries. As the patient's glucose is approaching normal levels and the anion gap is still open, requiring insulin infusion, the most appropriate next step is to stop normal saline infusion and begin infusion of 5% dextrose normal saline. In this way, hypoglycemia will be prevented and the insulin drip can continue. Once the diagnosis of ketoacidosis is made and ketones are initially demonstrated in the blood, it is not necessary to check repeat measurements. In fact, the primary ketone, β-hydroxybutyrate, is synthesized at three times the rate of the synthesis of acetoacetate, which is preferentially detected by commonly available assays. During its degradation process, β-hydroxybutyrate is converted to acetoacetate; thus, measured ketone levels may actually rise when diabetic ketoacidosis has been interrupted and is resolving.

DISEASE ASSOCIATIONS IN THE MULTIPLE ENDOCRINE NEOPLASIA (MEN) SYNDROMES

MEN 1	MEN 2	MIXED SYNDROMES
Parathyroid hyperplasia or adenoma Islet cell hyperplasia, adenoma, or carcinoma Pituitary hyperplasia or adenoma Pituitary hyperplasia or adenoma Other less common manifestations: foregut carcinoid, pheochromocytoma, subcutaneous or visceral lipomas	MEN 2A MTC Pheochromocytoma Parathyroid hyperplasia or adenoma Cutaneous lichen amyloidosis Hirschsprung disease Familial MTC MEN 2B MTC Pheochromocytoma Mucosal and gastrointestinal neuromas Marfanoid features	von Hippel–Lindau syndrome, pheochromocytoma, islet cell tumor, renal cell carcinoma, hemangioblastoma of central nervous system, retinal angioma Neurofibromatosis with features of MEN 1 or 2 Carney complex Myxomas of heart, skin, and breast Spotty cutaneous pigmentation Testicular, adrenal, and GH-producing pituitary tumors Peripheral nerve schwannoma

Note: MTC, medullary thyroid carcinoma.

54. and 55. The answers are D and E.

Discussion: *(Chap. 17)* Tight glycemic control with a hemoglobin A_{1C} of 7% or less has been shown in the Diabetes Control and Complications Trial (DCCT) in type 1 diabetic patients and the United Kingdom Prospective Diabetes Study (UKPDS) in type 2 diabetic patients to lead to improvements in microvascular disease. Notably, a decreased incidence of neuropathy, retinopathy, microalbuminuria, and nephropathy was shown in individuals with tight glycemic control. Interestingly, glycemic control had no effect on macrovascular outcomes. Instead, it was blood pressure control to at least moderate goals (142/88 mmHg) in the UKPDS that resulted in a decreased incidence of macrovascular outcomes, namely, DM-related death, stroke, and heart failure. Improved blood pressure control also resulted in improved microvascular outcomes.

56. The answer is E.

Discussion: *(Chap. 17)* Dyslipidemia is common among diabetic patients, and current recommendations are to screen aggressively for and treat abnormalities that are identified. The most common forms of dyslipidemia in diabetic patients are hypertriglyceridemia and reduced high-density lipoprotein (HDL) levels. Elevated levels of LDL cholesterol are not more common among diabetic patients; however, they are more atherogenic and are noted to be smaller and denser. LDL particles are more easily glycated and are more susceptible to oxidation in diabetic patients. This finding has led to the recommendation of many organizations, including the American Heart Association and the National Cholesterol Education Program, that patients with diabetes mellitus, regardless of their history of cardiovascular disease, have a goal LDL of less than 100 mg/dL. The American Heart Association also recommends the following targets: HDL >45 mg/dL in men and >55 mg/dL in women and triglycerides <150 mg/dL.

57. The answer is B.

Discussion: *(Chap. 17)* In the initial decision about which hypoglycemic agent to use, one must take into account the comorbidities of the patient and relative contraindications. Insulin secretagogues, α-glucosidase inhibitors, thiazolidinediones, biguanides, and insulin are all approved for monotherapy for diabetes. In light of the extensive clinical experience and generally acceptable safety profile, most patients are initially started on either a sulfonylurea or metformin. Although this regimen is generally very well tolerated, it is important to note that sulfonylureas are contraindicated for those with significant hepatic and liver dysfunction. Glipizide is primarily cleared by the liver and should be used preferentially in patients with mild to moderate renal dysfunction. Hypoglycemia is more common with sulfonylureas than it is with metformin. Metformin often causes gastrointestinal side effects with nausea, vomiting, and diarrhea. The most feared complication of metformin therapy is lactic acidosis. The risk of lactic acidosis is increased in patients with heart failure, liver disease, severe hypoxia, any form of acidosis, intravenous contrast administration, and renal insufficiency. Current recommendations are to avoid metformin in men with creatinine higher than 1.5 mg/dL and women with creatinine higher than 1.4 mg/dL. Thiazolidinediones reduce insulin resistance, and older generations of this class of drugs are associated with liver toxicity. The association of hepatotoxicity with rosiglitazone and pioglitazone is less well established; however, currently the U.S. Food and

Drug Administration (FDA) recommends avoiding the use of these drugs in patients with liver disease and frequent monitoring of liver function testing in patients who are taking them. They are associated with exacerbations of congestive heart failure and peripheral edema. Of note, metformin and thiazolidinediones have been shown to induce ovulation in women with polycystic ovarian syndrome, and premenopausal women should be warned about an increased incidence of pregnancy.

58. The answer is C.

Discussion: *(Chap. 17; Nathan, N Engl J Med 328:1676–1685, 1993.)* Nephropathy is a leading cause of death in diabetic patients. Diabetic nephropathy may be functionally silent for 10 to 15 years. Clinically detectable diabetic nephropathy begins with the development of microalbuminuria (30 to 300 mg of albumin per 24 h). The glomerular filtration rate actually may be elevated at this stage. Only after the passage of additional time will the proteinuria be overt enough (0.5 g/L) to be detectable on standard urine dipsticks. Microalbuminuria precedes nephropathy in patients with both non-insulin-dependent and insulin-dependent diabetes. An increase in kidney size also may accompany the initial hyperfiltration stage. Once the proteinuria becomes significant enough to be detected by dipstick, a steady decline in renal function occurs, with the glomerular filtration rate falling an average of 1 mL/min per month. Therefore, azotemia begins about 12 years after the diagnosis of diabetes. Hypertension clearly is an exacerbating factor for diabetic nephropathy.

59. The answer is E.

Discussion: *(Chaps. 23, 24, and 26)* The combination of hypocalcemia, hypophosphatemia, elevated serum parathyroid hormone levels, and bone fractures is consistent with a diagnosis of osteomalacia in this patient. In the absence of other gastrointestinal or renal abnormalities leading to malabsorption or increased renal loss of calcium or phosphorus, vitamin D deficiency is likely to be present. Inadequate intake of vitamin D and calcium together and limited exposure to the sun are common in this age group. Postmenopausal osteoporosis also is associated with vertebral and hip fractures, but laboratory abnormalities are not present. Primary hyperparathyroidism is associated with increased serum calcium concentration, as is ectopic parathyroid hormone secretion (although the existence of the latter has been questioned). Paget's disease of bone does not produce hypocalcemia, and it causes typical sclerotic changes on x-ray examination.

60. The answer is C.

Discussion: *(Chaps. 23 and 24)* Measurement of the serum concentration of 25(OH) vitamin D, the major circulating form of vitamin D, can be used to assess the adequacy of dietary intake and absorption of the vitamin. (Vitamin D also is made in the skin in the presence of sunlight.) Once ingested or synthesized, vitamin D is metabolized to 25(OH) vitamin D in the liver. This reaction is not tightly regulated, and an increase in dietary intake or endogenous production of vitamin D is reflected by linear elevations of serum 25(OH) vitamin D levels. Levels are reduced in patients with severe chronic parenchymal and cholestatic liver disease but usually are normal in patients with renal failure. Anticonvulsant drugs and glucocorticoids induce hepatic microsomal enzymes, which metabolize vitamin D and 25(OH) vitamin D into inactive products; this phenomenon, along with other complex effects on calcium metabolism, helps explain why these drugs cause osteopenia.

61. The answer is D.

Discussion: *(Chap. 4)* This patient has postpartum thyroiditis, which occurs in 5 to 9% of all postpartum women. Appropriate treatment is symptomatic because the hyperthyroidism is caused by the release of preformed thyroid hormone from a damaged thyroid gland. Therefore, therapies aimed at decreasing the formation of thyroid hormone, such as methimazole, or at inhibiting its release, such as SSKI, are ineffective. Radioactive iodine also is ineffective because it will not be taken up by the damaged thyroid gland (reflected in the 1% 24-h iodine uptake). In addition, the hyperthyroidism will resolve spontaneously. Aspirin and steroids are effective in treating subacute thyroiditis, which is characterized by a tender thyroid and often is preceded by a viral illness, but are not used for postpartum thyroiditis. Therapies, such as beta blockers, aimed at treating symptoms are the most effective treatment.

Postpartum thyroiditis is a form of lymphocytic thyroiditis, a painless inflammation of the thyroid that is thought to be autoimmune in etiology. About one-third of these patients enter a hypothyroid phase after experiencing hyperthyroidism. Eighty percent of these females recover normal thyroid function, but 20% remain hypothyroid and require indefinite replacement therapy. Therefore, serial thyroid function testing is indicated.

62. The answer is C.

Discussion: *(Chap. 21; Neufeld et al, Medicine 60:355–362, 1981.)* Polyglandular autoimmune syndrome type II (Schmidt's syndrome) is characterized by lymphocytic infiltration of the adrenal and thyroid glands along with type 1 diabetes mellitus in about half of affected families. Hypogonadism is also common. A few patients develop transient hypoparathyroidism caused by antibodies that compete with parathyroid hormone for binding to the parathyroid receptor. Mucocutaneous candidiasis does not occur as part of this syndrome. Instead, it occurs in most patients with polyglandular autoimmune syndrome type I. Patients who are found to have hypothyroidism should be checked for adrenal insufficiency before the initiation of thyroid replacement medication.

63. The answer is A.

Discussion: *(Chap. 14; Lue, N Engl J Med 342:1802–1813, 2000.)* Androgens increase libido, but their exact role in erectile dysfunction is unclear. Individuals with castrate levels of testosterone can still achieve erections from visual or sexual stimuli. Increased prolactin levels decrease libido by suppressing gonadotropin-releasing hormone (GnRH), which indirectly leads to a decreased serum testosterone level. Patients with diabetes mellitus have reduced amounts of nitric oxide synthase in both endothelial and neural tissues. Psychogenic erectile dysfunction is caused by a psychogenic stimulus to the sacral cord that inhibits reflexogenic responses. In addition, excess sympathetic stimulation may cause increased penile smooth muscle tone. Among the antihypertensive agents, the thiazide diuretics and beta blockers have been implicated most frequently. Calcium channel blockers and angiotensin converting-enzyme inhibitors are cited less frequently. Alpha blockers are less likely to be associated with erectile dysfunction.

64. The answer is B.

Discussion: *(Chap. 14; Lue, N Engl J Med 342:1802–1813, 2000; Goldstein et al, Sildenafil Study Group, N Engl J Med 338:1397–1404, 1998.)* Sildenafil has been proved to be effective in the treatment of erectile dysfunction. Sildenafil is a selective inhibitor of cyclic GMP–specific phosphodiesterase type V. This is the predominant isoenzyme that metabolizes cyclic GMP in the corpus cavernosum. The mechanism by which cyclic GMP stimulates relaxation in the smooth muscles has not been elucidated. Sildenafil has no effect on libido or sexual performance. Sildenafil is effective in the management of erectile dysfunction from a broad range of causes. These causes include psychogenic, diabetic, vasculogenic, postradical prostatectomy, and spinal cord injury. The onset of action is ~60 to 90 min; reduced initial doses should be considered for patients who are elderly or who have renal insufficiency. In addition, patients taking nitrates for coronary disease should avoid sildenafil. Side effects associated with sildenafil include headaches, facial flushing, dyspepsia, and nasal congestion. In addition, about 7% of men may experience a transient altered color vision (blue halo effect).

65. The answer is B.

Discussion: *(Chap. 10)* Pathologic gynecomastia develops when the effective ratio of testosterone to estrogen ratio is decreased owing to diminished testosterone production (as in primary testicular failure) or increased estrogen production. The latter may arise from direct estradiol secretion by a testis stimulated by LH or hCG or from an increase in peripheral aromatization of precursor steroids, most notably androstenedione. Elevated androstenedione levels may result from increased secretion by an adrenal tumor (leading to an elevated level of urinary 17-ketosteroids) or decreased hepatic clearance in patients with chronic liver disease. A variety of drugs, including diethylstilbestrol, heroin, digitalis, spironolactone, cimetidine, isoniazid, and tricyclic antidepressants, also can cause gynecomastia. In this patient, the history of paternity and the otherwise normal physical examination indicate that a karyotype is unnecessary, and the bilateral breast enlargement essentially excludes the presence of carcinoma and thus the need for biopsy. The presence of a low LH and testosterone suggests either estrogen or hCG production. Because of the normal testicular examination, a primary testicular tumor is not suspected. Carcinoma of the lung and germ cell tumors both can produce hCG, causing gynecomastia.

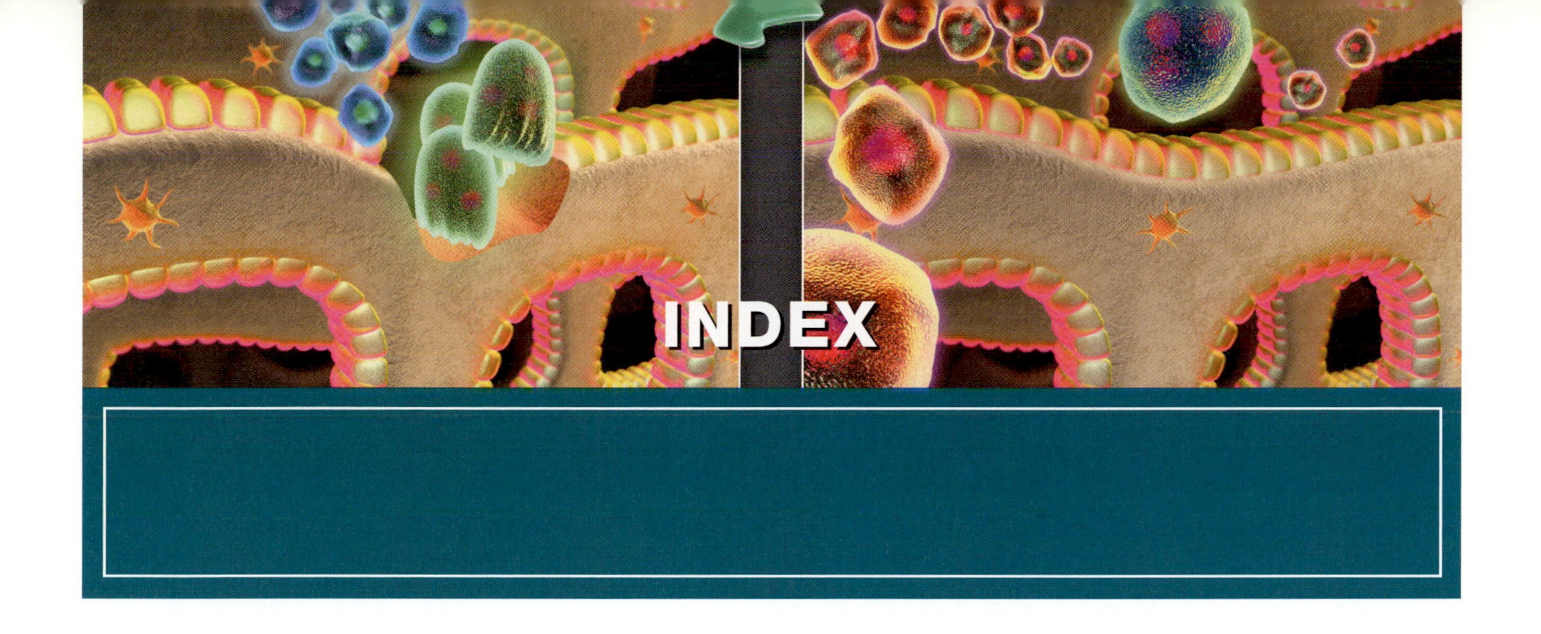

Bold number indicates the start of the main discussion of the topic; numbers with "f" and "t" refer to figure and table pages.